1007539685

Drug Abuse and Addiction in Medical Illness

Joris C. Verster • Kathleen Brady
Marc Galanter • Patricia Conrod
Editors

Drug Abuse and Addiction in Medical Illness

Causes, Consequences and Treatment

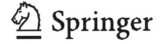 Springer

Editors
Joris C. Verster
Division of Pharmacology
Utrecht Institute for Pharmaceutical Sciences
Utrecht University
Utrecht, The Netherlands

Marc Galanter
Division of Alcoholism & Drug Abuse
School of Medicine
New York University
New York, NY, USA

Kathleen Brady
Department of Psychiatry
Medical University of South Carolina
Charleston, SC, USA

Patricia Conrod
National Addiction Centre
Institute of Psychiatry
King's College London
London, UK

ISBN 978-1-4614-3374-3 (Hardcover)   ISBN 978-1-4614-3375-0 (eBook)
ISBN 978-1-4614-8415-8 (Softcover)
DOI 10.1007/978-1-4614-3375-0
Springer New York Heidelberg Dordrecht London

Library of Congress Control Number: 2012940199

Printed on acid-free paper

Springer is part of Springer Science+Business Media (www.springer.com)

Preface

Drug abuse and addiction are common in clinical practice. Often they interfere with patient treatment or require an alternative approach. The volume *Drug Abuse and Addiction in Medical Illness: Causes, Consequences, and Treatment* discusses the causes and consequences of drug abuse and addiction in a systematic manner. We believe this volume is a gold standard book including current and cutting-edge information for all those working with drug abusing or addicted patients or for those interested in this topic from other research perspectives. The volume is a first of its kind book, rich yet comprehensive and focused (specifically to the designated area), and addresses the needs of the very active theoretical, basic, and clinical research in the field.

Leading experts in the field of addiction throughout the world have contributed to *Drug Abuse and Addiction in Medical Illness: Causes, Consequences, and Treatment*. This means the volume covers virtually every core, as well as contemporary, topic in the subject area, from the established theories to the most modern research and development in the field of drug abuse and addiction.

In brief, *Drug Abuse and Addiction in Medical Illness: Causes, Consequences, and Treatment* contains 46 chapters covering drugs of abuse and how they play a role in a wide range of medical illnesses. The volume starts with eight general chapters covering basic concepts of addiction research, research techniques, and major findings. Section II of the book is followed by 11 chapters discussing a variety of drugs of abuse, including cannabis, inhalants, alcohol, and cocaine. Section III discusses how, for some diseases, drug abuse will cause or enhance the progress of that disease/disorder, while other diseases may result in or enhance drug abuse. The chapters in Section III thus deal with this crucial, bidirectional relationship. Section IV of the book consists of ten chapters discussing current topics in addiction research such as the effects of drugs of abuse on traffic safety, prevention, and legal aspects of drug abuse. To aid educational usefulness of the volume as a text book, every chapter includes an abstract, and two boxes summarizing learning objectives and directions for future research. The chapters on individual drugs in Section II also include a box summarizing the pharmacokinetic properties of the drug.

Understanding drug abuse and addiction is of vital importance in clinical practice. We hope *Drug Abuse and Addiction in Medical Illness: Causes, Consequences, and Treatment* is of help to those who are involved in improving health and quality of life of their patients and others interested in this fascinating field of research.

Utrecht, The Netherlands   Joris C. Verster
Charleston, SC, USA   Kathleen Brady
New York, NY, USA   Marc Galanter
London, UK   Patricia Conrod

Credits and Acknowledgements

Composing this first of a kind comprehensive volume could not be realized without the enthusiastic help and effort of a great number of individuals. Many people were involved in the development of this new volume entitled *Drug Abuse and Addiction in Medical Illness: Causes, Consequences, and Treatment*. We want to thank all authors for contributing authoritative and up-to-date chapters. Because of their efforts, *Drug Abuse and Addiction in Medical Illness: Causes, Consequences, and Treatment* is a first class reference book for everybody who is interested in the impact of drug abuse and addiction in clinical practice. We also want to thank the editors at Springer for their support and guidance in developing this volume. Finally, we want to thank our friends and families for their patience and support.

Utrecht, The Netherlands	Joris C. Verster
Charleston, SC, USA	Kathleen Brady
New York, NY, USA	Marc Galanter
London, UK	Patricia Conrod

Contents

Contributors

Jean Philippe Azulay Clinical Neurosciences Department, Movement disorders Unit, CHU Timone, Marseille, France

Jane C. Ballantyne Penn Pain Medicine Center, Philadelphia, PA, USA

Sean P. Barrett Departments of Psychology and Psychiatry, Dalhousie University, Halifax, NS, Canada

David Belin INSERM European Associated Laboratory Psychobiology of Compulsive Habits, Pôle PBS, Poitiers

Department of Experimental Psychology, Downing stress, Cambridge

INSERM U1084 -LNEC & University of Poitiers, Pôle Biologie Santé, Poitiers, Cedex

Alyson Bond Department of Addiction, Institute of Psychiatry, King's College London, London, UK

Louisa M.C. Van den Bosch Psychiatric Hospital de Gelderse Roos, Arnhem, The Netherlands

Centre of Specific Psychotherapy, Oegstgeest, The Netherlands

Kathleen Brady Department of Psychiatry and Behavioral Sciences, Clinical Neurosciences Division, Medical University of South Carolina, Charleston, SC, USA

Thomas H. Brandon Tobacco Research & Intervention Program, H. Lee Moffitt Cancer Center, Tampa, FL, USA

Tibor Brunt Trimbos Institute, Utrecht, The Netherlands

John C.M. Brust Department of Neurology, Columbia University College of Physicians & Surgeons, New York, NY, USA

Paolo Calabresi Clinica Neurologica, Università degli Studi di Perugia, Perugia, Italy

R. Cappato Center of Clinical Arrhythmology and Electrophysiology, Istituto Policlinico San Donato, IRCCS, University of Milan, San Donato Milanese, Milan, Italy

Pieter-Jan Carpentier Reinier van Arkel groep, Hertogenbosch

Natalie Castellanos-Ryan Centre de recherche du CHU Ste-Justine, Université de Montréal, Montreal, Canada

Robey Champine Calhoun Cardiology Center, University of Connecticut Health center, Farmington, CT, USA

Albert E. Chudley Department of Pediatrics and Child Health, University of Manitoba, Winnipeg, MB, Canada

WRHA Program in Genetics and Metabolism, Health Sciences Centre, Winnipeg, MB, Canada

Patricia Conrod National Addiction Centre, Institute of Psychiatry, King's College London, London, UK

Department of Psychiatry, Université de Montréal, CHU Hôpital Ste Justine, Montreal, Canada

Letizia M. Cupini Centro Cefalee, Clinica Neurologica, Dipartimento Cranio Spinale, U.O.C. Neurologia, Ospedale S. Eugenio, Roma, Italy

Anne P. Daamen Division of Pharmacology, Utrecht Institute for Pharmaceutical Sciences, Utrecht University, Utrecht, The Netherlands

Jaffrey W. Dalley Department of Experimental Psychology, Behavioural and Clinical Neuroscience Institute, University of Cambridge, Cambridge, UK

L. De Ambroggi Center of Clinical Arrhythmology and Electrophysiology, Istituto Policlinico San Donato, IRCCS, University of Milan, San Donato Milanese, Milan, Italy

Joseph W. Ditre Department of Psychology, Texas A&M University, College Station, TX, USA

Tomas Drgon Molecular Neurobiology Branch, NIH-IRP (NIDA), Baltimore, MD, USA

Ahmed Elkashef Division of Pharmacotherapies and Medical Consequences of Drug Abuse, Department of Health and Human Services, National Institute on Drug Abuse(Retired), National Institutes of Health, Bethesda, MD, USA

Alexandre Eusebio Clinical Neurosciences Department, Movement Disorders Unit, CHU Timone, Marseille, France

Fabrizio Faggiano Department of Clinical and Experimental Medicine, Avogadro University, Novara, Italy

Matt Field School of Psychology, University of Liverpool, Liverpool, UK

Mark T. Fillmore Department of Psychology, University of Kentucky, Lexington, KY, USA

Julian D. Ford Department of Psychiatry, Division of Child and Adolescent Psychiatry, University of Connecticut Health Center, Farmington, CT, USA

F. Furlanello Center of Clinical Arrhythmology and Electrophysiology, Istituto Policlinico San Donato, IRCCS, University of Milan, San Donato Milanese, Milan, Italy

Bin Gao Division of Intramural Clinical and Biological Research, National Institute on Alcohol Abuse and Alcoholism, National Institutes of Health, Bethesda, MD, USA

A.E. Goudriaan Department of Psychiatry, Amsterdam Institute for Addiction Research, Academic Medical Center, University of Amsterdam, Amsterdam, The Netherlands

L. Gregg Division of Clinical Psychology, School of Psychological Sciences, University of Manchester, Manchester, UK

Vanessa L. Hamill Department of Psychology, The University of Western Ontario, London, ON, Canada

Megan Hancock Department of Psychology, The University of Western Ontario, London, ON, Canada

Bryan W. Heckman Tobacco Research & Intervention Program, H. Lee Moffitt Cancer Center, Tampa, FL, USA

Christopher Hess Department of Neurology, Columbia University College of Physicians and Surgeons, New York, NY, USA

Peter N.S. Hoaken Department of Psychology, The University of Western Ontario, London, ON, Canada

Jan B. Hoek Department of Pathology, Anatomy and Cell Biology, Thomas Jefferson University, Philadelphia, PA, USA

Jonathan A. Hollander Laboratory for Behavioral and Molecular Neuroscience, Department of Molecular Therapeutics, The Scripps Research Institute—Florida, Jupiter, FL, USA

Matthew O. Howard School of Social Work, The University of North Carolina at Chapel Hill, Chapel Hill, NC, USA

Gerry Jager Division of Human Nutrition, Wageningen University, Wageningen, The Netherlands

Brian Johnson Department of Psychiatry, Suny Upstate Medical University, Syracuse, NY, USA

Gen Kanayama Department of Psychiatry, Harvard Medical School, Boston, MA, USA

Paul J. Kenny Laboratory for Behavioral and Molecular Neuroscience, Department of Molecular Therapeutics, The Scripps Research Institute—Florida, Jupiter, FL, USA

Andrea R. Kilgour Department Clinical Health Psychology, University of Manitoba, Manitoba, Canada

Malcolm Lader Institute of Psychiatry, King's College, London, UK

Megan J. Lau Department of Psychology, The University of Western Ontario, London, ON, Canada

Erika B. Litvin Tobacco Research & Intervention Program, H. Lee Moffitt Cancer Center, Tampa, FL, USA

Clare J. Mackie National Addiction Centre, Institute of Psychiatry, King's College London, London, UK

Denis M. McCarthy Department of Psychological Sciences, University of Missouri, Columbia, MO, USA

Megan E. McLarnon Department of Psychology, Dalhousie University, Halifax, NS, Canada

Judith H. Miles Thompson Center for Autism and Neurodevelopmental Disorders, University of Missouri, Columbia, MO, USA

Tracy L. Monaghan Department of Psychology, Dalhousie University, Halifax, NS, Canada

Ivan Montoya Division of Pharmacotherapies and Medical Consequences of Drug Abuse, Department of Health and Human Services, National Institute on Drug Abuse(Retired), National Institutes of Health, Bethesda, MD, USA

Sebastian Mueller Department of Medicine and Center of Alcohol Research, Liver Disease and Nutrition, Salem Medical Center, University of Heidelberg, Heidelberg, Germany

Nicola C. Newton National Drug and Alcohol Research Centre, University of New South Wales, Randwick, NSW, Australia

Berend Olivier Division of Pharmacology, Utrecht Institute for Pharmaceutical Sciences, Utrecht University, Utrecht, The Netherlands

A.C. Parrott Department of Psychology, Swansea University, Swansea, Wales, UK

Renske Penning Division of Pharmacology, Utrecht Institute for Pharmaceutical Sciences, Utrecht University, Utrecht, The Netherlands

Naney M. Petry Calhoun Cardiology Center, University of Connecticut Health Center, Farmington, CT, USA

Harrison G. Pope Jr. Biological Psychiatry Laboratory, McLean Hospital, Belmont, MA, USA

Ty. A. Ridenour Center for Education and Drug Abuse Research, University of Pittsburgh, Pittsburgh, PA, USA

Timothy Roehrs Sleep Disorders and Research Center, Henry Ford Health System, Detroit, MI, USA

Department of Psychiatry and Behavioral Neurosciences, School of Medicine, Wayne State University, Detroit, MI, USA

Erin H. Ross Department of Psychology, The University of Western Ontario, London, ON, Canada

Thomas Roth Sleep Disorders and Research Center, Henry Ford Health System, Detroit, MI, USA

Department of Psychiatry and Behavioral Neurosciences, School of Medicine, Wayne State University, Detroit, MI, USA

Paola Sarchielli Clinica Neurologica, Università degli Studi di Perugia, Perugia, Italy

Rachel Saunders-Pullman Department of Neurology, Beth Israel Medical Center, New York, NY, USA

Department of Neurology, Albert Einstein College of Medicine, Bronx, NY, USA

Helmut K. Seitz Department of Medicine and Center of Alcohol Research, Liver Disease and Nutrition, Salem Medical Center, University of Heidelberg, Heidelberg, Germany

L. Vitali Serdoz Center of Clinical Arrhythmology and Electrophysiology, Istituto Policlinico San Donato, IRCCS, University of Milan, San Donato Milanese, Milan, Italy

Leo Sher James J. Peters Veterans' Administration Medical Center and Mount Sinai School of Medicine, New York, NY, USA

K.J. Sher University of Missouri-Columbia and Midwest Alcoholism Research Center, Columbia, MO, USA

Linda Simoni-Wastila Peter Lamy Center on Drug Therapy and Aging, School of Pharmacy, University of Maryland Baltimore, Baltimore, MD, USA

Valerie J. Slaymaker Butler Center for Research, Hazelden, Center City, MN, USA

Sherry H. Stewart Departments of Psychiatry, Psychology, and Community Health and Epidemiology, Dalhousie University, Halifax, NS, Canada

Jennifer L. Tapscott Department of Psychology, The University of Western Ontario, London, ON, Canada

Maree Teesson National Drug and Alcohol Research Centre, University of New South Wales, NSW, Australia

George R. Uhl Molecular Neurobiology Branch, NIH-IRP (NIDA), Baltimore, MD, USA

Haske van der Vorst Behavioural Science Institute, Radboud University Nijmegen, Nijmegen, The Netherlands

Margriet van Laar Trimbos Institute, Utrecht, The Netherlands

Janet Veldstra Faculty of Behavioural and Social Sciences, Section Experimental Psychology, University of Groningen, Traffic and Environmental Psychology, Groningen, The Netherlands

Roel Verheul Department of Clinical Psychology, University of Amsterdam, Amsterdam, The Netherlands

Viersprong Institute for Studies on Personality Disorders (VISPD), Center of Psychotherapy De, Viersprong, Halsteren, The Netherlands

Joris C. Verster Division of Pharmacology, Utrecht Institute for Pharmaceutical Sciences, Utrecht University, Utrecht, The Netherlands

Reinout Wiers University of Amsterdam, Amsterdam, The Netherlands

Bonnie B. Wilford Coalition on Physician Education in Substance Use Disorders (COPE) at Yale University School of Medicine, Easton, MD, USA

Tatiana Witjas Clinical Neurosciences Department, Movement Disorders Unit, CHU Timone, Marseille, France

Kim Wolff Addiction Science, Institute of Psychiatry, King's College London, London, UK

Stephen A. Wyatt Dual Diagnosis Program, Middlesex Hospital, Old Lyme, CT, USA

Hui-Wen Keri Yang Peter Lamy Center on Drug Therapy and Aging, School of Pharmacy, University of Maryland Baltimore, Baltimore, MD, USA

Samir Zakhari Division of Metabolism and Health Effects, National Institute on Alcohol Abuse and Alcoholism, National Institutes of Health, Bethesda, MD, USA

Part I

Drug Abuse and Addiction – An Overview

Epidemiology of Alcohol and Drug Use

Margriet van Laar

Abstract

This chapter describes trends in the prevalence and patterns of alcohol and illicit drug use. While methodological differences, imprecise estimates and lack of data preclude firm conclusions on the global situation and trends in substance use, the available data suggest that alcohol and illicit drug consumption varies widely between societies. Per capita alcohol consumption is highest in the European Union and lowest in the South-East Asian and Eastern Mediterranean regions. There is a general long-term trend towards harmonisation of alcohol consumption, with decreasing levels in regions with traditionally high levels and increasing levels in regions with low levels. Trend data from surveys showed an increase in heavy episodic drinking among pupils in many European countries in the past decade, especially among girls.

Prevalence rates of illicit drug use are generally lower in the European Union compared to the USA, Canada and Australia, for which most research data are available. However, there are large variations between EU countries. Cannabis is worldwide the most frequently used illicit drug. Prevalence rates among young people tend to stabilise or decline in the past years, after a general increasing trend in the 1990s. Annual cocaine prevalence is higher among the general population of the USA and Canada compared to Australia and the EU, while annual prevalence of ecstasy and amphetamine use is highest in Australia. Within Europe, cocaine generally dominates the stimulant markets in the Western and Southern regions, albeit restricted to a few large countries. Amphetamines are the main stimulants in North, Central and Eastern Europe. Injecting drug use increases the risk of transmission of blood-born infectious diseases, like HIV and hepatitis B and C. China, the USA and Russia have the largest numbers of drug injectors. In terms of (midpoint) prevalence, highest rates are found in Azerbaijan and lowest in Cambodia.

Learning Objectives
- There is no straightforward relation between the total amount of alcohol consumed in countries and the prevalence of alcohol use or alcohol use disorders.
- Cannabis prevalence increased in the 1990s in most western countries, and is generally stable or declining in the past years, especially among young people.
- School surveys show an increase in heavy episodic drinking in the past decade, especially among girls.

M. van Laar (✉)
Trimbos Institute, Da Costakade 45, PO Box 725,
3500 AS, Utrecht, The Netherlands
e-mail: mlaar@trimbos.nl

J.C. Verster et al. (eds.), *Drug Abuse and Addiction in Medical Illness: Causes, Consequences and Treatment*,
DOI 10.1007/978-1-4614-3375-0_1, © Springer Science+Business Media, LLC 2012

Issues that Need to Be Addressed by Future Research
- While cannabis is the most commonly used illicit drug, data on intensive use and on cannabis use disorders are scarce.
- Problem drug use may be defined differently across countries and (indirect) methods to estimate the number of problem drug users are available only for a limited number of countries.
- There should be more research attention paid to monitoring substance use in high risk groups, in addition to gathering data in the general population.

Introduction

This chapter gives an overview of trends in the prevalence and patterns of alcohol and illicit drug use, primarily in western countries. Data on alcohol use were mainly derived from the World Health Organisation (WHO). The European Monitoring Centre for Drugs and Drug Addiction (EMCDDA) served as a main source for data on the consumption of illicit drugs in the European Union. Well developed monitoring systems are available as well for other parts of the world, mainly the USA, Australia and Canada. Worldwide statistics of drug use are available from the United Nations Office of Drug Control (UNODC), but in spite of recent improvements data quality is still quite poor in many countries.

This chapter focuses on the most prevalent (classes of) substances: alcohol, cannabis, cocaine, amphetamines and ecstasy, and opioids. Many other drugs come and disappear on the market, sometimes gaining popularity in specific subpopulations, such as people in the nightlife settings (e.g. [1, 2]). Examples are GHB, ketamine, benzylpiperazine and poppers (alkyl nitrites). Collectively, these drugs may be referred to as "club drugs", of which only ecstasy has reached the stage of a relatively wide users group. However, consumption rates of most other drugs in the general population generally remain low.

For practical purposes, this chapter is organised by main substance. However, it should be realised that people who consume one substance often have also experience with using other substances. Occasionally substances are consumed together to enhance (or prolong) positive effects or to counteract negative side-effects. For example, the combined use of alcohol and cocaine is quite popular, among others because cocaine is said to have a sobering effect, permitting the user to drink more and for longer. Poly substance or poly drug use is common and may pose specific (health) risks to users [3, 4].

Estimates of substance use. Commonly, prevalence is measured in three ways, viz., lifetime (ever), last year (recent)

and last month (current). People who use a drug or alcohol at least once in their life will be included in the count of lifetime users. This practise may easily lead to misuse of statistics, with one-time and occasional users being lumped together with regular and problematic users. Moreover, as first substance use may have taken place a long time ago in someone's life, figures on lifetime prevalence do not give an actual picture, especially if they refer to a wide age group. Last year and last month prevalence better reflect the current situation, and are more likely to reflect regular use than experimenting.

Some people may experience social, physical or psychological problems related to the consumption of psychoactive substances. There is no universal definition of a problem alcohol or drug user. According to the EMCDDA, problem drug use is defined as "the injecting or long duration/regular use of opioids, cocaine and/or amphetamines". Problem drug use can also be defined according to clinical criteria for substance use disorders (e.g. abuse or dependence), such as provided in the Diagnostic and Statistical Manual on Mental Disorders (DSM) of the American Psychiatric Association or International Classification of Diseases and Related Disorders (ICD) of the WHO.

Whatever definition, survey data in the general population and youth underestimate problem drug use among marginalised populations, especially users of drugs like heroin, amphetamines (and crack) cocaine. On the one hand, problem drug users may be underrepresented, as they are less likely to be part of a conventional household setting targeted by population surveys. This is because they are relatively often homeless and institutionalised. On the other hand, illicit drug use may also not be disclosed due to perceived stigma associated with such use, especially when it is problematic. To estimate problem (hard) drug use, specific estimation methods can be applied, which also take into account the "hidden population" of drug users. Examples are capture–recapture and multiplier methods [2].

Commonly, the number of clients in treatment is reported as an (indirect) indicator of problem use. While an increase in the number of drug users seeking treatment may indeed reflect an increase in the extent of problem drug use, treatment statistics may also be heavily influenced by changes in quality and coverage of the registration, treatment capacity and availability and referral policies.

Comparability. Comparisons between and across countries are hampered by differences in the quality and nature of study design, data collection and analysis methods, and by variations in last monitoring year and the age range of respondents. The truthfulness of the answers may vary depending on how respondents perceive the protection of their privacy and the risk of acknowledging drug use. Even if respondents wish to respond honestly, the common self-report survey measures may incorrectly estimate both the frequencies of their drug use and the quantities they consume. Yet, several initiatives have been taken in the past decade to improve comparability of data at least at the methodological level. For example, the EMCDDA has developed standards for data collection for five epidemiological indicators. Moreover, several studies of the WHO and European studies (e.g. WMH surveys on mental disorders; HBSC, European School Survey Project on Alcohol and Drugs, ESPAD) have been conducted in which survey instruments are to a large extent harmonised. However, the stage of full methodological comparability has not been reached. This means that (small) differences between countries should be interpreted with caution.

Alcohol Use and Alcohol Use Disorders

Alcohol consumption in the population can be measured by analysing production and distribution statistics for alcoholic beverages. According to figures of the WHO, Europe is the heaviest drinking region of the world, with an average adult (15+) drinking 8.9 l of pure alcohol each year, which is well above world's average of 5.1 l of pure alcohol (WHO, Global Information System on Alcohol and Health; figures for 2001–2002). Figures for the European Union are even higher and point to an average almost 2.5 times above the world's average. Next to Europe comes the Pan American region with 6.7 l, followed by the Western Pacific region with 5.2 l, the African region with 4.5 l, and at distance the South-East Asian region and Eastern Mediterranean region with a per capita consumption of 0.5 and 0.2 l of pure alcohol, respectively.

Long-term trend data over the past 40 years show that consumption peaked in the early 1980s in the European region, the African region and the Pan American region, but throughout this period levels remained considerably higher in Europe compared to the other regions [5]. Except for the Eastern Mediterranean region, where most countries have a

majority of Muslim populations, there is a general trend towards harmonisation of consumption rates, with decreasing levels in regions with traditionally high levels and increasing levels in regions with low levels. To some extent increasing trends in alcohol consumption may parallel increasing levels of economic development. Note, however, that (trends in) consumption rates vary widely between countries, as illustrated in Figs. 1.1 and 1.2. For example, a steady decrease in the volume of alcohol consumption is visible in France since the 1960s, while an upward trend is apparent in the UK.

As far as beverage preference is concerned, worldwide some 37% of the alcohol comes from beer, 25% from wine and 33% from spirits. However, there are large inter-country and regional differences in the drink of choice. In the USA beer is by far most popular (54% of all alcohol consumption; 6% for wine and 30% for spirits). In general in northern European and Anglo-Saxon cultures, traditionally beer and spirits predominate, while in Southern Europe wine (as part of the diet, and often used during meals and in family settings) predominate. Yet, there are again large differences between European countries and a trend in the direction of harmonisation of beverage preference can also be observed [6].

These statistics are, however, based on recorded (taxed) amounts of alcohol production, which do not include alcohol that comes from smuggling, home production and cross-border shopping. Table 1.1 shows that within the EU-15, estimates of unrecorded consumption are fairly high in Sweden (3 l of pure alcohol per capita). In other European countries, relatively high levels (4 or more litres) are found in Lithuania, Hungary, Romania, Slovakia and Russia, with the Ukraine peaking with an unrecorded per capita alcohol consumption of 10.5 l. Taking both recorded and unrecorded alcohol consumption into account, Hungary is on top of the list with a consumption of almost 18 l pure alcohol per capita of 15+.

In general, average adult alcohol consumption tends to relate to the proportion of heavy drinkers in a population, as shown by high correlations between mean consumption and

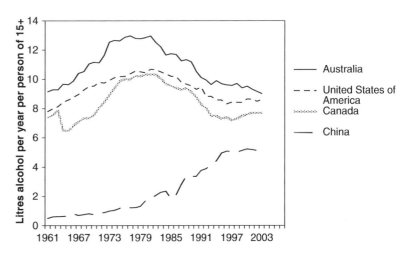

Fig. 1.1 Trends in recorded alcohol consumption per capita in the adult population of 15+ in Australia, USA, Canada and China (1961–2003). Source: WHO, Global Information System on Alcohol and Health

Fig. 1.2 Trends in recorded alcohol consumption per capita in the adult population of 15+ in several European countries (1961–2003). Source: WHO, Global Information System on Alcohol and Health

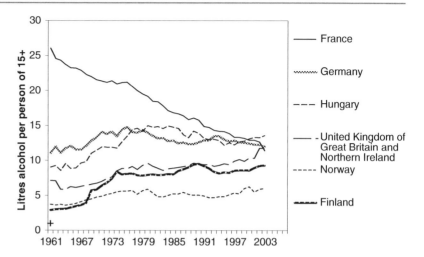

Table 1.1 Recorded and estimated unrecorded consumption of pure alcohol (litres per capita of 15+) and percentage of last year abstainers in selected countries in WHO regions

EU-27	Consumption			Percentage of last year abstainers		
	Recorded	Unrecorded	Total	Male	Female	Total
Hungary	13.6	4.0	17.6	9	26	18
Lithuania	9.9	4.9	14.8	10	28	20
Ireland	13.7	1.0	14.7	17	26	22
Luxembourg	15.6	−1.0[a]	14.6	1	4	2.5
Slovakia	10.4	4.0	14.4	4	10	8
Czech Republic	13.0	1.0	14.0	9	20	15
UK[b]	11.8	2.0	13.8	9	14	12
Romania	9.7	4.0	13.7	23	53	38
Denmark	11.0	2.0	13.0	2	4	3
Germany	12.0	1.0	13.0	4	6	5
Spain[c]	11.7	1.0	12.7	27	49	38
Portugal	11.5	1.0	12.5	7	24	16
Cyprus	11.5	1.0	12.5	1	15	8
France	11.4	1.0	12.4	4	9	7
Finland	10.5	1.9	12.4	7	8	7
Latvia	9.6	2.3	11.9	15	32	25
Austria	11.1	0.7	11.7	6	16	11
Poland	8.1	3.0	11.1	12	26	19
Belgium	10.6	0.2	10.8	12	26	19
Greece	9.0	1.8	10.8	1	15	8
Slovenia	6.7	3.6	10.4	12	36	24
The Netherlands	9.7	0.5	10.2	9	22	16
Estonia	9.0	1.0	10.0			
Sweden	6.6	3.0	9.6	8	15	11
Italy	8.0	1.5	9.5	36	13	25
Bulgaria	5.9	3.0	8.9	32	65	–
Malta	6.0	0.3	6.3	–	–	–
European region—other						
Israel	2.5	1.0	3.5	26	45	36
Ukraine[d]	6.1	10.5	16.6	15	27	23
Russian Federation	10.3	4.9	15.2	9	35	23
Pan American region						
USA	8.4	1.0	9.4	29	38	34
Colombia	5.7	2.0	7.7	5	21	15
Mexico	4.5	3	7.5	22	55	42

(continued)

Table 1.1 (continued)

EU-27	Consumption			Percentage of last year abstainers		
	Recorded	Unrecorded	Total	Male	Female	Total
Western Pacific region						
New Zealand	9.7	0.5	10.2	12	17	15
Japan	7.6	2.0	9.6	7	20	16
Australia	9.0	0.0	9.0	14	21	18
China	5.2	0.8	6.0	28	73	49
African region						
Nigeria[c]	10.6	3.5	14.1	51	90	76
South Africa	6.7	2.2	8.9	55	83	69
Eastern Mediterranean region						
Lebanon	3.2	0.5	3.7	67	87	77
Morocco	0.5	1.0	1.5	77	99	90
Egypt[d]	0.2	0.5	0.7	99	100	100
Afghanistan	0.0	0.0	0.0	–	–	–

Sources: WHO, Global Information System on Alcohol and Health; WHO Global Status Report on Alcohol. Figures on consumption refer to 2003, except for Denmark (2005 for recorded consumption), Finland (2005 for recorded and 2006 for unrecorded consumption), Sweden (2005 for recorded consumption), USA (2004 for recorded consumption), Mexico (2004 for recorded consumption). Data on abstainers refer to 1995–1999 in 15 countries (Lithuania, Luxembourg, Romania, Denmark, Portugal, Cyprus, France, Austria, Poland, Greece, Slovenia, Bulgaria, Russia, Mexico, South Africa) and 2000 or more recent in the remaining countries
[a] Negative unrecorded consumption due to sales to foreigners
[b] Great Britain and Northern Ireland
[c] Regional survey
[d] Abstinence rates pertain to lifetime prevalence

the prevalence of heavy drinking in several studies [6]. For example, in the USA the top 10% of heavy drinkers account for 60–70% of the total alcohol consumption. European figures are lower but still show that between a third and half of all alcohol consumption can be attributed to the top 10% of heavy users. Surprisingly, the total amount of alcohol consumed is commonly not correlated with the prevalence of the number of drinkers (or abstainers) or the prevalence of alcohol use disorders, and trends may be fairly independent [6, 7]. Other aspects of drinking behaviour, such as the amount of alcohol consumed per session (e.g. binge drinking) and context of use (e.g. drinking with meals and public drinking), may be better predictors of alcohol-related problems in a population [8–10].

Levels of Drinking

The injurious effects of excessive alcohol use are numerous. Alcohol use is related to over 60 disease conditions. For most of these, risk increases accordingly as more alcohol is consumed, although the pattern of drinking (e.g. heavy episodic drinking) is also relevant to the type of harm (refs). The above-mentioned way of quantifying alcohol use, i.e. the volume per capita, does not take into account the number of abstainers and differences between male and female drinkers. In the framework of the Global Burden of Disease Study, these variables were taken into account to estimate proportions

of "at risk drinkers" (see Table 1.2). Table 1.2 shows different categories of drinkers. Level II and III are considered as "heavy and hazardous drinking" [11].

Anderson and Baumberg (2006) extrapolated figures to the European Union, and found that about 14% of the EU population abstained from alcohol, which was generally defined as not having had a drink in the past year [6]. However, rates of abstinence vary widely between countries, both within and outside the European Union (Table 1.1).[1] These differences may be partly explained by variations in age groups, way of questioning, estimation methods (surveys and/or expert opinions) and widely varying reference years. Note also that data are fairly outdated in 15 of the listed countries. Nonetheless, a general finding across countries and cultures is the gender difference, in that women are more likely to abstain from alcohol than men. Noteworthy are also the large proportions of abstainers in Spain and Romania, while in other European countries like Luxembourg and

---

[1] For the EU, recent and more comparable figures are available from the Eurobarometer survey in 2006 [12]. This survey showed a last year prevalence of abstinence 25% (males 16%, females 32%) in the population of 15 years and above of the EU-25, with highest rates reported in Italy (40%), Hungary (38%), Portugal (37%) and Malta (35%), and lowest rates of abstinence in Denmark [13] and the Netherlands (10%). See also paragraph on binge drinking. Note, however, that precision of estimates owing to comparability of methods is partly offset by the fairly small sample (roughly 1,000 respondents per country, with some exceptions).

Table 1.2 Drinking levels and estimates for the adult European population (16+) in 2001

Drinking levels	Description	Definition (gram per day) Men	Women	Number of adults in EU[a]
Abstinent		0	0	53 million
Level I	Moderate to low risk drinking	>0–40	>0–20	263 million
Level II	Heavy, hazardous or excessive drinking	40–60	20–40	36 million
Level III	Alcohol-dependent or addictive drinking	>60	>40	22 million

[a]This estimate does not include Romania and Bulgaria, which joined the European Union in 2007 [11]

Spain almost every adult had drunk in the past year. Worldwide, highest abstinence rates are found in Africa and the Eastern Mediterranean region. To some extent these differences can be explained by religious factors, i.e. in countries with Islam as official religion abstinence rates are generally high. Note, however, that patterns of drinking and abstinence rates may also vary within subpopulations and across different regions of a particular country. For example, in Israel, overall lower levels of per capita alcohol consumption are reported compared to other Western countries. However, within the country, abstinence rates are highest among Arab Israelis, followed by Jewish Israelis and lowest among immigrants from the Former Soviet Union. These differences have been attributed to both socio-cultural and genetic factors [14].

Moderate or low-risk drinking is prevalent among seven in ten EU inhabitants. In general, low alcohol consumption is said to reduce the risk of cardiovascular illnesses [15]. It is unclear, however, whether this applies to all population groups. The exact degree of risk reduction and the amount of alcohol required to maximise this risk reduction are also still being debated. There are indications that light to moderate drinkers are less likely to die prematurely than non-drinkers or heavy drinkers. These associations appear only to apply to people who have a regular moderate drinking pattern, without episodes of heavy drinking. However, in a recent meta-analysis of the association between moderate alcohol use and death, it was concluded that the positive effects of moderate alcohol use were grossly overestimated in the past [16]. A major reason for this is that studies often listed people who had given up alcohol use as non-drinkers. Giving up drinking is also related to having poor health. Taking only those studies without this mistake, no significant difference in deaths was found between non-drinkers and moderate drinkers. Moreover, even low levels of alcohol consumption have been associated with the incidence of cancer [17].

Level II and III drinking is associated with many diseases, including certain types of cancer, cardiovascular disease, damage to the brain and nervous system as well as dependence [6]. Over 15% of the European population "drink too much",

which is defined as more than 20 g per day for women and 40 g per day for men, or roughly 2 and 4 drinks per day, respectively. The WHO collects data also in other countries, but comparisons are hampered due to major methodological differences (Country Profiles). The available data suggest wide variations in the prevalence of heavy drinking. Examples: in Ireland 30% of all males and 22% of all females (18 years and above) is a heavy drinker, defined as consuming >21 units per week for men and >14 units per week for women (data from a national survey). In contrast, in Spain only 2.6% of the population of 18 years and above (3.4 for males, 2.1% for females) is a heavy drinker (level II and III). In the Czech Republic, 26% of the drinking males and 13% of the drinking females is a heavy (level II and III) drinker (WHO GENACIS study). However, based on the World Health Survey rates of 5.8% among males and 2.2% among females in the total population of 18 years and above are reported. Taking into account the low rate of estimated last year abstainers (3% of males and 8% of females), the former survey seems to yield appreciably higher rates, despite age group differences.

Binge Drinking

Heavy episodic drinking or "binge drinking" lead to an increase in (un)intentional injuries (e.g. traffic accidents, falls, drowning) and many other medical conditions, including cardiovascular and cerebrovascular disease, dependence and atherosclerosis, even after adjustment for average volume of consumption [11, 18–20]. Generally, the higher the frequency of heavy drinking occasions and the greater the amount of alcohol consumed per occasion, the higher the alcohol-related disease burden. Binge drinking may be defined as drinking occasions which result in drunkenness or intoxication, although this outcome is of course not always planned. This subjective definition may have some advantages above a fixed quantity, given the wide inter-individual variations in the degree of drunkenness resulting from a certain amount of alcohol, which is partly related to factors like body weight, gender and tolerance. However, for research purposes binge drinking is often defined as a single drinking session that includes consumption above a given cut-off level of alcohol, while some definitions also include a time period for drinking this amount, for example 2 h.

A survey in 2006 carried out in the European Union (Eurobarometer) collected data on binge drinking using the same definition, that is "consuming 5 or more alcoholic drinks on one occasion" [12]. Data were collected in face-to-face interviews (generally computer-assisted). Figure 1.3 depicts the prevalence rates of "binge drinking" among last year drinkers (EU-25 prevalence 75%; see also footnote 1). About two in three Europeans who had drunk alcohol in the past year also had consumed 5 or more drinks on at least one occasion,

Fig. 1.3 Frequency of having had five or more drinks on one occasion during the past year (2006) among drinkers in the population of 15 years and above in the EU (percentage among those who had consumed alcohol at least once during previous 12 months). In 2006, Romania and Bulgaria were not yet member of the EU and their data are not included in the EU average. Source: [12])

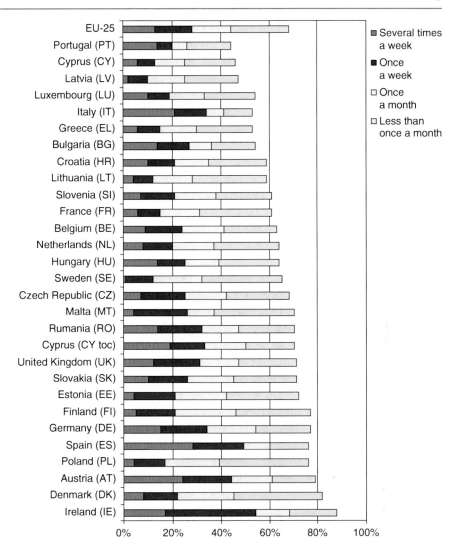

and 44% did so once per month or more frequent. Differences between Member States are large. Binge drinking *at least once per month* appears to be least common in Portugal, Cyprus and Latvia (25–26%) and most common in Ireland, Spain and Austria (60–68%). In Spain and Austria, even a quarter or more of the last year drinkers "binges" several times a week. Binge drinking at least once a month is more common among men than women (54% against 31%) and among younger compared to higher age groups, but it is certainly not exclusively a phenomenon among the young (e.g. 53% among 15–24 years old against 37% among age 55+).

Among last month drinkers (prevalence 65%), 10% indicated to have consumed 5 or more drinks on an occasion (same percentage for EU-25 and EU-15). A similar percentage was found for EU-15 in 2003. However, as the overall prevalence of last month alcohol consumption increased (from 61% to 67%), the actual number of people who drank 5 or more drinks has slightly increased.

Surveys in the USA and Australia also suggest that binge drinking is also quite common in these western countries. In the USA, an increase in binge drinking episodes among adults was reported between 1993 and 2001 [21]. Findings are from the Behaviour Risk Factor Surveillance System (BRFSS), a continuous telephone survey among the population of 18 years and above in all American states. While the prevalence of binge drinking, defined as consuming 5 or more alcoholic drinks on one occasion in the past month, among all US adults remained generally stable between 1993 and 2001 (14.3% in 2001; 22% for men, 7% for women), a significant increase in the total number of binge-drinking *episodes* was found in this period, from 1.2 to 1.5 billion. In 2001, among those who had consumed alcohol in the past month, 27% had "binged" at least once (36% for men; 27% for women).

Findings from the National Drugs Use and Health Survey showed that the prevalence of binge drinking (same definition as BRFSS) in the total U.S. population of 12 years and over remained stable as well between 2001 and 2007 (SAMSHA, 2008). This also applied when the definition was narrowed to heavy drinkers bingeing on at least 5 days in the past month. Peak levels for both binge drinking and heavy use

Fig. 1.4 Prevalence of last month (current) use of alcohol, binge drinking and heavy alcohol use by age group in the USA in 2007. For definitions of alcohol use see text. Groups of alcohol users are not mutually exclusive. Thus, heavy users are also included in the group of binge drinkers. Source: SAMSHA, 2008

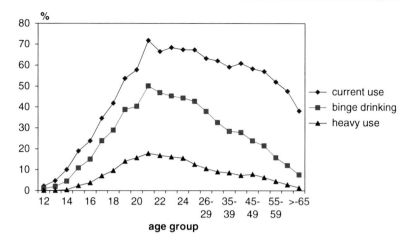

were found in age group 21–24 (see Fig. 1.4). No trends in binge drinking episodes were reported.

In Australia, measures of "risky drinking" in the general population remained fairly stable between 2001 and 2007 [22]. In the 2007 survey, 20% of the population of 14 years and above (24% for men, 17% for women) drank at levels considered to be risky or highly risky in the short term. This was defined as drinking at least 7 or more drinks per occasion for adult males and 5 or more per occasion or 7 or more per day for females, at least once per month. One in ten (10%, for both males and females) consumed alcohol at levels consider to be harmful in the long term (defined as drinking of 29 or more drinks per week for adult males and 15 or more drinks per week for adult females).

Prevalence of Drinking Among Young People

Alcohol consumption among young people has attracted much political attention in the past years. Early onset of alcohol use and drinking patterns are important predictors of later alcohol use problems. Moreover, research data point at negative effects of alcohol on adolescent brain development, although the evidence is not conclusive [23].

Several international studies provided comparable data on adolescent drinking. The Health Behaviour of School-Aged Children Survey (HBSC) in 2005/2006 of the WHO reported on weekly drinking and drunkenness among pupils of 11, 13 and 15 years in 41 countries. The results of this survey not only show that drinking and drunkenness are on average fairly common behaviours even among these young people, but also that there are wide differences between countries. On average one in four pupils (26%) of this age was a weekly drinker, with more boys (31%) than girls (21%) drinking. Highest levels are found in Ukraine (53%) and lowest in Finland (10%). At age 11, on average 5% of the pupils drank at least weekly (3% girls, 7% males) and increases in prevalence with increasing age are seen in virtually all countries, with the biggest change occurring between 13 and 15 years.

On average 15% of the pupils reported first drunkenness to occur as young as 13 years, with highest levels of early drunkenness reported among Esthonian boys (35%), followed by Lithuania, Austria, and England and Wales (boys between 23 and 29%, girls between 19 and 21%). Early drunkenness was least common in Italy, Israel and Greece (boys between 6 and 9%, girls between 3 and 5%). At age 15, even one in three pupils of 15 years (30% girls, 37% boys) had been drunk on at least twice, with highest levels in Denmark (57%) and lowest in Israel (15%). In most countries, drunkenness is more commonly reported among boys than girls. It should be noted that reports of drunkenness are subjective and sensitive to culture, and may refer to different levels of intoxication.

The European ESPAD survey among pupils of 15/16 years reported an increase in episodic heavy drinking (having 5 or more drinks on at least one occasion in the past month) between 1995 and 1999 and again between 2003 and 2007 [24]. The latter trend was found in over half of the participating countries and especially among females. In contrast, heavy episodic drinking (five or more drinks in a row during the prior 2-week interval) among American pupils shows a decreasing trend in the past years [25]. Longer-term trends resemble those of illicit drug use, with a peak in the early and mid-1980s, followed by a sharp decrease (e.g. prevalence decreased from 41% in 1983 to 28% in 1992 among 12th graders). This was followed by a slight increase in heavy episodic drinking until the mid-1990s, albeit much less than for illicit drug use, which slowly levelled off thereafter.

Alcohol Use Disorders

Chronic and excessive use of alcohol may lead to problems with health, personal relationships, and school or work. Surveys usually include alcohol dependence and alcohol abuse or harmful use, which are defined on the basis of clinical symptoms, rather than alcohol consumption patterns.

Table 1.3 Prevalence of DSM-IV alcohol use disorders in 2001–2003 among countries participating in the World Mental Health Survey initiative

	Alcohol abuse		Alcohol dependence*	
	Lifetime (%)	12-month (%)	Lifetime (%)	12-month (%)
The Americas				
Colombia	6.9	2.3	2.3	1.1
Mexico	14.5 (m), 1.3 (f)	4.3 (m), 0.2 (f)	6.2 (m), 0.7 (f)	2.0 (m), 0.2 (f)
USA	13.2	3.1	5.4	1.3
Africa				
Nigeria	1.9	0.6	0.3	0.2
South Africa	11.4	2.6	4.5	1.2
Eastern medit.				
Lebanon	1.5	1.2	0.4	0.3
European				
Belgium	7.8	1.7	1.7	0.3
France	6.7	–	1.6	–
Germany	6.3	1.0	1.5	0.3
Israel	4.0	1.1	0.4	<0.1
Italy	1.2	0.2	0.3	0.1
The Netherlands	8.4	1.8	1.5	0.4
Spain	3.6	0.7	0.6	0.1
Ukraine	10.0	3.7	3.5	2.1
	19.7 (m) 2.0 (f)	7.2 (m) 0.9 (f)	6.7 (m) 0.8 (f)	4.2 (m) 0.4 (f)
Western Pacific				
Japan	–	1.0	–	0.2
New Zealand	7.4	2.6	4.1	1.3
	10.7 (m) 4.3 (f)	3.7 (m), 1.6 (f)	5.6 (m) 2.6 (f)	1.7 (m) 0.9 (f)

Age ranges were 18 years and above in all countries, except for Colombia (18–65 years), Japan (20 years and above) and Mexico (18–65 years). Target response rates of 65% or above were not achieved in Belgium (51%), France (46%), Germany (57%), the Netherlands (56%) and Japan (56%)

[a] Prevalence rates may be underestimated (see text). Rates refer to people who also fulfilled a (lifetime) diagnosis of alcohol abuse. *m* males, *f* females. Sources: Kessler and Üstün [33]; [14], Oakley Browne et al. [34]; Bromet et al. [35]

The most common classification systems to define these disorders are the Diagnostic and Statistical Manuals of Mental Disorders of the American Psychiatric association (APA) and the International Classification of Diseases of the WHO [26]. The DSM is most widely used in research. Dependence is characterised by compulsion and a loss of self-control over alcohol use. A person abusing alcohol begins to disregard his/her responsibilities in school, at work, or socially because of alcohol use, and he/she may engage in dangerous activities while intoxicated. There is a hierarchy in that persons fulfilling criteria of both abuse and dependence are assigned the diagnosis dependence. In general, the diagnosis of dependence according to the latest versions of the DSM (III-R and IV) has shown to be reliable and valid. However, this does not apply to a diagnosis of alcohol abuse, which given the hierarchical rules can be considered as a "residual category" of alcohol use disorders. Moreover, an abuse diagnosis has been suggested to reflect a transitory pattern of maladaptive (risk) behaviour (especially common among young males), rather than a clinical disorder or form of psychopathology, given the low levels of co-morbidity with other mental disorders and relatively low impact on daily functioning and quality of life [27, 28]. Overall prevalence rates of alcohol use disorders in DSM-III-R and DSM IV are generally similar, but there may

be a shift towards higher abuse rates and lower dependence rates using DSM IV criteria [29].

For many years, comparisons of prevalence of alcohol use disorders between countries were hampered by large methodological differences. The World Mental Health Surveys, which were carried out in between 2001 and 2003 in 16 countries, aimed to improve this situation. These surveys are all based on the same instrument (CIDI 3.0) and methodologies are largely harmonised, although differences in age groups, response rates, may still affect comparability of findings. A disadvantage is that the prevalence rates of dependence may be slightly underestimated. In the early version of the CIDI 3.0, participants who did not report ever experiencing any symptom of abuse were not asked dependence questions. This may have resulted in an underestimation of dependence diagnoses, especially among women and ethnic minorities, although the impact of this "skip" is probably small [30–32]. Moreover, the CIDI remains a subjective instrument, which is sensitive to culture and context, and even within the same country and by using the same instruments, different studies may yield widely varying prevalence estimates [7].

With these reservations in mind, Table 1.3 gives the lifetime and 12-month prevalence rates for DSM IV alcohol abuse and dependence. Across all countries abuse diagnoses are (much) more common than dependence, although differences may be attenuated slightly when taking the possible underestimation of dependence diagnoses into account. More peculiar are, however, the widely varying prevalence rates for both disorders, with lifetime diagnoses of alcohol abuse peaking in the USA, South Africa and the Ukraine (10% and above), and being lowest in Lebanon, Italy and Nigeria (below 2%). Twelve-month prevalence abuse was also highest in the Ukraine and the USA (3.7 and 3.1%, respectively), followed by both South Africa and New Zealand (each 2.6%). Twelve-month diagnoses of alcohol abuse were least common in Italy, Spain and Nigeria (<1%). Twelve-month alcohol dependence is most frequently diagnosed in the Ukraine (2.1%), followed by intermediate rates in Colombia, Mexico, USA, South Africa and New Zealand (1.0–1.3%), and relatively low rates below 0.5% in the remaining countries.

Aggregated data from surveys in Belgium, France, Germany, the Netherlands and Spain (data gathered under the umbrella of the ESEMeD project) showed that alcohol use disorders were more common among men than women: 1.3 and 0.2%, respectively, for the 12-month prevalence of abuse and 0.4% and 0.1%, respectively, for the 12-month prevalence of dependence [36]. These differences are likely to reflect differences in drinking patterns, not decreased sensitivity as women may be more vulnerable to the negative effects of alcohol. Nonetheless, in the USA, gender differences in alcohol consumption, abuse, and dependence are decreasing over time [37]. The ESEMeD study also showed that 12-month prevalence rates of alcohol use disorders were highest in age group 18–24 years (2.2%). Rehm et al. (2005) note that in various European studies alcohol abuse tends to be more prevalent in younger age groups; no such clear picture emerges for alcohol dependence [7]. Yet, in New Zealand, peak levels for both abuse and dependence are seen in the younger age group (16–24 years) [34]. In the NESARC study in the USA, however, alcohol dependence clearly peaks in age group 18–29 years, while alcohol abuse rates are generally similarly high in age group 18–29 and 30–44 years.

Alcohol use disorders seem to be lowest among persons who are married or live with a partner, but this protective factor is common among most mental disorders [36]. Genetic factors greatly contribute to the development of alcohol dependence with heritability estimates in the range of 50–60% for both men and women [38]. For a review of risk factors for alcohol use disorders see Sher et al. [39].

As indicated before, the volume of alcohol consumption has been shown to be poorly correlated with the prevalence of alcohol use disorders [7], although different indicators of (problem) alcohol use for the Ukraine seems to be fairly consistent (e.g. high per capita consumption, high prevalence of binge drinking among adults and weekly drinking among youth, and high rates of alcohol use disorders).

Illicit Drug Use

Overall Picture

The United Nations estimates that worldwide the number of cannabis users is about ten times higher than the number of users of amphetamines, ecstasy, cocaine and opiates (Table 1.4) [40]. The number of opiate users equals the number of cocaine users. Due to low data quality, estimates for amphetamines and ecstasy are quite uncertain, as expressed in the wide range of the estimate. Within the group of amphetamines, it is estimated that some 54–59% relates to methamphetamine, 32–35% to amphetamine and 8–11% to other synthetic stimulants (e.g. pharmaceuticals).

Population surveys indeed show that in western countries cannabis is the most often used illicit drug (Table 1.5). With the methodological caveats in comparing and interpreting survey data in mind (see introduction), it can be concluded that experience with any drug as well as recent drug use is generally less prevalent in the EU than in the USA, Canada and Australia. However, there are large variations between individual EU countries, and prevalence rates in some EU countries equal or exceed those of the USA, Canada and Australia. Cannabis and cocaine use are more prevalent among the USA and Canada compared to Australia, while the use of ecstasy and amphetamines is far more prevalent in Australia (Table 1.5). Within Europe, cocaine generally dominates the stimulant markets in the Western and Southern regions, albeit restricted to a few large countries. Amphetamines are the main stimulants in North, Central and Eastern Europe.

Data from 17 countries collected in the framework of the World Mental Health Surveys (see "alcohol disorders") showed that illegal drug use was more likely among persons who had never been married or previously been married and among males compared to females. Yet, gender differences in initiating drug use were less consistent in younger age cohorts, suggesting that women may catch up to men, at least in some countries [43]. Drug use was also linked to income (higher income associated with higher prevalence), but this may be different for subgroups of problem drug users, who are more likely to have a lower socioeconomic status [44]. In general, there seems to be no straightforward relationship between drug use prevalence and drug policies [43, 45, 46].

Table 1.4 Estimated number of drug users (× million), worldwide[a]

Type of drug	Estimated number of people (× million)
Cannabis	142.6–190.3
Amphetamines	15.8–50.8
Ecstasy	11.6–23.5
Cocaine	15.6–20.8
Opiates	15.2–21.1

[a] Based on past year users. Source: UNODC [40]

Table 1.5 Lifetime and last year prevalence of drug use in the general population in the European Union (2004–2008)[a], USA (2008), Canada (2004) and Australia (2007)

	EU (age 15–64)	USA (age 12+)	Canada (age 15+)	Australia (age 14+)
Cannabis				
– Lifetime (%)	22 Range: 1.5–38.6	41	48.7	33.5
– Last year (%)	6.8 Range: 0.4–14.6	10.3	15.4	9.1
Cocaine/crack				
– Lifetime (%)	3.9 Range: 0.1–8.3	14.7	12.3	5.9
– Last year (%)	1.2 Range: 0.0–3.1	2.1	2.4	1.6
Ecstasy				
– Lifetime (%)	3.1 Range: 0.3–7.5	5.2	5.1	8.9
– Last year (%)	0.8 Range: 0.3–7.5	0.9	0.8	3.5
Amphetamines				
– Lifetime (%)	3.5 Range: 0.0–11.9	8.5[b]	6.1	6.3
– Last year (%)	0.5 Range: 0.0–1.3	1.1[b]	0.4	2.3

Sources: EMCDDA [2], Adlaf [41], SAMHSA [42], AIHW [22]

[a] Most surveys were conducted between 2004 and 2008. For the computation of the average: see EMCDDA, 2008, page 40. For the EU the standard age range 15–64 years was used in all countries, except in Czech Republic [19–65], Denmark [17–65], Germany [19–65], Hungary [19–65], Malta [19–65], Sweden [17–65] and UK [17–60]. In countries using wider age ranges, prevalence estimates may be slightly lower, and vice versa

[b] Category refers to nonmedical use of psychotherapeutics, stimulants and methamphetamine. Methamphetamine: lifetime 5%, last year 0.3%

Cannabis

It has been roughly estimated that in 2007 worldwide between 143 and 190 million people had used cannabis, with highest (absolute) numbers being reported for Africa, Asia and North America. In terms of percentage users of the population, highest values are found in North America, Oceania and Western and Central Europe [40].

In the European Union at least 23 million people had at least once used cannabis in the past year, which is about one-third of all lifetime users in the general population aged 15–64 years [2]. Highest prevalence rates of last year use are reported in Italy (15%), Spain (10%), the Czech Republic (9%) and France (9%), and lowest levels in Romania (0.4%), Malta (0.8%), Bulgaria (1.9%) Greece (1.7%) and Sweden (2%). In the USA, the absolute number of last year cannabis users is 26 million. Use is however disproportionally high among young people. Figure 1.5 depicts last year prevalence in EU countries both for the total population and among young people. In virtually all countries, prevalence rates clearly peak in age group 15–24 years. Highest levels are found in the Czech Republic, with almost three in ten young people reporting use of cannabis in the past year (28%), and lowest levels in Romania (1.6%) followed by, Greece and

Cyprus (3.6%). Male–female ratios of past year use range from 1/5 in Finland to 4.3 in Hungary.

Many people may try cannabis once or a few times or take the drug occasionally, such as less than once a month. Frequency of cannabis use is, however, not routinely included in surveys. According to the EMCDDA, in countries for which data are available 19–33% of the people who had used cannabis in the past month did so (at least near) daily, e.g., on 20 or more days a month [47]. This is 0.5–2.3% of the total population (1.2% on average, about four million Europeans).

Early adolescence seems to be an important period for the development of cannabis-related harm. Some studies indicate that the risk of adverse mental health effects, such as psychotic disorders, appear to be most pronounced among those who start using cannabis at a young age (before 16) [48–50]. Furthermore, an early age of onset is found to be associated with heavy use or problematic use of cannabis and other drugs at a later age [51]. Early users are also less likely to quit their habit than those beginning at later ages [52].

The HBSC study in 2005/2006 in 25 countries (see alcohol paragraph) shows that on average 12% of the students of 15 years were past-year users of cannabis. Half of this group only consumed cannabis once or twice ("experimenters"), 5% did so 3–39 times (regular users) and 1% was considered

Fig. 1.5 Last year prevalence of cannabis use in the general population of 15–64 years and among young people of 15–24 years in Member States of the EU and Norway. A standard age range of 15–64 years was used in all countries, except in Czech Republic [19–65], Denmark [17–65], Germany [19–65], Hungary [19–65], Malta [19–65], Sweden [17–65] and UK [17–60]. In countries using wider age ranges, prevalence estimates may be slightly lower, and vice versa. Source: EMCDDA [2]

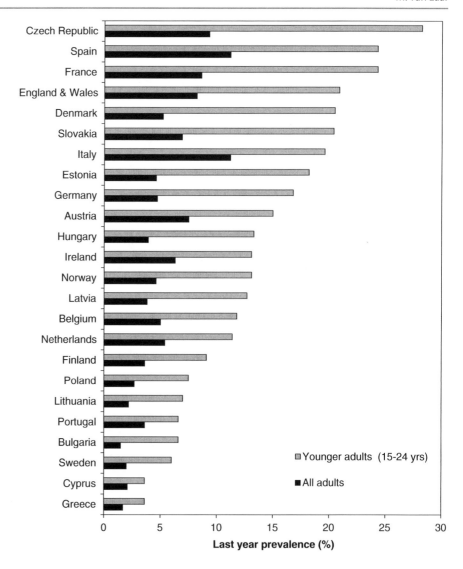

to be a heavy user (40 times or more in the past year). Differences between countries were big. Canada peaked on almost all indicators: 12-month prevalence 27%, 8% experimenters, 14% regular users and 5% experimenters. Spain and Switzerland are also on top of the list (23% last year prevalence; 11/10% of regular users and 4% heavy users). Lowest levels were reported in Iceland, TFYR Macedonia, Greece, Sweden and Israel (12-month prevalence 3% or below). Remarkably, in countries with higher prevalence rates, use among boys and girls tend to become more equal, although boys still tend to dominate in the heavy users group.

Trends in Cannabis Use

In general, figures point at stabilising or decreasing levels of cannabis use in recent years, although trends may diverge between countries. The USA have a longstanding tradition on monitoring drug use both among the general population and among students, allowing description of long-term trends. Cannabis consumption has evolved in two waves,

with use rates starting to increase in the 1960s, peaking mid and late 1970s, then dropped, and rose again although it did not reach the level of the first wave. More recent U.S. figures show a marginal decrease in last year prevalence in the population of 12 years and above from 11% in 2002 to 10% in 2007. This was mainly caused by a decrease in use between 2002 and 2005 among youth of 12–17 years [25].

The long-term trend in the USA is also seen in some European countries, although major differences between countries can be noted, with cannabis use starting to increase during the 1970s in Spain, during the 1980s in former West Germany and in the 1990s in Greece. Initially, cannabis use was probably much more bound to specific subgroups and subcultures than it was today [53, 54]. A general finding across almost all countries is the rise in cannabis use during the 1990s, especially among young people and pupils, which lasted at least till the early 2000s. Since 2001 trends are more divergent, but there is an overall tendency towards a stabilisation or decrease. In spite of slight increases in cannabis use

Table 1.6 Prevalence of cannabis use disorders in different population surveys

Population, age (years)	Year	Abuse		Dependence	
		Lifetime (%)	Last year (%)	Lifetime (%)	Last year (%)
U.S. population, 18+	2001/2002	7.2	1.1	1.3	0.3
Australian population, 18+	1998	–	0.7	–	1.5
German (Munich) population, 14–24	1995	2.8	–	1.2	–
New Zealand population, age 25	2002	–	–	13	–
Dutch population, 18–64	1996	1.2	0.4	1.0	0.5

In the first four studies, cases were classified according to DSM IV criteria; in the Dutch study DSM-III-R diagnoses were reported. Sources: USA [64]; Australia [65]; Germany/Munich [66]; New Zealand [67]; The Netherlands [68]

in Finland and Sweden, prevalence rates still remain low in these countries.

In Australia, last year prevalence of cannabis use among the population of 14 years and above increased from 13% in 1995 to 18% in 1998, and then strongly declined to 9% in 2007 [55]. Youth surveys point at declining or stabilising use, for example the HBSC studies in 2001/2002 and 2005/2006 among 15-year-old school students, although slight increases were seen in Estonia, Latvia and Malta [56]. The ESPAD surveys showed an overall increase in cannabis use between 1995 and 2003, which had come to a halt, if not decrease, in many countries in 2007 [24]. In some countries, decreases were quite dramatic. For example, the past month use of cannabis among 15/16-year-old pupils in the UK almost halved from 20% in 2003 to 11% in 2007.

Stabilising or decreasing trends are hard to explain. According to the EMCDDA, cannabis availability had not changed much for Europe as a whole and prices seem to be decreasing in most countries. Reasons for quitting cannabis use might be a "lack of interest", transitions in life phase and worries about the negative health effects of cannabis [53, 57, 58]. The reduction in cannabis use might also be secondary to a reduction in tobacco smoking, which share the same route of administration and are often consumed together in a joint, at least in Europe. Moreover, the seemingly waning popularity of cannabis among young people might be associated with increasing knowledge of the risks associated with the use of this drug [47].

Cannabis Use Disorders

According to the National Comorbidity Survey in the USA during the early 1990s, one in ten people who ever consume cannabis at least once will be dependent at some time in their life (10%) [59]. For alcohol and cocaine, these rates are 20% and 21%, respectively. Within 2 years after first cannabis use, 2–5% of the users fulfilled a diagnosis of cannabis dependence, and within 10 years this proportion has increased to 8%. Risk factors for the development of cannabis dependence include early age of onset of use, being male, low family income, use of three or more substances before starting

cannabis use, frequency of use (weekly or daily), antisocial behaviour, persistent tobacco smoking, death of a parent before age 15, low self-esteem and genetic predisposition [59–61]. Possibly also the potency of cannabis plays a role in the development of cannabis use disorders, but this depends on whether cannabis users adapt or titrate their cannabis use according to the concentration of THC, the main psychoactive component of cannabis [62].

Population data on cannabis use disorders are limited. Table 1.6 lists findings from studies providing DSM (III-R or IV) diagnoses of cannabis abuse and dependence in the general population of several countries. The data should be interpreted with caution. Apart from methodological differences, it is possible that data for the older studies are not representative for the current situation, due to for example, changes in cannabis consumption patterns (e.g. the strong decrease in prevalence in Australia) or cannabis potency (increases in the Netherlands).

The currently available data show that the prevalence of cannabis disorders varies between studies but a general finding is that they are generally most common among young adults. For example in the USA, last year prevalence rates of cannabis abuse and dependence in age group 18–29 were 3.3% and 1.1%, respectively. Corresponding lifetime prevalence rates were 9.5% and 2.7%, respectively. In Australia and the Netherlands, a similar age distribution is seen. Moreover, in all countries cannabis use disorders are far more common among men than women.

In the USA, one in four (25%) persons who had consumed cannabis in the past year fulfilled a diagnosis of cannabis abuse and 10% a diagnosis of dependence. In Australia, comparable figures were found, i.e. 21% and 11%, respectively. In the Netherlands, lower figures for abuse were found (9% among last year users) but a similar proportion for dependence (11%). Remind also that especially abuse diagnoses may be sensitive to culture and context of use, which might to contribute to differences between countries. For example, problems with police and justice in DSM IV (e.g. being arrested because of drug use) may depend on the legal status and law enforcement practises in a country.

In the USA, a slight increase in the overall prevalence of cannabis use disorders was seen from 1991/1992 to 2002/2002, whereas the prevalence of cannabis use remained stable [63]. The increase was especially seen in young black men and women and young Hispanic men. As quantity and frequency of cannabis consumption had not changed, it was suggested that the parallel increase in cannabis potency had contributed to the higher prevalence of cannabis use disorders. This explanation can, however, not account for differences in risks between ethnic groups.

Cocaine

The USA has been the dominant market for cocaine since the emergence of the modern cocaine epidemic in the 1980s. However, since the mid-1990s the European market for cocaine has expanded substantially, as reflected by increases in prevalence, seizures and treatment demand [69, 70]. As high use levels of cocaine are concentrated in a few countries, amphetamines still count as the second most commonly used drugs in most EU countries.

Cocaine can be used in different ways. Recreational or integrated users predominantly snort cocaine (hydrochloride) in powder form, whereas the more marginalised (problem) users consume cocaine by injecting or by smoking its base form, usually called "crack". Cocaine (injecting and smoking) is also common among opiate users. While both cocaine powder and crack cocaine are common drugs in the USA, crack use in Europe is concentrated to some subpopulations in several countries (and cities), such as Spain, the Netherlands, UK and Italy. Chronic cocaine use has been associated with a variety of health problems, especially cardiovascular and neurological diseases [70]. Risks associated with the route of administration include lung complications (coke lung, resulting from frequent crack use), damaged nostrils, resulting from frequent snorting, and infectious diseases an elevated overdose risk resulting from injecting cocaine.

In the USA, cocaine use peaked in the early 1980s, declined until the early 1990s and then showed a rise in again. However, recent surveys showed an overall stable level between 2002 and 2008, although a decrease in the youngest age group (12–17 years) and among pupils has been reported [25]. It is estimated that, approximately 5.3 million Americans aged 12 or older had used cocaine in 2008 (2.1%), with over one-fourth of that group smoking crack cocaine [25].

Estimates are lower in Europe, although indicators point at increasing use. In its 2009 Annual report, the EMCDDA reported that around four million Europeans of 15–64 years had used cocaine in the last year, which is about 1.2% on average. Use is mainly concentrated in young adults of 15–34 years (2.2%). However, there is considerable variation between European countries. Lowest rates of last year cocaine use in the general population of 15–64 years are reported in Romania, Greece, Poland, Latvia and the Czech Republic (0.2% or lower). Highest levels are found in Ireland (1.7%), Italy (2.2%), UK (2.3%) and Spain (3.1%), with levels over 5% among young adults of 15–34 years in Spain. The EMCDDA noted a strong increase in cocaine use since the late 1990s in the UK and Spain, with a less steep rise afterwards. More recent increases between 2002 and 2007 were also seen in Ireland, Latvia and Portugal. These trends were generally paralleled by a growing number of people entering treatment for cocaine problems in several countries, most prominently in Spain, Ireland and Italy. There were 61,000 cocaine clients in the EU in 2007. The proportion of cocaine clients among all drug clients increased from 13% in 2002 to 19% in 2007. Cocaine powder was the most common reason to enter treatment. While this may reflect differences in the extent of problem use between cocaine and crack, there are also indications that treatment needs of problem crack users may be more difficult to meet.

Data on the prevalence of cocaine use disorders are limited. In the USA, 0.6% of the general population of 18 years and above fulfilled DSM IV criteria for cocaine abuse and dependence, with most cases classified as dependence. This is one-fourth of all last year users. Prevalence rates of abuse and dependence were highest among age group 18–25 years (1.4%). A U.S. study also showed that 5–6% of the cocaine users fulfilled a diagnosis of dependence within 1 year after first cocaine use. Within 10 years, some 15–16% of the lifetime users are dependent (cf. 8% for cannabis) [71]. Moreover, the risk of being dependent 1 or 2 years after initiating cocaine use appears to be greater for crack users and cocaine injectors compared to snorters of cocaine [72]. These differences are consistent with variations in dependence risk, related amongst others to the more rapid onset of action and greater intensity of effects of the first two routes of administration [73].

General population surveys, as described above, may underestimate the number of problem users of cocaine/crack and other drugs, who are relatively often homeless or institutionalised (see introduction). In three European countries, specific methods have been used to estimate the number of problem cocaine users (defined as injection or long duration/regular use). In Spain (2001), there were between 4.5 and 6 problem cocaine users per 1,000 adult population (15–64 years) and in Italy (2006) between 3.7 and 4.5 per 1,000 [47]. In England, the population rate of problem *crack* use was 5.2–5.6 per 1,000 aged 15–64 years [74]. In the UK, this group overlaps to a large extent with those of the opiate users.

Availability and accessibility of cocaine-specific treatment programmes is generally low and there is as yet no effective pharmacological treatment for cocaine dependence, although some agents seem to be promising in clinical trials [47].

Amphetamines

The term amphetamines refers to a variety of psychostimulant drugs that are chemically related to amphetamine, such as dextroamphetamine or methamphetamine. Methamphetamine and amphetamine have similar behavioural effects, but methamphetamine is more potent and has longer-lasting effects on the central nervous system. Methamphetamine is mainly used in North America, Australia, New Zealand and East and South East Asia. Although amphetamine is the second most common illegal drug in many EU countries after cannabis, *meth-amphetamine* use is generally rare, except in the Czech Republic and to some extent Slovakia [2, 40]. At a global level, however, the number of methamphetamine users is estimated to be almost two times higher than the number of amphetamine users [40].

Amphetamines powder can be swallowed, snorted or injected; the crystalline form of methamphetamine (known as ice or crystal meth) may be smoked. Injection and smoking are the more harmful ways of using amphetamines. In the USA, smoking has become the most common route of administration of methamphetamine among those in treatment; injection is more common among dependent methamphetamine users in Australia [13, 75]. Chronic amphetamine use is associated with a range of (health) problems, including addiction, psychosis, mood disturbances, malnutrition and violent behaviour, whereas injection contributes to overdose and the spread of infectious diseases.

Worldwide, amphetamines use peaks in Oceania, with a last year prevalence rate of 2.6% among the population of 15–64 years, followed by North America (1.3%) and Central America (1.3%), the Caribbean (between 0.5% and 1%), East and South-East Asia (between 0.3% and 1.4%) and the EU (0.5%) [2, 40]. In Europe, last year prevalence rates vary from 0% in Greece, Romania and Malta to between 1.0 and 1.3% in the UK, Estonia, Denmark and Norway. Trends are mixed, with countries reporting either an increase, or a stabilisation or a decrease [2].

According to the 2007 ESPAD survey in 35 European countries, between 1% and 8% of the 15/16-year-old students had *ever* tried amphetamines. The lowest percentage of lifetime users (1% or less) was reported by Armenia, Faro islands, Finland, Norway, Romania, Russia and the Ukraine and highest percentages (6–8%) in Austria, Bulgaria, Latvia and the Slovak republic. By far the highest lifetime prevalence was reported for American students in the same age group, although a decreasing trend was observed from 16% in 1999 to 11% in 2007.

There are also some recent indications that in the USA, methamphetamine use might be over its top, which has been linked to a reduced availability due to strict precursor controls [40]. Whether this trend will persist is not known. The number of Americans aged 12 years or older reporting past-year methamphetamine use declined from 1.9 million (0.7%) in 2006 to 1.3 million (0.5%) in 2007 and 0.85 million (0.2%) in 2008. Yet, these declines are partially offset by increasing use in Mexico, which seems to take overproduction from the USA [40]. Moreover, methamphetamine use remains a serious problem, especially in the western American region, as indicated by data from treatment admissions, law enforcement agencies and county hospitals [13]. For the European region, amphetamine users make up a significant proportion of the overall treatment demand by drug users for drug use (16–34%) only in Latvia, Sweden and Finland. In Slovakia and the Czech Republic, methamphetamine users often feature in treatment statistics (25% and 61%, respectively, of all drug clients). While these data may point at a significant group of problem amphetamines users, the actual size remains unknown since not all problem users will come into contact with health care agencies and/or police, or are captured in population surveys.

There are little data from indirect estimation methods taking also into account the "hidden" population of problem amphetamines users. In Australia, such methods traditionally focused on dependent heroin users, who contribute to disease burden disproportionately to their numbers in the population. However, using multiplier methods the population of dependent methamphetamine users, most of whom inject the drug, has been estimated at 73,000 against approximately 45,000 regular heroin users [75].

In Europe, opioid users generally dominate the group of problem drug users. However, there are some exceptions. In Finland, the number of problem amphetamine users (12,000–22,000) was estimated to be four times higher than the number of problem opioid users [2]. In Slovakia, the number of problem users of methamphetamine was estimated in 2007 at 5,800–15,700 (or 1.5–4.0 cases per 1,000 population of 5–64 years). In the Czech Republic, the number of problem methamphetamine users was about 21,000 (about 2.8 per 1,000 population of 15–64 years), which was about twice the number of problem opioid users [2].

Ecstasy

The official name for ecstasy is 3,4-methylenedioxymethamphetamine (MDMA). This drug has both stimulant and so-called entactogenic effects, i.e. making people feel drawn to each other and make contact more easily. Ecstasy is most commonly consumed orally as tablet, which may have widely varying forms in terms of colours, weight and markings (such as a dove, E, yin/yang symbol, Mitsubishi symbol). Other substances that are chemically similar to MDMA (such as MDA, MDEA and MBDB)—but also substances that bear no resemblance to it—are also sold as ecstasy without the user being aware of the difference (e.g. benzylpiperazine or mCPP). In this chapter, unless otherwise indicated, "ecstasy" is understood to mean substances that are experienced or passed off as ecstasy.

The popularity of ecstasy increased strongly in the 1990s, mainly in Western and Central Europe, North America (especially the USA), and is closely linked to the dance and club scene, although its use has clearly spread beyond the night-life culture.

Worldwide ecstasy is less popular than amphetamines, although in various western countries the rank order is reversed. Oceania (notably Australia and New Zealand) accounts for the highest annual prevalence rate of ecstasy consumption of any region (between 3.6% and 4% among the population of 15–64 years), although it has the fewest users in absolute numbers [40]. At distance come North America (0.9%) and Central/Western Europe (0.8%). Lowest estimates are reported in Central and South America (<0.2%).

In Europe, the percentage of last year ecstasy users varies from less than 0.5% in Greece and Romania to between 1.5 and 1.7% in the UK, Estonia, Slovakia and Latvia, with an exceptionally high prevalence in the Czech Republic (3.5%). Trends are mixed, with countries reporting either an increase, or a stabilisation or a decrease [2]. Estimates are much higher among young people, with last year use of ecstasy among 15–24-year olds estimated at between 1.0% and 3.9% in the majority of European countries. However, there is a considerable difference between the lowest national estimate at 0.3% and the highest at 12% [2].

Among Australians of 14 years and older, ecstasy is the second most used illicit drug after cannabis (last year prevalence 3.5% and 9.1%, respectively [22]). Highest consumption rates were reported for age group 20–29 years (last year prevalence 11%). One in 12 users (8%) used ecstasy at least once a week; on average 1.6 pills were consumed per occasion.

On average, 4% of the pupils of 15 and 16 years in 25 European countries had ever tried ecstasy in 2007 [24]. Lifetime prevalence ranged from 1% in Norway and the Faroe Islands to 6 or 7% in Bulgaria, Estonia, Slovakia, Isle of Man and Russia (Moscow). Trend data available for 20 countries showed that overall lifetime prevalence remained stable between 1999 and 2007, but there were marked differences between countries.

Use levels among adolescents and young adults in recreational settings, notably dance parties and clubs, are commonly much higher, but comparable data from surveys in different countries are not available.

While animal studies suggest that MDMA may be a less potent reinforcer than other drugs, it clearly does have abuse and dependence potential [76]. In a large scale national population survey in the USA, 3.6% and 4.9% of the past year ecstasy users fulfilled criteria of DSM IV hallucinogen dependence and abuse, respectively [77]. Spending a lot of time using or getting over the effects of hallucinogens and

tolerance were the two most commonly reported symptoms by users. As ecstasy users also commonly use other hallucinogens (like PCP and LSD), these rates may overestimate substance use disorders due to MDMA use only. However, other studies suggest much higher rates of ecstasy dependence among users. For example, a study among 600 ecstasy users in different cities (Sydney, Miami and St Louis) revealed that 83% of moderate (100–499 pills lifetime) or heavy ecstasy users (500+ pills lifetime) and 43% of light ecstasy users (1–99 pills lifetime) fulfilled criteria of dependence [1]. These differences might be partly related to the fact that the study by Wu and colleagues followed the DSM IV, which does not recognise the "withdrawal" criterion to be present for hallucinogen dependence (to which ecstasy/MDMA "belongs"). Other studies also took withdrawal symptoms into account, which seem to occur at high rates among ecstasy users [1, 78]. It is, however, hard to tell whether these symptoms really comprise withdrawal symptoms or are just sub-acute drug effects [76].

Use of ecstasy is associated with a number of (other) adverse health and psychological problems, including memory disturbances, depression and impulsivity, and these symptoms may persist for quite a long time after cessation of use beyond the withdrawal phase. However, the contribution of other factors, such as pre-morbid diseases and the use of other substances, is often hard to exclude [79]. Nonetheless, these problems rarely seem to be a reason for users to seek treatment. In 2007, two-thirds of European countries reported that ecstasy clients comprised less than 1% of all drug clients seeking treatment for addiction problems [2]. There is no explanation for the apparent big difference between the proportion of ecstasy users with a use disorder and treatment demand. Possibly ecstasy users are relatively socially integrated users who may cope well with their use or cease use on their own accord (e.g. due to financial consequences or changes in life circumstances, like finding a job or new relationship [80]). Another explanation might be that (ex) ecstasy users do not find their way to specialised addiction services, as symptoms are often of medical or psychological nature, and may occur for quite some time after use has stopped. Moreover, ecstasy users often consume other substances like cocaine, alcohol and cannabis, and these substances are more frequently than ecstasy reported as primary reason for seeking treatment.

Opioids

The drug class of opioids (also referred to as opiates) comprises many substances. Some of these are known for their illegal use, such as heroin. Since the 1970s heroin use has been associated with relatively high rates of morbidity and mortality, especially when the drug is injected. However, in some

Fig. 1.6 Total number of problem drug users and number of problem opioid users per 1,000 population of 15–64 years in a number of EU countries. Source: EMCDDA [47]; Hay et al. [84]. Estimates refer to 2002–2007

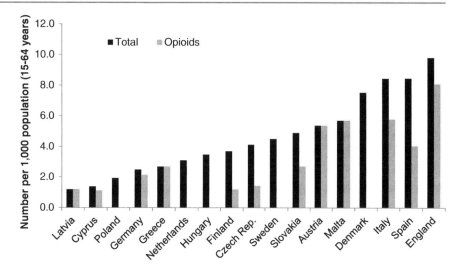

countries (e.g. the Netherlands, Germany and Switzerland) medical prescription of heroin to therapy-resistant registered drug addicts is possible, as standard regimen or within the framework of a medical trial [81, 82]. Other opioids are used for detoxification or as heroin substitutes during maintenance therapy, such as methadone and buprenorphine, Methadone, buprenorphine and a variety of other opioids (e.g. codeine, oxycodone) are also used therapeutically in medicine, amongst others, as pain relievers. While in the USA illicit drug use like cannabis and stimulants tend to decrease, especially among young people, the nonmedical use of prescription opioids, like OxyContin and Vicodin, has strongly increased in the past decade [25]. This trend also pertains to other psychotherapeutic drugs. Probably young people are less concerned about the dangers of using these drugs outside of medical regimen than they are about the dangers of using the illegal drugs, as suggested by the fact that the former are widely used for legitimate medical purposes [25].

Some degree of non-medical use of prescription opioids has been reported in Australia, Canada and several European countries as well, but comparisons are hampered by methodological differences [83]. In 2008, the EMCDDA also warned for possible increases in abuse of fentanyl, but this trend seems to be limited to the Baltic States [47].

According to estimates of the UNODC in 2009 there are worldwide roughly 15 and 21 million opioids users, with more than half of the world's opioids using population living in Asia. Highest population rates are found in Afghanistan along the main drug trafficking routes [40]. Europe holds the second largest population of (problem) opioids users, with 1.2–1.5 million estimated users living in West and Central Europe, and between 2.2 and 2.5 million living in Eastern and South Eastern Europe. However, these estimates are very rough as the underlying data sources are highly heterogeneous.

As indicated in the introduction, population surveys do not yield reliable estimates of the number of (problem) heroin users. The EMCDDA has issued guidelines for estimating problem drug use by using indirect estimation methods. Most commonly applied are the capture–re-capture and multiplier methods (http://www.emcdda.europa.eu/). These methods take into account that part of the problem drug users are in contact with treatment services, police or other organisations where they are registered, while another proportion is "hidden". Although the EMCDDA defines problem drug use as "injecting drug use or long-duration/regular use of opioids, cocaine and/or amphetamines", countries differ widely in the actual case definitions used for their estimates. For example, data in some countries allow a distinction between types of drugs (opioids, amphetamines, amphetamines) but in other countries no such distinction is made. Hence, the total number of problem drug users may be underestimated in some countries, unless of course the exclusion of amphetamines or cocaine may also reflect the drug situation in a particular country. In most countries, the group of problem drug users consist of heroin addicts, who often also consume a variety of other substances, like cocaine, alcohol, cannabis and benzodiazepines, but in some countries problem amphetamine or cocaine users are in the majority. Moreover, the application of different indirect estimation methods within the same country may yield varying results, and upper and lower ranges are often provided to indicate the degree of imprecision. For sake of comparisons between countries, Figure 1.6 gives a central estimate per country, but differences should be interpreted with caution.

In countries where specific estimates for problem opioids users are available, estimates range from about one per 1,000 inhabitants of 15–64 years in the Czech Republic, Poland, Latvia and Finland until about six or more per 1,000 inhabitants in this age group in Malta, Italy and England. In many countries the population of opioid users is growing older, as shown for example by increasing average age among opiate clients in treatment (average age 33 years). This may point at a decreasing influx of new (young) users, but recent data suggest that recruitment into heroin use still occurs. During the past decade several indicators, such as overdose fatalities, treatment demand and seizures suggested a stabilising or decreasing trend in heroin use. However, this trend seems to have halted in 2002/2003 and there are signs suggesting a worsening of the situation, although there are no indications of an epidemic spread of heroin use as seen in the 1980s and 1990s [2].

Infectious Diseases

The main routes of administration of heroin are injecting and smoking. Countries differ widely in the proportion of injecting heroin and other drug use, which is a risk factor for blood borne infectious diseases, like HIV/aids and hepatitis B and C. A review published in the Lancet suggests that worldwide on estimate 15.9 million (range 11.0–21.2 million) people inject drugs (not only heroin) [85]. As the quality of the data was often quite poor, estimates are generally not very precise, which is reflected in the wide ranges. The largest numbers of injectors were found in China, the USA and Russia. In terms of (midpoint) prevalence among the population of 15–64 years, estimated injecting drug use ranged from 0.02% in India and Cambodia till 5.2% in Azerbaijan. In most western European countries midpoint population estimates vary between 0.1% and 0.5%, except for Estonia (1.5%) (see also [2]). Injecting drug use was reported in 148 of the 200 countries included in the review, and this number seemed to have increased in the past decade [85]. Treatment data for EU countries, however, point at decreasing rates of injecting among opioid users, although there are great variations between countries [2].

Worldwide about three million people who inject drugs might be HIV positive but the estimate ranges from a lower limit of 0.8 to an upper limit of 6.6 million [85]. Prevalence of HIV among injecting drug users varied from 0.01% in eight countries to 72% in Estonia. Rates between 20% and 40% were found in five countries and rates over 40% in nine countries, with the largest numbers and concentrations of HIV-positive injecting drug users in Eastern Europe, East- and South-East Asia and Latin America. The spread of HIV has remained relatively low in Australia and New Zealand (1.5% and 1.6%, respectively) despite a higher prevalence of injecting (1.1% and 0.7%, respectively) compared to some other countries. This difference has been attributed to geographic isolation as well as the swift introduction of needle and syringe exchange programmes in the 1980s.

The incidence of HIV among injecting drug seems to diverge between European regions. Infection rates seem to have decreased or stabilised in most EU countries, following a peak in 2001–2002, which was due to outbreaks in Estonia, Latvia and Lithuania [86]. This positive trend is at least partly related to the increasing implementation of harm reduction measures, like needle and syringe exchange programmes and substitution treatment. However, in the former Soviet Republic the situation is worrying, as data suggest increasing incidence of HIV infection among people who inject drugs. In 2007, injecting drug users accounted for 57% of newly diagnosed HIV infections reported in this region.

A chronic hepatitis B or hepatitis C infection can cause serious forms of liver inflammation. Hepatitis C can virtually only be transmitted by direct blood to blood contact and is much more contagious than HIV. It can also be transmitted by sharing other contaminated (injecting) materials besides needles. The hepatitis B virus is transmitted by blood contact, for example by intravenous injecting with used needles, or through unprotected sexual contact. Data on hepatitis C are (also) not easily comparable between countries on account of differences in sources and methods of data collection. Nonetheless, the available data suggest that hepatitis C infection occurs usually with higher frequency among injecting drug users compared to HIV. A review in 2001 of 160 studies in 34 countries gave a weighted average hepatitis C prevalence of 70%, with North America and Asia having the highest rates [87]. A more recent review of 57 countries and 152 sub-national areas revealed prevalence rates of hepatitis C of at least 50% among injecting drug users in 49 countries or territories [88]. Worldwide, however, prevalence rates vary widely.

Among European countries, the variation in the rate of hepatitis B infection is greater than for hepatitis C. This may possibly be due to factors such as different vaccination strategies (universal versus risk groups). The most complete data available concern those having previously had a hepatitis B infection. The EMCDDA reported that in 2006–2007, three out of ten European countries reported that over 40% of injecting drug users had ever been infected with hepatitis B [2].

Conclusion

There are wide variations between countries and regions in substance use (problems). Differences are often hard to explain but contributing factors may include policies, availability, economic and (youth) cultural factors and the availability of preventive and harm reduction measures. Generally, (formal) drug policies are not strongly associated with prevalence of drug use, while the reverse is true for alcohol [45, 46, 89]. In terms of disease burden and societal costs, illicit drugs lag far behind alcohol. The Global Burden of Disease Study 2000 of the WHO estimated that worldwide alcohol accounts for 4% of the total burden of disability-adjusted life years (DALY's) and illicit drugs (mainly opiates) for 0.8%. Highest disease burden for both alcohol and illicit drug use can be attributed to developed regions, like North America, Europe, Australia en

New Zealand (12.2% for alcohol and 1.8% for illicit drugs) [90]. Moreover, economic costs are much higher for alcohol compared to illicit drugs. For example, in Australia 2004/2005 the total (direct and indirect) costs related to alcohol use were $15.3 billion against $8.2 billion for illicit drugs [91]. However, illicit drug use may have devastating effects on quality of life in some subpopulations, both for the afflicted persons themselves and their family and wider environment. In this regard, a positive development in the past decade concerns the increasing implementation of harm reduction policies, aiming to limit the negative health consequences of drug use. This trend can be observed in all regions of the world and has in fact become mainstream policy in many countries [69]. At same time knowledge of evidence-based treatments for substance use problems in general has strongly increased, which may be relevant at the individual level. Yet, the implementation of this knowledge in treatment practise remains to be improved in many countries. At societal level, alcohol use problems can be effectively reduced by various policy regulations, but differences between countries in the extent of implementation of these measures are large [89, 92].

References

1. Leung KS, Cottler LB. Ecstasy and other club drugs: a review of recent epidemiologic studies. Curr Opin Psychiatry. 2008;21: 234–41.
2. EMCDDA. Annual report: the state of the drugs problem in Europe. Lisbon: EMCDDA; 2009. p. 2009.
3. European Monitoring Centre for Drugs and Drug Addiction (EMCDDA). Selected Issue 2009: Polydrug use: patterns and responses. Luxembourg: Office for Official Publications of the European Communities; 2009.
4. European Monitoring Centre for Drugs and Drug Addiction (EMCDDA). EMCDDA 2002: Selected issue: polydrug use. Lisbon: EMCDDA; 2002.
5. World Health Organization. Global status report on alcohol 2004. Geneva: WHO; 2004.
6. Anderson P, Baumberg B. Alcohol in Europe: a public health perspective: a report for the European Commission. London: Institute of Alcohol Studies; 2006.
7. Rehm J, Room R, Van den Brink W, Kraus L. Problematic drug use and drug use disorders in EU countries and Norway: an overview of the epidemiology. Eur Neuropsychopharmacol. 2005;15(4):389–97.
8. Bobak M, Room R, Pikhart H, Kubinova R, Malyutina S, Pajak A, et al. Contribution of drinking patterns to differences in rates of alcohol related problems between three urban populations. J Epidemiol Community Health. 2004;58(3):238–42.
9. Gmel G, Room R, Kuendig H, Kuntsche S. Detrimental drinking patterns: empirical validation of the pattern values score of the Global Burden of Disease 2000 study in 13 countries. J Subst Use. 2007;12:337–58.
10. Rehm J, Rehn N, Room R, Monteiro M, Gmel G, Jernigan D, et al. The global distribution of average volume of alcohol consumption and patterns of drinking. Eur Addict Res. 2003;9(4):147–56.
11. Rehm J, Room R, Monteiro M, Gmel G, Graham K, Rehn N, et al. Alcohol use. In: Ezzati M, Lopez AD, Rodgers A, Murray CJL, editors. Comparative quantification of health risks global and regional burden of disease attributable to selected major risk factors. Geneva: WHO; 2004. p. 959–1108.
12. European Commission. Attitudes towards alcohol: special Eurobarometer 272. Brussel: European Commission; 2007.
13. Comminity Epidemiology Work Group. Epidemiologic Trends in Drug Abuse: Proceedings of the Community Epidemiology Work Group: Highlights and Executive Summary. Bethesda, MD: National Institute of Drug Abuse; 2008.
14. Neumark YD, Lopez-Quintero C, Grinshpoon A, Levinson D. Alcohol drinking patterns and prevalence of alcohol-abuse and dependence in the Israel National Health Survey. Isr J Psychiatry Relat Sci. 2007;44(2):126–35.
15. Rimm EB, Williams P, Fosher K, Criqui M, Stampfer MJ. Moderate alcohol intake and lower risk of coronary heart disease: meta-analysis of effects on lipids and haemostatic factors. BMJ. 1999; 319(7224):1523–8.
16. Fillmore KM, Kerr WC, Stockwell T, Chikritzhs T, Bostrom A. Moderate alcohol use and reduced mortality risk: systematic error in prospective studies. Addict Res Theory. 2006;14:101–32.
17. Lauer MS, Sorlie P. Alcohol, cardiovascular disease, and cancer: treat with caution. J Natl Cancer Inst. 2009;101(5):282–3.
18. Greenfield TK. Individual risk of alcohol-related disease and problems. In: Heather N, Peters T, Stockwell T, editors. International handbook of alcohol dependence and problems. New York: Wiley; 2001. p. 413–37.
19. Sundell L, Salomaa V, Vartiainen E, Poikolainen K, Laatikainen T. Increased stroke risk is related to a binge-drinking habit. Stroke. 2008;39(12):3179–84.
20. Deutsche Hauptstelle für Suchtfragen e.V.(DHS). Binge drinking and Europe. Hamm: DHS; 2008.
21. Naimi TS, Brewer RD, Mokdad A, Denny C, Serdula MK, Marks JS. Binge drinking among US adults. JAMA. 2003;289(1):70–5.
22. AIHW. National drug strategy household survey: detailed findings. Canberra: AIHW; 2007. p. 2008.
23. Clark DB, Thatcher DL, Tapert SF. Alcohol, psychological dysregulation, and adolescent brain development. Alcohol Clin Exp Res. 2008;32:375–85.
24. Hibell B, Guttormsson U, Ahlström S, Balakireva O, Bjarnason T, Kokkevi A, et al. The 2007 ESPAD report: substance use among students in 35 European countries. Stockholm: CAN; 2009.
25. Johnston LD, O'Malley PM, Bachman JG, Schulenberg JE. Monitoring the future: national results on adolescent drug use: overview of key findings, 2008. Bethesda, MD: National Institute on Drug Abuse; 2009.
26. Hasin D. Classification of alcohol use disorders. Alcohol Res Health. 2003;27(1):5–17.
27. De Graaf R, Bijl RV, Smit F, Vollebergh WA, Spijker J. Risk factors for 12-month comorbidity of mood, anxiety, and substance use disorders: findings from the Netherlands Mental Health Survey and Incidence Study. Am J Psychiatry. 2002;159(4):620–9.
28. Hasin DS, Stinson FS, Ogburn E, Grant BF. Prevalence, correlates, disability, and comorbidity of DSM-IV alcohol abuse and dependence in the United States: results from the National Epidemiologic Survey on Alcohol and Related Conditions. Arch Gen Psychiatry. 2007;64(7):830–42.
29. Grant BF. Toward an alcohol treatment model: a comparison of treated and untreated respondents with DSM-IV alcohol use disorders in the general population. Alcohol Clin Exp Res. 1996;20(2):372–8.
30. Grant BF, Compton WM, Crowley TJ, Hasin DS, Helzer JE, Li TK, et al. Errors in assessing DSM-IV substance use disorders. Arch Gen Psychiatry. 2007;64:379–80.
31. Cottler LB. Drug use disorders in the National Comorbidity Survey: have we come a long way? Arch Gen Psychiatry. 2007;64:380–1.
32. Kessler RC, Merikangas KR. Drug use disorders in the National Comorbidity Survey: have we come a long way? In reply. Arch Gen Psychiatry. 2007;64:381–2.
33. Kessler RC, Üstün TB. The WHO world mental health surveys: global perspectives on the epidemiology of mental disorders. New York: Cambridge University Press; 2008.

34. Oakley Browne MA, Wells JE, Scott KM. Te Rau Hinengaro: the New Zealand Mental Health Survey. Wellington: Ministry of Health; 2006.

35. Bromet EJ, Gluzman SF, Paniotto VI, Webb CP, Tintle NL, Zakhozha V, et al. Epidemiology of psychiatric and alcohol disorders in Ukraine: findings from the Ukraine World Mental Health survey. Soc Psychiatry Psychiatr Epidemiol. 2005;40(9):681–90.

36. Alonso J, Angermeyer MC, Bernert S, Bruffaerts R, Brugha TS, Bryson H, et al. Prevalence of mental disorders in Europe: results from the European Study of the Epidemiology of Mental Disorders (ESEMeD) project. Acta Psychiatr Scand Suppl. 2004;420:21–7.

37. Keyes KM, Grant BF, Hasin DS. Evidence for a closing gender gap in alcohol use, abuse, and dependence in the United States population. Drug Alcohol Depend. 2008;93(1–2):21–9.

38. Dick DM, Bierut LJ. The genetics of alcohol dependence. Curr Psychiatry Rep. 2006;8(2):151–7.

39. Sher KJ, Grekin ER, Williams NA. The development of alcohol use disorders. Annu Rev Clin Psychol. 2005;1:493–523.

40. United Nations Office On Drugs and Crime (UNODC). World Drug Report: 2009. Vienna: UNODC; 2009.

41. Adlaf EM, Begin P, Sawka E. Canadian Addiction Survey (CAS): a national survey of Canadians' use of alcohol and other drugs: Prevalence of use and related harms: Detailed report. Ottawa: Canadian Centre on Substance Abuse; 2005.

42. SAMHSA. Results from the 2007 National Survey on Drug Use and Health: National findings. Rockville, MD: Office of Applied Studies; 2008.

43. Degenhardt L, Chiu WT, Sampson N, Kessler RC, Anthony JC, Angermeyer M, et al. Toward a global view of alcohol, tobacco, cannabis, and cocaine use: findings from the WHO World Mental Health Surveys. PLoS Med. 2008;5(7):e141.

44. Furr-Holden CD, Anthony JC. Epidemiologic differences in drug dependence–a US-UK cross-national comparison. Soc Psychiatry Psychiatr Epidemiol. 2003;38(4):165–72.

45. Kilmer B. Do cannabis possession laws influence cannabis use? In: Spruit IP, editor. Cannabis 2002 report: a joint international effort at the initiative of the Ministers of Public Health of Belgium, France, Germany, The Netherlands, Switserland: technical report of the International Scientific Conference Brussels, Belgium, 25-02-2002. Brussels, Belgium: Ministry of Public Health; 2002. p. 119–42.

46. Simons-Morton B, Pickett W, Boyce W, Ter Bogt TF, Vollebergh W. Cross-national comparison of adolescent drinking and cannabis use in the United States, Canada, and the Netherlands. Int J Drug Policy. 2010;21(1):64–9.

47. EMCDDA. Annual report 2008: the state of the drugs problem in Europe. Lisbon: EMCDDA; 2008.

48. Arseneault L, Cannon M, Poulton R, Murray R, Caspi A, Moffitt TE. Cannabis use in adolescence and risk for adult psychosis: longitudinal prospective study. BMJ. 2002;325(7374):1212–3.

49. Stefanis NC, Delespaul P, Henquet C, Bakoula C, Stefanis CN, Van Os J. Early adolescent cannabis exposure and positive and negative dimensions of psychosis. Addiction. 2004;99(10):1333–41.

50. Fergusson DM, Horwood LJ, Swain-Campbell N. Cannabis use and psychosocial adjustment in adolescence and young adulthood. Addiction. 2002;97(9):1123–35.

51. Lynskey MT, Heath AC, Bucholz KK, Slutske WS, Madden PA, Nelson EC, et al. Escalation of drug use in early-onset cannabis users vs co-twin controls. JAMA. 2003;289(4):427–33.

52. DeWit DJ, Offord DR, Wong M. Patterns of onset and cessation of drug use over the early part of the life course. Health Educ Behav. 1997;24(6):746–58.

53. European Monitoring Centre for Drugs and Drug Addiction (EMCDDA). A cannabis reader: global issues and local experiences: perspectives on cannabis controversies, treatment and regulation in Europe, vol. 1. Lisbon: EMCDDA; 2008.

54. European Monitoring Centre for Drugs and Drug Addiction (EMCDDA). A cannabis reader: global issues and local experiences: perspectives on cannabis controversies, treatment and regulation in Europe, vol. 2. Lisbon: EMCDDA; 2008.

55. Australian Institute of Health and Welfare. 2007 National Drug Strategy Household Survey: first results. Canberra: AIHW; 2008.

56. Currie C, Gabhainn SN, Godeau E, Roberts C, Smith R, Currie D, et al. Inequalities in young people's health: HBSC international report from the 2005/2006 survey. Copenhagen: World Health Organisation, Europe; 2008.

57. Chen K, Kandel DB, Davies M. Relationships between frequency and quantity of marijuana use and last year proxy dependence among adolescents and adults in the United States. Drug Alcohol Depend. 1997;46(1–2):53–67.

58. Copersino ML, Boyd SJ, Tashkin DP, Huestis MA, Heishman SJ, Dermand JC, et al. Quitting among non-treatment-seeking marijuana users: reasons and changes in other substance use. Am J Addict. 2006;15(4):297–302.

59. Chen CY, O'Brien MS, Anthony JC. Who becomes cannabis dependent soon after onset of use? Epidemiological evidence from the United States: 2000-2001. Drug Alcohol Depend. 2005;79(1):11–22.

60. Coffey C, Carlin JB, Lynskey M, Li N, Patton GC. Adolescent precursors of cannabis dependence: findings from the Victorian Adolescent Health Cohort Study. Br J Psychiatry. 2003;182:330–6.

61. Von Sydow K, Lieb R, Pfister H, Hofler M, Wittchen HU. What predicts incident use of cannabis and progression to abuse and dependence? A 4-year prospective examination of risk factors in a community sample of adolescents and young adults. Drug Alcohol Depend. 2002;68(1):49–64.

62. Korf DJ, Benschop A, Wouters M. Differential responses to cannabis potency: a typology of users based on self-reported consumption behaviour. Int J Drug Policy. 2007;18(3):168–76.

63. Compton WM, Grant BF, Colliver JD, Glantz MD, Stinson FS. Prevalence of marijuana use disorders in the United States: 1991–1992 and 2001–2002. JAMA. 2004;291(17):2114–21.

64. Stinson FS, Ruan WJ, Pickering R, Grant BF. Cannabis use disorders in the USA: prevalence, correlates and co-morbidity. Psychol Med. 2006;36(10):1447–60.

65. Swift W, Hall W, Teesson M. Cannabis use and dependence among Australian adults: results from the National Survey of Mental Health and Wellbeing. Addiction. 2001;96(5):737–48.

66. Perkonigg A, Goodwin RD, Fiedler A, Behrendt S, Beesdo K, Lieb R, et al. The natural course of cannabis use, abuse and dependence during the first decades of life. Addiction. 2008;103(3):439–49.

67. Boden JM, Fergusson DM, Horwood LJ. Illicit drug use and dependence in a New Zealand birth cohort. Aust NZ J Psychiatry. 2006;40(2):156–63.

68. Van Laar M, Cruts G, Van Gageldonk A, Croes E, Van Ooyen-Houben M, Meijer R, et al. Drug situation 2006 the Netherlands: report to the EMCDDA. Utrecht: Trimbos Institute; 2007.

69. Reuter P, Trautmann F. A report on global illicit drugs markets 1998-2007: full report. Brussel: European Communities; 2009.

70. European Monitoring Centre for Drugs and Drug Addiction (EMCDDA). Cocaine and crack cocaine: a growing public health issue. Lisbon: EMCDDA; 2007.

71. Wagner FA, Anthony JC. From first drug use to drug dependence; developmental periods of risk for dependence upon marijuana, cocaine, and alcohol. Neuropsychopharmacology. 2002;26(4):479–88.

72. Chen CY, Anthony JC. Epidemiological estimates of risk in the process of becoming dependent upon cocaine: cocaine hydrochloride powder versus crack cocaine. Psychopharmacology (Berl). 2004;172(1):78–86.

73. Hatsukami DK, Fischman MW. Crack cocaine and cocaine hydrochloride. Are the differences myth or reality? JAMA. 1996;276(19): 1580–8.

74. Hay G, Gannon M, MacDougall J, Millar T, Williams K, Eastwood C, et al. National and regional estimates of the prevalence of opiate use and/or crack cocaine use 2006/07: a summary of key findings: research report 9. London: Home Office; 2008.

75. McKetin R, McLaren J, Kelly E, Hall W, Hickman M. Estimating the number of regular and dependent methamphetamine users in Australia. Sydney: National Drug and Alcohol Research Centre; 2005.

76. Degenhardt L, Bruno R, Topp L. Is ecstasy a drug of dependence? Drug Alcohol Depend. 2009;107:1–10.

77. Wu LT, Ringwalt CL, Mannelli P, Patkar AA. Hallucinogen use disorders among adult users of MDMA and other hallucinogens. Am J Addict. 2008;17(5):354–63.

78. Cottler LB, Womack SB, Compton WM, Ben-Abdallah A. Ecstasy abuse and dependence among adolescents and young adults: applicability and reliability of DSM-IV criteria. Hum Psychopharmacol. 2001;16(8):599–606.

79. Rogers G, Elston J, Garside R, Roome C, Taylor R, Younger P, et al. The harmful health effects of recreational ecstasy: a systematic review of observational evidence. Health Technol Assess. 2009;13(6):3–4.

80. Peters GJY, Kok G, Schaalma HP. Careers in ecstasy use: do ecstasy users cease of their own accord? Implications for intervention development. BMC Public Health. 2008;8:376.

81. Blanken P, Hendriks VM, Van Ree JM, Van den Brink W. Outcome of long-term heroin-assisted treatment offered to chronic, treatment-resistant heroin addicts in the Netherlands. Addiction. 2010;105(2): 300–8.

82. Uchtenhagen A. Heroin-assisted treatment in Switzerland: a case study in policy change. Addiction. 2010;105(1):29–37.

83. Gilson AM, Kreis PG. The burden of the nonmedical use of prescription opioid analgesics. Pain Med. 2009;10 Suppl 2:S89–100.

84. Hay G, Gannon M, MacDougall J, Millar T, Williams K, Eastwood C, et al. National and regional estimates of the prevalence of opiate use and/or crack cocaine use 2006/07: a summary of key findings. London: Home Office; 2008.

85. Mathers BM, Degenhardt L, Phillips B, Wiessing L, Hickman M, Strathdee SA, et al. Global epidemiology of injecting drug use and HIV among people who inject drugs: a systematic review. Lancet. 2008;372(9651):1733–45.

86. Wiessing L, Van de Laar MJ, Donoghoe MC, Guarita B. HIV among injecting drug users in Europe: increasing trends in the East. Eurosurveillance. 2008;13(50):11.

87. Crofts N. Going where the epidemic is. Epidemiology and control of hepatitis C among injecting drug users. Aust Fam Phys. 2001; 30(5):420–5.

88. Aceijas C, Rhodes T. Global estimates of prevalence of HCV infection among injecting drug users. Int J Drug Policy. 2007;18(5): 352–8.

89. Brand DA, Saisana M, Rynn LA, Pennoni F, Lowenfels AB. Comparative analysis of alcohol control policies in 30 countries. PLOS Med. 2007;4:752–9.

90. Rehm J, Taylor B, Room R. Global burden of disease from alcohol, illicit drugs and tobacco. Drug Alcohol Rev. 2006;25(6): 503–13.

91. Collins DJ, Lapsley HM. The costs of tobacco, alcohol and illicit drug abuse to Australian society in 2004/05: Summary version. Canberra: Commonwealth of Australia; 2008.

92. WHO. Evidence for the effectiveness and cost-effectiveness of interventions to reduce alcohol-related harm. Kopenhagen: WHO Regional Office for Europe; 2009.

Drug Abuse and Behavioral Disinhibition

2

Mark T. Fillmore

Abstract

Traditional models of drug abuse emphasize the drug's rewarding effects as reinforcing drug use to the point of physical dependence and addiction. However, the past several years have seen an increased focus on the role of cognitive disturbances both as temporary acute reactions to drugs and as enduring impairments owing to prolonged chronic drug abuse. This chapter focuses on impairments of impulse control and reviews several lines of research that point to the role of impaired control in the development and maintenance of drug abuse disorders. The sections describe how the concept of impaired control is embedded in diagnostic classifications of alcohol abuse disorders and how impaired control characterizes constructs, such as impulsivity and disinhibition, which are key aspects of personalities and psychopathologies commonly associated with drug abuse. Cognitive approaches to the concept of impaired self-control are also examined with the aim of identifying how specific impairments in the ability to inhibit an action can contribute to drug abuse, and possibly emerge as a consequence of prolonged drug abuse. The chapter concludes by highlighting areas for further research, such as gaining a better understanding of the role of deficient inhibitory control in drug abuse for more effective treatment development.

Learning Objectives
- Personality disorders and externalizing disorders that are characterized by impulsive or poorly controlled behaviors are considered risk factors for developing drug abuse disorders.
- Impulsivity and disinhibition are well recognized in diagnostic classifications of drug abuse disorders.
- A basic behavioral characteristic underlying impulsivity and disinhibition appears to be a deficit in the ability to inhibit inappropriate actions.
- CNS depressant drugs, such as alcohol and some psychostimulant drugs, can produce acute impairments of inhibitory control.
- Long-term chronic abusers of drugs display sustained deficits of inhibitory control which could reflect the neural insult owing to prolonged drug exposure.

M.T. Fillmore (✉)
Department of Psychology, University of Kentucky,
Lexington, KY 40506-0044, USA
e-mail: fillmore@uky.edu

J.C. Verster et al. (eds.), *Drug Abuse and Addiction in Medical Illness: Causes, Consequences and Treatment*,
DOI 10.1007/978-1-4614-3375-0_2, © Springer Science+Business Media, LLC 2012

Issues that Need to Be Addressed by Future Research

- Research is needed to determine if disinhibition/impulsivity better predicts risks for abuse of specific drugs (e.g., CNS depressants vs. psychostimulants) or if impulsivity represents a risk factor that is nonspecific with regards to types of drugs abused.
- Research needs to explore the possibility that uncontrolled excessive binge use of a drug can arise because of the drug's initial acute disinhibiting effects on the drug-user's behavior.
- Longitudinal studies are needed to understand the causal role of inhibitory control deficits as causal factors and/or behavioral consequences of drug use.
- Impaired self-control could impede the efficacy of drug abuse treatments, and so a better understanding of the role of deficient inhibitory control in drug abuse could help guide more effective treatment strategies.

Drug abuse represents a condition whereby drug-taking and drug-seeking come to dominate behavior to such a degree that drug use appears to usurp control over behavior that was once influenced by normal environmental reinforcers. For many individuals, the pattern of abusive drug use continues despite serious adverse effects and repeated efforts to abstain. The idea that drug abuse represents a loss of self-control has been a long-standing concept in the theory and treatment of addictions, particularly alcohol abuse disorders. Even before the "medicalization" of addiction, society viewed habitual alcohol use as a character flaw whose chief characteristic was a lack of will-power or self-control (e.g., [1]). Early medical accounts by E. M. Jellinek and Mark Keller, who pioneered research on alcoholism, did much to promote the concept of deficient self-control in the etiology of drug abuse [2, 3]. Most notable was Jellinek's notion of a "gamma" alcoholic whose chief, primary symptom was a "loss of control" such that the initial consumption of alcohol triggered an uncontrollable urge to consume more alcohol, leading to a binge. In its strictest interpretation, the loss of control concept failed to gain much empirical support. However, the concept of "reduced" or "impaired" self-control continues today in addiction research and theory. The role of impaired self-control in addiction is studied across a broad range of behavioral investigations, including studies in personality, psychopathology, behavioral neuroscience, and cognitive psychology. Much of the initial work on the etiological role of impaired control in drug abuse disorders concerns its role in alcoholism. As such, much of the theory and research evidence described in this chapter concerns alcohol abuse. The next two sections provide a brief overview of the relevance of impaired control as an important factor in the etiology of alcohol abuse. The sections describe how the concept of impaired control is embedded in diagnostic classifications of alcohol abuse disorders and how impaired control characterizes constructs, such as impulsivity and disinhibition, which are key aspects of personalities and psychopathologies commonly associated with drug abuse.

Impaired Control as Disinhibited Personality and Psychopathology

Much of the evidence for the involvement of impaired control in drug abuse has come from studies on personality [4]. This area of research has focused on broad-based personality traits generally labeled as "impulsivity" or "disinhibition." These traits refer to a pattern of under-controlled behavior in which the individual lacks the ability to delay gratification and acts without forethought or consideration of potential consequences. The traits are typically assessed by self-report instruments, some of which are designed specifically to assess the impulsivity-disinhibition trait, such as the Barratt Impulsivity Scale and the Eysenck Impulsivity Scale [5, 6]. The traits are also assessed by comprehensive personality inventories, such as the NEO-Five Factor Inventory [7], in which impulsivity-disinhibition is comprised within major dimensions of personality (e.g., extroversion, openness to experience).

Studies using these types of instruments have demonstrated reliable associations between impulsivity-disinhibition and drug use. Much of this work has concerned the relation between these traits and alcohol use. Studies find that impulsive or disinhibited individuals tend to drink more frequently and in larger amounts during drinking episodes [8–10]. Impulsive individuals are also more likely to binge drink [11]. That is, drink to the point of intoxication. Not surprisingly then, impulsivity and disinhibition also have been linked to actual substance and alcohol use disorders. For example, abusers of illicit drugs and individuals diagnosed with alcoholism tend to score higher on measures of impulsivity, disinhibition, and related traits, such as sensation-seeking [12–14]. Moreover, there is growing evidence that impulsivity might play an important causal role in drug abuse. Prospective studies have shown that impulsive characteristics often precede the onset of problem alcohol use. Longitudinal studies of children and adolescents have shown that impulsivity predicts early-onset drinking age and development of heavy drinking and alcohol dependence in young adults [15, 16]. Heritability studies of substance use disorders also point to the involvement of impulsivity-disinhibition. For example, studies of individuals with a familial risk for substance use disorder, such as children of alcoholics, find that these individuals also display increased impulsivity-disinhibition [17, 18].

Alcohol and other drug abuse disorders are considered by many investigators to be symptomatic of some disinhibitory psychopathology [4, 19–21]. This argument is based on findings from studies examining drug abuse in relation to impulsivity-disinhibition as a central characteristic of a psychopathology. For example, several studies have examined the link between DSM personality disorder clusters and drug abuse. The general finding from this research is that substance abuse disorders have a high comorbidity with cluster B personality disorders. This cluster includes antisocial, borderline, and histrionic disorders, which are all characterized by under-controlled, disinhibited, and impulsive patterns of behavior. By contrast, cluster type A "odd-eccentric" (e.g., schizotypical disorders) and cluster type C "anxiety-related" (e.g., obsessive–compulsive disorder) fail to demonstrate consistent relationships with substance use [14]. It is also well established that externalizing disorders in childhood and adolescence, such as Attention Deficit/Hyperactivity Disorder (ADHD) and Conduct Disorder (CD), also pose risk for developing substance abuse disorders [22–27]. Studies of adults with ADHD find lifetime rates of alcohol abuse disorders ranging between 21% and 53% [28, 29]. A hallmark characteristic of ADHD is disinhibited or under-controlled behavior. Accordingly, there is also growing suspicion that such disinhibition might be the common, core deficit of these disorders that mediates their risk potential for adolescent drug use [30].

Impaired Control in Diagnostic Criteria for Alcohol Abuse Disorders

Impaired or deficient self-control is also a criterion for diagnostic classifications of alcoholism. Early on it was recognized that alcoholism was a heterogeneous disorder. That is, alcoholics differed in their patterns of abusive drinking. For example, it was recognized that some alcoholics drink daily, never appear drunk or intoxicated, but would likely experience withdrawal effects should they stop drinking. By contrast, other drinkers would go days or even weeks without drinking, but once they began drinking, they drank excessively to the point of gross inebriation or loss of consciousness. For Jellinek, these two patterns of drinking behavior represented two different "species" of alcoholic [31]. Jellinek labeled the former species, "delta" and the latter, "gamma." The delta alcoholic drinks daily, is likely physically dependent, but can control the amount consumed during the drinking episode (i.e., does not binge drink). Aside from an inability to abstain from alcohol, this alcoholic functions well in society. In contrast, the gamma alcoholic appears able to abstain from alcohol for long periods of time, but once consumption begins, this alcoholic loses control over intake and drinks to excess (i.e., binges). Thus, a critical

distinction between these two primary typologies in Jellinek's schema is the aspect of drinking behavior for which the alcoholic has no control over: control over when to drink versus control over how much to drink.

The concept of impaired control continued to play a key role in later diagnostic classifications of alcoholism, whose typologies are still commonly used today. For example, based on prospective adoption studies, Cloninger [19] offered a genetic-based dichotomous classification of alcoholism: Type I and Type II. Type I alcoholics are said to drink primarily to relieve stress or negative effect, often referred to as "relief drinking." These individuals develop their abusive drinking patterns later in life (i.e., after age 25). They also continue to function fairly well, both vocationally and interpersonally. These drinkers are sometimes casually referred to as "functioning alcoholics." By contrast, Type II alcoholics demonstrate abusive drinking patterns early, before the age of 25, are typically male, are unable to abstain from alcohol for any extended period, and are physically dependent. Moreover, the Type II alcoholic is characterized by under-controlled, antisocial, or disinhibited behavior, especially during a drinking episode. This lack of controlled behavior often results in social and legal problems for the individual. Unlike Jellinek's early system, Cloninger's later classification scheme benefited from advances in personality assessment and application of DSM-based symptom criteria to establish evidence for under-controlled behavior. As such, the lack of control demonstrated in the Type II alcoholic was largely evident by the fact that these drinkers commonly met symptom criteria for comorbid diagnoses of antisocial personality disorder or conduct disorder. Similar to Cloninger's dichotomy, Babor described a distinction between Type A and Type B alcoholics [32]. Like Cloninger's Type I alcoholics, Type A alcoholics demonstrate a late onset of abusive drinking, have few social or legal problems, and show little or no comorbid psychopathology. Type B alcoholics resemble Cloninger's Type II alcoholic, in that these drinkers develop alcohol problems early on and tend to have a history of antisocial and conduct problems.

Based on the diagnostic classification systems described here, it is apparent that the concept of impaired control has played an important role in characterizing the heterogeneity of alcohol abuse disorders since the first systematic classification scheme offered by Jellinek. It is also important to note that the basic classification dichotomies of Cloninger and Babor have been successfully applied to other drug abuse as well (e.g., cocaine), suggesting that impaired self-control could be an important characteristic for subtyping drug abuse in general [33]. Although diagnostic typologies are sometimes criticized in favor of dimensional models of psychopathology and substance use disorders [34], such classification schemes are useful because they highlight groups or clusters of symptoms (e.g., impaired control, physical dependence) that could have a common etiology. With respect to disinhibition, the alcoholism subtypes characterized by this trait appear to represent the more severe form of alcoholism. Moreover, this behavioral characteristic could have a strong genetic component as evident by its association with early-onset drinking problems and comorbid psychopathology [35]. With regard to treatment, the recognition of distinct typologies enables treatments to be tailored specifically to the particular symptoms and behavioral problems in each subtype. For many behaviorally based alcohol interventions, the presence of disinhibited or under-controlled behavior is a key symptom area of behavioral management in the treatment of the disorder. As such, typology-specific diagnoses could aid in matching patients to specifically tailored treatment programs.

In sum, impulsivity-disinhibition is well recognized in diagnostic typologies for substance use disorders. Studies of personality and psychopathology provide compelling evidence for a link between disinhibition and substance abuse. The involvement of disinhibition is evident from studies of normal personality (i.e., trait impulsivity) and studies of impulsivity-disinhibition as expressed through externalizing disorders (e.g., ADHD) or personality disorders (e.g., antisocial personality disorder). From this research, several new questions have arisen in recent years. One question concerns the possibility that certain expressions of the impulsivity-disinhibition could be associated with risks for particular types of drug use (e.g., alcohol vs. stimulant abuse). For example, Flory et al. [23] found that extroversion was a stronger predictor of alcohol use, whereas openness to experience better predicted marijuana use. Others have also found some evidence for specificity between particular personality traits and the type of drug use they predict [36]. Another issue that has received considerable attention concerns the degree to which antisocial behavior accounts for much of the relationships between personality traits and drug abuse. Unquestionably, antisocial behavior is one of the strongest predictors of risk for drug abuse. As such, many investigators are concerned with the possibility that associations between certain personality traits with drug use might simply be accounted for by antisocial behavior [36–38]. Isolating the specific influence of antisocial behavior from personality traits is a major aim of current research.

Impaired Control as Deficient Response Inhibition

Although it is important to characterize the behavioral correlates of drug abuse in terms of complex traits and personality, there is also a need to identify specific behavioral mechanisms by which these traits might promote drug abuse. In particular, it is important to understand the basic behavioral mechanisms that underlie disinhibited or impulsive behavior. Cognitive neuroscience approaches the concept of impaired self-control with the aim of identifying and characterizing the basic neurocognitive mechanisms that underlie the regulation of behavior [39, 40]. Unlike personality or broad-based trait approaches, this approach breaks down these constructs to study their component mechanisms and identify disturbances in the basic "building blocks" of behavior. This section reviews some cognitive models that focus on inhibitory mechanisms of behavior and describes their current use in the study of drug abuse.

Behaviors are instigated or motivated by a host of factors, including internal states, such as hunger, and by external events, such as the rich array of environmental cues that signal biologically relevant stimuli (e.g., primary and secondary reinforcers). Without any means to control responses to these signals, an organism's behavior would be immediately responsive and completely determined by such events. However, it is widely recognized that higher organisms, such as humans and other mammals, can exert control over behavioral output to either delay, alter, or completely inhibit environmentally instigated responses. Several theories in cognitive neuroscience postulate that the control of behavior is governed by distinct inhibitory and activational systems [41–48].

Considerable research has focused on inhibitory mechanisms of behavioral control. This ability is thought to involve frontal lobe substrates that exert inhibitory influences over conditioned responses and reflexive behaviors [42, 43]. Studies in neuropharmacology and neuroanatomy have identified distinct neural systems that implicate separate inhibitory and activational mechanisms in the control of behavior [30, 49–51]. The orbitofrontal and medial prefrontal cortex contain neural substrates that subserve many ongoing activities that control and regulate behavior. The ability to inhibit or suppress an action enhances the organism's behavioral repertoire by affording it some control over when and where responses may be expressed. As such, the inhibition of behavior is an important function that sets the occasion for many other activities that require self-restraint and regulation of behavior. Not surprisingly then, deficient or impaired inhibitory control has been implicated in the display of impulsivity and disorders of self-control. Aggressive and impulsive behaviors that characterize disorders, such as antisocial personality, obsessive–compulsive, and ADHD, have been attributed to impaired inhibitory mechanisms [22, 52].

In recent years, several "model-based" assessments of inhibitory mechanisms have been used to characterize drug abusers (for a review, see [30, 53]). Stop-signal and cued go/no-go models evaluate control as the ability to activate and to inhibit prepotent (i.e., instigated) responses [45, 54, 55]. The tasks model behavioral control using a reaction time scenario that measures the countervailing influences of inhibitory and activational mechanisms. Individuals are required to quickly activate a response to a go-signal and to inhibit a response when a stop-signal occasionally occurs. Activation is typically measured as the speed of responding to go-signals and inhibition to stop-signals is assessed by the probability of suppressing the response or by the time needed to suppress the response. In these models, inhibition of a response is usually required in a context in which there is a strong tendency to respond to a stimulus (i.e., a prepotency), thus making inhibition difficult. The validity of these models is well documented. The models are sensitive to inhibitory deficits characteristic of brain injury [56, 57], trait-based impulsivity [58], and self-control disorders, such as ADHD [59–61].

Acute Drug-Induced Impairment of Inhibitory Control

Several recent studies using these tasks have provided consistent evidence that moderate doses of CNS depressant drugs, such as alcohol and benzodiazepines, selectively reduce the user's ability to inhibit behavior at doses that leave the ability to activate behavior relatively unaffected [62–66]. For example, Fillmore and Weafer [67] used a cued go no-go task to test the impairing effect of alcohol on drinkers' inhibitory control over their behavioral impulses. The cued go no-go task presented go and no-go targets to which subjects had to execute a response (go) or inhibit the response (no-go). Subjects' inhibitory control was tested on two occasions: following a placebo and following an active dose that was sufficient to raise a drinker's BAC to 0.08%. Compared with placebo, alcohol impaired inhibitory control by increasing the likelihood that drinkers would fail to inhibit responses to no-go targets. By contrast, no effect of alcohol at this dose was observed on the ability of drinkers to execute the responses to go targets as measured by their speed of responding.

What is particularly remarkable about findings such as these is the robust impairment that is evident in spite of the relatively simple nature of the inhibitory response tested. Typically, sensitivity to alcohol-induced impairment increases as a function of dose and task complexity [68]. However, the impairing effects of alcohol on the ability to inhibit behavior are often observed at blood alcohol concentrations at or below 0.08% [30]. The findings suggest that activities that require quick suppression of actions might be particularly vulnerable to the disruptive influences of alcohol.

In addition, alcohol-induced impairments of inhibitory mechanisms might actually exert considerable disruptive influence on higher-order, executive cognitive functions. Many fundamental cognitive and perceptual processes, such as inhibitory mechanisms, are considered to operate in a "bottom-up" fashion to exert increasing influence at each stage of higher-order attentional and cognitive functions. Thus, the alcohol-induced disturbances of basic control mechanisms, such as inhibitory processes, might actually result in much more pronounced impairments of the higher cognitive operations for which they serve (e.g., decision-making, planning, and goal maintenance).

The findings might also provide some account for the long-standing observation that alcohol intoxication is often characterized by increased impulsivity and aggression. Using the same types of tasks as those described here, deficits of inhibitory control have been identified in individuals with disorders characterized by aggressive or impulsive behaviors, such as ADHD and antisocial personality [22, 52]. In fact, the acute impairments of inhibitory control that are produced by alcohol closely resemble those inhibitory deficits that are assumed to be symptomatic of externalizing disorders [53]. This raises an intriguing possibility that alcohol temporarily disrupts cognitive functioning in a manner similar to the enduring cognitive disturbances that are characteristic of disorders, such as ADHD.

Evidence for the vulnerability of inhibitory mechanisms to alcohol effects also could offer important new insights into the development and maintenance of alcohol abuse. Although there is little dispute that reward mechanisms play an important role in abuse potential, the acute cognitive impairing effects of alcohol might also contribute to abuse by compromising mechanisms involved in the regulation and self-control of behavior and attention [30, 53]. In particular, inhibitory mechanisms likely play an important role in terminating alcohol use during an episode [30, 51, 53]. Many drinkers report intentions to limit their alcohol use to one or two drinks only to fail and instead drink excessively [69]. Such accounts have fueled the notion that alcohol reduces control over consumption in some individuals. Terminating a drinking episode requires inhibition of ongoing alcohol-administration behaviors and the reallocation of attention away from alcohol-related stimuli. Any impairment of normal inhibitory mechanisms resulting from an initial dose of alcohol could compromise the ability to stop additional alcohol administrations in a drinking situation. Thus, acute alcohol-induced impairment of inhibitory processes could represent an important behavioral mechanism by which an initial alcohol dose promotes subsequent self-administration. In fact, laboratory studies find that increased sensitivity to the acute disinhibiting effects of alcohol predicts heavy alcohol use in both humans [70] and laboratory animals [71].

Studies of inhibitory control have also examined the acute effects of psychostimulant drugs. Studies using stop-signal and cued go/no-go tasks have found that the stimulants, methylphenidate and D-amphetamine, can improve inhibitory control in children with ADHD and in healthy adults [72, 73]. It has been suggested that illicit use of the commonly abused stimulants, cocaine and amphetamine, might be motivated in part by a desire to self-medicate attentional deficits and hyperactive/impulsive tendencies (e.g., [74, 75]).

Drug-induced enhancement of inhibitory control might contribute to abuse potential by representing a desirable effect for the user that reinforces their use of stimulant drugs. However, evidence for facilitatory effects on inhibitory control is not entirely consistent. Some studies of cocaine and D-amphetamine have failed to demonstrate facilitatory effects on inhibitory control. In fact, studies of orally administered doses of cocaine HCl (50–150 mg) and D-amphetamine (5–20 mg) actually produced slight impairments of inhibitory control in stimulant abusers, as evidenced by a decreased ability to inhibit responses [76, 77]. However, in a study of adults with no history of stimulant abuse, D-amphetamine was found to have no effect on inhibitory control [78].

One factor that might be critical in determining facilitation of inhibitory control is dose. Some studies of methylphenidate in children with ADHD have reported U-shaped dose–response curves following methylphenidate [73, 79, 80]. In these studies methylphenidate improved childrens' inhibitory control in a dose-dependent fashion up to a point at which higher doses failed to produce any improvement. A study of adult stimulant drug abusers revealed a similar U-shaped dose–response curve in response to cocaine [81]. Lower doses of cocaine improved the subjects' inhibitory control but no beneficial effects of the drug were observed at higher doses. One speculation is that the facilitating effects of stimulant drugs on inhibitory control are limited to a range of intermediate doses, above which improvement is no longer evident and impairing effects could possibly emerge. Such a two-phasic dose–response function has implications for understanding how changes in inhibitory control could contribute to the abuse of stimulant drugs. An initial stimulant dose (i.e., a "rock" of cocaine) could restore or possibly enhance cognitive functioning. Moreover, such facilitation might represent a sought-after, restorative effect for the user. But, as additional doses are administered, inhibitory control could become impaired as brain levels increase, leading to behavioral impulsivity, perseverative responses, and possibly binge use of the drug.

Neuropsychological and brain imaging studies of cocaine users support a basic tenet of the restorative hypothesis, namely evidence of basal deficits in inhibitory control [30]. Compared with healthy controls, cocaine abusers show patterns of premature responding [82, 83] and perseverative behavior [84]. Brain imaging studies find evidence of hypoactivity in the cingulate and dorsolateral prefrontal cortical regions [85, 86] which are areas associated with inhibitory control of prepotent actions [87, 88]. The hypoactivity in these regions could reflect damage owing to long-term cocaine use [89, 90]. Recent studies of cocaine users also show enhanced sensitivity to stimulant drugs in these brain regions (i.e., heightened activation), possibly resulting from long-term cocaine abuse [91]. Such supra-sensitivity could lead to disinhibited or impulsive behavior in response to higher drug doses.

Chronic Drug-Induced Impairment of Inhibitory Control

As mentioned above, there is evidence that prolonged, chronic use of an abused drug, such as cocaine, can alter neural functioning, possibly leading to relatively permanent impairments of the user's cognitive abilities. Several studies have compared the neuropsychological test performance of chronic drug abusers to comparison controls (for reviews, see [49, 92, 93]). Much of this work has focused on alcoholics and abusers of stimulant drugs, such as cocaine and methamphetamine. With regard to alcohol, it has long been known that chronic abuse can result in sustained memory impairments, with the most severe form being Korsakoff's Syndrome. Currently, it is now recognized that prolonged abuse of alcohol is associated with widespread neuropsychological deficits, involving memory, attention, learning, problem solving, and perceptual motor speed [94–97]. Similarly, studies of stimulant abusers also demonstrate many of the same types of neuropsychological deficits [98]. Moreover, the deficits evident in these drug abusers do not appear to be acute effects of recent drug use, or acute withdrawal symptoms, because they have been shown to persist in detoxified, abstinent individuals for at least 1 year [99].

In addition to demonstrating general impairments in attention, memory and other global functions, more recent research has identified specific deficits in the inhibitory control of drug abusers. Studies using the stop-signal and cued go/no-go tasks find that cocaine users display deficits in the ability to inhibit responses, but no impairment in the ability to activate such behavior [100, 101]. Studies of abstinent alcoholics in treatment also find some evidence for deficient inhibitory control on the go/no-go task, which is most evident in the Type II subtype [102, 103].

It is important to recognize that such cross-sectional comparisons between drug abusers and control samples cannot establish a causal link between drug use and deficits of inhibitory control. Nonetheless, there are lines of evidence that suggest that such deficient inhibitory control among drug abusers could be due, in part, to prolonged exposure to abused drugs. First, the degree of inhibitory deficit is often related to the severity of drug abuse, such that those who have abused drugs more frequently, or for longer periods, tend to display the greatest deficits (e.g., [83, 104, 105]). Second, considerable work in neuroimaging has shed light on how drug abuse can alter neural systems underlying many neuropsychological functions, including inhibitory control [49, 106]. This approach examines both the neural changes that occur in response to the acute administration of an abused drug and the difference in neural functioning between drug abusers and healthy controls, presumably as a consequence of prolonged exposure. Much of this work examines individuals with histories of polydrug abuse (i.e., cocaine and alcohol abuse). The general aim of this approach is to understand how the neural responses to acute drug administration can eventually lead to permanent changes in neural functioning as a function of repeated drug use. Positron emission tomography (PET) and functional neural imaging techniques of polydrug abusers reveal altered dopamine functioning in brain areas associated with inhibitory control, such as the orbitofrontal cortex and cingulate gyrus [49, 51, 101, 106]. Impaired cognitive functions, such as reduced inhibitory control over approach behaviors, might result from a supraactivation of cortical D1-like receptor systems. A current working hypothesis is that individuals initially display elevated increases in dopamine (i.e., supraactivation) following drug use which, over repeated use, leads to neural adaptations that results in diminished dopaminergic activity in brain regions, leading to increased motivation for drugs and diminished impulse control [106].

A final line of evidence for a causal role between drug use and deficient inhibitory control comes from preclinical studies of laboratory animals. Studies of laboratory animals allow for a longitudinal approach in which neural and behavioral changes can be assessed before and following chronic exposure to a drug (for a review, see [107]). Preclinical studies provide considerable evidence for enduring neural and behavioral changes following chronic exposure to drugs. This body of literature is extensive and beyond the scope of this review. However, with regard to inhibitory control, studies of animals find that neural systems associated with inhibitory control are particularly vulnerable to neurotoxic insults from drug exposures, especially during critical developmental stages (e.g., [108]).

In sum, some interesting parallel effects have emerged in studies of acute and chronic drug effects on inhibitory control. As an acute reaction, an impaired ability to inhibit inappropriate responses has become well documented in response to some CNS depressant drugs, most notably, alcohol. It also appears that stimulant drugs, such as cocaine, are capable of reducing inhibitory control as an acute reaction, however, such effects might depend on the dose and the user's prior drug history. In terms of chronic use, several lines of evidence suggest that repeated abuse of stimulant drugs and alcohol can produce enduring changes in neural functioning that result in sustained deficits of impulse control.

Future Directions and Considerations

Traditional models of drug abuse emphasize the drug's rewarding effects as reinforcing drug use to the point of physical dependence and addiction. However, the past several years has seen an increased focus on the role of cognitive disturbances both as temporary acute reactions to drugs and as enduring impairments owing to prolonged chronic drug abuse. This chapter focused on impairments of impulse control and reviewed several lines of research that point to the role of impaired control in the development and maintenance of drug abuse disorders. There is considerable agreement among these lines of research that impaired self-control plays an important role in the risk for developing drug abuse disorders.

Cross-sectional identification of specific inhibitory deficits that may contribute to, or result from drug use will lay the foundation for longitudinal studies of drug use that track changes in inhibitory functioning in relation to drug use over time. Inhibitory deficits might directly contribute to the initiation of drug use, and thus operate as a specific behavioral risk factor. At the same time, inhibitory deficits might also arise as a result of neural insult owing to prolonged drug abuse. In such a case, inhibitory mechanisms might recover over a period of abstinence. Some research has already begun to examine changes in neuropsychological test performance as a function of varying periods of drug abstinence (e.g., [109]). Abstinence effects on specific inhibitory deficits have yet to be examined. Long-term observation of detoxified individuals could provide important information on the persistence of these deficits.

Finally, evidence for the involvement of impaired self-control also poses particular challenges for drug abuse treatment development, as treatment researchers come to recognize that poor impulse control and impaired cognitive functions, in general, can undermine the efficacy of many behaviorally based treatments. A better understanding of the role of deficient inhibitory control in drug abuse could help guide the development of pharmacological treatments for drug abuse as well. A sought-after effect of many candidate pharmacotherapies for drug abuse is the reduction of subjectively rewarding states produced by the drug. The concomitant disruption of neurocognitive control mechanisms has been afforded less attention as a mechanism of abuse. The possibility that some pharmacotherapies might operate to reduce drug use by strengthening inhibitory control has yet to be examined.

Acknowledgments This work was supported by grants R21 DA021027 and P50 DA005312 from the National Institute on Drug Abuse, and by grant R01 AA12895 from the National Institute on Alcohol Abuse and Alcoholism. The content is solely the responsibility of the author and does not necessarily represent the official views of the National Institutes of Health.

References

1. McCorkindale I. The Canadian lesson book on temperance and life. Toronto: Dominion Scientific Temperance Committee; 1926.
2. Jellinek EM. Current notes—phases of alcohol addiction. Q J Stud Alcohol. 1952;13:673–84.

3. Keller M. On the loss of control phenomenon in alcoholism. Br J Addict. 1972;67:153–66.

4. Widiger TA, Smith GT. Substance use disorder: abuse, dependence and dyscontrol. Addiction. 1994;89:267–82.

5. Eysenck SB, Pearson PR, Easting G, Allsopp JF. Age norms for impulsiveness, venturesomeness, and empathy in adults. Personal Individ Differ. 1985;6:613–9.

6. Patton JH, Stanford MS, Barratt ES. Factor structure of the Barratt Impulsiveness Scale. J Clin Psychol. 1995;51:768–74.

7. Costa PT, McCrae RR. Revised NEO Personality Inventory (NEO-PI-R) and NEO Five-Factor Inventory (NEO-FFI) professional manual. Obessa, FL: Psychological Assessment Resources; 1992.

8. Cherpitel CJ. Alcohol, injury, and risk-taking behavior: data from a national sample. Alcohol Clin Exp Res. 1993;17:762–6.

9. Goudriaan AE, Grekin ER, Sher KJ. Decision making and binge drinking: a longitudinal study. Alcohol Clin Exp Res. 2007;31:928–38.

10. Simons JS. Differential prediction of alcohol use and problems: the role of biopsychosocial and social-environmental variables. Am J Drug Alcohol Abuse. 2003;29:861–79.

11. Marczinski CA, Combs SW, Fillmore MT. Increased sensitivity to the disinhibiting effects of alcohol in binge drinkers. Psychol Addict Behav. 2007;21:346–54.

12. Bergman B, Brismar B. Hormone levels and personality traits in abusive and suicidal male alcoholics. Alcohol Clin Exp Res. 1994;18:311–6.

13. Sher KJ, Trull TJ, Bartholow BD, Vieth A. Personality and alcoholism: issues, methods, and etiological processes. In: Blane H, Leonard E, editors. Psychological theories of drinking and alcoholism. New York: Plenum; 1999. p. 54–105.

14. Trull TJ, Waudby CJ, Sher KJ. Alcohol, tobacco, and drug use disorders and personality disorder symptoms. Exp Clin Psychopharmacol. 2004;12:65–75.

15. August GJ, Winters KC, Realmuto GM, Fahnhorst T, Botzet A, Lee S. Prospective study of adolescent drug use among community samples of ADHD and non-ADHD participants. J Am Acad Child Adolesc Psychiatry. 2006;45:824–32.

16. Ernst M, Luckenbach DA, Moolchan ET, Leff MK, Allen R, Eshel N, London ED, Kimes A. Behavioral predictors of substance-use initiation in adolescents with and without attention-deficit/hyperactivity disorder. Pediatrics. 2006;117:2030–9.

17. Alterman AI, Bedrick J, Cacciola JS, Rutherford MJ, Searles JS, McKay JR, Cook TG. Personality pathology and drinking in young men at high and low familial risk for alcoholism. J Stud Alcohol. 1998;59:495–502.

18. Sher KJ. Children of alcoholics: a critical appraisal of theory and research. Chicago: University of Chicago Press; 1991.

19. Cloninger CR. Recent advances in family studies of alcoholism. Prog Clin Biol Res. 1987;241:47–60.

20. Finn PR, Kessler DN, Hussong AM. Risk for alcoholism and classical conditioning to signals for punishment: evidence for a weak behavioral inhibition system? J Abnorm Psychol. 1994;103:293–301.

21. Sher KJ, Trull TJ. Personality and disinhibitory psychopathology: alcoholism and antisocial personality disorder. J Abnorm Psychol. 1994;103:92–102.

22. Barkley R. Attention-deficit hyperactivity disorder: a handbook for diagnosis and treatment. 3rd ed. New York: Guilford; 2006.

23. Flory K, Milich R, Lynam DR, Leukefeld C, Clayton R. Relation between childhood disruptive behavior disorders and substance use and dependence symptoms in young adulthood: Individuals with symptoms of attention-deficit/hyperactivity disorder and conduct disorder are uniquely at risk. Psychol Addict Behav. 2003;17:151–8.

24. Flory K, Lynam DR. The relation between attention deficit hyperactivity disorder and substance abuse: what role does conduct disorder play? Clin Child Fam Psychol Rev. 2003;6:1–16.

25. Hartung CM, Milich R, Lynam DR, Martin CA. Understanding the relations among gender, disinhibition, and disruptive behavior in adolescents. J Abnorm Psychol. 2002;111:659–64.

26. Molina BSG, Smith BH, Pelham WE. Interactive effects of attention deficit hyperactivity disorder and conduct disorder on early adolescent substance use. Psychol Addict Behav. 1999;13:348–58.

27. Molina BSG, Pelham WE, Gnagy EM, Thompson AL, Marshal MP. Attention-deficit/hyperactivity disorder risk for heavy drinking and alcohol use disorder is age specific. Alcohol Clin Exp Res. 2007;31:643–54.

28. Barkley RA, Murphy KR, Kwasnik D. Motor vehicle driving competencies and risks in teens and young adults with attention deficit hyperactivity disorder. Pediatrics. 1996;98:1089–95.

29. Biederman J. Impact of comorbidity in adults with attention-deficit/hyperactivity disorder. J Clin Psychiatry. 2004;65:3–7.

30. Fillmore MT. Drug abuse as a problem of impaired control: current approaches and findings. Behav Cogn Neurosci Rev. 2003;2:179–97.

31. Jellinek EM. The disease concept of alcoholism. New Brunswick, NJ: Hillhouse; 1960.

32. Babor TF, Hofmann M, DelBoca FK, Hesselbrock VM, Meyer RE, Dolinsky ZS, Rounsaville B. Types of alcoholics: I. Evidence for an empirically derived typology based on indicators of vulnerability and severity. Arch Gen Psychiatry. 1992;49(8):599–608.

33. Ball SA, Carroll KM, Babor TF, Rounsaville BJ. Subtypes of cocaine abusers: support for a type A-type B distinction. J Consult Clin Psychol. 1995;63:115–24.

34. Widiger TA, Trull TJ. Plate tectonics in the classification of personality disorder: shifting to a dimensional model. Am Psychol. 2007;62:71–83.

35. Hesselbrock VM, Hesselbrock MN. Are there empirically supported and clinically useful subtypes of alcohol dependence? Addiction. 2006;101 Suppl 1:97–103.

36. Grekin ER, Sher KJ, Wood PK. Personality and substance dependence symptoms: modeling substance-specific traits. Psychol Addict Behav. 2006;20(4):415–24.

37. Miller JD, Lynam DR. Psychopathy and the Five-factor model of personality: a replication and extension. J Personal Assess. 2003;81:168–78.

38. Lynam DR, Leukefeld C, Clayton RR. The contribution of personality to the overlap between antisocial behavior and substance use/misuse. Aggress Behav. 2003;29(4):316–31.

39. Goschke T. Voluntary action and cognitive control from a cognitive neuroscience perspective. In: Massen S, Prinz W, Roth G, editors. Voluntary action: brains, minds, and sociality. New York, NY: Oxford University Press; 2003. p. 49–85.

40. Miller EK, Cohen JD. An integrative theory of prefrontal cortex function. Annu Rev Neurosci. 2001;24:167–202.

41. Fox E. Negative priming from ignored distractors in visual selection: a review. Psychonomic Bull Rev. 1995;2:145–73.

42. Fowles DC. Application of a behavioral theory of motivation to the concepts of anxiety and impulsivity. J Res Personal. 1987;21:417–35.

43. Gray JA. The behavioral inhibition system: a possible substrate for anxiety. In: Feldman MP, Broadhurst A, editors. Theoretical and experimental bases of behavior therapies. London: Wiley; 1976. p. 3–41.

44. Gray JA. Drug effects of fear and frustration. Possible limbic site of action of minor tranquilizers. In: Iverson LL, Iverson SD, Snyder SH, editors. Handbook of psychopharmacology, vol. 8. New York: Plenum; 1977. p. 433–529.

45. Logan GD, Cowan WB. On the ability to inhibit thought and action: a theory of an act of control. Psychological Review. 1984;91:295–327.

46. May CP, Kane MJ, Hasher L. Determinants of negative priming. Psychol Bull. 1995;118:35–54.

47. Patterson CM, Newman JP. Reflectivity and learning from aversive events: toward a psychological mechanism for the syndromes of disinhibition. Psychol Rev. 1993;100:716–36.

48. Quay HC. Inhibition and attention deficit hyperactivity disorder. J Abnorm Child Psychol. 1997;25:7–13.

49. Jentsch JD, Taylor JR. Impulsivity resulting from frontostriatal dysfunction in drug abuse: implication for the control of behavior by reward-related stimuli. Psychopharmacology. 1999;146:373–90.

50. Leigh RJ, Zee DS. The neurology of eye movements. 3rd ed. New York: Oxford University Press; 1999.

51. Lyvers M. "Loss of control" in alcoholism and drug addiction: a neuroscientific interpretation. Exp Clin Psychopharmacol. 2000;8: 225–49.

52. Nigg JT. What causes ADHD? Understanding what goes wrong and why. New York: Guilford; 2006.

53. Fillmore MT. Acute alcohol-induced impairment of cognitive functions: past and present findings. Int J Disabil Hum Dev. 2007;6: 115–25.

54. Logan GD. On the ability to inhibit thought and action: a user's guide to the stop-signal paradigm. In: Dagenbach D, Carr TH, editors. Inhibitory processes in attention, memory, and language. San Diego, CA: Academic; 1994.

55. Miller J, Schaffer R, Hackley SA. Effects of preliminary information in a go versus no-go task. Acta Psychol. 1991;76:241–92.

56. Cremona-Meteyard SL, Geffen GM. Event-related potential indices of visual attention following moderate to severe closed head injury. Brain Injury. 1994;8:541–58.

57. Malloy P, Bihrle A, Duffy J, Cimino C. The orbitomedial frontal syndrome. Arch Clin Neuropsychol. 1993;8:185–201.

58. Logan GD, Schachar RJ, Tannock R. Impulsivity and inhibitory control. Psychol Sci. 1997;8(1):60–4.

59. Tannock R. Attention deficit hyperactivity disorder: advances in cognitive, neurobiological, and genetic research. J Child Psychol Psychiatry. 1998;39:65–99.

60. Oosterlaan J, Sergeant JA. Inhibition in ADHD, aggressive, and anxious children: a biologically based model of child psychopathology. J Abnorm Child Psychol. 1996;24:19–37.

61. Schachar R, Tannock R, Marriott M, Logan G. Deficient inhibitory control in attention deficit hyperactivity disorder. J Abnorm Child Psychol. 1995;23:411–37.

62. de Wit H, Crean J, Richards JB. Effects of d-amphetamine and ethanol on a measure of behavioral inhibition in humans. Behav Neurosci. 2000;114:830–7.

63. Fillmore MT, Rush CR, Kelly HK, Hays L. Triazolam impairs inhibitory control of behavior in humans. Exp Clin Psychopharmacol. 2001;9:363–71.

64. Fillmore MT, Vogel-Sprott M. An alcohol model of impaired inhibitory control and its treatment in humans. Exp Clin Psychopharmacol. 1999;7:49–55.

65. Mulvihill LE, Skilling TA, Vogel-Sprott M. Alcohol and the ability to inhibit behavior in men and women. J Stud Alcohol. 1997;58: 600–5.

66. Marczinski CA, Fillmore MT. Pre-response cues reduce the impairing effects of alcohol on the execution and suppression of responses. Exp Clin Psychopharmacol. 2003;11:110–7.

67. Fillmore MT, Weafer J. Alcohol impairment of behavior in men and women (Target Article). Addiction. 2004;99:1237–46.

68. Maylor EA, Rabbitt PM, James GH, Kerr SA. Effects of alcohol, practice, and task complexity on reaction time distributions. Q J Exp Psychol Hum Exp Psychol. 1992;49:119–39.

69. Collins RL. Drinking restraint and risk for alcohol abuse. Exp Clin Psychopharmacol. 1993;1:44–54.

70. Weafer J, Fillmore MT. Individual differences in acute alcohol impairment of inhibitory control predict ad libitum alcohol consumption. Psychopharmacology. 2008;201(3):315–24.

71. Poulos CX, Parker JL, Le DA. Increased impulsivity after injected alcohol predicts later alcohol consumption in rats: evidence for 'loss-of-control drinking' and marked individual differences. Behav Neurosci. 1998;112(5):1247–57.

72. de Wit H, Engasser JL, Richards JB. Acute administration of d-amphetamine decreases impulsivity in healthy volunteers. Neuropsychopharmacology. 2002;27(5):813–25.

73. Tannock R, Schachar R, Logan G. Methylphenidate and cognitive flexibility: dissociated dose effects in hyperactive children. J Abnorm Child Psychol. 1995;23:235–67.

74. Khantzian E. The self-medication hypothesis of addictive disorders: focus on heroin and cocaine dependence. Am J Psychiatry. 1985;142:1259–64.

75. Schiffer F. Psychotherapy of nine successfully treated cocaine abusers: techniques and dynamics. J Subst Abuse Treat. 1988; 5:131–7.

76. Fillmore MT, Rush CR, Hays L. Acute effects of oral cocaine on inhibitory control of behavior in humans. Drug Alcohol Depend. 2002;67:157–67.

77. Fillmore MT, Rush CR, Marczinski CA. Effects of d-amphetamine on behavioral control in stimulant abusers: the role of prepotent response tendencies. Drug Alcohol Depend. 2003;71:143–52.

78. Fillmore MT, Kelly TH, Martin CA. Effects of d-amphetamine in human models of information processing and inhibitory control. Drug Alcohol Depend. 2005;77:151–9.

79. Bedard AC, Ickowicz A, Logan GD, Hogg-Johnson S, Schachar R, Tannock R. Selective inhibition in children with attention-deficit hyperactivity disorder off and on stimulant medication. J Abnorm Child Psychol. 2003;31(3):315–27.

80. Konrad K, Gunther T, Hanisch C, Herpertz-Dahlmann B. Differential effects of methylphenidate on attentional functions in children with attention-deficit/hyperactivity disorder. J Am Acad Child Adolesc Psychiatry. 2004;43(2):191–8.

81. Fillmore MT, Rush CR, Hays L. Acute effects of cocaine in two models of inhibitory control: implications of non-linear dose effects. Addiction. 2006;101:1323–32.

82. Bauer LO. Antisocial personality disorder and cocaine dependence: their effects on behavioral and electroencephalographic measures of time estimation. Drug Alcohol Depend. 2001;63:87–95.

83. Fillmore MT, Rush CR. Impaired inhibitory control of behavior in chronic cocaine users. Drug Alcohol Depend. 2002;66:265–73.

84. Lane SD, Cherek DR, Dougherty DM, Moeller FG. Laboratory measurement of adaptive behavior change in humans with a history of substance dependence. Drug Alcohol Depend. 1998;51(3):239–52.

85. Franklin TR, Acton PD, Maldjian JA, Gray JD, Croft JR, Dackis CA, O'Brian CP, Childress AR. Decreased gray matter concentration in the insular, orbitofrontal, cingulate, and temporal cortices of cocaine patients. Biol Psychiatry. 2002;51:134–42.

86. Kaufman JN, Ross TJ, Stein EA, Garavan H. Cingulate hypoactivity in cocaine users during a GO-NOGO task as revealed by event-related functional magnetic resonance imaging. J Neurosci. 2003;23(21):7839–43.

87. Aron AR, Robbins TW, Poldrack RA. Inhibition and the right inferior frontal cortex. Trends Cogn Sci. 2004;8:170–7.

88. Hester R, Fassbender C, Garavan H. Individual differences in error processing: a review and meta-analysis of three event-related fMRI studies using the GO/NOGO task. Cerebral Cortex. 2004;14: 986–94.

89. Volkow ND, Fowler JS, Wang GJ, Hitzemann R, Logan J, Schlyer DJ, Dewey SL, Wolf AP. Decreased dopamine D2 receptor availability is associated with reduced frontal metabolism in cocaine abusers. Synapse. 1993;14:169–77.

90. Volkow ND, Fowler JS, Wang GJ. Imaging studies on the role of dopamine in cocaine reinforcement and addiction in humans. J Psychopharmacol. 1999;13:337–45.

91. Volkow ND, Wang GJ, Ma Y, Fowler JS, Wong C, Ding YS, Hitzemann R, Swanson JM, Kalivas P. Activation of orbital and medial prefrontal cortex by methylphenidate in cocaine-addicted

subjects but not in controls: relevance to addiction. J Neurosci. 2005;25:3932–9.

92. Strickland TL, Stein R. Cocaine-induced cerebrovascular impairment: challenges to neuropsychological assessment. Neuropsychol Rev. 1995;5(1):69–79.

93. Bolla KI, Cadet JL, London ED. The neuropsychiatry of chronic cocaine abuse. J Neuropsychiatry Clin Neurosci. 1998;10(3):280–9.

94. Ardila A, Rosselli M, Strumwasser S. Neuropsychological deficits in chronic cocaine abusers. Int J Neurosci. 1991;57(1–2):73–9.

95. Bates ME, Bowden SC, Barry D. Neurocognitive impairment associated with alcohol use disorders: Implications for treatment. Exp Clin Psychopharmacol. 2002;10:193–212.

96. Beatty WW, Katzung VM, Moreland VJ, Nixon SJ. Neuropsychological performance of recently abstinent alcoholics and cocaine abusers. Drug Alcohol Depend. 1995;37(3):247–53.

97. O'Malley S, Adamse M, Heaton RK, Gawin FH. Neuropsychological impairment in chronic cocaine abusers. Am J Drug Alcohol Abuse. 1992;18(2):131–44.

98. Jovanovski D, Erb S, Zakzanis KK. Neurocognitive deficits in cocaine users: a quantitative review of the evidence. J Clin Exp Neuropsychol. 2005;27(2):189–204.

99. Toomey R, Lyons MJ, Eisen SA, Xian H, Chantarujikapong S, Seidman LJ, Faraone SV, Tsuang MT. A twin study of the neuropsychological consequences of stimulant abuse. Arch Gen Psychiatry. 2003;60(3):303–10.

100. Fillmore MT, Rush CR. Polydrug abusers display impaired discrimination-reversal learning in a model of behavioral control. J Psychopharmacol. 2006;20:24–32.

101. Hester R, Garavan H. Executive dysfunction in cocaine addiction: evidence for discordant frontal, cingulate, and cerebellar activity. J Neurosci. 2004;24(49):11017–22.

102. Bjork JM, Hommer DW, Grant SJ, Danube C. Impulsivity in abstinent alcohol-dependent patients: relation to control subjects and type 1-/type 2-like traits. Alcohol. 2004;34:133–50.

103. Dom G, De Wilde B, Hulstijn W, Van Den Brink W, Sabbe B. Behavioural aspects of impulsivity in alcoholics with and without a cluster-B personality disorder. Alcohol Alcohol. 2006;41(4):412–20.

104. Bolla KI, Funderburk FR, Cadet JL. Differential effects of cocaine and cocaine + alcohol on neurocognitive performance. Neurology. 2000;54(12):2285–92.

105. Verdejo-Garcia A, Rivas-Perez C, Lopez-Torrecillas F, Perez-Garcia M. Differential impact of severity of drug use on frontal behavioral symptoms. Addict Behav. 2006;31(8):1373–82.

106. Volkow ND, Fowler JS, Wang GJ. The addicted human brain viewed in the light of imaging studies: brain circuits and treatment strategies. Neuropharmacology. 2004;47 Suppl 1:3–13.

107. Perry JL, Carroll ME. The role of impulsive behavior in drug abuse. Psychopharmacology. 2008;200:1–26.

108. Crews F, He J, Hodge C. Adolescent cortical development: a critical period of vulnerability for addiction. Pharmacol Biochem Behav. 2007;86:189–99.

109. Di Sclafani V, Tolou Shams M, Price LJ, Fein G. Neuropsychological performance of individuals dependent on crack-cocaine, or crack-cocaine and alcohol, at 6 weeks and 6 months of abstinence. Drug Alcohol Depend. 2002;66(2):161–71.

Automatic and Controlled Processes in the Pathway from Drug Abuse to Addiction

3

Matt Field and Reinout Wiers

Abstract

Heavy drinking is associated with a cluster of cognitive processes, which we have termed controlled processes (rational decision-making and alcohol outcome expectancies), automatic processes (implicit memory associations and attentional bias) and executive dysfunction (which includes working memory and "impulsivity"). In this chapter, we review evidence which suggests that these different types of cognitions have a causal influence on future alcohol consumption and the development of alcohol problems. We highlight gaps in the evidence base which we hope will be tackled in future research. We also discuss recent research which suggests that it is important to consider interactions between these different types of cognitive processes when attempting to predict future alcohol problems, and we speculate on the relative importance of different types of cognitive processes at different stages of the alcohol addiction cycle, from controlled "social" drinking through to alcohol abuse and alcohol dependence.

Learning Objectives

- Alcohol consumption is influenced by *controlled* cognitive processes, such as rational decision-making and outcome expectancies for alcohol effects.
- Heavy drinking is associated with alterations in *automatic* cognitive processing, such as implicit memory associations and attentional bias. These processes may make unique contributions to future alcohol consumption, over and above those attributed to controlled cognitive processes.
- Heavy drinking is also associated with increased impulsivity and impaired *executive function*; this may reflect both a consequence of chronic alcohol exposure and a cause of loss of control over alcohol-seeking behaviour. Furthermore, it is likely to interact with controlled and automatic cognitive processes to produce further impairments in the loss of control over drinking.

M. Field (✉)
School of Psychology, University of Liverpool, Eleanor Rathbone Building, Bedford Street South, Liverpool L69 7ZA, UK
e-mail: mfield@liverpool.ac.uk

R. Wiers
University of Amsterdam, Amsterdam, The Netherlands

J.C. Verster et al. (eds.), *Drug Abuse and Addiction in Medical Illness: Causes, Consequences and Treatment*,
DOI 10.1007/978-1-4614-3375-0_3, © Springer Science+Business Media, LLC 2012

Issues that Need to Be Addressed by Future Research
- At what stage of the alcohol drinking "career" does the influence of controlled processes begin to wane and automatic processes come to predominate?
- What should we target during treatment: automatic processes, controlled processes, executive function or all three?
- How does executive function interact with controlled and automatic processes to influence alcohol-seeking behaviour?

Why do people drink alcohol? Why do some individuals progress from controlled "social" drinking through to alcohol abuse and ultimately to alcohol dependence? In this chapter we present an overview of these issues from a psychological perspective. Specifically, we focus on three distinct aspects of cognition which seem to be associated with individual differences in alcohol consumption, alcohol problems and alcohol dependence. These are (a) "controlled" cognitive processes, which are alcohol cognitions that people can consciously report to researchers through questionnaires or interviews; (b) "automatic" cognitive processes, which are alcohol cognitions that participants may not be able to directly report, but which can be inferred from measures such as reaction time when alcohol-related words or pictures are presented to participants and finally (c) executive dysfunction and impulsivity. This refers to the impaired ability to plan or regulate behaviour which seems to be a key feature of alcohol and other drug problems. We discuss the role of each of these aspects of cognition in relation to alcohol consumption and abuse, with a particular emphasis on causality: each type of alcohol cognition is clearly *associated* with individual differences in alcohol consumption and abuse, but additional types of evidence need to be considered before a causal relationship can be inferred. After considering each aspect of cognition in isolation, we consider the possible interactions between these different cognitions and we speculate on the role of each process in the transition from social drinking, through to alcohol abuse and dependence. Our chapter is focussed almost entirely on alcohol cognitions; however, most of the issues that we discuss are relevant for addictions to different substances as well and where relevant we discuss research relating to other drug classes, such as nicotine and cocaine.

Controlled Processes: Decision-Making, Alcohol Outcome Expectancies and Related Cognitions

To an extent, alcohol use is the outcome of a controlled decision-making process: individuals who perceive the beneficial effects of alcohol consumption to outweigh its negative consequences will drink alcohol more frequently or more intensively [1, 2]. The causal role of this controlled process is illustrated by a consideration of alcohol outcome expectancies (AOEs). AOEs are beliefs about the effects of alcohol that can be assessed with self-report questionnaires, such as the Alcohol Expectancy Questionnaire (AEQ) [3, 4], in which participants are asked whether they agree or disagree with a number of statements describing the effects of alcohol (e.g. "Alcohol makes me feel happy"). A variety of different AOEs have been described, including beliefs that alcohol increases positive affect (positive reinforcement expectancies), reduces negative affect (negative reinforcement expectancies), increases arousal and has negative consequences [5, 6]. Numerous cross-sectional and longitudinal studies demonstrate that individual differences in AOEs are associated with the level of alcohol consumption and with alcohol-related problems (for reviews see [5, 6]). In general, heavier drinkers are more likely to expect positive and arousing outcomes from drinking and less likely to expect negative outcomes, compared to lighter drinkers [5, 6]. Furthermore, the degree to which positive and arousing AOEs are endorsed is associated with the severity of alcohol-related problems [7], although negative reinforcement expectancies are particularly closely associated with alcohol problems [8–10].

Longitudinal studies have revealed that young people hold AOEs before they begin to use alcohol and individual differences in AOEs among youth predict the extent of their alcohol involvement at subsequent time points [11–13]. Additional research suggests that changes in AOEs may be an important mediator of the initiation into alcohol use among youth produced by other well-known causal factors, including peer influence [14], sensation-seeking [15], exposure to portrayals of alcohol use in the media and advertising [16] and a family history of alcoholism [17]. Furthermore, experimental work in which AOEs are experimentally manipulated provides more direct evidence for a causal role for AOEs on drinking behaviour. For example, in one study [18] participants were "primed" with either the positive or the negative consequences of drinking, and this manipulation influenced the amount of alcohol that participants opted to consume in the laboratory. Finally, there is evidence that after many years of heavy drinking, problem drinkers report an increase in their negative AOEs, and this is associated with abstinence or reduced alcohol consumption [6, 19, 20]. Therefore, increased negative AOEs, which presumably develop as a consequence of repeated experience of the negative aspects of heavy drinking, may lead to a reduction in alcohol consumption among heavy drinkers.

Self-reported "reasons for drinking" (RFD) are related to AOEs, although they may explain additional variance in alcohol consumption and alcohol problems [21]. RFD questionnaires require respondents to indicate the reasons why *they* drink, or the anticipated outcomes of drinking alcohol which motivate them to consume it [22, 23]. As might be expected based on the structure of AOEs, RFD can be separated into positive reinforcement motives (e.g. the desire to drink alcohol to elevate positive mood) and negative reinforcement motives (e.g. the desire to drink alcohol to alleviate negative mood). Although strong endorsement of any type of drinking motive is associated with alcohol consumption and alcohol problems, individuals who strongly endorse negative reinforcement motives in particular are more likely to drink heavily and be diagnosed with alcohol problems [22, 23], which mirrors the finding that strong endorsement of negative reinforcement AOEs is closely associated with alcohol problems [8–10].

The observed close association between AOEs/RFD and the quantity and frequency of alcohol consumed, both cross-sectionally, longitudinally and in experimental research, is consistent with the theory of planned behaviour [24] in that it suggests that alcohol consumption can be the outcome of a "controlled" decision-making process: alcohol involvement is largely dictated by individual differences in beliefs about the effects of alcohol consumption (AOEs) and in the perceived utility of those effects (RFD). However, closer inspection suggests that these controlled processes do not come close to explaining the majority of variance in alcohol consumption. Across all age groups, Jones et al. [6] have noted that, when previous drinking experience, age and gender are statistically controlled, individual differences in AOEs predict less than 5% of the variance in alcohol consumption using prospective designs. Furthermore, "expectancy challenge" manipulations, which lead to robust and seemingly permanent changes in AOEs (e.g. [25]), do not have consistent effects on alcohol consumption outside of the laboratory [6, 26], and any beneficial effects on alcohol consumption are not consistently mediated by changes in AOEs [27]. Perhaps more importantly, the ability of AOEs to predict subsequent drinking seems to diminish with age: although AOEs (particularly positive reinforcement AOEs) are a robust predictor of subsequent alcohol involvement in youth [11], their predictive utility is reduced in older age groups [13]. This may suggest that controlled processes such as AOEs and RFD are important determinants of the initiation into drinking among youth, but they may play a more limited role in alcohol use among older adults. As we discuss in the next section, automatic (rather than controlled) cognitive processes may be more important drivers of alcohol use among adults, i.e. those individuals who have extensive experience of alcohol use.

Automatic Processes: Implicit Memory Associations, Action Tendencies and Attentional Bias

Various experimental paradigms have been adapted to investigate spontaneous and relatively automatic ("implicit") [28] alcohol-related cognitions [29–31]. One way in which

to conceptualise this emerging body of research is as a complement to the research on self-report measures of alcohol cognitions such as AOEs, as described in the preceding section. The crucial difference is that indirect measures do not rely on participants' self-reports to make inferences about their cognitions. Instead, these measures rely on alternative responses, typically reaction time and spontaneous associations, to make inferences about the underlying cognitive processes.

For example, Stacy and colleagues [32–34] employed memory association tasks in which participants were asked to provide their first association to a variety of prime words that were ambiguously related to alcohol (e.g. "draft"). Findings indicated that the extent to which alcohol-related words were spontaneously generated in response to these ambiguous primes was a robust predictor of subsequent drinking, even when prior drinking and explicit measures were statistically controlled. Convergent findings were obtained in a study described by McCusker [29], in which heavy and light drinkers were asked if they would endorse various positive (e.g. "fun") and negative (e.g. "violent") associates of alcohol. Heavy drinkers endorsed more positive alcohol associates than light drinkers, although heavy and light drinkers did not differ in their endorsement of negative alcohol associates. However, the speed of endorsement was also measured in this study and analysis of reaction times yielded some particularly interesting findings: heavy drinkers were faster to endorse positive rather than negative alcohol associates, whereas for light drinkers the reverse was true. Findings such as these indicate that alcohol-related cognitions, particularly cognitions relating to the positive (rather than the negative) aspects of alcohol use, may be activated relatively automatically in heavy drinkers compared to lighter drinkers.

The implicit association test (IAT) is a different reaction time measure that has been used to probe individual differences in associations between alcohol and various target concepts (e.g. "positive" vs. "negative", or "arousal" vs. "sedation") [35]. On each trial of the task, participants rapidly categorise visually presented words by pressing keys on a computer keyboard. For example, they may be instructed to press the left response key when an alcohol-related word or a positive word is presented, but to press the right response key in response to alcohol-unrelated or negative words. The rationale for the task is that if participants automatically evaluate alcohol as positive rather than negative they should be quicker to respond when "alcohol" and "positive" words share the same response key (as in the example), compared to another block of the task where "alcohol" and "negative" words share the same response key. Given the previously discussed research into explicit alcohol-related cognitions (AOEs), which are generally more positive than negative in heavy drinkers, it is surprising that IAT studies have consistently demonstrated stronger alcohol-negative associations than alcohol-positive associations, in both heavy and light drinkers [35, 36]. This may be at least partially attributable to general (negative) social norms concerning alcohol use: the IAT may be detecting automatic negative alcohol associations (which should be present in everybody, irrespective of their experience with or beliefs about alcohol), and these may be masking positive alcohol associations, which one would expect to see in heavy drinkers only (see [30] for discussion). As such, heavy drinkers may have ambivalent alcohol associations (simultaneously positive and negative) which may influence their performance on a positive-negative IAT (see [37]). Support for this interpretation comes from studies that used a unipolar version of the IAT, in which positive and negative associations are assessed separately. Such studies have demonstrated that negative associations are stronger but unrelated to individual differences in alcohol consumption, whereas positive associations are weaker but positively correlated with individual differences in alcohol consumption [38, 39]. The latter finding is also supported by studies that used other types of reaction time paradigms to assess automatic alcohol-valence associations [40, 41].

The IAT has also been modified to assess the strength of automatic associations between alcohol and the concepts of arousal (versus sedation). Several studies demonstrated that heavy drinkers, but not light drinkers, have strong associations between alcohol and arousal [35, 38]. Similarly, the tendency to associate alcohol with approach concepts (rather than avoidance concepts) during an approach-avoidance IAT is associated with aspects of problem drinking including the frequency of binge drinking [42–44]. We have used related paradigms to investigate the speed at which individuals can direct approach versus avoidance movements towards alcohol-related and alcohol-unrelated pictorial cues. In these tasks, approach and avoidance elicited by alcohol-related cues was assessed either symbolically, by measuring the speed with which participants could move a manikin towards, or away from, an alcohol-related picture [45], or overt behavioural approach was measured, by measuring the speed at which participants could "pull" an alcohol-related picture towards themselves or "push" it away [46]. Results from both types of task demonstrate that heavy drinkers, but not light drinkers, are faster to approach rather than avoid alcohol-related pictures [45, 46]. Taken together, these findings suggest that heavy and problem drinkers automatically associate alcohol with arousal and behavioural approach, as well as with positive valence.

It is important to note that in many of the aforementioned studies (e.g. [33, 39, 40]), individual differences in implicit alcohol-related memory associations explained unique variance in alcohol consumption, over and above that explained by more "explicit" measures, such as AOE questionnaires. Therefore, although explicit measures such as AOEs and implicit measures such as IATs and related tasks are likely to be measuring the same underlying construct, to an extent

(see [47]), the associations between automatic cognitive processes and alcohol consumption may be stronger than the associations between controlled (or consciously reportable) cognitive processes and alcohol consumption. The challenge for implicit cognition researchers is to go beyond the current research, which mainly involves cross-sectional comparisons, to examine the causal role of implicit cognitive processes as determinants of future alcohol use and alcohol problems. For example, although implicit measures seem to predict future alcohol use over a short time period (e.g. 1 month), to a greater extent than that predicted by AOEs and other background variables [48], there are no published studies that explore the predictive utility of implicit measures over longer time periods. Three recent studies demonstrated that experimental manipulations of automatic alcohol cognitions led to alterations in drinking behaviour in the laboratory, which provides crucial support for their importance as determinants of alcohol-seeking [49–51]. Furthermore, one study demonstrated that experimental re-training of automatic approach tendencies leads to improvements in clinical outcome in alcohol-dependent inpatients [52]. The next decade will hopefully yield research findings that confirm these findings, and perhaps see the introduction of these types of training procedures into regular treatment programmes.

Heavy alcohol consumption and alcohol problems are also associated with "attentional bias" for alcohol-related cues: such cues tend to capture the attention in heavy drinkers [53]. For example, studies using the alcohol Stroop task have demonstrated that alcoholics and heavy social drinkers, but not light drinkers, are slow to name the colour in which alcohol-related pictures or words are presented [54–57]. This suggests that heavy drinkers find it difficult to disregard task-irrelevant alcohol-related cues, which leads to an impairment in the primary task (colour naming). Other studies have used the visual probe task, which provides a more direct measure of visuo-spatial attention. Results obtained from this task demonstrate that heavy drinkers, but not light drinkers, are faster to respond to probes that appear in the location of alcohol-related pictures compared to probes that appear in the location of control pictures, which suggests that heavy drinkers direct their spatial attention towards the location of the alcohol pictures [58, 59].

At present, there is no evidence to suggest that attentional biases operate below the threshold of conscious awareness [60, 61], although results obtained using the alcohol Stroop task suggests that distraction from alcohol-related cues occurs automatically, and it is difficult to control or impede [53, 57]. However, it is interesting to note that in visual probe task studies, heavy drinkers tend to show attentional biases for alcohol stimuli only when they are presented for relatively long exposure durations (500 ms or more; see [58, 59]) but not when they are presented briefly (e.g. 200 ms; see [58]). As such, attentional bias among heavy drinkers who are not seeking treatment may primarily reflect a bias in the mainte-nance of attention, or delayed disengagement of attention from alcohol-related cues [53]. By contrast, in alcohol-dependent inpatients (compared to non-alcoholic controls), attentional biases are seen for briefly presented (50 ms) alcohol-related stimuli, and the magnitude of this effect is related to the severity of alcohol dependence [62]. Also, among alcohol-dependent inpatients, if the stimuli are pre-sented for 500 ms or longer, attentional avoidance of those stimuli is seen [62–64]. This approach-avoidance pattern of attentional bias that is observed among treatment-seeking alcoholics may reflect motivational conflict or ambivalence: the initial orienting may reflect sensitisation of the incentive value of alcohol, whereas the subsequent avoidance may occur because alcohol-related cues are aversive when pre-sented in a treatment context. However, a recent meta-analysis [65] suggests that subjective craving is positively correlated with the latter component of attentional bias (delayed disengagement of attention), but not with the earlier component (rapid initial orienting). Given this, the approach-avoidance pattern of attentional bias among patients in treat-ment may actually reflect the aversive properties of alcohol cues in the treatment context (leading to rapid initial orient-ing towards alcohol cues) coupled with diminished subjec-tive craving (leading to a diminution or even reversal of the bias to maintain attention on alcohol-related cues).

The causal status of attentional bias is presently unclear. Theoretical accounts posit that attentional bias for alcohol-related cues reflects the (classically conditioned) incentive properties of those cues, which develop as a consequence of repeated alcohol consumption [66]. Other models extend these predictions by suggesting that, once established, atten-tional biases may increase the likelihood of alcohol self-administration, perhaps because an individual who is repeatedly distracted by alcohol-related cues in their envi-ronment will be more likely to experience alcohol craving, and then act on that craving and seek alcohol [53, 67, 68]. However, much of the present research on attentional bias involves cross-sectional comparisons: attentional bias seems to be present in heavy drinkers, relative to light drinkers or abstainers. These findings are consistent with the argument that attentional bias can contribute to heavy drinking, but of course there are myriad other explanations (e.g. attentional bias may occur solely as a consequence of heavy drinking, see [69]). However, more recently it has been demonstrated that individual differences in attentional bias among heavy drinkers can predict alcohol consumption several months later [70, 71]. Furthermore, attentional bias for alcohol cues is also related to treatment outcome among patients with alcoholism: in one study, attentional bias increased among patients who did not complete treatment, but there was no change among patients who did complete the treatment pro-gramme [72]. Similar findings have been reported in other addictions [73–75], although it should be noted that these effects are usually weak, and they have not always been rep-licated [76]. More direct evidence for a causal effect of atten-tional bias on alcohol consumption comes from a study [77] in which attentional bias for alcohol cues was experimentally manipulated by exposing participants to variants of a visual probe task in which their attentional bias was either increased ("attend alcohol" group) or decreased ("avoid alcohol" group). After this manipulation, it was observed that subjec-tive alcohol craving and ad-lib alcohol consumption were higher in the "attend alcohol" group compared to the "avoid alcohol" group. Despite this initial promising finding, the effects of experimental manipulation of attentional bias on ad-lib alcohol consumption could not be replicated in subse-quent studies [78, 79]. More recent attempts to study the effects of attentional bias modification on alcohol abusers have met with some success, in terms of either a reduction in alcohol consumption [80] or an earlier discharge from treatment [81], although the effects obtained were very small in one of these studies [81], and the other study lacked a suit-able control condition [80]. In summary then, attentional bias for alcohol-related cues is reliably associated with heavy drinking, and recent studies suggest that it may predict future alcohol use. However, unlike research into other aspects of automatic alcohol-related cognitions (e.g. implicit memory associations), it has not yet been established that attentional bias can predict variance in future alcohol consumption over and above that explained by controlled cognitive processes (e.g. AOEs), and neither has it been convincingly established that attentional bias plays a causal role in alcohol consump-tion in the short term.

Executive Dysfunction and "Impulsivity"

Executive function refers to a broad set of cognitive abilities that relate to goal-directed behaviour, including shifting from one environmental contingency to another, updating of work-ing memory in response to environmental changes and the suppression of inappropriate behavioural responses [82]. Arguably, working memory capacity is a core cognitive resource which is super-ordinate to, and ultimately deter-mines the level of, these diverse cognitive abilities [83]. Executive (dys)function is closely related to the psychologi-cal concept of "impulsivity", which is thought to underlie behaviours that are risky, poorly planned and result in unde-sirable consequences [84]. As such, it is implicated in a num-ber of psychiatric disorders, including substance abuse and addiction, and attention-deficit and conduct disorders in chil-dren [84]. Until fairly recently, impulsivity was considered as a form of personality trait, therefore rendering it suitable for assessment with questionnaires (e.g. [85]). More recently, behavioural measures of impulsivity and executive function have been developed. Much like our earlier distinction between "controlled" processes (which can be measured with self-report) and "automatic" processes (which are inferred from task performance, e.g. reaction time), behavioural measures of impulsivity and executive function directly assess behaviours that are implicated in definitions of executive function and impulsivity, such as the inability or unwillingness to delay gratification, the inability to withhold an inappropriate response or a propensity for risk-taking.

For example, in the delay discounting task (see [86]), participants are given a series of choices between two monetary rewards: a small amount of money available immediately, versus a larger amount of money that is available only after a delay. The size of the immediately available reward and the length of the delay before delivery of the delayed reward are typically varied in different experimental trials, and participants are asked to make a choice on each trial. Individual differences in "delay discounting" can then be calculated based on choice performance, with steeper discounting—a consistent preference for small immediate rewards over much larger delayed rewards—a measure of impulsive responding. The aspect of impulsivity that is assessed with delay discounting tasks has been termed "cognitive impulsivity" [87], and it can be contrasted with "motor impulsivity", which refers to the inability to inhibit a dominant motor response or failures of response inhibition [87]. In humans, motor impulsivity is typically assessed with tasks such as the Go/No-Go task or the stop-signal task [88] both of which are reaction time tasks in which participants learn to respond rapidly to certain target stimuli, but to withhold their response to targets under certain circumstances. In these tasks, the percentage of inappropriate responses to target stimuli (i.e. responses emitted on trials when the response should have been withheld) is taken as the index of motor impulsivity.

As recently reviewed by Verdejo-Garcia and colleagues [89], heavy use of and dependence on a variety of substances, including alcohol, is associated with elevated impulsivity and executive dysfunction, and this appears to be the case for a variety of impulsivity and executive function measures. For example, compared to controls, alcohol-dependent individuals perform worse on a variety of executive function tasks [90], they score higher on impulsivity questionnaires and have a higher rate of delay discounting [91], and they have a higher rate of response inhibition failures on a stop-signal task [92]. Furthermore, elevated impulsivity is not limited to alcohol-dependent patients: even heavy social drinkers, compared to light social drinkers, exhibit increased rates of delay discounting [93] and impaired response inhibition [94]. Therefore, "impulsivity" and executive dysfunction, broadly defined, are closely associated with alcohol consumption and alcohol abuse.

As with the other types of cognitive process that we discussed in the previous sections, the causal relationship between impulsivity, executive dysfunction and alcohol use appears to be bidirectional: high levels of impulsivity and impaired executive function may lead to heavy drinking, but chronic heavy drinking may lead to long-term increases in impulsivity and impairments in executive function, and so on. Firstly we consider the possible effects of executive dysfunction/impulsivity on heavy drinking. Within alcoholics some aspects of executive dysfunction are associated with relapse to drinking after treatment (see [89]). We also note that, in tobacco smokers, a high rate of delay discounting is a risk factor for relapse to smoking after a period of abstinence [95]. Perhaps more persuasive are the results from several large studies which demonstrate that in children, high levels of "neurobehavioural disinhibition", a broadly defined trait that shares many features with executive dysfunction (e.g. lack of planning, poor response inhibition, a desire for immediate gratification) is an important risk factor for the development of subsequent alcohol and drug problems in youth and early adulthood [96, 97]. Converging evidence comes from animal studies, which demonstrate that rats that are naturally impulsive will acquire cocaine self-administration more rapidly than their non-impulsive counterparts [98]. To return to a point that we made previously, the clearest test of the causal role of impulsivity or executive dysfunction on alcohol consumption requires impulsivity or executive function to be experimentally manipulated, and the effects of these manipulations on alcohol-seeking behaviour should be recorded. One recent study [99] demonstrates that such a manipulation (of inhibitory control) influences short-term drinking behaviour in the laboratory, although studies with longer-term follow-ups are required.

With regard to the effects of chronic heavy drinking and other drug use on executive function and impulsivity, some theoretical models [100, 101] suggest that chronic drug use leads to impaired functioning of the prefrontal cortex (PFC). As the PFC is the neural substrate of executive function and related processes, the clear implication from these models is that chronic drug and alcohol use are likely to lead to impaired executive function, increased impulsive responding and a general impairment in the ability to regulate behaviour. Cross-sectional comparisons of chronic drug users with drug-naïve volunteers reveal group differences in executive function/impulsivity that are of course consistent with the view that drug use caused these performance deficits, but they are equally compatible with the view that performance deficits predated drug/alcohol use and were the cause of extensive drug or alcohol involvement (see [98]). However, animal research has demonstrated that chronic administration of cocaine [102] and nicotine [103] can increase the rate of impulsive responding and these effects are independent of the acute effects of the drug. Therefore, there is some evidence to suggest that chronic drug use can cause impairments in executive function or increases in "impulsivity".

To briefly summarise: it is likely that the causal relationships between chronic drug use and impaired executive function/impulsivity are bi-directional. Of particular relevance here are findings which demonstrate that the damaging effects of binge alcohol consumption on the PFC are exacerbated among adolescent rats, compared to adult rats [104]. When considered in combination with findings which suggest that executive dysfunction during childhood seems to predate alcohol and drug involvement, and serves as a risk factor for alcohol and drug problems later on in life [96, 97], it seems that alcohol involvement during adolescence may be particularly devastating. Adolescents with relatively impaired executive function are more at risk for excessive drinking during adolescence, but drinking during adolescence is likely to be particularly damaging to the PFC, which should lead to further impairments in executive function and an inability to regulate alcohol consumption later on in life.

Interactions Between Controlled Processes, Automatic Processes and Executive Function

Most recently, investigators have begun to study how the prediction of future alcohol involvement and alcohol problems can be improved if *interactions* between the aforementioned cognitive processes are considered, rather than studying these processes in isolation. Firstly, a number of theoretical models suggest that the extent of executive dysfunction or impulsivity should be directly related to the perceived "salience" of drug-related cues [100, 101], which leads one to the prediction that individual differences in impulsivity should be correlated with individual differences in attentional bias (see [53]). As predicted, in a recent study [93], it was reported that attentional bias for alcohol-related words (as assessed with an alcohol Stroop task) was positively correlated with impulsive responding, as assessed with performance on a delay discounting task. Both attentional bias and impulsivity were associated with alcohol consumption in this adolescent sample.

Other models do not predict a direct relationship between measures of automatic alcohol cognitions and executive function, but they do suggest that the influence of controlled and automatic alcohol cognitions on subsequent alcohol consumption may be moderated by the degree of impairment to executive functioning. For example, in a recent model Wiers and colleagues [30] suggested that automatic or implicit alcohol cognitions should have the largest influence on subsequent alcohol-seeking among individuals with relatively impaired executive function. By contrast, controlled alcohol cognitions (such as AOEs) should have the largest influence on subsequent alcohol-seeking among individuals with relatively intact executive function. Evidence consistent with the model was recently reported. In one study [105], adolescents completed a measure of executive function (a working memory task), together with measures of controlled alcohol cognitions (an AOE questionnaire) and automatic alcohol cognitions (an alcohol IAT), before their alcohol consumption was recorded 1 month later. As predicted, among participants with low working memory capacity (i.e. executive dysfunction), IAT performance predicted prospective alcohol use, but there was no relationship between IAT performance and prospective alcohol use among participants with high working memory capacity. The reverse pattern was seen for AOEs: among participants with *high* working memory capacity, AOEs predicted prospective alcohol use, but there was no relationship between AOEs and prospective alcohol use among participants with low working memory capacity. Comparable findings were obtained in a later study which used different methods to assess automatic alcohol cognitions [106]. Furthermore, the moderating role of working memory capacity on the ability of controlled and automatic cognitive processes to predict future behaviour may be a general psychological phenomenon, which extends beyond the prediction of future substance use [107]; see [108] for a review. In future research, we hope that researchers can replicate and build on these findings, for example by examining whether attentional bias can predict future alcohol consumption among participants with varying working memory abilities, or whether the relationship between automatic alcohol cognitions and prospective alcohol use is moderated by other aspects of executive function, for example, impaired response inhibition [109].

The Transition from Recreational Use to Abuse and Dependence

Controlled cognitive processes, automatic cognitive processes and executive function and impulsivity are all associated with alcohol consumption. We believe that, although each of these processes are probably influenced by chronic alcohol use, they also play an important causal role in future alcohol consumption and the development of alcohol problems. Although each process seems to be important at each different stage of the developmental pathway from social drinking through to alcohol abuse and eventually to alcohol dependence, we suggest that some types of cognition may be more important at certain stages of the alcohol "career" than others. For example, controlled processes, such as AOEs, seem to develop relatively early on in life, and they are acquired before direct experience with alcohol. By contrast, automatic processes develop much more slowly, and their strength and impact on motivated behaviour are likely to increase in line with each experience of alcohol consumption (see [47]). Therefore, AOEs may be more important determinants of the level of alcohol involvement early on in life, but as individuals grow older and automatic processes grow in strength, their influence may come to predominate and the influence of controlled processes may begin to wane. Having said this, recent research suggests that there are important individual differences in the relative influence of controlled versus automatic processes on alcohol-seeking in youth: individuals with relatively intact executive function are more susceptible to the influence of controlled processes, but individuals with impaired executive function are more sensitive to the influence of automatic processes. One question for future research is whether the level of executive function plays a similar moderating role in older, severely dependent adults. One might predict that, if chronic alcohol or drug use leads to long-lasting executive dysfunction, the influence of controlled processes on alcohol or drug use may be negligible in severely dependent adult addicts, who have many years' experience of chronic drug use: among older adults, automatic alcohol cognitions may explain virtually all of the variance in future alcohol consumption. We hope that future research will provide the answers to many of these important questions.

Summary

Heavy drinking is associated with a cluster of changes in cognitive processes, which we have termed controlled processes (rational decision-making and AOEs), automatic processes (implicit memory associations and attentional bias) and executive function (which includes working memory and "impulsivity"). Each of these processes may change in response to chronic alcohol use, but importantly there is evidence that each process can influence future alcohol consumption. However, there are many gaps in the evidence base, and many outstanding questions, which we hope will be tackled in future research. Of particular interest are the many possible interactions between these different types of cognitive processes, and we suggest that a fuller understanding of the cognitions that underlie alcohol-seeking behaviour, and by extension those cognitions that influence the transition from controlled drinking through to alcohol abuse and dependence, will require a comprehensive understanding of the interactions and moderating influences between these different types of cognitive processes.

References

1. Heyman GM. Resolving the contradictions of addiction. Behav Brain Sci. 1996;19(4):561–610.
2. Boys A, Marsden J. Perceived functions predict intensity of use and problems in young polysubstance users. Addiction. 2003;98(7):951–63.
3. Brown SA, Christiansen BA, Goldman MS. The alcohol expectancy questionnaire: an instrument for the assessment of adolescent and adult alcohol expectancies. J Stud Alcohol. 1987;48(5):483–91.
4. Brown SA, Goldman MS, Inn A, Anderson LR. Expectations of reinforcement from alcohol: their domain and relation to drinking patterns. J Consult Clin Psychol. 1980;48(4):419–26.
5. Goldman MS, Christiansen BA, Brown SA, Smith GT. Alcoholism and memory: broadening the scope of alcohol-expectancy research. Psychol Bull. 1991;110(1):137–46.
6. Jones BT, Corbin W, Fromme K. A review of expectancy theory and alcohol consumption. Addiction. 2001;96(1):57–72.
7. Sher KJ, Wood MD, Wood PK, Raskin G. Alcohol outcome expectancies and alcohol use: a latent variable cross-lagged panel study. J Abnorm Psychol. 1996;105(4):561–74.
8. Carey KB, Carey MP. Reasons for drinking among psychiatric outpatients: relationship to drinking patterns. Psychol Addict Behav. 1995;9(4):251–7.
9. Carey KB, Correia CJ. Drinking motives predict alcohol-related problems in college students. J Stud Alcohol. 1997;58(1):100–5.
10. Cooper ML, Russell M, George WH. Coping, expectancies, and alcohol abuse: a test of social learning formulations. J Abnorm Psychol. 1988;97(2):218–30.
11. Aas HN, Leigh BC, Anderssen N, Jakobsen R. Two-year longitudinal study of alcohol expectancies and drinking among Norwegian adolescents. Addiction. 1998;93(3):373–84.
12. Christiansen BA, Goldman MS, Brown SA. The differential development of adolescent alcohol expectancies may predict adult alcoholism. Addict Behav. 1985;10(3):299–306.
13. Leigh BC, Stacy AW. Alcohol expectancies and drinking in different age groups. Addiction. 2004;99(2):215–27.
14. Wood MD, Read JP, Palfai TP, Stevenson JF. Social influence processes and college student drinking: the mediational role of alcohol outcome expectancies. J Stud Alcohol. 2001;62(1):32–43.
15. Henderson MJ, Goldman MS, Coovert MD, Carnevalla N. Covariance structure models of expectancy. J Stud Alcohol. 1994;55(3):315–26.
16. Austin EW, Pinkleton BE, Fujioka Y. The role of interpretation processes and parental discussion in the media's effects on adolescents' use of alcohol. Pediatrics. 2000;105(2):343–9.
17. Brown SA, Vik PW, Tate SR, Haas AL, Aarons GA. Modeling of alcohol use mediates the effect of family history of alcoholism on adolescent alcohol expectancies. Exp Clin Psychopharmacol. 1999;7(1):20–7.
18. Carter JA, McNair LD, Corbin WR, Black DH. Effects of priming positive and negative outcomes on drinking responses. Exp Clin Psychopharmacol. 1998;6(4):399–405.
19. Jones BT, McMahon J. Negative and positive alcohol expectancies as predictors of abstinence after discharge from a residential treatment program: a one-month and three- month follow-up study in men. J Stud Alcohol. 1994;55(5):543–8.
20. Jones BT, McMahon J. A comparison of positive and negative alcohol expectancy and value and their multiplicative composite as predictors of post-treatment abstinence survivorship. Addiction. 1996;91(1):89–99.
21. Cronin C. Reasons for drinking versus outcome expectancies in the prediction of college student drinking. Subst Use Misuse. 1997;32(10):1287–311.
22. Cooper ML. Motivations for alcohol use among adolescents: development and validation of a four-factor model. Psychol Assess. 1994;6(2):117–28.
23. Grant VV, Stewart SH, O'Connor RM, Blackwell E, Conrod PJ. Psychometric evaluation of the five-factor modified drinking

motives questionnaire—revised in undergraduates. Addict Behav. 2007;32(11):2611–32.

24. Godin G, Kok G. The theory of planned behavior: a review of its applications to health-related behaviors. Am J Health Promot. 1996;11(2):87–98.

25. Darkes J, Goldman MS. Expectancy challenge and drinking reduction: experimental evidence for a mediational process. J Consult Clin Psychol. 1993;61(2):344–53.

26. Wiers RW, Van De Luitgaarden J, Van Den Wildenberg E, Smulders FTY. Challenging implicit and explicit alcohol-related cognitions in young heavy drinkers. Addiction. 2005;100(6):806–19.

27. van de Luitgaarden J, Wiers RW, Knibbe RA, Candel MJJM. Single-session expectancy challenge with young heavy drinkers on holiday. Addict Behav. 2007;32(12):2865–78.

28. De Houwer J. What are implicit measures and why are we using them? In: Wiers RW, Stacy AW, editors. Handbook of implicit cognition and addiction. Thousand Oaks, CA: Sage; 2006. p. 11–28.

29. McCusker CG. Cognitive biases and addiction: an evolution in theory and method. Addiction. 2001;96(1):47–56.

30. Wiers RW, Bartholow BD, van den Wildenberg E, Thush C, Engels RCME, Sher KJ, et al. Automatic and controlled processes and the development of addictive behaviors in adolescents: a review and a model. Pharmacol Biochem Behav. 2007;86(2):263–83.

31. Rooke SE, Hine DW, Thorsteinsson EB. Implicit cognition and substance use: a meta-analysis. Addict Behav. 2008;33(10):1314–28.

32. Ames SL, Stacy AW. Implicit cognition in the prediction of substance use among drug offenders. Psychol Addict Behav. 1998;12(4):272–81.

33. Stacy AW. Memory activation and expectancy as prospective predictors of alcohol and marijuana use. J Abnorm Psychol. 1997;106(1):61–73.

34. Stacy AW, Ames SL, Sussman S, Dent CW. Implicit cognition in adolescent drug use. Psychol Addict Behav. 1996;10(3):190–203.

35. Wiers RW, Van Woerden N, Smulders FTY, De Jong PJ. Implicit and explicit alcohol-related cognitions in heavy and light drinkers. J Abnorm Psychol. 2002;111(4):648–58.

36. De Houwer J, Crombez G, Koster EHW, De Beul N. Implicit alcohol-related cognitions in a clinical sample of heavy drinkers. J Behav Ther Exp Psychiatry. 2004;35(4):275–86.

37. de Liver Y, van der Pligt J, Wigboldus D. Positive and negative associations underlying ambivalent attitudes. J Exp Soc Psychol. 2007;43(2):319–26.

38. Houben K, Wiers RW. Assessing implicit alcohol associations with the Implicit Association Test: fact or artifact? Addict Behav. 2006;31(8):1346–62.

39. Houben K, Wiers RW. Implicitly positive about alcohol? Implicit positive associations predict drinking behavior. Addict Behav. 2008;33(8):979–86.

40. De Houwer J, De Bruycker E. The identification-EAST as a valid measure of implicit attitudes toward alcohol-related stimuli. J Behav Ther Exp Psychiatry. 2007;38(2):133–43.

41. de Jong PJ, Wiers RW, van de Braak M, Huijding J. Using the Extrinsic Affective Simon Test as a measure of implicit attitudes towards alcohol: relationship with drinking behavior and alcohol problems. Addict Behav. 2007;32(4):881–7.

42. Ostafin BD, Palfai TP. Compelled to consume: the implicit association test and automatic alcohol motivation. Psychol Addict Behav. 2006;20(3):322–7.

43. Ostafin BD, Palfai TP, Wechsler CE. The accessibility of motivational tendencies toward alcohol: approach, avoidance, and disinhibited drinking. Exp Clin Psychopharmacol. 2003;11(4):294–301.

44. Palfai TP, Ostafin BD. Alcohol-related motivational tendencies in hazardous drinkers: assessing implicit response tendencies using the modified-IAT. Behav Res Ther. 2003;41(10):1149–62.

45. Field M, Kiernan A, Eastwood B, Child R. Rapid approach responses to alcohol cues in heavy drinkers. J Behav Ther Exp Psychiatry. 2008;39(3):209–18.

46. Wiers RW, Rinck M, Dictus M, Van Den Wildenberg E. Relatively strong automatic appetitive action-tendencies in male carriers of the OPRM1 G-allele. Genes Brain Behav. 2009;8(1):101–6.

47. Wiers RW, Stacy AW. Handbook on implicit cognition and addiction. Thousand Oaks, CA: Sage; 2006.

48. Thush C, Wiers RW, Ames SL, Grenard JL, Sussman S, Stacy AW. Apples and oranges? Comparing indirect measures of alcohol-related cognition predicting alcohol use in at-risk adolescents. Psychol Addict Behav. 2007;21(4):587–91.

49. Wiers RW, Rinck M, Kordts R, Houben K, Strack F. Retraining automatic action-tendencies to approach alcohol in hazardous drinkers. Addiction. 2010;105(2):279–87.

50. Houben K, Schoenmakers TM, Wiers RW. I didn't feel like drinking but I don't know why: the effects of evaluative conditioning on alcohol-related attitudes, craving and behavior. Addict Behav. 2010;35(12):1161–3.

51. Houben K, Havermans RC, Wiers RW. Learning to dislike alcohol: conditioning negative implicit attitudes toward alcohol and its effect on drinking behavior. Psychopharmacology. 2010;211(1):79–86.

52. Wiers RW, Eberl C, Rinck M, Becker ES, Lindenmeyer J. Re-training automatic action tendencies changes alcoholic patients' approach bias for alcohol and improves treatment outcome. Psychol Sci. 2011;22(4):490–7.

53. Field M, Cox WM. Attentional bias in addictive behaviors: a review of its development, causes, and consequences. Drug Alcohol Depend. 2008;97(1–2):1–20.

54. Bruce G, Jones BT. A pictorial Stroop paradigm reveals an alcohol attentional bias in heavier compared to lighter social drinkers. J Psychopharmacol. 2004;18(4):527–33.

55. Sharma D, Albery IP, Cook C. Selective attentional bias to alcohol related stimuli in problem drinkers and non-problem drinkers. Addiction. 2001;96(2):285–95.

56. Stormark KM, Laberg JC, Nordby H, Hugdahl K. Alcoholics' selective attention to alcohol stimuli: automated processing? J Stud Alcohol. 2000;61(1):18–23.

57. Cox WM, Fadardi JS, Pothos EM. The addiction-stroop test: theoretical considerations and procedural recommendations. Psychol Bull. 2006;132(3):443–76.

58. Field M, Mogg K, Zetteler J, Bradley BP. Attentional biases for alcohol cues in heavy and light social drinkers: the roles of initial orienting and maintained attention. Psychopharmacology. 2004;176(1):88–93.

59. Townshend JM, Duka T. Attentional bias associated with alcohol cues: differences between heavy and occasional social drinkers. Psychopharmacology. 2001;157(1):67–74.

60. Bradley B, Field M, Mogg K, De Houwer J. Attentional and evaluative biases for smoking cues in nicotine dependence: component processes of biases in visual orienting. Behav Pharmacol. 2004;15(1):29–36.

61. Field M, Mogg K, Bradley BP. Attention to drug-related cues in drug abuse and addiction: component processes. In: Wiers RW, Stacy AW, editors. Handbook on implicit cognition and addiction. Thousand Oaks, CA: Sage; 2006. p. 151–63.

62. Noel X, Colmant M, Van Der Linden M, Bechara A, Bullens Q, Hanak C, et al. Time course of attention for alcohol cues in abstinent alcoholic patients: the role of initial orienting. Alcohol Clin Exp Res. 2006;30(11):1871–7.

63. Stormark KM, Field NP, Hugdahl K, Horowitz M. Selective processing of visual alcohol cues in abstinent alcoholics: an approach-avoidance conflict? Addict Behav. 1997;22(4):509–19.

64. Townshend JM, Duka T. Avoidance of alcohol-related stimuli in alcohol-dependent inpatients. Alcohol Clin Exp Res. 2007;31(8): 1349–57.

65. Field M, Munafo MR, Franken IHA. A meta-analytic investigation of the relationship between attentional bias and subjective craving in substance abuse. Psychol Bull. 2009;135(4): 589–607.

66. Robinson TE, Berridge KC. The neural basis of drug craving: an incentive-sensitization theory of addiction. Brain Res Rev. 1993; 18(3):247–91.

67. Franken IHA. Drug craving and addiction: integrating psychological and neuropsychopharmacological approaches. Prog Neuropsychopharmacol Biol Psychiatry. 2003;27(4):563–79.

68. Ryan F. Detected, selected, and sometimes neglected: cognitive processing of cues in addiction. Exp Clin Psychopharmacol. 2002;10(2):67–76.

69. Field M, Duka T. Cues paired with a low dose of alcohol acquire conditioned incentive properties in social drinkers. Psychopharmacology. 2002;159(3):325–34.

70. Cox WM, Pothos EM, Hosier SG. Cognitive-motivational predictors of excessive drinkers' success in changing. Psychopharmacology. 2007;192(4):499–510.

71. Fadardi JS, Cox WM. Alcohol-attentional bias and motivational structure as independent predictors of social drinkers' alcohol consumption. Drug Alcohol Depend. 2008;97(3):247–56.

72. Cox WM, Hogan LM, Kristian MR, Race JH. Alcohol attentional bias as a predictor of alcohol abusers' treatment outcome. Drug Alcohol Depend. 2002;68(3):237–43.

73. Carpenter KM, Schreiber E, Church S, McDowell D. Drug Stroop performance: relationships with primary substance of use and treatment outcome in a drug-dependent outpatient sample. Addict Behav. 2006;31(1):174–81.

74. Marissen MAE, Franken IHA, Waters AJ, Blanken P, Van Den Brink W, Hendriks VM. Attentional bias predicts heroin relapse following treatment. Addiction. 2006;101(9):1306–12.

75. Waters AJ, Shiffman S, Sayette MA, Paty JA, Gwaltney CJ, Balabanis MH. Attentional bias predicts outcome in smoking cessation. Health Psychol. 2003;22(4):378–87.

76. Waters AJ, Shiffman S, Bradley BP, Mogg K. Attentional shifts to smoking cues in smokers. Addiction. 2003;98(10):1409–17.

77. Field M, Eastwood B. Experimental manipulation of attentional bias increases the motivation to drink alcohol. Psychopharmacology. 2005;183(3):350–7.

78. Schoenmakers T, Wiers RW, Jones BT, Bruce G, Jansen ATM. Attentional re-training decreases attentional bias in heavy drinkers without generalization. Addiction. 2007;102(3):399–405.

79. Field M, Duka T, Eastwood B, Child R, Santarcangelo M, Gayton M. Experimental manipulation of attentional biases in heavy drinkers: do the effects generalise? Psychopharmacology. 2007;192(4):593–608.

80. Fadardi JS, Cox WM. Reversing the sequence: reducing alcohol consumption by overcoming alcohol attentional bias. Drug Alcohol Depend. 2009;101(3):137–45.

81. Schoenmakers TM, de Bruin M, Lux IFM, Goertz AG, Van Kerkhof DHAT, Wiers RW. Clinical effectiveness of attentional bias modification training in abstinent alcoholic patients. Drug Alcohol Depend. 2010;109(1–3):30–6.

82. Miyake A, Friedman NP, Emerson MJ, Witzki AH, Howerter A, Wager TD. The nity and diversity of executive functions and their contributions to complex "frontal lobe" tasks: a latent variable analysis. Cogn Psychol. 2000;41(1):49–100.

83. Kane MJ, Engle RW. The role of prefrontal cortex in working-memory capacity, executive attention, and general fluid intelligence: an individual-differences perspective. Psychon Bull Rev. 2002;9(4):637–71.

84. Evenden JL. Varieties of impulsivity. Psychopharmacology. 1999;146(4):348–61.

85. Whiteside SP, Lynam DR, Miller JD, Reynolds SK. Validation of the UPPS impulsive behaviour scale: a four-factor model of impulsivity. Eur J Personal. 2005;19(7):559–74.

86. Bickel WK, Marsch LA. Toward a behavioral economic understanding of drug dependence: delay discounting processes. Addiction. 2001;96(1):73–86.

87. Olmstead MC. Animal models of drug addiction: where do we go from here? Q J Exp Psychol. 2006;59(4):625–53.

88. Logan GD, Cowan WB, Davis KA. On the ability to inhibit simple and choice reaction time responses: a model and a method. J Exp Psychol Hum Percept Perform. 1984;10(2):276–91.

89. Verdejo-Garcia A, Lawrence AJ, Clark L. Impulsivity as a vulnerability marker for substance-use disorders: review of findings from high-risk research, problem gamblers and genetic association studies. Neurosci Biobehav Rev. 2008;32(4):777–810.

90. Brown SA, Tapert SF, Granholm E, Delis DC. Neurocognitive functioning of adolescents: effects of protracted alcohol use. Alcohol Clin Exp Res. 2000;24(2):164–71.

91. Mitchell JM, Fields HL, D'Esposito M, Boettiger CA. Impulsive responding in alcoholics. Alcohol Clin Exp Res. 2005;29(12): 2158–69.

92. Goudriaan AE, Oosterlaan J, De Beurs E, Van Den Brink W. Neurocognitive functions in pathological gambling: a comparison with alcohol dependence, Tourette syndrome and normal controls. Addiction. 2006;101(4):534–47.

93. Field M, Christiansen P, Cole J, Goudie A. Delay discounting and the alcohol Stroop in heavy drinking adolescents. Addiction. 2007;102(4):579–86.

94. Colder CR, O'Connor R. Attention biases and disinhibited behavior as predictors of alcohol use and enhancement reasons for drinking. Psychol Addict Behav. 2002;16(4):325–32.

95. Yoon JH, Higgins ST, Heil SH, Sugarbaker RJ, Thomas CS, Badger GJ. Delay discounting predicts postpartum relapse to cigarette smoking among pregnant women. Exp Clin Psychopharmacol. 2007;15(2):176–86.

96. Tarter RE, Kirisci L, Mezzich A, Cornelius JR, Pajer K, Vanyukov M, et al. Neurobehavioral disinhibition in childhood predicts early age at onset of substance use disorder. Am J Psychiatry. 2003; 160(6):1078–85.

97. Giancola PR, Tarter RE. Executive cognitive functioning and risk for substance abuse. Psychol Sci. 1999;10(3):203–5.

98. Dalley JW, Fryer TD, Brichard L, Robinson ESJ, Theobald DEH, Laane K, et al. Nucleus accumbens D2/3 receptors predict trait impulsivity and cocaine reinforcement. Science. 2007;315(5816): 1267–70.

99. Jones A, Guerrieri R, Fernie G, Cole J, Goudie A, Field M. The effects of priming restrained versus disinhibited behaviour on alcohol-seeking in social drinkers. Drug Alcohol Depend. 2011; 113(1):55–61.

100. Goldstein RZ, Volkow ND. Drug addiction and its underlying neurobiological basis: neuroimaging evidence for the involvement of the frontal cortex. Am J Psychiatry. 2002;159(10):1642–52.

101. Jentsch JD, Taylor JR. Impulsivity resulting from frontostriatal dysfunction in drug abuse: implications for the control of behavior by reward-related stimuli. Psychopharmacology. 1999;146(4): 373–90.

102. Paine TA, Dringenberg HC, Olmstead MC. Effects of chronic cocaine on impulsivity: relation to cortical serotonin mechanisms. Behav Brain Res. 2003;147(1–2):135–47.

103. Dallery J, Locey ML. Effects of acute and chronic nicotine on impulsive choice in rats. Behav Pharmacol. 2005;16(1):15–23.

104. Crews FT, Braun CJ, Hoplight B, Switzer RC, Knapp DJ. Binge ethanol consumption causes differential brain damage in young

adolescent rats compared with adult rats. Alcohol Clin Exp Res. 2000;24(11):1712–23.

105. Thush C, Wiers RW, Ames SL, Grenard JL, Sussman S, Stacy AW. Interactions between implicit and explicit cognition and working memory capacity in the prediction of alcohol use in at-risk adolescents. Drug Alcohol Depend. 2008;94(1–3): 116–24.

106. Grenard JL, Ames SL, Wiers RW, Thush C, Sussman S, Stacy AW. Working memory capacity moderates the predictive effects of drug-related associations on substance use. Psychol Addict Behav. 2008;22(3):426–32.

107. Hofmann W, Gschwendner T, Friese M, Wiers RW, Schmitt M. Working memory capacity and self-regulatory behavior: toward an individual differences perspective on behavior determination by automatic versus controlled processes. J Personal Social Psychol. 2008;95(4):962–77.

108. Stacy AW, Wiers RW. Implicit cognition and addiction: a tool for explaining paradoxical behavior. Annu Rev Clin Psychol. 2010;6:551–75.

109. Houben K, Wiers RW. Response inhibition moderates the relationship between implicit associations and drinking behavior. Alcohol Clin Exp Res. 2009;33(4):626–33.

Personality and Substance Misuse: Evidence for a Four-Factor Model of Vulnerability

4

Natalie Castellanos-Ryan and Patricia Conrod

Abstract

The emphasis made on the significance of personality in the development of substance use problems has varied substantially through the years. Although early research has focused on identifying a single personality trait that conferred risk for substance use and misuse, recent research has highlighted the complex nature and heterogeneity of substance use behaviours and profiles, identifying a number of traits and risk pathways to substance use problems. This chapter reviews the evidence which provides support for the important aetiological role of a number of personality traits in the development and maintenance of substance use problems. Four personality-based causal pathways to substance misuse are proposed that help to explain some of the underlying mechanisms linking substance misuse with other mental disorders. Finally, implications for prevention and clinical practise are discussed.

Learning Objectives
- Four personality-related pathways to substance misuse, associated with the personality traits of impulsivity, sensation seeking, hopelessness and anxiety sensitivity, are proposed.
- Each personality trait is associated with distinct cognitive and motivational tendencies that render individuals vulnerable to substance use problems and, to some extent, the psychological disorders that co-occur with them.
- A personality-targeted approach in the prevention and/or early intervention of substance use problems, which focuses on the differential motivations for engaging in these behaviours, can improve current efforts in tackling both substance misuse and other co-occurring disorders.

N. Castellanos-Ryan (✉)
Centre de recherche du CHU Ste-Justine,
Université de Montréal, 3175 Chemin de la Côte Sainte-Catherine,
Montreal, H3T 1C5, Canada
e-mail: natalie.castellanos.ryan@umontreal.ca

P. Conrod, Ph.D.
National Addiction Centre, Institute of Psychiatry, King's College
London, 4 Windsor Walk, Denmark Hill, London SE5 8AF, UK

Department of Psychiatry, Université de Montréal,
CHU Hôpital Ste Justine, Montreal, Canada

J.C. Verster et al. (eds.), *Drug Abuse and Addiction in Medical Illness: Causes, Consequences and Treatment*,
DOI 10.1007/978-1-4614-3375-0_4, © Springer Science+Business Media, LLC 2012

Issues that Need to Be Addressed by Future Research

- Longitudinal studies that explore mediation effects are needed to further understand some of the causal mechanisms by which these personality dimensions convey risk for substance misuse.
- The impact of these personality-related pathways to substance use across different developmental periods (e.g. adolescence, early adulthood, late adulthood) and how these pathways can overlap require further examination.
- Gender differences in the mechanisms linking personality and substance use, as well as other comorbid disorders, need to be further examined.

It is common to hear the term "addictive personality" used to describe the character of someone prone to substance misuse, but can the personality of all drug users be narrowed down to one trait or even a particular set of traits? In fact, much research on this issue dating back to the 1970s failed to support this common view, and rather pointed to the possibility that a number of personality traits may be associated with vulnerability to substance use and misuse. Among the personality factors most commonly cited in the literature as being associated with alcohol and drug misuse are traits that fall within the two main overarching personality domains: the disinhibited and inhibited domains. These two domains of personality, respectively, correspond to the two main action tendencies of behaviour, approach and avoidance [1], which are manifestations of appetitive and aversive motivational tendencies [2, 3] and proneness toward positive and negative affective states [4]. Within the disinhibited personality domain, the two dimensions that have been most consistently implicated in substance use and misuse are: (a) impulsivity/disinhibition [5–7] and (b) extraversion/sociability/sensation seeking [8–11]. Within the inhibited domain, the personality dimensions that have been most associated with substance misuse are: (a) negative emotionality/introversion/hopelessness [8, 12–14] and (b) neuroticism, trait anxiety and anxiety sensitivity [7, 15–18].

However, it is important to note that the association between personality, substance use onset and substance misuse is not simple or straightforward. Findings from cross-sectional studies highlighting concurrent associations between personality and substance misuse sometimes differ from the associations found in longitudinal studies. Similarly, the personality traits that have often been found to characterise children of alcoholics or adolescent substance users are different from those that have been associated with clinical samples of substance misusers. Differences could be attributed to the fact that the strength of associations between personality and substance misuse becomes weaker or stronger at different developmental stages and at different stages in the course of the disorder,

with severe or chronic substance misuse possibly resulting in changes in negative affectivity and personality [10, 19].

This chapter will provide a selective review of the literature establishing personality factors as correlates of, as well as risk factors for, substance use and misuse. Prospective studies demonstrating temporal relationships between personality and substance use will be reviewed to delineate traits that are associated with future risk for substance use and those that might be considered particularly susceptible to the chronic effects of substance use. The chapter will then review some of the most cited aetiological models of substance misuse, placing particular emphasis on how personality traits are implicated in these aetiological models.

Disinhibited Personality

Disinhibition is often referred to a general inability to plan, control or regulate behaviour, especially behaviour that can be unduly risky or can sometimes result in negative consequences (see [20, 21] for reviews). Research carried out by Krueger and colleagues [22–24] on the structure of disinhibited behaviour and personality supports a hierarchical structure of disinhibited or externalising disorder symptoms and traits, with a latent externalising factor representing all disinhibited behaviour symptoms (including substance misuse and antisocial symptoms, as well as measures of disinhibited personality), and then two lower order factors representing more severe aggressive behaviour and drug use symptoms. While this line of research illustrates how disinhibited traits are closely linked to substance misuse and other externalising behaviour problems, and helps explain why substance misuse and other externalising symptoms like antisocial behaviour frequently co-occur, it also leaves open the possibility that multiple disinhibited personality traits contribute to these latent constructs in different ways.

Certainly, disinhibited tendencies have been referred to in a number of ways in the personality, behavioural and psychopathology literatures, from "acting without premeditation", "lack of planning", "excitement seeking", "low tolerance to boredome", "behavioural undercontrol" and impulsivity, among a number of constructs [20, 25, 26]. Consequently, measures labelled "disinhibition" or "impulsivity" may measure different constructs from each other. Indeed, although general factor models of personality typically identify only one factor for disinhibition/impulsivity, extensive research has been carried out on the differentiation between different dimensions of disinhibited personality [11, 27, 28], which usually results in between two and four subfactors of disinhibition. Using methodologies such as factor analysis, recent research in the field of personality have identified as many as four personality facets associated with impulsive-like behaviour: lack of planning, lack of persistence, urgency (acting rashly when upset or anxious) and sensation seeking [26, 29]. Laboratory studies using behavioural/cognitive measures of disinhibition have identified a minimum of two sub-factors of disinhibition [30–33]. Studies in both personality and behavioural fields agree that at least two clear sub-dimensions of disinhibition exist: one sub-dimension, which is referred to as impulsivity in this chapter, associated with a deficit in reflectiveness and planning, rapid decision making and action and a failure to inhibit a behaviour that is likely to result in negative consequences [34, 35], and another sub-dimension, which is referred to as sensation seeking, generally defined as a strong need for stimulation, a low tolerance to boredom and a willingness to take risks for the sake of having novel and varied experiences [36, 37].

Impulsivity

Impulsivity as a Correlate of Substance Misuse

Several disinhibited personality traits have been linked to alcohol and/or substance misuse, including impulsivity, thrill seeking and reduced harm avoidance [7, 14, 38]. It is clear from the literature on substance misuse in adolescent and adult samples that impulsive traits play a prominent role in addictive behaviour. Impulsivity has been often associated with substance misuse, specifically, quantity and frequency of drug use and early experimentation with drugs (e.g. [39]). Other studies have found that impulsivity (as measured by novelty seeking) is related to ecstasy use, but not polydrug use [40], and heroin use [41]. Although fewer studies have looked at the association between cannabis use and personality factors, some studies have found evidence of an association between impulsivity and cannabis use in undergraduates (as measure by Cloninger's novelty seeking; [42]) and cannabis abusers (as measured by the Barratt's impulsivity scale; [43]). Also, in their review of findings relating to personality traits and alcohol abuse and dependence, Sher and Thrull [44] concluded that impulsivity was the personality trait that was most consistently associated with alcohol use disorders.

Impulsivity as a Risk Factor for Substance Misuse

Studies on children of alcoholics, who are considered to have higher risk for future alcohol problems due to genetic vulnerability, have found that many of these children exhibit high levels of disinhibited personality and behaviours [45–47]. For example, Conrod and colleagues [48] conducted an investigation into multigenerational alcoholism and personality risk, using Eysenck's Personality Questionnaire (EPQ) [49]. Results showed that disinhibited personality, as measured by the psychoticism scale, was a significant correlate of increased drinking and mediated the relationship between family history of alcoholism and drinking behaviour.

Longitudinal studies have also implicated impulsivity/disinhibited traits in future substance misuse. For example, Sher, Bartholow and Wood [50] found that disinhibited traits in young adulthood, as measured by psychoticism, predicted alcohol use disorders 6 years later, but did not predict tobacco or drug use disorders. Similarly, several studies have found that impulsivity assessed in childhood was prospectively associated with substance misuse in adulthood. One of the first studies to assess the longitudinal nature between personality and substance use and misuse was carried out by Cloninger and colleagues [51] which assessed temperament traits of children aged 10–11 in Sweden and then assessed alcohol-related problems when they were aged 27 years. Boys who scored high on novelty seeking and low harm avoidance in childhood were 20 times more likely to report alcoholism at age 27 than boys who did not score high on these traits [51]. Masse and Tremblay [38] reported similar findings, which showed that high novelty-seeking and low harm avoidance scores in boys aged 6 were associated with a higher likelihood to initiate substance misuse in early adolescence. Findings from the Dunedin Study in New Zealand show that temperamental characteristics measured as early as 3 years of age, in particular that of "undercontrol", predicted alcohol use disorders at the age of 21 [52]. It is important to highlight that the prospective association between impulsive traits and substance misuse reported in these longitudinal studies were found for boys but not for girls. This said, Krueger and colleagues [53] showed that impulsivity, as measured by low constraint, assessed in participants of the Dunedin study at 18 years of age predicted alcohol abuse at age 21 in both men and women. More recently, Chassin and colleagues [54] found that parent's ratings of impulsivity in their young adolescent children, boys and girls alike, predicted increased drinking and drug use at ages 20 and 25. Similarly, Elkins, King, McGue and Iacono [55] found that low constraint in late adolescent boys and girls (aged 17) predicted alcohol use disorders 3 years later. Finally, a recent study carried out by Conrod, Castellanos-Ryan and Strang [56] which assessed personality and substance use from age 14 to age 16 in adolescents attending secondary schools in London found that impulsivity measured in adolescents aged 14 years predicted higher rates of onset of illicit substance use across adolescence and, using survival analysis, found that impulsivity was associated with a reduced likelihood of surviving adolescence without trying cocaine.

It is important to consider the possibility that the pathway from impulsivity to substance misuse might be bidirectional. Laboratory studies have shown that increased and persistent substance use may result in deficits in behavioural and/or cognitive measures of impulsivity such as response inhibition and decision making (e.g. [57, 58]), as well as increased levels of self-report trait impulsivity (e.g. [19]).

Finally, using a different statistical approach to understanding the relationship between personality and substance use, Littlefield, Sher and Wood [15] evaluated the extent to which changes in personality and changes in drinking behaviour co-vary and showed, using latent growth models, that changes in drinking behaviour from 18 to 35 years of age tend to co-occur with changes in neuroticism and impulsivity. While this analysis does not provide any insight into causal effects between these two factors, the findings suggest that the relationship between impulsivity and drinking behaviour might be slightly more complex than a simple causal relation, possibly reflecting a mutually exacerbating relationship.

Extraversion/Sociability/Sensation Seeking

Extraversion/Sensation Seeking as a Correlate of Substance Misuse

Findings on the association between traits related to extraversion and substance misuse in clinical samples have shown that adults with substance use disorders report similar levels of extraversion as controls (e.g. [10]). Similarly, findings on the association between extraversion and substance misuse in adult community samples have been somewhat inconsistent, but on average most studies have indicated a modest association (e.g. [59, 60]). In young adults, extraversion and sociability have been modestly associated with both drinking onset (e.g. [9]) and increased levels of alcohol use (e.g. [61, 62]).

A trait related to extraversion, namely, sensation seeking, has been shown to be more robustly related to substance misuse behaviours, especially heavy episodic drinking [7], and particularly in adolescents and young adults [14, 63–66]. For example, Woicik and colleagues [67] found that in a sample of drinking college students, sensation seeking explained a significant amount of variance in alcohol dependence symptoms, above and beyond that explained by the trait of extraversion as measured by the NEO-FFI.

Sensation Seeking as a Risk Factor for Substance Misuse

Longitudinal studies have shown extraversion/sensation seeking as an important risk factor for substance use behaviours. For example, Conrod and colleagues have found in both Canadian and British adolescents that sensation seeking was not only associated cross-sectionally with binge drinking [14] but could also predict growth in binge drinking rates during adolescence [68]. Krank and colleagues [69] also tested prospective associations between personality traits and substance misuse across a period of 1 year in adolescence, with findings confirming a prospective association between sensation seeking and alcohol use and binge drinking. This study also found a prospective association between this trait and marijuana, tobacco and hallucinogen

use. Other studies have also shown that extraversion measured in childhood or adolescence can prospectively predict the development of alcohol problems in adulthood [70, 71]. For example, Wennberg and Bohman [71] assessed temperament traits in children (aged 4) and correlated them to different substance use behaviours in adulthood, with findings showing that extraversion traits, such as activity level, predicted alcohol problems at age 36. Interestingly, Littlefield, Sher and Wood [15] did not find relationships between changes in drinking behaviour and changes in extraversion over the course of young adulthood, suggesting that it is the excitability, thrill seeking aspect of this broad personality trait, rather than sociability, which plays a role in earlier stages of substance use initiation.

Consistent with this are the findings from a number of studies showing that individuals high in sensation seeking generally drink or use substances for enhancement motives rather than for social motives or negatively reinforcing motives such as coping or conformity motives [63, 67, 72, 73].

Neuroticism/Inhibited Personality

Neuroticism is a broad personality construct that reflects negative emotionality, behavioural inhibition and anxiety [74]. Research on the structure of neurotic symptoms and neurotic personality generally supports a hierarchical structure of anxiety and mood disorder symptoms and traits, with negative affect representing a higher order factor common to all neurotic traits, and then two lower order factors, low positive affect and fear, accounting for unique variance in specific sets of traits and disorders [75]. This tripartite model of anxiety and depression also has relevance for understanding how neurotic/inhibited traits represent risk factors for substance misuse. For example, neuroticism appears to be inconsistently related to risk for substance use disorders (e.g. [76, 77]), but the lower order facets of neuroticism, particularly hopelessness and anxiety sensitivity, have been consistently shown to have specific relationships to particular aspects of substance use and we are now beginning to understand the functional nature of the relationships between these two sets of traits and substance-related behaviours.

First, with respect to the *broader trait of negative affect*, research has shown that individuals who experience depressed mood and anxiety drink more, and more often, particularly in negative situations [64, 78, 79]. Studies on clinical samples have shown that, compared to controls, individuals with substance use disorders score higher on measures of neuroticism and negative emotionality [12, 13, 80]. A link between negative emotionality and smoking has also been established (e.g. [81, 82]), with some studies showing that smokers who report increased levels of negative emotionality experience worse withdrawal symptoms [83] and are less successful at quitting smoking [84]. Although this association between emotional disorders and substance misuse has been shown in adult clinical samples [85], less support has been found in community-based samples, such as college students [12, 86] and adolescent samples [60, 64, 87, 88].

However, high scores on self-reported negative emotionality have been found in non-alcoholic adolescent children of alcoholics [89] suggesting that negative emotionality is not only a correlate of substance misuse but also a potential risk factor. This is confirmed by a number of prospective studies. For example, Krueger and colleagues [53] showed that negative emotionality assessed at age of 18 predicted alcohol abuse at age 21. Similarly, Jackson and Sher [12] were unable to find any directional effects between alcohol use disorders and psychological distress in a sample of 378 young adults but did reveal that the personality trait of neuroticism predicted both alcohol use disorders and depressive symptoms. Indeed, Sher and colleagues found that negative emotionality-related traits assessed at age 18 in this same sample of young adults was a modest but significant predictor of substance use disorders at age 24 [50] as well as at age 28 [12]. Moreover, Wills, Sandy and Shinar [90], who investigated the relationship between negative affect and the frequency of substance misuse in adolescents (12–15 years) over a 3-year period, found that those students who had the highest negative affect score at 12 years had the greatest increase in substance misuse across time.

Considering the hierarchical structure of neurotic traits and symptoms, it is also worth considering the association substance misuse has with the lower order facets of hopelessness and anxiety sensitivity.

Hopelessness as a Risk Factor for Substance Misuse

Conrod et al. [7] previously hypothesised that a lower order trait of negative affect, namely hopelessness or low positive affect, would be associated with a particular susceptibility to substance misuse patterns through a self-medication process involving analgesia-induced numbing of painful experiences and memories and reinstatement of previously extinguished reward behaviours. They then showed in a community-recruited sample of substance-dependent women that a personality factor reflecting introversion and hopelessness was associated with a substance misuse profile that involved higher rates of dependence on analgesics and greater comorbidity with recurrent depression and social phobia. In a follow-on study with college students and high schools students, Woicik et al. [67] showed that a similar dimension of personality was associated with higher rates of alcohol abuse and dependence, sedative (including analgesics) drug use, and self-report reasons for substance use linked to depression coping and numbing of painful memories. These researchers also showed that hopelessness, as measured by a brief 8-item self-report scale, showed incremental validity over and above the Five Factor

Inventory-Neuroticism Scale [91] with respect to accounting for alcohol dependence and abuse symptoms in college students. A concurrent association between hopelessness and alcohol use problems in youth attending vocational schools in Turkey has also been reported by Ilhan, Demirbas and Dogan [92]. Two studies carried by Bolland and colleagues [93, 94] showed significant cross-sectional as well as longitudinal associations between hopelessness and substance misuse in adolescents living in poor inner-city neighbourhoods in Alabama. Compared with adolescents with low levels of hopelessness, those with high levels of hopelessness were at least twice as likely to report smoking tobacco in the last month, drinking in the last week and using marijuana in the last month, as well as six times as likely to report cocaine use in the last month [93]. Using a longitudinal design, Bolland et al. [94] went on to show that adolescents from Caucasian ethnic backgrounds with high levels of hopelessness reported greater acceleration in their trajectories of tobacco use, alcohol use and marijuana use than those with low levels of hopelessness. More recently, this trait has been shown to be a robust predictor of future alcohol and illicit drug use in prospective studies with high school students in Canada and the UK [56, 68, 69]. The mechanisms by which this personality dimension conveys risk for substance misuse are not well understood, but there is some indication that it is mediated through the occurrence of depressive symptoms [95], and motivations for drinking that include coping with depression [96]. Interestingly, a recent study by Jaffee and Zurilla [97] showed that the association between hopelessness and lifetime alcohol and marijuana use in adolescence was mediated by reduced rational problem-solving skills, suggesting that problem solving might be an important mechanism underlying the link between this trait and substance misuse. The authors suggest that it is possible that in adolescence feelings of hopelessness and negative expectations might influence and impair the ability to effectively define and solve problems, which in turn, may lead to substance misuse in these individuals [97]. However, in line with motivational theories of substance misuse [64, 72], another possibility could be that deficient problem-solving skills could lead to adolescents experiencing higher number of negative outcomes which could lead to increased hopelessness, and, in turn, increased levels of substance misuse in order to cope with negative feelings. Further longitudinal studies are needed to confirm causal interpretations of these results.

Fear/Hyperarousal/Anxiety Sensitivity

Anxiety Sensitivity as a Correlate of Substance Misuse

Another lower order neurotic trait is anxiety sensitivity, described as a fear of anxiety-related physical sensations due to an unrealistic expectation that they could lead to loss of physical or mental control or other "catastrophic" consequences [98]. Like hopelessness, anxiety sensitivity is also associated with coping or negative reinforcement motives for substance use [99] and to high drinking levels [100, 101] and drinking problems [102] in adults. Several studies have linked anxiety sensitivity to misuse of a variety substances in adults, such as heroin [103], alcohol [18], nicotine [18, 104, 105] and anxiolytics [7], but not marijuana, hashish [18] or stimulants [7]. Other studies have also shown increased levels of anxiety sensitivity (AS) in individuals receiving treatment for substance use disorders (e.g. [106]). A number of studies have now demonstrated that AS is associated with self-report motivations for substance use that reflect self-medication of anxiety symptoms [99, 107] and a pharmacological sensitivity to the arousal dampening properties of alcohol [102, 108] and benzodiazepines [109]. AS has also been shown to predict reactivity to nicotine withdrawal [110, 111] and the tendency to rapidly return to smoking during quit attempts [112]. Often described as an arousal-accelerating factor [99, 113], AS appears to not only render individuals susceptible to high levels of arousal in normal stressful situations, but also in response to acute and chronic drug withdrawal, physiologic states that are easily dampened by the pharmacologic properties of alcohol and benzodiazepines [114].

Anxiety Sensitivity as a Risk Factor for Substance Misuse

Although there is some prospective evidence that anxiety symptoms in childhood or adolescence often precede substance use and misuse [115, 116], very few prospective studies on the association between anxiety sensitivity and substance misuse have been carried out and of those reported, the results are mixed or might suggest developmental and gender specificity. A study carried out by Pulkkinen and Pitkänen [117] found that anxiety/shyness assessed at the age of 8 predicted increased alcohol and other drug use 20 years later in women, but predicted reduced substance use in men. The previously mentioned longitudinal study carried out by Caspi and colleagues [52] showed that, together with under-controlled boys, inhibited boys—described as fearful, anxious and shy—were more likely to present alcohol-related problems. More recently, a study by Schmidt, Buckner and Keough [17] which assessed anxiety sensitivity and alcohol use disorders across 2 years in a community sample of young adults (mean age 19 years at baseline) showed that anxiety sensitivity was uniquely associated with the development of future alcohol use disorders. While Comeau, Stewart and Loba [63] found that high levels of anxiety sensitivity in adolescents were associated with high conformity motives for alcohol and marijuana use, and moderated the association between trait anxiety and coping motives for alcohol and

cigarette use, other studies have not confirmed a relationship between AS and early onset or higher severity of substance use in adolescents [56, 68]. Conrod, Pihl and Vassileva [102] showed that a community-recruited sample of high AS young men did not show higher levels of drinking quantity or frequency compared to an age-matched group of low AS young men, but they did report higher levels of coping motives for drinking and alcohol-related problems. Woicik et al. [67] examined the relationship between AS and substance use and misuse in high school and college-age students and showed a possible age-specific relationship between AS and such behaviours. In college students, AS was not shown to be related to quantity or frequency of alcohol use or alcohol problems, but was associated with high coping motives for drinking and higher rates of sedative drug use. In high school age participants, AS was only shown to be related to conformity motives for alcohol use. In a recent prospective study with younger high-school students in the UK (mean age 14 year), while AS was shown to predict maintenance of anxiety and panic symptoms over time [95, 118], there was no evidence of a cross-sectional or prospective relationship between AS and early alcohol or illicit drug use [56, 68].

When conceptualising AS as an arousal-accelerator, it is not surprising that prospective studies do not support the conclusion that AS is a risk factor for adolescent onset substance use. The evidence rather indicates that AS represents a specific risk profile predicting who will use substances to cope with stressors that produce physiologic arousal, such as drug withdrawal [119], trauma [79, 120] and severe negative life circumstances [121], but also those normative experiences such as social pressure to conform to peers substance use patterns [63]. Findings from a variety of studies suggesting that the relationship between AS and substance use in clinical [107] and high risk [95] samples is mediated by anxiety symptoms indicate that pathological anxiety and extreme levels of AS might directly lead to high enough levels of arousal and fear to stimulate substance use, without the need for stressful environmental input.

Aetiological Models of Substance Misuse and Personality

Although the associations between personality traits and substance misuse reviewed above highlight the important role personality plays in the onset and development of substance misuse, it is important to relate this information to established aetiological models, in order to explain how and why personality contributes to substance misuse.

A number of aetiological models of substance misuse are supported by the literature. These models include: the affect regulation models, the pharmacological vulnerability model, the deviance proneness model and the "psychological dysregulation" model. The first three models have been outlined previously by Sher and colleagues [85, 122, 123]. To these models, we have added the psychological dysregulation model, proposed and supported by Tarter and colleagues [124, 125] and Clark and colleagues [126–128], as, although not strictly an aetiological model of substance misuse, this model has gained substantial support in recent years as a model explaining the development of problem behaviour including substance misuse in adolescence and early adulthood. Finally, based on the literature reviewed above and expanding on models proposed by Conrod et al. [7], Phil and Peterson [47] and Woicik et al. [67], we propose a comprehensive model which includes four personality-specific pathways to substance use and misuse.

Affect Regulation

Several studies have shown that many individuals drink or use substances to regulate affect or emotional states. *Positive affect regulation* refers to when individuals drink or use substances for positive reinforcement or "enhancement" [129], which is strongly associated with positive expectancies for enhancement and personality traits such as reward and/or sensation seeking [7, 72]. The motivation for positive reinforcement from substances has been shown to be founded on the neuropharmacological effect substances have on the brain centres involved in basic reward mechanisms, i.e. substances stimulate mesolimbic dopamine activity [130] and increase activity in brain opioid systems [131] (this is further described in the next section on the pharmacological vulnerability model of substance misuse). Although disinhibited traits such as impulsivity and sensation seeking have both been associated with increased and problematic substance use [7, 14, 132], these traits have been shown to be related to substance misuse in different ways. While sensation seeking has consistently been associated with enhancement or reward-related motives for substance use [63, 67, 72], impulsivity has not been associated with a specific motive for substance misuse [64], but associated with a more disorganised and severe pattern of alcohol and drug abuse [67]. This was substantiated by a study carried out by Simons and colleagues [73] showing that while impulsivity was not associated with a specific motive for substance misuse, it was directly associated with marijuana and alcohol-related problems. Sensation seeking, on the other hand, was associated indirectly to alcohol problems through enhancement motives [73].

Conversely, some individuals use substances to relieve *negative affect*, i.e. depressed mood, stress and/or anxiety [72, 133, 134]. Also referred to as the "self-medication" hypothesis, many individuals report that they use substances to cope with negative affect and to forget about difficult situations [129]. Although the negative affect regulation model is one of the most enduring aetiological perspectives on SUDs [122], several researchers have concluded that this is highly dependent upon intra-individual factors such as personality, expectancies and genetics, as well as environmental factors, especially stress-inducing environments [64, 72, 133].

Inhibited traits have typically been implicated in models of negative affect regulation of substance misuse. Neuroticism/hopelessness has been argued to reflect sensitivity to punishment and has been linked to the development of alcohol use by using its analgesic properties to suppress feelings of negative affect [7]. Fitting with this profile of substance misuse are findings from Henderson and Gallen [135] who, assessing personality and substance misuse in a sample of male veterans attending treatment for a substance use disorder, found that substance misusers could be classified based on substance use severity measures and temperament. They found that one of the four groups identified was characterised by late onset substance misuse and low positive affect (similar to measures of hopelessness), which, in turn, had a higher incidence of depression, a greater tendency to use substances in solitary contexts and lower enhancement motives for alcohol. Anxiety sensitivity has also been associated with substance misuse for negative affect regulation, but specifically to relieve feelings of anxiety (see Stewart and Kushner [99] for a review of models of how anxiety sensitivity is associated to increased risk for substance misuse). Consistent with this are studies showing that anxiety sensitivity is associated generally with coping motives for alcohol use [63, 102] and that those high in anxiety sensitivity use substances specifically to avoid or escape anxiety symptoms [107]. Further confirmation comes from a study showing that risk for alcohol misuse results from elevated scores on anxiety sensitivity in combination with the belief that drinking alcohol can reduce tension (i.e. tension-reduction alcohol expectancies [136]).

Pharmacological Vulnerability

The pharmacological vulnerability model [85] proposes that individuals differ in their response to the effects of alcohol and other drugs, which can put certain individuals at risk in one of two ways: (1) individuals are at risk for substance misuse because they are especially sensitive to the reinforcing effects of substances and are therefore more likely to use substances as they experience greater effects from the substance and (2) some individuals are relatively insensitive to the reinforcement effects of substances and thus must consume larger amounts of the substance in order to achieve the desired effect, which can place them at risk for secondary drug-related harm and physiological dependence.

For example, many studies have showed that, compared to controls, individuals with a family history of alcoholism have a less intense subjective response to moderate doses of alcohol on scales primarily measuring sedative drug effects [137–140]. Using a longitudinal design, Schuckit and Smith [141] showed that this low subjective response to alcohol predicted the onset of alcohol dependence in young adults. However, others have found that heightened physiological sensitivity to substances is associated with risk (e.g. Conrod et al. [48]). For example, Peterson and colleagues [142] found that accelerated heart rate after alcohol consumption was associated with increased risk for alcoholism. Similarly, Gabbay [143] found that compared to controls, men with a family history of alcoholism experienced a heightened subjective stimulant response to amphetamine. Also, individuals who report heavy drinking have been shown to exhibit greater subjective stimulant effects of alcohol measured in the laboratory [144, 145]. In another study, college students with poor inhibitory control reported heavier drinking and exhibited enhanced subjective stimulation during the ascending limb of the blood alcohol curve [146]. These apparently contradictory findings may be explained by discrepancies in the methodology used in the different studies and the precise timing when the subjective response is measured. Specifically, participants with a positive family history of alcoholism exhibit an enhanced response when assessments are done as blood alcohol levels are rising (i.e. ascending limb of the alcohol curve), but display a less intense response when measurements are taken as those levels are decreasing (e.g. Newlin and Thomson [147]). Furthermore, Morzorati et al. [140] argued that an association between risk and enhanced response is more evident when measures of the subjectively positively reinforcing effects of alcohol (e.g. stimulation) are employed, compared to when measures of the negative effects (e.g. dizzy, clumsy) are used. Some researchers have suggested that individual differences in personality that were not taken into consideration in many of these studies might partly account for differing results. Consistent with this are studies showing that individuals who are high on disinhibited personality traits tend to be more sensitive to drug-induced reward [48, 50, 60, 146, 148] and display heightened heart rate response to alcohol (e.g. Brunelle et al. [148]), while individuals who are high on inhibited traits like anxiety sensitivity display reduced electrodermal activity to threat cues when moderate to high levels of alcohol have been consumed (e.g. Stewart and Pihl [149]). Brunelle et al. [148] showed that it was sensation seeking that was associated with a heightened heart rate response to alcohol and positive feelings after alcohol intoxication. As reviewed previously, heightened heart rate is associated, in turn, with increased risk for substance misuse, which could partly explain the association between sensation seeking and substance misuse [85]. Another possible explanation for the association between sensation seeking and substance misuse is offered by Leyton and colleagues [150]. Leyton et al. [150] found, in an exploratory study using posi-

tron emission tomography (PET), that sensation seeking (as measured by "exploratory-excitability", a sub-dimension of Cloninger's novelty seeking) was associated with greater amphetamine-induced dopamine release in the ventral striatum and drug wanting. The authors suggested that amphetamine consumption elicits a dopamine-mediated appetitive state which is stronger for those high in sensation seeking [150]. It is important to note that sensation seeking has also been linked to general or non-substance related measures of reward sensitivity, particularly in studies looking at gambling behaviour (e.g. Coventry and Constable [151]; McDaniel and Zuckerman [152]). Furthermore, a recent study by our research team showed that the association between sensation seeking and binge drinking in adolescence was partially mediated by reward sensitivity, as measured by a (monetary) rewarded go-no-go task, while impulsivity was not [153].

On the other side of the spectrum, inhibited traits such as AS and low positive affect have also been implicated in differential psychopharmacological effects of substances. As mentioned above, AS has been associated with experiencing increased withdrawal symptoms, particularly those related to tobacco [119], and thus poorer cessation outcomes [84]. Similarly, Leventhal et al. [154] found that it was low positive affect that uniquely, i.e. controlling for other traits or symptoms related to depression, predicted higher withdrawal symptoms in a sample of adults attending a smoking cessation clinic. In addition, low positive affect also predicted poorer outcomes incrementally to the other dimensions of depression, even when controlling for the level of nicotine dependence, smoking frequency and history of major depression.

Other studies which look at differences in alcohol response are studies assessing the stress response dampening effects of alcohol (e.g. Sher [134]). In general, studies have found that individuals with a family history of alcoholism have an increased sensitivity to the dampening effects of alcohol on stress response [155, 156] with findings showing that personality factors, particularly those related to anxiety (i.e. anxiety-sensitivity), also seem to play an important role [48, 149]. For example, Conrod, Pihl and Vassileva [102] found that men with higher self-reported levels of anxiety sensitivity experienced electrodermal response and heart rate dampening effects to aversive stimulation after alcohol administration, compared to low anxiety sensitive men, which the authors interpreted as a pharmacologic sensitivity that is produced by an interaction between sedative drug effects and anxious personality to produce a highly negatively reinforcing fear reduction.

Deviance Proneness

The last of the aetiological models for SUDs outlined by Sher [85] refers to substance use as part of a more general deviant pattern of behaviour, which generally begins in childhood, and can be attributed to poor socialisation. Several longitudinal studies looking at early onset alcohol problems show consistent associations between alcohol problems and a history of childhood antisocial behaviour, poor school achievement, poor interpersonal relationships, heightened activity or attentional problems during childhood, and inadequate parenting [157, 158]. One of the most prominent theories that seek to explain the association between early substance use and other problem behaviour is the problem behaviour theory initially proposed by Jessor and Jessor [159]. This theory, which highlights the importance of a person–environment interaction, states that a range of personality, family, peer and other environmental variables causally relate to involvement in a range of problem behaviours, of which alcohol and drug use are just one or two indicators of a broader factor of general deviance [160]. The theory involves the interplay and interdependence of three systems of variables: the behaviour system, the personality system and the perceived environmental system [161]. Although emphasis is placed on deficient socialisation as a major "instigator" or risk factor, this model also highlights the role temperament and personality traits have in socialisation and developmental processes [162].

Within this model, the trait of impulsivity has been the most widely and consistently implicated in deviant behaviour. Studies have shown that early "difficult temperament" characterised by high levels of disinhibition or impulsivity, in combination with poor parenting, lead to unsocialised behaviour (e.g. Tarter, Kabene, Escallier, Laird and Jacob [163]). Consistent with this model, impulsivity has been shown to be associated with substance misuse that is comorbid with antisocial behaviour, while other disinhibited traits like sensation seeking have not [7, 118, 164]. Indeed, recent findings from Mackie et al. [95] indicated that adolescents high in impulsivity showed their susceptibility to increased alcohol use through conduct disorder symptoms, whereas adolescents high in sensation seeking showed a direct susceptibility to increased alcohol use, and were only susceptible to conduct disorder symptoms as a consequence of their increased alcohol use. Furthermore, Castellanos-Ryan and Conrod [164] recently showed, using structural equation modelling, that while impulsivity was associated with an externalising behaviour factor, which accounted for the shared variance between measures of conduct disorder and substance misuse, as well as a specific conduct disorder factor, it was not associated with substance misuse that did not co-occur with other externalising behaviour problems in adolescence. Also consistent with this are findings from studies investigating the structure of psychiatric disorders showing that while traits related to sensation seeking (i.e. extraversion) and impulsivity (i.e. novelty seeking) were both associated with alcohol and drug dependence, only impulsivity accounted for some of the proportion of the

comorbidity between alcohol dependence and conduct disorder, as well as between drug dependence and conduct disorder [165]. These results, and the high rate of co-occurrence between substance misuse and antisocial behaviours, seem to lend support to the deviance proneness and the behavioural dysregulation (see section below) models of substance misuse and also suggest that impulsivity, but not other personality traits, may play a key role in these liability models.

The Psychological Dysregulation Theory

The psychological dysregulation theory is closely related to the deviance proneness model, as it also highlights the importance of the interplay or interaction between individual and environmental factors in the development of behavioural problems. However, while the deviance proneness model is firmly based on socio-psychological theory, the psychological dysregulation theory is based on psychobiological theory of human behaviour. Psychological dysregulation is defined as a deficiency in cognitive, behavioural and emotional domains when adapting to environmental challenges [128, 166]. This comprehensive model integrates several findings in the genetic, environmental and neuropsychiatry fields, to identify a "phenotype" (which is genetically predisposed) that reflects an individual's liability to substance misuse and related problems. Tarter et al. [124, 166] were the first to refer to the construct of psychological dysregulation, also termed neurobehavioural disinhibition, as an early (childhood) indicator of an individual's general liability of developing substance use problems. This model posits that for those with this liability, which may be transmitted from parent to child, difficult or adverse environmental factors often lead to the development of substance use disorders. Childhood manifestations of psychological dysregulation include irritability, behavioural impulsivity and conduct problems, as well as executive cognitive dysfunction. Studies have shown that childhood psychological dysregulation correlates with parental SUDs and prospectively predicts not only adolescent substance misuse, but other disorders as well, such as conduct disorder and affective disorders [22, 124, 167], and thus, has been considered as a potential factor which explains the high rates of co-occurrence between substance misuse and other disorders. Consistent with this model and the deviance proneness model described above are the recent findings from our lab showing that poor response inhibition, i.e. the inability to inhibit a prepotent response particularly when engaged in goal-directed behaviour as measured by the STOP task [168], partially mediates the association between impulsivity and externalising behaviours, including substance misuse and conduct disorder symptoms [153]. These results indicate that the link between impulsivity and substance misuse is, at least in part, explained by a deficit in response inhibition that makes impulsive individuals more prone to engage in externalising behaviour in general.

Supporting the notion of a common genetic liability for deviant or externalising behaviours are findings showing common genetic liability for conduct disorder, alcoholism and drug use [169, 170], conduct disorder, alcoholism and behavioural undercontrol [171, 172], as well as for the association between early measures of social deviance and later externalising disorders and substance misuse [173, 174]. Although it seems likely that over 100 genetic variants are implicated in externalising and substance use behaviours, support for this model has also been gained from molecular genetic studies, with some studies suggesting that a significant portion of the genetic contribution to early onset problem drinking and other drug use is mediated by personality [175, 176]. For example, while separate studies on substance misuse and conduct problems have both shown that the serotonin transporter (5HTT) and the low variant of the MAOA is implicated in substance use disorders and conduct disorder, it is particularly interesting that both these genes have also been associated with the personality trait of impulsivity [177, 178] and, in the case of MAOA, with neurocognitive measures of disinhibition [177, 179]. The serotonin transporter polymorphism (5-HTTLPR) has been shown to be associated with personality—both to neuroticism [180] and impulsivity [178]—and substance use [181, 182]. In addition, the D4 dopamine receptor (DRD4) has been shown to be associated with disinhibited personality [183] and substance misuse [60, 176, 184]. In line with the psychological dysregulation theory, these findings suggest the possibility that impulsivity/disinhibition is a common endophenotype shared by substance misuse and other problem behaviours. Supporting this notion also are studies showing that the DRD2 [185, 186] polymorphism is associated with neuro-cognitive and self-report measures of impulsivity, as well as substance use disorders [187–189].

A Four Factor Model of Personality Vulnerability to Substance Misuse

The development of substance misuse appears to be multi-determined and multiple risk factors for substance misuse have been identified, such as age of onset, genes, individual differences in sensitivity to the reinforcing effects of substances, the presence of deviant peers, as well as conduct and emotional problems. It is also clear that some young people, sometimes subjected to the same general risk factors, go on to experience substance abuse and dependence and some do not. Research seems to suggest that psychological factors such as personality traits and cognitive factors play an important role. Indeed, the cross-sectional and prospective studies reviewed above have shown that personality traits represent relevant

variables in the onset of substance misuse as well as in the development of substance use disorders and to some extent to the psychological disorders that co-occur with them. Recent findings further suggest that these personality traits might also be related to substance misuse through different motivational processes, and may even be associated with different patterns of substance use and misuse. For example, while findings support that sensation seeking seems to be associated with the initiation of substance use behaviours as well substance misuse through the mediation of reward sensitivity and the positive reinforcing effects of substances, anxiety sensitivity is associated with substance misuse through its association with the anxiolytic or stress dampening effects of substances. On the other hand, the findings seem to suggest that hopelessness is associated with substance misuse and mood disorders either through a motivation to cope with high levels of negative affect, or, alternatively, manage low levels of positive affect. Notably, certain personality traits could make individuals more likely to be exposed to other risk factors for substance misuse. That is, traits such as impulsivity or sensation seeking may make an individual more likely to interact with and be influenced by deviant peers, which in turn could place this individual at higher risk for initiating substance use or developing substance use disorders. Furthermore, although the aetiological models described in this chapter are theoretically distinct, they can overlap and several of these models can be of explanatory value not only in different cases of substance misuse, but also within an individual cluster or type of substance misuser. In this way, an individual with increased levels of disinhibition or impulsivity, for example, could have a liability towards substance misuse because of a genetic predisposition which implies deficits in motor inhibition and increased emotional reactivity, as posited by the psychological dysregulation theory, but also, in line with the deviant proneness model, because their socialisation processes could set them on a path for social deviance. Summarising the findings reviewed in this chapter and expanding on models proposed by Conrod et al. [7], Phil and Peterson [47] and Woicik et al. [67], Fig. 4.1 displays a tentative model of four distinct personality pathways to substance misuse, as well as other disorders often comorbid with substance misuse. Included in this figure are the distinct motivation profiles and/or underlying mechanisms that help explain the different ways in which these personality traits are related to substance misuse and psychopathology, which in turn, support one or more aetiologic models of substance misuse.

Figure 4.1 shows four personality traits—impulsivity, sensation seeking, hopelessness and anxiety sensitivity—organised along the two broad dimensions of inhibition/neuroticism and disinhibition. Each of these traits is represented by cognitive and motivational tendencies that render individuals sensitive to different reinforcing effects of drugs of abuse, which can then lead to substance misuse. Specifically, the trait of impulsivity,

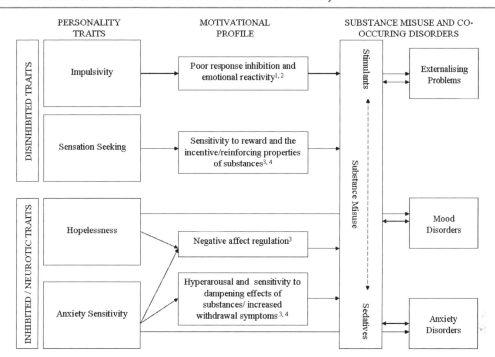

Fig. 4.1 A tentative model of four distinct personality pathways to substance misuse and comorbid psychopathology. Note: [1]supporting a deviance proneness model; [2]supporting a psychological dysregulation model; [3]supporting an affect regulation model; [4]supporting a psychopharmacological vulnerability model. This figure shows the personality traits of impulsivity, sensation seeking, hopelessness and anxiety sensitivity, organised along the two broad dimensions of neuroticism and disinhibition. Each of these traits is represented by cognitive and motivational tendencies that translate into different reinforcing effects of drugs of abuse, leading to substance misuse. That is, the trait of *impulsivity* is associated with a deficit in response inhibition, which in the context of substances that produce potent psycho-stimulant reward, individuals high on this trait are not protected by intact response inhibition system and more easily develop uncontrolled self-administration. Individuals high in *sensation seeking*, on the other hand, show a specific sensitivity to reward, including drug-induced reward, lowering the threshold for experiencing reward/psycho-stimulation from substances or developing drug-taking patterns to enhance psycho-stimulation (e.g. binging). Individuals high in *hopelessness* use substances to manage or reduced their negative affect, while individuals high in *anxiety sensitivity* use and misuse substances because of their sensitivity to the arousal dampening effects that are negatively reinforcing to these individuals. Finally, these personality traits are also associated with specific psychopathological disorders, which can lead directly to or further exacerbate substance misuse

while not associated uniquely with a sensitivity to reward, is associated with a deficit in response inhibition. This means that in the context of substances that produce potent psycho-stimulant reward, individuals high in impulsivity are not protected by an intact response inhibition system and more easily develop compulsive (or uncontrolled) self-administration. As reviewed earlier, this would be consistent with the psychological dysregulation model of substance use, which would identify these deficits in response inhibition and emotional regulation as risk factors for externalising behaviour in general. Individuals high in sensation seeking, on the other hand, show a specific sensitivity to reward, including drug-induced reward, lowering the threshold for experiencing reward/psycho-stimulation from substances not typically experienced as psycho-stimulants (e.g. alcohol) or developing drug-taking patterns to enhance psycho-stimulation (e.g. binge drinking). This personality path to substance misuse is therefore consistent with the psychopharmacological vulnerability model of addiction.

Under the inhibited domain, Fig. 4.1 shows that individuals high in hopelessness use substances in order to manage or reduce their negative affect, while individuals high in anxiety sensitivity use and misuse substances because of their sensitivity to the arousal dampening effects that are very negatively reinforcing to those who fear them. Both these personality paths to substance misuse could be considered to support the negative affect regulation model of addiction, with individuals using substances to regulate a negative affective state (i.e. negative mood in those high in hopelessness, and feelings of anxiety in those high in anxiety sensitivity). However, because those high in anxiety sensitivity have been shown to experience increased sensitivity to the dampening effects of substances, as well as increased withdrawal symptoms, this personality path to substance misuse is also consistent with the psychopharmacological vulnerability model of addiction. Finally, Fig. 4.1 shows that besides being associated with substance misuse, these personality traits are also associated with specific psychopathological symptoms or disorders (e.g. impulsivity with externalising problems such as antisocial behaviour), which have not only been identified as risk factors for developing substance use problems in their own right, but can also further exacerbate the substance misuse that is already present in the individuals high on these traits.

It is clear from the evidence reviewed in this chapter that personality traits play an integral part in the complex puzzle of biological, environmental and psychological factors involved in the onset and development of substance misuse, identifying them, in turn, as key targets for prevention and intervention efforts. Particularly in the case of the prevention of substance misuse, most approaches are universal in nature, with strategies targeting drinking and drug use behaviours directly. However, findings from the number of studies reviewed in this chapter (e.g. Conrod et al. [7, 14]; Smith et al. [29]) seem to indicate that interventions would logically want to target liability factors rather than behaviour. Prevention and treatment models that target liability like impulsive personality or anxiety sensitivity, rather than behaviour are relevant to those engaging not only in substance use behaviours but also in other maladaptive behaviours related to often co-occurring disorders, such as conduct disorder in the case of impulsivity, and anxiety disorders in the case of anxiety sensitivity. Notably, a personality-targeted approach has already been shown to be effective in the prevention/intervention of not only substance misuse in adolescence [14, 56, 68] and adults [190], but also of other personality-specific emotional and behavioural problems in youth [118]. That is, compared to personality-matched controls, adolescents who received the intervention targeting impulsivity were less likely to engage in antisocial behaviours such as shoplifting, while those who received the intervention targeting hopelessness reported reduced depression scores 6 months post-intervention. In this vein, it is clear that a personality-targeted approach in the prevention or early intervention of substance misuse, which focuses on specific personality risk factors and differential motivations for engaging in these behaviours, will improve current efforts in tackling both substance misuse and other disorders so prevalent in substance misusing populations.

References

1. Carver CS, Sutton SK, Scheier MF. Action, emotion, and personality: emerging conceptual integration. Person Social Psychol Bull. 2000;26(6):741–51.
2. Conway KP, et al. Personality, drug of choice, and comorbid psychopathology among substance abusers. Drug Alcohol Depend. 2002;65(3):225–34.
3. Matthews G, Gilliland K. The personality theories of H.J. Eysenck and J. A. Gray: a comparative review. Personal Individ Differ. 1999;26(4):583–626.
4. Sutton SK, Davidson RJ. Prefrontal brain asymmetry: a biological substrate of the behavioral approach and inhibition systems. Psychol Sci. 1997;8(3):204–10.
5. McGue M, et al. Personality and substance use disorders: I. Effects of gender and alcoholism subtype. Alcohol Clin Exp Res. 1997; 21(3):513–20.
6. Trull TJ, Waudby CJ, Sher KJ. Alcohol, tobacco, and drug use disorders and personality disorder symptoms. Exp Clin Psychopharmacol. 2004;12(1):65–75.
7. Conrod PJ, et al. Validation of a system of classifying female substance abusers on the basis of personality and motivational risk factors for substance abuse. Psychol Addict Behav. 2000;14(3):243–56.
8. Eysenck HJ. Normality-abnormality and the three-factor model of personality. In: Strack S, Lorr M, editors. Differentiating normal and abnormal personality. New York: Springer; 1994. p. 3–25.
9. Hill SY, et al. Factors predicting the onset of adolescent drinking in families at high risk for developing alcoholism. Biol Psychiatry. 2000;48(4):265–75.
10. Sher KJ, et al. Personality and alcoholism: issues, methods, and etiological processes. In: Leonard KE, Blane HT, editors. Theories of drinking and alcoholism. New York: Guilford; 1999. p. 54–105.
11. Zuckerman M. Good and bad humors: biochemical bases of personality and its disorders. Psychol Sci. 1995;6:325–32.
12. Jackson KM, Sher KJ. Alcohol use disorders and psychological distress: a prospective state-trait analysis. J Abnorm Psychol. 2003;112(4):599–613.
13. McGue M, Slutske W, Iacono WG. Personality and substance use disorders: II. Alcoholism versus drug use disorders. J Consult Clin Psychol. 1999;67(3):394–404.
14. Conrod PJ, et al. Efficacy of cognitive-behavioral interventions targeting personality risk factors for youth alcohol misuse. J Clin Child Adolesc Psychol. 2006;35(4):550–63.
15. Littlefield AK, Sher KJ, Wood PK. Is "maturing out" of problematic alcohol involvement related to personality change? J Abnorm Psychol. 2009;118(2):360–74.
16. McNally RJ. Anxiety sensitivity is distinguishable from trait anxiety. In: Rapee RM, editor. Current controversies in anxiety disorders. New York: Guilford; 1996. p. 214–27.
17. Schmidt NB, Buckner JD, Keough ME. Anxiety sensitivity as a prospective predictor of alcohol use disorders. Behav Modif. 2007;31(2):202–19.
18. Stewart SH, et al. Anxiety sensitivity and self-reported reasons for drug use. J Subst Abuse. 1997;9:223–40.
19. De Win MML, et al. A prospective cohort study on sustained effects of low-dose ecstasy use on the brain in new ecstasy users. Neuropsychopharmacology. 2007;32(2):458–70.
20. Evenden JL. Varieties of impulsivity. Psychopharmacology. 1999;146:348–61.
21. Iacono WG, Malone SM, McGue M. Behavioral disinhibition and the development of early-onset addiction: common and specific influences. Annu Rev Clin Psychol. 2008;4:325–48.
22. Krueger RF, et al. Etiologic connections among substance dependence, antisocial behavior, and personality: modeling the externalizing spectrum. J Abnorm Psychol. 2002;111:411–24.
23. Krueger RF, et al. Linking antisocial behavior, substance use, and personality: an integrative quantitative model of the adult externalizing spectrum. J Abnorm Psychol. 2007;116:645–66.
24. Krueger RF, et al. Externalizing psychopathology in adulthood: a dimensional-spectrum conceptualization and its implications for DSM-V. J Abnorm Psychol. 2005;114:537–50.
25. Depue RA, Collins PF. Neurobiology of the structure of personality: dopamine, facilitation of incentive motivation, and extraversion. Behav Brain Sci. 1999;22(3):491–517. discussion 518–69.
26. Whiteside SP, Lynam DR. The five factor model and impulsivity: using a structural model of personality to understand impulsivity. Personal Individ Differ. 2001;20:669–89.
27. Eysenck SBG, et al. Age norms for impulsiveness, venturesomeness and empathy in adults. Personal Individ Differ. 1985;6(5):613–9.
28. Patton JH, Stanford MS, Barratt ES. Factor structure of the Barratt impulsiveness scale. J Clin Psychol. 1995;51(6):768–74.
29. Smith GT, et al. On the validity and utility of discriminating among impulsivity-like traits. Assessment. 2007;14:155–70.

30. Lane SD, et al. Relationships among laboratory and psychometric measures of impulsivity: implications in substance abuse and dependence. Addict Disord Their Treat. 2003;2:33–40.

31. Olson S, Schilling E, Bates J. Measurement of impulsivity: construct coherence, longitudinal stability, and relationship with externalizing problems in middle childhood and adolescence. J Abnorm Child Psychol. 1999;27:151–65.

32. Reynolds B, et al. Dimensions of impulsive behavior: personality and behavioral measures. Personal Individ Differ. 2006;40:305–15.

33. Reynolds B, Penfold RB, Patak M. Dimensions of impulsive behavior in adolescents: laboratory behavioral assessments. Exp Clin Psychopharmacol. 2008;16:124–31.

34. Baumeister RF, Vohs KD. Handbook of self-regulation: research, Theory, and applications. New York: Guilford; 2004.

35. Schalling D. Psychopathy-related personlaity variables and the psychophysiology of socialization. In: Hare RD, Schalling D, editors. Psychopathic behaviour: approaches to research. New York: Wiley; 1978. p. 85–105.

36. Arnett J. Sensation seeking: a new conceptualization and a new scale. Personal Individ Differ. 1994;16(2):289–96.

37. Zuckerman M. Sensation seeking: beyond optimal level of arousal. Hillsdale, NJ: Erlbaum; 1979.

38. Masse LC, Tremblay RE. Behavior of boys in kindergarten and the onset of substance use during adolescence. Arch Gen Psychiatry. 1997;54(1):62–8.

39. Gerevich J, Bácskai E, Rózsa S. Usefulness of the temperament and character inventory among alcohol and drug using patients. Psychiatria Hung. 2002;17:182–92.

40. Dughiero G, Schifano F, Forza G. Personality dimensions and psychopathological profiles of Ecstasy users. Hum Psychopharmacol. 2001;16(8):635–9.

41. Le Bon O, et al. Personality profile and drug of choice; a multivariate analysis using Cloninger's TCI on heroin addicts, alcoholics, and a random population group. Drug Alcohol Depend. 2004; 73(2):175–82.

42. Agrawal A, et al. A twin study of early cannabis use and subsequent use and abuse/dependence of other illicit drugs. Psychol Med. 2004;34(7):1227–37.

43. Liraud F, Verdoux H. Which temperamental characteristics are associated with substance use in subjects with psychotic and mood disorders? Psychiatry Res. 2000;93(1):63–72.

44. Sher KJ, Trull TJ. Personality and disinhibitory psychopathology: alcoholism and antisocial personality disorder. J Abnorm Psychol. 1994;103(1):92–102.

45. Loukas A, et al. Parental alcoholism and co-occurring antisocial behavior: prospective relationships to externalizing behavior problems in their young sons. J Abnorm Child Psychol. 2001;29(2): 91–106.

46. Loukas A, et al. Developmental trajectories of disruptive behavior problems among sons of alcoholics: effects of parent psychopathology, family conflict, and child undercontrol. J Abnorm Psychol. 2003;112:119–31.

47. Pihl RO, Peterson JB. Alcoholism: the role of different motivational systems. J Psychiatry Neurosci. 1995;20(5):372–96.

48. Conrod PJ, Petersen JB, Pihl RO. Disinhibited personality and sensitivity to alcohol reinforcement: independent correlates of drinking behavior in sons of alcoholics. Alcohol Clin Exp Res. 1997;21(7):1320–32.

49. Eysenck HJ, Eysenck SBG. Manual of the Eysenck personality questionnaire. London: Hodder & Sthoughton; 1975.

50. Sher KJ, Bartholow BD, Wood MD. Personality and substance use disorders: a prospective study. J Consult Clin Psychol. 2000;68:818–29.

51. Cloninger CR, Sigvardsson S, Bohman M. Childhood personality predicts alcohol abuse in young adults. Alcohol Clin Exp Res. 1988;12(4):494–505.

52. Caspi A, et al. Behavioral observations at age 3 years predict adult psychiatric disorders. Longitudinal evidence from a birth cohort. Arch Gen Psychiatry. 1996;53(11):1033–9.

53. Krueger RF, Caspi A, Moffitt TE. Epidemiological personology: the unifying role of personality in population-based research on problem behaviors. J Personal. 2000;68:967–98.

54. Chassin L, Fora DB, King KM. Trajectories of alcohol and drug use and dependence from adolescence to adulthood: the effects of familial alcoholism and personality. J Abnorm Psychol. 2004; 113(4):483–98.

55. Elkins IJ, et al. Personality traits and the development of nicotine, alcohol, and illicit drug disorders: prospective links from adolescence to young adulthood. J Abnorm Psychol. 2006;115:26–39.

56. Conrod PJ, Castellanos-Ryan N, Strang J. Brief, personality-targeted coping skills interventions and survival as a non-drug user over a 2-year period during adolescence. Arch Gen Psychiatry. 2010;67:85–93.

57. Ersche KD, et al. Profile of executive and memory function associated with amphetamine and opiate dependence. Neuropsychopharmacology. 2006;31:1036–47.

58. Verdejo A, et al. Neuropsychological functioning in methadone maintenance patients versus abstinent heroin abusers. Drug Alcohol Depend. 2005;78(3):283–8.

59. Grau E, Ortet G. Personality traits and alcohol consumption in a sample of non-alcoholic women. Personal Individ Differ. 1999;27(6):1057–66.

60. Zuckerman M, Kuhlman DM. Personality and risk-taking: common biosocial factors. J Personal. 2000;68:999–1029.

61. Cook M, et al. Personality correlates of alcohol consumption. Personal Individ Differ. 1998;24(5):641–7.

62. Flory K, et al. The relations among personality, symptoms of alcohol and marijuana abuse, and symptoms of comorbid psychopathology: results from a community sample. Exp Clin Psychopharmacol. 2002;10(4):425–34.

63. Comeau N, Stewart SH, Loba P. The relations of trait anxiety, anxiety sensitivity, and sensation seeking to adolescents' motivations for alcohol, cigarette, and marijuana use. Addict Behav. 2001;26(6):803–25.

64. Cooper ML, Agocha VB, Sheldon MS. A motivational perspective on risky behaviors: the role of personality and affect regulatory processes. J Personal. 2000;68:1059–88.

65. Gerra G, et al. Substance use among high-school students: relationships with temperament, personality traits, and parental care perception. Subst Use Misuse. 2004;39(2):345–67.

66. Wills TA, Sandy JM, Yaeger A. Temperament and adolescent substance use: an epigenetic approach to risk and protection. J Personal. 2000;68:1127–51.

67. Woicik PA, et al. The substance use risk profile scale: a scale measuring traits linked to reinforcement-specific substance use profiles. Addict Behav. 2009;34:1042–55.

68. Conrod PJ, Castellanos N, Mackie C. Personality-targeted interventions delay the growth of adolescent drinking and binge drinking. J Child Psychol Psychiatry. 2008;49:181–90.

69. Krank M, et al. Structural, concurrent, and predictive validity of the substance use risk profile scale in early adolescence. Addict Behav. 2011;36(1–2):37–46.

70. Kilbey MM, Downey K, Breslau N. Predicting the emergence and persistence of alcohol dependence in young adults: the role of expectancy and other risk factors. Exp Clin Psychopharmacol. 1998;6(2):149–56.

71. Wennberg P, Bohman M. Childhood temperament and adult alcohol habits: a prospective longitudinal study from age 4 to age 36. Addict Behav. 2002;27(1):63–74.

72. Cooper ML, et al. Drinking to regulate positive and negative emotions: a motivational model of alcohol use. J Pers Soc Psychol. 1995;69(5):990–1005.

73. Simons J, et al. An affective-motivational model of marijuana and alcohol problems among college students. J Addict Behav. 2005;19:326–34.

74. Barlow DH. Unraveling the mysteries of anxiety and its disorders from the perspective of emotion theory. Am Psychol. 2000;55(11): 1247–63.

75. Clark LA, Watson D. Tripartite model of anxiety and depression: psychometric evidence and taxonomic implications. J Abnorm Psychol. 1991;100(3):316–36.

76. Zimmermann P, et al. Primary anxiety disorders and the development of subsequent alcohol use disorders: a 4-year community study of adolescents and young adults. Psychol Med. 2003;33(7): 1211–22.

77. Sutherland I. The development and application of a questionnaire to assess the changing personalities of substance addicts during the first year of recovery. J Clin Psychol. 1997;53(3):253–62.

78. Kushner, M.G.: Discussant's remarks in the symposium on "New research findings on anxiety sensitivity and risk for substance use and abuse". In: 34th annual meeting of the association for advancement of behavior therapy. 2000. New Orleans, LA.

79. Stewart SH, Samoluk SB, MacDonald AB. Anxiety sensitivity and substance use and abuse. In: Taylor S, editor. Anxiety sensitivity: theory, research, and treatment of the fear of anxiety. Mahwah, NJ: Erlbaum; 1999. p. 297–319.

80. Martin CS, et al. Gender differences and similarities in the personality correlates of adolescent alcohol problems. Psychol Addict Behav. 2000;14(2):121–33.

81. Kassel JD, Stroud LR, Paronis CA. Smoking, stress, and negative affect: correlation, causation, and context across stages of smoking. Psychol Bull. 2003;129(2):270–304.

82. Piasecki TM, et al. Listening to nicotine: negative affect and the smoking withdrawal conundrum. Psychol Sci. 1997;8(3):184–9.

83. Breslau N, Kilbey MM, Andreski P. Nicotine withdrawal symptoms and psychiatric disorders: findings from an epidemiologic study of young adults. Am J Psychiatry. 1992;149(4):464–9.

84. Anda RF, et al. Depression and the dynamics of smoking. A national perspective. JAMA. 1990;264(12):1541–5.

85. Sher KJ. Children of alcoholics: a critical appraisal of theory and research. Chicago: University of Chicago Press; 1991.

86. Hussong AM, et al. Specifying the relations between affect and heavy alcohol use among young adults. J Abnorm Psychol. 2001; 110(3):449–61.

87. Cloninger CR, et al. Personality antecedents of alcoholism in a national area probability sample. Eur Arch Psychiatry Clin Neurosci. 1995;245(4–5):239–44.

88. Earleywine M, et al. Factor structure and correlates of the Tridimensional Personality Questionnaire. J Stud Alcohol. 1992; 53(3):233–8.

89. Elkins IJ, et al. The effect of parental alcohol and drug disorders on adolescent personality. Am J Psychiatry. 2004;161(4):670–6.

90. Wills TA, Sandy JM, Shinar O. Cloninger's constructs related to substance use level and problems in late adolescence: a mediational model based on self-control and coping motives. Exp Clin Psychopharmacol. 1999;7(2):122–34.

91. Costa Jr PT, McCrae RR. Normal personality assessment in clinical practice: the NEO personality inventory. Psychol Assess. 1992; 4(1):5–13.

92. Ilhan IO, Demirbas H, Dogan YB. Psychosocial factors in alcohol use-related problems of working youth. Subst Use Misuse. 2007;42(10):1537–44.

93. Bolland JM. Hopelessness and risk behaviour among adolescents living in high-poverty inner-city neighbourhoods. J Adolesc. 2003;26(2):145–58.

94. Bolland JM, et al. Development and risk behavior among African American, Caucasian, and mixed-race adolescents living in high poverty inner-city neighborhoods. Am J Community Psychol. 2007;40(3–4):230–49.

95. Mackie C, Castellanos-Ryan N, Conrod PJ. Personality moderates the longitudinal relationship between psychological symptoms and alcohol use in adolescents. Alcohol Clin Exp Res. 2011;35(4): 703–16.

96. Grant VV, et al. Psychometric evaluation of the five-factor modified Drinking Motives Questionnaire–revised in undergraduates. Addict Behav. 2007;32(11):2611–32.

97. Jaffee WB, D'Zurilla TJ. Personality, problem solving, and adolescent substance use. Behav Ther. 2009;40(1):93–101.

98. Reiss S, et al. Anxiety sensitivity, anxiety frequency and the prediction of fearfulness. Behav Res Ther. 1986;24(1):1–8.

99. Stewart SH, Kushner MG. Introduction to the special issue on "Anxiety sensitivity and addictive behaviors". Addict Behav. 2001;26(6):775–85.

100. Stewart SH, Finn PR, Pihl RO. A dose-response study of the effects of alcohol on the perceptions of pain and discomfort due to electric shock in men at high familial-genetic risk for alcoholism. Psychopharmacology (Berl). 1995;119(3):261–7.

101. Stewart SH, Zvolensky MJ, Eifert GH. The relations of anxiety sensitivity, experiential avoidance, and alexithymic coping to young adults' motivations for drinking. Behav Modif. 2002; 26(2):274–96.

102. Conrod PJ, Pihl RO, Vassileva J. Differential sensitivity to alcohol reinforcement in groups of men at risk for distinct alcoholism subtypes. Alcohol Clin Exp Res. 1998;22(3):585–97.

103. Lejuez CW, et al. The association between heroin use and anxiety sensitivity among inner-city individuals in residential drug use treatment. Behav Res Ther. 2006;44(5):667–77.

104. Zvolensky MJ, et al. Anxiety sensitivity and anxiety and depressive symptoms in the prediction of early smoking lapse and relapse during smoking cessation treatment. Nicotine Tob Res. 2009; 11(3):323–31.

105. Zvolensky MJ, Schmidt NB, Stewart SH. Panic disorder and smoking. Clin Psychol Sci Pract. 2003;10(1):29–51.

106. Forsyth JP, Parker JD, Finlay CG. Anxiety sensitivity, controllability, and experiential avoidance and their relation to drug of choice and addiction severity in a residential sample of substance-abusing veterans. Addict Behav. 2003;28(5):851–70.

107. Kushner MG, et al. Anxiety mediates the association between anxiety sensitivity and coping-related drinking motives in alcoholism treatment patients. Addict Behav. 2001;26(6):869–85.

108. MacDonald AB, et al. Effects of alcohol on the response to hyperventilation of participants high and low in anxiety sensitivity. Alcohol Clin Exp Res. 2000;24(11):1656–65.

109. Stewart, S.H., et al.: Effects of lorazepam and anxiety sensitivity on response to hyperventilation challenge. In: 3rd World Congress of Behavioral and Cognitive Therapies. 2001. Vancouver, BC.

110. Zvolensky MJ, et al. Anxiety sensitivity: association with intensity of retrospectively-rated smoking-related withdrawal symptoms and motivation to quit. Cogn Behav Ther. 2004;33(3):114–25.

111. Brown RA, et al. Anxiety sensitivity: relationship to negative affect smoking and smoking cessation in smokers with past major depressive disorder. Addict Behav. 2001;26(6):887–99.

112. Zvolensky MJ, et al. Anxiety sensitivity and abstinence duration to smoking. J Mental Health. 2006;15:659–70.

113. Reiss S. Expectancy model of fear, anxiety, and panic. Clin Psychol Rev. 1991;11(2):141–53.

114. MacDonald AB, et al. The roles of alcohol and alcohol expectancy in the dampening of responses to hyperventilation among high anxiety sensitive young adults. Addict Behav. 2001;26(6): 841–67.

115. Rohde P, Lewinsohn PM, Seeley JR. Psychiatric comorbidity with problematic alcohol use in high school students. J Am Acad Child Adolesc Psychiatry. 1996;35(1):101–9.

116. Deas-Nesmith D, Brady KT, Campbell S. Comorbid substance use and anxiety disorders in adolescents. J Psychopathol Behav Assess. 1998;20(2):139–48.

117. Pulkkinen L, Pitkanen T. A prospective study of the precursors to problem drinking in young adulthood. J Stud Alcohol. 1994;55(5):578–87.

118. Castellanos N, Conrod P. Brief interventions targeting personality risk factors for adolescent substance misuse reduce depression, panic and risk-taking behaviours. J Mental Health. 2006;15(6):645–58.

119. Zvolensky MJ, et al. Affective style among smokers: understanding anxiety sensitivity, emotional reactivity, and distress tolerance using biological challenge. Addict Behav. 2001;26(6):901–15.

120. Stewart SH, et al. Posttraumatic stress disorder symptoms and situation-specific drinking in women substance abusers. Alcohol Treat Q. 2000;18(3):31–47.

121. Norton GR. Substance use/abuse and anxiety sensitivity: what are the relationships? Addict Behav. 2001;26(6):935–46.

122. Sher KJ, Grekin ER, Williams NA. The development of alcohol use disorders. Annu Rev Clin Psychol. 2005;1:493–523.

123. Sher KJ, Slutske WS. Disorders of impulse control. In: Stricker G, Widiger TA, editors. Handbook of psychology. New York: Wiley; 2003. p. 195–228.

124. Tarter R, et al. Neurobehavioral disinhibition in childhood predicts early age at onset of substance use disorder. Am J Psychiatry. 2003;160:1078–85.

125. Tarter R, Vanyukov M, Giancola P. Etiology of early age onset substance use disorder: a maturational perspective. Dev Psychopathol. 1999;11:657–83.

126. Clark DB, Thatcher DL, Tapert SF. Alcohol, psychological dysregulation, and adolescent brain development. Alcohol Clin Exp Res. 2008;32:375–85.

127. Clark DB, Winters KC. Measuring risks and outcomes in substance use disorders prevention research. J Consult Clin Psychol. 2002;70:1207–23.

128. Thatcher DL, Clark DB. Adolescents at risk for substance use disorders: role of psychological dysregulation, endophenotypes, and environmental influences. Alcohol Res Health. 2008;31(2):168–76.

129. Cooper ML, et al. Development and validation of a three-dimensional measure of drinking motives. Psychol Assess. 1992;4(2):123–32.

130. Koob G. Drug addiction. Neurobiol Dis. 2000;7(5):543–5.

131. Gianoulakis C. Implications of endogenous opioids and dopamine in alcoholism: human and basic science studies. Alcohol Alcohol Suppl. 1996;1:33–42.

132. Finn PR, et al. Early-onset alcoholism with conduct disorder: go/no go learning deficits, working memory capacity, and personality. Alcohol Clin Exp Res. 2002;26:186–206.

133. Greeley J, Oei T. Alcohol and tension reduction. In: Leonard KE, Blane HT, editors. Psychological theories of drinking and alcoholism. New York: Guilford; 1999. p. 14–53.

134. Sher KJ. Stress response dampening. In: Blane HT, Leonard KE, editors. Psychological theories of drinking and alcoholism. New York: Guilford; 1987. p. 227–71.

135. Henderson MJ, Galen LW. A classification of substance-dependent men on temperament and severity variables. Addict Behav. 2003;28(4):741–60.

136. O'Connor RM, Farrow S, Colder CR. Clarifying the anxiety sensitivity and alcohol use relation: considering alcohol expectancies as moderators. J Stud Alcohol Drugs. 2008;69(5):765–72.

137. Heath AC, Martin NG. Genetic differences in psychomotor performance decrement after alcohol: a multivariate analysis. J Stud Alcohol. 1992;53(3):262–71.

138. Schuckit MA. Alcoholism and genetics: possible biological mediators. Biol Psychiatry. 1980;15(3):437–47.

139. Schuckit MA. Subjective responses to alcohol in sons of alcoholics and control subjects. Arch Gen Psychiatry. 1984;41(9):879–84.

140. Morzorati SL, et al. Self-reported subjective perception of intoxication reflects family history of alcoholism when breath alcohol levels are constant. Alcohol Clin Exp Res. 2002;26(8):1299–306.

141. Schuckit MA, Smith TL. An 8-year follow-up of 450 sons of alcoholic and control subjects. Arch Gen Psychiatry. 1996;53(3):202–10.

142. Peterson JB, et al. Ethanol-induced change in cardiac and endogenous opiate function and risk for alcoholism. Alcohol Clin Exp Res. 1996;20:1542–52.

143. Gabbay FH. Family history of alcoholism and response to amphetamine: sex differences in the effect of risk. Alcohol Clin Exp Res. 2005;29:773–80.

144. Holdstock L, King AC, de Wit H. Subjective and objective responses to ethanol in moderate/heavy and light social drinkers. Alcohol Clin Exp Res. 2000;24(6):789–94.

145. King AC, et al. Biphasic alcohol response differs in heavy versus light drinkers. Alcohol Clin Exp Res. 2002;26(6):827–35.

146. Erblich J, Earleywine M. Behavioral undercontrol and subjective stimulant and sedative effects of alcohol intoxication: independent predictors of drinking habits? Alcohol Clin Exp Res. 2003;27:44–50.

147. Newlin DB, Thomson JB. Alcohol challenge with sons of alcoholics: a critical review and analysis. Psychol Bull. 1990;108(3):383–402.

148. Brunelle C, et al. Heightened heart rate response to alcohol intoxication is associated with a reward-seeking personality profile. Alcohol Clin Exp Res. 2004;28:394–401.

149. Stewart SH, Pihl RO. Effects of alcohol administration on psychophysiological and subjective-emotional responses to aversive stimulation in anxiety-sensitive women. Psychol Addict Behav. 1994;8(1):29–42.

150. Leyton M, et al. Amphetamine-induced increases in extracellular dopamine, drug wanting, and novelty seeking: a PET/[11C]raclopride study in healthy men. Neuropsychopharmacology. 2002;27:1027–35.

151. Coventry KR, Constable B. Physiological arousal and sensation-seeking in female fruit machine gamblers. Addiction. 1999;94(3):425–30.

152. McDaniel SR, Zuckerman M. The relationship of impulsive sensation seeking and gender to interest and participation in gambling activities. Personal Individ Differ. 2003;35(6):1385–400.

153. Castellanos-Ryan N, Rubia K, Conrod PJ. Response inhibition and reward response bias mediate the predictive relationships between impulsivity and sensation seeking and common and unique variance in conduct disorder and substance misuse. Alcohol Clin Exp Res. 2011;35(1):140–55.

154. Leventhal AM, et al. Dimensions of depressive symptoms and smoking cessation. Nicotine Tob Res. 2008;10(3):507–17.

155. Finn PR, Pihl RO. Men at high risk for alcoholism: the effect of alcohol on cardiovascular response to unavoidable shock. J Abnorm Psychol. 1987;96(3):230–6.

156. Finn PR, Zeitouni NC, Pihl RO. Effects of alcohol on psychophysiological hyperreactivity to nonaversive and aversive stimuli in men at high risk for alcoholism. J Abnorm Psychol. 1990;99(1):79–85.

157. Patock-Peckham JA, et al. A social learning perspective: a model of parenting styles, self-regulation, perceived drinking control, and alcohol use and problems. Alcohol Clin Exp Res. 2001;25(9):1284–92.

158. Zucker RA, Fitzgerald HE, Moses HD. Emergence of alcohol problems and the several alcoholisms: a developmental perspective on etiologic theory and life course trajectory. In: Cicchetti D, Cohen DJ, editors. Developmental psychopathology. New York: Wiley; 1995. p. 677–711.

159. Jessor R, Jessor SL. Problem behavior and psychosocial development: a longitudinal study of youth. New York: Academic; 1977.

160. Windle M, Davies PT. Depression and heavy alcohol use among adolescents: concurrent and prospective relations. Dev Psychopathol. 1999;11(4):823–44.

161. Jessor R, Donovan JE, Costa FM. Beyond adolescence: problem behavior and young adult development. New York: Cambridge University Press; 1991.

162. Petraitis J, Flay BR, Miller TQ. Reviewing theories of adolescent substance use: organizing pieces in the puzzle. Psychol Bull. 1995;117(1):67–86.

163. Tarter RE, et al. Temperament deviation and risk for alcoholism. Alcohol Clin Exp Res. 1990;14(3):380–2.

164. Castellanos-Ryan N, Conrod P. Personality correlates of the common and unique variance across conduct disorder and substance misuse symptoms in adolescence. J Abnorm Child Psychol. 2011; 39(4):563–76.

165. Khan AA, et al. Personality and comorbidity of common psychiatric disorders. Br J Psychiatry. 2005;186:190–6.

166. Tarter R, et al. Etiology of early age onset substance use disorder: a maturational perspective. Dev Psychopathol. 1999;11(4):657–83.

167. Clark DB, et al. Childhood risk categories for adolescent substance involvement: a general liability typology. Drug Alcohol Depend. 2005;77(1):13–21.

168. Logan GD. On the ability to inhibit thought and action: a users' guide to the stop signal paradigm. In: Dagenbach D, Carr TH, editors. Inhibitory processes in attention, memory, and language. San Diego: Academic Press; 1994. p. 189–239.

169. Button TM, et al. Examination of the causes of covariation between conduct disorder symptoms and vulnerability to drug dependence. Twin Res Hum Genet. 2006;9(1):38–45.

170. Button TMM, et al. The role of conduct disorder in explaining the comorbidity between alcohol and illicit drug dependence in adolescence. Drug Alcohol Depend. 2007;87:46–53.

171. Slutske WS, et al. Common genetic risk factors for conduct disorder and alcohol dependence. J Abnorm Psychol. 1998;107(3):363–74.

172. Slutske WS, et al. Personality and the genetic risk for alcohol dependence. J Abnorm Psychol. 2002;111(1):124–33.

173. McGue M, Iacono WG. The association of early adolescent problem behavior with adult psychopathology. Am J Psychiatry. 2005;162(6):1118–24.

174. McGue M, Iacono WG, Krueger R. The association of early adolescent problem behavior and adult psychopathology: a multivariate behavioral genetic perspective. Behav Genet. 2006;36(4):591–602.

175. McGue M, et al. Origins and consequences of age at first drink. II. Familial risk and heritability. Alcohol Clin Exp Res. 2001; 25:1166–73.

176. Laucht M, et al. Novelty seeking involved in mediating the association between the dopamine D4 receptor gene exon III polymorphism and heavy drinking in male adolescents: results from a high-risk community sample. Biol Psychiatry. 2007;61(1):87–92.

177. Manuck SB, et al. A regulatory polymorphism of the monoamine oxidase-A gene may be associated with variability in aggression, impulsivity, and central nervous system serotonergic responsivity. Psychiatry Res. 2000;95(1):9–23.

178. Twitchell G, et al. Serotonin transporter promoter polymorphism genotype is associated with behavioral disinhibition and negative affect in children of alcoholics. Alcohol Clin Exp Res. 2001;25: 953–9.

179. Meyer-Lindenberg A, et al. Neural mechanisms of genetic risk for impulsivity and violence in humans. Proc Natl Acad Sci USA. 2006;103(16):6269–74.

180. Caspi A, et al. Influence of life stress on depression: moderation by a polymorphism in the 5-HTT gene. Science. 2003;301(5631): 386–9.

181. Lichtermann D, et al. Support for allelic association of a polymorphic site in the promoter region of the serotonin transporter gene with risk for alcohol dependence. Am J Psychiatry. 2000; 157(12):2045–7.

182. Gerra G, et al. Association between low-activity serotonin transporter genotype and heroin dependence: behavioral and personality correlates. Am J Med Genet B Neuropsychiatr Genet. 2004; 126B(1):37–42.

183. Ebstein RP, et al. Dopamine D4 receptor (D4DR) exon III polymorphism associated with the human personality trait of novelty seeking. Nat Genet. 1996;12(1):78–80.

184. Laucht M, et al. Association of the DRD4 exon III polymorphism with smoking in fifteen-year-olds: a mediating role for novelty seeking? J Am Acad Child Adolesc Psychiatry. 2005;44(5): 477–84.

185. Berman SM, Noble EP. Reduced visuospatial performance in children with the D2 dopamine receptor A1 allele. Behav Genet. 1995;25(1):45–58.

186. Conner BT, et al. DRD2 genotypes and substance use in adolescent children of alcoholics. Drug Alcohol Depend. 2005;79(3): 379–87.

187. Contini V, et al. MAOA-uVNTR polymorphism in a Brazilian sample: further support for the association with impulsive behaviors and alcohol dependence. Am J Med Genet B Neuropsychiatr Genet. 2006;141B(3):305–8.

188. Verdejo-García A, Lawrence AJ, Clark L. Impulsivity as a vulnerability marker for substance-use disorders: review of findings from high-risk research, problem gamblers and genetic association studies. Neurosci Biobehav Rev. 2008;32:777–810.

189. Vanyukov MM, et al. Haplotypes of the monoamine oxidase genes and the risk for substance use disorders. Am J Med Genet B Neuropsychiatr Genet. 2004;125B(1):120–5.

190. Conrod PJ, et al. Efficacy of brief coping skills interventions that match different personality profiles of female substance abusers. Psychol Addict Behav. 2000;14(3):231–42.

Compulsive Drug Use and Brain Reward Systems

Jonathan A. Hollander and Paul J. Kenny

Abstract

Compulsive drug intake is a hallmark of addiction, yet the neurobiological mechanisms that contribute to the loss of control over drug consumption remain unclear. A better understanding of the mechanisms that drive compulsive drug taking may reveal targets for the development of novel therapeutics to alleviate this maladaptive behavioral state. Drug use is initiated primarily to obtain the stimulatory effects of addictive drugs on brain reward systems, an action that can be measured as drug-induced lowering of intracranial self-stimulation (ICSS) thresholds in rats and mice. Paradoxically, excessive drug intake can result in decreased activity of reward systems, reflected in elevated ICSS. Such drug-induced deficits in brain reward function likely reflect the engagement of compensatory mechanisms to counter drug effects. Recent evidence suggests that compulsive drug intake may develop in response to such adaptive decreases in brain reward systems. Further, environmental stimuli repeated paired with the actions of addictive drugs can attain "hedonic" salience to negatively regulate brain reward systems, and may thereby serve as a novel source of drug craving. The aim of this chapter is to review the impact of excessive drug consumption and drug-paired environmental stimuli on brain reward function, discuss the role for reward pathways in driving compulsive drug taking, and present potential neurobiological mechanisms that may underlie these processes.

Learning Objectives
- Intracranial self-stimulation (ICSS) and intravenous drug self-administration procedures are powerful behavioral techniques used to study the psychobiological effects of drugs of abuse.
- Many factors likely contribute to the development of compulsive drug intake, including genetic vulnerability and environment influences. Here, we will discuss the role for extended access to addictive drugs in the development of compulsive drug seeking and the potential involvement of brain reward systems in this process.

J.A. Hollander (✉) • P.J. Kenny
Laboratory for Behavioral and Molecular Neuroscience,
Department of Molecular Therapeutics, The Scripps Research
Institute—Florida, Jupiter, FL 33458, USA
e-mail: jholland@scripps.edu

Issues that Need to Be Addressed by Future Research

- Future research will be necessary to precisely delineate the impact of addictive drugs on brain reward systems and the role for these systems in the loss of control over drug-taking that characterizes addiction.
- Future pharmacotherapy for treatment of addiction may focus on reversing the reward deficit induced by overconsumption of addictive drugs and the altered reward processing induced by drug-paired environmental stimuli that may lead to drug craving.

Drug addiction is characterized by a transition from occasional to compulsive drug use, usually accompanied by a loss of control over the amount of drug consumed [1]. Use of drugs is initiated and sustained in large part by their hedonic actions. Indeed, as outlined below, all major drugs of abuse bypass much of the input side of conventional reinforcers such as food and water to artificially activate brain reward systems [2], an action that likely provides an important source of motivation to obtain and consume addictive drugs. Less clear, however, are the mechanisms contributing to the loss of control over drug intake and development of compulsive drug seeking (see Glossary). However, emerging evidence suggests that brain reward systems, and in particular dopamine-mediated transmission in reward-relevant brain regions, may play a central role in this process.

In contrast to their acute stimulatory effects, prolonged exposure to various classes of addictive drugs including opiates [3], psychomotor stimulants [4], and alcohol [5] decreases the baseline sensitivity of brain reward systems. This reaction in brain reward circuitries is hypothesized to reflect compensatory (homeostatic) adaptations to counteract their prolonged nonphysiological stimulation by drugs of abuse, and underlies the reward deficits associated with drug withdrawal [6]. Most recently, withdrawal-associated reward deficits were shown to be susceptible to classical (pavlovian) conditioning processes, such that exposure to withdrawal-paired environmental stimuli alone could decrease brain reward function [3, 7]. Reviewed here is the emerging evidence suggesting that disruption of basal reward processing through excessive drug consumption, or exposure to withdrawal-conditioned environmental stimuli, provides a crucial source of negative reinforcement that motivates compulsive drug intake.

Assessing Drug Intake in Laboratory Rodents: The Intravenous Self-Administration Procedure

In order to investigate the underlying neurobiology of compulsive drug use, it is necessary to employ an animal model that accurately recapitulates many aspects of this process

seen in human addicts. Loss of control over the amount of drug consumed marks the transition from controlled to the compulsive seeking that is a central feature of drug addiction. Importantly, periods of extended drug availability and resultant excessive drug consumption are likely critical factors that trigger the development of compulsive drug seeking in humans and a loss of control over intake [8–12]. Indeed, in human drug users a sudden increase in drug availability can precipitate the transition from low to high (and increasingly uncontrolled) levels of drug use [13–17].

The intravenous (IV) drug self-administration (SA) procedure is generally considered to be the most direct measure of the reinforcing effects of drugs of abuse in laboratory animals. In the SA procedure, experimental animals such as rats or mice are prepared with chronic indwelling IV catheters and trained to emit a response, typically to press a lever, to obtain IV drug infusions. The majority of drugs that are abused by humans are also self-administered by animals [18–24]. In addition, the laboratory animal drug SA procedure has several advantages over the use of human subjects for studying drug dependence. Besides ethical barriers impeding direct human study, the use of animals allows researchers to have precise control over drug history and potential environmental confounds, and facilitates invasive studies that can directly assess the neurobiological systems that regulate drug reinforcement. The validity of the SA procedure to model aspects of human drug addiction was recently demonstrated in an elegant study by Deroche-Gamonet and colleagues. In this study, rats with an extensive history of cocaine SA displayed many of the same "addiction-like" behaviors that are used to clinically diagnose substance abuse disorders in humans according to the criteria outlined in the Diagnostic and Statistical Manual of Mental Disorders (DSM-IV) [25]. In the drug SA procedure, drug availability and infusions are usually signaled by environmental stimuli (e.g., cue light, tone-houselight stimuli) so the subject can make the association between the required action and delivery of the drug. The experimenter typically imposes a schedule of reinforcement in which the animal must respond on the drug-paired lever a fixed number of times to obtain each drug infusion (fixed ratio schedule). In a more elaborate procedure, the investigator can establish a reinforcement schedule in which the number of responses that an animal must emit to obtain an infusion increases after each infusion is earned (progressive ratio schedule). Typically, an animal will respond under a progressive ratio schedule until the work necessary to obtain an infusion is no longer worth the effort to obtain the next infusion (i.e., the breakpoint). Thus, fixed ratio schedules of reinforcement are thought to best reflect the direct reinforcing effects of the drug, whereas responding under a progressive ratio is thought to better reflect the motivation to obtain the drug [26–28]. The relevance of the SA paradigm and use of different reinforcement schedules in laboratory animals to the study of compulsive drug use in humans is highlighted below.

Recent animal studies utilizing the drug SA procedure have shown that periods of extended access to cocaine and other addictive drugs may induce a loss of control over intake in rats similar to that observed in human drug users, resulting in a gradual escalation in daily cocaine intake [11, 15, 25, 29]. Specifically, it has been shown that animals permitted restricted (1-h) daily access to IV cocaine SA results in the establishment of regular and stable patterns of consumption [11]. However, in common with human drugs users, rodents can also demonstrate "escalating" levels of drug intake when offered extended daily access (6–18 h per day) to cocaine [11], heroin [30], nicotine [31], or methamphetamine [32]. This apparent loss of control over drug intake associated with extended drug access in rats is reminiscent of that observed in human drug users during the development of dependence. In addition, it has been shown that prolonged access to cocaine results in the development of drug-seeking responses (lever presses) resistant to the suppressant effects of a noxious stimulus (a cue previously associated with the delivery of aversive electric foot-shocks) [29]. However, the same noxious stimulus was shown to decrease cocaine-seeking responses in rats with a history of restricted access to the drug [29]. This observation in rats is evocative of drug-seeking observed in human addicts that persists even in the face of negative social, economic and/or health consequences associated with their drug habit [1]. Furthermore, rats with a history of very prolonged cocaine exposure (3 months) persist in their drug-taking behavior even when drug delivery was paired with a punishing electric shock [25]. In particular, those rats that demonstrated the most rapid escalation of intake during extended daily sessions were the most impervious to the inhibitory effects of negative outcome on drug seeking [25]. Thus, a history of extended drug access can manifest an addiction-like state in rats, characterized by a loss of control over the amounts of drug consumed (reflected in escalating daily intake) [11, 15, 25, 29], and drug seeking that is impervious to negative outcome [9, 12, 33].

Recent studies have sought to understand the mechanisms that may contribute to the compulsive-like escalation in drug intake observed in rats with extended drug access. Wee and colleagues found that rats with prolonged daily cocaine access exhibited higher breakpoint values for the drug under a progressive-ratio schedule of reinforcement compared with animals with restricted (1 h per day) access [34]. This observation suggests that the development of escalated drug intake is associated with increased motivation to obtain and consume the drug. This finding is intuitively appealing, as it is clear that the motivational value is increased in human drug users after the transition from controlled to compulsive drug taking has been established. Recent evidence suggests that noradrenergic neurotransmission, a key component of brain stress pathways, may regulate the increased breakpoints for cocaine observed in cocaine-escalated animals.

Specifically, it was found that prazosin (an α_1 receptor antagonist) reduced the higher breakpoints found in cocaine-escalated rats compared with controls [34]. In addition to noradrenergic transmission, other components of brain stress systems also appear to be engaged during the development of escalated levels of cocaine taking in rats with extended access to the drug [35]. Indeed, Weiss and colleagues have shown that cocaine-escalated rats had increased reactivity to a stressor (electric shock), and that these effects were attenuated by the metabotropic glutamate 2/3 receptor (mGluR2/3) agonist LY379268 [36]. Moreover, Specio and colleagues found that the selective corticotrophin-releasing factor (CRF) receptor 1 antagonist antalarmin reduced the escalated levels of cocaine-taking in rats with extended daily access to the drug [37]. Taken together, these findings suggest that brain stress pathways may be corrupted by extensive drug intake, and that this corruption in stress pathways may contribute to the development of escalated levels of drug-taking in rats with extended daily drug access.

Assessing Brain Reward Systems in Laboratory Rodents: Intracranial Self-Stimulation Thresholds

Electrical intracranial self-stimulation (ICSS) of certain brain areas, such as the lateral hypothalamus (LH) or ventral tegmental area (VTA), is powerfully rewarding for humans [38] and for laboratory animals such as dogs, rats, and mice. The powerfully rewarding properties of ICSS are reflected in the fact that subjects will readily learn to self-administer brief electrical pulses to their own brains, and endure painful stimuli such as electrical stock to the feet to obtain ICSS [39]. The high reward value of ICSS suggests that it directly activates brain circuitries that regulate the rewarding effects of more conventional reinforcers such as food, water and/or sex [39]. The minimal stimulation intensity that maintains ICSS behavior, termed the reward threshold [40], demonstrates little change in rats during extended or repeated testing sessions. As such, the ICSS threshold procedure provides a sensitive measure of the activity of brain reward systems in vivo, with lowering of reward thresholds interpreted as increased brain reward function and threshold elevations interpreted as decreased reward function. The ICSS procedure has proved particularly useful for monitoring the effects of addictive drugs on brain reward systems. Indeed, intravenous self-administration of relatively low amounts of cocaine [41], heroin [3], or nicotine [42] was shown to lower ICSS thresholds. This threshold lowering likely arises because of drug-induced amplification of reward signals in the brain, resulting in a potentiation of the rewarding properties of ICSS. Such drug-induced increases in the activity of brain reward systems may play an important role in establishing and perpetuating drug self-administration behavior [41, 42]. Conversely, withdrawal from chronic exposure to drugs of abuse usually elevates ICSS thresholds in rats. This withdrawal-associated elevation of reward thresholds likely reflects the engagement of inhibitory adaptations in brain reward systems to counter their over-stimulation by addictive drugs. However, during drug withdrawal the inhibitory adaptations in reward systems are no longer counterbalanced by the stimulatory actions of the drug, resulting in decreased activity of brain reward systems and reduced sensitivity to the reward effects of ICSS. The relevance of such compensatory adaptations in the basal sensitivity of brain reward systems to compulsive drug seeking is discussed below.

Compulsive Drug Use and Brain Reward Systems

The acute stimulatory effects of addictive drugs on brain reward systems are hypothesized to contribute to the establishment and maintenance of drug-taking behavior. More recently, it was hypothesized that drug-induced dysregulation of the same reward systems and the emergence of a state of reward hypofunction may motivate compulsive drug taking [6, 43]. Specifically, it has been argued that compensatory decreases in the activity of brain reward systems induced by excessive consumption of addictive drugs trigger the transition from casual to compulsive drug seeking by continuously motivating drug intake to alleviate this persistent state of diminished reward [9, 12, 15, 44].

Consistent with the above hypothesis, it has been shown that restricted daily access to cocaine, which produced low and stable patterns of intake [15], did not alter basal reward thresholds assessed 1 h before or 3 h after each daily SA session [15]. In contrast, reward thresholds became progressively more elevated (i.e., reward systems became progressively less functional) in rats with extended access to cocaine, in which there was also a gradual escalation of intake across days. Crucially, this reward deficit temporally preceded and was highly correlated with the magnitude by which cocaine intake was escalated [15]. Furthermore, this reward deficit persisted for at least 8 days after extended cocaine access was no longer available, demonstrating the durability of this phenomenon [15]. Most recently, the effects on reward thresholds of restricted or extended daily access to heroin self-administration were also examined [3]. In the restricted rats, reward thresholds assessed immediately after heroin consumption were lowered [3]. However, daily heroin intake and baseline ICSS thresholds assessed immediately before each self-administration session were stable and unaltered across days [3]. In contrast, rats with extended (23 h) daily heroin access demonstrated progressive elevations of reward thresholds, coupled with a gradual escalation of intake across

days [3], effects that were closely time-locked. Thus, excessive cocaine or heroin intake profoundly decreased the excitability of reward systems, an effect that may motivate consumption of ever-increasing amounts of drug, perhaps to alleviate this reward deficit. Paradoxically, increased drug consumption further worsened the underlying reward deficit and motivated even greater levels of intake. Thus, as heroin or cocaine dependence develops, a new source of motivation may emerge in which the drug is consumed not only for its acute rewarding effects, but also to counter persistent reward deficits. This interpretation is supported by a recent pharmacokinetic/pharmacodynamic modeling study of intravenous drug self-administration [9]. In this study, simulating an elevation of baseline reward thresholds recapitulated the alterations in self-administration behavior seen in rats with prolonged access to cocaine or heroin [9]. Interestingly, extended (12 h) daily access to nicotine for 20 consecutive days did not result in escalated intake, nor were there progressive elevations of ICSS thresholds [42]. This may reflect the fact that rats self-administered far less nicotine (~1.36 mg/kg per day base) than was previously shown to induce dependence and withdrawal-associated reward deficits when administered passively via osmotic minipumps (~3.16 mg/kg per day base) [45]. Thus, more prolonged periods of exposure to self-administered nicotine (>20 days) may be necessary to induce cocaine or heroin-like reward deficits and thereby motivate escalation of intake. Nevertheless, the above observations suggest that the emergence of a negative reinforcement dimension to drug consumption is likely a key dynamic in the development of compulsive drug intake.

In addition to a negative reinforcement interpretation of the above findings in which drugs are consumed to alleviate persistent reward deficits, a number of additional mechanisms by which drug-induced reward deficits may contribute to compulsive drug seeking should also be highlighted. It has been hypothesized that drug withdrawal may serve as a motivational state that enhances the incentive value of a drug analogous to the increased incentive value of food during periods of hunger [46]. Indeed, repeatedly consuming food while in a hungry state may facilitate the development of compulsive eating behavior [47–49]. Hence, persistent reward deficits may contribute to compulsive drug seeking at least partly by persistently increasing the incentive value of the drug analogous to the role of hunger in motivating compulsive food consumption. In addition, recent conceptualizations regarding the transition from occasional to compulsive drug use support that this process may be less dependent upon the rewarding effects of addictive drugs, and more related to a gradual shift from action-outcome (goal-directed) to stimulus–response (habit) responding with repeated drug exposure, primarily at the level of the dorsal striatum [50]. It is an interesting possibility that persistent drug-induced reward deficits, as described above in rats with extended daily access to cocaine or heroin, may facilitate the transition to habit-like responding for drugs [50]. Recent studies have shown that chronic amphetamine exposure that resulted in locomotor sensitization increased the progression from goal-directed to habit-based responding in rats [51], supporting the notion that drug-induced plasticity may indeed contribute to the emergence of habitual behaviors.

As outlined above, disruption of hedonic stability through excessive drug consumption likely contributes to the development of compulsive drug seeking. An important question, then, is what are the neurobiological mechanisms by which excessive drug consumption disrupts reward processing? Recently, Ahmed and colleagues utilized high-density oligonucleotide arrays to assess alterations in gene expression throughout the brains of rats with a history of restricted (1 h) or extended (6 h) daily access to cocaine self-administration [52]. In rats with a history of extended cocaine access, the most robust alterations in gene expression were found in the lateral hypothalamus (regions examined also included the prefrontal cortex, nucleus accumbens, septum, amygdala, and ventral tegmental area) [52]. The lateral hypothalamus is a major component of brain reward systems and the site at which rats responded for rewarding ICSS in the majority of the studies described in this review. Thus, functional alterations in the lateral hypothalamus may play an important role in drug-induced disruption of reward processing. However, more extensive studies will be required to determine the precise role of the lateral hypothalamus and the contribution of other cortical, hypothalamic, limbic, and basal ganglia regions to compulsive drug intake. Recently, the effects of the dopamine receptor antagonist *cis*-flupenthixol on drug intake were examined in rats with restricted or extended daily cocaine access [53]. Lower doses of the *cis*-flupenthixol increased drug intake whereas higher doses decreased intake in restricted rats, and the dose–response function was shifted leftward in extended rats [53]. Furthermore, Mantsch and colleagues observed increased levels of dopamine D2 receptor mRNA transcripts in the nucleus accumbens of rats with extended daily cocaine access relative to restricted rats [54]. Intriguingly, these dopaminergic changes in the nucleus accumbens may be a part of a larger synaptic reorganization or "rewiring" of the brain reward circuitry following extended access to cocaine. For example, Ferrario and colleagues found increased density of dendritic spines on medium spiny neurons in the core of the nucleus accumbens [55]. Nevertheless, in light of its important role in modulating the sensitivity of brain reward systems [56], these data suggest that drug-induced alterations in dopaminergic neurotransmission may contribute to the enduring deficits in brain reward function associated with excessive cocaine consumption.

Conditioning and Brain Reward Systems

There is considerable evidence that learning and memory systems may be corrupted by drugs of abuse; for detailed discussion of the role of reward-related learning in addiction see [57–64]. In human addicts environmental stimuli repeatedly associated with the effects of addictive drugs can attain motivational significance through classical conditioning processes, and evoke cravings and motivate drug seeking [65, 66]. The powerful motivational significance of drug-paired conditioned stimuli (CS) supports the notion that drug seeking becomes more habitual and compulsive, and less subject to executive control, as drug dependence evolves [50]. Aspects of withdrawal from various drugs of abuse may also become conditioned to environmental stimuli through classical conditioning processes [67, 68], and subsequent exposure to withdrawal-associated CS can induce a "conditioned withdrawal" state. Indeed, presentation of CS previously paired with experimenter-administered cocaine or morphine injections lowered ICSS thresholds in rats [69, 70]. Thus, stimuli repeatedly paired with the rewarding effects of addictive drugs may increase the activity of brain reward systems in a manner similar to unconditioned effects of addictive drugs. Such an action likely contributes to the high motivational significance attained by drug-associated CS [50]. Considering the importance of CS in motivating drug intake, recent studies have accessed if withdrawal-associated reward deficits are susceptible to conditioning processes. It was previously shown that neutral stimuli (flashing light and tone) alone could elevate reward thresholds after being repeatedly paired with precipitated withdrawal in rats made morphine dependent via subcutaneously implanted pellets [7]. Thus, withdrawal-associated reward deficits may be conditioned to environmental stimuli, providing a potential source of conditioned negative reinforcement that motivates compulsive drug intake. However, little empirical evidence has been generated in support of a role for conditioned withdrawal in motivating drug intake in humans or animals [71, 72]. Indeed, the role of withdrawal and conditioned withdrawal in provoking drug intake has been a contentious issue for many years [73–75]. Therefore, more recent studies have sought to determine the significance of conditioned reward deficits in motivating drug intake. It was shown that naloxone (30 µg) increased heroin intake and reversed heroin-induced lowering of reward thresholds in rats with restricted (1 h) daily access to heroin, but did not elevate reward thresholds above baseline levels (i.e., did not precipitate withdrawal) [3], actions of naloxone that were not susceptible to classical conditioning. Thus, in restricted rats naloxone simply reversed the pharmacological actions of heroin. However, in rats with extended (23 h) access to heroin, which demonstrated progressive elevations of basal reward thresholds and a time-locked escalation of heroin intake [3], naloxone elevated reward thresholds (i.e., precipitated withdrawal) above their already elevated baseline levels and increased heroin intake by magnitude far greater than that observed in restricted rats. Most importantly, CS repeatedly paired with naloxone administration elevated reward thresholds and provoked significant increases in heroin consumption in extended rats. Importantly, Hellemans and colleagues have shown that withdrawal-associated CS motivate heroin intake only in rats that previously had access to the drug during withdrawal-cue conditioning sessions, and could thereby learn the contingency between heroin consumption and alleviation of withdrawal [76]. Overall, these findings suggest that CS predicting the onset of withdrawal-associated reward deficits attain motivational significance as drug dependence develops and can provoke drug intake. Thus, craving for drugs may be elicited not only by environmental cues associated with the pleasurable effects of drugs, but also by cues associated with the aversive consequences of drug abstinence.

Considering the important role that drug-paired CS may play in motivating drug-seeking behaviors, the recent findings of Lee and colleagues demonstrating the "labile" nature of drug-associated memories are of particular interest [77, 78]. It has been shown that previously encoded memories can return to a labile state when reactivated during retrieval, and that inhibition of protein synthesis after memory reactivation may produce selective amnesia for recalled memories by blocking their reconsolidation [79]. Most recently, Lee and colleagues have shown that intra-amygdala infusions of antisense oligonucleotides against the immediate early gene product Zif268 (which plays a role in reconsolidating processes) prior to exposure to a cocaine-paired CS abolished the motivational significance of the CS, reflected in the fact that the CS could no longer facilitate acquisition of a new drug-seeking response [77], maintain responding under a second-order schedule of reinforcement [78], or reinstate extinguished cocaine-seeking responses [78]. Importantly, there is extensive overlap in the neurobiological substrates that regulate formation and expression drug-CS and withdrawal-CS associations [80]. Thus, it is an interesting possibility that blockade of reconsolidation processes may also abolish the motivational significance of withdrawal-paired CS.

Challenges for Future Research

As described above, deficits in brain reward function associated with excessive consumption of addictive drugs or induced by withdrawal-paired environmental stimuli may contribute to the development of compulsive drug taking. Importantly, emerging evidence suggests that variability in various domains of "personality" may increase vulnerability in particular individuals to developing compulsive drug-taking

behavior. For example, it was recently shown that high levels of impulsivity in rats, as measured by high rates of premature responding in a five choice serial reaction time task (5-CSRTT), was highly correlated with the development of compulsive-like drug-seeking responses characterized by resistance to environmental adversity [81]. Thus, it appears that very different domains of behavior, including responsiveness to reward, impulsive behavior and even propensity to develop habit-like responding for drugs (see [50, 82]), may impact the development of compulsive-like drug-seeking responses in rats. A major change for future research will be to understand how these apparently different behavioral domains are linked, and the mechanisms through which they may impact vulnerability to addiction. With this in mind, it is interesting to consider the recent findings of Everitt, Robbins and colleagues in this regard. It was found that high levels of trait impulsivity predicted the development of compulsive-like drug-seeking responses [81]. However, high levels of trait impulsivity were also correlated with low levels of striatal dopamine D2/3 receptors [83]. Importantly, striatal D2/3 receptor levels are known to be decreased in humans following excessive consumption of drugs of abuse [84–87]. Further, a genetic polymorphism in the human D2 dopamine receptor referred to as the Taq1A allele results in significantly decreased striatal D2 receptor density [88]. Individuals harboring this allele are over-represented in populations that abuse alcohol [89], cocaine [90], and opiates [91]. Moreover, individuals harboring the Taq1A allele display reduced dorsal striatum activation in response to palatable food, indicating a blunted reward response [92]. Indeed, striatal dopamine D2 receptors are considered important positive regulators of reward responsiveness [56, 93–96]. These data suggest that reductions in D2 dopamine receptor signaling may arise through genetic predisposition and/or over consumption of addictive drugs. Interestingly, the D2 dopamine receptor plays a central role in regulating the activity of brain reward systems. Thus, genetic or drug-induced deficits in striatal D2 receptor signaling simultaneously could contribute to the impulsive-like behaviors often observed in human drug addiction, and also contribute to the drug-induced reward deficits that may motivate escalating levels of drug-taking behavior. Future studies will be necessary to determine the precise role for dopamine D2 receptors in compulsive drug taking and also to understand how various neurobiological substrates that may contribute to the development of compulsive drug taking interact with one another.

Concluding Remarks

The findings reviewed here suggest that reward deficits associated with excessive drug consumption or precipitated by exposure to withdrawal-paired environmental stimuli may provide an important source of motivation that contributes to compulsive drug consumption. Nevertheless, a number of outstanding questions remain. Most importantly, what are the neurobiological mechanisms by which drugs of abuse persistently decrease brain reward function, and can these reward deficits be reversed? Moreover, will reversal of persistent deficits in brain reward function alleviate compulsive drug-seeking behaviors? The above findings increase our understanding of the reward mechanisms and motivational drives that contribute to compulsive drug seeking. More importantly, these findings may ultimately facilitate efforts to develop therapeutics for the treatment of substance abuse disorders. In particular, novel therapeutics that selectively reverse persistent drug-induced deficits in reward function or block the effects of drug-paired conditioned stimuli on reward systems may prove efficacious for the treatment of compulsive drug use. Such an approach would represent a conceptual advance in the design of treatment agents for addiction compared with the majority of currently available agents, the majority of which are designed simply as drug replacement therapies (nicotine patch for tobacco smoking, methadone for opiate addiction).

Acknowledgements J.A.H. was supported by a postdoctoral fellowship from the National Institute on Drug Abuse (NIDA) (DA 024932). P.J.K. was supported by grants from NIDA (DA020686; DA023915; DA025983).

Glossary

Reinforcer Reinforcer is an object or event that is obtained or that occurs in response to a particular behavior, is contiguous with that behavioral response in a temporal and spatial manner, and is associated with an increased probability that the behavior response will occur again. Put simply, a reinforcer is anything that increases the likelihood that a given response will be repeated.

Classical conditioning Classical conditioning was originally characterized by the Russian physiologist Ivan Pavlov, and involves the learning process in which a previously neutral environmental cue (conditioned stimulus; CS) can attain motivational salience and elicit a conditioned response (CR) after being repeatedly associated with an intrinsically salient stimulus (unconditioned stimulus; US) that induces an automatic response (unconditioned response; UR). In our experiments, a CS (previously neutral flashing light and tone) is repeatedly paired with a US, usually a drug of abuse or a receptor antagonist that precipitates withdrawal in drug-dependent animals (see below), during daily conditioning sessions. The CS can eventually elicit responses similar to those induced by the US.

Intracranial self-stimulation (ICSS) Intracranial self-stimulation (ICSS) is a behavioral procedure that provides a sensitive measure of the effects of addictive drugs on brain reward systems. Rats turn a response wheel to receive electrical pulses directly into their brain via indwelling stimulating electrodes located within components of the brain's reward system. In our experiments, the stimulating electrode is located within the posterior lateral hypothalamus, targeting the medial forebrain bundle. The intensity of the electrical pulse is varied (according to the method of limits) such that the minimal electrical intensity (termed the "reward threshold") for which the animal is prepared to respond can be identified for each rat. Acute administration of major drugs of abuse lowers the reward threshold, whereas withdrawal from addictive drugs after chronic administration usually elevates the reward threshold.

Action-outcome (goal-directed) responding Action-outcome (goal-directed) responding is behavior directed toward achieving a goal, and is under voluntary control (i.e., sensitive to the relative value of the goal). Action-outcome responding is dependent upon the animal learning the causal relationship between its actions and the likelihood of achieving the goal.

Stimulus–response (habit) responding Stimulus–response (habit) responding usually emerges after goal-directed responding has been repeated on many occasions until such responding becomes more habitual and sensitive to goal-associated conditioned stimuli, and less under voluntary control (i.e., insensitive to the relative value of the goal).

Precipitated withdrawal Precipitated withdrawal is the process by which withdrawal may be transiently "precipitated" in drug-dependent animals (or humans) by administration of a compound that antagonizes the actions of that particular drug. For example, withdrawal may be precipitated in opiate dependent rats by administration of the opioid receptor antagonist naloxone.

Escalation of drug intake Escalation of drug intake in rats is the process by which extended daily access to a drug results in the gradual increase of drug intake over time, a process reminiscent of the loss of control over intake usually observed in human drug addicts.

References

1. Association AP. Diagnostic and statistical manual of mental disorders. 4th ed. Washington: American Psychiatric Press; 1994.
2. Nesse RM, Berridge KC. Psychoactive drug use in evolutionary perspective. Science. 1997;278(5335):63–6.
3. Kenny PJ, Chen SA, Kitamura O, Markou A, Koob GF. Conditioned withdrawal drives heroin consumption and decreases reward sensitivity. J Neurosci. 2006;26(22):5894–900.
4. Markou A, Koob GF. Postcocaine anhedonia. An animal model of cocaine withdrawal. Neuropsychopharmacology. 1991;4(1):17–26.

5. Schulteis G, Markou A, Cole M, Koob GF. Decreased brain reward produced by ethanol withdrawal. Proc Natl Acad Sci USA. 1995;92(13):5880–4.

6. Koob GF, Le Moal M. Plasticity of reward neurocircuitry and the 'dark side' of drug addiction. Nat Neurosci. 2005;8(11):1442–4.

7. Kenny PJ, Markou A. Conditioned nicotine withdrawal profoundly decreases the activity of brain reward systems. J Neurosci. 2005;25(26):6208–12.

8. Wikler A. A psychodynamic study of a patient during experimental self-regulated re-addiction to morphine. Psychiatr Q. 1952;26(2): 270–93.

9. Ahmed SH, Koob GF. Transition to drug addiction: a negative reinforcement model based on an allostatic decrease in reward function. Psychopharmacology (Berl). 2005;180(3):473–90.

10. Ahmed SH. Imbalance between drug and non-drug reward availability: a major risk factor for addiction. Eur J Pharmacol. 2005; 526(1–3):9–20.

11. Ahmed SH, Koob GF. Transition from moderate to excessive drug intake: change in hedonic set point. Science. 1998;282(5387): 298–300.

12. Kenny PJ. Brain reward systems and compulsive drug use. Trends Pharmacol Sci. 2007;28(3):135–41.

13. Gawin FH, Ellinwood Jr EH. Cocaine dependence. Annu Rev Med. 1989;40:149–61.

14. Kramer JC, Fischman VS, Littlefield DC. Amphetamine abuse. Pattern and effects of high doses taken intravenously. JAMA. 1967;201(5):305–9.

15. Ahmed SH, Kenny PJ, Koob GF, Markou A. Neurobiological evidence for hedonic allostasis associated with escalating cocaine use. Nat Neurosci. 2002;5(7):625–6.

16. Siegel RK. Changing patterns of cocaine use: longitudinal observations, consequences, and treatment. NIDA Res Monogr. 1984; 50:92–110.

17. Ferri CP, Gossop M, Laranjeira RR. High dose cocaine use in Sao Paulo: a comparison of treatment and community samples. Subst Use Misuse. 2001;36(3):237–55.

18. Griffiths RR, Balster RL. Opioids: similarity between evaluations of subjective effects and animal self-administration results. Clin Pharmacol Ther. 1979;25(5 Pt 1):611–7.

19. Griffiths RR, Brady JV, Bigelow GE. Predicting the dependence liability of stimulant drugs. NIDA Res Monogr. 1981;37:182–96.

20. Weeks J. Experimental morphine addiction: methods for automated intravenous injections in unrestrained rats. Science. 1962;138:143–4.

21. Criswell HE, Ridings A. Intravenous self-administration of morphine by naive mice. Pharmacol Biochem Behav. 1983;18(3): 467–70.

22. Risner ME, Jones BE. Self-administration of CNS stimulants by dog. Psychopharmacologia. 1975;43(3):207–13.

23. Wilson MC, Schuster CR. The effects of chlorpromazine on psychomotor stimulant self-administration in the rhesus monkey. Psychopharmacologia. 1972;26(2):115–26.

24. Donny EC, Caggiula AR, Knopf S, Brown C. Nicotine self-administration in rats. Psychopharmacology (Berl). 1995;122(4): 390–94.

25. Deroche-Gamonet V, Belin D, Piazza PV. Evidence for addiction-like behavior in the rat. Science. 2004;305(5686):1014–7.

26. Markou A, Weiss F, Gold LH, Caine SB, Schulteis G, Koob GF. Animal models of drug craving. Psychopharmacology (Berl). 1993;112(2–3):163–82.

27. Richardson NR, Roberts DC. Progressive ratio schedules in drug self-administration studies in rats: a method to evaluate reinforcing efficacy. J Neurosci Methods. 1996;66(1):1–11.

28. Pickering C, Avesson L, Lindblom J, Liljequist S, Schioth HB. To press or not to press? Differential receptor expression and response

to novelty in rats learning an operant response for reward. Neurobiol Learn Mem. 2007;87(2):181–91.

29. Vanderschuren LJ, Everitt BJ. Drug seeking becomes compulsive after prolonged cocaine self-administration. Science. 2004; 305(5686):1017–9.

30. Ahmed SH, Walker JR, Koob GF. Persistent increase in the motivation to take heroin in rats with a history of drug escalation. Neuropsychopharmacology. 2000;22(4):413–21.

31. George O, Ghozland S, Azar MR, Cottone P, Zorrilla EP, Parsons LH, O'Dell LE, Richardson HN, Koob GF. CRF-CRF1 system activation mediates withdrawal-induced increases in nicotine self-administration in nicotine-dependent rats. Proc Natl Acad Sci USA. 2007;104(43):17198–203.

32. Kitamura O, Wee S, Specio SE, Koob GF, Pulvirenti L. Escalation of methamphetamine self-administration in rats: a dose-effect function. Psychopharmacology (Berl). 2006;186(1):48–53.

33. Koob GF, Ahmed SH, Boutrel B, Chen SA, Kenny PJ, Markou A, O'Dell LE, Parsons LH, Sanna PP. Neurobiological mechanisms in the transition from drug use to drug dependence. Neurosci Biobehav Rev. 2004;27(8):739–49.

34. Wee S, Mandyam CD, Lekic DM, Koob GF. Alpha 1-noradrenergic system role in increased motivation for cocaine intake in rats with prolonged access. Eur Neuropsychopharmacol. 2008;18(4):303–11.

35. Koob GF. Neuroadaptive mechanisms of addiction: studies on the extended amygdala. Eur Neuropsychopharmacol. 2003;13(6): 442–52.

36. Aujla H, Martin-Fardon R, Weiss F. Rats with extended access to cocaine exhibit increased stress reactivity and sensitivity to the anxiolytic-like effects of the mGluR 2/3 agonist LY379268 during abstinence. Neuropsychopharmacology. 2008;33(8):1818–26.

37. Specio SE, Wee S, O'Dell LE, Boutrel B, Zorrilla EP, Koob GF. CRF(1) receptor antagonists attenuate escalated cocaine self-administration in rats. Psychopharmacology (Berl). 2008;196(3): 473–82.

38. Bishop MP, Elder ST, Heath RG. Intracranial self-stimulation in man. Science. 1963;140:394–6.

39. Olds J. Self-stimulation of the brain. Science. 1958;127:315–24.

40. Kornetsky C, Esposito RU. Euphorigenic drugs: effects on the reward pathways of the brain. Fed Proc. 1979;38(11):2473–6.

41. Kenny PJ, Polis I, Koob GF, Markou A. Low dose cocaine self-administration transiently increases but high dose cocaine persistently decreases brain reward function in rats. Eur J Neurosci. 2003;17(1):191–5.

42. Kenny PJ, Markou A. Nicotine self-administration acutely activates brain reward systems and induces a long-lasting increase in reward sensitivity. Neuropsychopharmacology. 2006;31(6):1203–11.

43. Koob GF, Le Moal M. Drug abuse: hedonic homeostatic dysregulation. Science. 1997;278(5335):52–8.

44. Koob GF, Le Moal M. Addiction and the brain antireward system. Annu Rev Psychol. 2008;59:29–53.

45. Epping-Jordan MP, Watkins SS, Koob GF, Markou A. Dramatic decreases in brain reward function during nicotine withdrawal. Nature. 1998;393(6680):76–9.

46. Hutcheson DM, Everitt BJ, Robbins TW, Dickinson A. The role of withdrawal in heroin addiction: enhances reward or promotes avoidance? Nat Neurosci. 2001;4(9):943–7.

47. Wardle J. Compulsive eating and dietary restraint. Br J Clin Psychol. 1987;26(Pt 1):47–55.

48. Colantuoni C, Schwenker J, McCarthy J, Rada P, Ladenheim B, Cadet JL, Schwartz GJ, Moran TH, Hoebel BG. Excessive sugar intake alters binding to dopamine and mu-opioid receptors in the brain. Neuroreport. 2001;12(16):3549–52.

49. Avena NM, Hoebel BG. A diet promoting sugar dependency causes behavioral cross-sensitization to a low dose of amphetamine. Neuroscience. 2003;122(1):17–20.

50. Everitt BJ, Robbins TW. Neural systems of reinforcement for drug addiction: from actions to habits to compulsion. Nat Neurosci. 2005;8(11):1481–9.

51. Nelson A, Killcross S. Amphetamine exposure enhances habit formation. J Neurosci. 2006;26(14):3805–12.

52. Ahmed SH, Lutjens R, van der Stap LD, Lekic D, Romano-Spica V, Morales M, Koob GF, Repunte-Canonigo V, Sanna PP. Gene expression evidence for remodeling of lateral hypothalamic circuitry in cocaine addiction. Proc Natl Acad Sci USA. 2005; 102(32):11533–8.

53. Ahmed SH, Koob GF. Changes in response to a dopamine receptor antagonist in rats with escalating cocaine intake. Psychopharmacology (Berl). 2004;172(4):450–4.

54. Mantsch JR, Yuferov V, Mathieu-Kia AM, Ho A, Kreek MJ. Effects of extended access to high versus low cocaine doses on self-administration, cocaine-induced reinstatement and brain mRNA levels in rats. Psychopharmacology (Berl). 2004;175(1): 26–36.

55. Ferrario CR, Gorny G, Crombag HS, Li Y, Kolb B, Robinson TE. Neural and behavioral plasticity associated with the transition from controlled to escalated cocaine use. Biol Psychiatry. 2005; 58(9):751–9.

56. Elmer GI, Pieper JO, Levy J, Rubinstein M, Low MJ, Grandy DK, Wise RA. Brain stimulation and morphine reward deficits in dopamine D2 receptor-deficient mice. Psychopharmacology (Berl). 2005;182(1):33–44.

57. Redish AD. Addiction as a computational process gone awry. Science. 2004;306(5703):1944–7.

58. Wise RA. Drive, incentive, and reinforcement: the antecedents and consequences of motivation. Nebr Symp Motiv. 2004;50: 159–95.

59. Kelley AE. Memory and addiction: shared neural circuitry and molecular mechanisms. Neuron. 2004;44(1):161–79.

60. Schultz W. Neural coding of basic reward terms of animal learning theory, game theory, microeconomics and behavioural ecology. Curr Opin Neurobiol. 2004;14(2):139–47.

61. Montague PR, Hyman SE, Cohen JD. Computational roles for dopamine in behavioural control. Nature. 2004;431(7010):760–7.

62. Hyman SE, Malenka RC, Nestler EJ. Neural mechanisms of addiction: the role of reward-related learning and memory. Annu Rev Neurosci. 2006;29:565–98.

63. Hyman SE. Addiction: a disease of learning and memory. Am J Psychiatry. 2005;162(8):1414–22.

64. Berke JD, Hyman SE. Addiction, dopamine, and the molecular mechanisms of memory. Neuron. 2000;25(3):515–32.

65. Childress A, Ehrman R, McLellan AT, O'Brien C. Conditioned craving and arousal in cocaine addiction: a preliminary report. NIDA Res Monogr. 1988;81:74–80.

66. Monti PM, Rohsenow DJ, Rubonis AV, Niaura RS, Sirota AD, Colby SM, Abrams DB. Alcohol cue reactivity: effects of detoxification and extended exposure. J Stud Alcohol. 1993;54(2): 235–45.

67. Wikler A. Dynamics of drug dependence. Implications of a conditioning theory for research and treatment. Arch Gen Psychiatry. 1973;28(5):611–6.

68. O'Brien CP, Testa T, O'Brien TJ, Brady JP, Wells B. Conditioned narcotic withdrawal in humans. Science. 1977;195(4282): 1000–2.

69. Hayes RJ, Gardner EL. The basolateral complex of the amygdala mediates the modulation of intracranial self-stimulation threshold by drug-associated cues. Eur J Neurosci. 2004;20(1): 273–80.

70. Kenny PJ, Koob GF, Markou A. Conditioned facilitation of brain reward function after repeated cocaine administration. Behav Neurosci. 2003;117(5):1103–7.

71. Shaham Y, Rajabi H, Stewart J. Relapse to heroin-seeking in rats under opioid maintenance: the effects of stress, heroin priming, and withdrawal. J Neurosci. 1996;16(5):1957–63.

72. Shaham Y, Shalev U, Lu L, De Wit H, Stewart J. The reinstatement model of drug relapse: history, methodology and major findings. Psychopharmacology (Berl). 2003;168(1–2):3–20.

73. Stewart J, Wise RA. Reinstatement of heroin self-administration habits: morphine prompts and naltrexone discourages renewed responding after extinction. Psychopharmacology (Berl). 1992; 108(1–2):79–84.

74. Childress AR, McLellan AT, O'Brien CP. Assessment and extinction of conditioned withdrawal-like responses in an integrated treatment for opiate dependence. NIDA Res Monogr. 1984;55:202–10.

75. Childress AR, McLellan AT, Ehrman R, O'Brien CP. Classically conditioned responses in opioid and cocaine dependence: a role in relapse? NIDA Res Monogr. 1988;84:25–43.

76. Hellemans KG, Dickinson A, Everitt BJ. Motivational control of heroin seeking by conditioned stimuli associated with withdrawal and heroin taking by rats. Behav Neurosci. 2006;120(1):103–14.

77. Lee JL, Di Ciano P, Thomas KL, Everitt BJ. Disrupting reconsolidation of drug memories reduces cocaine-seeking behavior. Neuron. 2005;47(6):795–801.

78. Lee JL, Milton AL, Everitt BJ. Cue-induced cocaine seeking and relapse are reduced by disruption of drug memory reconsolidation. J Neurosci. 2006;26(22):5881–7.

79. Nader K, Schafe GE, Le Doux JE. Fear memories require protein synthesis in the amygdala for reconsolidation after retrieval. Nature. 2000;406(6797):722–6.

80. Schulteis G, Ahmed SH, Morse AC, Koob GF, Everitt BJ. Conditioning and opiate withdrawal. Nature. 2000;405(6790): 1013–4.

81. Belin D, Mar AC, Dalley JW, Robbins TW, Everitt BJ. High impulsivity predicts the switch to compulsive cocaine-taking. Science. 2008;320(5881):1352–5.

82. Robbins TW, Everitt BJ. Drug addiction: bad habits add up. Nature. 1999;398(6728):567–70.

83. Dalley JW, Fryer TD, Brichard L, Robinson ES, Theobald DE, Laane K, Pena Y, Murphy ER, Shah Y, Probst K, Abakumova I, Aigbirhio FI, Richards HK, Hong Y, Baron JC, Everitt BJ, Robbins TW. Nucleus accumbens D2/3 receptors predict trait impulsivity and cocaine reinforcement. Science. 2007;315(5816):1267–70.

84. Volkow ND, Fowler JS, Wang GJ, Swanson JM, Telang F. Dopamine in drug abuse and addiction: results of imaging studies and treatment implications. Arch Neurol. 2007;64(11):1575–9.

85. Melis M, Spiga S, Diana M. The dopamine hypothesis of drug addiction: hypodopaminergic state. Int Rev Neurobiol. 2005;63: 101–54.

86. Volkow ND, Fowler JS, Wang GJ, Hitzemann R, Logan J, Schlyer DJ, Dewey SL, Wolf AP. Decreased dopamine D2 receptor availability is associated with reduced frontal metabolism in cocaine abusers. Synapse. 1993;14(2):169–77.

87. Hietala J, West C, Syvalahti E, Nagren K, Lehikoinen P, Sonninen P, Ruotsalainen U. Striatal D2 dopamine receptor binding characteristics in vivo in patients with alcohol dependence. Psychopharmacology (Berl). 1994;116(3):285–90.

88. Noble EP. Addiction and its reward process through polymorphisms of the D2 dopamine receptor gene: a review. Eur Psychiatry. 2000;15(2):79–89.

89. Noble EP, Zhang X, Ritchie TL, Sparkes RS. Haplotypes at the DRD2 locus and severe alcoholism. Am J Med Genet. 2000; 96(5):622–31.

90. Noble EP, Blum K, Khalsa ME, Ritchie T, Montgomery A, Wood RC, Fitch RJ, Ozkaragoz T, Sheridan PJ, Anglin MD, et al. Allelic association of the D2 dopamine receptor gene with cocaine dependence. Drug Alcohol Depend. 1993;33(3):271–85.

91. Lawford BR, Young RM, Noble EP, Sargent J, Rowell J, Shadforth S, Zhang X, Ritchie T. The D(2) dopamine receptor A(1) allele and opioid dependence: association with heroin use and response to methadone treatment. Am J Med Genet. 2000;96(5):592–8.

92. Stice E, Spoor S, Bohon C, Small DM. Relation between obesity and blunted striatal response to food is moderated by TaqIA A1 allele. Science. 2008;322(5900):449–52.

93. Nakajima S, O'Regan NB. The effects of dopaminergic agonists and antagonists on the frequency-response function for hypothalamic self-stimulation in the rat. Pharmacol Biochem Behav. 1991;39(2):465–8.

94. Ranaldi R, Beninger RJ. The effects of systemic and intracerebral injections of D1 and D2 agonists on brain stimulation reward. Brain Res. 1994;651(1–2):283–92.

95. Knapp CM, Kornetsky C. Bromocriptine, a D2 receptor agonist, lowers the threshold for rewarding brain stimulation. Pharmacol Biochem Behav. 1994;49(4):901–4.

96. Durieux PF, Bearzatto B, Guiducci S, Buch T, Waisman A, Zoli M, Schiffmann SN, de Kerchove d'Exaerde A. D(2)R striatopallidal neurons inhibit both locomotor and drug reward processes.Nat Neurosci. 2009;12(4):393–5.

Animal Models in Addiction Research

David Belin and Jeffrey W. Dalley

Abstract

Animal models have provided valuable insights into the brain mechanisms of drug addiction, including the elucidation of neural substrates that support the primary reinforcing effects of widely abused drugs such as cocaine and heroin and the long-term consequences of drug addiction for neurocognitive functioning. In recent years, considerable progress has been made in developing animal models that closely resemble the clinical features of drug addiction according to published diagnostic guidelines especially in the domain of compulsive drug use which represents the final stage of a progressive series of neural and psychological alterations induced by chronic drug exposure. In this chapter, we review a number of animal models used in addiction research and discuss their relevance and explanatory utility to the different stages of the addiction cycle.

Learning Objectives
- To understand how animal models can be used to investigate the psychobiological bases of the pathways to addiction
- To gain an appreciation of the behavioural constructs used to define compulsive drug seeking and taking in animal models of addiction
- To appreciate the evolution of such models from theoretical and clinical standpoints
- To recognise how different animal models can help inform our understanding of the different components of the drug addiction cycle

D. Belin (✉)
INSERM European Associated Laboratory Psychobiology of Compulsive Habits, Pôle PBS,
bâtiment B36 1 rue Georges Bonnet, 86022 Poitiers
e-mail: david.belin@inserm.fr

Department of Experimental Psychology, Downing stress, CB2 3EB, Cambridge

INSERM U1084 -LNEC & University of Poitiers, Pôle Biologie Santé, 1 rue Georges Bonnet, 86022 Poitiers, Cedex

J.W. Dalley
Behavioural and Clinical Neuroscience Institute, Department of Experimental Psychology, University of Cambridge, Downing St, Cambridge, CB2 3EB, UK

Department of Psychiatry, Addenbrooke's Hospital, University of Cambridge, Hill's Road, Cambridge, CB2 2QQ, UK

Issues that Need to Be Addressed for Future Research
- Neural and psychological substrates underlying the shift from initial drug exposure to habitual, compulsive patterns of drug intake
- Comparative effects of stimulant and opiate drugs on neurocognitive functioning
- Strategies to investigate compulsive heroin and cocaine drug self-administration in animal models
- The significance of behavioural traits (e.g. novelty seeking, impulsivity) to the emergence of compulsive drug self-administration

J.C. Verster et al. (eds.), *Drug Abuse and Addiction in Medical Illness: Causes, Consequences and Treatment*,
DOI 10.1007/978-1-4614-3375-0_6, © Springer Science+Business Media, LLC 2012

Introduction

Drug addiction is a complex brain disease [1, 2], affecting the motivational [3], learning [4, 5] and behavioural control systems of the brain [6, 7]. Despite considerable research we still do not understand why individuals become dependent on drugs nor do we have effective treatments to reduce the substantial social and economic burden of this disorder [8].

Animal models provide a valuable means to investigate the different stages of the drug addiction cycle including especially the initiation of drug taking, the maintenance phase, which is often accompanied by bouts of drug binge-ing and escalation, and finally the switch to compulsive drug intake defined operationally by an increased motiva-tion to take the drug, an inability to inhibit drug seeking and continued drug use despite negative or adverse consequences.

Two strategies are generally used when designing animal models of drug addiction. First, the model can address a specific symptom, a neurobiological or psychological feature or a behavioural construct associated with the pathology. These models have been widely developed over the last 40 years and have provided substantial information about the molecular targets of addictive drugs as well as the neurobio-logical and psychological adaptations resulting from either acute or chronic drug exposure. Indeed, models that focus on defined features of drug addiction provide a powerful heuris-tic framework for determining the brain mechanisms underly-ing the pathology in question. However, they rarely allow for other clinical dimensions of the disorder such as behavioural predictive factors or interactions between different symptoms of the pathology. Thus, the second type of models are those that try to incorporate several symptoms of the pathology in humans, thereby providing powerful tools for longitudinal studies or even testing pharmacological treatments, but are somewhat limited in the identification of underlying mecha-nisms. Indeed, the behavioural complexity of these models makes it difficult to implement causal investigative studies where the end point is well defined. We discuss the general utility and application of both modelling approaches as complementary tools to investigate the neurobiological and psychological mechanisms of drug addiction and its vulnerability.

Necessity for Animal Models in Drug Addiction Research

The case for animal experimentation in addiction research is compelling. Studies in human addicts are often prone to interpretative issues not least due to inter-subject variability in drug exposure, the frequent co-abuse of several drugs often in combination with alcohol, cannabis and nicotine; the regular occurrence of co-morbid brain disorders such as depression, conduct disorder and attention-deficit/hyperac-tivity disorder (ADHD) and the difficulty in controlling pre-morbid cognitive and intellectual abilities. Whilst animal models can never reproduce the complex social and often personal reasons why people abuse drugs they nevertheless provide a rigorous means to precisely control drug exposure as well as assessing behavioural and cognitive performance prior to drug administration. They also enable controlled neural manipulations to be made (e.g. using selective neuro-toxins) and so establish the causal influences of putative neu-ral loci and, in turn, the cellular and molecular substrates of drug addiction.

The seminal discovery by Olds and Milner of intra-cranial self-stimulation (ICSS) in 1954 marked a major turning point for research on the neural mechanisms of addiction [9]. The discovery that dopaminergic projections from the ventral tegmental area (VTA) to limbic cortico-striatal structures (nucleus accumbens, olfactory tubercle, amygdala, orbitof-rontal cortex, medial prefrontal cortex) were effective sub-strates for ICSS sparked considerable interest in the brain dopamine systems as neural substrates for the rewarding properties of both natural (food) and drug incentives. A few years later Weeks developed an operant procedure to deliver intravenous morphine infusions to relatively unrestrained rats [10], a method still widely used in many pre-clinical research laboratories today. That research continued on the opioid drugs morphine and heroin for some considerable time, thereafter, was no surprise given the strong emphasis at that time in the DSM-III on the symptomatology of opioid dependence and withdrawal.

Based on work over a number of years it has now been established that a broad range of psychoactive substances abused by humans are reinforcing in many lower species including planarian [11] and flies [12, 13] as well as many vertebrate species including mice [14–18], rats [19–22], dogs [23] and non-human primates [24–33]. However, it remains unclear the extent to which these findings help inform our understanding of drug addiction in humans since it is a brain disorder that is clearly far removed from primary reinforce-ment mechanisms. Indeed, even after the publication of the DSM-IV in 1994 and the new diagnostic criteria for compul-sive drug use that now form the hallmark of the clinical fea-tures of drug addiction many, if not all, of the early animal models focused on the "rewarding" properties of addictive drugs and their acute and chronic neurobiological effects. Only until relatively recently, however, have animal models been developed to measure loss of control over drug intake [34, 35] and compulsive drug self-administration [36–40]. It is therefore important to briefly define the purpose and valid-ity of animal models, and especially animal models of drug addiction.

Validity Criteria of Animal Models

An animal model is a preparation in one organism that allows for the study of one or several aspects of a human condition. Thus, a model of drug addiction must provide insights into the neurobiological, psychological or etiological mechanisms of the pathology in humans, at least mimicking some aspects of the pathology.

A model is usually composed of an independent variable and a dependent variable. The independent variable is the causal manipulation whereas the dependent variable refers to the phenotype under investigation [41, 42]. The selection of both variables is generally based upon theoretical aspects relative to the aetiology of the pathology (independent variable), and diagnostic criteria or psychological and neurobehavioural constructs (dependent variable). The independent variable in animal models can be very broad, from a specific lesion of the brain to the modification of a particular gene. Similarly the dependent variable can belong to different levels of investigation, such as behaviour, neural systems (dopamine levels, for example), gene expression (as measured with quantitative PCR or in situ hybridisation) or electrical activity of single neurons. Thus, animal models provide standardised tools to investigate the different levels of integration of the brain and therefore represent precious tools for the investigation of the cellular and molecular substrates of the disease under investigation, and especially addiction. However, animal models of psychiatric disorders present limitations that are worth keeping in mind. First standard housing conditions in laboratory facilities do not reflect ethological conditions; second the subjective aspects of a psychopathology such as drug addiction are unlikely to be addressed in non-human species. For this it has been suggested that drug addiction is a pathology unique to humans [43].

The validation of animal models of addiction is based upon the same principles that have been established for models in general, namely fulfilling standard criteria amongst which reliability and predictive validity are the most important [41]. However, there are other criteria that have been used widely in validating animal models of drug addiction, including face validity and construct validity [41]. Briefly, *Reliability* refers to the consistency and stability with which the independent and the dependent variables are measured. Thus, a reliable model of drug addiction must allow for a precise and reproducible manipulation of the independent variable and an objective and reproducible measure of the dependent variable in standard conditions. A further key criterion for the validation of an animal model is its *predictive validity*. A valid animal model should predict either the therapeutical potential of a compound in humans (pharmacological isomorphism) or a variable that may influence both the dependent variable of the model and the process under investigation in humans.

Face validity refers to the similarities between the dependent variable of the model, i.e. behaviour in the case of drug addiction, and the human condition, i.e. the symptoms of the pathology. Thus, face validity may be important in designing the model but is unlikely an objective criterion to actually assess its validity. Indeed, it is very difficult if not impossible to provide an objective criterion to evaluate the similarities between the behavioural output of a rat preparation and drug addiction in humans when the behavioural repertoire of the two species is so different. Construct validity has been increasingly considered in animal models of drug addiction. It refers to the ability of a model to take into account psychological or neurobiological constructs that characterise the specific pathological processes in humans. Thus, incentive sensitisation, habit formation or top-down prefrontal executive control failure are examples of constructs which have been investigated in animal models.

Reinforcing Effects of Drugs of Abuse, Abuse Liability

As previously mentioned all addictive substances show reinforcing properties in animals. Indeed, the abuse liability of a substance is often measured by its ability to support self-administration and a conditioned place preference (CPP) [44]. In this section, we briefly review the experimental designs that have been developed to investigate the reinforcing properties of addictive drugs. These procedures, combined with molecular biology and pharmacology, have been crucial in the identification and functional characterisation of the molecular targets of addictive drugs.

Reinforcement-Associated Learning Mechanisms

Addictive substances exert powerful effects on primary and secondary (i.e. conditioned) reinforcement mechanisms. As instrumental reinforcers they strongly encourage behaviours that lead to the availability of a drug, a process subserved by stimulus–response associative mechanisms (instrumental conditioning). Abused drugs also facilitate Pavlovian conditioning whereby previously neutral stimuli in the environment become conditioned to the drug, and can predict it, or even act as conditioned reinforcers. In operational terms, a reinforcer is a stimulus that increases the probability of a response consequent upon its presentation. Thus, all addictive drugs are reinforcers since they are self-administered by animals and humans and support CPP (a form of contextual Pavlovian conditioning). Pavlovian conditioned reinforcers can have powerful motivational effects and support long sequences of instrumental drug-seeking behaviour by bridging delays to future drug reinforcement [5, 45–47].

Conditioned Place Preference

CPP has been used extensively to probe the psychological [48] and neurobiological [11, 49] mechanisms underlying the rewarding properties of addictive drugs [49], as well as negative emotional states associated with drug withdrawal [50]. Indeed, through Pavlovian conditioning, the negative affective state caused by drug withdrawal can induce a reliable conditioned place aversion [50, 51]. The first study based on the modern paradigm of CPP was reported by Rossi and Reid in 1976 [52] although earlier demonstrations of preference for a drug-paired environment was published as early as the 1940s [49].

In this procedure, two different unconditioned stimuli (US) are paired with two distinct environments. These contextual cues differ in their spatial configuration, colour, flooring and sometimes even olfactory cues. Briefly, the CPP procedure involves injecting animals with either the drug in question or a control solution, each being administered in a different environment often over successive days. The conditioning phase may combine several pairings, ideally according to a Latin square and unbiased design such that every pairing does not predict subsequent pairings, and that any spontaneous bias or preference for a compartment is initially controlled for. CPP is then tested during a drug-free choice phase where subjects are given access to both compartments. Preference for the drug-paired environment is indicative of the rewarding properties of the drug. CPP can be established not only for addictive drugs [53] but also for natural rewards such as food, water, sexual partner and novelty [49]. Based on a plethora of studies it is widely accepted that increased dopamine transmission is necessary for the establishment of CPP [54]. Although some authors suggest that CPP is a model of drug-seeking behaviour (or drug craving), being essentially dependent upon Pavlovian associations, CPP alone cannot account for the instrumental nature of drug-seeking and drug-taking behaviour, which is perhaps better modelled by drug self-administration procedures.

Drug Self-Administration Models

Drug self-administration procedures lie at the core of the most sophisticated preclinical models of drug addiction that have been developed over the last 20 years, ranging from relapse to drug taking [22, 55], to loss of control over intake [34] and compulsive drug taking [37, 39, 40] (see "Transition from Controlled to Pathological Drug-Seeking and Drug-Taking Behaviour" section).

Addictive drugs act as reinforcers, in that they increase the probability of a behavioural response that leads to their presentation, through instrumental conditioning. Thus, animals can readily detect the contingency between an instrumental response and the delivery of a particular drug (e.g. an intravenous infusion of heroin, cocaine, nicotine or THC or a small volume of alcohol in a magazine) and respond in an instrumental manner to obtain such drugs. The acquisition of drug self-administration is a behavioural marker of its reinforcing properties[1] and abuse liability [44]. Indeed, apart from LSD, all drugs abused by humans are self-administered by animals.

Drugs of abuse can be self-administered by a variety of routes across preclinical models, including intramuscular, intranasal, oral and intravenous [56]. Drug self-administration was initially developed in non-human primates; however since the pioneering work of Weeks [10], rats have extensively been used to investigate the psychological, neural and cellular mechanisms underlying drug self-administration.

Self-administration procedures can be arranged according to different schedules of reinforcement. In fixed ratio schedules, the drug is delivered after the completion of a fixed number of responses by the animal, thereby providing a direct relationship between the actual response and drug delivery. By contrast, in fixed interval schedules, the animal is trained to seek the drug for prolonged periods of time under the control of contingent presentations of drug-associated stimuli. Different schedules allow for the investigation of different processes of drug-taking or drug-seeking behaviour which are beyond the scope of this chapter. However, insightful descriptions of, and discussions about, these schedules can be found in [47, 56–59].

The acquisition of psychostimulant self-administration is widely considered to depend on the functional integrity of the olfactory tubercle and the shell of the nucleus accumbens [5]. An important role for mesolimbic dopamine in this process was inferred by findings in freely moving rats that dopamine concentration is greatly increased in the striatum, and especially the nucleus accumbens, following the self-administration of drugs commonly abused by humans [60]. This important study supported the influential hypothesis at that time that addictive drugs exert their primary reinforcing effects and addictive properties through activation of the mesolimbic dopamine system [61–63]. Although it is now clear that increased dopamine release in the nucleus accumbens does not provide a sufficient account for the addictive properties of drugs such as cocaine, alcohol and heroin, dopamine still remains one of the most important neurotransmitters in the aetiology of drug addiction, a role underscored by its proposed involvement in salience detection and learning [5, 64–73].

---

[1] A positive reinforcer is a stimulus that increases the probability of a behaviour which results in the presentation of the stimulus. Thus, addictive drugs act as positive reinforcers, supporting instrumental responses over prolonged periods of time.

In its classic form the drug self-administration paradigm has provided valuable insights into the brain substrates mediating drug-taking behaviour, which differ somewhat according to the particular drug under investigation [19, 20, 74]. Addictive drugs not only influence the function of the mesolimbic dopamine system [60] but they also trigger a variety of between-systems neuroadaptations and changes in gene transcription and function in a number of brain systems [75–78], including the nucleus accumbens [79, 80], dorsal striatum [81] and prefrontal cortex [79], with important effects on stress responsivity [44, 82–84] and epigenetic processes in the limbic system [85–88].

When one considers working on drug addiction one has to keep in mind that studying drug taking behaviour is not a way of studying drug addiction. Indeed, as already stated by Wise and Bozart [89] and quoted by Robinson and Berridge [90]: "To assert that all addictive drugs are reinforcers is to do little more than redefine the phenomenon of addiction." … "To identify a drug as reinforcing goes no further than to identify the drug as addicting"; indeed, there is an obvious gulf between taking a drug on a social basis, as most of us often do, at least when one considers a glass of wine, and compulsively taking drugs. Thus, animal models of this complex disorder have evolved in recent years to distinguish between the ability of most, if not all, addictive drugs, to support self-administration and the development of dependence and compulsive forms of drug taking, which apparently only occurs in a small subset of the population [91].

Psychomotor Sensitisation

Behavioural sensitisation is a long-lasting adaptive response to psychostimulants, opiates and other classes of drugs [90] characterised by an increased locomotor response to the same dose of a given drug after repeated intermittent injections. Behavioural sensitisation forms the basis of a prominent theory of drug addiction, namely incentive sensitisation [90].

Formally described by Segal and colleagues [92], behavioural sensitisation has been well characterised for opiates, PCP and other drugs of abuse [90]. Interestingly, behavioural sensitisation facilitates the acquisition of low-dose amphetamine self-administration [93] and CPP [94, 95], as well as the escalation of cocaine self-administration, [96]. These findings indicate that sensitisation not only increases the motivational properties of addictive drugs but also facilitates loss of control over drug intake, a hallmark of drug addiction.

At the neurophysiological level, repeated exposure to psychostimulants induces a neurochemical sensitisation of the dopaminergic system, characterised by a progressive enhancement of drug-induced dopamine release after repeated exposure to the same dose of cocaine or amphetamine [97–101]. This long-lasting neuroadaptation has been reported to be measurable in cocaine addicts [102] and is associated with an increased behavioural response to drug challenge which in turn correlates with cellular and molecular adaptations in the nucleus accumbens [98, 103].

The sensitised dopamine response to psychostimulant administration has been suggested to contribute to the narrowing of the behavioural repertoire of drug addicts who focus on drug-seeking and drug-taking behaviours at the expense of other sources of reward. Thus, superimposed on the decreased basal dopamine levels in the striatum that accompanies withdrawal from stimulants [44], a sensitised dopamine response to the drug may ultimately become an important mechanism enabling an optimal level of reinforcement in the brain, thereby providing stimulant, and perhaps other, addictive drugs with the ability to increase dopamine transmission sufficiently to maintain drug-seeking behaviour [6].

At the psychological level, behavioural sensitisation has been suggested to reflect maladaptive learning mechanisms, whereby repeated exposure to psychostimulants impacts upon Pavlovian incentive mechanisms dependent upon the ventral striatum, leading to increased incentive properties of drug-associated stimuli and pathological "wanting", as distinct from other subjective states such as drug "liking" [3, 90, 104–106].

Sensitisation of the dopaminergic system has strongly been argued to play a role in the pathophysiology of psychostimulant addiction [3, 90], but the nature of the psychological processes affected by this neuroadaptation is still a matter of debate. The "incentive sensitisation" theory emphasises Pavlovian mechanisms that influence motivational states, potentially via Pavlovian-instrumental transfer (PIT) effects, suggested to be one manifestation of drug "wanting" [107]. However, amphetamine or cocaine sensitisation also facilitate the development of habitual responding for food [108, 109], thus indicating that behavioural sensitisation may also reflect adaptations within the cortico-dorsal striatal circuitry that controls instrumental performance [45, 66]. Additionally, the demonstration that repeated cocaine exposure fails to induce behavioural sensitisation in Pitx3-deficient mice lacking a nigrostriatal pathway [110] suggests that the dorsal striatum, the locus of stimulus–response learning mechanisms [111, 112], may be an important substrate for the establishment of a neurobiological process that has been considered previously to mainly involve the ventral striatum.

Transition from Controlled to Pathological Drug Intake

During the last 10 years, pre-clinical research in drug addiction has attempted to better integrate one or more clinical features of drug addiction according to the DSM-IV diagnostic criteria. New phenotypes have been identified based on a loss of control over drug taking [34], reinstatement [113] or relapse to drug seeking [114], compulsive cocaine seeking and taking [38, 40], and individual vulnerability to drug addiction [36–38].

Craving and Relapse

Drug addicts show a high propensity to relapse, even after protracted abstinence [115]. This hallmark feature of addiction can be modelled in animals using two main procedures: extinction–reinstatement and abstinence–relapse. Reinstatement of responding for drug can be induced by stress, low doses of the drug itself and by the presentation of drug-associated cues [55, 113, 116–118]. In the extinction-reinstatement procedure [22, 119], animals experience a series of extinction sessions following a short period of drug self-administration, leading to a progressive decline in responding. Following extinction, responding for drug is reinstated by a stressful stimulus, a priming injection of drug injection, presentation of a conditioned stimulus (CS) or by placing the animal in a drug-associated environment. In the abstinence-relapse procedure [120], animals are given a forced abstinence period after a brief period of drug self-administration. They are then maintained in their home cage until they are exposed again to the self-administration chamber where they are tested under extinction.

Escalation of Drug Taking

The first well-established animal model of loss of control over drug intake, namely escalation of drug self-administration, is based on the fourth diagnostic criterion of drug addiction and was developed by Serge Ahmed and George Koob in 1998 [34]. Short access ("ShA") to addictive drugs generally results in stable levels of self-administration such that plasma drug levels are controlled within an optimal level of reinforcement. As mentioned previously, this pattern of self-administration does not account for the clinical features of drug addiction in humans. Ahmed and Koob thus gave extended access to cocaine to a group of animals ("LgA", or long access) following a period of moderate exposure (ShA, fixed ratio 1, one hour a day). A second group of rats received short access to cocaine throughout the experiment.

Introduction of the long access was immediately associated with higher drug intake, as compared to ShA rats. In other words, the LgA rats escalating their rate of cocaine self-administration compared with ShA rats, which maintained a constant level of cocaine intake. LgA rats also exhibited higher rates of cocaine self-administration during the first hour of each session associated with the initial loading phase. Escalation has also been reported for heroin [121] and has been associated with an upward shift in the intra-cranial

self-administration threshold (ICSS), indicative of reward dysfunction [34]. Interestingly, escalation of cocaine self-administration is not associated with psychomotor sensitisation but, instead, with a sensitisation of the incentive motivational properties of cocaine [122], thereby suggesting a dissociation between addiction-like behaviour and behavioural sensitisation. Escalation of drug intake has been associated with higher resistance to shock-induced suppression of drug self-administration and conditioned suppression [39, 40], and is suggested to be an important contributing factor to the subsequent development of compulsive or habitual forms of drug seeking and taking (see below).

Second-Order Schedules of Drug Reinforcement

Second-order schedules of cocaine and heroin self-administration were initially developed by Goldberg and colleagues in non-human primates to assess the influence of environmental stimuli on drug self-administration [57, 123, 124]. In second-order schedules of reinforcement, the conditioned stimulus (CS) is presented response-contingently under a fixed ratio schedule, during an overall fixed interval or fixed ratio schedule for the primary reinforcer. The effect of CS presentation is often dramatic, increasing as it does responding under a second-order schedule of reinforcement for long periods of time. Under such a schedule of reinforcement, a strong contingency exists between the instrumental response (controlled by a fixed ratio) and the presentation of the CS that completely overshadows the relatively weak contingency that is arranged between the instrumental performance and the outcome (the drug) that is reinforced only after completion of the first ratio after each interval has elapsed. Such schedules therefore facilitate the instantiation of stimulus–response control over instrumental response which is separable from the drug itself. In addition, it has been shown that omission of CS presentation in second-order schedules of reinforcement disrupts cocaine seeking more than food-seeking behaviour [125], suggesting that prolonged psychostimulant seeking is particularly dependent upon conditioned reinforcement. Thus, instrumental responding during the first interval of a second-order schedule of reinforcement shows face and construct validity with respect to drug seeking in humans, which is strongly stimulus bound and seemingly dissociated from the unconditioned effects of the drug [126].

The establishment of a second-order schedule of reinforcement is described by Arroyo and colleagues [127]. Rats were initially trained to self-administer cocaine under a continuous schedule of reinforcement (i.e. FR1). After stabilisation of responding (5–7 daily 2 h sessions), a second-order schedule with fixed ratio components of the type $FR_x(FR_y:S)$ was introduced, with initial values of x and y set to 1, so that each active lever press resulted in the presentation of the CS and the delivery of 0.25 mg of cocaine. Then x and y values were progressively increased with increments in response requirements starting with x, i.e. FR5(FR1:S) and FR10(FR1:S), then y, i.e. FR10(FR2:S), FR10(FR4:S), FR10(FR7:S) and FR10(FR10:S). After stabilisation of responding under this FR10(FR10:S) schedule that requires 100 active lever presses and 10 one second presentations of the CS to obtain a cocaine infusion, a final fixed interval schedule FI15(FR10:S) was introduced such that a cocaine infusion was delivered only following the tenth active lever press that occurred when the 15-min interval had elapsed. Finally, rats were allowed to perform cocaine-seeking behaviour under this schedule for ten days. This acquisition procedure produced robust and stable contingent CS-dependent rates of responding under a second-order schedule of reinforcement [127] and has been used extensively to probe the neural mechanisms involved in the acquisition and performance of cue-controlled cocaine seeking [128–131].

Some recent refinements have been made to the establishment of a second-order schedule of drug reinforcement. For example, in a study by Lee et al. [132] it was shown the acquisition period can be reduced to just 11 days. In this case, the training phase consisted of three days of FR1 training, 2 h daily sessions, 30 infusions (0.25 mg cocaine/infusion) followed by the introduction of interval schedules, with daily increments: FI 1 min, FI 2 min, FI 4 min, FI 8 min, FI 10 min, FI 15 min. After three days of training under the FI15 schedule, contingent presentations of the CS were introduced under a FR10 schedule such that rats now trained under a FI15(FR10:S) second-order schedule of reinforcement. This acquisition procedure provides a direct measure of the potentiation of responding during interval schedules by the contingent presentation of the CS since they are introduced only when responding under a fixed interval schedule had stabilised. Thus, although the average response rate is 50–70 during the first interval of a FI 15 schedule, it reaches 150–200 when the CS is contingently presented, as described by Belin and Everitt in a study addressing intra-striatal mechanisms involved in habitual cocaine seeking [128]. Indeed, short- and long-term training under second-order schedules of reinforcement for cocaine have been critical tools for the establishment of the neural mechanisms involved in the transition from newly acquired to well established or habitual cue-controlled cocaine seeking.

Cue-Controlled Cocaine Seeking

The acquisition of cue-controlled cocaine seeking depends upon the basolateral nucleus of the amygdala (BLA) [133–135], the AcbC [130, 136] and orbitofrontal cortex [137, 138]. Performance of cue-controlled cocaine seeking depends upon the VTA [139] and interactions between the BLA and AcbC [136]. In addition, the nucleus accumbens

shell mediates the dopamine-dependent potentiating effects of cocaine over cue-controlled cocaine seeking [130]. When cue-controlled cocaine seeking becomes well established, or habitual, i.e. after several weeks of training under a FI second-order schedule of reinforcement, contingent presentations of CSs increase extracellular dopamine concentration in the dorsolateral striatum (DLS) but not in the AcbC or in the AcbS [129]. Moreover, bilateral dopamine receptor blockade in the DLS selectively reduces cocaine-seeking habits in rats [128, 131].

Therefore, the acquisition and maintenance of cue-controlled cocaine seeking involves an apparent shift in the locus of control from the nucleus accumbens to the dorsolateral striatum, which, we have hypothesised, reflects the development of habitual drug seeking [5, 45]. We have established that this progressive ventral to dorsal striatum shift depends upon intra-striatal and serial dopamine-dependent connectivity, linking the AcbC to the DLS [140–142], that has been proposed to be an anatomical substrate for integrative mechanisms linking incentive motivation to cognitive processes [140, 141]. We have recently demonstrated that disconnecting the AcbC and impairing dopamine transmission in the DLS impairs habitual cue-controlled cocaine seeking to the same extent as bilateral dopamine receptor blockade in the DLS alone [128]. This asymmetric manipulation does not impair general operant responding when instrumental performance for either a natural reward or cocaine is still under instrumental goal-directed control (Belin D., Besson M. and Everitt B.J., unpublished observations). Based on this evidence we speculate that after extended training under the second order of cocaine reinforcement, cocaine seeking becomes established as an incentive habit whereby the Pavlovian incentive influences exerted by the BLA over the AcbC, eventually in turn, enable control to be subsumed by dopamine-dependent habit mechanisms in the dorsal striatum.

Although incentive habits may play an important role in the pathophysiology of drug addiction, they do not account for the different behavioural aspects of the pathology, and especially compulsive drug use, i.e. maintained drug use despite adverse consequences, which is a hallmark of drug addiction [143]. Only recently have preclinical models of compulsive drug self-administration been developed, based on the premise that compulsive drug seeking or taking can be operationalised as persistent instrumental responding despite aversive consequences such as punishment and which only emerges after extended drug access.

Compulsive Drug Taking

A hallmark feature of drug addiction is the development of compulsive drug use defined as the continuing abuse of drugs despite negative or adverse consequences. To establish whether cocaine seeking devolves eventually to a compulsive habit, Vanderschuren and Everitt [40] developed a method to evaluate whether animals would continue to seek drug (in this case cocaine) in the presence of an aversive stimulus (i.e. a stimulus previously associated with mild electric foot shock). Animals were trained under a "seeking-taking heterogeneous chain of reinforcement such that responses on one lever—the 'seeking' lever"—enabled access to a drug "taking" lever. When compulsive drug seeking was assessed, the aversive stimulus was presented during drug-seeking sequences. It was found that cocaine seeking was suppressed following short access to cocaine by not following protracted access to cocaine.

This procedure was recently adapted by Pelloux and colleagues [39], who introduced a contingent punishment schedule of the seeking responses to measure compulsive cocaine seeking. When compulsive drug seeking was assessed in this study, 50% of the responses on the seeking lever resulted in the presentation of mild electric foot-shock; the remaining responses resulted in the presentation of the taking lever. This study demonstrated important individual differences in the development of resistance to punishment, confirming that only a small subgroup of rats exposed to extended access to cocaine develop compulsive drug seeking.

Animal Models of Addiction-Like Behaviour

There are two main strategies when developing preclinical models of drug addiction. The first category refers to models developed to understand the psychobiological, neurological, cellular and molecular processes involved in a particular aspect of the pathology. Therefore, these models specifically address one aspect of the pathology, whether a diagnostic criterion, such as escalation of intake, resistance to punishment, high motivation for the drug, habitual instrumental performance, vulnerability to relapse or impaired cognitive flexibility. They may also be relevant to influential theories such as behavioural sensitisation [3, 71, 90, 104] and hedonic allostasis [82, 83]. Such models generally assume that drug exposure triggers rather similar behavioural, neural or molecular effects in all the subjects tested. The animal models of habitual or compulsive drug seeking we have discussed so far are good illustrations of this strategy. Nevertheless, it is likely that the best example of such animal models remains the escalation model [34, 35].

However, these models cannot address other aspects of drug addiction, such as *inter-individual* differences in the vulnerability to develop the pathology and their behavioural and biological correlates. They also fail to capture the multi-symptomatic nature of drug addiction. Thus, the second category of animal models of drug addiction takes into account both inter-individual differences and the complementary strategy of meeting diagnostic criteria of the pathology in humans according to the DSM-IV. Thus, to be diagnosed as "addicted" an individual must fulfil three out of seven diagnostic criteria of drug abuse over the last 12 months. This clinical judgement forms the basis of a new pre-clinical animal model based on vulnerability to addiction-like behaviour in the rat [36, 37].

In this model, three diagnostic criteria, namely (1) an inability to refrain from drug seeking, (2) high motivation for the drug and (3) maintained drug use despite negative consequences, have been operationalised by, respectively, (1) drug seeking during periods when the drug is not available and signalled as such, (2) break points during progressive ratio schedules of reinforcement and (3) persistence of self-administration despite punishment by contingent electric foot-shocks. For each of these three addiction-like criteria animals are ranked according to their score. If a rat's score is included in the 40% highest percentile of the distribution, this rat is considered positive for that addiction-like criterion and is given an arbitrary criterion score of 1. Then the arbitrary criteria scores for each of the three addiction-like criteria are added, and consequently four distinct groups are identified according to the number of positive scores: 0 criteria, 1 criterion, 2 criteria and 3 criteria rats (Fig. 6.1a–c).

This model is based on the comparison of three criteria and 0 criteria rats. 3 criteria rats show high scores for each of the three addiction-like criteria and are therefore considered "addicted", whereas 0 criteria rats are considered resistant to addiction. 3 criteria rats represent approximately 20% of the population exposed to cocaine (Fig. 6.1d), an a percentage remarkably similar to that reported in humans [91]. Although 3 criteria rats do not differ significantly from 0 criteria rats in terms of initial rates of cocaine self-administration (Fig. 6.1e) [38], 3 criteria rats eventually develop higher motivation for the drug, an inability to refrain from drug seeking, and resistance to punishment [36–38]. They also show escalation of cocaine self-administration when given long access exposure to the drug (Fig. 6.1f) and therefore fulfil a fourth criterion of addiction, namely an inability to control drug intake [38]. 3 criteria rats also show a high vulnerability to relapse in response to non-contingent infusions of cocaine (Fig. 6.1g) or contingent presentations of a drug-associated stimulus [36]. Thus, even though selected on three addiction-like criteria, after chronic exposure to cocaine, 3 criteria rats display important features of clinical addiction as defined in the DSM-IV. Moreover, since addiction-like behaviour emerges in 3 criteria rats only after extended exposure to the drug, these results highlight the importance of the *interaction* between a vulnerable phenotype and chronic drug exposure in the development of compulsive drug self-administration.

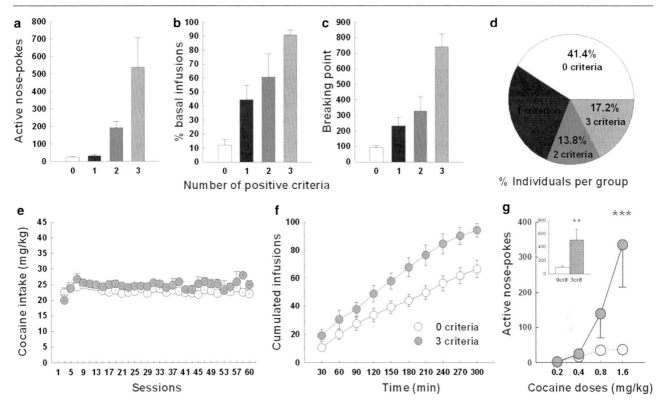

Fig. 6.1 Addiction-like behaviour in the rat. A modelling approach for the investigation of addiction-like behaviour in the rat. A key feature of this model is that some, but not all animals chronically exposed to drug self-administration eventually develop one of more behavioural features resembling clinical drug addiction as defined in the DSM-IV. Thus, we have operationally defined three addiction-like criteria, namely, (1) an inability to refrain from drug seeking (**a**), (2) maintained drug use despite aversive consequences (**b**) and (3) increased motivation to take the drug (**c**). Rats showing none of these criteria ("0 criteria" rats) are resistant to addiction whereas rats that show all three criteria ("3 criteria" rats) are considered "addicted", and represent 15–20% of the population initially exposed to cocaine (**d**). Importantly, these behavioural differences are not due to differential rates of cocaine self-administration (**e**). However, when provided with longer access to cocaine 3crit rats exhibit an inability to limit drug intake (**f**) and a higher vulnerability for relapse, as measured by reinstatement of cocaine-seeking behaviour induced by the non-contingent administration of cocaine (**g**). (**a–e**) after Deroche-Gamonet, Belin and Piazza 2004, (**f–g**) after Belin, Balado, Piazza and Deroche-Gamonet 2009

Vulnerability to Drug Addiction

Like many other psychiatric disorders, we are not all equally vulnerable to develop drug addiction. Epidemiological studies have revealed that between 15 and 35% of the population exposed to addictive drugs will develop compulsive drug use [91]. The results described in the previous section illustrate very well that inter-individual differences in vulnerability to develop compulsive cocaine self-administration can also be observed in rats. Thus, in any given population of rats exposed to cocaine only some develop addiction-like behaviour, thereby demonstrating that animal models provide a realistic estimate of risk for addiction in humans. The underlying aetiology of the different pathways to addiction is likely to involve interactions between a vulnerable phenotype, environmental influences and, of course, drug exposure itself (Fig. 6.2) [8, 148]. Epidemiological studies in human populations have revealed striking associations

between drug use [149, 150] and certain behavioural traits [151–166], such as anxiety [167–171], impulsivity [155, 172, 173] and sensation seeking [158, 166, 174–177]. The relevance of these traits for animal models of addiction is discussed below.

Anxiety

Anxiety can be assessed in preclinical models using various procedures which include the elevated plus maze (EPM) [178, 179]. During the classic 5-min test session on the EPM, a variety of behaviours are measured including the ratio of open and closed arms entries, time spent in the open and closed arms as well as self-grooming which are all indices of anxiety. High levels of anxiety including high grooming behaviour and a low percentage of time spent in the open arms of the EPM have been associated with an enhanced

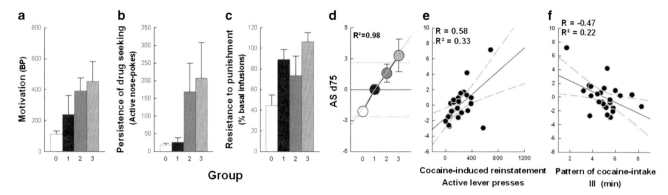

Fig. 6.2 Predictive markers of the vulnerability to shift from controlled to compulsive cocaine self-administration. The identification of behavioural vulnerability markers underlying the switch from controlled to compulsive drug use holds the key to understanding the progressive development of drug addiction in susceptible individuals and thus in developing novel therapies. For this purpose we have established an addiction severity index in rats (AS) (**d**) that takes into account the quantitative severity of each of the addiction-like criteria (see main text and [36] for more details). Based on this analysis 0 criteria rats show negative scores, thereby illustrating their resistance to addiction whereas 3 criteria rats show high addiction severity scores that exceed one standard deviation of the sampling distribution. The AS may reflect the addiction severity index in humans [144–147] and carry utility in dimensional analyses to investigate relationships between addiction-like behaviour and potential predictive markers. The AS also predicts cocaine-induced reinstatement, a putative measure of craving (**e**) and binge-like cocaine self-administration (**f**) [36]

propensity to acquire cocaine CPP [180] as well as an increased motivation to self-administer cocaine [181], but see [182]. Trait anxiety has also been associated with an enhanced preference for alcohol [183, 184], consistent with the notion that alcohol use may self-medicate underlying mood disorders related to anxiety and stress [185, 186].

Sensation Seeking/Novelty Seeking

Sensation- and novelty-seeking traits have been the focus of a large number of pre-clinical studies on addiction vulnerability (for review, see [187]). The pioneering work of Piazza and colleagues was the first to investigate the role of sensation seeking in this context by measuring the locomotor response of rats to an inescapable novel environment [93]. In this model, rats are placed for 2 h in a new environment and their horizontal activity is monitored. Based on inter-individual differences in locomotor response animals are either selected as high (HR) or low responders (LR) according to a median division [93]. HR rats show a greater propensity to acquire psychostimulant self-administration [93] since they more readily self-administer low doses of amphetamine than LR rats [37, 93]. Moreover, HR rats are more vulnerable to the induction of behavioural sensitisation produced by repeated injections of amphetamine than LR rats. They also show a greater propensity for drug-induced neural plasticity [188] and increased stress-evoked dopamine release in the nucleus accumbens [189].

However, sensation seeking does not predict the acquisition of CPP for addictive drugs, which instead is predicted by novelty seeking [49, 187, 190], a behavioural trait which is dissociable from sensation seeking [48, 191]. Novelty seeking

is normally assessed by measuring the preference of rats for a novel versus familiar compartment using a procedure quite similar to CPP [192]. Animals selected as novelty seekers are those that fall in the upper quartile range. Unlike animals selected from the lower quartile of the population, high novel seekers readily develop a CPP to amphetamine [193].

At the neurobiological level, novelty-seeking behaviour has been shown to depend on dopamine receptor function. Thus, novelty preference is blocked by the dopamine receptor antagonist haloperidol [192] and by the selective dopamine D1 receptor antagonist SCH23390 [194]. Additionally, studies in humans have revealed that high sensation/novelty seekers, as assessed using the Zuckerman sensation seeking scale [195, 196], have lower platelet monoamine oxidase levels than low novelty seekers, suggested that other monoamines, in addition to dopamine, may underlie inter-individual differences in novelty seeking [197].

Impulsivity

A popular paradigm used to assess impulsivity in rodents is the 5-choice serial reaction time task (5-CSRTT), which was developed originally as an analogue of the human continuous performance task of sustained attention [198]. The 5-CSRTT requires animals to detect brief flashes of light presented pseudo-randomly in one of five holes and to make a nose-poke response in the correct spatial location in order to receive a food reward. The rat is thus required to monitor a horizontal array of apertures and to withhold from responding until the onset of the stimulus. Generally, the accuracy of stimulus discrimination provides an index of attentional capacity, while premature responses—made before the presentation of the stimulus—are regarded as a form of impulsive behaviour and hence a failure in impulse control [199, 200]. The neural and neurochemical basis of impulsivity on the 5-CSRTT has been extensively investigated, involving important contributions from the anterior cingulate cortex, infralimbic cortex, nucleus accumbens, medial striatum and by the ascending monoaminergic systems [201, 202]. More recently, the 5-CSRTT has been used to screen for spontaneously high levels of impulsivity in rats, a phenotype associated with increased cocaine and nicotine self-administration [203, 204] and an increased propensity to develop compulsive cocaine seeking and taking [37]. Interestingly, we have shown using microPET brain imaging that high impulsive rats have lower dopamine D2/3-binding levels in the ventral striatum as compared to low impulsive littermates [203], thereby suggesting that alteration of dopamine D2/3 receptors in the nucleus accumbens may contribute to high impulsivity and vulnerability to drug addiction (Figs. 6.3 and 6.4).

Predicting the Switch from Controlled to Compulsive Drug Use

We have used the animal model of addiction-like behaviour described in previous sections to investigate potential behavioural markers of vulnerability to develop compulsive cocaine taking behaviour. For this we have developed an

"addiction severity scale" in rats [36, 37], which we suggest corresponds to the addiction severity index in human addicts [144–147, 170, 207]. This "addiction severity scale" allows for simple dimensional studies such as correlation

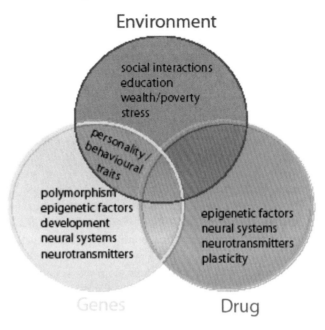

Fig. 6.3 Triad of influences underlying vulnerability to drug addiction. A number of interacting influences are hypothesised to influence the pathway to addiction, including biological determinants (genes), drug exposure and the environment. Genetic influences may account for up to 40% of the vulnerability for drug addiction (for review see [44])

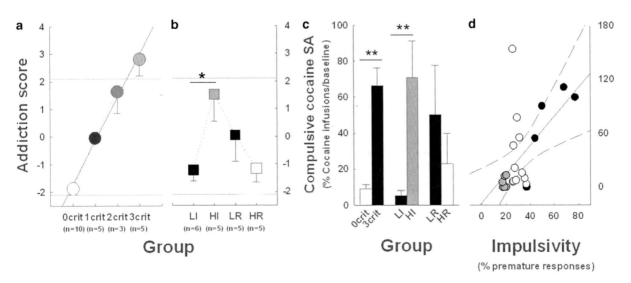

Fig. 6.4 A shift occurs from impulsivity to compulsivity in the development of addiction. High impulsivity can be assessed using the 5-choice serial reaction time test, a sustained visual attentional test in which subjects are required to wait for a visual stimulus before making a response. The selection of high impulsive rats on this task is based on the performance of well-trained rats on three challenge sessions comprising a longer waiting interval before the onset of the trigger stimulus [37, 203, 205]. A small proportion of rats (<30%) display high level of

premature responses (i.e. they respond before the stimulus) and are thereby deemed to be high impulsive (HI). We have demonstrated that after protracted cocaine self-administration (**a**) HI rats displayed higher addiction scores than low impulsive (LI) rats [93]). HI rats also develop compulsive cocaine self-administration unlike rats exhibiting high and low levels of locomotor activity in a novel environment (HR and LR phenotypes, [93, 206]) (**b**). Moreover, at the population level, impulsivity predicts compulsive cocaine self-administration ($R = 0.42$)

and regression, and is therefore a useful tool to address predictive factors in compulsive drug use.

Although differential drug exposure is not necessary for the development of addiction-like behaviour, we have identified that the early pattern of cocaine self-administration (measured by inter-infusion intervals), and sensitivity to the incentive properties of cocaine (measured as sensitivity to cocaine-induced reinstatement [208]), predict the subsequent development and severity of addiction-like behaviour. Thus, 3 criteria rats develop two important features of cocaine addiction [209, 210] soon after the initiation of cocaine self-administration, namely a "binge-like" pattern of self-administration and increased drug-induced "craving", the latter measured in animal models using the drug-induced reinstatement procedure [113, 122, 211, 212].

We have also established that addiction-like behaviour is predicted by impulsivity [37], but not the locomotor response to novelty, an animal model of sensation seeking [213] related to the vulnerability to acquire drug self-administration [93]. Thus, highly impulsive rats, identified on the basis of their level of premature responses during long inter-trial intervals in the five choice serial reaction time test [199], show much higher scores than low impulsive littermates in the rat addiction severity scale after chronic cocaine self-administration. This difference is attributable to the development of compulsive behaviour in high impulsive rats, since these animals maintain cocaine self-administration despite punishment by contingent mild electric foot shocks [37]. However, high impulsive and low impulsive animals do not differ in their locomotor response to a new environment, nor in their propensity to acquire cocaine self-administration, a behavioural feature that is instead predicted by the high locomotor response to novelty [37, 93].

This evidence suggests that the predisposition to initiate drug use is independent of the vulnerability to shift from controlled to compulsive drug taking, and therefore provides new insights into the various behavioural and psychological factors that influence the pathways to addiction. In particular, the demonstration that the high impulsive trait predicts the shift to compulsive drug taking behaviour is of major interest since a shift from impulse control failure to compulsivity has been suggested to play a major role in the development of drug addiction in humans [82, 83].

Contribution of Animal Models to the Understanding of Drug Addiction

Animal models of drug addiction have proven particularly useful for understanding brain mechanisms associated with vulnerability as well as numerous and complex adaptations that occur in the brain in response to acute or chronic exposure to the drug. Indeed, addictive drugs produce a range of effects on brain structures [76, 85, 86, 88, 214–220] and functions [101, 137, 221–233] which are widely suggested to contribute to the development of addictive states.

Based on this broad set of data animal models of drug addiction have been developed either from a Pavlovian point of view, as it is the case for the incentive sensitisation theory [3, 90, 104, 234] which provides an explanation of the high motivation that addicts have for the drug, an instrumental point of view, as suggested by the habit hypothesis [4, 5, 45, 46, 71], or a negative-reinforcement view as suggested by the hedonic allostatis theory of drug addiction [44, 82–84, 235]. A detailed discussion of these neuropsychobiological theories is beyond the scope of this chapter but a very important notion is that they are far from being exclusive. Thus, one may consider that drug addiction develops as the result of within and between systems adaptations [5, 44], with modulatory effects on positive and negative reinforcement processes and impaired incentive mechanisms. Collectively, these neural and psychological sequelae are widely hypothesised to be exacerbated by drug-induced impairment in top-down executive control [5] (Fig. 6.5).

Treatment with stimulant drugs that sensitise DA transmission also facilitates the development of habits over goal-directed instrumental responses for natural rewards [108, 109], while orally ingested drug rewards such as alcohol and cocaine engage stimulus–response habits more rapidly than do natural reinforcers [238, 239]. Moreover in the course of cocaine self-administration, neurobiological alterations initially restricted to the ventral striatum eventually spread to encompass the dorsal striatum in non-human primates [240, 241]. These data resonate well with the apparent shift from the ventral to the dorsolateral striatum in the locus of control over cocaine seeking under a second-order schedule of reinforcement [128, 131]. Thus, drug-seeking habits progressively come to dominate drug-seeking behaviour and are strongly influenced by Pavlovian incentive mechanisms. Hence in the development of drug addiction, drug seeking may be viewed as an *incentive habit* [45]. Belin and Everitt argue that incentive habits depend at least in part upon serial processing between the BLA, the AcbC and the ascending dopaminergic systems. Incentive habits can be triggered by drug-associated stimuli, withdrawal-associated stimuli or internal states that influence the motivational value of these stimuli. Therefore, by generating an increased incentive value of drug-associated stimuli or a withdrawal (including conditioned withdrawal) induced drive towards drug taking, incentive sensitisation [3, 90, 104–106] and negative affective states [44, 82–84, 235] may play an important role in the establishment and persistence of incentive habits (Fig. 6.5).

However, incentive habits alone cannot account for the compulsive nature of drug addiction (i.e. drug use that persists despite negative consequences) [143]. It is instead

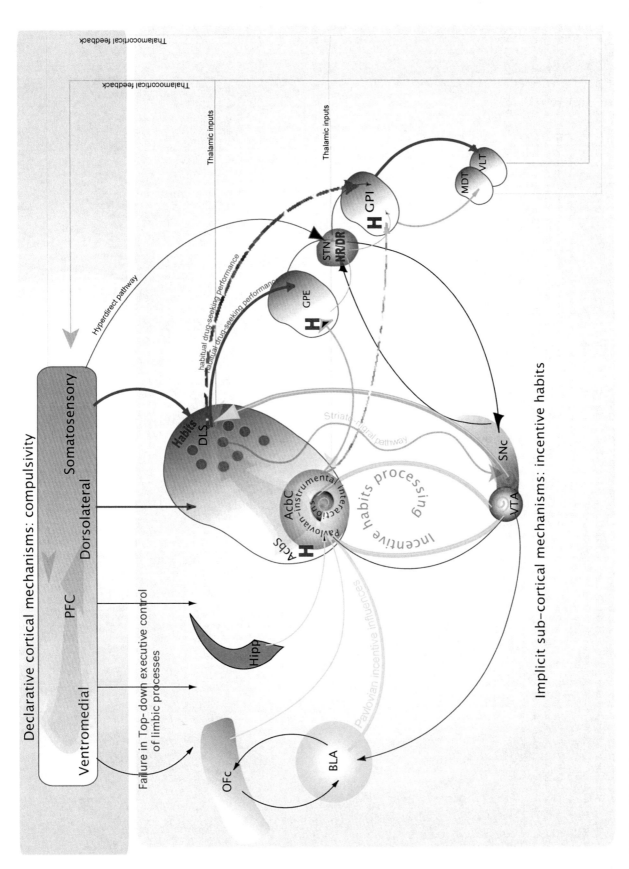

Fig. 6.5 Neurobiological substrates of the development of drug addiction: an incentive habit hypothesis. Simplified schema showing the neural substrates and mechanisms underlying the development and persistence of drug addiction. The reinforcing and possibly hedonic (H) effects of psychostimulants depend upon the shell of the nucleus accumbens (AcbS), the olfactory

Fig. 6.5 (continued) tubercle and the ventral pallidum, whereas the motivational balance between natural and drug rewards (NR/DR) may depend upon the subthalamic nucleus (STN). Exposure to addictive drugs triggers adaptive changes in neural networks involved in implicit sub-cortical and declarative cortical mechanisms. At the subcortical level, addictive drugs alter both Pavlovian and instrumental learning mechanisms. (1) Addictive drugs enhance Pavlovian incentive influences mediated by the basolateral nucleus of the amygdala (BLA) and core of the nucleus accumbens (AcbC) and alter Pavlovian incentive processing between the BLA and the orbitofrontal cortex (OFc) thereby resulting in an increased incentive salience of drugs and environmental stimuli associated with them. Alterations of hippocampal function may also contribute to an enhanced incentive control of contextual cues over drug-seeking and drug-taking behaviour. (2) Addictive drugs also facilitate the instantiation of habitual responding whereby drug-seeking behaviour is no longer under the direct control of the motivational properties of the drug itself, but instead, governed by stimuli in the environment. The development of habitual drug-seeking and drug-taking behaviour may be related to a ventral to dorsal striatal shift in the locus of control over behaviour (), which depends at least in part upon ascending DA-dependent circuitry linking the ventral to the dorsolateral striatum (DLS) via recurrent connections with the dopaminergic neurons in the ventral tegmental area (VTA) and substantia nigra pars compacta (SNc) in the ventral midbrain [141]. Thus, maladaptive, drug-focused Pavlovian incentive processes that control "drug-oriented incentive impulses" in the AcbC eventually influence the dorsal striatum-dependent stimulus–response, or "habit" system, thereby leading to incentive habits. In parallel, exposure to addictive drugs may produce a progressive shift from ventromedial to dorsolateral prefrontal cortex leading to deficiencies in top-down executive control over instrumental behaviour and exemplified by cognitive inflexibility and impaired decision-making [4, 5, 45, 46, 66, 236, 237]. Collectively, these mechanisms encourage the development of incentive habits and compulsive drug use. After Belin and Everitt, Handbook of the Basal Ganglia, 2009 (In Press)

hypothesised that the development of compulsive drug use may reflect a loss of prefrontal executive control over incentive habits that underlie drug seeking and taking [5, 71, 242]. Indeed, repeated exposure to drugs of abuse is associated with cognitive and behavioural deficits related to the PFC including those in visual attention, delay discounting, reversal learning, impulsivity or decision making in both humans [155, 243, 244] and in animal models of addiction [232, 245–251].

Therefore, protracted exposure to addictive drugs may diminish the influence of top-down executive control by the PFC, thereby facilitating the impact of Pavlovian motivational influences on instrumental drug-seeking responses [232, 236, 237, 252]. Additionally, by subverting orbitofrontal-dependent decision-making processes [242, 253], drugs of abuse may bias individual choices towards drugs and diminish sensitivity to negative feedback, thereby promoting compulsive drug seeking [5]. This view is further supported by data in non-human primates self-administering cocaine [254] in which drug-induced neurobiological alterations observed in the ventromedial prefrontal cortex after acute exposure to the drug spread to eventually encompass the dorsolateral prefrontal cortex. Such findings are clearly consistent with parallel alterations in striatal DA function discussed earlier and together likely contribute to the emergence of compulsive drug use.

Conflict of Interest The authors declare they have no competing interests.

Acknowledgements DB is funded by the INSERM, the IREB, the FRM and an INSERM AVENIR Grant, and this work was supported by the IREB. JW Dalley acknowledges support from the UK Medical Research Council. The authors would like to thank Pr Barry J. Everitt for insightful discussions and constructive comments on previous versions of this Ms.

References

1. Leshner AI. Addiction is a brain disease, and it matters. Science. 1997;278:45–7.
2. Leshner AI. Addiction is a brain disease. Issues in Science and Technology 2001;17(3). http://www.issues.org/17.3/leshner.htm.
3. Robinson T, Berridge K. The psychology and neurobiology of addiction: an incentive-sensitization view. Addiction. 2000;95: S91–S117.
4. Everitt BJ, Dickinson A, Robbins TW, The neuropsychological basis of addictive behaviour. Brain Res Rev. 2001;36(2–3): 129–38.
5. Everitt BJ, Robbins TW, Neural systems of reinforcement for drug addiction: from actions to habits to compulsion. Nat Neurosci. 2005;8:1481–9.
6. Goldstein R, Volkow N. Drug addiction and its underlying neurobiological basis: neuroimaging evidence for the involvement of the frontal cortex. Am J Psychiatry. 2002;159(10):1642–52.
7. Volkow N, Fowler J. Addiction, a disease of compulsion and drive: involvement of the orbitofrontal cortex. Cereb Cortex. 2000;10(3):318–25.
8. Kreek M, Laforge K, Butelman E. Pharmacotherapy of addictions. Nat Rev Drug Discov. 2002;1:710–26.
9. Olds J, Milner P. Positive reinforcement produced by electrical stimulation of septal area and other regions of rat brain. J Comp Physiol Psychol. 1954;47:419–27.
10. Weeks JR. Experimental morphine addiction: method for automatic intravenous injections in unrestrained rats. Science. 1962;138(3537):143–4.
11. Kusayama T, Watanabe S. Reinforcing effects of methamphetamine in planarians. Neuroreport. 2000;11:2511–3.
12. Li H, Chaney S, Roberts IJ, Forte M, Hirsh J. Ectopic G-protein expression in dopamine and serotonin neurons blocks cocaine sensitization in Drosophila melanogaster. Curr Biol. 2000;10:211–4.
13. Wolf F, Heberlein U. Invertebrate models of drug abuse. J Neurobiol. 2002;54:161–78.
14. Carney JM, Landrum RW, Cheng MS, Seale TW. Establishment of chronic intravenous drug self-administration in the C57BL/6J mouse. Neuroreport. 1991;2:477–80.
15. Grahame NJ, Phillips TJ, Burkhart-Kasch S, Cunningham CL. Intravenous cocaine self-administration in the C57BL/6J mouse. Pharmacol Biochem Behav. 1995;51:827–34.
16. Highfield DA, Mead AN, Grimm JW, Rocha BA, Shaham Y. Reinstatement of cocaine seeking in 129X1/SvJ mice: effects of cocaine priming, cocaine cues and food deprivation. Psychopharmacology (Berl). 2002;161:417–24.
17. Rocha BA, Scearce-Levie K, Lucas JJ, et al. Increased vulnerability to cocaine in mice lacking the serotonin-1B receptor. Nature. 1998;393:175–8.
18. van der Veen R, Koehl M, Abrous DN, de Kloet ER, Piazza PV, Deroche-Gamonet V. Maternal environment influences cocaine intake in adulthood in a genotype-dependent manner. PLoS ONE. 2008;3:e2245.
19. Ettenberg A, Pettit HO, Bloom FE, Koob GF. Heroin and cocaine intravenous self-administration in rats: mediation by separate neural systems. Psychopharmacology. 1982;78(3):204–9.
20. Pettit HO, Ettenberg A, Bloom FE, Koob GF. Destruction of dopamine in the nucleus accumbens selectively attenuates cocaine but not heroin self-administration in rats. Psychopharmacology (Berl). 1984;84:167–73.
21. Pickens R, Harris WC. Self-administration of d-amphetamine by rats. Psychopharmacologia. 1968;12:158–63.
22. De Wit H, Stewart J. Reinstatement of cocaine-reinforced responding in the rat. Psychopharmacology (Berl). 1981;75:134–43.
23. Risner ME, Goldberg SR. A comparison of nicotine and cocaine self-administration in the dog: fixed-ratio and progressive-ratio schedules of intravenous drug infusion. J Pharmacol Exp Ther. 1983;224:319–26.
24. Deneau G, Yanagita T, Seevers MH. Self-administration of psychoactive substances by the monkey. Psychopharmacologia. 1969;16:30–48.
25. Goldberg SR, Woods JH, Schuster CR. Morphine: conditioned increases in self-administration in rhesus monkeys. Science. 1969;166(3910):1306–7.
26. Kelleher RT, Goldberg SR. Fixed-interval responding under second-order schedules of food presentation or cocaine injection. J Exp Anal Behav. 1977;28:221–31.
27. Hoffmeister F. Progressive-ratio performance in the rhesus monkey maintained by opiate infusions. Psychopharmacology (Berl). 1979;62:181–6.
28. Rowlett JK, Wilcox KM, Woolverton WL. Self-administration of cocaine-heroin combinations by rhesus monkeys: antagonism by naltrexone. J Pharmacol Exp Ther. 1998;286:61–9.
29. Panlilio LV, Goldberg SR, Gilman JP, Jufer R, Cone EJ, Schindler CW. Effects of delivery rate and non-contingent infusion of cocaine on cocaine self-administration in rhesus monkeys. Psychopharmacology (Berl). 1998;137:253–8.

30. Nader MA, Green KL, Luedtke RR, Mach RH. The effects of ben-zamide analogues on cocaine self-administration in rhesus mon-keys. Psychopharmacology (Berl). 1999;147:143–52.

31. Tanda G, Munzar P, Goldberg SR. Self-administration behavior is maintained by the psychoactive ingredient of marijuana in squirrel monkeys. Nat Neurosci. 2000;3:1073–4.

32. Nader M, Morgan D, Gage H, et al. PET imaging of dopamine D2 receptors during chronic cocaine self-administration in monkeys. Nat Neurosci. 2006;9:1050–6.

33. Panlilio LV, Thorndike EB, Schindler CW. Cocaine self-administration under variable-dose schedules in squirrel monkeys. Pharmacol Biochem Behav. 2006;84:235–43.

34. Ahmed SH, Koob G. Transition from moderate to excessive drug intake: change in hedonic set point. Science. 1998;282(5387):298–300.

35. Ahmed SH, Koob G. Long-lasting increase in the set point for cocaine self-administration after escalation in rats. Psychophar-macology. 1999;146(3):303–12.

36. Belin D, Balado E, Piazza PV, Deroche-Gamonet V. Pattern of intake and drug craving predict the development of cocaine addic-tion-like behavior in rats. Biol Psychiatry. 2009;65:863–8.

37. Belin D, Mar A, Dalley JW, Robbins TW, Everitt BJ. High impul-sivity predicts the switch to compulsive cocaine-taking. Science. 2008;320:1352–5.

38. Deroche-Gamonet V, Belin D, Piazza P. Evidence for addiction-like behavior in the rat. Science. 2004;305:1014–7.

39. Pelloux Y, Everitt BJ, Dickinson A. Compulsive drug seeking by rats under punishment: effects of drug taking history. Psychopharmacology (Berl). 2007;194:127–37.

40. Vanderschuren L, Everitt BJ. Drug seeking becomes compulsive after prolonged cocaine self-administration. Science. 2004;305(5686):1017–9.

41. Geyer MA, Markou A, Bloom FE, Kupfer DJ. Animal models in psychatric disorders. Psychoparmacology: the fourth generation of progress. New York: Raven; 1995. p. 787–98.

42. Geyer MA, Markou A, Kenneth LD, Dennis C, Joseph TC, Charles N. The role of preclinical models in the development of psycho-tropic drugs. In: Davis KL, Charney D, Coyle JT, Nemeroff C, editors. Neuropsychopharmacology: the fifth generation of prog-ress. New York: Lippincott Williams and Wilkins; 2002. p. 446–57.

43. Le Moal M. Modèles et psychopathologie Aspects théoriques. Encyclopédie Médico-Chirurgicale (Paris), Psychiatrie 1992; 37-040-C-10.

44. Koob GF, Moal ML. Neurobiology of addiction. London: Academic Press; 2005.

45. Belin D, Jonkman S, Dickinson A, Robbins TW, Everitt BJ. Parallel and interactive learning processes within the basal gan-glia: relevance for the understanding of addiction. Behav Brain Res. 2008;199(1):89–102.

46. Everitt BJ, Belin D, Economidou D, Pelloux Y, Dalley JW, Robbins TW. Review: Neural mechanisms underlying the vulner-ability to develop compulsive drug-seeking habits and addiction. Philos Trans R Soc Lond B Biol Sci. 2008;363(1507):3125–35.

47. Everitt BJ, Robbins TW. Second-order schedules of drug rein-forcement in rats and monkeys: measurement of reinforcing efficacy and drug-seeking behaviour. Psychopharmacology. 2000;153:17–30.

48. Pelloux Y, Costentin J, Duterte-Boucher D. Differential effects of novelty exposure on place preference conditioning to amphet-amine and its oral consumption. Psychopharmacology. 2004; 171:277–85.

49. Bardo M, Bevins RA. Conditioned place preference: what does it add to our preclinical understanding of drug reward? Psychopharmacology (Berl). 2000;153:31–43.

50. Frenois F, Cador M, Caille S, Stinus L, Le Moine C. Neural cor-relates of the motivational and somatic components of naloxone-precipitated morphine withdrawal. Eur J Neurosci. 2002;16: 1377–89.

51. Frenois F, Le Moine C, Cador M. The motivational component of withdrawal in opiate addiction: role of associative learning and aversive memory in opiate addiction from a behavioral, anatomi-cal and functional perspective. Rev Neurosci. 2005;16:255–76.

52. Rossi NA, Reid LD. Affective states associated with morphine injections. Physiol Psychol. 1976;4:269274.

53. Tzschentke TM. Measuring reward with the conditioned place preference (CPP) paradigm: update of the last decade. Addict Biol. 2007;12:227–462.

54. Tzschentke T. Behavioral pharmacology of buprenorphine, with a focus on preclinical models of reward and addiction. Psychopharmacology. 2002;161:1–16.

55. Bossert JM, Ghitza UE, Lu L, Epstein DH, Shaham Y. Neurobiology of relapse to heroin and cocaine seeking: an update and clinical implications. Eur J Pharmacol. 2005;526:36–50.

56. Spealman RD, Goldberg SR. Drug self-administration by labora-tory animals: control by schedules of reinforcement. Annu Rev Pharmacol Toxicol. 1978;18:313–39.

57. Goldberg SR, Kelleher RT, Morse WH. Second-order schedules of drug injection. Fed Proc. 1975;34:1771–6.

58. Schindler CW, Panlilio LV, Goldberg SR. Second-order schedules of drug self-administration in animals. Psychopharmacology (Berl). 2002;163:327–44.

59. Stafford D, LeSage MG, Glowa JR. Progressive-ratio schedules of drug delivery in the analysis of drug self-administration: a review. Psychopharmacology. 1998;139(3):169–84.

60. Di Chiara G, Imperato A. Drugs abused by humans preferentially increase synaptic dopamine concentrations in the mesolimbic system of freely moving rats. Proc Natl Acad Sci USA. 1988;85: 5274–8.

61. Wise RA. The role of reward pathways in the development of drug dependence. Pharmacol Ther. 1987;35:227–63.

62. Wise RA, Bozarth MA. Brain mechanisms of drug reward and euphoria. Psychiatr Med. 1985;3:445–60.

63. Wise RA, Bozarth MA. Brain substrates for reinforcement and drug self-administration. Prog Neuropsychopharmacol. 1981;5:467–74.

64. Berridge KC, Robinson TE, Aldridge JW. Dissecting components of reward: 'liking', 'wanting', and learning. Curr Opin Pharmacol. 2009;9(1):65–73.

65. Berridge KC. The debate over dopamine's role in reward: the case for incentive salience. Psychopharmacology (Berl). 2007;191: 391–431.

66. Everitt BJ, Wolf ME. Psychomotor stimulant addiction: a neural systems perspective. J Neurosci. 2002;22(9):3312–20.

67. Di Chiara G, Tanda G, Bassareo V, et al. Drug addiction as a dis-order of associative learning. Role of nucleus accumbens shell/extended amygdala dopamine. Ann NY Acad Sci. 1999;877: 461–85.

68. Everitt BJ, Parkinson JA, Olmstead CM, Arroyo M, Robledo P, Robbins TW. Associative processes in addiction and reward. The role of amygdala-ventral striatal subsystems. Ann NY Acad Sci. 1999;877:412–38.

69. Hyman SE, Malenka RC, Nestler EJ. Neural mechanisms of addiction: the role of reward-related learning and memory. Annu Rev Neurosci. 2006;29:565–98.

70. Jones S, Bonci A. Synaptic plasticity and drug addiction. Curr Opin Pharmacol. 2005;5:20–5.

71. Robbins TW, Everitt BJ. Drug addiction: bad habits add up. Nature. 1999;398:567–70.

72. Thomas MJ, Kalivas P, Shaham Y. Neuroplasticity in the mesolim-bic dopamine system and cocaine addiction. Br J Pharmacol. 2008;154:327–42.

73. Volkow ND, Fowler JS, Wang GJ, Goldstein RZ. Role of dop-amine, the frontal cortex and memory circuits in drug addiction:

insight from imaging studies. Neurobiol Learn Mem. 2002; 78:610–24.

74. Kelly PH, Roberts DC. Effects of amphetamine and apomorphine on locomotor activity after 6-OHDA and electrolytic lesions of the nucleus accumbens septi. Pharmacol Biochem Behav. 1983; 19:137–43.

75. Robinson T, Kolb B. Alterations in the morphology of dendrites and dendritic spines in the nucleus accumbens and prefrontal cortex following repeated treatment with amphetamine or cocaine. Eur J Neurosci. 1999;11:1598–604.

76. Robinson T, Kolb B. Structural plasticity associated with exposure to drugs of abuse. Neuropharmacology. 2004;47 Suppl 1:33–46.

77. Robinson T, Kolb B. Persistent structural modifications in nucleus accumbens and prefrontal cortex neurons produced by previous experience with amphetamine. J Neurosci. 1997;17:8491–7.

78. Robinson T, Kolb B. Morphine alters the structure of neurons in the nucleus accumbens and neocortex of rats. Synapse. 1999;33:160–2.

79. Kolb B, Gorny G, Li Y, Samaha AN, Robinson T. Amphetamine or cocaine limits the ability of later experience to promote structural plasticity in the neocortex and nucleus accumbens. Proc Natl Acad Sci USA. 2003;100:10523–8.

80. Chang L, Alicata D, Ernst T, Volkow N. Structural and metabolic brain changes in the striatum associated with methamphetamine abuse. Addiction. 2007;102 Suppl 1:16–32.

81. Jedynak J, Uslaner J, Esteban J, Robinson T. Methamphetamine-induced structural plasticity in the dorsal striatum. Eur J Neurosci. 2007;25:847–53.

82. Koob G, Le Moal M. Drug addiction, dysregulation of reward, and allostasis. Neuropsychopharmacology. 2001;24:97–129.

83. Koob G, Le Moal M. Plasticity of reward neurocircuitry and the 'dark side' of drug addiction. Nat Neurosci. 2005;8:1442–4.

84. Koob G, Le Moal M. Addiction and the brain antireward system. Annu Rev Psychol. 2008;59:29–53.

85. Nestler EJ. The neurobiology of cocaine addiction. Sci Pract Perspect. 2005;3:4–10.

86. Nestler EJ. Is there a common molecular pathway for addiction? Nat Neurosci. 2005;8:1445–9.

87. Nestler EJ. Review. Transcriptional mechanisms of addiction: role of DeltaFosB. Philos Trans R Soc Lond B Biol Sci. 2008;363: 3245–55.

88. Nestler EJ. Epigenetic mechanisms in psychiatry. Biol Psychiatry. 2009;65:189–90.

89. Wise RA, Bozarth MA. A psychomotor stimulant theory of addiction. Psychol Rev. 1987;94:469–92.

90. Robinson T, Berridge K. The neural basis of drug craving: an incentive-sensitization theory of addiction. Brain Res Rev. 1993;18(3):247–91.

91. Anthony JC, Warner LA, Kessler RC. Comparative epidemiology of dependence on tobacco, alcohol, controlled substances, and inhalants: basic findings from the National comorbidity Survey. Exp Clin Psychopharmacol. 1994;2(3):244–68.

92. Segal DS, Weinberger SB, Cahill J, McCunney SJ. Multiple daily amphetamine administration: behavioral and neurochemical alterations. Science. 1980;207:904–7.

93. Piazza PV, Deminiere JM, Le Moal M, Simon H. Factors that predict individual vulnerability to amphetamine self-administration. Science. 1989;245:1511–3.

94. Lett BT. Repeated exposures intensify rather than diminish the rewarding effects of amphetamine, morphine, and cocaine. Psychopharmacology (Berl). 1989;98:357–62.

95. Zarrindast MR, Ebrahimi-Ghiri M, Rostami P, Rezayof A. Repeated pre-exposure to morphine into the ventral pallidum enhances morphine-induced place preference: involvement of dopaminergic and opioidergic mechanisms. Behav Brain Res. 2007;181:35–41.

96. Ferrario C, Robinson T. Amphetamine pretreatment accelerates the subsequent escalation of cocaine self-administration behavior. Eur Neuropsychopharmacol. 2007;17:352–7.

97. Belin D, Deroche-Gamonet V, Jaber M. Cocaine-induced sensitization is associated with altered dynamics of transcriptional responses of the dopamine transporter, tyrosine hydroxylase, and dopamine D2 receptors in C57Bl/6 J mice. Psychopharmacology (Berl). 2007;193:567–78.

98. Pierce R, Kalivas P. A circuitry model of the expression of behavioral sensitization to amphetamine-like psychostimulants. Brain Res Rev. 1997;25(2):192–216.

99. Robinson T, Becker JB. Behavioral sensitization is accompanied by an enhancement in amphetamine-stimulated dopamine release from striatal tissue in vitro. Eur J Pharmacol. 1982;85:253–4.

100. Robinson T, Becker JB, Presty SK. Long-term facilitation of amphetamine-induced rotational behavior and striatal dopamine release produced by a single exposure to amphetamine: sex differences. Brain Res. 1982;253:231–41.

101. Robinson T, Jurson PA, Bennett JA, Bentgen KM. Persistent sensitization of dopamine neurotransmission in ventral striatum (nucleus accumbens) produced by prior experience with (+)-amphetamine: a microdialysis study in freely moving rats. Brain Res. 1988;462:211–22.

102. Schlaepfer TE, Pearlson GD, Wong DF, Marenco S, Dannals RF. PET study of competition between intravenous cocaine and [11C] raclopride at dopamine receptors in human subjects. Am J Psychiatry. 1997;154:1209–13.

103. Vanderschuren L, Kalivas P. Alterations in dopaminergic and glutamatergic transmission in the induction and expression of behavioral sensitization: a critical review of preclinical studies. Psychopharmacology. 2000;151(2–3):99–120.

104. Robinson T, Berridge K. Incentive-sensitization and addiction. Addiction. 2001;96:103–14.

105. Robinson TE, Berridge KC. Addiction. Annu Rev Psychol. 2003;54:25–53.

106. Robinson TE, Berridge KC. Review. The incentive sensitization theory of addiction: some current issues. Philos Trans R Soc Lond B Biol Sci. 2008;363:3137–46.

107. Wyvell CL, Berridge K. Incentive sensitization by previous amphetamine exposure: increased cue-triggered "wanting" for sucrose reward. J Neurosci. 2001;21:7831–40.

108. Nelson A, Killcross S. Amphetamine exposure enhances habit formation. J Neurosci. 2006;26:3805–12.

109. Nordquist RE, Voorn P, de Mooij-van Malsen JG, Joosten RN, Pennartz CM, Vanderschuren LJ. Augmented reinforcer value and accelerated habit formation after repeated amphetamine treatment. Eur Neuropsychopharmacol. 2007;17:532–40.

110. Beeler J, Cao Z, Kheirbek M, Zhuang X. Loss of cocaine locomotor response in Pitx3-deficient mice lacking a nigrostriatal pathway. Neuropsychopharmacology. 2008;34(5):1149–61.

111. Yin H, Knowlton B, Balleinc B. Lesions of dorsolateral striatum preserve outcome expectancy but disrupt habit formation in instrumental learning. Eur J Neurosci. 2004;19(1):181–9.

112. Yin H, Knowlton B, Balleine B. Inactivation of dorsolateral striatum enhances sensitivity to changes in the action–outcome contingency in instrumental conditioning. Behav Brain Res. 2006;166:189–96.

113. Shaham Y, Shalev U, Lu L, De Wit H, Stewart J. The reinstatement model of drug relapse: history, methodology and major findings. Psychopharmacology. 2003;168:3–20.

114. Fuchs R. Different neural substrates mediate cocaine seeking after abstinence versus extinction training: a critical role for the dorsolateral caudate-putamen. J Neurosci. 2006;26:3584–8.

115. O'Brien CP. A range of research-based pharmacotherapies for addiction. Science. 1997;278(5335):66–70.

116. Capriles N, Rodaros D, Sorge RE, Stewart J. A role for the prefrontal cortex in stress- and cocaine-induced reinstatement of

cocaine seeking in rats. Psychopharmacology (Berl). 2003; 168:66–74.

117. Fuchs R, Tran-Nguyen LT, Specio SE, Groff RS, Neisewander JL. Predictive validity of the extinction/reinstatement model of drug craving. Psychopharmacology (Berl). 1998;135:151–60.

118. Kalivas P, Mcfarland K. Brain circuitry and the reinstatement of cocaine-seeking behavior. Psychopharmacology (Berl). 2003; 168:44–56.

119. De Wit H, Stewart J. Drug reinstatement of heroin-reinforced responding in the rat. Psychopharmacology (Berl). 1983;79:29–31.

120. See R, Elliott J, Feltenstein M. The role of dorsal vs ventral striatal pathways in cocaine-seeking behavior after prolonged abstinence in rats. Psychopharmacology. 2007;194:321–31.

121. Ahmed SH, Walker JR, Koob G. Persistent increase in the motivation to take heroin in rats with a history of drug escalation. Neuropsychopharmacology. 2000;22(4):413–21.

122. Ahmed S, Cador M. Dissociation of psychomotor sensitization from compulsive cocaine consumption. Neuropsychopharmacology. 2006;31:563–71.

123. Goldberg SR. Comparable behavior maintained under fixed-ratio and second-order schedules of food presentation, cocaine injection or d-amphetamine injection in the squirrel monkey. J Pharmacol Exp Ther. 1973;186:18–30.

124. Goldberg SR, Morse WH, Goldberg DM. Behavior maintained under a second-order schedule by intramuscular injection of morphine or cocaine in rhesus monkeys. J Pharmacol Exp Ther. 1976;199:278–86.

125. Goldberg SR, Kelleher RT, Goldberg DM. Fixed-ratio responding under second-order schedules of food presentation or cocaine injection. J Pharmacol Exp Ther. 1981;218:271–81.

126. Tiffany ST. A cognitive model of drug urges and drug-use behavior: role of automatic and nonautomatic processes. Psychol Rev. 1990;97:147–68.

127. Arroyo M, Markou A, Robbins TW, Everitt BJ. Acquisition, maintenance and reinstatement of intravenous cocaine self-administration under a second-order schedule of reinforcement in rats: effects of conditioned cues and continuous access to cocaine. Psychopharmacology (Berl). 1998;140:331–44.

128. Belin D, Everitt BJ. Cocaine-seeking habits depend upon dopamine-dependent serial connectivity linking the ventral with the dorsal striatum. Neuron. 2008;57:432–41.

129. Ito R, Dalley JW, Robbins TW, Everitt BJ. Dopamine release in the dorsal striatum during cocaine-seeking behavior under the control of a drug-associated cue. J Neurosci. 2002;22:6247–53.

130. Ito R, Robbins TW, Everitt BJ. Differential control over cocaine-seeking behavior by nucleus accumbens core and shell. Nat Neurosci. 2004;7:389–97.

131. Vanderschuren L. Involvement of the dorsal striatum in cue-controlled cocaine seeking. J Neurosci. 2005;25:8665–70.

132. Lee J. Reconsolidation and extinction of conditioned fear: inhibition and potentiation. J Neurosci. 2006;26:10051–6.

133. Burns LH, Robbins T, Everitt B. Differential effects of excitotoxic lesions of the basolateral amygdala, ventral subiculum and medial prefrontal cortex on responding with conditioned reinforcement and locomotor activity potentiated by intra-accumbens infusions of D-amphetamine. Behav Brain Res. 1993;55:167–83.

134. Cador M, Robbins TW, Everitt BJ. Involvement of the amygdala in stimulus-reward associations: interaction with the ventral striatum. Neuroscience. 1989;30(1):77–86.

135. Everitt BJ, Cador M, Robbins TW. Interactions between the amygdala and ventral striatum in stimulus-reward associations: studies using a second-order schedule of sexual reinforcement. Neuroscience. 1989;30:63–75.

136. Di Ciano P. Direct interactions between the basolateral amygdala and nucleus accumbens core underlie cocaine-seeking behavior by rats. J Neurosci. 2004;24:7167–73.

137. Everitt BJ, Hutcheson D, Ersche K, Pelloux Y, Dalley JW, Robbins TW. The orbital prefrontal cortex and drug addiction in laboratory animals and humans. Ann NY Acad Sci. 2007;1121:576–97.

138. Hutcheson DM, Everitt BJ. The effects of selective orbitofrontal cortex lesions on the acquisition and performance of cue-controlled cocaine seeking in rats. Ann NY Acad Sci. 2003; 1003:410–1.

139. Di Ciano P, Everitt BJ. Contribution of the ventral tegmental area to cocaine-seeking maintained by a drug-paired conditioned stimulus in rats. Eur J Neurosci. 2004;19:1661–7.

140. Haber S. The primate basal ganglia: parallel and integrative networks. J Chem Neuroanat. 2003;26:317–30.

141. Haber S, Fudge JL, McFarland NR. Striatonigrostriatal pathways in primates form an ascending spiral from the shell to the dorsolateral striatum. J Neurosci. 2000;20(6):2369–82.

142. Ikemoto S. Dopamine reward circuitry: two projection systems from the ventral midbrain to the nucleus accumbens–olfactory tubercle complex. Brain Res Rev. 2007;56:27–78.

143. DSM-IV APA. Diagnostic and statistical manual of mental disorders. Washington, DC: American Psychiatric Association; 2000.

144. Cacciola J, Alterman A, O'Brien CP, Mclellan A. The addiction severity index in clinical efficacy trials of medications for cocaine dependence. NIDA Res Monogr. 1997;175:182–91.

145. Kampman KM, Volpicelli JR, McGinnis DE, et al. Reliability and validity of the cocaine selective severity assessment. Addict Behav. 1998;23:449–61.

146. Mclellan A, Kushner H, Metzger D, Peters R. The fifth edition of the addiction severity index. J Subst Abuse Treat. 1992;9(3): 199–213.

147. Rikoon S, Cacciola J, Carise D, Alterman A, Mclellan A. Predicting DSM-IV dependence diagnoses from addiction severity index composite scores. J Subst Abuse Treat. 2006;31:17–24.

148. Kreek M, Nielsen D, Butelman E, Laforge K. Genetic influences on impulsivity, risk taking, stress responsivity and vulnerability to drug abuse and addiction. Nat Neurosci. 2005;8:1450–7.

149. Teichman M, Barnea Z, Rahav G. Sensation seeking, state and trait anxiety, and depressive mood in adolescent substance users. Int J Addict. 1989;24:87–99.

150. Teichman M, Barnea Z, Ravav G. Personality and substance use among adolescents: a longitudinal study. Br J Addict. 1989;84: 181–90.

151. Adams JB, Heath AJ, Young SE, Hewitt JK, Corley RP, Stallings MC. Relationships between personality and preferred substance and motivations for use among adolescent substance abusers. Am J Drug Alcohol Abuse. 2003;29:691–712.

152. Conway K, Swendsen JD, Rounsaville BJ, Merikangas KR. Personality, drug of choice, and comorbid psychopathology among substance abusers. Drug Alcohol Depend. 2002;65:225–34.

153. Khantzian EJ. Psychiatric illness in drug abusers. N Engl J Med. 1980;302:869–70.

154. Kilpatrick DG, Sutker PB, Roitzsch JC, Miller WC. Personality correlates of polydrug abuse. Psychol Rep. 1976;38:311–7.

155. Moeller FG, Dougherty DM, Barratt ES, et al. Increased impulsivity in cocaine dependent subjects independent of antisocial personality disorder and aggression. Drug Alcohol Depend. 2002;68:105–11.

156. Moss HB. Psychopathy, aggression, and family history in male veteran substance abuse patients: a factor analytic study. Addict Behav. 1989;14:565–70.

157. Pomerleau CS, Pomerleau OF, Flessland KA, Basson SM. Relationship of Tridimensional Personality Questionnaire scores and smoking variables in female and male smokers. J Subst Abuse. 1992;4:143–54.

158. Sarramon C, Verdoux H, Schmitt L, Bourgeois M. Addiction and personality traits: sensation seeking, anhedonia, impulsivity. Encephale. 1999;25:569–75.

159. Schinka JA, Curtiss G, Mulloy JM. Personality variables and self-medication in substance abuse. J Pers Assess. 1994;63:413–22.
160. Scourfield J, Stevens DE, Merikangas KR. Substance abuse, comorbidity, and sensation seeking: gender differences. Compr Psychiatry. 1996;37:384–92.
161. Sher KJ, Bartholow BD, Wood MD. Personality and substance use disorders: a prospective study. J Consult Clin Psychol. 2000; 68:818–29.
162. Skinstad AH, Swain A. Comorbidity in a clinical sample of substance abusers. Am J Drug Alcohol Abuse. 2001;27:45–64.
163. Wills TA, Vaccaro D, McNamara G. Novelty seeking, risk taking, and related constructs as predictors of adolescent substance use: an application of Cloninger's theory. J Subst Abuse. 1994;6:1–20.
164. Zuckerman M. Sensation seeking and the endogenous deficit theory of drug abuse. NIDA Res Monogr. 1986;74:59–70.
165. Zuckerman M. P-impulsive sensation seeking and its behavioral, psychophysiological and biochemical correlates. Neuropsychobiology. 1993;28:30–6.
166. Zuckerman M, Neeb M. Sensation seeking and psychopathology. Psychiatry Res. 1979;1:255–64.
167. Forsyth J. Anxiety sensitivity, controllability, and experiential avoidance and their relation to drug of choice and addiction severity in a residential sample of substance-abusing veterans. Addict Behav. 2003;28:851–70.
168. O'Leary TA, Rohsenow DJ, Martin R, Colby SM, Eaton CA, Monti PM. The relationship between anxiety levels and outcome of cocaine abuse treatment. Am J Drug Alcohol Abuse. 2000; 26:179–94.
169. Roberts A. Psychiatric comorbidity in white and African-American illicit substance abusers: evidence for differential etiology. Clin Psychol Rev. 2000;20:667–77.
170. Thomas McLellan A, Cacciola J, Alterman A, Rikoon S, Carise D. The addiction severity index at 25: origins, contributions and transitions. Am J Addict. 2006;15:113–24.
171. Zilberman ML, Tavares H, Hodgins DC, el-Guebaly N. The impact of gender, depression, and personality on craving. J Addict Dis. 2007;26:79–84.
172. Hanson KL, Luciana M, Sullwold K. Reward-related decision-making deficits and elevated impulsivity among MDMA and other drug users. Drug Alcohol Depend. 2008;96:99–110.
173. Petry NM. Discounting of delayed rewards in substance abusers: relationship to antisocial personality disorder. Psychopharmacology (Berl). 2002;162:425–32.
174. Franques P, Auriacombe M, Tignol J. Addiction and personality. Encephale. 2000;26:68–78.
175. Chandra PS, Krishna VA, Benegal V, Ramakrishna J. High-risk sexual behaviour & sensation seeking among heavy alcohol users. Indian J Med Res. 2003;117:88–92.
176. Zuckerman M. Sensation seeking and behavior disorders. Arch Gen Psychiatry. 1988;45:502–4.
177. Zuckerman M. The psychophysiology of sensation seeking. J Personal. 1990;58:313–45.
178. Hogg S. A review of the validity and variability of the elevated plus-maze as an animal model of anxiety. Pharmacol Biochem Behav. 1996;54:21–30.
179. Pellow S, Chopin P, File SE, Briley M. Validation of open:closed arm entries in an elevated plus-maze as a measure of anxiety in the rat. J Neurosci Methods. 1985;14:149–67.
180. Pelloux Y, Costentin J, Duterte-Boucher D. Anxiety increases the place conditioning induced by cocaine in rats. Behav Brain Res. 2009;197:311–6.
181. Homberg J, Van Den Akker M, Raaso H, et al. Enhanced motivation to self-administer cocaine is predicted by self-grooming behaviour and relates to dopamine release in the rat medial prefrontal cortex and amygdala. Eur J Neurosci. 2002;15: 1542–50.
182. Bush D, Vaccarino F. Individual differences in elevated plus-maze exploration predicted progressive-ratio cocaine self-administration break points in Wistar rats. Psychopharmacology. 2007;194:211–9.
183. Henniger MS, Spanagel R, Wigger A, Landgraf R, Holter SM. Alcohol self-administration in two rat lines selectively bred for extremes in anxiety-related behavior. Neuropsychopharmacology. 2002;26:729–36.
184. Spanagel R, Montkowski A, Allingham K, et al. Anxiety: a potential predictor of vulnerability to the initiation of ethanol self-administration in rats. Psychopharmacology (Berl). 1995;122: 369–73.
185. Chakroun N, Doron J, Swendsen J. Substance use, affective problems and personality traits: test of two association models. Encephale. 2004;30:564–9.
186. Stewart SH, Karp J, Pihl RO, Peterson RA. Anxiety sensitivity and self-reported reasons for drug use. J Subst Abuse. 1997;9:223–40.
187. Bardo M, Donohew RL, Harrington NG. Psychobiology of novelty seeking and drug seeking behavior. Behav Brain Res. 1996;77(1–2):23–43.
188. Hooks MS, Jones GH, Smith AD, Neill DB, Justice JB. Individual differences in locomotor activity and sensitization. Pharmacol Biochem Behav. 1991;38:467–70.
189. Piazza PV, Rouge-Pont F, Deminiere JM, Kharoubi M, Le Moal M, Simon H. Dopaminergic activity is reduced in the prefrontal cortex and increased in the nucleus accumbens of rats predisposed to develop amphetamine self-administration. Brain Res. 1991;567: 169–74.
190. Misslin R, Cigrang M. Does neophobia necessarily imply fear or anxiety? Behav Process. 1986;12:45–50.
191. Klebaur JE, Bevins RA, Segar TM, Bardo M. Individual differences in behavioral responses to novelty and amphetamine self-administration in male and female rats. Behav Pharmacol. 2001;12(4):267–75.
192. Bardo M, Neisewander JL, Pierce R. Novelty-induced place preference behavior in rats: effects of opiate and dopaminergic drugs. Pharmacol Biochem Behav. 1989;32:683–9.
193. Klebaur JE, Bardo M. Individual differences in novelty seeking on the playground maze predict amphetamine conditioned place preference. Pharmacol Biochem Behav. 1999;63:131–6.
194. Bardo MT, Bowling SL, Robinet PM, Rowlett JK, Lacy M, Mattingly BA. Role of dopamine D1 and D2 receptors in novelty-maintained place preference. Exp Clin Psychopharmacol. 1993;1:101–9.
195. Zuckerman M, Link K. Construct validity for the sensation-seeking scale. J Consult Clin Psychol. 1968;32:420–6.
196. Zuckerman M, Bone RN, Neary R, Mangelsdorff D, Brustman B. What is the sensation seeker? Personality trait and experience correlates of the Sensation-Seeking Scales. J Consult Clin Psychol. 1972;39:308–21.
197. Schooler C, Zahn TP, Murphy DL, Buchsbaum MS. Psychological correlates of monoamine oxidase activity in normals. J Nerv Ment Dis. 1978;166:177–86.
198. Beck LH, Bransome ED, Mirsky AF, Rosvold HE, Sarason I. A continuous performance test of brain damage. J Consult Psychol. 1956;20:343–50.
199. Bari A, Dalley JW, Robbins TW. The application of the 5-choice serial reaction time task for the assessment of visual attentional processes and impulse control in rats. Nat Protoc. 2008; 3(5):759–67.
200. Robbins TW. The 5-choice serial reaction time task: behavioural pharmacology and functional neurochemistry. Psychopharmacology. 2002;163(3–4):362–80.
201. Dalley JW, Cardinal R, Robbins JW. Prefrontal executive and cognitive functions in rodents: neural and neurochemical substrates. Neurosci Biobehav Rev. 2004;28:771–84.

202. Dalley JW, Mar A, Economidou D, Robbins TW. Neurobehavioral mechanisms of impulsivity: fronto-striatal systems and functional neurochemistry. Pharmacol Biochem Behav. 2008;90: 250–60.

203. Dalley JW, Fryer T, Brichard L, et al. Nucleus accumbens D2/3 receptors predict trait impulsivity and cocaine reinforcement. Science. 2007;315:1267–70.

204. Diergaarde L, Pattij T, Poortvliet I, et al. Impulsive choice and impulsive action predict vulnerability to distinct stages of nicotine seeking in rats. Biol Psychiatry. 2008;63:301–8.

205. Economidou D, Pelloux Y, Robbins TW, Dalley JW, Everitt BJ. High impulsivity predicts relapse to cocaine-seeking after punishment-induced abstinence. Biol Psychiatry. 2009;65(10):851–6.

206. Deminiere JM, Piazza PV, Le Moal M, Simon H. Experimental approach to individual vulnerability to psychostimulant addiction. Neurosci Biobehav Rev. 1989;13:141–7.

207. O'Brien CP, Mclellan A. Myths about the treatment of addiction. Lancet. 1996;347:237–40.

208. Stewart J, De Wit H. Reinstatement of drug taking behaviour as a method of assessing incentive motivational properties of drugs. In: Bozarth MA, editor. Assessing drug reinforcement. New York: Springer; 1987. p. 12.

209. Gawin FH. Cocaine abuse and addiction. J Fam Pract. 1989;29: 193–7.

210. Gawin FH. Cocaine addiction: psychology and neurophysiology. Science. 1991;251:1580–6.

211. Lenoir M, Ahmed S. Heroin-induced reinstatement is specific to compulsive heroin use and dissociable from heroin reward and sensitization. Neuropsychopharmacology. 2007;32:616–24.

212. Shalev U, Grimm JW, Shaham Y. Neurobiology of relapse to heroin and cocaine seeking: a review. Pharmacol Rev. 2002; 54(1):1–42.

213. Piazza PV, Deminiere JM, Maccari S, Mormede P, Le Moal M, Simon H. Individual reactivity to novelty predicts probability of amphetamine self-administration. Behav Pharmacol. 1990; 1:339–45.

214. Koob GF. Neurobiological substrates for the dark side of compulsivity in addiction. Neuropharmacology. 2009;56 Suppl 1:18–31.

215. Shen H, Toda S, Moussawi K, Bouknight A, Zahm D, Kalivas P. Altered dendritic spine plasticity in cocaine-withdrawn rats. J Neurosci. 2009;29:2876–84.

216. Sarti F, Borgland SL, Kharazia VN, Bonci A. Acute cocaine exposure alters spine density and long-term potentiation in the ventral tegmental area. Eur J Neurosci. 2007;26:749–56.

217. Lee KW, Kim Y, Kim AM, Helmin K, Nairn AC, Greengard P. Cocaine-induced dendritic spine formation in D1 and D2 dopamine receptor-containing medium spiny neurons in nucleus accumbens. Proc Natl Acad Sci USA. 2006;103:3399–404.

218. Li Y, Acerbo M, Robinson T. The induction of behavioural sensitization is associated with cocaine-induced structural plasticity in the core (but not shell) of the nucleus accumbens. Eur J Neurosci. 2004;20:1647–54.

219. Norrholm SD, Bibb JA, Nestler EJ, Ouimet CC, Taylor JR, Greengard P. Cocaine-induced proliferation of dendritic spines in nucleus accumbens is dependent on the activity of cyclin-dependent kinase-5. Neuroscience. 2003;116:19–22.

220. Robinson T, Gorny G, Mitton E, Kolb B. Cocaine self-administration alters the morphology of dendrites and dendritic spines in the nucleus accumbens and neocortex. Synapse. 2001;39:257–66.

221. Koob GF, Nestler EJ. The neurobiology of drug addiction. J Neuropsychiatry Clin Neurosci. 1997;9:482–97.

222. Volkow ND, Wang GJ, Fowler JS, et al. Decreased striatal dopaminergic responsiveness in detoxified cocaine-dependent subjects. Nature. 1997;386:830–3.

223. Koob G, Weiss F. Neuropharmacology of cocaine and ethanol dependence. Recent Dev Alcohol. 1992;10:201–33.

224. Arnsten AF, Li BM. Neurobiology of executive functions: catecholamine influences on prefrontal cortical functions. Biol Psychiatry. 2005;57:1377–84.

225. Bassareo V, Tanda G, Di Chiara G. Increase of extracellular dopamine in the medial prefrontal cortex during spontaneous and naloxone-precipitated opiate abstinence. Psychopharmacology (Berl). 1995;122:202–5.

226. Bechara A, Damasio H. Decision-making and addiction (part I): impaired activation of somatic states in substance dependent individuals when pondering decisions with negative future consequences. Neuropsychologia. 2002;40:1675–89.

227. Bechara A, Dolan S, Hindes A. Decision-making and addiction (part II): myopia for the future or hypersensitivity to reward? Neuropsychologia. 2002;40:1690–705.

228. Briand LA, Flagel S, Garcia-Fuster MJ, et al. Persistent alterations in cognitive function and prefrontal dopamine D2 receptors following extended, but not limited, access to self-administered cocaine. Neuropsychopharmacology. 2008;33(12):2969–80.

229. Koya E, Uejima JL, Wihbey KA, Bossert JM, Hope BT, Shaham Y. Role of ventral medial prefrontal cortex in incubation of cocaine craving. Neuropharmacology. 2009;56 Suppl 1:177–85.

230. Porrino L, Lyons D. Orbital and medial prefrontal cortex and psychostimulant abuse: studies in animal models. Cereb Cortex. 2000;10:326–33.

231. Porrino L, Domer FR, Crane AM, Sokoloff L. Selective alterations in cerebral metabolism within the mesocorticolimbic dopaminergic system produced by acute cocaine administration in rats. Neuropsychopharmacology. 1988;1:109–18.

232. Schoenbaum G, Saddoris MP, Ramus SJ, Shaham Y, Setlow B. Cocaine-experienced rats exhibit learning deficits in a task sensitive to orbitofrontal cortex lesions. Eur J Neurosci. 2004;19: 1997–2002.

233. Winstanley CA, LaPlant Q, Theobald DE, et al. DeltaFosB induction in orbitofrontal cortex mediates tolerance to cocaine-induced cognitive dysfunction. J Neurosci. 2007;27:10497–507.

234. Berridge KC, Robinson TE. What is the role of dopamine in reward: hedonic impact, reward learning, or incentive salience? Brain Res Brain Res Rev. 1998;28:309–69.

235. Koob G, Moal ML. Drug abuse: hedonic homeostatic dysregulation. Science. 1997;278(5335):52–8.

236. Schoenbaum G, Roesch M, Stalnaker T. Orbitofrontal cortex, decision-making and drug addiction. Trends Neurosci. 2006;29:116–24.

237. Schoenbaum G, Shaham Y. The role of orbitofrontal cortex in drug addiction: a review of preclinical studies. Biol Psychiatry. 2008;63(3):256–62.

238. Dickinson A, Wood N, Smith J. Alcohol seeking by rats: action or habit? Q J Exp Psychol Sect B. 2002;55:331–48.

239. Miles F, Everitt B, Dickinson A. Oral cocaine seeking by rats: action or habit? Behav Neurosci. 2003;117:927–38.

240. Porrino L. Cocaine self-administration produces a progressive involvement of limbic, association, and sensorimotor striatal domains. J Neurosci. 2004;24:3554–62.

241. Letchworth SR, Nader MA, Smith HR, Friedman DP, Porrino L. Progression of changes in dopamine transporter binding site density as a result of cocaine self-administration in rhesus monkeys. J Neurosci. 2001;21:2799–807.

242. Jentsch JD, Taylor JR. Impulsivity resulting from frontostriatal dysfunction in drug abuse: implications for the control of behavior by reward-related stimuli. Psychopharmacology. 1999;146(4): 373–90.

243. Hester R, Garavan H. Executive dysfunction in cocaine addiction: evidence for discordant frontal, cingulate, and cerebellar activity. J Neurosci. 2004;24:11017–22.

244. Kirby KN, Petry NM. Heroin and cocaine abusers have higher discount rates for delayed rewards than alcoholics or non-drug-using controls. Addiction. 2004;99:461–71.

245. Black Y. Altered attention and prefrontal cortex gene expression in rats after binge-like exposure to cocaine during adolescence. J Neurosci. 2006;26:9656–65.
246. Calu D, Stalnaker T, Franz T, Singh T, Shaham Y, Schoenbaum G. Withdrawal from cocaine self-administration produces long-lasting deficits in orbitofrontal-dependent reversal learning in rats. Learn Mem. 2007;14:325–8.
247. Dalley J, Lääne K, Pena Y, Theobald D, Everitt B, Robbins T. Attentional and motivational deficits in rats withdrawn from intravenous self-administration of cocaine or heroin. Psychopharmacology. 2005;182:579–87.
248. Dalley J, Theobald D, Berry D, et al. Cognitive sequelae of intravenous amphetamine self-administration in rats: evidence for selective effects on attentional performance. Neuropsychopharmacology. 2005;30:525–37.
249. George O, Mandyam C, Wee S, Koob G. Extended access to cocaine self-administration produces long-lasting prefrontal cortex-dependent working memory impairments. Neuropsychopharmacology. 2008;33:2474–82.
250. Paine T, Olmstead M. Cocaine disrupts both behavioural inhibition and conditional discrimination in rats. Psychopharmacology (Berl). 2004;175:443–50.
251. Paine TA, Dringenberg HC, Olmstead MC. Effects of chronic cocaine on impulsivity: relation to cortical serotonin mechanisms. Behav Brain Res. 2003;147:135–47.
252. Schoenbaum G. Cocaine makes actions insensitive to outcomes but not extinction: implications for altered orbitofrontal-amygdalar function. Cereb Cortex. 2004;15:1162–9.
253. Bolla KI, Eldreth DA, London ED, et al. Orbitofrontal cortex dysfunction in abstinent cocaine abusers performing a decision-making task. NeuroImage. 2003;19:1085–94.
254. Porrino L, Smith HR, Nader MA, Beveridge TJ. The effects of cocaine: a shifting target over the course of addiction. Prog Neuropsychopharmacol Biol Psychiatry. 2007;31:1593–600.

Genetic Contributions to Individual Differences in Vulnerability to Addiction and Abilities to Quit

George R. Uhl and Tomas Drgon

Abstract

Individuals differ in their vulnerabilities to becoming dependent on one or more abused substances. Not all of the individuals who have opportunities to use addictive substances do in fact use them, not all users become regular users or abusers and not all regular users or abusers become dependent or addicted. Abundant evidence from family, adoption, and twin studies point to large genetic contributions to individual differences in vulnerability to develop dependence on addictive substances. Twin data suggests that much of this genetic vulnerability is shared by individuals who are dependent on a variety of addictive substances, though some is likely to be substance specific.

Substance-dependent individuals also differ in their abilities to quit use of addictive substances and to maintain abstinence. Twin data for abilities to quit smoking provide some of the best evidence for genetic influences on abilities to achieve and maintain abstinence on an addictive substance.

These estimates for overall genetic contributions still leave open a variety of possibilities concerning the "genetic architectures" that underlie these "addiction vulnerability" and "quit success" phenotypes. Current molecular genetic data relevant to each of these phenotypes fit with the idea that each displays largely polygenic influences. Major gene effects have been identified for alcohol dependence in Asians with the flushing syndrome and for low-level cigarette use ("chippers") with modest signs of physiological nicotine dependence at a chromosome 15 nicotinic receptor locus. Genes identified in molecular genetic studies of "addiction vulnerability" and "quit success" phenotypes partially overlap, as we would expect from classical genetic studies, and fall into several functional classes more than expected by chance. These data provide a substrate to improve understanding of substance dependence and the ability to quit smoking. With better understanding of genetic influences on these phenotypes, we may be better positioned to improve understanding of the large environmental influences on these phenotypes, to personalize treatments, and even to personalize prevention strategies for individuals at especial risk.

G.R. Uhl (✉) • T. Drgon
Molecular Neurobiology Branch, NIH-IRP (NIDA), Suite 3510,
333 Cassell Drive, Baltimore, MD 21224, USA
e-mail: guhl@intra.nida.nih.gov

J.C. Verster et al. (eds.), *Drug Abuse and Addiction in Medical Illness: Causes, Consequences and Treatment*,
DOI 10.1007/978-1-4614-3375-0_7, © Springer Science+Business Media, LLC 2012

Learning Objectives

1. To understand the relative roles of genetic and environmental influences in vulnerability to addictions and abilities to quit smoking.
2. To understand the few large effects at single gene loci.
3. To understand the concept of polygenic genetic influences, the large roles that they play in addiction vulnerability and quit success and the difficulties that such genetic architecture poses for developing certainty about the involvement of specific genes.
4. To understand the ways in which groups of genetic influences, taken together, can make powerful contributions to our understanding of addictions and quit success and ability to personalize prevention and treatments.

Issues that Need to Be Addressed by Future Research

1. To identify the molecular and biochemical ways in which variants in addiction associated and quit-success associated genes alter the brain in ways that alter addiction and quitting behaviors.
2. To understand the ways in which addiction-related gene variants also exert influences on addiction-associated phenotypes (pleiotropic influences).
3. To understand the roles of epigenetic marks in contributing to individual differences in addiction vulnerability and ability to quit.
4. To use genetic information to help match individuals to the prevention and treatment strategies that are likely to work best for them.
5. To control for genetic influences in ways that expand the power of studies of the environmental influences on addiction vulnerability and ability to quit.

Current Views of the "Genetic Architecture" for Substance Dependence Phenotypes

Current models for the genetic architecture for dependence on addictive substances in the population are based on the information from (1) family study data (in which risk to relatives of addicted individuals is compared to risks in members of the general population), (2) adoption study data (in which adoptees' similarities to biological relatives vs. adoptive family members are compared), and (3) twin study data (in which concordance in genetically identical monozygotic vs. genetically half-identical dizygotic twins are compared).

These data are complemented and supplemented by overall results from molecular genetic studies, including (1) linkage studies that assess the ways that traits and genetic markers move together through families and (2) association studies of the ways in which traits and genetic markers move together through "unrelated" members of the population.

Support for the idea that vulnerability to addictions is a complex trait with strong genetic influences that are largely shared by abusers of different legal and illegal addictive substances [1–4] comes from such classical genetic studies. Family studies document that first-degree relatives (e.g., sibs) of addicts display greater risk for developing substance dependence than more distant relatives [1, 5]. Adoption studies find greater similarities between levels of substance abuse between adoptees vs. biological relatives than adoptees vs. members of the adoptive families [1]. In twin studies, differences in concordance between genetically identical and fraternal twins also support substantial heritability for vulnerability to addictions [3, 6–12]. Twin data allows quantitation of the amount, about half, of addiction vulnerability that is heritable. Twin data also supports the idea that the environmental influences on addiction vulnerability that are not shared among members of twin pairs are much larger than those that are shared by members of twin pairs. Analyses of these data fractionate the similarity between twins in ways that attempt to segregate additive genetic influences (a), common environmental influences shared by sibs (c) and unique environmental influences that are not necessarily shared by sibs (e). In this terminology, e^2 is $\gg c^2$ in virtually every such study, supporting the idea that many of the environmental influences on human addiction vulnerability are thus likely to come from outside of the immediate family environment.

Not all environments allow the genetic vulnerabilities to become dependent on a substance to be expressed. A striking example of a shift from a less to more permissive environment comes from studies of the apparent heritability of smoking in Scandinavian twin pairs sampled from different birth cohorts. Studies of twins raised in late nineteenth- to twentieth century Swedish environments document the progressively greater emergence of apparent heritable influences on smoking in women over this time period [13]. During this time, the initially strong social constraints against smoking in women were relaxed. Interestingly, heritability estimates in men were similar through this same time period. The allelic variants that predispose modern Swedish women to smoke are likely to be virtually identical to those present in their grandmothers who were environmentally constrained against smoking [13]. This work thus provides one of the most striking examples of influences that a strongly nonpermissive environment can have on the expression of an underlying genetic vulnerability.

We are also fortunate to have data from studies of identical vs. fraternal twin pairs that evaluate the degree to which one twin's dependence on a substance enhances the chance that his or her co-twin will become dependent on a substance of a different class. Results of these analyses document that many (and probably most) of the genetic influences on addiction vulnerability are common to dependence on multiple different substances, though others do appear to be substance specific [2, 9, 10].

Data from linkage studies can identify large effects at single gene loci with good sensitivity and specificity in ways that are highly reproducible. When effects at each single locus are small, however, different linkage-based studies display results that replicate at about the rates expected by chance alone. When we assemble linkage data for dependence on alcohol in individuals with Asian genetic backgrounds, there is a robust effect of chromosome 4 markers at the alcohol dehydrogenase/acetaldehyde dehydrogenase locus that are associated with the protective effect of "flushing syndrome" variants in members of these populations. However, there have been no other gene variants which reproducibly provide such large single-gene influences on vulnerabilities to addictions in members of other populations. Our view of the genetic architecture of addiction vulnerability in Asian individuals is thus that it is composed of the large effect of these chromosome 4 variants and more modest effects of variants at other loci, while there is no single gene variant that appears to provide such a strong influence in individuals with African or European heritages.

Data from association studies of addiction, per se, provides little evidence for any very large effect of any single gene. However, in studies of the quantity of cigarettes that smokers use, a variety of studies have now identified robust effects of variants at a chromosome 15 locus that contains a number of nicotinic acetylcholine receptor genes (see below).

Current Views of the "Genetic Architecture" for Cessation Success Phenotypes

Data from classical genetic studies of individual differences in abilities to quit are sparser than data from studies of vulnerability to become dependent. Nevertheless, twin studies do identify substantial differences between monozygotic- and dizygotic-twin similarities for the ability to quit smoking. Twin data from several studies strongly support the idea that ability to quit smoking can display a robust heritable component, accounting for about half of the individual differences in this phenotype in recent twin datasets [14]. It is likely that these genetic influences display modest overlap with those that influence development of dependence, though support for this idea is more indirect [14].

Potential Molecular Genetic Configurations for Substance Dependence and Quit Success

One way in which to frame the actual molecular genetics of substance dependence and quit success is to consider some of the ways in which different genetic and environmental components might combine to produce overall vulnerabilities with about half genetic and about half environmental influences.

Small vs. large effects of most allelic variants that contribute to vulnerability. It was conceivable, prior to molecular genetic studies, that large effects of variants at a relatively few genes could provide the genetic contributions to addiction vulnerability and abilities to quit smoking. If this were so, linkage studies would provide major signals based on the ways in which these phenotypes moved together with chromosomal markers within pedigrees. Unfortunately, most linkage data in this field does not provide such reproducible signals, with the exception of data for the chromosome 4 ADH/ALDH locus in Asians. Based on this largely negative information, our attention is turned toward consideration of relatively small contributions from individual allelic variants.

Many vs. relatively few allelic variants that contribute to vulnerability. It was conceivable, prior to molecular genetic studies, that allelic variants at a relatively small number of chromosomal loci could contribute to addiction vulnerability and ability to quit smoking. Under these circumstances, many or even most of the individuals whose addiction or quit success received genetic contributions would be influenced by many or even most of the same allelic variants. Under such circumstances, many of the allelic variants that influence these phenotypes in the general population would be represented in each individual with these phenotypes. These circumstances provide the most opportune setting for genome-wide association. They also provide the most opportune setting in which we could use genotypes to predict individual vulnerabilities. The simple form of this model demands that the variants should be similar in individuals from each current racial/ethnic group. Such variants should thus be "old" in the sense that they need to have (a) arisen prior to separation of the modern racial/ethnic groups and (b) to have been maintained in the populations that arose from these ancestral humans through balancing selection or similar mechanisms [15]. Unfortunately, data from genome-wide association studies supports only modest number of allelic variants with such properties, though they may well provide contributions to both quit success and addiction vulnerability phenotypes.

Additive vs. interactive effects of most allelic variants. It is conceivable that the influences of many individual allelic variants, and those of many individual environmental contributions, sum in additive fashion, to at least a first approximation. Indeed, most current analyses of twin data use mathematical formulations that identify additive genetic components, supporting the idea that much of the genetic influence on addiction vulnerability and quit success can be fit, again to a first approximation, by additive models. Such an overall fit, however, is not able to exclude numbers of interactions between (a) the effects of individual allelic genetic variants and (b) genetic and environmental features. Indeed, the twin data cited above that documents increasing evidence for heritability for smoking in Scandinavian women as the environment became increasingly permissive for such smoking support a strong G×E interaction between genetic and environmental components.

Relatively "old" vs. relatively "new" variants. Addiction vulnerability and ability to quit smoking could be influenced by allelic variants that arose relatively recently in the course of human history, and/or those that arose in the more distant past. In general, "older" variants are more likely to be common in human population, and to be present in individuals of each of the current racial/ethnic groups. By contrast, "newer" variants may be present at strikingly different frequencies in individuals from different current racial/ethnic groups. "*Common disease/common allele*" models [16] would support roles for common variants in these common phenotypes. However, for variants that have been maintained in the population for long periods of time, we must consider how *genetic selection* might have acted in environments that include the early African environments experienced small groups of early humans. No study of these early environments finds any strong evidence for the presence of any potent addictive substance, to our knowledge. We thus need to consider the ways in which selective processes might have operated in the absence of both addictive substances and in the absence of selective evolutionary pressures that can be attributed to use of addictive substances. For such variants to exert substantial effects, it thus also seems likely that many allelic variants that influence addiction vulnerability must have provided *balancing selection*. Balancing selection provides one of the few theoretical means for maintaining common allelic variants over extended periods of time. "In the era of molecular population genetics, … balancing selection (refers to) loci (that display) levels of nucleotide polymorphism that exceed neutral expectation" [17]. We think of balancing selection as providing influences that are favorable in some individuals or organs or circumstances and unfavorable in other individuals or organs or circumstances.

Genetic vs. epigenetic influences. Addiction vulnerability and ability to quit smoking are both likely to receive contributions from both classical DNA sequence variations passed through the population in classical ways and also from epigenetic marks, including imprinted marks that are passed from specific parents to offspring. As family studies improve in their resolution, parent of origin effects might help to reveal influences of this variety of epigenetic effect. However, it is likely that elucidation of most epigenetic influences will require studies of their molecular genomic bases.

Relatively large vs. relatively small DNA changes. DNA differences from individual to individual include single nucleotide polymorphisms (SNPs), insertions/deletions of as few as a single base, simple sequence length polymorphisms, typically of two, three, or four base pairs repeated many times, variable number tandem repeats, often of ca 40 bp, and copy number variations, of at least 1,000 bp but typically much longer. Large differences in DNA and small-sized differences in DNA are each present when we compare any two unrelated individuals. Presumably, differences of each of these molecular types are likely to contribute to the allelic variants that contribute to the heritable elements in the population that alter vulnerability to addiction vulnerability and ability to quit smoking.

Haplotypes vs. single DNA changes. The DNA differences from individual to individual that are present in the population are inherited as parts of haplotype "blocks," in which multiple DNA variations are inherited together. The allelic variation at a specific locus that contributes to a phenotypes can thus be considered as a single DNA change (such as a change that produces missense variations in the encoded protein) or as a haplotype, in which multiple nearby DNA variants contribute, as a group, to the phenotype.

Simple allelic variation vs. allelic heterogeneity. At any single gene locus, it is possible that traits can be influenced by only single variants. However, allelic heterogeneity provides a mechanism whereby multiple different DNA differences at the same locus can each contribute to a phenotype. Different missense variations in the CFTR gene can all lead to cystic fibrosis, for example [18]. It seems likely that at least some of the genes in which one variant can provide a basis for balancing selection and for addiction vulnerability will also manifest other distinct allelic variants that provide the same features.

Approaches: Genome-Wide Association

Genome-wide association (GWA or GWAS) is now a principal method of choice for identifying allelic variants that contribute to complex genetic disorders, especially those with polygenic genetic bases (e.g., derived from effects at many gene loci, each with modest effects, as well as from environmental determinants) [19–35]. In current applications of genome-wide association, alleles at one million SNP markers are assessed in cases and controls. These experiments thus ask how phenotypes and genetic markers (genotyped approximately every 1/1,000,000th of the genome) are found together in nominally unrelated individuals (although we are all distantly related to each other, of course). We and others have developed these methods, relying on the increasing densities of SNP markers that can be assessed using "SNP chip" microarrays of increasing sophistication [28–32, 34, 35]. Genome-wide association gains power, as densities of genomic markers increase. Association identifies much smaller chromosomal regions than linkage-based approaches. Association thus allows us to identify variants in specific genes rather than in large chromosomal regions. Genome-wide association fosters pooling strategies that preserve confidentiality and reduce costs [28–31, 36–42]. Genome-wide association provides ample genomic controls. Proper genomic controls can minimize the chances that disease vs. control differences are confounded by occult stratification, such as the stratification that might arise from unintended occult ethnic mismatches between disease and control samples.

Substance dependence was one of the first complex phenotypes for which replicated association-based genome scanning data was reported [21, 28–30, 43, 44]. There is now a torrent of information from genome-wide association studies of both substance dependence and other brain-based heritable phenotypes that co-occur with addictions more than expected by chance and are thus good candidates to display genetic overlaps with addiction (reviewed in [45]).

Actual Molecular Genetic Observations for Substance Dependence

Oligogenic effect of chromosome 15 haplotypes on FTND dependence among smokers. The largest single addiction-related molecular genetic effects in non-Asians is found in data that compares heavy smokers with high FTND scores to smokers without evidence for dependence by FTND criteria. Markers in the chromosome 15 gene cluster that encodes the α3, α5 and β4 nicotinic acetylcholine receptors display different allelic frequencies between these heavy vs. light smokers in each of several studies [21, 33, 46]. This chromosome 15 locus is likely to provide a good example of "secondary" pharmacogenomics, since (1) it is identified in relation to this quantity–frequency related phenotype, (2) it has not been identified as prominently in comparisons between FTND dependent and control, nonsmokers and (3) it has not been associated as reproducibly with dependence on other substances [45]. Markers in this chromosomal location have now been associated with differences between light and heavy smokers (and/or with lung cancers whose cell types are intimately associated with smoking histories) in samples from several international sites, though most of these samples are from European genetic backgrounds [44, 47–51].

Smaller effects of variants at other loci on DSM dependence. No GWA or linkage study provides evidence for any other effect of this magnitude of variants at any single locus on DSM dependence on any substance. On the other hand, comparisons of dependent individuals with control individuals with modest or no lifetime smoking identify polygenic effects of genes at a variety of gene loci.

In analyzing data from addiction vulnerability samples, we focus here and in recent reviews [45] on clusters of genomic marker SNPs whose allele frequencies distinguish control individuals from those with substance dependence or addiction-related phenotypes. We identify chromosomal regions that contain clusters of such nominally positive results in replicate samples for addiction vulnerability. In the analyses presented in this chapter, we focus on addiction-associated allelic variants that lie in genes. Evolutionarily old common haplotypes (e.g., groups of nearby variants that travel together through generations) that lie within genes are among the most likely to be tagged by SNP markers that are represented on current microarrays. Haplotypes that involve genes are thus among the most likely variants to exist in currently reported datasets. It seems reasonable to postulate that many of these allelic variants that lie within genes provide regulatory variants that alter expression or regulation. Other variants are likely to alter mRNA half-lives or mRNA splicing. Variants that alter mRNA splicing could occur at the locus of the affected gene (*cis*) or at genes at different loci that alter generic mRNA splicing processes (*trans*). It seems likely that only a minority of the addiction-associated variants will involve missense effects on expressed proteins.

It also seems likely that many addiction-associated variants will lie outside of genes, at least as we currently understand them. Loci reproducibly associated with diabetes/body mass, for example, lack conventional hallmarks of "genes," such as expressed sequences [25]. While the analyses in this chapter focus on the identification of variants within genes, we should also remain alert for roles for "intergenic" variations in chromosomal regions that lie between the currently understood genes.

Samples for genome studies of human addiction vulnerability. As we have recently reviewed [45], genome-wide association data for addiction vulnerability samples from European, African and Asian genetic heritages are now available. These data come from European-American research volunteers, African-American research volunteers, Asian individuals who largely presented to emergency facilities with methamphetamine psychosis and matched controls, dependent and

Table 7.1 Genes likely to contain variants that influence addiction vulnerability based on their identification by at least three GWA analyses [45] from six 500k to 1M GWA datasets shown (p values from Monte Carlo simulations, not corrected for repeated testing)

Gene	chr	bp:start	NIDA IM	NIDA 600k	NIH	ECA	JGIDA	Taiw	p-Value
AGBL4	1	48,822,129	6			3		3	0.0026
PBX1	1	162,795,561	5		4		3		0.0036
PRKCE	2	45,732,547	3			7		3	0.0145
GRM7	3	6,877,927	3	3		3	11		0.0119
ZNF659	3	21,437,651	3				9	6	0.0033
FHIT	3	59,710,076	5	3	15	24	20	8	0.0032
GRIK2	6	101,953,675	3	1	4				0.0261
SYNE1	6	152,484,516	3			7	20		0.0025
PDE1C	7	31,795,772	3	3	9		4		0.0036
CSMD1	8	2,782,789	10	15	14	29	25	18	0.0011
XKR4	8	56,177,571	3	5			4	5	0.0045
FKBP15	9	114,967,620	4				4	4	0.0008
FRMD4A	10	13,725,718	3			3	3	5	0.0142
MPP7	10	28,382,994	3	3			5		0.0065
PCDH15	10	55,250,866	3			11	3		0.0128
CTNNA3	10	67,349,937	3	4	4	2	3		0.0283
C10orf11	10	77,212,525	3		9			5	0.0128
PARVA	11	12,355,679	4	1			3		0.0033
LDLRAD3	11	35,922,188	3			3		4	0.0116
GRM5	11	87,880,626	5			3	9		0.0043
ETV6	12	11,694,055	3				4	3	0.0118
SLC2A13	12	38,435,090	6			4	14		0.0001
ABCC4	13	94,470,090	4	3			3		0.0048
PRKCH	14	60,858,268	5			7	9		0.0006
NRXN3	14	77,939,846	3		1		6		0.0694
THSD4	15	69,220,842	3		4	3			0.0236
CDH13	16	81,218,079	3	6	14	18	17	18	0.0009
FHOD3	18	32,131,700	3		8		3		0.0092
C20orf133	20	13,924,269	3				21	6	0.0271
DSCAM	21	40,306,213	4	3			9	6	0.0046

nonsmokers, largely of European ancestries and individuals sampled as parts of epidemiological studies.

These data can be compared to data from studies of individuals of European ancestries with alcohol dependence compared to nondependent controls recruited from the same areas.

Substance-dependent individuals, when compared to control individuals, reproducibly display association signals of modest sizes that identify genes [45, 52]. Monte Carlo simulations provide a basis for assessing how often their reproducible association signals might be found by chance. In comparison of the data from a number of samples, these simulations identify convergent data that is virtually never found by chance (reviewed in [45]).

These analyses provide some of the strongest molecular genetic support for the classical genetic studies of addiction vulnerability. They also provide substantial support for the idea that many of the allelic variants that predispose to addiction vulnerability are evolutionarily "old," since strongly convergent findings are found in comparing substance-dependent to control individuals of European-, African- and Asian genetic backgrounds. These analyses also provide support for the idea that dependence on substances of different classes is influenced by substantially overlapping genetic influences. We have identified overlaps that are much greater than chance for dependence on a number of illegal substances (including methamphetamine), alcohol and nicotine ([32, 34, 35] and reviewed in [45]). None of the results that compare substance-dependent vs. control individuals identifies any gene's allelic variants that appear to provide large effects. These observations are consistent with the failure of linkage-based studies for substance dependence to identify any highly reproducible loci, even though similar DSM and Fagerstrom diagnoses were used for linkage.

We list some of the genes that are identified by these reproducible findings in Table 7.1. It is important to note that few of these genes are identified by results from each study and that few display Monte Carlo p value that withstand rigorous corrections for multiple testing. While the entire list of genes shown in Table 7.1 is very unlikely to have been identified by chance, many of the individual genes in this list are likely to have been identified by chance. These results

Table 7.2 Functional genomic results from evaluating the classes of "addiction vulnerability" genes over- and under-represented in Gene Ontology categories [MNB GWA studies, hyprgeomertic tests, BioBase (http://helixweb.nih.gov/biobase, TD, GRU (2009) unpublished data)]

GO identifier	GO term	# Hits in group	Group size	Over(+)/under(−) representation	p-Value
GO:0007268	Synaptic transmission	26	336	+	2.45777E-06
GO:0007155	Cell adhesion	49	898	+	4.07463E-06
GO:0019226	Transmission of nerve impulse	27	377	+	6.71324E-06
GO:0009058	Biosynthetic process	78	4,046	−	4.09647E-05

from polygenic underlying genetic architectures are likely to result in continuing debate concerning influence of many of these genes by workers in the field. However, we can make increasingly confident statements about the properties of these sets of genes as a group, even though the nature of these individual genes is likely to be complex for many readers of this chapter. For example, bioinformatic methods now allow statistically valid comparisons of the frequencies with which we identify genes that fall into certain functional classes in comparison to the degree to which we might have identified these classes by chance. These genome-wide functional enrichment analyses provide evidence for overrepresentation of genes of specific functional classes related to brain connectivities and neurotransmitter function, as shown in Table 7.2.

Actual Molecular Genetic Observations for Smoking Cessation

Smoking cessation molecular genetics is a more recent area in which studies of small numbers of individuals who participated in smoking cessation trials are now complemented by increasing numbers of studies of individual from larger samples who report current smoking vs. those who report former smoking and successful abstinence.

We have recently reported data from genome-wide association in (a) three samples of smokers who were successful, compared to those who were unsuccessful, in clinical trials conducted in Philadelphia, Washington DC, Buffalo, Providence, and Durham [35]. These subjects for clinical trials were treated with nicotine replacement or with bupropion, accompanied by standardized behavioral counseling; (b) a sample of smokers, ascertained at the NIH, who were successful vs. unsuccessful in quitting in the community [53]; (c) a sample of smokers who were successful vs. unsuccessful in quitting in a trial of denicotinized cigarettes [54]; and (d) a sample of smokers who were successful vs. unsuccessful in quitting in a study of the effects of different doses of "prequit date" NRT (and denicotinized cigarettes) (Uhl et al (2009), submitted). We have completed additional analyses for smoking cessation in a UK general practice setting and in a randomized controlled clinical trial of pre-cessation

nicotine replacement. Caporaso and colleagues have also recently reported several SNPs that display the most nominal significance in comparisons of former to current smokers in cancer cohorts [55]. In pregnant smokers, there is also recent data that the chromosome 15 locus variants alter ability to quit [56].

There is remarkably convergent data from comparisons of the initial three "smoking cessation success" GWA datasets. Nominally positive clustered SNPs from successful vs. unsuccessful quitter comparisons from these samples cluster together on small chromosomal regions to extents much greater than chance [35]. The Monte Carlo p values for the replication for these samples, taken two at a time, were 0.00054, 0.0016, and 0.00063, respectively.

Among the smokers identified in the NIH samples described above [53, 57], we were also able to compare data from individuals who reported lifetime nicotine dependence and current smoking when interviewed vs. individuals who reported having been nicotine dependent at some time in their lives but who achieved abstinence [53]. The "current smokers" started to smoke at age 17 (±4), smoked for 18 (±13) years, consumed 20 (±13) cigarettes per day and continued to smoke when interviewed, while the "quitters" starting smoking at 17 (±3) years of age, smoked an average of 20 (±13) cigarettes per day for 13 (±11) years but subsequently maintained abstinence for 16 (±12) years by the time of interviews.

Remarkably, the data from these "community quitter" comparison overlapped significantly with data from quit success in two of the three clinical trial samples in [35] ($p \leq 0.0001$). Genes that we have identified by clusters of nominally positive SNPs in both clinical trial and community-based samples for the ability to successfully quit smoking include ataxin 2-binding protein 1, CUB and Sushi multiple domain 1, Down syndrome cell adhesion molecule, protocadherin 15, and the retinoic acid receptor β. As for a number of the other comparisons noted here, a disproportionate number of these genes thus represent cell adhesion molecules.

The data for clustered, nominally positive SNPs from the UK samples also provide significant overlap with data from prior samples. Overlaps between the clusters of nominally positive SNPs from this dataset with previously reported results from the initial three quit success samples [35] identified 100, 217 and 183 clusters of nominally positive SNPs, respectively ($p < 0.0001$ for each comparison). The clustered positive SNPs from this work also displayed a significant overlap with clustered, nominally positive SNPs from NIH research volunteer samples [53]. Overlaps with these data identified 78 clusters of nominally positive SNPs ($p < 0.0001$). Finally, the clusters from the current samples identify 68 clusters from comparisons between successful and unsuccessful quitters studied in the clinical trials of denicotinized cigarettes [54]. The overlaps between the clustered, nominally positive SNPs from the 25k results from the current sample and the clustered, nominally positive SNPs from at least one other sample of successful vs. unsuccessful quitters and/or nicotine dependence identify 245 chromosomal regions.

There were two SNPs that displayed nominally significant differences with the most significant p values in the work of Caporaso and colleagues [55]; there were nominally positive SNPs from our work that lay within 40 kb of each of these SNPs.

When we seek convergence between genes identified by multiple samples that include recent work with J Rose and colleagues, we identify a number of genes. Again, the statistical odds that this entire list of genes is due to chance are very low despite the fact that a number of the genes on this list are likely to reflect false positives (Table 7.3). As a group, these genes are also expressed in brain more than we could expect by chance and provide more representation of specific Gene Ontology classes than would be expected by chance using hypergeometric tests (Table 7.4).

Table 7.3 Genes likely to contain variants that influence ability to quit smoking based on their identification by at least three GWA analyses that include recent data [45] from 500k to 1M GWA datasets (p values from Monte Carlo simulations, not corrected for repeated testing)

Gene	ch	bp: start	R II	PIP	V	H	L	R I	B	Bi	p-Value
KIF1B	1	10,193,418	5	16		8					0.0005
DAB1	1	57,236,167	9	93			7		2	3	0.0021
DNM3	1	170,077,261	7	17			3			1	0.0095
ASTN	1	175,096,826	6	12				2	1		0.0082
CTNNA2	2	79,593,634	6	57				2	2	7	0.0066
TCF7L1	2	85,214,245	5	1				2			0.0122
RAPGEF4	2	173,308,853	10	6						1	0.0052
RBMS3	3	29,297,947	4	11					2	8	0.0068
FHIT	3	59,710,076	11	105		7		2		2	0.0033
EEFSEC	3	129,355,003	6	17					2		0.0077
SLC9A9	3	144,466,754	4	33				2		5	0.0099
TP73L	3	190,831,910	3	4			1			1	0.0145
LEPREL1	3	191,157,316	9	11				4	2		0.0010
FGF12	3	193,342,413	5	5				3	2		0.0175
RNASEN	5	31,436,926	6	1		1					0.0094
PDE4D	5	58,302,468	4	15						1	0.0428
SLC22A5	5	131,733,343	6	8					1		0.0039
SLIT3	5	168,025,857	6	24	5	3		3		1	0.0012
KCNIP1	5	169,713,459	5	23						3	0.0088
KIAA1900	6	97,479,324	6	6						1	0.0125
GRIK2	6	101,953,675	2	16				2	2	1	0.0139
UST	6	149,110,157	6	41						4	0.0039
PARK2	6	161,689,661	6	91				6	2	8	0.0044
DGKB	7	14,153,770	4	38				1			0.0262
MAGI2	7	77,484,310	6	51					2	1	0.0314
SEMA3A	7	83,428,426	12					2		1	0.0024
CSMD1	8	2,782,789	6	191	4	10		10	5	12	0.0015
DLC1	8	12,985,243	5	17					2		0.0169
PSD3	8	18,432,343	18	23						1	0.0013
TG	8	133,948,387	4	11					3		0.0123
ST3GAL1	8	134,540,312	5	9				2	1		0.0042
ZNF406	8	135,559,213	4	21						3	0.0072
COL22A1	8	139,669,660	6	21						1	0.0119
PTPRD	9	8,307,268	4	42				2	8	2	0.0026
KIAA1797	9	20,648,309	5	5						2	0.0214

(continued)

Table 7.3 (continued)

Gene	ch	bp: start	R II	PIP	V	H	L	R I	B	Bi	p-Value
PIP5K1B	9	70,510,436	4	51						1	0.0030
GABBR2	9	100,090,187	4	19					5		0.0101
DIP2C	10	311,432	8	7	3					1	0.0043
BICC1	10	59,942,910	4	8						2	0.0244
NRAP	10	115,338,573	1	11					1	1	0.0057
CASP7	10	115,428,925	11	10					1	2	0.0004
SLC1A2	11	35,229,329	7	34				3	3		0.0004
SOX5	12	23,576,498	10	48			2		2		0.0053
MYBPC1	12	100,512,878	8	4						1	0.0047
GPR133	12	130,004,790	4	26						1	0.0090
NBEA	13	34,414,456	9	5						1	0.0206
LMO7	13	75,092,571	5	23					2		0.0076
GPC5	13	90,848,930	1	25					2	1	0.1015
GPC6	13	92,677,096	17	40					1	4	0.0013
STK24	13	97,902,414	4	22			1				0.0075
NPAS3	14	32,478,200	16	70				5	1		<0.0001
RGS6	14	71,469,586	32	15					1	4	<0.0001
WDR72	15	51,594,652	7	14					2	2	0.0021
HMOX2	16	4,466,447	4		1				2		0.0113
A2BP1	16	6,009,133	6	181		3	14		12	13	<0.0001
CDH13	16	81,218,079	7	160	5		8	3	7	2	<0.0001
PRKCA	17	61,729,388	9	21				4		1	0.0036
SLC14A2	18	41,448,764	10	11	4						0.0002
MYO18B	22	24,468,120	5	32				5	3	1	0.0015

Table 7.4 Functional genomic results from evaluating the classes of "quit success" genes over-represented in Gene Ontology categories [MNB GWA studies, hyprgeometric tests, BioBase (http://helixweb.nih.gov/biobase, TD, GRU (2009) unpublished data)]

GO identifier	GO term	# Hits in group	Group size	Over(+)/under(−) representation	p-Value
GO:0007154	Cell communication	150	4,357	+	9.13404E-06
GO:0007165	Signal transduction	137	3,996	+	0.00003875
GO:0015914	Phospholipid transport	5	18	+	6.91349E-05
GO:0007155	Cell adhesion	42	898	+	0.000107121
GO:0050808	Synapse organization and biogenesis	8	61	+	0.000152339

Conclusions

It is an exciting time to be able to summarize and review the rapidly emerging data on the complex genetics of human addiction vulnerability, ability to quit and related phenotypes. Genome-wide association results for dependence on several classes of addictive substances converge with each other in striking fashion that is highly unlikely, overall, to be due to chance. These data fit a genetic architecture for addiction and ability to quit smoking that is based on polygenic contributions from common allelic variants. Such a genetic architecture is quite consistent with data from family, adoption and twin classical genetic studies. As we note here, there are limitations to our current understanding. Few, if any, other individual genes are likely to display such reproducible findings as those exerted by the ADH/ALDH observations in Asians and the chromosome 15 cholinergic receptor gene cluster findings for smoking quantity/chipper phenotypes. Although we have confidence in the overall data from groups of genes, small effects at other gene loci are likely to provide limited confidence in results for some time. It is nevertheless reassuring that genes which are likely to contain variants that influence both addiction vulnerability and quit success, such as cadherin 13, have been identified reproducibly in many of our studies and those of others, suggesting that variants in a number of genes whose effects are polygenic but reproducible will be generally accepted as addiction association in the relatively near future.

Acknowledgments We are very grateful for the subjects for each of these samples, and to collaborators who include Jed Rose, Caryn Lerman, Ray Niaura, Sean David, Marcus Munafo, Elaine Johnstone, Catherine Johnson, Paul Aveyard, the Japanese Genetic Initiative on Drug Abuse (JGIDA) and the Taipei methamphetamine study group (SK Lin and collaborators), and financial support from NIH IRP (NIDA).

References

1. Uhl GR, Elmer GI, Labuda MC, Pickens RW. Genetic influences in drug abuse. In: Gloom FE, Kupfer DJ, editors. Psychopharmacology: the fourth generation of progress. New York: Raven; 1995. p. 1793–2783.

2. Tsuang MT, Lyons MJ, Meyer JM, Doyle T, Eisen SA, Goldberg J, et al. Co-occurrence of abuse of different drugs in men: the role of drug-specific and shared vulnerabilities. Arch Gen Psychiatry. 1998;55(11):967–72.

3. Karkowski LM, Prescott CA, Kendler KS. Multivariate assessment of factors influencing illicit substance use in twins from female-female pairs. Am J Med Genet. 2000;96(5):665–70.

4. True WR, Heath AC, Scherrer JF, Xian H, Lin N, Eisen SA, et al. Interrelationship of genetic and environmental influences on conduct disorder and alcohol and marijuana dependence symptoms. Am J Med Genet. 1999;88(4):391–7.

5. Merikangas KR, Stolar M, Stevens DE, Goulet J, Preisig MA, Fenton B, et al. Familial transmission of substance use disorders. Arch Gen Psychiatry. 1998;55(11):973–9.

6. Woodward CE, Maes HH, Silberg JL, Meyer JM, Eaves LJ. Tobacco, alcohol and drug use in 8-16 year old twins. NIDA Res Monogr. 1996;162:309.

7. Tsuang MT, Lyons MJ, Eisen SA, Goldberg J, True W, Lin N, et al. Genetic influences on DSM-III-R drug abuse and dependence: a study of 3,372 twin pairs. Am J Med Genet. 1996;67(5):473–7.

8. Kendler KS, Prescott CA. Cocaine use, abuse and dependence in a population-based sample of female twins. Br J Psychiatry. 1998; 173:345–50.

9. Kendler KS, Aggen SH, Tambs K, Reichborn-Kjennerud T. Illicit psychoactive substance use, abuse and dependence in a population-based sample of Norwegian twins. Psychol Med. 2006;36(7): 955–62.

10. Agrawal A, Neale MC, Prescott CA, Kendler KS. A twin study of early cannabis use and subsequent use and abuse/dependence of other illicit drugs. Psychol Med. 2004;34(7):1227–37.

11. Grove WM, Eckert ED, Heston L, Bouchard Jr TJ, Segal N, Lykken DT. Heritability of substance abuse and antisocial behavior: a study of monozygotic twins reared apart. Biol Psychiatry. 1990;27(12): 1293–304.

12. Gynther LM, Carey G, Gottesman II, Vogler GP. A twin study of non-alcohol substance abuse. Psychiatry Res. 1995;56(3):213–20.

13. Kendler KS, Thornton LM, Pedersen NL. Tobacco consumption in Swedish twins reared apart and reared together. Arch Gen Psychiatry. 2000;57(9):886–92.

14. Broms U, Silventoinen K, Madden PA, Heath AC, Kaprio J. Genetic architecture of smoking behavior: a study of Finnish adult twins. Twin Res Hum Genet. 2006;9(1):64–72.

15. Uhl GR, Drgon T, Johnson C, Liu QR. Vulnerability to substance abuse. In: Johnson BA, editor. Addiction medicine: science and practice. Heidelberg: Springer; 2010.

16. Lander ES. The new genomics: global views of biology. Science. 1996;274(5287):536–9.

17. Mitchell-Olds T, Willis JH, Goldstein DB. Which evolutionary processes influence natural genetic variation for phenotypic traits? Nat Rev Genet. 2007;8(11):845–56.

18. Zielenski J. Genotype and phenotype in cystic fibrosis. Respiration. 2000;67(2):117–33.

19. WellcomeTrustConsortium. Genome-wide association study of 14,000 cases of seven common diseases and 3,000 shared controls. Nature. 2007;447(7145):661–78.

20. Baum AE, Akula N, Cabanero M, Cardona I, Corona W, Klemens B, et al. A genome-wide association study implicates diacylglycerol kinase eta (DGKH) and several other genes in the etiology of bipolar disorder. Mol Psychiatry. 2007;13(2):197–207.

21. Bierut LJ, Madden PA, Breslau N, Johnson EO, Hatsukami D, Pomerleau OF, et al. Novel genes identified in a high-density genome wide association study for nicotine dependence. Hum Mol Genet. 2007;16(1):24–35.

22. Coon KD, Myers AJ, Craig DW, Webster JA, Pearson JV, Lince DH, et al. A high-density whole-genome association study reveals that APOE is the major susceptibility gene for sporadic late-onset Alzheimer's disease. J Clin Psychiatry. 2007;68(4):613–8.

23. Li H, Wetten S, Li L, St Jean PL, Upmanyu R, Surh L, et al. Candidate single-nucleotide polymorphisms from a genomewide association study of Alzheimer disease. Arch Neurol. 2007;65(1): 45–53.

24. Dudbridge F, Gusnanto A, Koeleman BP. Detecting multiple associations in genome-wide studies. Hum Genomics. 2006;2(5):310–7.

25. Frayling TM. Genome-wide association studies provide new insights into type 2 diabetes aetiology. Nat Rev Genet. 2007;8(9): 657–62.

26. Seshadri S, DeStefano AL, Au R, Massaro JM, Beiser AS, Kelly-Hayes M, et al. Genetic correlates of brain aging on MRI and cognitive test measures: a genome-wide association and linkage analysis in the Framingham Study. BMC Med Genet. 2007;8 Suppl 1:S15.

27. Gottlieb DJ, O'Connor GT, Wilk JB. Genome-wide association of sleep and circadian phenotypes. BMC Med Genet. 2007;8 Suppl 1:9.

28. Liu QR, Drgon T, Johnson C, Walther D, Hess J, Uhl GR. Addiction molecular genetics: 639,401 SNP whole genome association identifies many "cell adhesion" genes. Am J Med Genet B Neuropsychiatr Genet. 2006;141(8):918–25.

29. Liu QR, Drgon T, Walther D, Johnson C, Poleskaya O, Hess J, et al. Pooled association genome scanning: validation and use to identify addiction vulnerability loci in two samples. Proc Natl Acad Sci USA. 2005;102(33):11864–9.

30. Uhl GR, Liu QR, Walther D, Hess J, Naiman D. Polysubstance abuse-vulnerability genes: genome scans for association, using 1,004 subjects and 1,494 single-nucleotide polymorphisms. Am J Hum Genet. 2001;69(6):1290–300.

31. Johnson C, Drgon T, Liu QR, Walther D, Edenberg H, Rice J, et al. Pooled association genome scanning for alcohol dependence using 104,268 SNPs: validation and use to identify alcoholism vulnerability loci in unrelated individuals from the collaborative study on the genetics of alcoholism. Am J Med Genet B Neuropsychiatr Genet. 2006;141(8):844–53.

32. Uhl GR, Liu QR, Drgon T, Johnson C, Walther D, Rose JE. Molecular genetics of nicotine dependence and abstinence: whole genome association using 520,000 SNPs. BMC Genet. 2007; 8(1):10.

33. Saccone SF, Hinrichs AL, Saccone NL, Chase GA, Konvicka K, Madden PA, et al. Cholinergic nicotinic receptor genes implicated in a nicotine dependence association study targeting 348 candidate genes with 3713 SNPs. Hum Mol Genet. 2007;16(1):36–49.

34. Uhl GR, Drgon T, Liu QR, Johnson C, Walther D, Komiyama T, et al. Genome-wide association for methamphetamine dependence: convergent results from 2 samples. Arch Gen Psychiatry. 2008;65(3):345–55.

35. Uhl GR, Liu QR, Drgon T, Johnson C, Walther D, Rose JE, et al. Molecular genetics of successful smoking cessation: convergent genome-wide association study results. Arch Gen Psychiatry. 2008; 65(6):683–93.

36. Meaburn E, Butcher LM, Liu L, Fernandes C, Hansen V, Al-Chalabi A, et al. Genotyping DNA pools on microarrays: tackling the QTL

problem of large samples and large numbers of SNPs. BMC Genomics. 2005;6(1):52.

37. Meaburn E, Butcher LM, Schalkwyk LC, Plomin R. Genotyping pooled DNA using 100K SNP microarrays: a step towards genomewide association scans. Nucleic Acids Res. 2006;34(4):e27.

38. Butcher LM, Meaburn E, Dale PS, Sham P, Schalkwyk LC, Craig IW, et al. Association analysis of mild mental impairment using DNA pooling to screen 432 brain-expressed single-nucleotide polymorphisms. Mol Psychiatry. 2005;10(4):384–92.

39. Butcher LM, Meaburn E, Knight J, Sham PC, Schalkwyk LC, Craig IW, et al. SNPs, microarrays and pooled DNA: identification of four loci associated with mild mental impairment in a sample of 6000 children. Hum Mol Genet. 2005;14(10):1315–25.

40. Butcher LM, Meaburn E, Liu L, Fernandes C, Hill L, Al-Chalabi A, et al. Genotyping pooled DNA on microarrays: a systematic genome screen of thousands of SNPs in large samples to detect QTLs for complex traits. Behav Genet. 2004;34(5):549–55.

41. Sham P, Bader JS, Craig I, O'Donovan M, Owen M. DNA Pooling: a tool for large-scale association studies. Nat Rev Genet. 2002;3(11):862–71.

42. Pearson JV, Huentelman MJ, Halperin RF, Tembe WD, Melquist S, Homer N, et al. Identification of the genetic basis for complex disorders by use of pooling-based genomewide single-nucleotide-polymorphism association studies. Am J Hum Genet. 2007;80(1):126–39.

43. Hung RJ, McKay JD, Gaborieau V, Boffetta P, Hashibe M, Zaridze D, et al. A susceptibility locus for lung cancer maps to nicotinic acetylcholine receptor subunit genes on 15q25. Nature. 2008;452(7187):633–7.

44. Thorgeirsson TE, Geller F, Sulem P, Rafnar T, Wiste A, Magnusson KP, et al. A variant associated with nicotine dependence, lung cancer and peripheral arterial disease. Nature. 2008;452(7187):638–42.

45. Uhl GR, Drgon T, Johnson C, Li CY, Contoreggi C, Hess J, et al. Molecular genetics of addiction and related heritable phenotypes: genome-wide association approaches identify "connectivity constellation" and drug target genes with pleiotropic effects. Ann NY Acad Sci. 2008;1141:318–81.

46. Berrettini W, Yuan X, Tozzi F, Song K, Francks C, Chilcoat H, et al. Alpha-5/alpha-3 nicotinic receptor subunit alleles increase risk for heavy smoking. Mol Psychiatry. 2008;13(4):368–73.

47. Amos CI, Wu X, Broderick P, Gorlov IP, Gu J, Eisen T, et al. Genome-wide association scan of tag SNPs identifies a susceptibility locus for lung cancer at 15q25.1. Nat Genet. 2008;40(5):616–22.

48. Lips EH, Gaborieau V, McKay JD, Chabrier A, Hung RJ, Boffetta P, et al. Association between a 15q25 gene variant, smoking quantity and tobacco-related cancers among 17 000 individuals. Int J Epidemiol. 2009;39(2):563–77.

49. Broderick P, Wang Y, Vijayakrishnan J, Matakidou A, Spitz MR, Eisen T, et al. Deciphering the impact of common genetic variation on lung cancer risk: a genome-wide association study. Cancer Res. 2009;69(16):6633–41.

50. Schwartz AG, Cote ML, Wenzlaff AS, Land S, Amos CI. Racial differences in the association between SNPs on 15q25.1, smoking behavior, and risk of non-small cell lung cancer. J Thorac Oncol. 2009;4(10):1195–201.

51. Wu C, Hu Z, Yu D, Huang L, Jin G, Liang J, et al. Genetic variants on chromosome 15q25 associated with lung cancer risk in Chinese populations. Cancer Res. 2009;69(12):5065–72.

52. Treutlein J, Cichon S, Ridinger M, Wodarz N, Soyka M, Zill P, et al. Genome-wide association study of alcohol dependence. Arch Gen Psychiatry. 2009;66(7):773–84.

53. Drgon T, Montoya I, Johnson C, Liu QR, Walther D, Hamer D, et al. Genome-wide association for nicotine dependence and smoking cessation success in NIH research volunteers. Mol Med. 2009;15(1–2):21–7.

54. Drgon T, Johnson C, Walther D, Albino AP, Rose JE, Uhl GR. Genome-wide association for smoking cessation success: participants in a trial with adjunctive denicotinized cigarettes. Mol Med. 2009;15(7–8):268–74.

55. Caporaso N, Gu F, Chatterjee N, Sheng-Chih J, Yu K, Yeager M, et al. Genome-wide and candidate gene association study of cigarette smoking behaviors. PLoS One. 2009;4(2):e4653.

56. Freathy RM, Ring SM, Shields B, Galobardes B, Knight B, Weedon MN, et al. A common genetic variant in the 15q24 nicotinic acetylcholine receptor gene cluster (CHRNA5-CHRNA3-CHRNB4) is associated with a reduced ability of women to quit smoking in pregnancy. Hum Mol Genet. 2009;18(15):2922–7.

57. Lueders KK, Hu S, McHugh L, Myakishev MV, Sirota LA, Hamer DH. Genetic and functional analysis of single nucleotide polymorphisms in the beta2-neuronal nicotinic acetylcholine receptor gene (CHRNB2). Nicotine Tob Res. 2002;4(1):115–25.

Pharmacotherapy of Addiction

8

Ahmed Elkashef and Ivan Montoya

Abstract

Addiction is a very serious and very costly public health problem. FDA-approved medications are available for alcohol, nicotine, and opiate addiction but not for stimulants or cannabis addictions. The focus of this chapter is on the medications to treat illicit substances, mainly heroin, stimulants, and cannabis. Currently, psychotherapy is still the primary mode of treatment for stimulants and cannabis addiction; however, relapse rates remain high. The search for effective pharmacological treatments has yielded some positive signals in proof of concept trials. Medications that are being tested in confirmatory trials for stimulants addiction include bupropion, topiramate, modafinil, disulfiram, ondansetron, and methylphenidate. For cannabis addiction there have been proof of concept trials that have shown efficacy, such as buspirone, nefazadone, and marinol. Early preclinical and clinical data suggest that some new molecular entities would be promising for multiple addictions, e.g., CB1 antagonists, D3 partial agonists, and CRF antagonists.

Learning Objectives

- Pharmacotherapy strategies to treat addiction
- Disulfiram, modafinil, topiramate, and ondansetron are promising medications for cocaine addiction
- Bupropion, methylphenidate, modafinil, and naltrexone are promising medications for methamphetamine addiction
- Buspirone, nefazadone, marinol, and flouextine are promising medications for cannabis addiction

Issues that Need to Be Addressed by Future Research

- The role of CB1 antagonist, CRF antagonist, and D3 partial agonist in addiction treatment
- Subgroup response and biomarkers
- Validation of preclinical model and clinical data

Background/Introduction

Over the past two decades, there has been a significant improvement over our understanding of the addictive processes which impacted our approach to pharmacological treatment.

Data emerging from preclinical and clinical studies imply that specific medications in the addictive process take on a selective role. This would suggest that certain medications could be targeted for a specific function involved in the addictive process or at a specific phase of treatment.

A. Elkashef, M.D. (✉) • I. Montoya, M.D.
Division of Pharmacotherapies and Medical Consequences of Drug Abuse, Department of Health and Human Services, National Institute on Drug Abuse (Retired), National Institutes of Health,
6001 Executive Boulevard, Room 4151, Bethesda, MD 20892, USA
e-mail: ahmedelkashef@me.com

J.C. Verster et al. (eds.), *Drug Abuse and Addiction in Medical Illness: Causes, Consequences and Treatment*,
DOI 10.1007/978-1-4614-3375-0_8, © Springer Science+Business Media, LLC 2012

For example:

1. Withdrawal phase to ameliorate or reduce symptom severity.
2. Active use phase to facilitate abstinence.
3. Abstinence maintenance to prevent relapse by modulating stress, cue reactivity, and priming effects.
4. Improving cognition (strategic thinking) and strengthening frontal inhibitory mechanisms (impulse control and decision making).

There are two caveats worth highlighting on the road to medication discovery. The first being preclinical animal models of addiction, e.g., self-administration, reinstatement, and cue reactivity. These are commonly used to screen compounds for their potential as medications. Although these models are helpful in selecting compounds, they have very limited predictive validity especially for stimulants. This is a critical issue and will not be fully resolved until an effective medication is found that can be tested in animals for model validation. Second, using human laboratory studies to assess safety and to test medication effects on the illicit drug of abuse subjective effects or self-administration is also burdened with the limitations of the artificiality of the lab setting, and the fact that patients recruited for these studies are not treatment seekers or motivated to quit. In order to advance compounds for further development, these limitations need to be considered. This shifts the burden to the costly outpatient proof of concept trials for proof of efficacy. In order to maximize success of these trials, a priori hypotheses for subgroup response and the use of biomarkers are greatly stressed.

Clinical and preclinical data are emerging and would suggest that some marketed medications, e.g., naltrexone, lofexidine, and topiramate, and some new molecular entities, e.g., corticotropin-releasing factor (CRF) antagonists, CB-1 antagonists, and D3 partial agonists, could be efficacious in targeting the neurobiological processes underlying addiction regardless of the illicit drug used. Naltrexone, already approved for alcohol and opiate addiction, has shown efficacy in proof of concept studies for cocaine [1] and methamphetamine [2]. Topiramate dual mechanism of action as a GABA agonist and AMPA antagonist has shown efficacy in early trials for alcohol, nicotine, food, and cocaine addictions [3]. Preclinical data suggest a role for lofexidine—already approved for opiate withdrawal [4] in Europe—for stress-induced relapse to stimulants use [5] and in human lab studies for cannabis withdrawal and relapse [6].

Preclinical data for the role of CRF in drug addiction is very important especially for relapse [7–9]. CRF appears to be a mediator of stress-induced reinstatement in rodent models. This effect was found not to be unique to only cocaine in the rat models of stress-induced relapse [10, 11] but has also been shown in heroin [11, 12] and alcohol [13]. These data support the well-known notion that stress is a major precipitant of relapse in abstaining patients.

Dopamine D3 receptors, cloned in 1990 [14], are located mainly in the accumbens. This dopamine receptor subtype was found to be upregulated in postmortem brains of patients with cocaine addiction who died of cocaine overdose [15]. D3 agonists exhibit cocaine-like effects in rodents and primates [14, 15]. D3 partial agonists have been shown to block cue-induced cocaine reinstatement [16, 17], cocaine-primed cocaine seeking [17, 18], and footshock-induced reinstatement of cocaine self-administration in rats [19], overall suggesting a potential role for D3 antagonists in preventing the three triggers of relapse.

The cannabinoid-1 (CB-1) receptor antagonists have been shown in different animal models to have a potential to treat multiple addictions [20, 21]. CB-1 antagonists act either by blocking the subjective/rewarding effects of drugs like THC or by blocking the ability of conditioned cues to promote reinstatement of drug-seeking behavior in animals, presumably through the endocannabinoid system. Taken together, results suggest a role for the cannabinoid system for polysubstance addiction.

Numerous marketed medications have been evaluated for efficacy in treating stimulants and cannabis addiction. Below we review the data for published trials for stimulants and cannabis addiction.

Pharmacotherapy of Heroin/Opiates Addiction

Opioid addiction, in the form of heroin or prescription opioid addiction is a public health priority. According to the National Survey on Drug Use and Health of 2007, it has been estimated that in the USA there were approximately 1.7 million persons classified with dependence on or abuse of opioid analgesics and 213,000 with dependence on or abuse of heroin. Approximately 6% of young adults aged 18–25 used prescription analgesics nonmedically. Population estimates on receiving treatment for drug addiction show that 558,000 individuals received treatment for addiction to pain relievers and 335,000 for heroin addiction. This appears to be the tip of the iceberg, because many more people who are in need of treatment do not receive treatment. According to the NSDUH estimates, of the illicit drug users who need treatment, only 17.8% actually receive treatment [22].

The treatment of opioid addiction may intend to (a) alleviate the signs and symptoms of opioid withdrawal, (b) reduce the craving for opioids, (c) prevent or reduce the use of illicit opioids, (d) prevent opioid use relapse, and (e) prevent the psychosocial and medical complications associated with illicit opioid use. From the pharmacological perspective, opioid addiction can be treated with opioid agonists, opioid antagonists, and nonopioid medications. The Food and Drug Administration (FDA) has given approval to methadone (opioid agonist), buprenorphine (partial opioid agonist) alone and in combination with naloxone (opioid antagonist), levomethadyl acetate (LAAM) (opioid agonist), and naltrexone (opioid antagonist). Other medications that have been investigated for the treatment of opioid addiction include alpha2 agonists (i.e., clonidine and lofexidine), N-methyl-D-aspartate (NMDA) receptor antagonists, tramadol, and corticotropin-releasing hormone (CRH) antagonists.

Methadone

Methadone is a synthetic opioid agonist that has been used for the treatment of opioid addiction since the 1960s [23]. Methadone can alleviate the signs and symptoms of opioid withdrawal, as well as reduce the craving and illicit use of opioids. Furthermore, the treatment with methadone can improve the medical and psychosocial consequences, and mortality associated with illicit opioid use [24–27].

Doses of methadone of 20 mg/day orally and higher have been shown effective. However, it has been suggested that the dose of methadone should be determined on a case-by-case basis. For opioid withdrawal, the initial dose is 15–30 mg orally and then adjust based upon control of withdrawal. For maintenance, it should be determined based on the dose that is effective in preventing opioid withdrawal signs or symptoms. Usually, the dose ranges from 80 to 120 mg/day, but some patients may require even higher doses.

Methadone is contraindicated in individuals with bronchial asthma, known or suspected paralytic ileus, respiratory depression, and hypersensitivity to methadone hydrochloride. Patients should not drink alcohol while receiving treatment with methadone. Side effects of methadone include diaphoresis, constipation, nausea, vomiting, asthenia, dizziness, lightheadedness, sedation, respiratory depression, and cardiovascular problems. Methadone has a black box warning from the FDA indicating that only approved hospitals and pharmacies can dispense oral methadone for the treatment of narcotic addiction and that QT interval prolongation and serious arrhythmias (torsades de pointes) have been observed during treatment with methadone (although most cases involve patients being treated with doses greater than 200 mg/day).

Some concomitant medications that may increase methadone's risk to prolong QT interval include amitriptyline, desipramine, sertraline, fluvoxamine, fluoxetine, nortriptyline, erythromycin, levofloxacin, moxifloxacin, rifampin, sparfloxacin, haloperidol, mesoridazine, pimozide, prochlorperazine, quetiapine, thioridazine, ziprasidone, as well as laxatives, steroids, diuretics. Other medications that may interact with methadone include opioid agonists and antagonists, antiretroviral medications, anticonvulsants, and monoaminoxidase inhibitors. Despite its potential risks, when methadone is prescribed under good medical supervision, it is a safe and cost-effective medication for the treatment of opioid addiction.

Methadone is widely used for the treatment of opioid-dependent pregnant and lactating women, although it is not approved for this population. Methadone is an FDA Pregnancy Category C. This means that studies in animals have revealed adverse effects on the fetus, and there are no controlled studies in women. The medication should be given only if the potential benefit justifies the potential risk to the fetus. The psychosocial and medical benefits have been well documented. Patients stabilized on methadone before pregnancy should remain on it. Opioid-dependent patient who requires methadone treatment can start with a dose of 10–30 mg/day with additional doses of 5–10 mg every 4–6 h if signs or symptoms of withdrawal syndrome appear. Methadone is also recommended for the treatment of opioid dependence during the postpartum period. The dose of methadone doses should be similar to the one received prior to pregnancy, which is often lower than the dose received during the last trimester of pregnancy. Methadone is also recommended for opioid-dependent women who are breast-feeding. The benefits of breastfeeding well exceed the risks of methadone. Additionally, methadone may help to reduce the severity of neonatal abstinence syndrome [28, 29].

Buprenorphine

Buprenorphine is a partial agonist at the mu opiate receptor that has less subjective effects and produces less withdrawal syndrome than morphine, and can block the subjective responses of up morphine. Due to its first-pass effects, the route administration of buprenorphine for the treatment opioid dependence is sublingual [30–32].

An article published in 1989 suggested that buprenorphine could be a pharmacotherapy for opioid dependence. The first double-blind clinical trial that compared sublingual buprenorphine 8 mg/day vs. oral methadone 20 and 60 mg/day was published in 1992. The results showed that buprenorphine was superior to 20 mg/day of methadone in retention in treatment and reduction of illicit opiate use [33]. Then, in 1998 a study showed that buprenorphine 8 mg/day produced significant reduced illicit opiate use and drug craving [34]. Given the potential abuse liability and diversion of buprenorphine alone, it was decided to develop a new formulation of the combination of buprenorphine and the opioid antagonist naloxone.

In October 2002, the FDA approved sublingual buprenorphine tablets and buprenorphine/naloxone tablets for the treatment of opiate dependence. Subutex® (buprenorphine hydrochloride) and Suboxone® tablets (buprenorphine hydrochloride and naloxone hydrochloride) treat opiate addiction by preventing symptoms of withdrawal from heroin and other opiates [35]. Buprenorphine is a Schedule III medication of the US Controlled Substances Act classification. The Drug Abuse Treatment Act of 2000 allows qualified physicians prescribe Schedule III, IV, and V opiates for the treatment of opiate dependence. Therefore, prescription of buprenorphine is limited to physicians who meet certain qualifying requirements and have notified the Secretary of Health and Human Services (HHS) of their intent to prescribe this product for the treatment of opioid dependence [35].

The appropriate dose and formulation of buprenorphine are based on the goals of the treatment and the clinical characteristics of the individual patient. In general, buprenorphine alone is indicated for the induction into buprenorphine, the treatment of opioid withdrawal, and for patients with high levels of opioid dependence. This formulation appears to be better tolerated by patients in the first several days of treatment and has less risk of precipitating opioid withdrawal. Patients treated with this formulation should have close supervision because of the risk of abuse and diversion of this formulation. The initial dose of sublingual buprenorphine alone is 12–16 mg/day, adjusting the dose in 2–4 mg/day increments/decrements depending on the level of opioid withdrawal symptoms.

The combination of buprenorphine and naloxone is the preferred medication for maintenance treatment because the opioid antagonist effects of naloxone help to deter intravenous abuse by persons dependent on other opiates. This is also the preferred formulation when clinical use includes unsupervised administration. The daily dose of this formulation is 12 mg or higher depending on the patient's level of opioid withdrawal. The dose should be adjusted in 2–4 mg/day increments/decrements to a level that prevents the emergence of opioid withdrawal syndrome. Depending on the individual, the usual daily dose of the combination of buprenorphine and naloxone is from 4 to 24 mg/day [36].

There is little research about the safety and efficacy of buprenorhine for the treatment of opioid-dependent pregnant and postpartum women. As with any opioid agonist, buprenorphine use during pregnancy is expected to be associated with neonatal abstinence syndrome (NAS), retardation of growth, and respiratory depression (Hytinantti et al. 2008; Lee 1994; Cunningham et al. 1993). It is recommended that buprenorphine be used during pregnancy only if the benefit outweighs the potential risk to the fetus. Buprenorphine is also being investigated for the treatment of opioid NAS.

The safety and efficacy of new formulations of buprenorphine that appear to provide long-term buprenorphine delivery are being investigated for the treatment of opioid dependence. Probuphine, a subcutaneous implant of buprenorphine, is reported to provide 6 months of stable medication blood levels [37, 38].

Naltrexone

Naltrexone is an opioid antagonist that is approved by the FDA for the treatment of opioid dependence. The clinical evaluation of naltrexone was published in 1978 [39], but it is not widely used by clinicians. Naltrexone should be considered an adjunct to social and psychological assistance in rehabilitation. It appears most efficacious in patients who are short-term opioid users, for example, adolescents, opioid-dependent patients who have been abstinent from opioids risk (e.g., released prisoners), patients who recently underwent medically supervised detoxification, and patients who are highly motivated to stop opioid use. The initiation of naltrexone should be after opioid-dependent patients have been opioid-free for 7–10 days and do not show clinical manifestation of opioid withdrawal. Multiple induction schedules with methadone or buprenorphine have been tested. The treatment should be started with a dose of 25 mg the first day, 50 mg the second day, and then continue with this daily dose. Alternate dose schedules are available. Side effects of naltrexone include dysphoria, depression, deep venous thrombosis, liver damage, and, if the patient did not have an appropriate detoxification, a naltrexone-precipitated opioid withdrawal.

The clinical effectiveness of oral naltrexone has been unsatisfactory because patients frequently do not adhere to the prescribed medication dose regimen. To improve medications adherence new formulations of Naltrexone has been investigated. Depot naltrexone "vivitrol" was recently approved for the treatment of alcohol dependence and opioid relapse prevention. Naltrexone implants are still being investigated in clinical trials for safety and efficacy [40–43].

LAAM

In the 1970s, studies showed that LAAM administered three times a week was effective for the treatment of opioid dependence [44], and studies conducted in the 1990s supported its FDA approval [45, 46]. The recommended dose is 20–40 mg three times weekly, which may be adjusted by increments of 5–10 mg, depending on the clinical observation of opioid withdrawal. In 2001, postmarketing reports showed that LAAM can induce prolongation of the QT interval in the electrocardiogram, arrhythmias, torsades de pointes, and other cardiac side effects. The same year, the manufacturer discontinued the sale and distribution of LAAM in the USA and LAAM was also removed from the European market. Currently, LAAM has a "black box" warning from the FDA.

Tramadol

Tramadol is an analgesic with moderate mu agonist opioid action that appears to have low abuse potential. It is not approved by the FDA for the treatment of opioid dependence but given its pharmacological properties it may help to treat opioid withdrawal with a low risk of opioid physical dependence. At a dose of 200–400 mg/day, tramadol appears to suppress opioid withdrawal signs and symptoms [47].

Nonopioid Medications

Alpha2 adrenergic agonists have been widely used and are being investigated for the treatment of opioid dependence. Medications such as lofexidine and clonidine appear effective for the treatment of opioid withdrawal, without the risks of opioid agonists such as perpetuating opioid dependence, illicit opioid use, medication diversion, and, in particular, the cardiac risks of methadone. Currently they are not approved by the FDA for this indication. Compared to clonidine, lofexidine may have the advantage of producing less hypotension [48, 49]. A recently published Phase III clinical trial showed that lofexidine can be safely used and is more efficacious than placebo for the treatment of opioid withdrawal symptoms in inpatients undergoing medically supervised opioid detoxification [48].

The N-methyl-D-aspartate (NMDA) receptor antagonists are being investigated for the treatment of opioid dependence because they appear to prevent the development of tolerance and dependence to the analgesic effects of morphine. For example, memantine has been shown to reduce opioid craving and the reinforcing effects of heroin. Further research is needed to determine the role of NMDA antagonists for the treatment of opioid addiction. Thus, NMDA antagonists may be useful adjunct medications for the treatment of opioid addiction [50, 51].

Pharmacotherapy of Cocaine Addiction

Leading the list for marketed medications tested so far for cocaine addiction are disulfiram, topiramate, modafinil, and ondansetron with regard to effect sizes and/or consistent findings in multiple trials. These four medications are currently being pursued in larger phase III confirmatory studies. The efficacy of disulfiram is thought to be related to its ability to inhibit the enzyme dopamine B-hydroxlase responsible for the conversion of dopamine to norepinephrine, in turn making more dopamine available. This may help in restoring the depleted dopamine stores following chronic cocaine use. The ongoing work with disulfiram is exploring the different DBH phenotypes and their link to response to disulfiram. However, disulfiram also inhibits the plasma esterase that metabolizes cocaine to BE and leads to an increase in cocaine blood levels when coadministered with cocaine [52]. This leads to an increase in HR and BP and makes disulfiram an undesirable medication to pursue for cocaine treatment.

Modafinil was tested for cocaine addiction because of its stimulant effect, and positive effects on improving impulse control [53] and decision making [54]. A very similar finding to the earlier pilot data conducted by Dackis et al. [55] was discovered in a recently completed multisite trial of modafinil for cocaine [56] showed an effect only in the nonalcohol cocaine-addicted patients and no effect in the codependent cocaine alcoholic patients. To date, there are two more trials for modafinil in progress. The data from these trials will help shed more light on the role of modafinil in cocaine addiction.

Ondansetron is approved for nausea and is mostly prescribed for cancer patients receiving chemotherapy. It is thought to decrease dopamine release through the 5HT3 receptor system in the accumbens. It has been shown to be efficacious in alcohol addiction [57]. The proof of concept study [58] showed that the 8-mg dose was superior to other lower doses and placebo in helping patients achieve abstinence from cocaine. Currently, ondansetron is being studied in larger trials to study its effects on combined cocaine and alcohol addiction.

Topiramate, a GABA agonist and AMPA antagonist antiseizure medication, showed positive effects in treating alcohol and nicotine addiction. It is also known to cause weight loss. The dual mechanism of action makes it unique among other GABA agonists in that it may not only reduce dopamine release through its GABA effect but it may also help reduce carvings and cue-induced relapse which has been shown with other AMPA antagonists [59]. The proof of concept trial conducted in cocaine [60] showed topiramate to have a therapeutic effect in the subgroup of patients who were able to stop using cocaine for a few days prior to randomization. This makes it a potential medication for low-to-moderate users with mild withdrawal symptoms and possibly for cuc-induced relapse prevention. In addition, topiramate's therapeutic effect in alcohol-dependent patients would also make it a candidate for dually dependent patients or for polysubstance addiction. These questions will be answered by the ongoing larger confirmatory trials.

Table 8.1 summarizes most of the conducted double-blind controlled trials in the past decade for cocaine addiction.

Amantadine and propranolol have shown efficacy in helping patients with severe withdrawal symptoms, as assessed by the Cocaine Symptom Severity Assessment scale (CSSA) devised by Kyle Kampman [63]. In a follow-up placebo-controlled study of either medication alone or

Table 8.1 Summary of data on published double-blind, placebo-controlled medication trials for cocaine dependence

Author/title	Study	Results
[59] A double-blind, placebo-controlled trial of modafinil for cocaine dependence.	62 randomized received a single morning dose of modafinil (400 mg) or matched placebo. The primary efficacy measure was cocaine abstinence based on urine BE levels. Secondary measures were craving, cocaine withdrawal, retention, and AEs.	Subjects treated with modafinil provided significantly more cocaine-negative urine samples when compared to those of the placebo group.
[61] Effectiveness of propranolol for cocaine-dependence treatment may depend on cocaine withdrawal symptom severity.	108 randomized received 100-mg propranolol or matched placebo. Quantitative urinary BE levels were the primary outcome measure. Secondary included treatment retention, ASI results, cocaine craving, mood and anxiety Sx, cocaine withdrawal Sx, and AEs.	No difference overall between the two groups with the exception of cocaine withdrawal Sxs in the propranolol subjects. However, propranolol-treated subjects with more severe cocaine withdrawal Sxs responded better than their placebo counterparts.
[62] A double-blind, placebo-controlled trial of amantadine, propranolol, and their combination for the treatment of cocaine dependence in patients with severe cocaine withdrawal symptoms.	199 randomized received 300 mg/day of amantadine, 100 mg/day of propranolol, a combination of 300 mg/day, or matching placebo. Cocaine abstinence was the primary outcome measure.	The odds of cocaine abstinence improved significantly over time in propranolol-treated subjects that were highly adherent to study medication but not in placebo-treated subjects.
[62] A pilot trial of topiramate for the treatment of cocaine dependence.	40 randomized titrating up to 200 mg daily of topiramate. Cocaine abstinence was the primary outcome measure verified by twice weekly urine BE.	Compared to placebo, the topiramate-treated subjects were more likely to be abstinent from cocaine compared to placebo-treated subjects.
[63] Tiagabine increases cocaine-free urines in cocaine-dependent methadone-treated patients: results of a randomized pilot study.	45 randomized to 12 or 24 mg of tiagabine or matched placebo. Reduction of use as measured by cocaine-free urines.	In weeks 9 and 10, cocaine-free urines increased from baseline by 33% in subject taking 24 mg/day, by 14 % (12 mg/day), by 14% (12 mg/day), and decreased by 10% with placebo-treated subjects.
[64] Treatment of cocaine and alcohol dependence with psychotherapy and disulfiram.	122 randomized with 250–500 mg of disulfiram vs. psychotherapy control (1 of 5 treatments). Duration of continuous abstinence from cocaine or alcohol; frequency and quantity of cocaine and alcohol use by week, verified by urine toxicology and breathalyzer screens.	Disulfiram treatment was associated with better retention in treatment as well as longer duration of abstinence from alcohol and cocaine use. The two active psychotherapies (CBT and TSF) reduced cocaine use over time compared to the supportive (CM).
[65] Disulfiram vs. placebo for cocaine dependence in buprenorphine-maintained subjects: a preliminary trial.	20 randomized to 250 mg of disulfiram vs. matched placebo. Duration of abstinence from cocaine verified by urine test.	The total number of weeks abstinent from cocaine was higher in the disulfiram group vs. placebo-treated subjects.
[66] Disulfiram treatment for cocaine dependence in methadone-maintained opioid addicts.	67 randomized to 250 mg disulfiram vs. matched placebo. Weekly assessments of the frequency and quantity of drug and alcohol use, weekly urine toxicology screens and breathalyzer readings.	Cocaine use was significantly decreased in quantity and frequency in subjects treated with disulfiram as compared to placebo-treated subjects.
[67] Efficacy of disulfiram and cognitive behavior therapy in cocaine-dependent outpatients: a randomized placebo-controlled trial.	121 randomized to 250 mg/day of disulfiram or matched placebo. Random regression analyses of self-reported frequency of cocaine use and results of urine toxicology screens.	Disulfiram treated subjects reduced their cocaine use more than placebo-treated subjects.
[68] Desipramine and contingency management for cocaine and opiate dependence in buprenorphine-maintained patients.	160 randomized to 150 mg/day or matched placebo (with and without contingency management). Cocaine abstinence as verified by urine test.	Cocaine-free and combined opiate and cocaine-free urines increased over time in those treated with either desipramine or contingency management and those receiving both had more drug-free urines (50%).
[69] Six-month trial of bupropion with contingency management for cocaine dependence in a methadone-maintained population.	106 randomized to 300 mg/day of bupropion or matched placebo (with and without voucher control and contingency management). Reduction of cocaine use as tested by thrice-weekly urine toxicologic test results for cocaine and heroin.	Overall, voucher-based control and bupropion had fewer cocaine-positive urine drug screens than had the other groups.
[70] Nefazodone treatment of cocaine dependence with comorbid depressive symptoms.	69 randomized to 200 mg (b.i.d) of nefazodone or matching placebo. Cocaine use measured by urine BE and self-report.	Median weekly BE declined in the nefazadone group and scores for strength of cocaine craving decreased compared to placebo.

(continued)

Table 8.1 (continued)

Author/title	Study	Results
[71] A double-blind, placebo-controlled trial of reserpine for the treatment of cocaine dependence.	119 randomized to 0.5 mg/day of reserpine or matching placebo. Cocaine use as determined by self-report confirmed with urine BE, cocaine craving, ASI, and CGI scores.	No significant differences between reserpine and placebo.
[72] A double-blind, placebo-controlled trial of tiagabine for the treatment of cocaine dependence.	140 randomized to 20 mg/day of tiagabine or matching placebo. Cocaine use as determined by self-report confirmed with urine BE, qualitative and quantitative urine toxicology measures.	Qualitative urine toxicology results suggest a possible weak signal for tiagabine in reducing cocaine use.
[73] Multicenter trial of baclofen for abstinence initiation for severe cocaine dependence.	160 randomized to 60 mg of baclofen (max dose). Cocaine use as determined by self-report confirmed by urine BE.	No significant effect between baclofen over placebo-treated subjects.
Randomized, placebo-controlled trial of cabergoline for the treatment of cocaine dependence.	70 randomized to 0.5 mg/wk of cabergoline or matched placebo. Retention, self-report, cocaine use verified by urine drug screen, HAM-D, cocaine craving, and CGI rating.	Cabergoline reduced craving ratings over placebo-treated subjects.
[74] Double-blind, placebo-controlled trial of selegiline transdermal system (STS) for the treatment of cocaine dependence.	300 subjects to 20 mg of selegiline. Self-reported cocaine use substantiated by urine BE.	There was no effect of selegiline over placebo-treated subjects.
[75] Citalopram combined with behavioral therapy reduces cocaine use: a double-blind, placebo-controlled trial.	76 randomized to 20 mg/day of citalopram or matched placebo (with cognitive management and cognitive behavioral therapy). Reduction in cocaine-positive urines.	Cocaine-treated subjects showed a significant reduction in positive urines during treatment as compared to placebo-treated subjects.
[58] A preliminary randomized double-blind, placebo-controlled study of the safety and efficacy of ondansetron in the treatment of cocaine dependence.	Cocaine use by urine BE.	The 8 mg/day group had the lowest drop out and greater rate of negative urine BE ($p=0.02$) compared to placebo. Ondansetron was well tolerated with no serious adverse events.

their combination, only propranolol showed efficacy in the medication adherent group analysis and not the intent-to-treat analysis. The combination did not prove to be superior to either alone [64].

Clinical Trials in Methamphetamine Addiction

In contrast to cocaine, methamphetamine enters the presynaptic neurons where it exerts its main action of reversing the vesicular monoamine transporter-2 (VMAT), thus impeding the incorporation/packaging of neurotransmitters into vesicles and causing the rapid efflux of intravesicular monoamines causing extremely high concentrations of cytosolic monoamines and release into the extracellular space. Methamphetamine also has a weak inhibitory effect on monoamine oxidase (MAO) thereby interfering with monoamine metabolism.

Bupropion has been shown in two clinical studies (Table 8.2) to be efficacious in facilitating abstinence in mild-to-moderate methamphetamine addicts, further confirmatory studies are underway. Modafinil has shown efficacy in a small double-blind, placebo-controlled trial at a dose of 200 mg/day in methamphetamine addicts [87]. Another double-blind, placebo-controlled study [88] showed an effect on maximum days abstinent in patients who were compliant with their medication. Methylphenidate (concerta) has been shown in a small pilot study to reduce amphetamine use [89]. Naltrexone has been shown to facilitate abstinence in patients with amphetamine addiction. These four medications are being studied in large confirmatory studies.

The unique effect of MA on the VMAT2 makes lobeline, a VMAT2 inhibitor, a candidate for testing. Indeed preclinical studies showed that lobeline blocks methamphetamine self-administration [90].

Table 8.2 Summary of data on published double-blind, placebo-controlled medication trials for methamphetamine dependence

Author/title	Study	Results
[76] Bupropion reduces methamphetamine-induced subjective effects and cue-induced craving.	26 participants were enrolled and 20 completed ($n = 10$ placebo and $n = 10$ bupropion), parallel groups design. To assess the impact of bupropion treatment on the subjective effects produced by MA in the laboratory, and to assess the effects of bupropion treatment on craving elicited by exposure to videotaped MA cues.	Bupropion treatment was associated with reduced ratings of "any drug effect" ($p < 0.02$) and "high" ($p < 0.02$) following MA administration. There was also a significant bupropion-by-cue exposure interaction on General Craving Scale total score ($p < 0.002$) and on the Behavioral Intention subscale ($p < 0.001$). Overall, data revealed that bupropion reduced acute MA-induced subjective effects and reduced cue-induced craving.
[77] A controlled trial of imipramine for the Tx of methamphetamine dependence.	31 subjects randomized two-dose study of either 10 or 150 mg/day of imipramine for 180 days. Test efficacy of imipramine as a Tx for MA dependence and establish feasibility of conducting controlled clinical trial at the clinic.	Retention in Tx was significantly longer for subjects treated with 150 mg of imipramine compared to control (median days: 33.0 vs. 10.5). No consistent differences in percent of urine samples positive for MA, Beck Depression Inventory scores, or craving.
[78] Randomized, placebo-controlled trial of baclofen and gabapentin for the treatment of methamphetamine dependence.	16-week, randomized, placebo-controlled, double-blind trial of two GABAergic medications, baclofen (20 mg tid) and gabapentin (800 mg tid). Baclofen ($n = 25$) gabapentin ($n = 26$), placebo ($n = 37$), clinic thrice weekly with psychosocial counseling, complete assessments, and urine samples.	No statistically significant main effects for baclofen or gabapentin in reducing methamphetamine use were observed using a generalized estimating equation (GEE). A significant Tx effect was found in post hoc analyses for baclofen relative to placebo, but not gabapentin, among participants who reported taking a higher percentage of study meds (significant Tx group by medication adherence in GEE model of MA use).
[79] Randomized, placebo-controlled trial of sertraline and contingency management for the treatment of methamphetamine dependence.	Participants completed a 2-week, nonmedication baseline, randomized to one of four conditions for 12 weeks: sertraline plus CM ($n = 61$), sertraline only ($n = 59$), matching placebo plus CM ($n = 54$), or matching placebo-only ($n = 55$). Thrice weekly clinic visits for data collection, medication dispensing, and relapse prevention groups. 1. Evaluate the efficacy of sertraline (50 mg bid) and contingency management (CM) for the Tx of MA dependency. 2. MA urine drug screening and self-reported days of use, retention, drug craving, and mood symptoms.	No statistically significant main or interaction effects for sertraline or CM in reducing methamphetamine use were observed using a generalized estimating equation (GEE), although post hoc analyses showed the sertraline-only condition had significantly poorer retention than other conditions (chi-sq (3) = 8.40, $p < 0.05$). Sertraline conditions produced significantly more adverse events than placebo conditions. Significantly higher proportion of participants in CM conditions achieved three consecutive weeks of MA abstinence than those in the non-CM conditions.
[80] A preliminary randomized, double-blind, placebo-controlled study of the safety and efficacy of ondansetron in the treatment of methamphetamine dependence.	150 methamphetamine-dependent men and women received ondansetron (0.25 mg, 1 mg, or 4 mg b.i.d.) or placebo over 8 weeks. Subjects provided urine three times weekly and were enrolled in cognitive behavioral therapy three times weekly. Primary outcome was number of methamphetamine nonuse days as assessed by urine analysis. Secondary outcomes include decreasing methamphetamine use, withdrawal, craving, and ASI.	Ondansetron was well tolerated. No group differences were statistically significant between any of the three doses of ondansetron and placebo on the primary or secondary outcomes.
[81] Effects of acute topiramate dosing on methamphetamine-induced subjective mood.	Tested in 10 meth-dependent individuals (3 females) whether low- or high-dose (15 or 30 mg i.v.) meth-induced positive subjective effects and reinforcement can be antagonized by low- or high dose (100 or 220 mg orally). Hypothesis is that mechanistically, topiramate's therapeutic effects are due to inhibition of cortico-mesolimbic dopamine function, the primary substrate that governs the acquisition, maintenance, and reinstatement of goal-directed behavior toward seeking abused drugs.	MA administration was associated with orderly, prototypical, and significant increases on measures of stimulation, euphoria, craving, and reinforcement. Some dysphoric symptoms emerged. Topiramate alone showed nonsignificant trend toward mild reductions in positive mood and reinforcement. Topiramate appeared to accentuate the appreciation of MA-induced stimulation and euphoria significantly, but not for craving or reinforcement. Combination of topiramate and MA appeared to be safe and well tolerated. Few adverse events. Acute dosing with up to 200 mg topiramate appeared to enhance, rather than attenuate the positive subjective effects of MA.
[82] A comparison of aripiprazole, methylphenidate, and placebo for amphetamine dependence.	53 randomly assigned to receive aripiprazole (15 mg/day), slow-release methylphenidate (54 mg/day) or placebo for 20 weeks. Intent-to treat analysis. Outcome measure was the proportion of amphetamine-positive urine samples.	Study terminated prematurely due to unexpected results of interim analysis. Patients allocated to aripiprazole had significantly more amphetamine-positive urine samples than patients in the placebo group (odds ratio = 3.77, 95%CI = 1.55–9.18), whereas patients who received methylphenidate had significantly fewer amphetamine positive urine samples than patients who had received placebo (odds ratio = 0.46, 95% CI = 0.26–0.81).

(continued)

Table 8.2 (continued)

Author/title	Study	Results
[83] Methamphetamine-amlodipine interactions: preliminary analysis.	Nine subjects (6 males and 3 females) underwent 2 two-day sessions in each of which they received 30-mg immediate release oral-d methamphetamine hydrochloride after premedication with amlodipine 20 mg or placebo. To examine the subjective and physiological effects of oral-D-methamphetamine after acute premedication with amlodipine.	MA produced significant increases over time in systolic and diastolic blood pressure, heart rate, ARCI, MBG and A scores and POMS Vigor, Arousal, and Positive Mood scores. No other treatment-related differences emerged in subjective responses such as euphoria hyperactivity, with the exception of significantly higher POMS arousal scores in the amlodipine group; levels did not differ in the two groups.
[84] Methamphetamine quantitative urine concentrations during a controlled trial of fluoxetine treatment: preliminary analysis.	Eight-week randomized, controlled, parallel group design with a 1-week single-blind placebo lead-in followed by 7 weeks of double-blind fluoxetine 40 mg per day or placebo. Mean age was 35, 42 (70%) were males, and 9 (15%) were HIV seropositive. Subjects had used MA an average of 7.1 years. Urine MA and amphetamine concentrations, measured by gas chromatography, were available for the first 30 subjects. Evaluate the use of quantitative urine MA concentrations as the primary outcome measure in pharmacotherapy trials in MA dependence. Attempted to answer the following questions: Characteristics of quantitative urine MA levels in outpatients undergoing pharmacotherapy research. Is quantitative urine MA a valid measure of MA use? Does it correlate with self-reports of use, and with what self-reports does urine MA best correlate?	Mean urine MA concentrations at each assessment point ranged from 647 to 23,676 ng/ml, and individual sample values ranged from 0 to 336,559 ng/ml. Analysis of the relationship between urine methamphetamine levels and various self-reported measures of MA use showed significant and strong correlations between MA levels and self-reported measures of MA use (nonparametric Kendall's tau, $p < 0.05$). Correlations were significant for self-reported days, grams, and dollars worth of MA used at intake and in each of the 8 weeks of the clinical trial. Kendall's correlations ranged from 0.33 to 0.84, and averaged 0.63 for these measures.
[85] Effects of Naltrexone on the subjective response to amphetamine in healthy volunteers.	Used the visual analog scales assessing subjective effects over 7 h. Assessed effects of opioid antagonist, naltrexone's subjective response to an oral dose of dexamphetamine (30 mg) in 12 healthy volunteers in double-blind, placebo-controlled design. Study measurements included: visual analog scale, monitoring of blood pressure, heart rate, skin conduction, and speed of reading. To evaluate the effect of pretreatment with naltrexone on the subjective response to amphetamine.	Preliminary evidence indicate that naltrexone is well tolerated in healthy human subjects and may reduce the reinforcing effects of amphetamine via modulation of the opioid system.
[2] Naltrexone for the treatment of amphetamine dependence. A randomized, placebo-controlled trial	12 weeks of treatment. 80 participants were randomized to placebo or (50 mg) naltrexone. Subjects visited the clinic twice weekly to receive medication and relapse prevention therapy and provide urine samples. The main outcome measure was abstinence from amphetamine use as indicated by the total number of negative amphetamine urine samples during the 12 weeks of treatment.	This trial demonstrated the efficacy of naltrexone in reducing amphetamine use in amphetamine dependent individuals.
[86] Bupropion for the treatment of methamphetamine dependence.	12 weeks of treatment and a 30-day follow-up. 72 participants were randomized to placebo and 79 to bupropion Sustained Release 150 mg twice daily. Patients were asked to come to the clinic three times per week for assessments, urine drug screens, and 90-minute group psychotherapy. The primary outcome was the change in proportion of participants having a methamphetamine-free week. Secondary outcomes included: urine for quantitative methamphetamine, self-report of methamphetamine use, subgroup analyses of balancing factors and comorbid conditions, addiction severity, craving, risk behaviors for HIV, and use of other substances.	The GEE regression analysis showed that overall, the difference between bupropion and placebo groups in the probability of a nonuse week over the 12-week treatment period was not statistically significant ($p = 0.09$). Mixed model regression was used to allow adjustment for baseline factors in addition to those measured (site, gender, level of baseline use, and level of symptoms of depression). This subgroup analysis showed that bupropion had a significant effect compared to placebo, among males who had a lower level of methamphetamine use at baseline ($p < 0.0001$). Co-morbid depression and ADHD did not change the outcome.
Modafinil for the treatment of methamphetamine dependence.	210 patients randomized to modafinil 200mg, 400mg, or placebo for 12 weeks. The primary outcome measure was methamphetamine non-use week.	Regression analysis showed no significant difference between either modafinil group (200 or 400mg) However, an ad-hoc analysis of medication compliance, did find a significant difference in maximum duration of abstinence (23 days vs. 10 days, p=0.003), between those having the top quartile of compliance (>85% of urines were positive for modafinil, N=36), and the lower three quartiles of modafinil 200 and 400mg groups (N=106).

Pharmacotherapy of Cannabis Addiction

Tetrahydrocannabinol (THC) is the most clinically significant of all the cannabinoids. It exerts its effects through the CB1 and CB2 receptors. CB1 receptors are located mainly in brain, spinal cord, and peripheral tissue, while CB2 are mainly in immune cells [91]. The effects on the CB1 can be blocked by the CB1-selective antagonist SR-141716 [92, 94].

Clinical studies for cannabis addiction have focused on the treatment of the well-documented withdrawal symptoms [94–96] of anxiety, depression, irritability, marijuana craving, decreased quantity and quality of sleep, and decreased food intake compared to baseline conditions. This effort has been led by Haney and others in a human lab setting to the effects of medications on marijuana withdrawal symptoms. Medications tested in this paradigm included marinol, bupropion, valproic acid, and nefazadone.

Recent research has focused on the development of a human laboratory studies designed to characterize and test the effects of potential treatment medications on marijuana dependence and relapse [6].

The cannabinoid agonist, dronabinol/marinol, was tested, and compared to placebo, oral THC significantly improved anxiety, misery, chills, self-reported sleep disturbance, and reversed the anorexia and the weight loss associated with marijuana withdrawal with no intoxicating effects. Sustained-release bupropion (0, 300 mg/day) substantially *worsened* mood ratings (irritability, depression) and ratings of sleep compared to maintenance on placebo [97]. Similarly, the mood stabilizer, divalproex (1,500 mg/day), significantly worsened mood ratings (irritability, edginess, anxiety), sleep, and cognitive performance in marijuana smokers [98, 99]. These data do not support the use of either bupropion or divalproex to treat marijuana withdrawal.

Nefazodone (0, 450 mg/day), an antidepressant that effectively treats anxiety and has sedative side effects, was found to significantly decrease ratings of anxiety and muscle pain compared to placebo, but had no effect on other symptoms of withdrawal, such as irritability [100].

Two clinical studies with the CB1-cannabinoid receptor antagonist, rimonabant, showing blockade of the "drug high," "stoned," and "drug strength" and reduction in heart rate, suggest that THC effects are mainly CB1 mediated [101].

It is too early to tell whether an agonist or antagonist approach will prove to be more beneficial in the management of marijuana dependence; however, it is possible that each will have a role in treatment, where an agonist may be indicated initially to control withdrawal symptoms and facilitate abstinence and an antagonist will be mainly used for relapse prevention, similar to the methadone/naltrexone approach for the treatment of heroin addiction.

Other medications tested include buspirone administered in an open label fashion to 11 subjects undergoing treatment for marijuana dependence [102]. Participants reported using marijuana on 76.9% of days prior to treatment and 38.9% of days while on buspirone ($p=0.004$). Large-scale double-blind studies are underway to test the pilot findings.

Lithium (500 mg, bid) was administered to 20 adolescent marijuana abusers in an impatient setting for up to 7 days. Decreased anger, improved mood, and decreased anxiety were reported [103]. Interestingly, there is evidence that lithium modulated the cannabis withdrawal syndrome via an oxytocin release mechanism [104].

A subgroup analysis of depressed marijuana smokers in a double-blind, placebo-controlled trial of the antidepressant fluoxetine noted that the placebo group had almost 20 times the amount of marijuana uses as the fluoxetine group [105].

The data from these pilot studies suggest that more rigorous double-blind, placebo-controlled studies with fluoxetine and lithium should be performed.

Conclusions/Summary

Progress in stimulants pharmacotherapy has made some strides over the past two decades. Multiple marketed medications are in confirmatory trials for stimulants and cannabis addiction. Many other new molecules are in early development and hold promise for polysubstance addiction.

Patient demographics and clinical characteristics including patterns of use seem to be an important factor in predicting outcome. Baseline use has always been thought of as one of the strongest predictors of outcome, this was very obvious in the data from the cocaine topiramate study and the bupropion study for methamphetamine dependence where burpropion was found to be efficacious only in the group with low-to-moderate use at baseline. More recently data from alcohol and nicotine studies highlight the role of pharmacogenomics as a very promising tool in predicting outcome [106, 107].

Genetic and clinical biomarkers predicting outcome could only improve our results and are being incorporated in many ongoing addiction trials to help elucidate subgroup response.

In this age of personalized medicine pharmacogenomics and biomarkers are a must in every clinical trials.

Recent data from cocaine studies suggest that the effect of the medication could be synergized when combined with contingency management (CM). Two separate studies, one using bupropion and one using desipramine, in opiate-dependent cocaine abusing population showed an enhanced effect of the combination of medication plus CM than each treatment arm alone [99, 100].

Although most drug addicts would cite a drug of choice, most use more than one drug. This could be good or bad news.

Having a polysubstance dependence could lead to treatment resistance as in the case of the recently completed modafinil study for cocaine addiction where the alcohol/cocaine-codependent group showed no response to modafinil.

On the other hand the good news is that medications that address common mechanisms in addiction could help polysubstance addicted patients. Further studies will tell.

References

1. Oslin DW, Pettinati HM, Volpicelli JR, Wolf AL, Kampman KM, O'Brien CP. The effects of naltrexone on alcohol and cocaine use in dually addicted patients. J Subst Abuse Treat. 1999;16(2): 163–7.

2. Jayaram-Lindstrom N, Hammarbert A, Beck O, Franck J. Naltrexone for the treatment of amphetamine dependence: a randomized, placebo-controlled trial. Am J Psychiatry. 2008; 165(11):1442–8.

3. Johnson BA, Rosenthal N, Capece JA, Wiegand F, Mao L, Beyers K, et al. Topiramate for treating alcohol dependence: a randomized controlled trial. JAMA. 2007;298(14):1641–51.

4. Yu E, Miotto K, Akerele E, Montgomery A, Elkashef A, Walsh R, Montoya I, et al. A phase 3 placebo-controlled, double-blind, multi-site trial of the alpha-s-adrenergic agonist, lofexidine, for opioid withdrawal. Drug Alcohol Depend. 2008;97(1–2): 158–68.

5. Erb S, Hitchcott PK, Phil D, Heshmat R, Mueller D, Shaham Y, et al. Alpha-2 adrenergic receptor agonists block stress-induced reinstatement of cocaine seeking. Neuropsychopharmacology. 2000;23(2):138–50.

6. Haney M. The marijuana withdrawal syndrome: diagnosis and treatment. Curr Psychiatry Rep. 2005;7(5):360–6.

7. Koob GF. Stress, corticotrophin-releasing factor, and drug addiction. Ann NY Acad Sci. 1999;897:27–45.

8. Stewart J. Pathways to relapse: the neurobiology of drug- and stress-induced relapse to drug-taking. J Psychiatry Neurosci. 2000;25(2):125–36.

9. Sarnyai Z, Shaham Y, Heinrichs SC. The role of corticotropin-releasing factor in drug addiction. Phamacol Rev. 2001;53(2): 209–43.

10. Erb S, Shaham Y, Stewart J. The role of corticotropin-releasing factor and corticosterone in stress- and cocaine-induced relapse to cocaine seeking in rats. J Neurosci. 1998;18(4):4429–5536.

11. Shaham Y, Erb S, Leung S, Buczek Y, Stewart J. CP-154-526, a selective, non-peptide antagonist of the corticotropin-releasing factor1 receptor attenuates stress-induced relapse to drug seeking cocaine- and heroin-trained rats. Psychopharmacology (Berl). 1998;137(2):184–90.

12. Shaham Y, Funk D, Erb S, Brown TJ, Walker CD, Stewart J. Corticotropin-releasing factor, but not corticosterone, is involved in stress-induced relapse to heroin-seeking in rats. J Neurosci. 1997;17(7):2605–14.

13. Le AD, Harding S, Juzytsch W, et al. The role of corticotrophin-releasing factor in stress-induced relapse to alcohol-seeking behavior in rats. Psychopharmacology (Berl). 2000;150(3): 317–24.

14. Acri JB, Carter SR, Alling K, Geter-Douglass B, Dijkstra D, Wikstrom H, et al. Assessment of cocaine-like discriminative stimulus effects of dopamine D3 receptor ligands. Eur J Pharmacol. 1995;281(2):R7–9.

15. Spealcocainen RD. Dopamine D3 receptor agonists partially reproduce the discriminative stimulus effects of cocaine in squirrel monkeys. J Pharmacol Exp Ther. 1996;278(3):1128–37.

16. Pilla M, Perachon S, Sautel F, Garrido F, Mann A, Wermuth CG, et al. Selective inhibition of cocaine-seeking behaviour by a partial dopamine D3 receptor agonist. Nature. 1999;400(6742):371–5.

17. Di Ciano P, Underwood RJ, Hagan JJ, Everitt BJ. Attenuation of cue-controlled cocaine-seeking by a selective D3 dopamine receptor antagonist SB-277011-A. Neuropsychopharmacology. 2003;28(2):329–38.

18. Gilbert JG, Newman AH, Gardner EL, Ashby Jr CR, Heidreder CA, Pak AC, et al. Acute administration of SB-277011A, NGB 2904, or BP 897 inhibits cocaine cue-induced reinstatement of drug-seeking behavior in rats: role of dopamine D3 receptors. Synapse. 2005;57(1):17–28.

19. Xi ZX, Gilbert J, Campos AC, Kline N, Ashby Jr CR, Hagan JJ, et al. Blockade of mesolimbic dopamine D3 receptors inhibits stress-induced reinstatement of cocaine-seeking rats. Psychopharmacology (Berl). 2004;176(1):57–65.

20. Le Foll B, Goldberg SR. Cannabinoid CB1 receptor antagonists as promising new medications for drug dependence. J Pharmacol Exp Ther. 2005;312(3):875–83.

21. Beardsley PM, Thococaines BF. Current evidence supporting a role of cannabinoid CB1 receptor (CB1R) antagonists as potential pharcocainecotherapies for drug abuse disorders. Behav Pharmacol. 2005;16(5–6):275–96.

22. Substance Abuse and Mental Health Services Administration. Results from the 2007 National Survey on Drug Use and Health: National findings. 2008. Rockville, MD: Office of Applied Studies; NSDUH Series H-34, DHHS Publication No. SMA 08-4343.

23. Dole V, Nyswander M. A medical treatment for diacetylmorphine (heroin) addiction: A clinical trial with methadone hydrochloride. JAMA. 1965;193:646–50.

24. Gronbladh L, Gunne L. Methadone-assisted rehabilitation of Swedish heroin addicts. Drug Alcohol Depend. 1989;24(1):31–7.

25. Ball JC, Corty E, Petroski SP, Bond H, Tommasello A, Graff H. Treatment effectiveness: medical staff and services provided to 2,394 patients at methadone programs in three states. NIDA Res Monogr. 1987;76:175–81.

26. Ball JC, Lange WR, Myers CP, Friedman SR. Reducing the risk of AIDS through methadone maintenance treatment. J Health Soc Behav. 1988;29(3):214–26.

27. Kleber HD. Methadone maintenance 4 decades later: thousands of lives saved but still controversial. JAMA. 2008;300(19):2303–5.

28. Jones HE, Martin PR, Heil SH, Kaltenbach K, Selby P, Coyle MG, et al. Treatment of opioid-dependent pregnant women: clinical and research issues. J Subst Abuse Treat. 2008;35(3):245–59.

29. Finnegan LP. Treatment issues for opioid-dependent women during the perinatal period. J Psychoactive Drugs. 1991;23(2): 191–201.

30. Bickel WK, Stitzer ML, Bigelow GE, Liebson IA, Jasinski DR, Johnson RE. Buprenorphine: dose-related blockade of opioid challenge effects in opioid dependent humans. J Pharmacol Exp Ther. 1988;247(1):47–53.

31. Jasinski DR, Fudala PJ, Johnson RE. Sublingual versus subcutaneous buprenorphine in opiate abusers. Clin Pharmacol Ther. 1989;45(5):513–9.

32. Martin WR, Eades CG, Thompson JA, Huppler RE, Gilbert PE. The effects of morphine- and nalorphine-like drugs in the nondependent and morphine-dependent chronic spinal dog. J Pharmacol Exp Ther. 1976;197(3):517–32.

33. Johnson RE, Jaffe JH, Fudala PJ. A controlled trial of buprenorphine treatment for opioid dependence. JAMA. 1992;267(20): 2750–5.

34. Ling W, Charuvastra C, Collins JF, Batki S, Brown Jr LS, Kintaudi P, et al. Buprenorphine maintenance treatment of opiate dependence: a multicenter, randomized clinical trial. Addiction. 1998;93(4):475–86.

35. US Food and Drug Administration Center for Drug Evaluation and Research Drug Information. Subutex (buprenorphine

hydrochloride) and Suboxone tablets (buprenorphine hydrochloride and naloxone hydrochloride). http://www.fda.gov/cder/drug/infopage/subutex_suboxone/default.htm. 2008.

36. Johnson RE, McCagh JC. Buprenorphine and naloxone for heroin dependence. Curr Psychiatry Rep. 2000;2(6):519–26.

37. Sigmon SC, Wong CJ, Chausmer AL, Liebson IA, Bigelow GE. Evaluation of an injection depot formulation of buprenorphine: placebo comparison. Addiction. 2004;99(11):1439–49.

38. Liu KS, Kao CH, Liu SY, Sung KC, Kuei CH, Wang JJ. Novel depots of buprenorphine have a long-acting effect for the management of physical dependence to morphine. J Pharm Pharmacol. 2006;58(3):337–44.

39. Clinical evaluation of naltrexone treatment of opiate-dependent individuals. Report of the National Research Council Committee on Clinical Evaluation of Narcotic Antagonists. Arch Gen Psychiatry. 1978; 35(3):335–40.

40. Comer SD, Sullivan MA, Hulse GK. Sustained-release naltrexone: novel treatment for opioid dependence. Expert Opin Investig Drugs. 2007;16(8):1285–94.

41. Ngo HT, Tait RJ, Hulse GK. Comparing drug-related hospital morbidity following heroin dependence treatment with methadone maintenance or naltrexone implantation. Arch Gen Psychiatry. 2008;65(4):457–65.

42. Kruptisky EM, Burakov AM, Tsoy MV, Egorova VY, Slavina TY, Grinenko AY, et al. Overcoming opioid blockade from depot naltrexone (Prodetoxon). Addiction. 2007;102(7):1164–5.

43. Hulse GK, Tait RJ, Comer SD, Sullivan MA, Jacobs IG, Arnold-Reed D. Reducing hospital presentations for opioid overdose in patients treated with sustained release naltrexone implants. Drug Alcohol Depend. 2005;79(3):351–7.

44. Ling W, Charuvastra C, Kaim SC, Klett CJ. Methadyl acetate and methadone as maintenance treatments for heroin addicts. A veterans administration cooperative study. Arch Gen Psychiatry. 1976;33(6):709–20.

45. Eissenberg T, Bigelow GE, Strain EC, Walsh SL, Brooner RK, Stitzer ML, et al. Dose-related efficacy of levomethadyl acetate for treatment of opioid dependence. A randomized clinical trial. JAMA. 1997;277(24):1945–51.

46. Jones HE, Strain EC, Bigelow GE, Walsh SL, Stitzer ML, Eissenberg T, et al. Induction with levomethadyl acetate: safety and efficacy. Arch Gen Psychiatry. 1998;55(8):729–36.

47. Lofwall MR, Walsh SL, Bigelow GE, Strain EC. Modest opioid withdrawal suppression efficacy of oral tramadol in humans. Psychopharmacology (Berl). 2007;194(3):381–93.

48. Yu E, Miotto K, Akerele E, Montgomery A, Elkashef A, Walsh R, et al. A Phase 3 placebo-controlled, double-blind, multi-site trial of the alpha-2-adrenergic agonist, lofexidine, for opioid withdrawal. Drug Alcohol Depend. 2008;97(1–2):158–68.

49. Walsh SL, Strain EC, Bigelow GE. Evaluation of the effects of lofexidine and clonidine on naloxone-precipitated withdrawal in opioid-dependent humans. Addiction. 2003;98(4):427–39.

50. Akerele E, Bisaga A, Sullivan MA, Garawi F, Comer SD, Thomas AA, et al. Dextromethorphan and quinidine combination for heroin detoxification. Am J Addict. 2008;17(3):176–80.

51. Comer SD, Sullivan MA. Memantine produces modest reductions in heroin-induced subjective responses in human research volunteers. Psychopharmacology (Berl). 2007;193(2):235–45.

52. McCance-Katz EF, Kosten TR, Jatlow P. Disulfiram effects on acute cocaine administration. Drug Alcohol Depend. 1998;52(1):27–39.

53. Turner DC, Clark L, Dowson J, Robbins TW, Sahakian BJ. Modafinil improves cognition and response inhibition in adult attention-deficit/hyperactivity disorder. Biol Psychiatry. 2004;55(10):1031–40.

54. Turner DC, Robbins TW, Clark L, Aron AR, Dowson J, Sahakian BJ. Cognitive enhancing effects of modafinil in healthy volunteers. Psychopharm (Berl). 2003;165(3):260–9.

55. Dackis CA, Kampman KM, Lynch KG, Pettinati HM, O'Brien CP. A double-blind, placebo-controlled trial of modafinil for cocaine dependence. Neuropsychopharmacology. 2005;30(1):205–11.

56. Anderson AL, Reid MS, Li SH, Holmes T, Shemanski L, Slee A, Smith EV, Kahn R, Chiang N, Vocci F, Ciraulo D, Dackis C, Roache JD, Salloum IM, Somoza E, Urschel HC 3rd, Elkashef AM. Modafinil for the treatment of cocaine dependence. Drug Alcohol Depend. 2009 Jun 25.

57. Johnson BA, Campling GM, Griffiths P, Cowen PJ. Attenuation of some alcohol-induced mood changes and the desire to crink by 5-HT3 receptor blockade: a preliminary study in healthy male volunteers. Psychopharm (Berl). 1993;112(1):142–4.

58. Johnson BA, Roache JD, Ait-Daoud N, Javors MA, Harrison JM, Elkashef A, Mojsiak J, et al. A preliminary randomized, double-blind, placebo-controlled study of the safety and efficacy of ondansetron in the treatment of cocaine dependence. Drug Alcohol Depend. 2006;84:256–63.

59. Volkow ND, Wang GJ, Telang F, Fowler JS, Logan J, Childress AR, et al. Cocaine cues and dopamine in dorsal striatum: mechanism of craving in cocaine addiction. J Neurosci. 2006;26(24):6583–8.

60. Kampman KM, Pettinati H, Lynch KG, Dackis C, Sparkman T, Weigley C, et al. A pilot trial of topiramate for the treatment of cocaine dependence. Drug Alcohol Depend. 2004;75(3):233–40.

61. Kampman KM, Volpicelli JR, Mulvaney F, Alterman AI, Cornish J, Gariti P, et al. Effectiveness of propranolol for cocaine dependence treatment may depend on cocaine withdrawal symptom severity. Drug Alcohol Depend. 2001;63(1):69–78.

62. Kampman KM, Dackis C, Lynch KG, Pettinati H, Tirado C, Gariti P, et al. A double-blind, placebo-controlled trial of amantadine, propranolol, and their combination for the treatment of cocaine dependence in patients with severe cocaine withdrawal symptoms. Drug Alcohol Depend. 2006;85(2):129–37.

63. Gonzalez G, Sevarion K, Sofuoglu M, Poling J, Oliveto A, Gonsai K, et al. Tiagabine increases cocaine-free urines in cocaine-dependent methadone-treated patients: results of a randomized pilot study. Addiction. 2003;98(11):1625–32.

64. Carroll KM, Nich C, Ball SA, McCance E, Rounsaville BJ. Treatment of cocaine and alcohol dependence with psychotherapy disulfiram. Addiction. 1998;93(5):713–27.

65. George TP, Chawarski MC, Pakes J, Carroll KM, Kosten TR, Schottenfeld RS. Disulfiram versus placebo for cocaine dependence in buprenorphine-maintained subjects: a preliminary trial. Biol Psychiatry. 2000;47(12):1080–6.

66. Petrakis IL, Carroll KM, Nich C, Gordon LT, McCance-Katz EF, Frankforter T, et al. Disulfiram treatment for cocaine dependence in methadone-maintained opioid addicts. Addiction. 2000;95(2):219–28.

67. Carroll KM, Fenton LR, Ball SA, Nich C, Frankforter TL, Shi J, et al. Efficacy of disulfiram and cognitive behavior therapy in cocaine-dependent outpatients: a randomized placebo-controlled trial. Arch Gen Psychiatry. 2004;61(3):264–72.

68. Kosten T, Oliveto A, Feingold A, Poling J, Sevarino K, McCance-Katz E, et al. Desipramine and contingency management for cocaine and opiate dependence in buprenorphine-maintained patients. Drug Alcohol Depend. 2003;70(3):P315–325.

69. Poling J, Oliveto A, Petry N, Sofuoglu M, Gonsai K, Gonzalez G, et al. Six-month trial of bupropion with contingency management for cocaine dependence in a methadone-maintained population. Arch Gen Psychiatry. 2006;63(2):219–28.

70. Ciraulo DA, Knapp C, Rotrosen J, Sarid-Segal O, Ciraulo A, LoCastro J, et al. Nefazodone treatment of cocaine dependence with comorbid depressive symptoms. Addiction. 2005;100 Suppl 1:23–31.

71. Winhusen T, Somoza E, Sarid-Segal O, Goldsmith RJ, Harrer JM, Coleman FS, et al. A double-blind, placebo-controlled trial of

reserpine for the treatment of cocaine dependence. Drug Alcohol Depend. 2007;91:205–12.

72. Winhusen T, Somoza E, Ciraulo D, Harrer JM, Goldsmith RJ, Grabowski J, Coleman FS, et al. A double-blind, placebo-controlled trial of tiagabine for the treatment of cocaine dependence. Drug Alcohol Depend. 2007;91:141–8.

73. Kahn R, Biswas K, Childress A, Shoptaw S, Fudala PJ, Gorgon L, Montoya I, et al. Multi-center trial of baclofen for abstinence initiation for severe cocaine dependence. Drug Alcohol Depend. 2009;103(1–2):59–64.

74. Elkashef A, Fudala PJ, Gorgon L, Li SH, Kahn R, Chiang N, et al. Double-blind, placebo-controlled trial of selegiline transdermal system (STS) for the treatment of cocaine dependence. Drug Alcohol Depend. 2006;85(3):191–7.

75. Moeller FG, Schmitz JM, Steinbert JL, Green CM, Reist C, Lai LY, et al. Citalopram combined with behavioral treatment reduces cocaine use: a double-blind, placebo-controlled trial. Am J Drug Alcohol Abuse. 2007;33(3):367–78.

76. Newton TF, Roache JD, De La Garza 2nd R, Fong T, Wallace CL, Li SH, et al. Bupropion reduces methamphetamine-induced subjective effects and cue-induced craving. Neuropsychopharmacology. 2006;31(7):1537–44.

77. Galloway G, Newmeyer J, Knapp T, Stalcup SA, Smith D. A controlled trial of imipramine for the treatment of methamphetamine dependence. J Subst Abuse. 1996;13(6):493–7.

78. Heinzerling KG, Shoptaw S, Peck JA, Yang X, Liu J, Roll J, et al. Randomized, placebo-controlled trial of baclofen and gabapentin for the treatment of methamphetamine dependence. Drug Alcohol Depend. 2006;85(3):177–84.

79. Shoptaw S, Hubert A, Peck J, Yang X, Liu J, Dang J, et al. Randomized, placebo-controlled trial of sertraline and contingency management for the treatment of methamphetamine dependence. Drug Alcohol Depend. 2006;85(1):12–8.

80. Johnson BA, Ait-Daoud N, Elkashef AM, Smith EV, Kahn R, Vocci F, et al. A preliminary randomized, double-blind, placebo-controlled study of the safety and efficacy of ondansetron in the treatment of methamphetamine dependence. Int J Neuropsychopharmacol. 2008;11:1–14.

81. Johnson BA, Roache JD, Ait-Daoud N, Wells LT, Wallace CL, Dawes MA, et al. Effects of acute topiramate dosing on methamphetamine-induced subjective mood. Int J Neuropsychopharmacol. 2007;10(1):85–98.

82. Tiihonen J, Kuoppasalmi K, Fohr J, Tuomola P, Kuikanmaki O, Vorma H, et al. A comparison of aripiprazole, methylphenidate, and placebo for amphetamine dependence. Am J Psychiatry. 2007;164(1):160–2.

83. Batki SL, Bui L, Mendelson J, Benowitz N, Bradley JM, Jones RT, et al. Methamphetamine-amlodipine interactions: preliminary analysis. Poster Session 2002 College on Problems of Drug Dependency (CPDD), 2002.

84. Batki SL, Moon J, Delucchi K, Bradley M, Hersh D, Smolar S, Mengis M, Lefkowitz E, Sexe D, Morello L, Evenhart T, Jones RT, Jacob 3rd P. Methamphetamine quantitative urine concentrations during a controlled trial of fluoxetine treatment: preliminary analysis. Ann NY Acad Sci. 2000;909:260–3.

85. Jayaram-Lindstrom N, Wennberg P, Hurd YL, Franck J. Effects of naltrexone on the subjective response to amphetamine in healthy volunteers. J Clin Psychopharmacol. 2004;24(6):655–9.

86. Elkashef AM, Rawson RA, Anderson AL, Li SH, Holmes T, Smith EV, et al. Bupropion for the treatment of methamphetamine dependence. Neuropsychopharmacology. 2008;33(5):162–70.

87. Shearer J, Darke S, Rodgers C, Slade T, van Beek I, Lewis J, Brady D, McKetin R, Mattick RP, Wodak A. A double-blind, placebo-controlled trial of modafinil (200 mg/day) for methamphetamine dependence. Addiction. 2009;104(2):224–33

88. Anderson AL, Li SH, Biswas K, McSherry F, Holmes T, Iturriaga E, et al. Modafinil for the treatment of methamphetamine dependence. Drug Alcohol Depend. 2012;120(1–3):135–41. Epub 2011 Aug 12.

89. Tiihonen J, Kuoppasalmi K, Fohr J, Kuikanmaki O, Vorma H, et al. A comparison of aripiprazole, methylphenidate, and placebo for amphetamine dependence. Am J Psychiatry. 2007;164:160–2.

90. Harrod SB, Dwoskin LP, Crooks PA, Klebaur JE, Bardo MT. Lobeline attenuates d-methamphetamine self-administration in rats. J Pharmacol Exp Ther. 2001;298(1):172–9.

91. Matsuda LA, Lolait SJ, Brownstein MJ, Young AC, Bonner TI. Structure of a cannabinoid receptor and functional expression of the cloned DNA. Nature. 1990;346(6284):561–4.

92. Huestis MA, Gorelick DA, Heishman SJ, Preston KL, Nelson RA, Moolchan ET, Frank RA. Blockade of effects of smoked marijuana by the CB1-selective cannabinoid receptor antagonist SR141716. Arch Gen Psychiatry. 2001;58:322–8.

93. Tanda G, Munzar P, Goldberg SR. Self-administration behavior is maintained by the psychoactive ingredient of marijuana in squirrel monkeys. Nat Neurosci. 2000;3(11):1073–4.

94. Dishion T, Kavanagh K. Intervening in adolescent problem behavior: a family-centered approach. New York, NY: Guilford; 2003.

95. Stanger C, Budney AJ, Kamon J. Abstinence-based vouchers and parent-directed contingency management enhance outcomes for adolescent marijuana abuse. Abstract at International Society for Addiction Medicine, Annual Meeting, Oporto, Portugal; 2006.

96. Moore BA, Budney AJ. Relapse in outpatient treatment for marijuana dependence. J Subst Abuse Treat. 2003;25:85–9.

97. Haney M, Ward AS, Comer SD, et al. Bupropion SR worsens mood during marijuana withdrawal in humans. Psychopharmacology. 2001;155:171–9.

98. Haney M, Hart CL, Vosburg SK, Nasser J, Bennett A, Zubaran C, et al. Marijuana withdrawal in humans: effects of oral THC and divalproex. Neuropsychopharmacology. 2004;29:158–70.

99. Levin F, McDowell D, Evans S, Nunes E, Akerele E, Donovan S, Vosburg SK. Pharmacotherapy for marijuana dependence: a double-blind, placebo-controlled pilot trial of divalproex sodium. Am J Addict. 2004;13(1):21–32.

100. Haney M, Hart CL, Ward AS, et al. Nefazodone decreases anxiety during marijuana withdrawal in humans. Psychopharmacology. 2003;165:157–65.

101. Gorelick DA, Heishman SJ, Preston KL, Nelson RA, Moolchan ET, Huestis MA. The cannabinoid CB1 receptor antagonist rimonabant attenuates the hypotensive effect of smoked marijuana in male smokers. Am Heart J. 2006;151(3):754.e1–5.

102. McRae AL, Brady KT, Carter RE. Buspirone for treatment of marijuana dependence: a pilot study. Am J Addict. 2006;15:404.

103. Winstock A, Lea T, Copeland J. Cannabis withdrawal treatment options, including results from an in-patient trial of lithium. Presented at the Australasian Professional Society on Alcohol and Other Drugs meeting in Cairns, Australia, November 2006.

104. Cui SS, Bowen RC, Gu GB, Hannesson DK, Yu PH, Zhang X. Prevention of cannabinoid withdrawal syndrome by lithium: involvement of oxytocinergic neuronal activation. J Neurosci. 2001;21:9867–76.

105. Cornelius JR, Salloum IM, Haskett RF, Ehler JG, Jarrett PJ, Thase ME, Perel JM. Fluoxetine versus placebo for the marijuana use of depressed alcoholics. Addict Behav. 1999;24(1):111–4.

106. David SP, Munafo MR, Murphy MFG, Proctor M, Walton RT, Johnstone EC. Genetic variation in the dopamine D4 receptor (DRD4) gene and smoking cessation: follow-up of a randomized clinical trial of transdermal nicotine patch. Pharmacogenomics J. 2008;8:122–8.

107. Rutter JL. Symbiotic relationship of pharmacogenetics and drugs of abuse. AAPS J. 2006;8(1):174–84.

Alcohol

A.E. Goudriaan and K.J. Sher

Abstract

This chapter first discusses the prevalence of alcohol use and the patterns of alcohol use in different countries worldwide. Criteria for alcohol use disorders (AUDs; alcohol abuse and dependence) are described. The acute and chronic effects of alcohol on the human peripheral and central nervous system are outlined. Unintentional and intentional injuries due to alcohol use are a considerable part of the disease burden of alcohol use, and comprise traffic accidents, alcohol poisoning, cancer, and liver disorders. Chronic heavy alcohol use is associated with negative health effects such as gastrointestinal abnormalities, and with structural and functional brain abnormalities. These negative health effects are higher when heavier alcohol use is present. Negative effects on cognitive functions have been reported for heavy alcohol use, but results are less evident for moderate alcohol use. The potential beneficial effects of light alcohol use (mostly defined as a maximum of 7 drinks per week, spread evenly) are suggested to have some health benefits. Risk factors associated with AUDs are discussed at the genetic, psychological, and environmental level. Effective psychosocial and pharmacological interventions for AUDs are outlined.

Learning Objectives
- Alcohol use has a high spread of regular use across the world.
- Alcohol use disorders (AUDs) are most prevalent in older adolescents and young adults; however, a small percentage of individuals with AUDs have chronic (intermittent) alcohol problems across the lifetime.

- Heavy alcohol use has been related to increased health problems (gastrointestinal, brain abnormalities, and cognitive functions), whereas light alcohol use has been related to some beneficial health effects. Mixed evidence is present regarding moderate alcohol use, and amount and patterns of drinking influence health effects.
- Risk factors associated with AUDs exist on a genetic, psychological, and environmental level, and interactions between risk factors influence the development of alcohol use patterns and AUDs.
- Effective treatment for alcohol dependence generally consists of psychosocial interventions, or a combination of psychosocial and pharmacological interventions.

A.E. Goudriaan Ph.D. (✉)
Department of Psychiatry, Amsterdam Institute for Addiction
Research, Academic Medical Centre, University of Amsterdam,
Amsterdam, The Netherlands
e-mail: agoudriaan@gmail.com; A.E.Goudriaan@amc.uva.nl

K.J. Sher
University of Missouri-Columbia and Midwest Alcoholism
Research Center, Columbia, MO 65211, USA

J.C. Verster et al. (eds.), *Drug Abuse and Addiction in Medical Illness: Causes, Consequences and Treatment*,
DOI 10.1007/978-1-4614-3375-0_9, © Springer Science+Business Media, LLC 2012

Background

Alcohol has been consumed as a beverage since antiquity and continues to be used in diverse cultures in industrialized and nonindustrialized countries. Beer was brewed in Egypt about 3700 years BC. Unger [1] notes that in the middle ages, beer was consumed more than water, since it was cleaner than water and less likely to transmit diseases or cause poisoning. In the middle ages, the process of distillation was invented [2], and spirits (beverages with very high ethanol concentrations) could be consumed. In the eighteenth century, alcohol use was seen as a large social problem in London, England, where the "gin epidemic" broke loose, after prices for distilled drinks were lowered considerably [3].

Thus alcohol consumption can be viewed as an enduring and global issue. When attempting to quantify alcohol consumption across populations, it is useful to have metrics to aid comparisons. First, persons can be defined as alcohol users, or nonusers (abstainers). Among users, there can be considerable variability in patterns of consumption and with negative consequences of consumption. From a clinical and public health perspective, it is useful to consider AUDs, syndromes associated with problematic consumption. The risk factors for excessive consumption, negative consequences, and AUDs are diverse and include both individual factors (e.g., ethanol metabolism, personality, and beliefs about alcohol) and environmental factors ranging from prenatal exposures to broad social influences. In this chapter, alcohol use, its actions on the human body, AUDs, and associated risk factors are discussed.

Alcohol Use

In most Western countries, either in Europe or in North America, a high percentage of people have consumed alcohol in their lifetime, or have done so in the last year. For instance, in the USA, past year alcohol consumption level lies at 70% of the adult population [4], whereas in European countries like Germany, Denmark, and France, about 90–97% of the adult population used alcohol in the previous year; in the UK, Ireland, Italy, and Sweden, these numbers were 80–90%. Initiation of alcohol use usually occurs in adolescence: In the USA, approximately two-thirds of 18- to 20-year olds report alcohol consumption in the past year. In European countries, proportions of alcohol use among 15-year olds differ widely: from 50% of 15-year olds in the UK, Denmark, and the Netherlands, to 10–20% of 15-year olds in Ireland, France, Sweden, and the Baltic countries [5]. Considerable variation exists between persons in how frequently they consume alcohol and the amount of alcohol they consume on each occasion. Frequency and quantity of consumption can be defined as the consumption of pure ethanol per year per person; however, individuals often differ in patterns of use, leading some researchers to measure volume/variability in order to resolve further an individual's drinking pattern, by using "graduated frequency" approaches (1–2 drinks, 3–4 drinks, 5–6 drinkers, etc.) [6].

Total volume of alcohol consumption (pure alcohol) in those who consume alcohol lies at 8.5 L in the USA, 12.6 L in the European union varying from 8–10 L in Italy and Sweden, to 15–20 L in many eastern European countries, e.g., Hungary, Lithuania, Latvia, and Slovakian Republic. Consumption lies lower in Asian, African, Pacific, and African regions, with higher income countries consuming more alcohol than lower income countries, and countries with a majority Muslim population consuming less alcohol [5, 7].

Heavy alcohol use can generally be defined as alcohol use exceeding a certain standard of moderate drinking (e.g., exceeding a certain daily volume or a certain quantity per occasion). Definitions of heavy alcohol use differ between surveys, and are therefore not always comparable. In the USA, 6.4% of men and 5% of women who drink can be defined as heavy drinkers (drinking more than 40 g of pure alcohol per day for men, and 20 g of pure alcohol per day for women; [7]). Using the same definition of heavy drinking, higher rates are present in countries like Germany (11.2% in males and 11.3% in females), France (16.6% in males and 7.8% in females), Japan (16.9% in men, 9.3% in women), Brazil (17.8% in males, 18.2% in females), the Czech Republic (25.7% in males, 12.5% in females), and comparable rates are present in countries like Israel (5.9% in males, 4.7% in females) and Finland (5.8% in males, 3.4% in females), and lower rates are present in less-developed countries in Africa (e.g., Ghana: 1.9%), India: 1.4%, and Dominican Republic: 2.1% [7].

Alcohol Use Disorders: Definition and Prevalence

The Fourth edition of the Diagnostic and Statistical Manual (DSM-IV) of American Psychiatric Association [8] describes two major forms of AUDs: (1) alcohol abuse and (2) alcohol dependence. Alcohol dependence is defined by a maladaptive pattern of [alcohol] use, leading to clinically significant impairment or distress, as manifested by three (or more) of the following symptoms occurring during the same 12-month period: (1) tolerance, (2) withdrawal, (3) drinking alcohol in larger amounts or over a longer period than intended, (4) a persistent desire or unsuccessful efforts to cut down or control alcohol use, (5) spending a great deal of time obtaining alcohol, using it, or recovering from its effects, (6) important social, occupational, or recreational activities are given up or reduced because of substance use, (7) continued use of alcohol despite knowledge that alcohol either causes or exacerbates a persistent or recurrent physical or psychological problem. A diagnosis of alcohol abuse is met when a maladaptive drinking pattern characterized by one of the following is present: (1) a failure to fulfill major role obligations at work, school, or home, (2) recurrent alcohol use in situations in which it is physically hazardous, (3) recurrent alcohol-related legal problems, and (4) continued alcohol use despite having persistent or recurrent social or interpersonal problems caused or exacerbated by alcohol. Within the DSM-IV, alcohol abuse is a residual category that is superseded by a current or past diagnosis of alcohol dependence.

In the USA, prevalence studies on AUDs have been conducted in the last 25 years. In the USA, AUDs show a peak prevalence in late adolescence and early adulthood, suggesting that AUDs can be considered a developmental disorder of young adulthood, for the larger part of those with AUDs [9]. The most recent study the National Epidemiologic Survey on Alcohol and Related Conditions, or NESARC [10–12], indicates a 30.3% lifetime and 8.5% past year prevalence of AUDs. In many European countries, past-year prevalence of alcohol dependence is estimated at 4–5% for most countries, but has been reported to be higher in France (8.7%); past-year prevalence of alcohol dependence in Canada was estimated at 2.6%; AUDs in China are estimated at 5% and in Israel at 4.2% [13–17]. The high prevalence of AUDs places them among the most common mental disorders in the general population of many countries.

Acute Effects of Alcohol: Alcohol as a Drug

Alcohol Use: Absorption, Distribution, and Breakdown

An alcoholic beverage contains ethanol, commonly known as alcohol. The chemical structure of ethanol is depicted in Fig. 9.1. For reasons of clarity, we will refer to alcohol when discussing the absorption, distribution, and breakdown of ethanol.

Alcohol absorption in the body takes place in the stomach and intestines. Through uptake in the bloodstream, alcohol is dispersed throughout the body and affects both the peripheral and the central nervous system. The speed of distribution of alcohol in the body depends on the speed of drinking alcoholic beverages, and the relative alcohol content in the beverage. Additional effects that influence the absorption rate are stomach contents (when alcohol is consumed on a full stomach, absorption in the blood stream is slowed down compared to alcohol consumption on an empty stomach) and previous alcohol use pattern. Alcohol is a psychoactive drug with a depressant effect. This means that alcohol dampens perception, slows reaction times, and diminishes accurate motor responding. The blood alcohol concentration (BAC) that results from consuming a certain amount of alcohol depends on the amount of body fluid and body weight: less body fluid results in a higher BAC. Because women have a relatively lower proportion of body fluid compared to their body weight than men, a similar amount of alcohol affects a woman more than a man, when they have a similar body weight. BAC is often expressed in % or ‰, where the level of alcohol is expressed as a mass of alcohol per volume of blood, e.g., 1/1000 (‰) g/mL = 1 mg/mL, or 1/100 (%) g/mL = 1 cg/mL. Because 1 mL of blood is equivalent to 1.06 g, units by volume

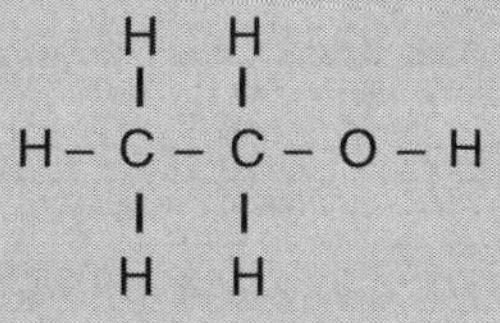

$$
\begin{array}{ccc}
\text{H} & \text{H} \\
| & | \\
\text{H} - \text{C} - \text{C} - \text{O} - \text{H} \\
| & | \\
\text{H} & \text{H}
\end{array}
$$

Fig. 9.1 Ethanol

(continued)

(continued)

are similar but not identical to units by mass. A BAC rating of 0.2% reflects serious intoxication, and 0.40% is the LD_{50}, the dose that is lethal for 50% of adults.

Alcohol is metabolized primarily in the liver. The breakdown of one standard drink (please note that standard drinks vary across countries: in the USA, a standard drink contains 14 g of pure alcohol, UK: 7.9 g, Australia: 10 g, and France: 12 g) alcoholic beverage takes about 1–1.5 h (about 0.017%/h), but can be quicker or slower primarily depending upon individual differences in ethanol metabolism. The process of alcohol metabolism cannot be enhanced by drinking coffee or eating. About 95% of excretion of alcohol in the human body takes places through metabolism in the liver, 1–3% is excreted in urine, and 1–5% is evaporated through the breath. A minimal amount is excreted through sweating. Metabolism of alcohol starts as soon as alcohol is absorbed in the stomach and liver. Alcohol is first broken down into acetaldehyde by alcohol dehydrogenase (ADH). Acetaldehyde is a toxic substance, which is metabolized into (nontoxic) acetyl-CoA by acetaldehyde dehydrogenase. Alcohol is also metabolized in non-liver tissues by the enzymes cytochrome P450 (CYP450) and catalase, for instance in the brain. Alcohol is metabolized at a constant rate, since alcohol saturates the enzymes' capacity to breakdown alcohol fully (even when only one alcoholic beverage is consumed).

Effects on Health

Alcohol Use: Acute and Chronic Effects on the Central Nervous System

Alcohol affects several of the major neutrotransmitter systems in the brain, including catecholaminergic systems (e.g., the dopamine system), GABAergic systems, glutaminergic systems, serotonergic systems, and neuropeptides such as opioid peptides, endorphins, and enkephalins. Most of its intoxicating effects can be related to effects on one or more of these systems, with an initial action at ligand-gated ion channel receptors such as GABA and glutamate. In addition, protracted alcohol use disturbs the homeostasis of intracellular processes, resulting in a long-term dysregulation of glutamatergic, opioid peptide, and dopaminergic neurotransmission and the brain antistress neuropeptide Y (NPY) system [18–21].

Dopamine, serotonin, GABA, and endogenous opiates are thought to be associated with the reinforcing effects of alcohol [22]. Alcohol's effect on GABA, the primary inhibitory neurotransmitter in the human brain, is related to the anxiolytic, sedative, and motor impairment effects of alcohol [23, 24]. Glutamate is a major excitatory neurotransmitter in the central nervous system, and alcohol impairs memory, cognition, and motor functioning through glutamatergic actions affecting N-methyl-D-aspartate (NMDA) and α-amino-3-hydroxy-5-methyl-4-isoxazole propionic acid (AMPA) receptor sites [25–27].

Most of the chronic effects of alcohol on the different neurotransmitter systems are in the opposite direction of their acute effects. For example, while alcohol acutely increases activity in the dopamine, serotonin, GABA, and opiate systems and decreases activity in the glutamate system, chronic effects reflecting neuroadaptation tend to be the reverse [21, 28]. Upregulation of NMDA receptors in response to chronic inhibition by alcohol to withdrawal has been related to cognitive deficits associated with alcohol dementia and Wernicke–Korsakoff syndrome, and cell death through chronic augmentation of postsynaptic neurons (an effect known as excitotoxicity) [29].

Acute Effects
Unintentional and Intentional Injury

Alcohol is associated with a higher risk of both unintentional injuries (e.g., fatal and nonfatal motor vehicle traffic crashes, and falls) and intentional injuries (e.g., physical aggression, and suicidal and parasuicidal behavior). Increases in the risk of injury are already present at low BACs: measurable decrements in driving performance were reported at levels as low as 0.01 g/100 mL [30]. The risk of injuries increases exponentially when BACs increase, with male drivers having a higher risk compared to female drivers, and younger drivers having higher risks compared to older drivers [31, 32]. Recent meta-analyses and review articles indicate that alcohol use is associated with high levels of traffic injuries, both fatal and nonfatal: 40% of motor vehicle accidents and 30–50% of accidental drowning accidents are associated with alcohol use in the USA, Canada, and Australia [7, 33–36]. Intentional injuries and their relation to alcohol use are harder to estimate, since subjective expectations regarding alcohol and aggression influence the effect of alcohol on aggressiveness [37]. Studies on alcohol use and violence have repeatedly shown an association between violence preceded by alcohol use, with higher BACs associated with more severe forms of violence [38–40]. More detailed discussions of the relation between alcohol and unintended and intended injury can be found in Chapters 38 (Drug Use and Abuse and Human Aggressive Behavior), 39 (Suicidal Behavior in Alcohol and Drug Abuse), and 44 (Drugs of Abuse and Traffic Safety) of this book.

Alcohol Poisoning

Alcohol poisoning is characterized by mental confusion, unconsciousness, or coma; vomiting; seizures; slow or irregular breathing; hypothermia; and pale or blue skin color. Toxicity of alcohol poisoning is due to a build-up of metabolic products of ADH and aldehyde dehydrogenase.

Alcohol poisoning or an alcohol overdose can lead to irreversible brain damage. Patients of alcohol poisoning need continued care, which can include a variety of treatments and tests, such as monitoring for clear airways to prevent choking, oxygen therapy to dilute alcohol in the body, IV and vitamins to keep the patient hydrated, and a kidney dialysis to prevent permanent kidney damage. Alcohol poisoning has risen steeply from the 1970s until 2002 in Eastern European countries and Russia [41, 42]. The influence of level of alcohol consumption patterns on acute risk of fatal injuries and alcohol poisoning is not well known at present.

Chronic Effects

Alcohol Use: Chronic Effects on Gastrointestinal Functions

Alcohol use is associated with more than 60 medical conditions, and for most of these, the risk increases with increased alcohol consumption [43, 44]. Moderate and heavy alcohol use affects the stomach, liver, and intestines. Heavy use is associated with damage to the mucous membrane of the stomach, the liver, and the brain. Chances for developing liver disorders and cancer of the throat, esophagus, stomach, liver, and intestines increase with heavier alcohol use (see Chap. 35 on alcohol and cancer). The relation between cirrhosis mortality and population drinking levels is well established [45]. Alcohol use during pregnancy can lead to abnormal development of the fetus, birth defects, and fetal alcohol syndrome (see Chap. 36 on alcohol and fetal alcohol spectrum disorders). Alcohol affects the action of many drugs (both illegal substances and prescription drugs), and caution should be taken when alcohol is combined with medication use.

Positive effects of light alcohol use (one standard drink every 2 days) have also been reported. Light to moderate alcohol use appears to decrease the risk of coronary artery diseases, type 2 diabetes [46–48], and ischemic stroke [49], compared to that in abstainers. These positive effects seem to be present only when light alcohol use is spread evenly, and drinking large amounts in short periods is avoided [43, 44].

Worldwide, alcohol use is associated with 4% of the global disease burden, and the diseases and deaths that are associated with alcohol use are comparable to the global disease burden for smoking (4.1%) and high blood pressure (4.4%) [44].

Heavy Alcohol Use: Effects on Brain Structure

Numerous studies have associated prolonged alcohol abuse and dependence with cerebral gray and white matter abnormalities: Alcohol dependence is associated with larger volumes of cortical sulci and lateral and third ventricles, and reductions in gray and white matter volume compared to that in healthy controls, and this relation holds for both men and women with AUDs [50, 51]. The dorsolateral prefrontal cortex, an area related to regulation of emotions and behavior, or executive functions, is especially affected [50–52]. Gray matter reductions are present in nontreatment-seeking AUD groups and in heavy drinkers, whereas white matter abnormalities seem to be present more often in treatment-seeking alcohol dependent populations [52–57]. Direct comparisons of alcohol-dependent groups in treatment and heavy drinkers suggest that the degree of brain atrophy and neuronal and membrane injury in alcohol-dependent patients in treatment is more severe than that of alcohol-dependent persons in the general population [58]. Smoking interacts with the effects of alcohol use on the brain; smoking heavy drinkers have higher gray matter reductions than nonsmoking heavy drinkers [53, 59], and smoking adversely affects cerebral perfusion in alcohol-dependent patients [60]. Studies on the effects of light to moderate alcohol use are scarce: one MRI study reported increased gray matter volumes and decreased white matter volumes in a large MRI study of male light alcohol users (mean of 7–8 drinks a week), but not for female light alcohol users [61].

There is both preclinical [62–65] and clinical research [66, 67] suggesting that adolescence is a period of heightened vulnerability to alcohol-related brain damage. Clinical studies in adolescents with AUDs show that diminished gray matter in prefrontal cortex, thalamus, hippocampus, and abnormalities of the corpus callosum are associated with heavy alcohol use in adolescence [68–70]. Subgroups at high risk for developing AUDs (e.g., high on externalizing symptoms; family history positive for alcoholism) also show abnormalities in gray matter volumes of the frontal, cingulate, and parahippocampal gyri; amygdala; thalamus; and cerebellum [71, 72], indicating that some of the abnormalities in gray matter volume may be a pre-existing risk factor for the development of alcohol dependence.

Effects on Cognitive Brain Functions

The effects of light and moderate alcohol use on cognitive functions have been studied in a couple of studies in older adults predominantly. In adults over the age of 70 years, light alcohol use (one drink a day or less) was associated with better neurocognitive functions in women [73, 74], but not in men [73]; however, another study found positive effects of similar amounts of alcohol in a sample of male veterans [75]. Light to moderate alcohol use in middle age and at an older age seems to be related to better episodic memory, psychomotor speed, and executive function, especially in nonsmokers [76]. In a review of the literature, Parsons and Nixon conclude that increasing negative cognitive effects of alcohol use are present, starting from some cognitive deficits at five to six US standard drinks a day, to mild cognitive deficits when 7–9 standard drinks are used, to moderate and severe cognitive deficits, comparable to those with alcohol dependence, at levels of 10 or more drinks a day [77].

The effects of chronic heavy alcohol use and of AUDs on cognitive functions have been well established. Chronic alcohol use is associated with diminished neurocognitive performance in persons with AUDs [51, 78–81]; in general memory functions, visuospatial learning executive functions such as attention, planning, inhibition, and cognitive flexibility are affected in persons with AUDs [82]. The effects of alcohol dependence can be exacerbated by smoking history [79].

Korsakoff's Syndrome

Korsakoff's syndrome is a chronic brain disease characterized by retrograde amnesia (inability to recall remote memories) and anterograde amnesia (inability to develop new memories). Korsakoff's syndrome is related to nutritional deficiencies such as thiamine deficiency and vitamin B deficiency that accompany chronic heavy alcohol use, when insufficient other nutrients are taken besides alcohol [83–85]. Korsakoff's syndrome often occurs together with Wernicke encephalopathy, a disorder characterized by neurological signs such as ataxia, nystagmus, and confusion. Improved nutrition, including vitamin supplementation and abstinence of alcohol, will help in reducing some of the signs of both Wernicke's and Korsakoff's syndrome, but the amnesia associated with Korsakoff's syndrome resolves in only about 20% of the patients [84], and it therefore is a condition with severe consequences for daily life and the ability to live independently.

Etiology

Risk Factors for Developing Alcohol Use Disorders: Biopsychosocial Influences

Personality and Comorbidity

There is no specific relation between alcohol use or AUDs and a specific constellation of personality traits. However, several personality traits have been associated with the development of alcohol use and AUDs. Three personality dimensions that are frequently discussed in the literature on alcohol

and personality are neuroticism/negative emotionality, impulsivity/disinhibition, and extraversion/sociability.

The relation between alcohol-dependent patients in treatment and neuroticism/negative emotionality has been established in several lines of research. High rates of anxiety and depression are found in alcohol-dependent samples [86–88], and individuals with AUDs tend to score higher on self-report measures of neuroticism and negative emotionality than nonalcoholic controls, both in cross-sectional and in prospective studies [89–93].

Individuals who meet AUD criteria score high on both self-report and behavioral (laboratory) measures of impulsivity [94–98]. In addition, alcohol-dependent persons have higher rates of Cluster B personality disorders, such as antisocial [99, 100] and borderline personality disorder [101–103], and it seems likely that there are reciprocal influences between consumption and personality pathology. Genetic variance in behavioral undercontrol accounts for a significant proportion of the genetic variance in alcohol dependence [104]. Disinhibition and impulsivity have also been related to high-risk subgroups; e.g., children of alcohol-dependent parents exhibit high levels of externalizing and disinhibited behaviors [105, 106]. In addition, disinhibited traits were related prospectively to AUDs in high-risk samples [107–109].

Extraversion/sociability has been related to age of onset of alcohol use, rather than to AUDs [110] and to alcohol consumption among social drinkers [111–113].

Persons with AUDs are at a higher risk for a variety of Axis I and Cluster B Axis II disorders, but the relative strength of this association differs as a complex function of age and transitional life events [114]; comorbidity is higher when it concerns alcohol dependence than when alcohol abuse is involved, and comorbidity is lower in college student samples [115, 116].

Genetics

Genetic vulnerability factors are not specific for AUDs, but are related to substance dependence in general, and even seem to extend to "behavioral addictions" such as pathological gambling [117–120]. The strong familial relation of AUDs has long been established in twin and adoption studies (for a review, see [121]). Multiple genes are responsible for the genetic effect, but the nature of the genetic vulnerability is not clear yet. A recent quantitative linkage study indicated that genes on chromosomes 1, 2, and 10 were related to alcohol dependence [119, 122]. Genetic influences on AUDs seem to be mediated by individual differences that relate to ethanol metabolism. Genes related to the breakdown of alcohol (ADH2, ADH3, ALDH2 genes) are related to diminished risk for AUDs in Asian populations [123, 124] and have recently also been related to diminished risk for AUDs in African Americans [125]. It is unclear at present how this genetic variation is relevant in other populations, since the prevalence of this gene is very low in Caucasians, for example.

Other genes that have been proposed as candidate genes related to AUDs are genes that influence neurotransmitter functioning, such as genes related to GABA transmission (GABRA2, GABRG1). Specifically, the GABRA2 gene has been related to a higher risk for AUDs in adults and for the onset of AUD symptoms in young adulthood [126–128]. The GABRA2 gene has been related to subjective and objective effects of alcohol (e.g., body sway, motor coordination, and hedonic value of alcohol), and this gene may be related to AUDs through this biobehavioral mechanism [129, 130]. The GABRG1 gene has been suggested to be related to AUDs both dependent on the GABRA2 haplotype [131] and independent of the GABRA2 genotype [132]. Other genes, such as those related to NMDA receptors (an excitatory glutamate receptor known to be extremely sensitive to alcohol in physiological doses), cyclic AMP genes, serotonine and dopamine transporter genes, and genes relating to the metabolism of serotonine and dopamine (e.g., COMT and MAO), have been proposed [133–137]. The recent studies indicating the GABRA2 and GABRG1 genes in relation to AUD risk in several independent studies seem to be important clues for future research into the relation between brain function and AUD risk.

Endophenotypes have been proposed as a promising approach for understanding the genetics of AUDs. Endophenotypes are biological markers lying in between genotype and a behavioral phenotype (e.g., heavy alcohol or drug use and dependence). It has been proposed that the study of endophenotypes will provide a link between genotype and related phenotypes. Recent studies have linked endophenotypes such as functional brain responses to addiction-related cues to specific genetic markers. For example, Hutchison and colleagues [138] examined the role of the D_4 dopamine receptor gene (DRD4) in relation to craving and responses to alcohol and tobacco (or related cues), and reported individual differences in alcohol-related craving, which was associated with different variants of the DRD4 gene for both substances. In another study, Filbey and colleagues investigated brain responses in a functional magnetic resonance imaging (fMRI) study [139]. Alcohol cues prior to alcohol priming resulted in a larger orbitofrontal, anterior cingulate, and striatal brain response in individuals with the DRD4 VNTR >7 repeat allele (DRD4.L), compared to that in individuals with DRD4 <7 repeats (DRD4.S). In addition, individuals with at least one copy of the OPRM1 + 118 G allele had greater brain responses in mesocorticolimbic areas both before and after alcohol priming compared with homozygous OPRM1 + 118 A allele individuals, and both in DRD4.L and OPRM1 + 118 G groups, striatal brain responses correlated with greater frequency and quantity of alcohol use.

These findings provide intriguing data on the relevance of specific genes for influencing responsivity to alcohol cues, and alcohol consumption, which influence alcohol (and other drug) seeking. Clinical studies show that in substance-dependent patients, higher brain responsivity to drug cues, and lower prefrontal brain activity during a decision-making task can predict relapse in substance dependence with a high accuracy [140, 141]. A recent study by Wrase and colleagues indicated that smaller amygdala volumes were related to a higher relapse rate in alcohol-dependent patients [142]. These studies show that the study of endophenotypes and their relation to genotypes is a promising area for future research on factors that influence alcohol and drug sensitivity, cue reactivity, and relapse. Future research may result in developing risk profiles of genotypes and endophenotypes.

Environment

Environmental influences on AUDs can be distal influences such as peer influences and parenting practices, and proximal influences such as prenatal exposure to alcohol, or the effects of drinking contexts on acute alcohol use. For the effects of prenatal alcohol exposure, we refer to Chap. 36 (Fetal Alcohol Spectrum Disorder). Below, we discuss the effects of familial environment (parental substance use and parenting practices) and peer influences on alcohol use and AUDs.

Familial Environmental Influences

It is well known that children of parents with AUDs (children of alcoholics; COAs) are at a higher risk to develop AUDs in adolescence and adulthood. About half of this association, however, is not determined by environment, but by genetic vulnerability (Kapprio et al. 2002; Rose et al. 2001; Viken et al. 1999). Twin research shows that the majority of these environmental influences are unique, and thus, not shared between offspring, and thus, the role of shared familial environment on COAs' alcohol use patterns and alcohol problems remains unclear. Gene–environment interactions have been established for AUDs. A study in offspring of twins reported that environmental influence of growing up in a family with a parent with an AUD influences the AUDs in offspring, dependent on their genetic vulnerability for AUDs [143]. Environmental influences on drinking behavior of COAs seem to be partially related to modeling of alcohol use behavior, since research findings on the influence of active drinking behavior of parents or active AUDs versus remitted AUDs and influences on AUDs in offspring have been mixed [144–146].

Parenting practices have been associated with alcohol use in adolescents and young adults, at several levels. For instance, at the level of specific alcohol parenting practices, Spijkerman and colleagues found in a study among 1,344 adolescents and their parents that applying strict rules about alcohol use and constructively discussing alcohol use are associated with lower heavy drinking patterns, whereas parental alcohol use promotes adolescents' alcohol use [147]. Several studies on general parenting practices indicate that higher behavioral control is related to alcohol-specific rule enforcement [148] and that authoritative parenting style (characterized by high warmth and behavioral control) protects adolescents from negative outcomes such as the development of alcohol and substance use problems [149, 150]. Poor parental monitoring has also been found to put children at risk for association with substance-using peers, and association with substance-abusing peers is a critical risk factor for early onset alcohol use and the development of AUDs [151].

Peer Influences

When children grow older, the influence of peers on behaviors like alcohol use increases, whereas parental influence decreases. Socialization, the shaping of alcohol use by influence from peers or a peer group, is one factor in peer influences on alcohol use. For instance, affiliations with alcohol-using peers encourage alcohol use through social learning, peer group pressure, modeling, and social facilitation [152–155]. Another factor in peer influences is selection: this occurs when adolescents seek affiliation with peers who display similar patterns of substance use or deviant behavior (self-selection), or when environmental selection occurs, such as in transitioning from high school into college [153, 155]. Studies show that involvement with peers who use alcohol and engage in deviant behavior is a predictor of the development of AUDs in adolescence [156]. Coming from a disadvantaged environment or a disrupted family, and having a predisposition toward antisocial behavior predict AUDs, and these factors are also associated with selection into deviant peer groups, a risk factor for AUDs in itself [157–159].

Treatment of Alcohol Use Disorders

In general, treatment for substance dependence involves a combination of several psychosocial interventions, which can be combined with pharmacological interventions. Treatment of AUDs can be preceded by a detoxification, depending on severity of alcohol dependence. Personality and Substance Misuse and Pharmacotherapy of Addiction are discussed in depth in Chapters 4 and 8. A short description and discussion of psychological and pharmacological interventions in AUDs are presented below.

Detoxification: Symptoms, Medication

The first stage of treatment for alcohol dependence often consists of alcohol detoxification, in order to prevent complications during detoxification, and to diminish symptoms and adverse effects associated with detoxification. Symptoms can develop within several hours after last alcohol use, and usually show a peak 24–36 h after abstinence. Symptoms that can be experienced during alcohol detoxification are anxiety, restlessness, sleeplessness, sweating, nausea, vomiting, tremors, heightened blood pressure, and an increased heart rate [20]. Alcohol detoxification is estimated to take a week, although sleep disturbances and psychological withdrawal symptoms can persist much longer [160].

Monitoring of alcohol-dependent patients during detoxification is especially relevant because serious effects as delirium, epileptic insults, or dehydration can be present. If an alcoholic delirium occurs (usually after 3–5 days of abstinence), it is characterized by severe sympathetic hyperactivity (e.g., severe perspiration, fever, tachycardia, and hypertension). Medications used in detoxification usually consist of slow-acting benzodiazepines (e.g. diazepam, clorazepine, or chlordiazepoxide), which are dosed based on symptoms or according to a fixed dose [161–165]. Dosage of benzodiazepines depends on the severity of the detoxification symptoms, and should take in consideration that benzodiazepines can build up in persons with diminished liver functioning. When severe liver dysfunctioning is present, benzodiazepines with a short half-time should therefore be considered (e.g., oxazepam and lorazepam) [160, 166]. Next to benzodiazepines, haloperidol is used to diminish restlessness and to lower the chance of epileptic insults. Thiamine and vitamin B suppletion is used to avoid the development of Wernicke's syndrome [167], and should be continued for a longer period after detoxification (1 month to 3 months), depending on thiamine and vitamin B deficiencies.

Psychosocial Interventions for Alcohol Use Disorders

A range of psychosocial interventions has been implemented in the treatment of AUDs. These interventions range from brief interventions by primary health care providers to intensive residential treatment. Brief interventions for AUDs are effective in reducing drinking levels, and regarding cost-effectiveness of brief interventions tends to be very high [168–170]. A recently developed type of brief intervention, motivational interviewing [MI], is designed to enhance the readiness of individuals to change their behavior on their own and/or undertake more formal treatment. MI can be a useful intervention for drinkers who have not yet recognized the problematic nature of their drinking. There is a long history of behavioral approaches to alcohol treatment, and contingency management is a new promising approach that seems to be more effective in promoting abstinence, compared to other treatment methods (for a review, see [171]).

In cognitive behavior therapy (CBT), the focus is to learn new skills to cope with problems and to change harmful behavior patterns by employing a wide range of behavioral and cognitive techniques, although it is not clear what specific factors account for treatment effectiveness [172]. CBT focuses on processes such as learning adaptive behavioral strategies to cope with alcohol craving and with stressful situations that result in a high chance of relapse (e.g., distraction strategies, leaving the situation, or calling a friend), and identifying and reducing irrational, erroneous, or self-defeating thought patterns about alcohol use. One type of CBT that has received considerable support is relapse prevention training where there is a strong explicit focus on situations most likely to result in relapse [173, 174].

Like cognitive behavioral therapies, twelve-step models provide a range of coping behaviors but view alcohol dependence as a spiritual disease and medical disease. Twelve-step programs outline 12 consecutive activities that individuals with AUDs should achieve during the recovery process. Twelve-step models view alcoholism as a disease which can be controlled, but can never be cured, and therefore, twelve-step models focus on abstinence, rather than diminishing alcohol use. Similarities between twelve-step models and CBT lie in the development of coping skills to resist alcohol craving and urges. The combination of a twelve-step program combined with CBT has not been studied extensively in randomized control trials: one study found that a combination of professional treatment and a twelve-step program led to better treatment results than a twelve-step program alone [175]. A nonrandomized trial found that a twelve-step approach was more effective [176]. Twelve-step models seem to be more effective compared to CBT and motivational enhancement therapy in a subgroup of individuals with AUDs who have a social network which is highly supportive of drinking [177]. This interaction is likely related to the fact that twelve-step models provide an alternative social network not supportive of drinking. More randomized controlled trials have to be done to compare potential differences in treatment effectiveness of twelve-step models and other psychosocial treatments [178].

Family and couple therapy is sometimes employed in the treatment of AUDs, in order to engage the immediate social environment as a support system for change, and to address interpersonal communication and the role it has in the addictive behavior. A recent review reported that behavioral couple therapy was associated with better outcome (frequency of use, consequences of use, and relationship satisfaction) than individual behavioral therapy, especially at follow-up [179].

Pharmacological Interventions for Alcohol Dependence

Anticraving Medication (Naltrexone, Acamprosate, Topiramate)

Two anticraving medications (acamprosate, oral naltrexone, and the once-monthly injectable, extended release naltrexone) have received approval for the treatment of alcohol dependence in the USA and European countries [180]. Acamprosate is thought to act by normalizing protracted dysregulation of NMDA-mediated glutamatergic neurotransmission, a result of chronic heavy alcohol use and withdrawal. The safety and efficacy of acamprosate have been established in several clinical trials (for a review, see [181, 182]), although not all studies find positive effects: a large clinical trial did not find any effects of acamprosate alone, or in combination with naltrexone and/or CBT, compared to placebo [183]. Naltrexone is an opioid antagonist which is thought to reduce alcohol craving by blocking the mu-opioid receptors, and thereby reducing the rewarding properties of alcohol and other psychoactive substances [184]. Naltrexone has been shown to be effective in reducing relapse and diminishing percent of drinking days, when combined with several interventions, ranging from medical management to CBT ([183], for a review, see [185]). A promising off-label pharmacological intervention for alcohol dependence is topiramate, which is thought to reduce the reinforcing effects of alcohol by facilitating gamma-aminobutyric acid function and inhibiting glutaminergic pathways in the corticomesolimbic system. Several clinical trials show the efficacy of topiramate above placebo [186–188]. Another off-label pharmacological intervention for AUDs that recently has been studied is baclofen, a GABA-B receptor agonist. Some first studies show effectiveness of baclofen over placebo [189, 190], but null-findings are reported as well [191]. Therefore, the effectiveness of baclofen has to be studied in large clinical trials to demonstrate clearly the efficacy of baclofen and to ascertain whether efficacy is influenced by certain AUD characteristics such as severity and alcohol dependence subtype [192].

Aversive Medication

Disulfiram is an FDA-approved aversive medication for treatment of alcohol dependence. It inhibits the action of aldehyde dehydrogenase, thus preventing the breakdown of alcohol into acetate, resulting in nausea, vomiting, headache, and chestpain when alcohol is taken. The mechanism of disulfiram thus is an aversive response to alcohol consumption, even at a low level of alcohol consumption. Nonadherence tends to be high to very high in clinical trials of disulfiram, and reviews suggest that supervised prescription of disulfiram is needed to increase adherence [180, 193]. A severe side effect of disulfiram is the rare and idiosyncratic but potentially fatal hepatotoxicity that can occur with disulfiram [194]. For a more recent discussion on the use of disulfiram in AUDs, see [195–198].

References

1. Unger RW. Beer in the middle ages and the renaissance. Philadelphia, PA: University of Pennsylvania Press; 2007.
2. Patrick CH. Alcohol, culture, and society. Durham, NC: Duke University Press; 1952. Reprint edition by AMS Press, New York, 1970 edn.
3. Abel EL. The gin epidemic: much ado about what? Alcohol Alcohol. 2001;36(5):401–5.
4. Grant BF, Moore TC, Shepard J, Kaplan K. Source and accuracy statement: Wave 1 National Epidemiologic Survey on Alcohol and Related Conditions (NESARC). Bethesda, MD: National Institute on Alcohol Abuse and Alcoholism; 2003.
5. World Health Organisation. Country Reports. 2004. http://www.eurocare org/resources/country_profiles. Accessed 7 Nov 2008.
6. Greenfield TK. Ways of measuring drinking patterns and thedifference they make: experience with graduated frequencies. J Subst Abuse. 2000;12:33–49.
7. World Health Organisation. Global status report on alcohol 2004. Geneva: World Health Organisation Department of Mental Health and Substance Abuse; 2004.
8. American Psychiatric Association. Diagnostic and statistical manual of mental disorders. 4th ed. Washington, DC: American Psychiatric Press; 1994.
9. Sher KJ, Gotham HJ. Pathological alcohol involvement: a developmental disorder of young adulthood. Dev Psychopathol. 1999;11:933–56.
10. Grant BF, Harford TC, Muthen BO, Yi HY, Hasin DS, Stinson FS. DSM-IV alcohol dependence and abuse: further evidence of validity in the general population. Drug Alcohol Depend. 2007; 86(2–3):154–66.
11. Grant BF, Stinson FS, Dawson DA, Chou SP, Ruan WJ, Pickering RP. Co-occurrence of 12-month alcohol and drug use disorders and personality disorders in the United States: results from the National Epidemiologic Survey on Alcohol and Related Conditions. Arch Gen Psychiatry. 2004;61(4):361–8.
12. Grant BF, Dawson DA, Stinson FS, Chou SP, Dufour MC, Pickering RP. The 12-month prevalence and trends in DSM-IV alcohol abuse and dependence: United States, 1991-1992 and 2001-2002. Drug Alcohol Depend. 2004;74(3):223–34.
13. Alonso J, Lepine JP. Overview of key data from the European Study of the Epidemiology of Mental Disorders (ESEMeD). J Clin Psychiatry. 2007;68 Suppl 2:3–9.
14. Cnossen S. Alcohol taxation and regulation in the European Union. The Netherlands, The Hague: CPB Netherlands Bureau for Economic Policy Analysis; 2006. Report No.: 76.
15. Kim JH, Lee S, Chow J, Lau J, Tsang A, Choi J, et al. Prevalence and the factors associated with binge drinking, alcohol abuse, and alcohol dependence: a population-based study of Chinese adults in Hong Kong. Alcohol Alcohol. 2008;43(3):360–70.
16. Neumark YD, Lopez-Quintero C, Grinshpoon A, Levinson D. Alcohol drinking patterns and prevalence of alcohol-abuse and dependence in the Israel National Health Survey. Isr J Psychiatry Relat Sci. 2007;44(2):126–35.
17. Tjepkema M. Alcohol and illicit drug dependence. Health Rep. 2004;15(Suppl):9–19.
18. Nestler EJ. Molecular neurobiology of addiction. Am J Addict. 2001;10(3):201–17.
19. Nestler EJ. Molecular basis of long-term plasticity underlying addiction. Nat Rev Neurosci. 2001;2(2):119–28.
20. Koob GF, Le Moal M. Alcohol. In: Koob GF, Le Moal M, editors. Neurobiology of addiction. San Diego: Elsevier Academic; 2006. p. 173–241.
21. Vengeliene V, Bilbao A, Molander A, Spanagel R. Neuropharmacology of alcohol addiction. Br J Pharmacol. 2008; 154(2):299–315.
22. Kranzler HR, Anton RF. Implications of recent neuropsychopharmacologic research for understanding the etiology and development of alcoholism. J Consult Clin Psychol. 1994;62(6):1116–26.
23. Jia F, Pignataro L, Harrison NL. GABAA receptors in the thalamus: alpha4 subunit expression and alcohol sensitivity. Alcohol. 2007;41(3):177–85.
24. Korpi ER. Role of GABAA receptors in the actions of alcohol and in alcoholism: recent advances. Alcohol Alcohol. 1994;29(2): 115–29.
25. Lovinger DM, White G, Weight FF. Ethanol inhibition of neuronal glutamate receptor function. Ann Med. 1990;22(4):247–52.
26. Weight FF. Cellular and molecular physiology of alcohol actions in the nervous system. Int Rev Neurobiol. 1992;33:289–348.
27. Nagy J. Alcohol related changes in regulation of NMDA receptor functions. Curr Neuropharmacol. 2008;6(1):39–54.
28. Fromme K, D'Amico EJ. Neurobiological bases of alcohol's psychological effects. In: Leonard KE, Blane HT, editors. Psychological theories of drinking and alcoholism.New York: Guilford Press; 1999. p. 422–55.
29. Tsai G, Gastfriend DR, Coyle JT. The glutamatergic basis of human alcoholism. Am J Psychiatry. 1995;152(3):332–40.
30. Roehrs T, Beare D, Zorick F, Roth T. Sleepiness and ethanol effects on simulated driving. Alcohol Clin Exp Res. 1994;18(1): 154–8.
31. Zador PL, Krawchuk SA, Voas RB. Alcohol-related relative risk of driver fatalities and driver involvement in fatal crashes in relation to driver age and gender: an update using 1996 data. J Stud Alcohol. 2000;61(3):387–95.
32. Zador PL. Alcohol-related relative risk of fatal driver injuries in relation to driver age and sex. J Stud Alcohol. 1991;52(4): 302–10.
33. Rehm J, Monteiro M. Alcohol consumption and burden of disease in the Americas: implications for alcohol policy. Rev Panam Salud Publica. 2005;18(4–5):241–8.
34. Rehm J, Taylor B, Patra J. Volume of alcohol consumption, patterns of drinking and burden of disease in the European region 2002. Addiction. 2006;101(8):1086–95.
35. Rehm J, Giesbrecht N, Patra J, Roerecke M. Estimating chronic disease deaths and hospitalizations due to alcohol use in Canada in 2002: implications for policy and prevention strategies. Prev Chronic Dis. 2006;3(4):A121.
36. Rehm J, Taylor B, Room R. Global burden of disease from alcohol, illicit drugs and tobacco. Drug Alcohol Rev. 2006;25(6): 503–13.
37. Gmel G, Rehm J. Harmful alcohol use. Alcohol Res Health. 2003;27(1):52–62.
38. Bye EK. Alcohol and violence: use of possible confounders in a time-series analysis. Addiction. 2007;102(3):369–76.
39. Caetano R, McGrath C, Ramisetty-Mikler S, Field CA. Drinking, alcohol problems and the five-year recurrence and incidence of male to female and female to male partner violence. Alcohol Clin Exp Res. 2005;29(1):98–106.
40. Bushman BJ, Cooper HM. Effects of alcohol on human aggression: an integrative research review. Psychol Bull. 1990;107(3): 341–54.
41. Kotwica M, Czerczak S. Acute poisonings registered since 1970: trends and characteristics. Analysis of the files collected in the National Poison Information Centre, Lodz, Poland. Int J Occup Med Environ Health. 2007;20(1):38–43.
42. Stickley A, Leinsalu M, Andreev E, Razvodovsky Y, Vagero D, McKee M. Alcohol poisoning in Russia and the countries in the

European part of the former Soviet Union, 1970–2002. Eur J Public Health. 2007;17(5):444–9.

43. Anderson P, Baumberg B. Alcohol in Europe: a public health perspective: a report for the European Commission. London: Institute of Alcohol Studies; 2006.

44. Room R, Babor T, Rehm J. Alcohol and public health. Lancet. 2005;365(9458):519–30.

45. Norstrom T, Ramstedt M. Mortality and population drinking: a review of the literature. Drug Alcohol Rev. 2005;24(6):537–47.

46. Koppes LL, Twisk JW, Van MW, Snel J, Kemper HC. Cross-sectional and longitudinal relationships between alcohol consumption and lipids, blood pressure and body weight indices. J Stud Alcohol. 2005;66(6):713–21.

47. Koppes LL, Dekker JM, Hendriks HF, Bouter LM, Heine RJ. Moderate alcohol consumption lowers the risk of type 2 diabetes: a meta-analysis of prospective observational studies. Diabetes Care. 2005;28(3):719–25.

48. Sierksma A, Van der Gaag MS, van TA, James RW, Hendriks HF. Kinetics of HDL cholesterol and paraoxonase activity in moderate alcohol consumers. Alcohol Clin Exp Res. 2002;26(9):1430–5.

49. Elkind MS, Sciacca R, Boden-Albala B, Rundek T, Paik MC, Sacco RL. Moderate alcohol consumption reduces risk of ischemic stroke: the Northern Manhattan Study. Stroke. 2006; 37(1):13–9.

50. Pfefferbaum A, Rosenbloom M, Deshmukh A, Sullivan E. Sex differences in the effects of alcohol on brain structure. Am J Psychiatry. 2001;158(2):188–97.

51. Chanraud S, Martelli C, Delain F, Kostogianni N, Douaud G, Aubin HJ, et al. Brain morphometry and cognitive performance in detoxified alcohol-dependents with preserved psychosocial functioning. Neuropsychopharmacology. 2007;32(2):429–38.

52. Fein G, Di S, Cardenas VA, Goldmann H, Tolou-Shams M, Meyerhoff DJ. Cortical gray matter loss in treatment-naive alcohol dependent individuals. Alcohol Clin Exp Res. 2002;26(4): 558–64.

53. Durazzo TC, Cardenas VA, Studholme C, Weiner MW, Meyerhoff DJ. Non-treatment-seeking heavy drinkers: effects of chronic cigarette smoking on brain structure. Drug Alcohol Depend. 2007;87(1):76–82.

54. Cardenas VA, Studholme C, Meyerhoff DJ, Song E, Weiner MW. Chronic active heavy drinking and family history of problem drinking modulate regional brain tissue volumes. Psychiatry Res. 2005;138(2):115–30.

55. Jang DP, Namkoong K, Kim JJ, Park S, Kim IY, Kim SI, et al. The relationship between brain morphometry and neuropsychological performance in alcohol dependence. Neurosci Lett. 2007;428(1): 21–6.

56. Mechtcheriakov S, Brenneis C, Egger K, Koppelstaetter F, Schocke M, Marksteiner J. A widespread distinct pattern of cerebral atrophy in patients with alcohol addiction revealed by voxel-based morphometry. J Neurol Neurosurg Psychiatry. 2007; 78(6):610–4.

57. Taki Y, Kinomura S, Sato K, Goto R, Inoue K, Okada K, et al. Both global gray matter volume and regional gray matter volume negatively correlate with lifetime alcohol intake in non-alcohol-dependent Japanese men: a volumetric analysis and a voxel-based morphometry. Alcohol Clin Exp Res. 2006;30(6):1045–50.

58. Gazdzinski S, Durazzo TC, Weiner MW, Meyerhoff DJ. Are treated alcoholics representative of the entire population with alcohol use disorders? A magnetic resonance study of brain injury. Alcohol. 2008;42(2):67–76.

59. Gazdzinski S, Durazzo TC, Studholme C, Song E, Banys P, Meyerhoff DJ. Quantitative brain MRI in alcohol dependence: preliminary evidence for effects of concurrent chronic cigarette smoking on regional brain volumes. Alcohol Clin Exp Res. 2005;29(8):1484–95.

60. Gazdzinski S, Durazzo T, Jahng GH, Ezekiel F, Banys P, Meyerhoff D. Effects of chronic alcohol dependence and chronic cigarette smoking on cerebral perfusion: a preliminary magnetic resonance study. Alcohol Clin Exp Res. 2006;30(6):947–58.

61. Sachdev PS, Chen X, Wen W, Anstry KJ. Light to moderate alcohol use is associated with increased cortical gray matter in middle-aged men: a voxel-based morphometric study. Psychiatry Res. 2008;163(1):61–9.

62. Blizard DA, Vandenbergh DJ, Jefferson AL, Chatlos CD, Vogler GP, McClearn GE. Effects of periadolescent ethanol exposure on alcohol preference in two BALB substrains. Alcohol. 2004;34(2–3):177–85.

63. Schulteis G, Archer C, Tapert SF, Frank LR. Intermittent binge alcohol exposure during the periadolescent period induces spatial working memory deficits in young adult rats. Alcohol. 2008; 42(6):459–67.

64. Crews FT, Mdzinarishvili A, Kim D, He J, Nixon K. Neurogenesis in adolescent brain is potently inhibited by ethanol. Neuroscience. 2006;137(2):437–45.

65. Crews FT, Nixon K. Mechanisms of neurodegeneration and regeneration in alcoholism. Alcohol Alcohol. 2009;44(2): 115–27.

66. Crews F, He J, Hodge C. Adolescent cortical development: a critical period of vulnerability for addiction. Pharmacol Biochem Behav. 2007;86(2):189–99.

67. Monti PM, Miranda Jr R, Nixon K, Sher KJ, Swartzwelder HS, Tapert SF, et al. Adolescence: booze, brains, and behavior. Alcohol Clin Exp Res. 2005;29(2):207–20.

68. De B, Narasimhan A, Thatcher DL, Keshavan MS, Soloff P, Clark DB. Prefrontal cortex, thalamus, and cerebellar volumes in adolescents and young adults with adolescent-onset alcohol use disorders and comorbid mental disorders. Alcohol Clin Exp Res. 2005;29(9):1590–600.

69. De B, Van VE, Hooper SR, Gibler N, Nelson L, Hege SG, et al. Diffusion tensor measures of the corpus callosum in adolescents with adolescent onset alcohol use disorders. Alcohol Clin Exp Res. 2008;32(3):395–404.

70. De Bellis MD, Clark DB, Beers SR, Soloff PH, Boring AM, Hall J, et al. Hippocampal volume in adolescent-onset alcohol use disorders. Am J Psychiatry. 2000;157(5):737–44.

71. Benegal V, Antony G, Venkatasubramanian G, Jayakumar PN. Gray matter volume abnormalities and externalizing symptoms in subjects at high risk for alcohol dependence. Addict Biol. 2007;12(1):122–32.

72. Hill SY, De B, Keshavan MS, Lowers L, Shen S, Hall J, et al. Right amygdala volume in adolescent and young adult offspring from families at high risk for developing alcoholism. Biol Psychiatry. 2001;49(11):894–905.

73. McGuire LC, Ajani UA, Ford ES. Cognitive functioning in late life: the impact of moderate alcohol consumption. Ann Epidemiol. 2007;17(2):93–9.

74. Stampfer MJ, Kang JH, Chen J, Cherry R, Grodstein F. Effects of moderate alcohol consumption on cognitive function in women. N Engl J Med. 2005;352(3):245–53.

75. Reid MC, Van Ness PH, Hawkins KA, Towle V, Concato J, Guo Z. Light to moderate alcohol consumption is associated with better cognitive function among older male veterans receiving primary care. J Geriatr Psychiatry Neurol. 2006;19(2):98–105.

76. Ngandu T, Helkala EL, Soininen H, Winblad B, Tuomilehto J, Nissinen A, et al. Alcohol drinking and cognitive functions: findings from the Cardiovascular Risk Factors Aging and Dementia (CAIDE) Study. Dement Geriatr Cogn Disord. 2007;23(3): 140–9.

77. Parsons OA, Nixon SJ. Cognitive functioning in sober social drinkers: a review of the research since 1986. J Stud Alcohol. 1998;59(2):180–90.

78. Friend KB, Malloy PF, Sindelar HA. The effects of chronic nicotine and alcohol use on neurocognitive function. Addict Behav. 2005;30(1):193–202.

79. Durazzo TC, Rothlind JC, Gazdzinski S, Banys P, Meyerhoff DJ. A comparison of neurocognitive function in nonsmoking and chronically smoking short-term abstinent alcoholics. Alcohol. 2006;39(1):1–11.

80. Goudriaan AE, Oosterlaan J, de BE, Van den BW. Neurocognitive functions in pathological gambling: a comparison with alcohol dependence, Tourette syndrome and normal controls. Addiction. 2006;101(4):534–47.

81. Liappas I, Theotoka I, Kapaki E, Ilias I, Paraskevas GP, Soldatos CR. Neuropsychological assessment of cognitive function in chronic alcohol-dependent patients and patients with Alzheimer's disease. In Vivo. 2007;21(6):1115–8.

82. Giancola PR, Moss HB. Executive cognitive functioning in alcohol use disorders. Recent Dev Alcohol. 1998;14:227–51.

83. Victor M, Adams RD, Collins GH. The Wernicke-Korsakoff syndrome. A clinical and pathological study of 245 patients, 82 with post-mortem examinations. Contemp Neurol Ser. 1971;7:1–206.

84. Victor M. Persistent altered mentation due to ethanol. Neurol Clin. 1993;11(3):639–61.

85. Victor M. Alcoholic dementia. Can J Neurol Sci. 1994;21(2): 88–99.

86. Hesselbrock VM, Hesselbrock MN. Are there empirically supported and clinically useful subtypes of alcohol dependence? Addiction. 2006;101 Suppl 1:97–103.

87. Gratzer D, Levitan RD, Sheldon T, Toneatto T, Rector NA, Goering P. Lifetime rates of alcoholism in adults with anxiety, depression, or co-morbid depression/anxiety: a community survey of Ontario. J Affect Disord. 2004;79(1–3):209–15.

88. Weitzman ER. Poor mental health, depression, and associations with alcohol consumption, harm, and abuse in a national sample of young adults in college. J Nerv Ment Dis. 2004;192(4):269–77.

89. Jackson KM, Sher KJ. Alcohol use disorders and psychological distress: a prospective state-trait analysis. J Abnorm Psychol. 2003;112(4):599–613.

90. Elkins IJ, King SM, McGue M, Iacono WG. Personality traits and the development of nicotine, alcohol, and illicit drug disorders: prospective links from adolescence to young adulthood. J Abnorm Psychol. 2006;115(1):26–39.

91. James LM, Taylor J. Impulsivity and negative emotionality associated with substance use problems and Cluster B personality in college students. Addict Behav. 2007;32(4):714–27.

92. Malouff JM, Thorsteinsson EB, Rooke SE, Schutte NS. Alcohol involvement and the Five-Factor model of personality: a meta-analysis. J Drug Educ. 2007;37(3):277–94.

93. Mortensen EL, Jensen HH, Sanders SA, Reinisch JM. Associations between volume of alcohol consumption and social status, intelligence, and personality in a sample of young adult Danes. Scand J Psychol. 2006;47(5):387–98.

94. Bjork JM, Hommer DW, Grant SJ, Danube C. Impulsivity in abstinent alcohol-dependent patients: relation to control subjects and type 1-/type 2-like traits. Alcohol. 2004;34(2–3):133–50.

95. Chen AC, Porjesz B, Rangaswamy M, Kamarajan C, Tang Y, Jones KA, et al. Reduced frontal lobe activity in subjects with high impulsivity and alcoholism. Alcohol Clin Exp Res. 2007;31(1):156–65.

96. Dom G, Hulstijn W, Sabbe B. Differences in impulsivity and sensation seeking between early- and late-onset alcoholics. Addict Behav. 2006;31(2):298–308.

97. MacKillop J, Mattson RE, Anderson Mackillop EJ, Castelda BA, Donovick PJ. Multidimensional assessment of impulsivity in undergraduate hazardous drinkers and controls. J Stud Alcohol Drugs. 2007;68(6):785–8.

98. Magid V, Maclean MG, Colder CR. Differentiating between sensation seeking and impulsivity through their mediated relations with alcohol use and problems. Addict Behav. 2007;32(10):2046–61.

99. Bottlender M, Preuss UW, Soyka M. Association of personality disorders with Type A and Type B alcoholics. Eur Arch Psychiatry Clin Neurosci. 2006;256(1):55–61.

100. Compton WM, Conway KP, Stinson FS, Colliver JD, Grant BF. Prevalence, correlates, and comorbidity of DSM-IV antisocial personality syndromes and alcohol and specific drug use disorders in the United States: results from the national epidemiologic survey on alcohol and related conditions. J Clin Psychiatry. 2005;66(6):677–85.

101. Thatcher DL, Cornelius JR, Clark DB. Adolescent alcohol use disorders predict adult borderline personality. Addict Behav. 2005;30(9):1709–24.

102. Stepp SD, Trull TJ, Sher KJ. Borderline personality features predict alcohol use problems. J Personal Disord. 2005;19(6): 711–22.

103. Tragesser SL, Sher KJ, Trull TJ, Park A. Personality disorder symptoms, drinking motives, and alcohol use and consequences: cross-sectional and prospective mediation. Exp Clin Psychopharmacol. 2007;15(3):282–92.

104. Slutske WS, Heath AC, Madden PA, Bucholz KK, Statham DJ, Martin NG. Personality and the genetic risk for alcohol dependence. J Abnorm Psychol. 2002;111(1):124–33.

105. Loukas A, Krull JL, Chassin L, Carle AC. The relation of personality to alcohol abuse/dependence in a high-risk sample. J Personal. 2000;68(6):1153–75.

106. Puttler LI, Zucker RA, Fitzgerald HE, Bingham CR. Behavioral outcomes among children of alcoholics during the early and middle childhood years: familial subtype variations. Alcohol Clin Exp Res. 1998;22(9):1962–72.

107. Sher KJ, Bartholow BD, Wood MD. Personality and substance use disorders: a prospective study. J Consult Clin Psychol. 2000;68(5):818–29.

108. Schuckit MA. Biological, psychological and environmental predictors of the alcoholism risk: a longitudinal study. J Stud Alcohol. 1998;59(5):485–94.

109. Caspi A, Moffitt TE, Newman DL, Silva PA. Behavioral observations at age 3 years predict adult psychiatric disorders. Longitudinal evidence from a birth cohort. Arch Gen Psychiatry. 1996; 53(11):1033–9.

110. Hill SY, Shen S, Lowers L, Locke J. Factors predicting the onset of adolescent drinking in families at high risk for developing alcoholism. Biol Psychiatry. 2000;48(4):265–75.

111. Hussong AM. Social influences in motivated drinking among college students. Psychol Addict Behav. 2003;17(2):142–50.

112. Jackson CP, Matthews G. The prediction of habitual alcohol use from alcohol related expectancies and personality. Alcohol Alcohol. 1988;23(4):305–14.

113. Edward AM, Schork MA, Harburg E, Moll PP, Burns TL, Ozgoren F. Sources of variability in quantitative levels of alcohol use in a total community: sociodemographic and psychosocial correlates. Int J Epidemiol. 1986;15(1):82–90.

114. Dawson DA, Grant BF, Stinson FS, Chou PS. Maturing out of alcohol dependence: the impact of transitional life events. J Stud Alcohol. 2006;67(2):195–203.

115. Dawson DA, Grant BF, Stinson FS, Chou PS. Psychopathology associated with drinking and alcohol use disorders in the college and general adult populations. Drug Alcohol Depend. 2005;77(2):139–50.

116. Dawson DA, Grant BF, Stinson FS, Chou PS, Huang B, Ruan WJ. Recovery from DSM-IV alcohol dependence: United States, 2001-2002. Addiction. 2005;100(3):281–92.

117. Bierut LJ, Schuckit MA, Hesselbrock V, Reich T. Co-occurring risk factors for alcohol dependence and habitual smoking. Alcohol Res Health. 2000;24(4):233–41.

118. Kendler KS, Schmitt E, Aggen SH, Prescott CA. Genetic and environmental influences on alcohol, caffeine, cannabis, and nicotine use from early adolescence to middle adulthood. Arch Gen Psychiatry. 2008;65(6):674–82.

119. Agrawal A, Hinrichs AL, Dunn G, Bertelsen S, Dick DM, Saccone SF, et al. Linkage scan for quantitative traits identifies new regions of interest for substance dependence in the Collaborative Study on the Genetics of Alcoholism (COGA) sample. Drug Alcohol Depend. 2008;93(1–2):12–20.

120. Black DW, Monahan PO, Temkit M, Shaw M. A family study of pathological gambling. Psychiatry Res. 2006;141(3):295–303.

121. McGue M. A behavioral-genetic perspective on children of alcoholics. Alcohol Health Res World. 1997;21(3):210–7.

122. Bierut LJ, Saccone NL, Rice JP, Goate A, Foroud T, Edenberg H, et al. Defining alcohol-related phenotypes in humans. The Collaborative Study on the Genetics of Alcoholism. Alcohol Res Health. 2002;26(3):208–13.

123. Reich T, Edenberg HJ, Goate A, Williams JT, Rice JP, Van EP, et al. Genome-wide search for genes affecting the risk for alcohol dependence. Am J Med Genet. 1998;81(3):207–15.

124. Peng GS, Chen YC, Tsao TP, Wang MF, Yin SJ. Pharmacokinetic and pharmacodynamic basis for partial protection against alcoholism in Asians, heterozygous for the variant ALDH2*2 gene allele. Pharmacogenet Genomics. 2007;17(10):845–55.

125. Scott DM, Taylor RE. Health-related effects of genetic variations of alcohol-metabolizing enzymes in African Americans. Alcohol Res Health. 2007;30(1):18–21.

126. Kramer JR, Chan G, Dick DM, Kuperman S, Bucholz KK, Edenberg HJ, et al. Multiple-domain predictors of problematic alcohol use in young adulthood. J Stud Alcohol Drugs. 2008;69(5):649–59.

127. Bauer LO, Covault J, Harel O, Das S, Gelernter J, Anton R, et al. Variation in GABRA2 predicts drinking behavior in project MATCH subjects. Alcohol Clin Exp Res. 2007;31(11):1780–7.

128. Lind PA, MacGregor S, Agrawal A, Montgomery GW, Heath AC, Martin NG, et al. The role of GABRA2 in alcohol dependence, smoking, and illicit drug use in an Australian population sample. Alcohol Clin Exp Res. 2008;32(10):1721–31.

129. Lind PA, MacGregor S, Montgomery GW, Heath AC, Martin NG, Whitfield JB. Effects of GABRA2 variation on physiological, psychomotor and subjective responses in the alcohol challenge twin study. Twin Res Hum Genet. 2008;11(2):174–82.

130. Haughey HM, Ray LA, Finan P, Villanueva R, Niculescu M, Hutchison KE. Human gamma-aminobutyric acid A receptor alpha2 gene moderates the acute effects of alcohol and brain mRNA expression. Genes Brain Behav. 2008;7(4):447–54.

131. Covault J, Gelernter J, Jensen K, Anton R, Kranzler HR. Markers in the 5′-region of GABRG1 associate to alcohol dependence and are in linkage disequilibrium with markers in the adjacent GABRA2 gene. Neuropsychopharmacology. 2008;33(4):837–48.

132. Enoch MA, Hodgkinson CA, Yuan Q, Albaugh B, Virkkunen M, Goldman D. GABRG1 and GABRA2 as independent predictors for alcoholism in two populations. Neuropsychopharmacology. 2009;34(5):1245–54.

133. Bowirrat A, Oscar-Berman M. Relationship between dopaminergic neurotransmission, alcoholism, and Reward Deficiency syndrome. Am J Med Genet B Neuropsychiatr Genet. 2005;132B(1):29–37.

134. Edenberg HJ, Foroud T. The genetics of alcoholism: identifying specific genes through family studies. Addict Biol. 2006;11(3–4):386–96.

135. Kohnke MD. Approach to the genetics of alcoholism: a review based on pathophysiology. Biochem Pharmacol. 2008;75(1):160–77.

136. Soyka M, Preuss UW, Hesselbrock V, Zill P, Koller G, Bondy B. GABA-A2 receptor subunit gene (GABRA2) polymorphisms and risk for alcohol dependence. J Psychiatr Res. 2008;42(3):184–91.

137. Enoch MA, Schuckit MA, Johnson BA, Goldman D. Genetics of alcoholism using intermediate phenotypes. Alcohol Clin Exp Res. 2003;27(2):169–76.

138. Hutchison KE, McGeary J, Smolen A, Bryan A, Swift RM. The DRD4 VNTR polymorphism moderates craving after alcohol consumption. Health Psychol. 2002;21(2):139–46.

139. Filbey FM, Ray L, Smolen A, Claus ED, Audette A, Hutchison KE. Differential neural response to alcohol priming and alcohol taste cues is associated with DRD4 VNTR and OPRM1 genotypes. Alcohol Clin Exp Res. 2008;32(7):1113–23.

140. Paulus MP, Tapert SF, Schuckit MA. Neural activation patterns of methamphetamine-dependent subjects during decision making predict relapse. Arch Gen Psychiatry. 2005;62(7):761–8.

141. Kosten TR, Scanley BE, Tucker KA, Oliveto A, Prince C, Sinha R, et al. Cue-induced brain activity changes and relapse in cocaine-dependent patients. Neuropsychopharmacology. 2006;31(3):644–50.

142. Wrase J, Makris N, Braus DF, Mann K, Smolka MN, Kennedy DN, et al. Amygdala volume associated with alcohol abuse relapse and craving. Am J Psychiatry. 2008;165(9):1179–84.

143. Jacob T, Waterman B, Heath A, True W, Bucholz KK, Haber R, et al. Genetic and environmental effects on offspring alcoholism: new insights using an offspring-of-twins design. Arch Gen Psychiatry. 2003;60(12):1265–72.

144. Chassin L, Rogosch F, Barrera M. Substance use and symptomatology among adolescent children of alcoholics. J Abnorm Psychol. 1991;100(4):449–63.

145. Chassin L, Pitts SC, DeLucia C, Todd M. A longitudinal study of children of alcoholics: predicting young adult substance use disorders, anxiety, and depression. J Abnorm Psychol. 1999;108(1):106–19.

146. Ellis DA, Zucker RA, Fitzgerald HE. The role of family influences in development and risk. Alcohol Health Res World. 1997;21:218–26.

147. Spijkerman R, van den Eijnden RJ, Huiberts A. Socioeconomic differences in alcohol-specific parenting practices and adolescents' drinking patterns. Eur Addict Res. 2008;14(1):26–37.

148. Zundert V, Van d V, Vermulst AA, Engels RC. Pathways to alcohol use among Dutch students in regular education and education for adolescents with behavioral problems: the role of parental alcohol use, general parenting practices, and alcohol-specific parenting practices. J Fam Psychol. 2006;20(3):456–67.

149. Patock-Peckham JA, Cheong J, Balhorn ME, Nagoshi CT. A social learning perspective: a model of parenting styles, self-regulation, perceived drinking control, and alcohol use and problems. Alcohol Clin Exp Res. 2001;25:1284–92.

150. Adalbjarnardottir S, Hafsteinsson LG. Adolescents' perceived parenting styles and their substance use: concurrent and longitudinal analyses. J Res Adolesc. 2001;11:401–23.

151. Hawkins JD, Catalano RF, Miller JY. Risk and protective factors for alcohol and other drug problems in adolescence and early adulthood: implications for substance abuse prevention. Psychol Bull. 1992;112(1):64–105.

152. Bahr SJ, Hoffmann JP, Yang X. Parental and peer influences on the risk of adolescent drug use. J Prim Prev. 2005;26(6):529–51.

153. Borsari B, Carey KB. How the quality of peer relationships influences college alcohol use. Drug Alcohol Rev. 2006;25(4):361–70.

154. Dick DM, Pagan JL, Viken R, Purcell S, Kaprio J, Pulkkinen L, et al. Changing environmental influences on substance use across development. Twin Res Hum Genet. 2007;10(2):315–26.

155. Read JP, Wood MD, Capone C. A prospective investigation of relations between social influences and alcohol involvement during the transition into college. J Stud Alcohol. 2005;66(1):23–34.

156. Westling E, Andrews JA, Hampson SE, Peterson M. Pubertal timing and substance use: the effects of gender, parental monitoring and deviant peers. J Adolesc Health. 2008;42(6):555–63.

157. Ellickson SL, Tucker JS, Klein DJ, McGuigan KA. Prospective risk factors for alcohol misuse in late adolescence. J Stud Alcohol. 2001;62(6):773–82.

158. Fergusson DM, Woodward LJ, Horwood L. Childhood peer relationship problems and young people's involvement with deviant peers in adolescence. J Abnorm Child Psychol. 1999;27:357–69.

159. Li F, Duncan TE, Hops H. Examining developmental trajectories in adolescent alcohol use using piecewise growth mixture modeling analysis. J Stud Alcohol. 2001;62(2):199–210.

160. Miller NS, Gold MS. Management of withdrawal syndromes and relapse prevention in drug and alcohol dependence. Am Fam Physician. 1998;58(1):139–46.

161. Center for Substance Abuse Treatment (CSAT). A Guide to Substance Abuse Services for Primary Care Clinicians. Rockville (MD): Substance Abuse and Mental Health Services Administration (US); 1997. (Treatment Improvement Protocol (TIP) Series, No. 24.) Appendix A—Pharmacotherapy.

162. Daeppen JB, Gache P, Landry U, Sekera E, Schweizer V, Gloor S, Yersin B. Symptom-triggered vs fixed-schedule doses of benzodiazepine for alcohol withdrawal: a randomized treatment trial. Arch Intern Med. 2002;162(10):1117–21.

163. Holbrook AM, Crowther R, Lotter A, Cheng C, King D. Meta-analysis of benzodiazepine use in the treatment of acute alcohol withdrawal. CMAJ. 1999b;160(5):649–55.

164. Mayo-Smith MF. Pharmacological management of alcohol withdrawal. A meta-analysis and evidence-based practice guideline. American Society of Addiction Medicine Working Group on Pharmacological Management of Alcohol Withdrawal. JAMA. 1997;278(2):144–51.

165. Saitz R, Friedman LS, Mayo-Smith MF. Alcohol withdrawal: a nationwide survey of inpatient treatment practices. J Gen Intern Med. 1995;10(9):479–87.

166. Holbrook AM, Crowther R, Lotter A, Cheng C, King D. Diagnosis and management of acute alcohol withdrawal. CMAJ. 1999a; 160(5):675–80.

167. Mayo-Smith MF. Pharmacological management of alcohol withdrawal. A meta-analysis and evidence-based practice guideline. American Society of Addiction Medicine Working Group on Pharmacological Management of Alcohol Withdrawal. JAMA. 1997;278(2):144–51.

168. Mundt MP. Analyzing the costs and benefits of brief intervention. Alcohol Res Health. 2006;29(1):34–6.

169. Fleming MF, Mundt MP, French MT, Manwell LB, Stauffacher EA, Barry KL. Brief physician advice for problem drinkers: long-term efficacy and benefit-cost analysis. Alcohol Clin Exp Res. 2002;26(1):36–43.

170. Grossberg PM, Brown DD, Fleming MF. Brief physician advice for high-risk drinking among young adults. Ann Fam Med. 2004;2(5):474–80.

171. Prendergast M, Podus D, Finney J, Greenwell L, Roll J. Contingency management for treatment of substance use disorders: a meta-analysis. Addiction. 2006;101(11):1546–60.

172. Miller WR, Wilbourne PL, Hettema JE. What works? A summary of treatment outcome research. Handbook of alcoholism treatment approaches: effective alternatives. 3rd ed. Needham Heights, MA: Allyn & Bacon; 2003. p. 13–63.

173. McCrady BS. Alcohol use disorders and the Division 12 Task Force of the American Psychological Association. Psychol Addict Behav. 2000;14(3):267–76.

174. Bennett GA, Withers J, Thomas PW, Higgins DS, Bailey J, Parry L, et al. A randomised trial of early warning signs relapse prevention training in the treatment of alcohol dependence. Addict Behav. 2005;30(6):1111–24.

175. Walsh DC, Hingson RW, Merrigan DM, Levenson SM, Cupples LA, Heeren T, et al. A randomized trial of treatment options for alcohol-abusing workers. N Engl J Med. 1991;325(11):775–82.

176. Ouimette PC, Finney JW, Moos RH. Twelve-step and cognitive–behavioral treatment for substance abuse: a comparison of treatment effectiveness. J Consult Clin Psychol. 1997;65(2):230–40.

177. Wu J, Witkiewitz K. Network support for drinking: an application of multiple groups growth mixture modeling to examine client-treatment matching. J Stud Alcohol Drugs. 2008;69(1):21–9.

178. Kaskutas LA. Alcoholics anonymous effectiveness: faith meets science. J Addict Dis. 2009;28(2):145–57.

179. Powers MB, Vedel E, Emmelkamp PM. Behavioral couples therapy (BCT) for alcohol and drug use disorders: a meta-analysis. Clin Psychol Rev. 2008;28(6):952–62.

180. Garbutt JC. The state of pharmacotherapy for the treatment of alcohol dependence. J Subst Abuse Treat. 2009;36(1):S15–23.

181. Mason BJ. Acamprosate in the treatment of alcohol dependence. Expert Opin Pharmacother. 2005;6(12):2103–15.

182. Mason BJ, Crean R. Acamprosate in the treatment of alcohol dependence: clinical and economic considerations. Expert Rev Neurother. 2007;7(11):1465–77.

183. Anton RF, O'Malley SS, Ciraulo DA, Cisler RA, Couper D, Donovan DM, et al. Combined pharmacotherapies and behavioral interventions for alcohol dependence: the COMBINE study: a randomized controlled trial. JAMA. 2006;295(17):2003–17.

184. Anton RF. Pharmacologic approaches to the management of alcoholism. J Clin Psychiatry. 2001;62 Suppl 20:11–7.

185. Roozen HG, de WR, van der Windt DA, van den BW, de Jong CA, Kerkhof AJ. A systematic review of the effectiveness of naltrexone in the maintenance treatment of opioid and alcohol dependence. Eur Neuropsychopharmacol. 2006;16(5):311–23.

186. Johnson BA, Rosenthal N, Capece JA, Wiegand F, Mao L, Beyers K, et al. Topiramate for treating alcohol dependence: a randomized controlled trial. JAMA. 2007;298(14):1641–51.

187. Johnson BA. Recent advances in the development of treatments for alcohol and cocaine dependence: focus on topiramate and other modulators of GABA or glutamate function. CNS Drugs. 2005;19(10):873–96.

188. Ma JZ, It-Daoud N, Johnson BA. Topiramate reduces the harm of excessive drinking: implications for public health and primary care. Addiction. 2006;101(11):1561–8.

189. Addolorato G, Leggio L, Ferrulli A, Cardone S, Vonghia L, Mirijello A, et al. Effectiveness and safety of baclofen for maintenance of alcohol abstinence in alcohol-dependent patients with liver cirrhosis: randomised, double-blind controlled study. Lancet. 2007;370(9603):1915–22.

190. Addolorato G, Caputo F, Capristo E, Domenicali M, Bernardi M, Janiri L, et al. Baclofen efficacy in reducing alcohol craving and intake: a preliminary double-blind randomized controlled study. Alcohol Alcohol. 2002;37(5):504–8.

191. Garbutt JC, Kampov-Polevoy AB, Gallop R, Kalka-Juhl L, Flannery BA. Efficacy and safety of baclofen for alcohol dependence: a randomized, double-blind, placebo-controlled trial. Alcohol Clin Exp Res. 2010;34(11):1849–57.

192. Leggio L, Garbutt JC, Addolorato G. Effectiveness and safety of baclofen in the treatment of alcohol dependent patients. CNS Neurol Disord Drug Targets. 2010;9(1):33–44.

193. Brewer C. Controlled trials of Antabuse in alcoholism: the importance of supervision and adequate dosage. Acta Psychiatr Scand Suppl. 1992;369:51–8.

194. Chick J. Safety issues concerning the use of disulfiram in treating alcohol dependence. Drug Saf. 1999;20(5):427–35.

195. Fuller RK, Gordis E. Does disulfiram have a role in alcoholism treatment today? Addiction. 2004;99(1):21–4.

196. Ehrenreich H, Krampe H. Does disulfiram have a role in alcoholism treatment today? Not to forget about disulfiram's psychological effects. Addiction. 2004;99(1):26–7.

197. Poikolainen K. The disulfiram-ethanol reaction (DER) experience. Addiction. 2004;99(1):26–8.

198. Chick J. Disulfiram: cautions on liver function; how to supervise. Addiction. 2004;99(1):25–8.

Nicotine

10

Erika B. Litvin, Joseph W. Ditre, Bryan W. Heckman,
and Thomas H. Brandon

Abstract

Tobacco use is the leading cause of preventable mortality worldwide, and nicotine (a small tertiary amine consisting of a pyridine and pyrrolidine ring) is the primary psychoactive constituent in tobacco. When inhaled, nicotine reaches the brain within 7–10 s, with peak blood levels occurring within a few minutes. In the USA, the prevalence of smoking among adults is just under 20%, although over half of all ever-smokers have now quit. Nicotine dependence is characterized by tolerance, withdrawal symptoms (e.g., irritability, depression, restlessness, insomnia, anxiety, hunger and poor concentration, as well as craving), and compulsive use. Tobacco use and dependence are more prevalent among psychiatric patients and persons with certain medical conditions, including HIV and chronic pain. Smokers often report that cigarettes enhance both their mood state and their cognitive functioning (e.g., attention); however, it is difficult to determine if these are actual nicotine onset effects, relief of nicotine withdrawal effects, or psychological expectancy (i.e., placebo) effects. Treatments for tobacco use include seven FDA-approved pharmacotherapies (nicotine gum, patch, nasal spray, inhaler, and lozenge, plus bupropion, and varenicline) with roughly similar efficacies. In addition, behavioral counseling enhances efficacy rates. Even minimal counseling, such as brief physician advice, significantly increases the odds of cessation, but more intensive counseling produces greater effects. Other options include self-help and telephone quitlines.

Learning Objectives
- Tobacco use is the leading cause of preventable mortality worldwide, killing over five million people annually.
- Tobacco smoking is associated with increased risk of lung and other cancers, coronary heart disease, peripheral vascular disease, chronic lung disease, stroke, and pneumonia.
- Approximately 20% of US adults continue to smoke.
- Nicotine is the addictive agent in tobacco. The essential features of nicotine dependence are tolerance, withdrawal symptoms, and compulsive use.
- Nicotine typically acts as a stimulant within the central and peripheral nervous system, but large doses can produce effects similar to a depressant.
- Nicotine dependence is associated with several psychiatric disorders, including major depression, anxiety, substance abuse, and schizophrenia.
- Although acute effects of nicotine include apparent cognitive and affective enhancement, it is difficult

E.B. Litvin • B.W. Heckman • T.H. Brandon (✉)
Tobacco Research & Intervention Program, H. Lee Moffitt
Cancer Center, University of South Florida, 4115 E.
Fowler Avenue, Tampa FL 33617, USA
e-mail: Thomas.Brandon@Moffitt.org

J.W. Ditre
Department of Psychology, Texas A&M University,
College Station, TX 77843, USA

J.C. Verster et al. (eds.), *Drug Abuse and Addiction in Medical Illness: Causes, Consequences and Treatment*,
DOI 10.1007/978-1-4614-3375-0_10, © Springer Science+Business Media, LLC 2012

to rule out simple reversal of withdrawal-induced deficits in these areas.

- For comprehensive, empirically based recommendations on smoking cessation strategies, see the U.S. Public Health Service's Clinical Practice Guideline on Treating Tobacco Use and Dependence.
- The seven FDA-approved pharmacotherapies for treating tobacco dependence include five nicotine replacement therapies (gum, patch, nasal spray, inhaler, and lozenge), plus bupropion and varenicline.
- Behavioral counseling improves the efficacy of pharmacotherapy in a dose–response manner. However, even minimal interventions, such as brief physician advice, significantly increase abstinence rates.

Issues That Need to Be Addressed by Future Research

- Parsing the degree to which acute nicotine effects (e.g., cognitive and affective enhancement) are the product of (a) direct nicotine onset; (b) offset of nicotine withdrawal; and (c) psychological expectancy effects.
- Determining if the comorbidity of nicotine dependence and psychiatric disorders represents self-medication for specific psychiatric symptoms, and the development of targeted treatments for these smokers.
- The development of personalized medicine for treating nicotine dependence, based on genetic, physiological, or psychological individual differences.
- The development of novel behavioral interventions, particularly those that complement or synergize with pharmacotherapy effects.

Nicotine is believed to be the primary psychoactive constituent in tobacco smoke [1]. Whereas the psychoactive effects of nicotine are more subtle than other drugs of abuse, ironically the likelihood of the development of dependence and the morbidity and mortality associated with tobacco products is far greater. Although tobacco use rates have declined steadily since the 1960s, nicotine remains one of the most heavily used substances in the USA, and tobacco use is the leading preventable cause of death worldwide [2]. This chapter reviews the use and abuse of nicotine, including long-term consequences of use, prevalence of use and the development of tolerance and dependence, acute physiological and psychological effects, and treatment considerations. Given that cigarette smoking is by far the most widely used

method for nicotine delivery, the majority of this chapter focuses on smoked tobacco.

Nicotine and Tobacco Preparations

Although cigarette smoking has been the most popular method of nicotine self-administration since the early twentieth century, nicotine is also commonly derived from the smoke of other tobacco preparations (e.g., cigars, pipes, hookahs, bidis, and kreteks) and from smokeless tobacco (e.g., chewing tobacco and snuff). Hookahs (or water pipes) have been gaining in popularity among young adults in the USA. Hookahs vary in size, shape, and composition, and hookah tobacco is available in a variety of flavors [3]. Bidis are small, hand-rolled cigarettes that consist of tobacco wrapped in the leaves of plants native to Asia [4]. Kreteks (or clove cigarettes) typically contain a combination of tobacco, cloves, and other additives [5]. Both bidis and kreteks have been found to contain higher concentrations of nicotine, tar, and carbon monoxide than conventional cigarettes [4, 5]. With respect to smokeless preparations, chewing tobacco is commonly used in a loose leaf form, whereas snuff is finely ground tobacco that may be dry, moist, or delivered in pouches. Although snuff can be inhaled through the nose, most users place the tobacco between their cheek and gum.

Tobacco-Related Mortality

Tobacco use is the single most preventable cause of death in the world today, killing an average of more than five million people each year [2]. Furthermore, worldwide smoking-related mortality is estimated to reach ten million annually by 2030, with 70% of these deaths occurring in developing countries [6]. In the USA, tobacco smoking accounts for an estimated 443,000 deaths each year, including about 38,000 from secondhand (or environmental) tobacco smoke exposure [7, 8]. Thus, US mortality data indicate that tobacco use is responsible for more annual American deaths than HIV, motor vehicle injuries, illegal drug use, alcohol use, murders, and suicides combined [7, 9]. On average, smokers die 13–14 years earlier than nonsmokers [7], and for every person who dies of a smoking-related disease, 20 more people develop at least one serious smoking-related illness [10]. Excluding deaths from residential fires and adult deaths from secondhand smoke, tobacco smoking accounts for approximately 5.1 million years of potential life lost each year [8]. Tobacco use is also associated with tremendous societal costs, including about $193 billion in annual medical expenses and lost productivity, or about $3,750 per adult smoker [8, 11]. Healthcare costs associated with exposure to secondhand smoke average $10 billion annually [12].

Tobacco-Related Health Effects

Tobacco Smoking

Tobacco smoking harms nearly every organ of the body and causes a wide range of diseases, including several forms of cancer [6, 13]. Diseases causally linked with tobacco use include: chronic obstructive pulmonary disease, coronary heart disease, peripheral vascular disease, chronic lung disease, peptic ulcers, stroke, abdominal aortic aneurysm, cataract, pneumonia, and periodontitis [6]. Relative to nonsmokers, smokers are ten times more likely to develop peripheral vascular disease [14]; twice as likely to suffer from a stroke [15]; and up to four times more likely to develop coronary heart disease [16]. Smoking is also known to cause cancers of the oral cavity, larynx, pharynx, esophagus, cervix, bladder, kidney, lung, pancreas, and stomach, as well as acute myeloid leukemia. Tobacco smoking is responsible for about 85% of all lung cancer deaths, and the risk of dying from lung cancer is about 23 times greater for male smokers and about 13 times greater for female smokers relative to male and female never-smokers [13]. Rates of tobacco-related cancer vary considerably by race and ethnicity but are generally greatest among African-American men [17]. It is important to note that many adverse health effects of tobacco smoking are considered reversible, with treatments for smoking cessation identified as some of the most cost effective of all healthcare interventions [6].

Smokeless Tobacco and Secondh and Smoke Exposure

Smokeless tobacco contains numerous carcinogens and is known to increase the risk for developing cancer of the oral cavity [18]. In addition, several oral health problems (e.g., leukoplakia and recession of the gums) are strongly associated with smokeless tobacco use [19]. Secondhand smoke exposure is known to have immediate adverse effects on the cardiovascular system and is a causal agent in the development of coronary heart disease [20]. Secondhand smoke has also been found to cause lung cancer among never-smokers, with approximately 3,000 lung cancer deaths attributable to secondhand smoke exposure each year [20].

Prevalence of Tobacco Use

Tobacco Smoking

Despite treatment advances and the widely known health consequences of tobacco use, approximately 20.6% of all U.S. adults (46 million people) continue to smoke cigarettes [21]. Furthermore, about 20% of America's youth are classified as current smokers by the time they complete high school [22]. The prevalence of tobacco smoking by age is estimated to be 21.4% for persons 18–24, 23.7% for persons 25–44, 22.6% for persons 45–64, and 9.3% for persons 65 or older [21]. Smoking rates also vary by gender, ethnicity, education, and income [21]. For example, tobacco smoking is more prevalent among men (23.1%) than women (18.3%), and among American Indians/Alaska Natives (32.4%), relative to Caucasians (22.0%), African Americans (21.3%), Hispanics/Latinos (15.8%), and Asian Americans (9.9%). The prevalence of smoking is also inversely related to educational attainment and economic status. Whereas 41.3% of adults with only a General Education Development (GED) diploma smoke, only 5.7% of those with a graduate college degree do. Likewise, the prevalence of smoking for those with incomes below versus above the poverty line is 31.5% versus 19.6%, respectively.

Smokeless Tobacco

Although smokeless tobacco use is much less prevalent than smoking, adolescents who use smokeless tobacco are more likely to become regular cigarette smokers [19]. An estimated 3.5% of US adults are current smokeless tobacco users, including 6.8% of men and 0.4% of women [23]. Smokeless tobacco use is most common among American Indians/Alaska Natives (5.4%), followed by Caucasians (4.5%), African Americans (1.4%), Hispanics/Latinos (1.1%), and Asian Americans (1.1%). In addition, approximately 8% of high school students and 4% of middle school students are classified as current smokeless tobacco users [22].

Comorbid Psychiatric Disorders

Psychiatric disorders are more common among smokers than in the general population [24]. Persons diagnosed as nicotine dependent are more likely to present with major depression, anxiety, and substance abuse/dependence disorders [25, 26]. In fact, it has been estimated that individuals with psychiatric or substance use disorders account for approximately 44% of all cigarettes smoked in the USA [27]. Of all persons seeking treatment for tobacco dependence, about 30–60% of persons report a history of depression [28, 29]. In addition, tobacco smokers account for up to 80% of all individuals who abuse drugs and alcohol [30–32]. Specifically, tobacco smoking has been associated with increased rates of alcohol, cannabis, and cocaine dependence [33, 34]. Finally, personality disorders (e.g., schizotypal and borderline) are also significantly more common among tobacco users [35].

Comorbid Medical Disorders

The recently updated U.S. Department of Health and Human Services' Clinical Practice Guidelines for Treating Tobacco Dependence identified smokers with comorbid medical conditions (e.g., cancer, cardiac disease, chronic obstructive pulmonary disease, diabetes, and asthma) as important targets for tobacco cessation because smoking is known to exacerbate these conditions [29]. It has been suggested that clinicians treating smokers with these conditions should consider integrating tobacco dependence interventions into chronic disease management programs because patients may benefit from this "teachable-moment" or "window of opportunity" [29, 36]. In addition, both HIV-positive individuals [37, 38] and persons who live with chronic pain [39–42] are more likely to smoke tobacco than the general population. HIV-positive smokers have higher mortality rates and report lower quality of life than HIV-positive nonsmokers [43, 44], and chronic pain patients who smoke present with more maladaptive pain behaviors than treatment-seeking nonsmokers [41].

Nicotine and Tobacco Dependence

Course

Although the prevalence of tobacco use in the USA has been closely monitored, less is known about the epidemiology of nicotine *dependence* [45]. Greater than 80% of adult smokers initiate tobacco use prior to age 18 [46]. Common correlates of daily smoking and lifetime/current nicotine dependence among young adults include: low education, parental and peer smoking, novelty seeking, early age of smoking onset, pleasurable initial smoking experiences, and Hispanic ethnicity [45]. On the other end of the spectrum, although 70% of adult smokers report a desire to quit using tobacco [47], only about 40% of smokers attempt to quit each year (with younger smokers more likely to try) [48]. Unfortunately, relapse is the most common outcome of these quit attempts, with 95–98% of those who quit on their own [49] and 70–85% of those who receive psychological and/or pharmacological treatment [29] resuming tobacco use within 1 year.

There is no consensus as to whether current tobacco smokers may be more tobacco dependent than earlier populations of smokers [50]. However, a recent report indicates that nicotine dependence has reached a 15-year high, with nearly 75% of persons currently seeking treatment for tobacco dependence categorized as highly nicotine dependent [51]. Consistent with this conclusion, analyses of published clinical trials of smoking cessation interventions have revealed a steady drop in cessation rates over the past two decades, suggesting that smokers are becoming increasingly difficult to treat [52, 53].

Taken together, cessation data indicate that few tobacco users achieve permanent abstinence during an initial quit attempt, but that most users cycle through periods of remission and relapse for many years [29]. Thus, nicotine and tobacco dependence may best be conceptualized as a chronic relapsing disorder that requires consistent, ongoing care.

Tolerance and Withdrawal

Nicotine dependence and withdrawal can develop with use of all tobacco preparations (e.g., cigarettes, chewing tobacco, snuff, pipes, and cigars) and nicotine replacement medications [54]. The relative capacity for these products to produce dependence or withdrawal is primarily dependent on the amount of nicotine they contain and how rapidly the nicotine is delivered to the brain. The essential features of nicotine dependence as described in both the ICD-10 and the DSM-IV are tolerance (i.e., smoking more over time to obtain the same effects), withdrawal symptoms (e.g., irritability, depression, restlessness, insomnia, anxiety, hunger, and poor concentration), and compulsive drug taking [54, 55]. Withdrawal symptoms have been observed as early as 30 min after the last cigarette [56]. Although withdrawal typically peaks within the first few days of abstinence, and subsides over the following 2 weeks, considerable deviation from this pattern has been found for a substantial subset of smokers [57].

Psychology of Nicotine Dependence

Multiple psychological constructs have been proposed to account for tobacco use and dependence [58]. Among the most prominent constructs included in models of tobacco and other drug use are basic learning principles such as positive reinforcement from the pleasurable effects of smoking, negative reinforcement from withdrawal relief and other stress relief, and classical conditioning, which involves the association of smoking with stimuli that are often paired with smoking.

Classical conditioning models of addiction suggest that during self-administration of substances such as nicotine, cues reliably paired with substance use or withdrawal may come to elicit craving and a variety of physiological, psychological, and behavioral responses capable of motivating ongoing drug use and increasing the probability of relapse [59–61]. Considering that tobacco use occurs in a variety of situations and contexts, an extensive array of cues may potentially become associated with nicotine self-administration. Cues that are most commonly associated with tobacco use include paraphernalia such as cigarettes, lighters, and ashtrays. However, cues that may come to trigger tobacco use can also be more distal (e.g., environments in which tobacco consumption commonly occurs) and internal (e.g., withdrawal symptoms, mood states, somatic sensations). In terms of tobacco research, cue reactivity assessments enable researchers to examine tobacco users' physiological and subjective reactions to cues and situations that are considered high risk for relapse [62, 63]. Indeed, research indicates that the extent to which a tobacco user experiences cue-elicited reactivity may be predictive of cessation success and posttreatment relapse to smoking [64–66].

Additionally, cognitive models have stressed the role of automatic processes involved with drug use, suggesting that the experienced smoker requires very little controlled cognitive effort to seek out and smoke a cigarette [67]. An influential motivational construct in the addiction field has been outcome expectancies, which refer to the user's expected consequences from consuming a substance. Expectancies are posited to represent a fundamental causal link involved with drug use initiation, maintenance, cessation, and relapse, and they do not necessarily function in conscious awareness [68, 69]. With respect to smoking, commonly held and motivationally potent expectancies include those related to positive reinforcement (e.g., positive mood, social facilitation), negative reinforcement (e.g., reduction of negative mood), and appetite/weight control [70].

Acute Physiological Effects of Nicotine

Nicotine produces complex, dose-related acute physiological consequences on both the central and peripheral nervous systems as a result of nicotine binding to nicotinic acetylcholine receptors (nAChRs), which are found in the central nervous system (CNS) as well as the autonomic ganglia, the neuromuscular junction, and several non-neuronal tissues [71]. The nAChRs are ligand-gated ion channels comprised of five individual subunits joined together to form a central pore consisting primarily of alpha and beta type subunits. Alpha type subunits can be further differentiated into nine isoforms (α2 to α10) and beta subunits into three isoforms (β2 to β4), leading to an assortment of subunit combinations within the brain [72]. At least 12 unique types of nAChRs have been identified. The heteromic α4β2 receptor subtype is the most abundant type, and these receptors may be the primary site of action mediating nicotine dependence. In addition to receptor subtype, receptor subunit location (presynaptic, axonal, and postsynaptic) and composition are also determining factors for how nicotine will affect neurotransmitter release and contribute to the complexity of the effects of nicotine [73].

Depending on the amount consumed, nicotine can act as a stimulant or depressant. Low doses produce arousal and an increase in heart rate or blood pressure, indicating central or peripheral nervous system stimulation. On the other hand, bradycardia and hypotension can be a result of high doses of nicotine. Physiological tolerance to nicotine can develop rapidly, beginning with consumption of the first cigarette. For example, many smokers will develop a partial tolerance to the acceleration of heart rate produced by nicotine within 1 day [74].

Central Nervous System

Nicotine stimulates presynaptic nAChRs throughout the brain, including regions of the thalamus, amygdala, hippocampus, midbrain, cingulated cortex, basal ganglia, cerebellum, and various other areas in the cerebral cortex [75]. As nicotine binds to these sites, positively charged ions (primarily sodium, potassium, and calcium) are allowed to enter the cell. These cations then activate voltage-dependent calcium channels, resulting in further influx of calcium and subsequently altered electrical activity, which increases the probability of depolarization and neurotransmitter release [73].

Nicotine may influence the action of a variety of neurotransmitters, including acetylcholine, dopamine, norepinephrine, serotonin, glutamate and γ-aminobutyric acid (GABA), as well as endorphins. Dopamine is thought to be of particular importance to the understanding of nicotine dependence. Nicotine leads to dopamine release in the corpus striatum, frontal cortex, and mesolimbic pathway. More specifically, nicotine-induced increases in dopamine within the ventral tegmental area of the midbrain, and the nucleus accumbens appear to be critical to the rewarding effects of nicotine [73, 76]. Activation of dopaminergic neurons within this system is further modulated by the effects of nicotine on inhibitory GABA and excitatory glutamate inputs [77].

Imaging techniques have been instrumental for aiding in the understanding of the acute effects of nicotine in the brain (e.g., functional magnetic resonance imaging, positron emission, single photon emission computed tomography, and autoradiography). Researchers have reliably demonstrated that nicotine administration leads to a decrease in global brain activity in human cigarette smokers [78, 79]. With respect to the effects of nicotine on regional activity in smokers, studies have commonly found relative increases in activity in the prefontal cortex (including the dorsolateral prefrontal cortex, medial frontal, and orbitofrontal gyri), thalamus, and visual system (see [80]). These findings are consistent with the idea that nicotine activates cortico-basal ganglia-thalamic circuitry [81], which may play a critical role in the subjective effects of smoking. Animal studies have provided convergent evidence concerning these effects of nicotine on brain activity [80].

Peripheral Nervous System

Nicotine is primarily responsible for the hemodynamic effects of smoking [82]. A sympathomimetic drug, nicotine leads to increased plasma levels of catecholamines, including norepinephrine and epinephrine [83]. This release of catecholamines locally by neurons and systemically from the adrenal gland contributes to increases in heart rate up to 15 bpm and increases in systolic blood pressure up to 5–10 mmHg following nicotine administration [82]. Additionally, myocardial contractility is amplified as nicotine is consumed. Together, these alterations in heart rate, blood pressure, and contractility result in changes in myocardial work, increasing coronary blood flow by up to 40% in healthy individuals [84]. Additionally, acute nicotine administration can lead to vasodilation or vasoconstriction, depending on the vascular bed location. For example, vasodilation occurs in skeletal muscle, whereas vasoconstriction occurs in the skin [82].

Acute Psychological Effects of Nicotine

As previously mentioned, tobacco users hold strong expectancies, or beliefs, that acute nicotine administration confers psychological benefits (e.g., mood and cognitive performance enhancement). In contrast to users' beliefs, studies that have investigated the *actual* acute psychological effects of nicotine have produced inconsistent results that are difficult to summarize briefly. A variety of methodological challenges and controversies complicate the interpretation of these findings. For example, many studies have lacked placebo control conditions, have not assessed pre-nicotine administration (i.e., baseline) status, and have employed small sample sizes resulting in possibly inadequate statistical power [85, 86]. Additional procedural considerations include the amount and timing of nicotine dosing and the route of administration (i.e., cigarette, intravenous, subcutaneous, patch, nasal spray, or gum), whether dosing is standardized or individualized, how mood is manipulated and measured, task difficulty and complexity, and other situational factors [85–88]. Finally, individual participant variables, such as the strength of their preexisting expectancies about the effects of nicotine, which may exert a placebo effect, variation in nicotine exposure history, pre-existing differences in mood and/ or cognitive abilities in smokers versus never-smokers, personality traits and psychological disorders, and baseline psychological state (e.g., baseline level of negative affect) may influence outcomes [85, 86, 89].

Importantly, many studies have not controlled for nicotine withdrawal status, and therefore it has been difficult to disentangle the absolute effects of nicotine from reversal of withdrawal-induced deficits. Studies that have included non-deprived smokers and nonsmokers have provided a more direct test of the effects of nicotine [85, 86, 90]. However, even these designs are not without controversy, as null results may indicate ceiling effects or that benefits only occur after tolerance is acquired [86]. Newer imaging technologies that have begun to reveal the physiological effects of nicotine that underlie psychological responses may help resolve some of this controversy [86, 88, 91].

Cognitive Performance

Consistent with smokers' self-reports, nicotine withdrawal is often characterized by objectively quantifiable decreases in attention and concentration (e.g., [92, 93]) that may emerge in as little as 30 min after smoking [56]. More specifically, nicotine deprivation appears to impair sensory abilities such as critical flicker frequency (highest frequency at which an individual can detect flicker in a flickering light source), simple psychomotor speed (i.e., finger tapping), and accuracy and reaction time in tests of sustained attention. Nicotine administration effectively reverses these deficits [85, 94, 95].

Above and beyond withdrawal-reversal, chronic nicotine consumption is consistently negatively associated with cognitive performance, whereas experimental human studies indicate that acute doses of nicotine may enhance performance in some domains [87, 90]. A recent meta-analysis demonstrated evidence for acute absolute enhancement effects of nicotine on fine motor abilities (e.g., finger tapping), attentional capabilities including accuracy and reaction time in alerting attention as well as reaction time in orienting attention, accuracy of short-term episodic memory recall, and reaction time in working memory tasks [90]. Nicotine does not appear to have a strong impact on accuracy of responding in timed tasks or on logical reasoning, problem solving, arithmetic, or other types of memory tasks [87], and effects that have been found in these higher order domains may be mediated by effects on attention [96]. However, not all studies have found this pattern of effects, with some studies finding no effects or even that nicotine may impair performance in some areas, and absolute enhancement effects may differ for nonsmokers lacking previous nicotine exposure versus experienced smokers who have developed a tolerance to nicotine (for reviews, see [85, 87, 90]). Furthermore, the clinical significance of these effects, and whether they represent direct effects or effects mediated by other factors such as general arousal or mood (see [89]), remains under debate [85, 87, 88].

One contemporary view is that nicotine may result in cognitive improvements among individuals with nicotine-relevant cognitive deficits, which may in part account for null and even negative findings among normal populations [88, 96, 97]. For example, it is well documented that individuals with disorders that affect attentional control, such as attention-deficit hyperactivity disorder (ADHD) [98, 99] and schizophrenia [100], smoke at much higher rates and are more severely nicotine dependent than the general population. Growing empirical evidence suggests that nicotine may confer differential benefits on these individuals such that nicotine use effectively serves as a form of self-medication that ameliorates attentional control-related deficits [88, 97, 101]. Subclinical individual differences in cognitive abilities (e.g., [102]) and schizophrenia-spectrum traits (for a review see [88]), as well as genetic differences in dopamine function (e.g., [103]) ultimately may be the substantive source of nicotine effects on cognition among people with these disorders.

The relationship between nicotine use and age-related cognitive impairments has also been explored. Tobacco smoking is consistently identified as a protective factor in the development of Parkinson's disease, a movement disorder that often includes cognitive symptoms [104]. Early studies also suggested a protective effect of smoking on Alzheimer's disease and other dementias, but a recent meta-analysis indicated that smoking is associated with an increased risk of dementia [105].

Many of the drugs currently being examined in relation to mild cognitive impairments and dementias associated with aging involve nicotine-related compounds (i.e., drugs that act on nicotine acetylcholine receptors). Treatment with nicotine via a skin patch or gum may have limited acute benefits for individuals with cognitive disorders, including Parkinson's, Alzheimer's, ADHD, and schizophrenia, but many studies have been small and uncontrolled. Whether the benefits persist in the long-term, especially considering other data suggesting that chronic nicotine use is associated with cognitive decline, remains to be demonstrated [96, 97, 106, 107].

Mood and Other Subjective Effects

A recent extensive systematic review and meta-analysis were conducted regarding the subjective effects of various forms of nicotine [86, 108]. The conclusions drawn from these reviews indicated that smoking a cigarette with an intermediate nicotine yield produces positive effects such as pleasure and enjoyment in significantly deprived (i.e., greater than 2 h) smokers; however, in this case withdrawal relief cannot be distinguished from absolute effects. Across methods of nicotine administration, there was some evidence for a linear dose–response relationship for arousal, head rush, and euphoria among deprived smokers. Somewhat surprisingly and inconsistent with smokers' beliefs, there was far less

evidence for relaxing, calming, or tension-reducing effects. Additionally, some studies found no effects of nicotine, and adverse effects tended to be found at intermediate and high doses and with certain forms of nicotine. Among minimally deprived smokers, these reviews revealed few effects of nicotine on subjective experience, although there were far fewer studies in this area and methodological problems prevented firm conclusions. In contrast to findings among smokers, nicotine produced mainly aversive subjective effects in nicotine-naive individuals. Never-smokers who received intravenous nicotine reported fatigue, dysphoria, and decreased alertness and calmness. Nicotine nasal spray and gum produced a mix of effects including head rush, euphoria, increased tension and confusion, and decreased relaxation and vigor Nicotine patch, a slower method of absorption, appeared to have less impact on subjective experience in never-smokers, with two studies reporting some evidence for improved mood.

The relationship between tobacco use and negative affect is complex, may be reciprocal, and is not yet fully understood [109]. In any discussion about the effects of nicotine on negative affect, it is important to also acknowledge the reverse; that is, the effects of negative affect on smoking behavior. Depression, negative life experiences, and life stress have been found to predict initiation of tobacco use, progression to daily smoking, and the development of nicotine dependence (for a review, see [109]). Smokers also generally report higher levels of stressful life events and negative affect than nonsmokers and are more likely to suffer from depression and some anxiety disorders than nonsmokers. Negative affect is even more tightly linked to cessation outcomes, as both acute negative affect (e.g., stressful situation) and chronic negative affect (e.g., depression) are robust predictors of smoking relapse [110–113]. These findings may be largely attributable to smokers' aforementioned expectancies about the stress-relieving properties of cigarette smoking [114, 115].

Despite smokers' beliefs and self-reports, there is less clarity about (1) whether acute, situational increases in negative affect *actually* prompt smoking behavior among continuing (i.e., not trying to quit) smokers [116, 117], and conversely, (2) whether nicotine reduces negative affect independent of withdrawal relief [109, 118]. With respect to the first question, both experimental and naturalistic studies have produced mixed results on the role of negative affect motivating smoking behavior. However, these divergent findings might be reconciled if smokers use cigarettes to fend off anticipated or early signs of negative affect, and if they often detect negative affect preconsciously [119]. As to the second question, placebo-controlled studies (i.e., comparing responses to regular cigarettes vs. denicotinized cigarettes) have determined that self-reported reduction in negative affect can be attributed to both the pharmacological effects of nicotine and to smokers' expectations that smoking will improve their mood [120, 121]. Variation in procedures used to induce and measure negative affect also influences study results [122]. Furthermore, other non-pharmacological factors such as the ritual of lighting and holding the cigarette and deep breathing during puffing may have calming properties and contribute to subjectively experienced negative affect relief.

Contemporary views suggest that nicotine may also serve as a form of self-medication for individuals with emotional disorders [91]. About 40–50% of individuals with major depressive disorder (MDD), bipolar disorder, panic disorder, generalized anxiety disorder (GAD), and postraumatic stress disorder (PTSD) are current cigarette smokers, compared to only 20% of the general population [27]. Some evidence suggests that nicotine may reduce feelings of depression and anxiety in both smokers and nonsmokers diagnosed with these disorders (for a review, see [91]).

In summary, a broad survey of relevant literatures, including both animal and human brain and behavioral studies, suggests that nicotine may enhance some aspects of cognition [88, 90] and subjective experience [86]. These benefits may more pronounced and constitute self-medication in individuals with attentional and emotional difficulties [91]. Ultimately, the attentional and mood-enhancing effects of nicotine may converge, as there is evidence that nicotine may contribute to the relief of negative affect by narrowing attentional focus onto competing stimuli and away from aversive internal states such as stress and anxiety [123–127].

Treatment of Nicotine Dependence

There are an increasing number of options available for the treatment of nicotine dependence. As noted above, nicotine dependence is a chronic, relapsing disorder, and treatment should be approached from this perspective. The U.S. Public Health Service's Clinical Practice Guideline on Treating Tobacco Use and Dependence [29] is a comprehensive review of smoking cessation research, with recommendations based on numerous meta-analyses. It is the best resource for evaluating currently available treatments, and therefore it is the basis for most of the conclusions that we present here.

Pharmacotherapies

To date, there are seven FDA-approved medications that reliably increase long-term abstinence rates. These include five nicotine replacement therapies (NRT) (gum, transdermal patch, inhaler, nasal spray, and lozenge), and two non-nicotine medications (bupropion SR, and varenicline). NRTs are designed to wean smokers gradually off nicotine in a manner that reduces the severity of withdrawal symptoms and cravings to smoke. They are typically used during the first 8–12 weeks of tobacco abstinence. Although the products vary in their routes of nicotine delivery (with the patch providing the most consistent delivery and stable blood levels), their efficacy levels are roughly equivalent, with odds ratios of approximately 2.0 compared to placebo, producing 6-month abstinence rates of approximately 20–25% [29]. Thus, choice of NRT can be based on patient preference and availability (gum, patch, and lozenge are available over the counter). These products have relatively mild side-effect profiles that are primarily related to their route of administration (e.g., skin irritation from the patch, nasal passage irritation from the spray).

Bupropion, which is also prescribed as an antidepressant, appears to function by inhibiting the neuronal reuptake of dopamine and norepinephrine. Unlike NRTs, the smoker begins taking bupropion 1 week prior to the target quit-smoking day. Contraindications include a history of seizure disorders or factors known to increase the risk of seizures (e.g., bulimia or anorexia nervosa, serious head trauma, alcoholism). The efficacy of bupropion is similar to the NRTs [29].

Varenicline is a partial nAChR agonist. It reduces withdrawal symptoms and cravings, and it may also reduce the satisfaction obtained from smoking. As with bupropion, the patient begins varenicline use approximately 1 week prior to quitting smoking. Odds ratios for varenicline to date are higher than for the other smoking cessation medications, with this drug approximately tripling the odds of quitting smoking [128–130]. Although the primary side effect of varenicline is nausea, the drug is receiving renewed scrutiny due to post-marketing reports of changes in behavior, agitation, depressed mood, suicidal ideation, and actual suicidal behavior. Consequently, the FDA issued a *Boxed Warning* in 2009 [131], and product labeling was revised to alert patients and healthcare providers to the possibility of these neuropsychiatric effects. Then in 2009, the FDA issued an advisory for both varenicline and bupropion and required boxed warnings about neuropsychiatric symptoms on both products. Follow-up studies are ongoing to quantify the frequency of these adverse reactions. Meanwhile, physicians and patients must weigh the potential health benefits associated with the greater efficacy of this product against the serious but apparently rare potential risks that have been reported.

Recent research reviewed in the Clinical Practice Guideline also supports the use of combination pharmacotherapy. Specifically, evidence supports the use of the nicotine patch combined with either another NRT or bupropion SR, which might be considered for highly nicotine-dependent patients or those unable to quit with a single medication (e.g., [132, 133]).

Behavioral Counseling

An unfortunate consequence of the progress over the past 25 years in the development of pharmacotherapies for treating nicotine dependence has been that both patients and providers increasingly fail to recognize the benefits of counseling. The most recent Clinical Practice Guideline [29] clarifies that the highest rates of cessation tend to be achieved with a combination of medication and counseling. These two strategies tend to complement each other, with medication reducing the severity of withdrawal symptoms and nicotine cravings, while counseling teaches information and cessation-related skills, as well as providing social support and motivational enhancement.

Counseling approaches can be ordered by level of intensity, ranging from very brief physician advice, through very intensive multi-session individual or group counseling. In general, there is a monotonic relationship between the level of intensity and the efficacy of counseling interventions [29]. Nevertheless, even as few as 3 min of physician advice and assistance can produce significant increases in cessation rates (with 6-month abstinence of approximately 13–14%), which may cumulatively produce dramatic effects at the population level. See the Clinical Practice Guidelines for specifics about the "5 A's" of brief counseling: Ask, Advise, Assess, Assist, and Arrange Follow-up [29].

At the most intensive end of the counseling continuum, smoking cessation clinics often provide 4–8 weeks of counseling that involves: teaching smokers the nature of nicotine addiction, including the symptoms and time course of nicotine withdrawal; training in recognizing and avoiding high-risk situations that "trigger" urges to smoke; training in cognitive and behavioral skills to cope with cravings to smoke; and training in how to respond to an initial smoking slip or "lapse" should it occurs, so that it does not progress to a full relapse to regular smoking. In addition, intensive counseling usually includes valued social support and motivational encouragement. Intensive counseling without pharmacotherapy can produce abstinence rates in the range of 15–25% [29]. Treatment manuals are available [134].

Two nontraditional modalities for providing behavioral counseling include self-help and telephone quitlines. Self-help refers to the provision of informational materials (traditionally in the form of pamphlets and brochures, but increasingly provided via video or Internet websites). In general, self-help interventions for smoking cessation have produced very low efficacy [135], but there is emerging evidence that increasing the focus of self-help materials may enhance their efficacy. For example, self-help booklets written specifically for individuals who had recently quit smoking, with a goal of reducing smoking relapse, have been found to be efficacious and highly cost effective [136, 137]. Moreover, interventions that are computer tailored to the demographic and psychological characteristics of each individual smoker usually show slightly superior efficacy compared to standard, untailored self-help materials [135].

Telephone quitlines represent the second nontraditional counseling modality. These quitlines are now available in each state and can be accessed through a single telephone number (1-800-QUITNOW). Individual quitlines differ in the services that they provide (e.g., provision of materials, local referrals, and pharmacotherapy), but they all offer some degree of counseling [138]. Two recent meta-analyses concluded that quitlines were efficacious, which translates into differential long-term abstinence rates of at least 3–5% [29, 139].

Although the less intensive forms of counseling (including brief physician advice, self-help, and telephone quitlines) produce lower cessation rates than more intensive behavioral counseling, this must be balanced against the much higher potential reach of these interventions. Therefore, with sufficient dissemination, such minimal intervention may nevertheless produce significant public health impact.

Conclusions

Tobacco exacts the greatest personal and economic toll in our society of any addictive drug. Fortunately, the prevalence of tobacco use has been declining over the last half century in the USA, although the remaining smokers may be more tobacco dependent and challenging to treat. Smokers perceive various acute benefits of tobacco use, such as cognitive and mood enhancements, but these are difficult to disentangle from the relief of nicotine withdrawal symptoms caused by smoking itself. There has also been substantial progress in the development of treatments for nicotine dependence, particularly in the area of pharmacotherapy. Although these medications tend to double or triple abstinence rates, quitting success can be further enhanced with some form of behavioral counseling. Thus, healthcare providers should regularly advise smokers to quit, and then either provide counseling or refer their smoking patients to a local cessation specialist or a telephone quitline. The cumulative public health impact of such consistent actions would be substantial.

Box: Pharmacokinetics of Nicotine

Absorption and Distribution

Nicotine is a small tertiary amine consisting of a pyridine and pyrrolidine ring [1]. It can readily dissolve in both fatty and water-based substances enabling rapid absorption and distribution [2]. Nicotine can be absorbed into the bloodstream through buccal mucosa (e.g., chew, nicotine gum, cigars), nasal mucosa (e.g., snuff, nasal spray), the skin (e.g., nicotine patch), or through alveoli within the lungs (e.g., cigarettes). About 80% of the inhaled nicotine is absorbed in the lungs [3], with the average cigarette yielding approximately 1–2 mg of nicotine [4]. Following absorption in the lungs, nicotine enters the pulmonary venous circulation leading to the heart. It then enters the arterial circulation and a concentrated bolus of nicotine (mass of nicotine in the blood) travels to the brain, where it readily crosses the blood–brain barrier. This process is rapid and efficient with nicotine reaching the brain within 7–10 s from the time of inhalation, and peak blood levels occurring within a few minutes [2, 5].

When nicotine is consumed via routes other than inhalation, the absorption and distribution process occurs more slowly. For example, smokeless tobacco will result in comparable levels of nicotine blood levels, but this will take up to 20 min [2, 5]. These other routes also tend to yield greater initial distribution across the body, resulting in a less concentrated nicotine bolus, which also reaches the brain more slowly.

Although initial nicotine levels may be some six to ten times higher in arterial versus venous blood following smoking [6], these levels are diluted by about 90% within a few minutes [7]. As the blood continues to circulate, nicotine can also be absorbed by the liver, kidneys, and fatty tissues. Within 10–30 min, venous blood levels of nicotine decrease by about 50% (i.e., initial or redistribution half-life).

Action and Elimination

Nicotine is eliminated primarily by hepatic metabolism, but the lungs and other organs also assist. For example, the kidneys are responsible for approximately 10–20% of nicotine excretion [2]. Metabolism of nicotine within the liver results in cotinine, which is further metabolized into trans-3'-hydroxycotinine (3HC), and a number of other chemicals. The liver enzyme CYP2A6 is primarily responsible for these transformations, but glucorinidation (via UGT) also contributes to the process [8]. Although nicotine has a terminal half-life of approximately 2 h, this takes much longer

for cotinine, averaging about 16 h. The stability and ease at which cotinine can be measured (e.g., blood, urine, and saliva) make it a useful marker of consumption [1].

There is wide individual variability in the rate of nicotine metabolism. Caucasians and Hispanics metabolize nicotine on average more quickly than Asians and African Americans [9, 10]. It also appears that women metabolize nicotine faster than men, and estrogen-containing oral contraceptives lead to even faster metabolism [11].

References

References to Chapter

1. Benowitz NL. Nicotine addiction. Prim Care. 1999;26(3): 611–31.
2. World Health Organization. WHO Report on the Global Tobacco Epidemic, 2008: the MPOWER package. Geneva: World Health Organization; 2008.
3. Knishkowy B, Amitai Y. Water-pipe (narghile) smoking: an emerging health risk behavior. Pediatrics. 2005;116(1):e113–9.
4. Watson CH, Polzin GM, Calafat AM, Ashley DL. Determination of tar, nicotine, and carbon monoxide yields in the smoke of bidi cigarettes. Nicotine Tob Res. 2003;5(5):747–53.
5. Malson JL, Lee EM, Murty R, Moolchan ET, Pickworth WB. Clove cigarette smoking: biochemical, physiological, and subjective effects. Pharmacol Biochem Behav. 2003;74(3):739–45.
6. Fagerstrom K. The epidemiology of smoking: health consequences and benefits of cessation. Drugs. 2002;62 Suppl 2:1–9.
7. CDC. Annual smoking-attributable mortality, years of potential life lost, and productivity losses—United States, 1997–2001. MMWR Morb Mortal Wkly Rep. 2005;54:625–8.
8. CDC. Smoking-attributable mortality, years of potential life lost, and productivity losses—United States, 2000–2004. MMWR Morb Mortal Wkly Rep. 2008;57(45):1226–8.
9. McGinnis JM, Foege WH. Actual causes of death in the United States. JAMA. 1993;270(18):2207–12.
10. CDC. Cigarette Smoking-Attributable Morbidity—United States, 2000. MMWR Morb Mortal Wkly Rep. 2003;53.
11. CDC. Best practices for comprehensive tobacco control programs—2007. Atlanta, GA: Department of Health and Human Services, Centers for Disease Control and Prevention, National Center for Chronic Disease Prevention and Health Promotion, Office on Smoking and Health; 2007.
12. Behan DF, Eriksen MP, Lin Y. Economic effects of environmental tobacco smoke Report. Schaumburg, IL: Society of Actuaries; 2005 [cited 2008 November 14]; Available from: http://www.soa.org/research/life/research-economic-effect.aspx.
13. USDHHS. The health consequences of smoking: A Report of the Surgeon General. Atlanta, GA: U.S. Department of Health and Human Services, Centers for Disease Control and Prevention, National Center for Chronic Disease Prevention and Health Promotion, Office on Smoking and Health; 2004.
14. Fielding JE, Husten CG, Eriksen MP. Tobacco: health effects and control. In: Maxcy KF, Rosenau MJ, Last JM, Wallace RB,

Doebbling BN, editors. Public health and preventive medicine. New York: McGraw-Hill; 1998. p. 817–45.

15. Ockene IS, Miller NH. Cigarette smoking, cardiovascular disease, and stroke: a statement for healthcare professionals from the American Heart Association. American Heart Association Task Force on Risk Reduction. Circulation. 1997;96(9):3243–7.

16. USDHHS. Reducing the health consequences of smoking—25 years of progress: a report of the Surgeon General. Atlanta, GA: U.S. Department of Health and Human Services, CDC; 1989. DHHS Pub. No. (CDC) 89-8411.

17. Novotny TE, Giovino GA. Tobacco Use. In: Brownson RC, Remington PL, Davis JR, editors. Chronic disease epidemiology and control. Washington, DC: American Public Health Association; 1998.

18. Boffetta P, Hecht S, Gray N, Gupta P, Straif K. Smokeless tobacco and cancer. Lancet Oncol. 2008;9(7):667–75.

19. USDHHS. Preventing tobacco use among young people: a report of the Surgeon General. Atlanta, GA: U.S. Department of Health and Human Services, Public Health Service, CDC, National Center for Chronic Disease Prevention and Health Promotion, Office on Smoking and Health; 1994.

20. Moritsugu KP. The 2006 Report of the Surgeon General: the health consequences of involuntary exposure to tobacco smoke. Am J Prev Med. 2007;32(6):542–3.

21. CDC. Cigarette smoking among adults and trends in smoking cessation—United States, 2008. MMWR Morb Mortal Wkly Rep. 2009;58(44):1227–32.

22. Johnston LD, O'Malley PM, Bachman JG, Schulenberg JE. Monitoring the future national results on adolescent drug use: overview of key findings, 2004. Bethesda, MD: NIH. NIH Publication No 05-5726; 2005.

23. SAMHSA. Results from the 2008 National Survey on Drug Use and Health: national findings. Rockville, MD: Office of Applied Studies, NSDUH Series H-36, HHS Publication No. SMA 09-4434; 2009.

24. Ziedonis D, Hitsman B, Beckham JC, Zvolensky M, Adler LE, Audrain-McGovern J, et al. Tobacco use and cessation in psychiatric disorders: National Institute of Mental Health report. Nicotine Tob Res. 2008;10(12):1691–715.

25. Breslau N. Psychiatric comorbidity of smoking and nicotine dependence. Behav Genet. 1995;25(2):95–101.

26. Williams JM, Ziedonis D. Addressing tobacco among individuals with a mental illness or an addiction. Addict Behav. 2004;29(6):1067–83.

27. Lasser K, Boyd JW, Woolhandler S, Himmelstein DU, McCormick D, Bor DH. Smoking and mental illness: a population-based prevalence study. JAMA. 2000;284(20):2606–10.

28. Anda RF, Williamson DF, Escobedo LG, Mast EE, Giovino GA, Remington PL. Depression and the dynamics of smoking. A national perspective. JAMA. 1990;264(12):1541–5.

29. Fiore MC, Jaen CR, Baker TB, Bailey WC, Benowitz NL, Curry SJ, et al. Treating Tobacco Use and Dependence: 2008 Update. Clinical Practice Guideline. Rockville, MD: U.S. Department of Health and Human Services. Public Health Service; 2008.

30. Hurt RD, Offord KP, Croghan IT, Gomez-Dahl L, Kottke TE, Morse RM, et al. Mortality following inpatient addictions treatment. Role of tobacco use in a community-based cohort. JAMA. 1996;275(14):1097–103.

31. Kalman D, Morissette SB, George TP. Co-morbidity of smoking in patients with psychiatric and substance use disorders. Am J Addict. 2005;14(2):106–23.

32. Romberger DJ, Grant K. Alcohol consumption and smoking status: the role of smoking cessation. Biomed Pharmacother. 2004;58(2):77–83.

33. Breslau N, Kilbey M, Andreski P. Nicotine dependence, major depression, and anxiety in young adults. Arch Gen Psychiatry. 1991;48(12):1069–74.

34. Barrett SP, Tichauer M, Leyton M, Pihl RO. Nicotine increases alcohol self-administration in non-dependent male smokers. Drug Alcohol Depend. 2006;81(2):197–204.

35. Kolliakou A, Joseph S. Further evidence that tobacco smoking correlates with schizotypal and borderline personality traits. Pers Individ Dif. 2000;29(1):191–4.

36. Sabido M, Sunyer J, Masuet C, Masip J. Hospitalized smokers: compliance with a nonsmoking policy and its predictors. Prev Med. 2006;43(2):113–6.

37. Burkhalter JE, Springer CM, Chhabra R, Ostroff JS, Rapkin BD. Tobacco use and readiness to quit smoking in low-income HIV-infected persons. Nicotine Tob Res. 2005;7(4):511–22.

38. Gritz ER, Vidrine DJ, Lazev AB, Amick 3rd BC, Arduino RC. Smoking behavior in a low-income multiethnic HIV/AIDS population. Nicotine Tob Res. 2004;6(1):71–7.

39. Ditre JW, Brandon TH. Pain as a motivator of smoking: effects of pain induction on smoking urge and behavior. J Abnorm Psychol. 2008;117(2):467–72.

40. Fishbain DA, Lewis JE, Cole B, Cutler RB, Rosomoff HL, Rosomoff RS. Variables associated with current smoking status in chronic pain patients. Pain Med. 2007;8(4):301–11.

41. Jamison RN, Stetson BA, Parris WC. The relationship between cigarette smoking and chronic low back pain. Addict Behav. 1991;16(3–4):103–10.

42. Michna E, Ross EL, Hynes WL, Nedeljkovic SS, Soumekh S, Janfaza D, et al. Predicting aberrant drug behavior in patients treated for chronic pain: importance of abuse history. J Pain Symptom Manage. 2004;28(3):250–8.

43. Crothers K, Griffith TA, McGinnis KA, Rodriguez-Barradas MC, Leaf DA, Weissman S, et al. The impact of cigarette smoking on mortality, quality of life, and comorbid illness among HIV-positive veterans. J Gen Intern Med. 2005;20(12):1142–5.

44. Turner J, Page-Shafer K, Chin DP, Osmond D, Mossar M, Markstein L, et al. Adverse impact of cigarette smoking on dimensions of health-related quality of life in persons with HIV infection. Aids Patient Care STDS. 2001;15(12):615–24.

45. Hu MC, Davies M, Kandel DB. Epidemiology and correlates of daily smoking and nicotine dependence among young adults in the United States. Am J Public Health. 2006;96(2):299–308.

46. Henningfield JE, Jude NR. Prevention of nicotine addiction: neuropsychopharmacological issues. Nicotine Tob Res. 1999;1 Suppl 1:S41–8.

47. Centers for Disease Control and Prevention. Cigarette smoking among adults–United States, 2000. MMWR Morb Mortal Wkly Rep. 2002;51:642–5.

48. CDC. Cigarette Smoking Among Adults—United States, 2007. MMWR Morb Mortal Wkly Rep. 2008;57(45):1221–6.

49. Hughes JR, Keely J, Naud S. Shape of the relapse curve and long term abstinence among untreated smokers. Addiction. 2004;99(1):29–38.

50. Warner KE, Burns DM. Hardening and the hard-core smoker: concepts, evidence, and implications. Nicotine Tob Res. 2003;5(1):37–48.

51. Sachs DPL, editor. Improving treatment outcome in the face of increasingly severe nicotine dependence in patients seeking tobacco-dependence treatment. Philadelphia, PA: American College of Chest Physicians; 2008.

52. Irvin JE, Brandon TH. The increasing recalcitrance of smokers in clinical trials. Nicotine Tob Res. 2000;2(1):79–84.

53. Irvin JE, Hendricks PS, Brandon TH. The increasing recalcitrance of smokers in clinical trials II: Pharmacotherapy trials. Nicotine Tob Res. 2003;5(1):27–35.

54. American Psychiatric Association. Diagnostic and statistical manual of mental disorders. 4th ed. Washington, DC: American Psychiatric Association; 1994.

55. World Health Organization. International classification of diseases and related health problems. 10th ed. Geneva: World Health Organization; 1995.

56. Hendricks PS, Ditre JW, Drobes DJ, Brandon TH. The early time course of smoking withdrawal effects. Psychopharmacology. 2006;187(3):385–96.

57. Piasecki TM, Fiore MC, Baker TB. Profiles in discouragement: two studies of variability in the time course of smoking withdrawal symptoms. J Abnorm Psychol. 1998;107:238.

58. Baker TB, Brandon TH, Chassin L. Motivational influences on cigarette smoking. Annu Rev Psychol. 2004;55:463–91.

59. Drobes DJ. Cue reactivity in alcohol and tobacco dependence. Alcohol Clin Exp Res. 2002;26(12):1928–9.

60. Chiamulera C. Cue reactivity in nicotine and tobacco dependence: a "multiple-action" model of nicotine as a primary reinforcement and as an enhancer of the effects of smoking-associated stimuli. Brain Res Brain Res Rev. 2005;48(1):74–97.

61. Carter BL, Tiffany ST. Cue-reactivity and the future of addiction research. Addiction. 1999;94(3):349–51.

62. Abrams DB. Transdisciplinary concepts and measures of craving: commentary and future directions. Addiction. 2000;95 Suppl 2:S237–46.

63. Hutchison KE, Monti PM, Rohsenow DJ, Swift RM, Colby SM, Gnys M, et al. Effects of naltrexone with nicotine replacement on smoking cue reactivity: preliminary results. Psychopharmacology. 1999;142(2):139–43.

64. Niaura RS, Abrams D, Demuth B, Pinto R, Monti P. Responses to smoking-related stimuli and early relapse to smoking. Addict Behav. 1989;14(4):419–28.

65. Abrams DB, Monti PM, Carey KB, Pinto RP, Jacobus SI. Reactivity to smoking cues and relapse: two studies of discriminant validity. Behav Res Ther. 1988;26(3):225–33.

66. Payne TJ, Smith PO, Adams SG, Diefenbach L. Pretreatment cue reactivity predicts end-of-treatment smoking. Addict Behav. 2006;31(4):702–10.

67. Tiffany ST. A cognitive model of drug urges and drug-use behavior: role of automatic and nonautomatic processes. Psychol Rev. 1990;97(2):147–68.

68. Brandon TH, Juliano LM, Copeland AC. Expectancies for tobacco smoking. In: Kirsch I, editor. How expectancies shape experience. Washington, DC: American Psychological Association; 1999. p. 263–99.

69. Goldman MS. Expectancy operation: Cognitive-neural models and architectures. In: Kirsch I, editor. How expectancies shape experience. Washington, DC: American Psychological Association; 1999. p. 41–63.

70. Brandon TH, Baker TB. The smoking consequences questionnaire: the subjective expected utility of smoking in college students. Psychol Assess. 1991;3(3):484–91.

71. Benowitz NL. Nicotine and postoperative management of pain. Anesth Analg. 2008;107(3):739–41.

72. Mineur YS, Picciotto MR. Genetics of nicotinic acetylcholine receptors: relevance to nicotine addiction. Biochem Pharmacol. 2008;75(1):323–33.

73. Dani JA, De Biasi M. Cellular mechanisms of nicotine addiction. Pharmacol Biochem Behav. 2001;70(4):439–46.

74. Benowitz NL. Clinical pharmacology of nicotine: implications for understanding, preventing, and treating tobacco addiction. Clin Pharmacol Ther. 2008;83(4):531–41.

75. Gaimarri A, Moretti M, Riganti L, Zanardi A, Clementi F, Gotti C. Regulation of neuronal nicotinic receptor traffic and expression. Brain Res Rev. 2007;55(1):134–43.

76. Nestler EJ. Is there a common molecular pathway for addiction? Nat Neurosci. 2005;8(11):1445–9.

77. Mansvelder HD, McGehee DS. Cellular and synaptic mechanisms of nicotine addiction. J Neurobiol. 2002;53(4):606–17.

78. Domino EF, Minoshima S, Guthrie SK, Ohl L, Ni L, Koeppe RA, et al. Effects of nicotine on regional cerebral glucose metabolism in awake resting tobacco smokers. Neuroscience. 2000;101(2): 277–82.

79. Stapleton JM, Gilson SF, Wong DF, Villemagne VL, Dannals RF, Grayson RF, et al. Intravenous nicotine reduces cerebral glucose metabolism: a preliminary study. Neuropsychopharmacology. 2003;28(4):765–72.

80. Brody AL. Functional brain imaging of tobacco use and dependence. J Psychiatr Res. 2006;40(5):404–18.

81. Alexander GE, Crutcher MD, DeLong MR. Basal ganglia-thalamocortical circuits: parallel substrates for motor, oculomotor, "prefrontal" and "limbic" functions. Prog Brain Res. 1990; 85:119–46.

82. Benowitz NL. Cigarette smoking and cardiovascular disease: pathophysiology and implications for treatment. Prog Cardiovasc Dis. 2003;46(1):91–111.

83. Benowitz NL, Gourlay SG. Cardiovascular toxicity of nicotine: implications for nicotine replacement therapy. J Am Coll Cardiol. 1997;29(7):1422–31.

84. Czernin J, Waldherr C. Cigarette smoking and coronary blood flow. Prog Cardiovasc Dis. 2003;45(5):395–404.

85. Heishman SJ, Taylor RC, Henningfield JE. Nicotine and smoking: a review of effects on human performance. Exp Clin Psychopharmacol. 1994;2(4):345–95.

86. Kalman D. The subjective effects of nicotine: methodological issues, a review of experimental studies, and recommendations for future research. Nicotine Tob Res. 2002;4:25.

87. Belanger HG, Simmons VN, Schinka JA. Nicotine. In: Kalechstein A, Van Gorp WG, editors. Neuropsychology and substance use: state-of-the-art and future directions. New York: Psychology Press; 2007.

88. Evans DE, Drobes DJ. Nicotine self-medication of cognitive-attentional processing. Addiction Biol 2008:14(1):32–42.

89. Waters A, Andrews J, Sutton S. Direct and indirect effects of nicotine/smoking on cognition in humans. Addict Behav. 2000;25:29.

90. Heishman SJ, Kleykamp BA, Singleton EG. Meta-analysis of the acute effects of nicotine and smoking on human performance. Psychopharmacology. 2010;210(4):453–69.

91. Gehricke JG, Loughlin SE, Whalen CK, Potkin SG, Fallon JH, Jamner LD, et al. Smoking to self-medicate attentional and emotional dysfunctions. Nicotine Tob Res. 2007;9 Suppl 4:S523–36.

92. Snyder FR, Davis FC, Henningfield JE. The tobacco withdrawal syndrome: performance decrements assessed on a computerized test battery. Drug Alcohol Depend. 1989;23(3):259–66.

93. Leventhal AM, Waters AJ, Moolchan ET, Heishman SJ, Pickworth WB. A quantitative analysis of subjective, cognitive, and physiological manifestations of the acute tobacco abstinence syndrome. Addict Behav. 2010;35(12):1120–30.

94. Bell SL, Taylor RC, Singleton EG, Henningfield JE, Heishman SJ. Smoking after nicotine deprivation enhances cognitive performance and decreases tobacco craving in drug abusers. Nicotine Tob Res. 1999;1(1):45–52.

95. Snyder FR, Henningfield JE. Effects of nicotine administration following 12 h of tobacco deprivation: assessment on computerized performance tasks. Psychopharmacology. 1989;97(1):17–22.

96. Newhouse PA, Potter A, Singh A. Effects of nicotinic stimulation on cognitive performance. Curr Opin Pharmacol. 2004;4(1):36–46.

97. Newhouse P, Singh A, Potter A. Nicotine and nicotinic receptor involvement in neuropsychiatric disorders. Curr Top Med Chem. 2004;4(3):267–82.

98. Pomerleau OF, Downey KK, Stelson FW, Pomerleau CS. Cigarette smoking in adult patients diagnosed with attention deficit hyperactivity disorder. J Subst Abuse. 1995;7(3):373–8.

99. Wilens TE, Vitulano M, Upadhyaya H, Adamson J, Sawtelle R, Utzinger L, et al. Cigarette smoking associated with attention deficit hyperactivity disorder. J Pediatr. 2008;153(3):414–9.

100. de Leon J, Diaz FJ. A meta-analysis of worldwide studies demonstrates an association between schizophrenia and tobacco smoking behaviors. Schizophr Res. 2005;76(2–3):135–57.

101. Kumari V, Postma P. Nicotine use in schizophrenia: the self medication hypotheses. Neurosci Biobehav Rev. 2005;29(6):1021–34.

102. Poltavski DV, Petros T. Effects of transdermal nicotine on attention in adult non-smokers with and without attentional deficits. Physiol Behav. 2006;87(3):614–24.

103. Jacobsen LK, Pugh KR, Mencl WE, Gelernter J. C957T polymorphism of the dopamine D2 receptor gene modulates the effect of nicotine on working memory performance and cortical processing efficiency. Psychopharmacology. 2006;188(4):530–40.

104. Allam MF, Campbell MJ, Hofman A, Del Castillo AS, Fernandez-Crehuet Navajas R. Smoking and Parkinson's disease: systematic review of prospective studies. Mov Disord. 2004;19(6):614–21.

105. Anstey KJ, von Sanden C, Salim A, O'Kearney R. Smoking as a risk factor for dementia and cognitive decline: a meta-analysis of prospective studies. Am J Epidemiol. 2007;166(4):367–78.

106. Quik M, O'Leary K, Tanner CM. Nicotine and Parkinson's disease: implications for therapy. Mov Disord. 2008;23(12):1641–52.

107. Lopez-Arrieta JLA, Sanz FJ. Nicotine for Alzheimer's disease. Cochrane Database Syst Rev. 2008(4).

108. Kalman D, Smith SS. Does nicotine do what we think it does? A meta-analytic review of the subjective effects of nicotine in nasal spray and intravenous studies with smokers and nonsmokers. Nicotine Tob Res. 2005;7(3):317–33.

109. Kassel JD, Stroud LR, Paronis CA. Smoking, stress, and negative affect: correlation, causation, and context across stages of smoking. Psychol Bull. 2003;129(2):270–304.

110. Covey LS. Tobacco cessation among patients with depression. Primary Care. 1999;26(3):691–706.

111. Kenford SL, Smith SS, Wetter DW, Jorenby DE, Fiore MC, Baker TB. Predicting relapse back to smoking: contrasting affective and physical models of dependence. J Consult Clin Psychol. 2002;70(1):216–27.

112. Brandon TH, Tiffany ST, Obremski KM, Baker TB. Postcessation cigarette use: the process of relapse. Addict Behav. 1990; 15(2):105–14.

113. Shiffman S, Paty JA, Gnys M, Kassel JA, Hickcox M. First lapses to smoking: within-subjects analysis of real-time reports. J Consult Clin Psychol. 1996;64(2):366–79.

114. Brandon TH. Negative affect as motivation to smoke. Curr Dir Psychol Sci. 1994;3:33–7.

115. Copeland AL, Brandon TH, Quinn EP. The smoking consequences questionnaire-adult: measurement of smoking outcome expectancies of experienced smokers. Psychol Assess. 1995;7:484–94.

116. Payne TJ, Schare ML, Levis DJ, Colletti G. Exposure to smoking-relevant cues: effects on desire to smoke and topographical components of smoking behavior. Addict Behav. 1991;16(6):467–79.

117. Shiffman S, Gwaltney CJ, Balabanis MH, Liu KS, Paty JA, Kassel JD, et al. Immediate antecedents of cigarette smoking: an analysis from ecological momentary assessment. J Abnorm Psychol. 2002;111(4):531–45.

118. Parrott A. Does cigarette smoking cause stress? Am Psychol. 1999;54:817.

119. Baker TB, Piper ME, McCarthy DE, Majeskie MR, Fiore MC. Addiction motivation reformulated: an affective processing model of negative reinforcement. Psychol Rev. 2004;111(1):33–51.

120. Juliano LM, Brandon TH. Effects of nicotine dose, instructional set, and outcome expectancies on the subjective effects of smoking in the presence of a stressor. J Abnorm Psychol. 2002;111(1): 88–97.

121. Kelemen WL, Kaighobadi F. Expectancy and pharmacology influence the subjective effects of nicotine in a balanced-placebo design. Exp Clin Psychopharmacol. 2007;15(1):93–101.

122. Perkins KA, Karelitz JL, Conklin CA, Sayette MA, Giedgowd GE. Acute negative affect relief from smoking depends on the affect situation and measure but not on nicotine. Biol Psychiatry. 2010;67(8):707–14.

123. Gilbert DG. The situation x trait adaptive response (STAR) model of drug use, effects, and craving. Hum Psychopharmacol. 1997;12:89–102.

124. Gilbert DG, Rabinovich NE, Malpass D, Mrnak J, Riise H, Adams L, et al. Effects of nicotine on affect are moderated by stressor proximity and frequency, positive alternatives, and smoker status. Nicotine Tob Res. 2008;10(7):1171–83.

125. Kassel J. Smoking and attention: a review and reformation of the stimulus-filter hypothesis. Clin Psychol Rev. 1997;17:451.

126. Kassel J, Shiffman S. Attentional mediation of cigarette smoking's effect on anxiety. Health Psychol. 1997;16(4):359–68.

127. Kassel JD, Unrod M. Smoking, anxiety, and attention: support for the role of nicotine in attentionally-mediated anxiolysis. J Abnorm Psychol. 2000;109(1):161–6.

128. Gonzales D, Rennard SI, Nides M, Oncken C, Azoulay S, Billing CB, et al. Varenicline, an alpha4beta2 nicotinic acetylcholine receptor partial agonist, vs sustained-release bupropion and placebo for smoking cessation: a randomized controlled trial. JAMA. 2006;296(1):47–55.

129. Jorenby DE, Hays JT, Rigotti NA, Azoulay S, Watsky EJ, Williams KE, et al. Efficacy of varenicline, an alpha4beta2 nicotinic acetylcholine receptor partial agonist, vs placebo or sustained-release bupropion for smoking cessation: a randomized controlled trial. JAMA. 2006;296(1):56–63.

130. Cahill K, Stead LF, Lancaster T. Nicotine receptor partial agonists for smoking cessation. Cochrane Database Syst Rev. 2008(3): CD006103.

131. FDA. Information for Healthcare Professionals: Varenicline (marketed Chantix) and Bupropion (marketed as Zyban, Wellbutrin, and generics). Silver Spring: U.S. Food and Drug Administration; 2009. http://www.fda.gov/Drugs/DrugSafety/PostmarketDrugSafetyInformationforPatientsandProviders/DrugSafetyInformationforHeathcareProfessionals/ucm169986.htm. Accessed 28 Sept 2010.

132. Smith SS, McCarthy DE, Japuntich SJ, Christiansen B, Piper ME, Jorenby DE, et al. Comparative effectiveness of 5 smoking cessation pharmacotherapies in primary care clinics. Arch Intern Med. 2009;169(22):2148–55.

133. Piper ME, Smith SS, Schlam TR, Fiore MC, Jorenby DE, Fraser D, et al. A randomized placebo-controlled clinical trial of 5 smoking cessation pharmacotherapies. Arch Gen Psychiatry. 2009;66(11):1253–62.

134. Perkins KA, Conklin CA, Levine MD. Cognitive-behavioral therapy for smoking cessation: a practical guidebook to the most effective treatments. New York: Routledge; 2007.

135. Lancaster T, Stead LF. Self-help interventions for smoking cessation. Cochrane Database Syst Rev. 2005(3):CD001118.

136. Brandon TH, Collins BN, Juliano LM, Lazev AB. Preventing relapse among former smokers: a comparison of minimal interventions through telephone and mail. J Consult Clin Psychol. 2000;68(1):103–13.

137. Brandon TH, Meade CD, Herzog TA, Chirikos TN, Webb MS, Cantor AB. Efficacy and cost-effectiveness of a minimal intervention

to prevent smoking relapse: dismantling the effects of amount of content versus contact. J Consult Clin Psychol. 2004;72(5):797–808.

138. Cummings SE, Bailey L, Campbell S, Koon-Kirby C, Zhu S. Tobacco cessation quitlines in North America: a descriptive study. Tob Control. 2007;16:9–15.

139. Stead LF, Perera R, Lancaster T. Telephone counselling for smoking cessation. Cochrane Database Syst Rev. 2006;(3): CD002850.

References to Boxes

1. Benowitz NL. Pharmacology of nicotine: addiction, smoking-induced disease, and therapeutics. Annu Rev Pharmacol Toxicol. 2009;49:57–71.

2. Benowitz NL. Pharmacology of nicotine: addiction and therapeutics. Annu Rev Pharmacol Toxicol. 1996;36:597–613.

3. Armitage AK, Dollery CT, George CF, Houseman TH, Lewis PJ, Turner DM. Absorption and metabolism of nicotine from cigarettes. Br Med J. 1975;4(5992):313–6.

4. Federal Trade Commission. "Tar," nicotine, and carbon monoxide of the smoke of 1294 varieties of domestic cigarettes for the year 1998. Washington, DC: FTC; 2000.

5. Hoffmann D, Djordjevic MV, Hoffmann I. The changing cigarette. Prev Med. 1997;26(4):427–34.

6. Henningfield JE, Stapleton JM, Benowitz NL, Grayson RF, London ED. Higher levels of nicotine in arterial than in venous blood after cigarette smoking. Drug Alcohol Depend. 1993;33(1):23–9.

7. Kozlowski LT, Henningfield JE, Brigham J. Cigarettes, nicotine, & health: a biobehavioral approach. Thousand Oaks, CA: Sage; 2001.

8. Hukkanen J, Jacob 3rd P, Benowitz NL. Metabolism and disposition kinetics of nicotine. Pharmacol Rev. 2005;57(1):79–115.

9. Benowitz NL, Perez-Stable EJ, Herrera B, Jacob 3rd P. Slower metabolism and reduced intake of nicotine from cigarette smoking in Chinese-Americans. J Natl Cancer Inst. 2002;94(2):108–15.

10. Perez-Stable EJ, Herrera B, Jacob 3rd P, Benowitz NL. Nicotine metabolism and intake in black and white smokers. JAMA. 1998;280(2):152–6.

11. Benowitz NL, Lessov-Schlaggar CN, Swan GE, Jacob 3rd P. Female sex and oral contraceptive use accelerate nicotine metabolism. Clin Pharmacol Ther. 2006;79(5):480–8.

Cannabis

11

Gerry Jager

Abstract

Cannabis is the world's most widely used illicit drug with 5–15% of young people in many western countries being regular cannabis users. Until the 1990s, the prevailing medical opinion was that cannabis use was nonaddictive and caused no long-term harm to health, brain, and brain function. This attitude has changed since, and current consensus is that regular cannabis use can result in dependence, increases the risk of using other illicit drugs, and is associated with increased mental health problems. However, it is still uncertain if these relationships are causal. There is, however, a steady increase in the number of people seeking help for cannabis-related problems. The increase in treatment demands has been linked to the high potency of nowadays cannabis products which may increase the risk of abuse and dependence. Cannabis affects the brain by interacting with the endogenous cannabinoid system which exists of cannabinoid receptors and their endogenous ligands. Acute intoxication with cannabis causes marked changes in subjective mental status (feeling high) and impairs cognition. These effects are accompanied by a number of bodily effects such as increased heart rate. The acute effects of cannabis on behavior, mood, and cognition are dose-dependent and biphasic (e.g., U-shaped pattern). There is still controversy regarding the persistence of effects of cannabis use on behavior, cognition, brain, and brain function once drug use has stopped. There is some evidence for subtle persisting effects, but these effects have predominantly been observed in certain vulnerable populations, i.e., individuals with either very long and very heavy exposure and/or very early onset of cannabis use, and/or comorbid conditions such as psychopathology.

Learning Objectives
- Cannabis has an addictive potential with cannabis dependence being a formal DSM-IV diagnosis
- Acute cannabis intoxication results in marked changes in subjective mental status (feeling high), mood, and cognition that affect everyday activities such as driving a car, operating machinery, and school performance
- The evidence for long-term effects of cannabis use that persist after prolonged abstinence is still controversial
- Frequent cannabis use is associated with increased risk for abuse and dependence, increased use of other illicit drug, and increased risk for mental health problems. Whether these relationships are causal is not yet clear
- Cannabis is not only a potentially harmful drug but also a potentially useful remedy in the treatment of a series of neurological and other diseases

G. Jager, Ph.D. (✉)
Division of Human Nutrition, Wageningen University,
Room 302A, Bomenweg 2, 6703 HD Wageningen, The Netherlands

Division of Human Nutrition, Wageningen University,
Courier 62, PO Box 8129, 6700 EV Wageningen, The Netherlands
e-mail: gerry.jager@wur.nl

J.C. Verster et al. (eds.), *Drug Abuse and Addiction in Medical Illness: Causes, Consequences and Treatment*,
DOI 10.1007/978-1-4614-3375-0_11, © Springer Science+Business Media, LLC 2012

Issues that Need to Be Addressed by Future Research

- Future research into the addictive potential of cannabis must focus on factors that affect the transition from occasional use to abuse and dependence
- Additional research is needed on risk and protective factors (genetic profile, age, gender, ethnicity, lifestyle, use of other substances, etc.) that may enhance or reduce the negative consequences of cannabis use
- Longitudinal and prospective studies are needed to resolve the controversy on persisting effects of cannabis use after prolonged abstinence
- Preclinical and clinical research into the therapeutic properties of both plant-derived and synthetic cannabinoids is valuable as these substances may provide lead compounds for development of future psychopharmacological interventions for many CNS disorders

Introduction

The popularity of drugs is subject to trends, and their popularity waxes and wanes. Some drugs, however, never disappear completely and boast an ancient tradition. Cannabis is certainly one of them, being a natural drug that has been used for thousands of years across many cultures. The drug has been employed in religious rites and as a medicine in the ancient Middle East. Much later, in the nineteenth century it reached a position of prominence within Western Medicine, but then fell in disgrace in the twentieth century when concern about the dangers of abuse led in 1937 to the banning of cannabis for further medicinal use in the USA [1–3]. Despite worldwide suppression, recreational cannabis use has regained enormous popularity since the 1960s and the drug has remained easily obtainable in most countries ever since [4]. Until the 1990s, the prevailing medical opinion was that smoking cannabis was nonaddictive and caused no long-term harm to health. This attitude has changed since, and in the past two decades cannabis has re-emerged not only as a potentially harmful drug but also as a potentially useful remedy. The result is intense debate on the one hand on the negative consequences of cannabis use for mental health, the brain and brain function, and its addictive potential. On the other hand, cannabis has been rediscovered as a drug with therapeutic potential in the treatment of a series of neurological and other diseases [5–8].

This chapter will review use and abuse of cannabis, its addictive potential, how cannabis works in the brain, and how the drug affects brain function and behavior. The effects of cannabis on physical and mental illnesses will only be touched upon where relevant, as these topics are covered elsewhere in this book. There will be, however, a brief outline of cannabis as a medicine and its therapeutic potential.

Use and Abuse of Cannabis

From all psychoactive substances, cannabis has the disreputable status of being the third most used substance worldwide, after alcohol and tobacco. In Europe, it is conservatively estimated that cannabis has been used at least once (lifetime prevalence) by approximately one quarter of the adult population (i.e., more than 70 million European adults). In the USA, Canada and Australia, these figures are even higher as they reach about 40% of the adult population (see Tables 11.1a and 11.1b) [9]. Cannabis use is notably high among young people. In the 15- to 24-year age range, prevalence estimates range from 25 to 45% for most countries (for details see EMCCA Annual Report 2007 [14]). Rates of lifetime and last-year use of cannabis have been consistently rising since the 1990s, with disproportionate strong increases in juveniles. Some of the more recent data available from surveys suggest that this upward trend is now leveling off, albeit at historical high levels [9, 14].

Special Groups

As mentioned above, in the general population, use of cannabis is more prevalent among adolescents and young adults. As with many drugs of abuse, cannabis is used more often by males than by females, although this distinction tends to disappear among the younger users. Geographically, cannabis use occurs more often in urban compared to rural areas, which has very likely to do with accessibility.

In distinct groups of the general population, cannabis use seems to be the rule rather than the exception. These groups include the homeless, the detained, people with a (specific) mood, anxiety or alcohol disorder, and special groups of juveniles and young adults, such as marginalized youth, young drifters, school dropouts, and juveniles in detention [9].

Use, Abuse, and Dependence

With regard to patterns of cannabis use it is a general trend that many users restrict themselves to occasional use and discontinue after a short experimental period, usually during adolescence or young adulthood, and rates of use generally decline as individuals grow older. Of more concern is the number of individuals that continues use after this initial period and progresses from chronic regular use to abuse and finally to cannabis-related substance use disorders. Currently,

Table 11.1a Cannabis use in the general population of a number of EU-15 member states and Norway: age group 15–64 years

Country	Year	Ever use (%)	Recent use (%)	Current use (%)
Spain	2003	29	11	8
France	2000	23	8	4
Netherlands	2005	23	5	3
Ireland	2002/2003	18	5	3
Austria	2005	20	8	4
N. Ireland	2002/2003	17	5	–
Luxembourg	1998	13	–	–
Finland	2004	13	3	2
Norway	2004	16	5	2
Belgium	2001	11	–	3
Greece	2004	9	2	1
Portugal	2001	8	3	

A precise comparison between countries is hampered by differences in survey year, measuring methods, and sampling. Percentage of ever users, recent (past year), and current (past month). – not measured

Table 11.1b Cannabis use in the general population of a number of EU-15 member states and Canada, the USA and Australia: other age groups[a]

Country	Year	Age (years)	Ever use (%)	Recent use (%)	Current use (%)
Canada	2004	15+	45	14	–
USA	2005	12+	40	10	6
Australia	2004	14+	34	11	7
Denmark	2000	16–64	31	6	3
UK	2004	?	30	10	6
Germany	2003	18–59	25	7	3
Italy	2003	15–54	22	7	5
Sweden	2005	16–64	12	2	1

Source: NDM Annual Report 2006 [9]
A precise comparison between countries is hampered by differences in survey year, measuring methods, and sampling. Percentage of ever users, recent (past year), and current (past month)
[a]Drug use is relatively low in the youngest [10–13] and oldest age groups (>64). Consumption figures in studies with respondents younger and/or older than the EMCDDA standard may be lower than figures in studies that do use the EMCDDA standard. The opposite is true for studies with a more limited age span. – not measured

there is little information on the continuation rates for cannabis use, but the following figures illustrate the extent of the problem. A crude estimation made by EMCDDA in 2004 suggests that around 1% of European adults, or about three million people, are daily or almost daily cannabis users [15]. Estimates from 2004 and 2005 indicate that 1.7% of the U.S. population met DSM-IV (Diagnostic and Statistical Manual of Mental Disorders, fourth edition) criteria for cannabis abuse or dependence during the year preceding the survey [10]. Others estimated that in the United States, 9.1% of the people that reported lifetime use of cannabis transitioned to dependence [11]. The transition from occasional use to abuse and dependence is affected by many different and complex factors. Yet, there is a clear need to better understand the factors associated with continuing (or discontinuing use of cannabis.

The distinction between frequent use, abuse and cannabis dependence is somewhat blurred, but according to the international psychiatric classification system DSM-IV, both abuse and dependence are associated with a pattern of use and intoxication that interferes with normal everyday functioning (i.e., problems at school or work, risk-taking behavior such as driving when intoxicated, legal and financial problems, and social, psychological and health problems). In addition to these cannabis use-associated problems, cannabis dependence is characterized by a context of compulsive use, the inability to stop or regulate use despite negative consequences, and withdrawal symptoms. The addictive potential of cannabis is low, compared to nicotine, alcohol, and other drugs of abuse. However, the risk of dependence increases with duration and frequency of use, consumption of cannabis products with high potency (i.e., high concentrations of delta9-tetrahydrocannabinol (THC)), and co-use of other substances. Unlike cannabis dependence which is included in the DSM-IV as a diagnostic category, there is still controversy regarding the existence of a clinically significant cannabis withdrawal syndrome. The syndrome, however, has been described by several authors as a separate entity that is characterized by restlessness, loss of appetite, irritability and insomnia that begins less than 24 h after discontinuation of the drug, peaks between 2 and 4 days after cessation, and lasts for 7–10 days [12, 13, 16].

In recent years, concern is growing about the increase in the number of people seeking help for cannabis-related problems. Data on treatment demands for Europe, the USA, and Australia (surveys 2005) indicate that cannabis was the primary reason for entering treatment in about 20% of all cases. When comparing these rates to those from older surveys (1999), the total numbers of cannabis treatment demands have approximately trebled. The increase in treatment demands has been linked to the stronger potency of nowadays cannabis products which may increase the risk of abuse and dependence. Potency is determined by the content of THC, and in recent years increasingly potent forms of weed and hashish have been on the market, with percentages of THC up to 20% (compared to about 7% in 2000). However, when looking at the characteristic profile of people nowadays entering outpatient treatment for cannabis use, i.e., young, male, still in education, it seems unlikely that increased potency is the only factor affecting treatment demands [9, 14].

How Cannabis Works in the Brain

The Endocannabinoid System

Our current understanding of how cannabis affects the brain started in the early 1960s with the identification of the chemical structure of delta9-tetrahydrocannabinol (THC), the major psychoactive ingredient in cannabis [17]. This discovery stimulated the development of a whole range of structurally similar compounds [18]. Studies of the neurobiological effects of THC and its analogs [19, 20] and the availability of a radioligand that allowed mapping of cannabinoid receptors in the brain [21], eventually led to the subsequent identification of an orphan G-protein-coupled receptor as the site of action for both plant-derived and synthetic cannabinoids. This receptor was later named the cannabinoid 1 (CB1) receptor [22]. To date, two cannabinoid receptors have been identified and cloned, the CB1 receptor, which constitutes the most abundant receptor in the mammalian brain and is the primary site of action for THC. A second cannabinoid receptor (CB2) is primarily expressed in peripheral tissues, mainly in the immune system. Over the years, pharmacological evidence is accumulating that one or

more additional receptors do exist [23, 24]. The discovery of the cannabinoid receptors prompted a search for their endogenous agonists, i.e., naturally occurring THC-like molecules or endocannabinoids. The best known endocannabinoids so far are anandamide (arachidonoylethanolamide) and 2-AG (2-arachidonylglecerol) but there are several others, including noladin ether, virodhamine, and N-arachidonoyldopamine [25].

Endocannabinoids represent a new class of neurotransmitters, also referred to as neuromodulators. Unlike other neurotransmitters, endocannabinoids are not stored in cell vesicles but rather synthesized by the cell on demand. They are released from the postsynaptic neuron, and then diffuse retrogradely across the synaptic cleft to stimulate CB1 receptors on the presynaptic neuron, where they inhibit the release of fast-acting amino acid neurotransmitters, predominantly GABA (γ-aminobutyric acid) and glutamate [2, 8]. Endocannabinoids are synthesized by principal outcome neurons, such as pyramidal neurons in the hippocampus and the neocortex, dopaminergic neurons in the midbrain, medium spiny neurons in the striatum, and Purkinje cells in the cerebellum. It is thought that endocannabinoid retrograde signaling allows these neurons to "fine-tune" their own excitatory (glutamatergic) and inhibitory (GABA-ergic) inputs [26–28].

It is important to mention that unlike the subtle and locally restricted effects of endocannabinoids, acute administration of exogenous cannabinoids such as THC activates CB1 receptors in a massive nonlocalized way. Consequently, acute administration of THC and other exogenous cannabinoids markedly disrupts, or indeed floods, normal CB1-receptor-mediated neuronal signaling, resulting in the psychological, cognitive, and behavioral effects of cannabis.

Rewarding and Reinforcing Properties

The rewarding and reinforcing properties of most drugs that are abused by humans can be easily demonstrated in animals using the techniques of drug-induced conditioned place preference; a behavioral test paradigm in which laboratory animals, when given a choice, prefer one compartment in a box above another when this compartment has been repeatedly paired with the experience of receiving the drug under investigation. Another technique used is drug self-administration, where the animals are willing to work, for example by pressing levers, to self-administer the drug intravenously or by intracranial self-stimulation. Initially, these phenomena could not be shown in animals for THC, which led to the belief that cannabinoids were nonaddictive. However, it now appears that the initial negative studies were lacking the appropriate conditions to demonstrate the rewarding and reinforcing properties of cannabinoids. For example, the first exposure to THC, especially in high doses, often involves aversive reactions that mask its rewarding effects. Therefore, a key factor in animal experiments may be the use of low THC doses, and under these conditions it has been demonstrated that animals reliably will self-administer THC [29–31]. Other studies have found that THC can produce conditioned place preference in mice and rats [32, 33], but that in mice the rewarding properties of THC could only be demonstrated after the mice had been preexposed to THC at least once in their home cage. Thus, under appropriate conditions it can be demonstrated that THC and related cannabinoid agonists have an addictive potential and fulfill the reward-related behavioral criteria for drugs of abuse.

Another key feature of all addictive drugs is their ability to increase dopamine levels in the mesolimbic dopaminergic reward pathway, which is part of the brain reward circuitry and is involved in the rewarding and reinforcing effects of addictive drugs.

In animals, it has been demonstrated that THC increases striatal dopamine neurotransmission [34]. Whether this is also true for humans is still debated, but a recent imaging study yielded supportive evidence by demonstrating that THC inhalation in human volunteers indeed induced dopamine release in the striatum [35]. Taken together, evidence is accumulating that THC shares a potentially addictive property with other drugs of abuse.

Tolerance

For many drugs of abuse, regular use quickly leads to powerful tolerance as well as physical and psychological dependence. Animal studies have shown that repeated administration of THC or other cannabinoid agonists also induces profound tolerance for the drug's physiological and behavioral effects [31]. This tolerance has been mainly attributed to functional and pharmacodynamic adaptations of the central nervous system that reflect a decreased sensitivity to the effects of the drug, such as desensitization and reduction in density of CB1 receptors [36]. Interestingly, animal studies show that tolerance rapidly develops for many effects of cannabinoids, such as the hypothermic, analgesic, and locomotor effects, but not to all [31]. For example, in an animal study, rats showed tolerance to several central effects of THC but not to the behavioral effects of THC in a working memory test (T-maze performance) [37]. There are similar reports in humans. It has been demonstrated that the pleasurable effects of cannabis (the subjective "high") remained similar in heavy or frequent users compared to light or infrequent users, whereas the chronic users were much less affected than the infrequent users by the sedative effects of the drug [38]. Together, preclinical and clinical findings indicate that tolerance to the effects of THC can develop differentially, depending on the brain area, the function, and the behavioral effects under investigation.

Dependence and Withdrawal

The belief that cannabis had no addictive potential was, in part, based on observations that withdrawal of the drug did not result in spontaneous physical withdrawal symptoms either in animals or in humans. However, epidemiological surveys showed that approximately one in nine cannabis users meet the clinical criteria for dependence as described by the International Classification of Mental Disorders 10 (ICD 10) or DSM-IV [39].

In recent years, attitudes have changed markedly. Researchers recognized that the absence of withdrawal symptoms might have been due to the long elimination half-life of THC, that is, the slow and gradual break down of THC in the body. As a result, cannabinoid receptors remain partially occupied for a significant period of time even after termination of drug administration [40]. After the development of the CB1 antagonist SR141716A (Rimonabant), a drug that blocks and inactivates the CB1 receptors, thereby preventing the action of lingering cannabinoids, the existence of dependence and withdrawal symptoms in animals could be demonstrated convincingly through the approach of precipitated withdrawal. In precipitated withdrawal, animals are treated chronically with THC for some time, and then are challenged with SR141716 at the same time THC administration is ended. Administration of the antagonist immediately blocks all CB1 receptors, despite the continued presence of THC, and results in relapse [41] or in an abstinence syndrome in the animals [42, 43].

In summary, based on the latest insights cannabis should be considered as a drug with an addictive potential; albeit the conditions for this addictive potential to emerge are somewhat different than those known from the "typical" addictive drugs such as amphetamines and opiates where tolerance, dependence and withdrawal are robust phenomena after repeated use.

Effects of Cannabis on Behavior, Mood, Cognition, and Brain Function

Any summary of the acute and long-term effects of cannabis on behavior, mental status, and cognitive function is necessarily an oversimplification. Many of the central nervous system effects of THC and other cannabinoids are biphasic and bidirectional, meaning they depend on dose, time frame, the user's prior experience with the drug, the user's expectations of the drug, degree of tolerance, mode of administration, personality, and various other environmental and individual factors. This can explain why the acute subjective effects in normal subjects can range from euphoria, relaxation, heightened perception, and hyperactivity to depressed mood, anxiety, paranoia, sedation, perceptual disorganization, and motor deficits. It is beyond the scope of this chapter to fully cover the diversity of effects of cannabis under various conditions and at different doses. For the interested reader, I recommend some books and book chapters dedicated to these topics [44–47]. The aim of the present chapter is to present an overview of the "typical" effects of cannabis on behavior, mood, cognition, and brain function, where the reader has to keep in mind that these typical effects may vary according to the context in which cannabis use takes place.

Distinction Acute and Nonacute

When discussing the effects of cannabis use, a distinction can be made between the acute, pharmacological effects (i.e., when someone is under the influence of THC), and the nonacute effects (i.e., when subjects are sober). However, the distinction between acute and nonacute effects of cannabis use is not straightforward and merely a matter of definition. The psychotropic effects of THC wear off after approximately 4 h after administration (see Box 11.1), but THC and its metabolites, some of which are also psychoactive, can linger in the body for some period of time. THC is soluble in fat and thus is stored in adipose tissue after repeated use with slow release into the bloodstream afterwards and, therefore, slow elimination. Presence of THC and its metabolites can vary from a couple of days (after single administration in naive users) up to 2–3 weeks (in chronic daily users) [48]. Whether this residue also remains in the central nervous system and whether it is still psychoactive is largely unknown. Apart from the remaining residue, assessment of residual effects of cannabis on mood, behavior, and cognition is also complicated by withdrawal symptoms that may be experienced by chronic users and can persist for several days. Withdrawal symptoms likely affect mood, behavior, and cognitive functioning of recently abstinent cannabis users, and may cause them to get temporarily worse before they get better [49].

Acute Effects of Cannabis Use

Mood, Behavior, and Bodily Sensations

Acute intoxication with cannabis causes marked changes in subjective mental status. As summarized in Iversen (2000) [1], there are four stages: the "buzz," the "high," "being stoned," and "the come-down." The buzz is a short initial period during which the user may feel lightheaded or slightly dizzy, and tingling sensations in the extremities and other body parts can be experienced. The "high" is characterized by euphoria, exhilaration and unrestrained behavior, for example, giggling. The "high" progresses into "being stoned" when the user usually feels relaxed, calm, happy, and in a dreamlike state. When used in a social setting, the "high" is often accompanied by infectious laughter, talkativeness, and increased sociability [50–52]. After approximately 4 h, these sensations diminish and the "come-down" sets in [1, 40].

The effects on mood are accompanied by a number of bodily effects, such as an increase in heart rate, a decrease in blood pressure when standing (postural hypotension; which may explain the initial feeling of "light-headedness"), and increases in the release of various catecholamine neurotransmitters, among which norepinephrine (adrenalin), responsible for phenomena like a dry mouth, pupil dilatation, and redness of the retina due to vasodilation of small vessels in the eye [53].

Unpleasant psychological reactions after cannabis intoxication are reported less often but do occur, ranging from a feeling of anxiety or depressed mood, dizziness, to full-blown panic attacks. These effects are most often reported by naive or inexperienced users who are unfamiliar with the effects of cannabis. For example, in healthy young users the cardiovascular effects such as increased heart rate and postural hypotension are unlikely to be of any clinical significance, but they may increase discomfort and anxiety if they are misinterpreted as symptoms of a serious adverse event (i.e., fear of going mad or getting a heart attack), which may trigger a panic attack.

Psychotic symptoms, such as delusions and hallucinations do occur only at rare occasions, usually at very high doses of THC. In susceptible individuals, i.e., with comorbid conditions, these serious adverse events can occur at lower doses [54].

Acute Effects of Cannabis on Cognition

The most consistently demonstrated effect of acute cannabis intoxication on cognition is memory impairment. Specifically, when subjects are presented with new information when intoxicated, they show deficits in their ability to spontaneously recall (both immediately and after a delay) the information. In contrast, their ability to recall information that was presented prior to cannabis use (i.e., when sober) is typically intact. Similarly, no deficits are found in recalling remote events or semantic knowledge [50, 55]. Intriguingly, across all memory paradigms tested, whether they involve wordlists, prose, or nonverbal stimuli, subjects under the influence of THC display a tendency to produce more intrusion and false-positive errors when recalling information [55]. This could be related to a loosening of association induced by cannabis intoxication, which may result in becoming lost in reverie and fantasy.

Acute effects of cannabis use on other cognitive functions include impaired decision-making, increased impulsivity, impaired sustained attention, and impairments in motor skills, reaction time and motor coordination, for example in studies investigating tracking and driving skills. The results, however, remain somewhat mixed, as some of the reported effects could not be replicated. Also, effects are dependent on dose, with higher doses of THC (i.e., 15 mg oral dose), but not lower doses (i.e., 7.5 mg) producing poorer performance on several tasks [56–59]. Interestingly, it has been shown that significant prior cannabis use may reduce the acute adverse cognitive effects of cannabis, implicating that experienced frequent users develop behavioral, in this case cognitive tolerance to some extent [60].

Acute Effects of Cannabis on Brain Function

A whole range of investigations has been conducted to examine the acute effects of cannabis on brain functioning, using various neuroimaging techniques such as single photon emission computer tomography (SPECT), positron emission tomography (PET), and functional magnetic resonance imaging (fMRI). Together, these studies have yielded several consistent findings. With regard to brain metabolism and perfusion, findings indicate increases in cerebral blood flow (CBF) and brain metabolism throughout the cortex during acute cannabis intoxication. When looking at regional effects, increased regional CBF is reported most often in frontal, limbic, paralimbic, and cerebellar brain regions. These regional changes in brain perfusion and metabolism are broadly consistent with the cognitive, behavioral and subjective effects of acute cannabis intoxication, as these brain areas are critically involved in memory and executive functioning, locomotor functions, and mood regulation [50, 61, 62]. Studies examining the acute effects of THC on neurocognitive functioning during a cognitive challenge, i.e., when subjects are engaged in specific cognitive tasks, are still very few. O'Leary and colleagues [63] performed a PET study in which subjects were asked to perform a dichotic listening task after cannabis administration. The results showed typical patterns of increased CBF in frontal, limbic and cerebellar regions, but decreased CBF in temporal regions important for auditory attention, whereas task performance was not affected [63]. Recently, the first pharmacological functional MRI studies on the neural basis of THC-mediated changes in cognitive brain function were published [64, 65]. Pharmacological fMRI is a powerful tool to assess the effects of a direct pharmacological challenge on cognitive brain function. In case of cannabis research, functional MRI is used to probe brain function in volunteers after a double-blind crossover administration of THC or placebo. Phan and colleagues [64] found that THC administration reduced brain activity in relevant brain regions, i.e., amygdala, in response to social signals of threat, i.e., pictures of angry and fearful faces. These findings support the notion that THC

and other cannabinoids may have an anxiolytic effect which is reflected on the level of brain activity. Borgwardt and colleagues [65] showed that compared to placebo, THC administration attenuated brain activity in regions that mediate response inhibition, i.e., the inferior frontal and anterior cingulate cortex, without substantially affecting performance accuracy on a response inhibition task (go–nogo), indicating that THC may alter brain activation patterns related to impulse regulation. The expectation is that in the near future other studies employing the promising technique of pharmacological fMRI will further extend our knowledge on the neural systems underlying the subjective effects and neuropsychological impairments associated with acute cannabis intoxication.

Nonacute Effects

Despite decades of research, consensus on the nonacute effects of cannabis has not yet been achieved, and the evidence for long-term effects that persist after prolonged abstinence is still controversial. One possible explanation for the discrepancy in reported findings in cannabis users could be that cannabis use affects some populations more than others. Vulnerable populations are either groups of individuals with very long and heavy exposure and/or very early exposure to the drug, i.e., initiation of cannabis use early in adolescence [49, 66] and/or comorbid conditions, such as existing psychopathology [67–69]. Another explanation for inconsistent findings is that cannabis research in humans faces a series of methodological challenges which hamper the reliability and interpretability of reported findings. For example, cannabis research in humans is often confined to retrospective and cross-sectional study designs, i.e., comparing individuals with a history of cannabis use with nonusers on behavioral, cognitive, and/or brain function indices after a single measurement. Ideally, one would opt for assigning healthy individuals randomly into groups that are administered varying amounts of cannabis for a long period of time in a supervised and controlled setting and later test them after different periods of abstinence. It is clear, however, that for obvious ethical reasons this is not possible in humans. Instead, studies investigating the nonacute effects of cannabis often employ groups of participants that differ substantially on factors as length of abstinence, amount, frequency and duration of use, and the presence of comorbid conditions, such as use of other drugs, psychiatric disorders, or other confounding factors. However, different outcomes may then depend, for example, on what time point after last use participants were tested, that is, within a couple of days after abstinence when withdrawal symptoms may be present, after withdrawal symptoms have subsided but with THC and its metabolites still present in the body (residual effects), or after several weeks has elapsed after last use (long-term or persistent effects) [49, 50, 70]. It is, therefore, important to keep those methodological issues in mind when reading the overview of nonacute effects of cannabis use below.

Nonacute Effects on Cognition

There is a large body of research on the nonacute effects of cannabis on cognitive functioning, and many excellent reviews are available [1, 45, 50, 71–73]. Taken together, studies on long-term effects of cannabis on cognition have failed to find proof of gross abnormalities, but there is some evidence for mild cognitive impairments, particularly in the domain of memory and learning [49, 50, 73]. This is supported by a meta-analysis, conducted in 2003 by Grant and colleagues [74] that reported quantitative estimates (effect sizes) of potential long-term effects of cannabis use on eight cognitive domains, i.e., simple reaction time, attention, verbal/language, executive functioning, perceptual motor function, simple motor function, learning, and forgetting/retrieval. With the exception of learning and forgetting (i.e., memory), no statistically reliable long-term effects were observed across studies included in the meta-analysis. As for the "residual cannabis effect" on memory, albeit statistical significant it was of small magnitude ($d=-0.15$), suggesting that cannabis users' memory performance was about one-fifth of a standard deviation worse than controls. To conclude, there is some evidence for subtle persisting effects of cannabis use on memory function, but as this effect is of small magnitude, the clinical relevance remains to be determined. In addition, alternative explanations for these subtle decrements in memory function cannot be excluded and need further investigation, such as the impact of preexisting genetic or neurobehavioral risk factors, or of residual confounders that hamper the interpretation of previous studies. For example, despite efforts on good matching between cannabis users and controls, users may differ on other factors besides cannabis use from the control group that cannot easily be controlled for (lifestyle, use of other substances, cultural divergence, premorbid differences in cognitive abilities, differences in educational and vocational career, etc.). Each of these factors may add to or interact with cannabis-induced effects.

Nonacute Effects of Cannabis on Cognitive Brain Function: Neuroimaging Studies

Whereas most work on the residual effects of cannabis on cognitive functioning concerns the application of neuropsychological tests, recently modern neuroimaging techniques have entered the field, in particular functional magnetic resonance imaging (fMRI). FMRI is an important tool to visualize "the brain in action," that is, measuring brain activity in subjects who are engaged in a cognitive task. A commonly used technique is blood-oxygen-level dependent (BOLD) fMRI, which can be described as follows: fMRI images are obtained using an MRI scanner, which is basically a large magnet. Changes in neuronal activity are accompanied by changes in blood flow, causing the oxygen level in the blood to rise in brain regions that are active. As oxygenated hemoglobin is diamagnetic, i.e., it exerts little effect on the regional magnetic field, and deoxygenated blood is paramagnetic, i.e., it disturbs the magnetic field, the changes in relative levels of oxygen in the blood can be effectively measured with fMRI and are reflected in changes in the BOLD signal [75]. A strength of fMRI is that it combines behavioral (task performance) and brain activity measures. Thus, fMRI can reveal abnormalities in the organization of brain networks involved in cognitive processing, which may occur as an adaptive (compensatory) response to brain damage and which may be difficult to detect in behavior (task performance) alone.

Recent review papers have summarized the main findings from previous fMRI studies that compared abstinent cannabis users and controls on several higher cognitive functions, such as (working) memory, attention, and response inhibition. Taken together, these studies in abstinent chronic cannabis users reveal alterations in the activation of brain networks responsible for higher cognitive functions, including areas in the prefrontal, parietal and temporal lobes, but often without impaired task performance [50, 61, 62]. These changes in brain activation may signify neuroadaptation in response to chronic cannabis use and, as is often argued, compensatory mechanisms reflecting stronger neuronal "effort" in cannabis users' brains to maintain normal task performance. Yet, some caution is warranted. There are few studies with sufficiently long abstinence periods to rule out withdrawal symptoms or effects of lingering cannabis residues. In addition, the absence of functional consequences in terms of impaired task performance leaves open the possibility that other (noncognitive) factors may explain or contribute to the observed alterations in brain activation [76]. For example, chronic cannabis use may induce persisting changes in neurochemistry or brain perfusion, and this may in turn affect the BOLD signal [77].

In conclusion, functional neuroimaging studies indicate alterations in the activation of brain networks involved in cognitive functions in cannabis users, but it is not yet certain whether these changes are reversible with prolonged abstinence or whether they truly signify clinical relevant cognitive effects.

Cannabis: Friend or Foe?

"Historically, some societies have idealized cannabis whereas others have demonized it and, recently, Western society has tended to oscillate between the two. In reality, as cannabis derivatives have the potential for causing both good and harm, the important question for society is how to maximize the former and minimize the latter" (cited from "Cannabis, the mind and society: the harsh realities" by Murray and colleagues [78]).

Cannabis and Mental Illness

The majority of recreational cannabis users does not experience serious adverse reactions and is able to regulate their use. However, a minority of frequent or long-term users will develop problems. Abuse and dependence have already been discussed, as well as potential long-term consequences of chronic use for cognitive brain function. But another problem that drew much attention in recent years is the steady increase in mental health problems associated with cannabis use. As other chapters in this book deal with this topic in more detail, I will only give a short overview here.

Most of the interest concerning cannabis and mental health issues has focused on psychosis and schizophrenia. Here, the core question is whether cannabis plays an etiological role in schizophrenia, i.e., does cannabis use cause schizophrenia. A causal relationship between cannabis and schizophrenia is qualitatively different from an association acting in two directions, that is, cannabis use is a risk factor for as well as a consequence of schizophrenia [68]. Nowadays, the association between cannabis use and psychosis and schizophrenia is well-established. For one, epidemiological studies have shown that frequent cannabis use is associated with a greater risk of suffering from psychotic symptoms or of developing schizophrenia and this is particularly prominent in those who started cannabis use at an early age [79]. Once the disease has manifested itself, continued cannabis use can trigger more severe psychotic symptoms and relapse, and is associated with poorer clinical outcome [80, 81]. Second, the proportion of schizophrenic patients that abuses cannabis is much higher than in the general population [81]. Overall, the available evidence strongly suggests that cannabis use may precipitate the development of schizophrenia in vulnerable people, increases the symptoms, and reduces the likelihood to recover from the disease. But the hypothesis that cannabis use causes schizophrenia has not been proven yet. Moreover, we should keep in mind that schizophrenia is a very complex multifactor condition with multiple causes in which a great number of environmental factors interact with (genetic) predispositions to cause this disease [67, 78, 82].

Compared with schizophrenia, there is less evidence of cannabis playing a role in the etiology of other mental disorders, including depression, bipolar disorder, and anxiety disorder. Similar to schizophrenia, there seems to be a link between affective disorders and elevated rates of cannabis use, but the number of studies investigating the exact nature of this relationship is still limited and until now, has not resulted in a consistent picture [67, 69].

Cannabinoids as a Medicine

The focus of this chapter is on the potential negative consequences of cannabis use, i.e., abuse, dependence and addiction, persistent effects on mood, behavior, brain and brain function, and increased mental health problems. With this in mind, it seems odd to include a paragraph on the therapeutic properties of cannabinoids. Yet, this is an issue that should not be ignored, as cannabinoid pharmacology in medicine is a rapidly expanding and exciting field of research. I will not go into detail about the apparent paradoxical mechanisms by which cannabinoids may induce both detrimental and therapeutic effects, but for the interested reader there are some excellent reviews on this topic from Sarne and colleagues [83, 84].

Cannabis as a therapeutic drug is not new. It has been of medicinal and social significance for millennia, and it even was listed on the US Pharmacopeia until 1944. Then, it was removed owing to political pressure to ban its social use in the USA [85]. It has never been reinstated since, but in 1986 the Food and Drug Administration authorized the use of THC for specific medical purposes. Legislation of medical use of THC and some other cannabinoids has followed, also in other countries. Now, several cannabinoids are commercially available, such as Marinol® (dronabinol; a pure isomer from THC), Cesamet® (nabilone; a synthetic form of THC), and Sativex® (containing THC and cannabidiol (CBD), a nonpsychoactive component from *Cannabis sativa*). Approved indications are treatment for nausea and vomiting induced by chemotherapy in cancer patients, to relieve AIDS-associated anorexia and physical wasting, and pain reduction in patients with neuropathic and multiple sclerosis-related pain [7, 85, 86]. However, the therapeutic potential of cannabinoids has been recognized for many other medical conditions and includes muscle relaxation in diseases causing muscle spasms, anti-inflammatory and anti-allergic effects, improvement of mood, lowering of intraocular pressure (treatment of glaucoma), bronchodilatation, anticonvulsive, and neuroprotective effects [87]. Many of these potential applications are still tested in the preclinical stage (animal research) or in the stage of experimental clinical trials in humans.

One major drawback of cannabinoids that hampers their clinical use is the unavoidable psychotropic effects exhibited by many of them. In most conditions, these effects are considered as unwanted side-effects. In this context, much attention is currently focused on cannabidiol (CBD) that is, like THC, a main constituent of *C. sativa*. Due to its lack of any cognitive and psychoactive side-effects, CBD is a promising future candidate for clinical utilization [88]. Finally, interest is growing in the role of the body's own (endogenous) cannabinoid brain system and the role this system may play in the pathophysiology of several psychiatric disorders. For example, in rodents it has been shown that administration of a chemical denoted URB597, which inhibits the breakdown of the endocannabinoid anandamide, resulted in amplification of the effects of anandamide on neuronal signaling. This produced antidepressant-like effects in mice [69, 89]. It will probably take several years of additional preclinical and clinical research, but these studies show that cannabidiol and the endocannabinoids may provide valuable lead compounds for development of future psychopharmacological interventions for many psychiatric and CNS disorders.

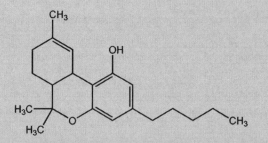

Fig. 11.1 Chemical structure of delta9-tetrahydrocannabinol (THC), the primary psychoactive ingredient in the cannabis plant

distribution, in accordance with the high lipophilicity of THC, resulting in a rapid clearance from the plasma and a rapid penetration into target tissues containing cannabinoid receptors, such as the brain. Psychotropic effects start within seconds to a few minutes, peak after 15–30 min, and then gradually decline within 2–4 h. Following oral ingestion, absorption is delayed, and psychotropic effects set in after 30–90 min, reach their maximum after 2–3 h and persist for about 4–12 h, depending on dose and specific effect. THC is metabolized by hydroxylation in 11-OH-THC (11-hydroxy-THC), which is still psychoactive, and then further oxidized to 11-Nor-9-carboxy-THC (THC-COOH). Metabolism primarily occurs in the liver by enzymes of the cytochrome P450 (CYP) complex. Elimination by metabolism is relatively slow. The main reason for this is the high lipophilicity of THC, resulting in a slow rediffusion of THC from body fat and other tissues back into the blood, so that it can be metabolized in the liver. The main route of excretion of THC metabolites is via the feces (55%) and urine (20%). After a single occasion of smoking THC, metabolites such as THC-COOH can be detected in urine for several days (range 2–7 days) depending on the dose.

Box 11.1 Pharmacokinetics of Cannabis

Cannabis (marijuana) is a psychoactive product of the plant *Cannabis sativa*. The herbal form (weed) of the drug consists of dried mature flowers and tops of the female plants, whereas the resinous form, known as hashish, consists primarily of fine glandular outgrowths (trichomes) collected from the same plant material. The main psychoactive compound in cannabis is delta9-tetrahydrocannabinol, commonly referred to as THC (Fig. 11.1), but the plant is known to contain about 60 different cannabinoids, the major ones including cannabidiol (CBD), cannabigerol, and cannabichomene [44]. However, from all the purified compounds tested in animals and humans, only THC shows psychotropic activity [52]. Natural cannabinoids, including THC, are usually inhaled (smoking marijuana cigarettes, water pipe or hookah) or taken orally. Various other routes of administration have been tested for therapeutic purposes (i.e., rectal route with suppositories or skin patches). The pharmacokinetics (absorption, distribution, effects, and elimination) vary depending on the route of administration and are dose-dependent. Pharmacokinetic–pharmacodynamic (PK–PD) modeling studies in humans have shown that pulmonary administration of a cumulative dose of 8 mg THC induces clear subjective and central nervous system (CNS) effects that corresponds to the effects of smoking one or two marijuana cigarettes. Absorption of THC after inhalation is fast and causes maximum blood plasma concentrations within minutes. This is followed by a rapid

(continued)

References

1. Iversen LL. The science of marijuana. Oxford, UK: Oxford University Press; 2000.
2. Howlett AC, Breivogel CS, Childers SR, Deadwyler SA, Hampson RE, Porrino LJ. Cannabinoid physiology and pharmacology: 30 years of progress. Neuropharmacology. 2004;47 Suppl 1:345–58.
3. Mackie K. Cannabinoid receptors as therapeutic targets. Annu Rev Pharmacol Toxicol. 2006;46:101–22.
4. UNODC. World Drug Report 2008. Vienna: United Nations Office on Drugs and Crime; 2008.
5. Katona I, Freund TF. Endocannabinoid signaling as a synaptic circuit breaker in neurological disease. Nat Med. 2008;14(9):923–30.

6. Kogan NM, Mechoulam R. Cannabinoids in health and disease. Dialogues Clin Neurosci. 2007;9(4):413–30.

7. Hosking RD, Zajicek JP. Therapeutic potential of cannabis in pain medicine. Br J Anaesth. 2008;101(1):59–68.

8. Pertwee RG. Ligands that target cannabinoid receptors in the brain: from THC to anandamide and beyond. Addict Biol. 2008; 13(2):147–59.

9. NDM. NDM annual report 2006. Utrecht: Trimbos Instituut; 2007.

10. SAMHSA. The national survey on drug use and health. Rockville, MD: Substance Abuse and Mental Health Services Administration (SAMHSA); 2005.

11. NIDA. Research report series marijuana abuse. Lexington, KY: National Institute on Drug Abuse; 2005.

12. Budney AJ, Novy PL, Hughes JR. Marijuana withdrawal among adults seeking treatment for marijuana dependence. Addiction. 1999;94(9):1311–22.

13. Budney AJ, Hughes JR, Moore BA, Novy PL. Marijuana abstinence effects in marijuana smokers maintained in their home environment. Arch Gen Psychiatry. 2001;58(10):917–24.

14. EMCDDA. Annual report 2007. Lisbon: European Monitoring Centre for Drugs and Drug Addiction; 2007.

15. EMCDDA. Annual report 2004. Lisbon: European Monitoring Centre for Drugs and Drug Addiction; 2004.

16. Copersino ML, Boyd SJ, Tashkin DP, Huestis MA, Heishman SJ, Dermand JC, et al. Cannabis withdrawal among non-treatment-seeking adult cannabis users. Am J Addict. 2006;15(1):8–14.

17. Mechoulam R, Hanus L. A historical overview of chemical research on cannabinoids. Chem Phys Lipids. 2000;108(1–2):1–13.

18. Howlett AC, Barth F, Bonner TI, Cabral G, Casellas P, Devane WA, et al. International Union of Pharmacology. XXVII. Classification of cannabinoid receptors. Pharmacol Rev. 2002;54(2): 161–202.

19. Hollister LE. Structure-activity relationships in man of cannabis constituents, and homologs and metabolites of delta9-tetrahydrocannabinol. Pharmacology. 1974;11(1):3–11.

20. Jones G, Pertwee RG, Gill EW, Paton WD, Nilsson IM, Widman M, et al. Relative pharmacological potency in mice of optical isomers of delta 1-tetrahydrocannabinol. Biochem Pharmacol. 1974;23(2):439–46.

21. Herkenham M, Lynn AB, Johnson MR, Melvin LS, de Costa BR, Rice KC. Characterization and localization of cannabinoid receptors in rat brain: a quantitative in vitro autoradiographic study. J Neurosci. 1991;11(2):563–83.

22. Matsuda LA, Lolait SJ, Brownstein MJ, Young AC, Bonner TI. Structure of a cannabinoid receptor and functional expression of the cloned cDNA. Nature. 1990;346(6284):561–4.

23. Begg M, Pacher P, Batkai S, Osei-Hyiaman D, Offertaler L, Mo FM, et al. Evidence for novel cannabinoid receptors. Pharmacol Ther. 2005;106(2):133–45.

24. Pacher P, Batkai S, Kunos G. The endocannabinoid system as an emerging target of pharmacotherapy. Pharmacol Rev. 2006;58(3): 389–462.

25. Piomelli D. The molecular logic of endocannabinoid signalling. Nat Rev Neurosci. 2003;4(11):873–84.

26. Freund TF, Katona I, Piomelli D. Role of endogenous cannabinoids in synaptic signaling. Physiol Rev. 2003;83(3):1017–66.

27. Mackie K. Cannabinoid receptor homo- and heterodimerization. Life Sci. 2005;77(14):1667–73.

28. de Rodriguez FF, Del A, Bermudez-Silva FJ, Bilbao A, Cippitelli A, Navarro M. The endocannabinoid system: physiology and pharmacology. Alcohol Alcohol. 2005;40(1):2–14.

29. Justinova Z, Tanda G, Redhi GH, Goldberg SR. Self-administration of delta9-tetrahydrocannabinol (THC) by drug naive squirrel monkeys. Psychopharmacology (Berl). 2003;169(2):135–40.

30. Justinova Z, Goldberg SR, Heishman SJ, Tanda G. Self-administration of cannabinoids by experimental animals and human marijuana smokers. Pharmacol Biochem Behav. 2005;81(2):285–99.

31. Tanda G, Goldberg SR. Cannabinoids: reward, dependence, and underlying neurochemical mechanisms–a review of recent preclinical data. Psychopharmacology (Berl). 2003;169(2):115–34.

32. Braida D, Iosue S, Pegorini S, Sala M. Delta9-tetrahydrocannabinol-induced conditioned place preference and intracerebroventricular self-administration in rats. Eur J Pharmacol. 2004;506(1):63–9.

33. Valjent E, Maldonado R. A behavioural model to reveal place preference to delta9-tetrahydrocannabinol in mice. Psychopharmacology (Berl). 2000;147(4):436–8.

34. Zangen A, Solinas M, Ikemoto S, Goldberg SR, Wise RA. Two brain sites for cannabinoid reward. J Neurosci. 2006;26(18): 4901–7.

35. Bossong MG, van Berckel BN, Boellaard R, Zuurman L, Schuit RC, Windhorst AD, et al. Delta9-tetrahydrocannabinol induces dopamine release in the human striatum. Neuropsychopharmacology. 2009;34(3):759–66.

36. Maldonado R. Study of cannabinoid dependence in animals. Pharmacol Ther. 2002;95(2):153–64.

37. Nava F, Carta G, Colombo G, Gessa GL. Effects of chronic Delta(9)-tetrahydrocannabinol treatment on hippocampal extracellular acetylcholine concentration and alternation performance in the T-maze. Neuropharmacology. 2001;41(3):392–9.

38. Kirk JM, de WH. Responses to oral delta9-tetrahydrocannabinol in frequent and infrequent marijuana users. Pharmacol Biochem Behav. 1999;63(1):137–42.

39. Swift W, Hall W, Teesson M. Characteristics of DSM-IV and ICD-10 cannabis dependence among Australian adults: results from the National Survey of Mental Health and Wellbeing. Drug Alcohol Depend. 2001;63(2):147–53.

40. Meyer JS, Quenzer LF. Marijuana and the cannabinoids. In: Psychopharmacology, Drugs, the brain, and behavior. Massachusetts, USA: Sinauer Associates; 2005. p. 327–46.

41. Justinova Z, Munzar P, Panlilio LV, Yasar S, Redhi GH, Tanda G, et al. Blockade of THC-seeking behavior and relapse in monkeys by the cannabinoid CB(1)-receptor antagonist rimonabant. Neuropsychopharmacology. 2008;33(12):2870–7.

42. Aceto MD, Scates SM, Lowe JA, Martin BR. Dependence on delta 9-tetrahydrocannabinol: studies on precipitated and abrupt withdrawal. J Pharmacol Exp Ther. 1996;278(3):1290–5.

43. Wilson DM, Varvel SA, Harloe JP, Martin BR, Lichtman AH. SR 141716 (Rimonabant) precipitates withdrawal in marijuana-dependent mice. Pharmacol Biochem Behav. 2006;85(1):105–13.

44. Paton WDM, Pertwee RG. The actions of cannabis in man. In: Mechoulam R, editor. Marijuana. New York: Academic; 1973. p. 287–333.

45. Solowij N. Cannabis and cognitive functioning. Cambridge: Cambridge University Press; 1998.

46. Heishman SJ. Effects of marijuana on human performance and assessment of driving impairment. In: Onaivi ES, editor. Biology of marijuana: from gene to behavior. New York: Taylor and Francis; 2002. p. 308–32.

47. Castle D, Murray R, editors. Marijuana and madness: psychiatry and neurobiology. Cambridge: Cambridge University Press; 2004.

48. Grotenhermen F. Pharmacokinetics and pharmacodynamics of cannabinoids. Clin Pharmacokinet. 2003;42(4):327–60.

49. Pope HG, Yurgelun-Todd D. Residual cognitive effects of long-term cannabis use. In: Castle D, Murray R, editors. Marijuana and madness: psychiatry and neurobiology. Cambridge: Cambridge University Press; 2004. p. 198–210.

50. Gonzalez R. Acute and non-acute effects of cannabis on brain functioning and neuropsychological performance. Neuropsychol Rev. 2007;17(3):347–61.

51. Green B, Kavanagh D, Young R. Being stoned: a review of self-reported cannabis effects. Drug Alcohol Rev. 2003;22(4):453–60.

52. Wachtel SR, ElSohly MA, Ross SA, Ambre J, de WH. Comparison of the subjective effects of Delta(9)-tetrahydrocannabinol and marijuana in humans. Psychopharmacology (Berl). 2002;161(4):331–9.

53. Ameri A. The effects of cannabinoids on the brain. Prog Neurobiol. 1999;58(4):315–48.
54. Thomas H. A community survey of adverse effects of cannabis use. Drug Alcohol Depend. 1996;42(3):201–7.
55. Ranganathan M, D'Souza DC. The acute effects of cannabinoids on memory in humans: a review. Psychopharmacology (Berl). 2006;188(4):425–44.
56. McDonald J, Schleifer L, Richards JB, de WH. Effects of THC on behavioral measures of impulsivity in humans. Neuropsychopharmacology. 2003;28(7):1356–65.
57. Lane SD, Cherek DR, Tcheremissine OV, Lieving LM, Pietras CJ. Acute marijuana effects on human risk taking. Neuropsychopharmacology. 2005;30(4):800–9.
58. Ramaekers JG, Kauert G, van RP, Theunissen EL, Schneider E, Moeller MR. High-potency marijuana impairs executive function and inhibitory motor control. Neuropsychopharmacology. 2006;31(10):2296–303.
59. Curran HV, Brignell C, Fletcher S, Middleton P, Henry J. Cognitive and subjective dose-response effects of acute oral Delta 9-tetrahydrocannabinol (THC) in infrequent cannabis users. Psychopharmacology (Berl). 2002;164(1):61–70.
60. Hart CL, van GW, Foltin RW, Fischman MW. Effects of acute smoked marijuana on complex cognitive performance. Neuropsychopharmacology. 2001;25(5):757–65.
61. Quickfall J, Crockford D. Brain neuroimaging in cannabis use: a review. J Neuropsychiatry Clin Neurosci. 2006;18(3):318–32.
62. Chang L, Chronicle EP. Functional imaging studies in cannabis users. Neuroscientist. 2007;13(5):422–32.
63. O'Leary DS, Block RI, Koeppel JA, Flaum M, Schultz SK, Andreasen NC, et al. Effects of smoking marijuana on brain perfusion and cognition. Neuropsychopharmacology. 2002;26(6):802–16.
64. Phan KL, Angstadt M, Golden J, Onyewuenyi I, Popovska A, de WH. Cannabinoid modulation of amygdala reactivity to social signals of threat in humans. J Neurosci. 2008;28(10):2313–9.
65. Borgwardt SJ, Allen P, Bhattacharyya S, Fusar-Poli P, Crippa JA, Seal ML, et al. Neural basis of Delta-9-tetrahydrocannabinol and cannabidiol: effects during response inhibition. Biol Psychiatry. 2008;64(11):966–73.
66. Jager G, Ramsey NF. Long-term consequences of adolescent cannabis exposure on the development of cognition, brain structure and function: an overview of animal and human research. Curr Drug Abuse Rev. 2008;1:114–23.
67. Moore TH, Zammit S, Lingford-Hughes A, Barnes TR, Jones PB, Burke M, et al. Cannabis use and risk of psychotic or affective mental health outcomes: a systematic review. Lancet. 2007;370(9584):319–28.
68. Di FM, Morrison PD, Butt A, Murray RM. Cannabis use and psychiatric and cognitive disorders: the chicken or the egg? Curr Opin Psychiatry. 2007;20(3):228–34.
69. Leweke FM, Koethe D. Cannabis and psychiatric disorders: it is not only addiction. Addict Biol. 2008;13(2):264–75.
70. Pope Jr HG. Cannabis, cognition, and residual confounding. JAMA. 2002;287(9):1172–4.
71. Pope Jr HG, Gruber AJ, Yurgelun-Todd D. The residual neuropsychological effects of cannabis: the current status of research. Drug Alcohol Depend. 1995;38(1):25–34.
72. Solowij N, Stephens RS, Roffman RA, Babor T, Kadden R, Miller M, et al. Cognitive functioning of long-term heavy cannabis users seeking treatment. JAMA. 2002;287(9):1123–31.
73. Solowij N, Battisti R. The chronic effects of cannabis on memory in humans: a review. Curr Drug Abuse Rev. 2008;1:81–98.
74. Grant I, Gonzalez R, Carey CL, Natarajan L, Wolfson T. Non-acute (residual) neurocognitive effects of cannabis use: a meta-analytic study. J Int Neuropsychol Soc. 2003;9(5):679–89.
75. Nair DG. About being BOLD. Brain Res Brain Res Rev. 2005;50(2):229–43.
76. Jager G, Van Hell HH, De Win MM, Kahn RS, Van Den Brink W, Van Ree JM, et al. Effects of frequent cannabis use on hippocampal activity during an associative memory task. Eur Neuropsychopharmacol. 2007;17(4):289–97.
77. Sneider JT, Pope Jr HG, Silveri MM, Simpson NS, Gruber SA, Yurgelun-Todd DA. Altered regional blood volume in chronic cannabis smokers. Exp Clin Psychopharmacol. 2006;14(4):422–8.
78. Murray RM, Morrison PD, Henquet C, Di FM. Cannabis, the mind and society: the harsh realities. Nat Rev Neurosci. 2007;8(11):885–95.
79. Sundram S. Cannabis and neurodevelopment: implications for psychiatric disorders. Hum Psychopharmacol. 2006;21(4):245–54.
80. Grech A, van OJ, Jones PB, Lewis SW, Murray RM. Cannabis use and outcome of recent onset psychosis. Eur Psychiatry. 2005;20(4):349–53.
81. Boydell J, van OJ, Caspi A, Kennedy N, Giouroukou E, Fearon P, et al. Trends in cannabis use prior to first presentation with schizophrenia, in South-East London between 1965 and 1999. Psychol Med. 2006;36(10):1441–6.
82. Rathbone J, Variend H, Mehta H. Cannabis and schizophrenia. Cochrane Database Syst Rev 2008;(3):CD004837.
83. Sarne Y, Keren O. Are cannabinoid drugs neurotoxic or neuroprotective? Med Hypotheses. 2004;63(2):187–92.
84. Sarne Y, Mechoulam R. Cannabinoids: between neuroprotection and neurotoxicity. Curr Drug Targets CNS Neurol Disord. 2005;4(6):677–84.
85. Walsh D, Nelson KA, Mahmoud FA. Established and potential therapeutic applications of cannabinoids in oncology. Support Care Cancer. 2003;11(3):137–43.
86. Fogarty A, Rawstorne P, Prestage G, Crawford J, Grierson J, Kippax S. Marijuana as therapy for people living with HIV/AIDS: social and health aspects. AIDS Care. 2007;19(2):295–301.
87. Pertwee RG. The therapeutic potential of drugs that target cannabinoid receptors or modulate the tissue levels or actions of endocannabinoids. AAPS J. 2005;7(3):E625–54.
88. Scuderi C, Filippis DD, Iuvone T, Blasio A, Steardo A, Esposito G. Cannabidiol in medicine: a review of its therapeutic potential in CNS disorders. Phytother Res. 2009;23(5):597–602.
89. Bortolato M, Mangieri RA, Fu J, Kim JH, Arguello O, Duranti A, et al. Antidepressant-like activity of the fatty acid amide hydrolase inhibitor URB597 in a rat model of chronic mild stress. Biol Psychiatry. 2007;62(10):1103–10.

Cocaine

12

Anne P. Daamen, Renske Penning, Tibor Brunt,
and Joris C. Verster

Abstract

After cannabis, cocaine is the most commonly used illicit drug in Europe. An estimated 13 million Europeans have used it at least once in their lifetime. Also, in the USA cocaine is one of the most prevalent illicit drugs, with an annual prevalence of seven million people. Cocaine is a well-known addictive stimulant drug and scientific literature concerning its various pharmacological properties dates back to the nineteenth century. This chapter describes the mechanism of action of cocaine, how addiction and tolerance develop, and the physiological and psychological risks of cocaine use. Finally, pharmacotherapy and psychosocial interventions available to treat cocaine dependence are discussed. It is concluded that none of these interventions have been proven sufficiently effective to reduce craving and maintain abstinence in all patients.

Learning Objectives
- Cocaine is a highly addictive psychostimulant drug
- Cocaine inhibits the dopamine transporter, thereby causing phasic accumulation of dopamine at the postsynaptic terminals
- The intensity and time of onset of cocaine's effects depend on the route of administration
- Cocaine is associated with several physical and psychological adverse effects, with acute cardiovascular pathology among the most critical described

Issues that Need to Be Addressed by Future Research
- Pharmacotherapy for cocaine addiction holds promise, especially combined with psychosocial treatments. But a better insight into the precise efficacious combination of therapies needs to be developed
- In treating cocaine dependence and adverse effects, the many interactions of cocaine with other drugs should be taken into account more. Cocaine is often used in combination with medication and/or alcohol
- The mechanism through which cocaine works in the brain needs to be clarified even more, so that potential new candidates for pharmacotherapy can be developed

A.P. Daamen • R. Penning • J.C. Verster (✉)
Division of Pharmacology, Utrecht Institute for Pharmaceutical
Sciences, Utrecht University, Universiteitsweg 99, 3584CG Utrecht,
The Netherlands
e-mail: j.c.verster@uu.nl

T. Brunt
Trimbos Institute, Da Costakade 45, 3521 VS Utrecht,
Utrecht, The Netherlands

Introduction

Cocaine is an extract from leaves of the cocaplant (*Erythroxylum coca*), which grows abundantly in the Andes Mountains. Its leaves contain 0.1–0.9% of cocaine.

J.C. Verster et al. (eds.), *Drug Abuse and Addiction in Medical Illness: Causes, Consequences and Treatment*,
DOI 10.1007/978-1-4614-3375-0_12, © Springer Science+Business Media, LLC 2012

For centuries, local people chew coca leaves against altitude sickness and to provide more energy to function at high altitudes. In the sixteenth century, the Spanish introduced cocaine in Europe. It lasted 200 years before cocaine was extracted from the leaves of the coca plant [1]. One of the first publications on cocaine was "Über Coca" by Sigmund Freud. Freud argued that cocaine abuse could lead to less moral notion, but that the medical usefulness of cocaine should not be underestimated [2]. For example, it was discovered that cocaine was effective as a local anesthetic. In the wake of Freud's publication, more and more products with cocaine appeared. The most popular of these was Coca Cola [3]. Today, the small amount of cocaine that the drink initially contained has been replaced by caffeine. In the 1920s, cocaine became illegal in most countries which tempered its popularity among the general public [4]. However, since its use was prohibited cocaine remained a popular recreational drug among different subgroups including musicians (since the 1950s), yuppies (since the 1980s), and partygoers (since the 1990s) [5, 6]. After cannabis, cocaine is currently the most frequently used illicit drug in Europe.

Globally, in 2007 about 4.9% (208 million people) of people between the age of 15 and 64 had used cocaine at least one time in their lives. About 0.6% of them uses cocaine frequently and can be regarded as problematic users. Worldwide, the number of people who used in 2006 and 2007 equaled 16 million, i.e. about 0.4% of the global population [7]. Most cocaine users live in North America (7.1 million), followed by Europe (4 million). Cocaine use is lowest in Africa (1 million) and Asia and Oceania (0.3 million).

Mechanism of Action

Cocaine is a stimulant drug. The pharmacokinetic characteristics of cocaine are summarized in Table 12.1.

Cocaine (benzoylmethylecgonine) is an ester of methylecgonine and benzoic acid and for the most part (90%) metabolized by nonspecific plasma cholinesterase and tissue esterases. This results in urinary excretion of the inactive metabolites ecgonine methyl ester, benzoylecgonine, and ecgonine. In the presence of ethanol, which is frequently used together with cocaine, carboxylesterase catalyzes the formation of cocaethylene, a substance with comparable pharmacologic properties as cocaine but presumably with higher toxicity. About 10% of cocaine is metabolized by CYP3A4 and forms norcocaine. This pharmacologically active N-demethylated cocaine metabolite is further metabolized to N-hydroxynorcocaine and the presumably hepatotoxic norcocaine nitroxide [11–14]. The plasma half-life of cocaine is dose dependent and ranges between 0.7 and 1.5 h [15].

Table 12.1 The (pharmacokinetic) characteristics of cocaine [7–10]

Name	Cocaine
Structure	
Formulae	$C_{17}H_{21}NO_4$ (clark)
Chemical name	Methyl-[1R-(exo,exo)]-3-(benzoyloxy)-8–methyl–8–azabicyclo[3.2.1]-octane–2–carboxylate (clark)
Mass	303.4 (clark)
pK_a	8.61 (drugbank)
log P experimental	2.3 (drugbank)
Melting point	195°C (drugbank)
Density	1.216 g/cm³ (chemical database)
V_d (l/kg)	2.7
Cl_T (ml/min/kg)	20–30
Cl_R (% of total)	1
$t_{1/2}$ (h)	0.8

Cocaine's main pharmacological action is to inhibit monoamine transporters, in particular the dopamine transporter (DAT). To a lesser extent, cocaine is also able to inhibit the serotonin transporter (SERT) and the norepinephrine transporter (NET). Normally after dopamine release, there is presynaptic dopamine reuptake by the DAT. Inhibition of the DAT causes dopamine to remain longer in the synapse where its concentration accumulates. The fast blocking of dopamine reuptake and the large amount of transporter is thought to cause the euphoric effect reported by cocaine users [16, 17]. The effect on serotonin, mainly 5-HT$_2$, may contribute to the hyperlocomotor effects associated with cocaine use [18]. Increased dopamine concentrations due to DAT inhibition are seen especially in the limbic system. The nucleus accumbens (NAc), part of the mesolimbic dopamine pathway, is involved in feelings of pleasure and reward. The buildup of dopamine in this system causes a powerful feeling of euphoria and happiness, much more powerful than feelings caused by natural incentives such as food or sex [16, 17]. For example, some experiments showed that animals preferred cocaine over food [19]. This process, referred to as sensitization, is caused by an enhanced dopaminergic response in the NAc after repeated exposure to stimulant drugs. Whether this process is similar in humans is unclear [20]. A decreased inhibition from the medial prefrontal cortex (mPFC) to the ventral tegmental area (VTA)

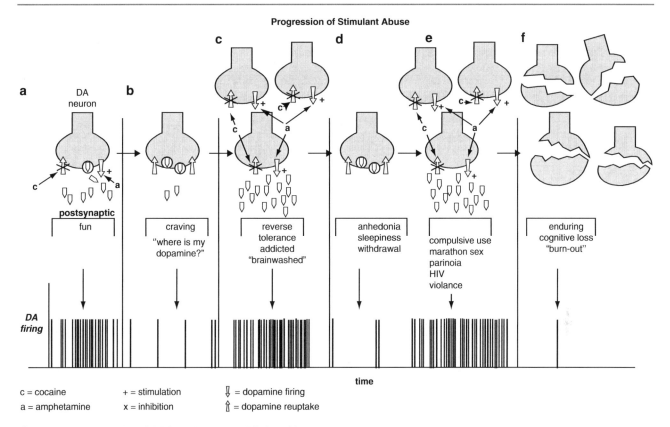

Fig. 12.1 Progression from initial cocaine use to addiction [16]

and NAc is involved in cocaine sensitization, and is probably regulated via gamma-amino-butyric-acid (GABA) and glutamate neurotransmitter systems [21]. The central amygdala plays a role in the incubation of cocaine craving effects over time, partially via glutaminergic and extracellular signal-regulated kinases. Glutamate is considered to play a major role in processes of learning, memory, and reward systems involved in addiction [22, 23].

Besides the effects on catecholamines and their uptake, cocaine has also an effect on voltage-gated sodium channels in the neuronal membrane by reversibly blocking these channels. It binds to sites within the sodium channel, thereby blocking the increase of sodium in the neuronal cells. The blocking of the sodium increase inhibits depolarization and thus the generation of an action potential [5, 24].

Addiction, Tolerance, and Craving

Cocaine addiction is relatively uncommon. Surveys suggest that only a small percentage (16%) of users become addicted. Why not every user becomes addicted is currently unknown. Because drug seeking and craving make them lose control over their behavior, people who do become addicted are at great risk for different kinds of personal harm (e.g. job loss,

family problems, medical problems, and even death) (Fig. 12.1) [25].

After the first time of use, cocaine causes a phasic dopamine release which gives a pleasurable and euphoric feeling. After repeated use, dopamine release is less phasic and thus less pleasure is experienced. Higher doses are needed to give the same pleasurable feeling of phasic dopamine firing that was experienced after first using cocaine. How this process of tolerance develops is not completely understood yet. However, it has been hypothesized that pharmacodynamic factors have a major role in the development of tolerance. A combination of three mechanisms is assumed to be important. Repeated cocaine use (1) reduces the basal dopamine concentration, (2) inhibits the release of dopamine by cocaine stimulation, and (3) changes the sensitivity of receptors or the intracellular pathway [16, 25–27]. Eventually, the dopamine neurons may be damaged or irreversible changed.

When abstaining from use, "craving," i.e. the desire for using cocaine, can be experienced. This desire seems to develop in the (para)limbic regions of the brain [28–30]. During craving, symptoms such as anhedonia and sleepiness are often reported. When cocaine is used, these symptoms rapidly diminish, but gradually higher dosages are needed to achieve the same high [16].

Fig. 12.2 Subjective responses to the different administration routes of cocaine [36]

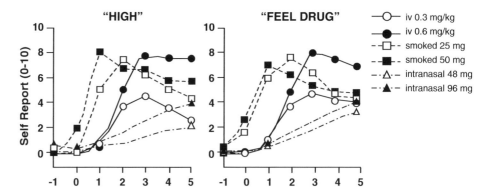

This effect, called tolerance, is the phenomenon whereby a drug user becomes physically accustomed to a particular dose and requires increasing dosages in order to obtain the same effects.

Routes of Administration

Snorting cocaine hydrochloride powder is the most popular way of using cocaine. On average, cocaine powders contain 59% pure cocaine, but this may vary from 1% to 99%. Generally, pure cocaine is mixed with inactive compounds such as baking powder or sugars (mannitol or lactose) [31]. In addition, various pharmacologically active compounds are added that may increase or mimic cocaine's effects. Main reason for mixing cocaine with other compounds is reducing of the production costs. This way, cocaine users can be misled that the powder contains a higher percentage of pure cocaine than it actually does. For example, lidocaine is sometimes added because like cocaine it produces local anesthetic effects on gums and teeth [32].

In addition to snorting, cocaine can also be dissolved in water and administered by intravenous injection [5, 33, 34]. Cocaine hydrochloride cannot be smoked, because of its high melting point and decomposition when burned. However, the so-called "free base cocaine" and "crack" can be smoked [5, 25]. To produce free base, cocaine hydrochloride is dissolved in water together with a base such as ammonia. Ether is added to dissolve the cocaine base. Afterwards, the free base cocaine can be extracted from the ether by evaporation. To produce crack cocaine, cocaine hydrochloride is also dissolved in water, but sodium bicarbonate or baking soda is added [5, 35]. Through heating, the substance becomes a soft mass that turns into a rock-like substance after drying. The end product, crack cocaine, can be smoked. Sometimes cocaine is mixed with heroin, to form a so-called speedball [5].

The magnitude and time of onset of cocaine's effects depend on the route of administration (see Fig. 12.2; Table 12.2).

Table 12.2 Absorption characterizations of cocaine [37, 38]

	Route of administration		
	Intranasal	Smoked	Oral
F (ratio)	0.8	0.57–0.70 (variable)	0.33
T_{max} (h)	0.17	0.05	0.75

It seems that smoking free base or crack induces the fastest administration to the brain and thereby the fastest effects (3–6 s). After intravenous injection, slightly more time is needed to reach the brain where cocaine can induce its effects [25, 39]. A study by Cone et al. [38] shows that both smoked and intravenous injected cocaine produce almost immediate effects on heart rate and blood pressure. However, subjective feelings like euphoria have a more rapid and more intense onset after smoking cocaine [39].

Cocaine is also well absorbed in the mucus layer of the nasal cavity, with even higher total absorption rates then after smoking the drug.

Due to the vasoconstrictive effects of cocaine, the amount that is absorbed by the nasal mucosa differs between individuals [25, 39]. It is likely that some amount of the snorted cocaine is swallowed and enters the gastrointestinal tract. After the rapid blood concentration peak produced by snorting, a second concentration peak is seen, when cocaine is absorbed by gastrointestinal mucus layers [37, 40]. After snorting it takes approximately 3–5 min to induce the first euphoric effects, but these effects seems to continue longer then after smoking or injecting the drug [5, 25]. Therefore, it is not surprising that snorting is the most popular way of cocaine use.

The Effects and Risks of Cocaine Use

Most people use cocaine for its pleasurable psychological effects, such as euphoria, increased alertness and energy, and increased confidence. The drug has also laxative properties and diminishes the user's appetite. These last effects are sometimes used for establishing weight loss. Another important pharmacological effect of cocaine is its local anesthetic effect, due to the blockage of sodium channels in neuronal cells [5, 24, 25, 34].

Besides the desired effects, cocaine use has also been associated with both negative physical and psychological effects which may be compromising to the user's health.

Cardiovascular Risks

Cocaine use is often accompanied by adverse hematologic and cardiovascular effects. These effects are due to cocaine's effect on the norepinephrine and dopamine reuptake in the presynaptic adrenergic terminals. This results in a buildup of these catecholamines near their receptors (mainly α_2-adrenerge) which leads to a powerful sympathomimetic effect. Cocaine's blocking of sodium channels leads to decreased action potential generation, which leads in turn to antidysrhythmic effects. Cocaine also affects levels of endothelin-1 (a vasoconstrictor) and nitric oxide (a vasodilator) [5, 41, 42]. These effects may also result in intense coronary vasoconstriction and platelet activation. Autopsy reports on young cocaine abusers report about atherosclerosis. Therefore, cocaine abusers are at serious risk for developing cardiovascular diseases. However, a sizable proportion of cocaine addicts already show uncovered vascular abnormalities, which could worsen the negative effects of cocaine itself. Therefore, this should be taken into consideration when cocaine addicts are being investigated [41, 43, 44].

Myocardial ischemia, myocardial infarction, and arrhythmias are commonly seen as cardiovascular complications in cocaine abusers [41, 44]. Chronic users can also develop dilated cardiomyopathy, but this is usually reversible. Its sympathicomimetic effects can also lead to hypertension (through vasoconstriction and a larger cardiac output), which, together with the positive ionotropic and chronotropic cardiac effects, can lead to aortic dissection. The risk for these events is the highest in the first hours after administration, but can last till a week after taking cocaine [44].

Pulmonary Risks

Besides cardiovascular complications cocaine users are also at risk to develop pulmonary complications, whereby smoking cocaine causes the highest risk for developing these problems [25, 45]. Cocaine users may suffer from pulmonary edema, which can be a result of the cardiac problems, but there is also a great risk for noncardiogenic pulmonary edema. How these administration routes can cause pulmonary edema is not clear, although there are theories about the

direct toxic effect on the alveolar-capillary membrane and immune response activation. Pulmonary alveolar hemorrhage is often seen after cocaine use, especially after smoking crack [44–46].

Neurological Risks

Cerebrovascular effects are the most important in the drug-related neurotoxic complications. Cerebrovascular strokes, either hemorrhage or ischemic, can occur after all forms of cocaine administration [34, 44]. Beside the cerebrovascular effects intracranial hemorrhage is a great issue in cocaine use, since cocaine use can lead to hypertension and therefore to intracranial hemorrhage. Many of the preexisting vascular damages mentioned earlier were seen in 50% of the cocaine-related intracranial hemorrhage patients [44]. Hypertension as a result of cocaine use can also cause posterior reversible encephalopathy syndrome (PRES). Chronic use of cocaine can further cause cerebral atrophy, ischemia or infarctions and vascular headaches [25, 44].

Cocaine-related seizures are seen mostly in chronic users, but can also occur after first time using and are another risk for cocaine users. These seizures can develop in all users, but those with preexisting disorders have a twofold risk [25, 34]. Seizures are probably caused by high serotonin concentrations in the brain. The rise of serotonin concentrations is caused by the reuptake blocking effect of cocaine and stimulation of muscarine and sigma receptors in the brain. However, they can also occur due to cocaine-induced hyperthermia or acidosis. Most cocaine-induced seizures are generalized tonic–clonic, but focal seizures can also occur [5, 34, 47].

Cocaine can also induce movement disorders due to dopamine accumulation not only in the synaptic clefts of mostly the basal ganglia, but also in other brain regions. This buildup can cause movement disorders like Tourette syndrome and tardive dyskinesia [34].

Renal Risks

Acute renal failure has been noted in cocaine abusers. However the most important cause of renal failure is rhabdomyolysis, which damages tubular functioning. Vasoconstriction, renal infarction, and atherosclerosis are named as factors that can produce such injury. Hypertension due to cocaine use can be a complicating factor in cocaine-induced renal failure and has been associated with hypertensive nephrosclerosis and chronic kidney disease. Symptoms of renal failure include changed serum creatine kinase levels, electrolyte abnormalities, and urinary myoglobin [25, 43, 48].

Other Risks

Other risks of cocaine use include hyperthermia, ischemia of bowel tissue, gastric ulcerations, retroperitoneal fibrosis, and visceral infarction are among the gastrointestinal conditions in which cocaine has been implicated [43, 49]. The administration routes themselves may also cause problems for the user's health, especially when cocaine is administrated intravenously. Intravenous cocaine users are at risk of developing endocarditis. This is the result of bacteremia, caused by using nonsterile injection needles. The use of nonsterile needles produces also an increased risk for catching infectious diseases, such as HIV [25, 44].

Snorting cocaine can cause perforation of the nasal septum, but there is also chance of necrosis in other structures. Epiglottises, aspiration, sinusitis, and bronchitis are conditions which are associated with cocaine snorting [43, 44].

Finally, cocaine can be a complicating factor in pregnant users, whom are at risk for placenta abruption, having a baby with low birth weight or with neurological or psychological problems [43, 50].

Psychological Risks

Psychiatric illnesses such as depression, bipolar diseases, attention-deficit disorders, and schizophrenia are commonly seen in cocaine users [51, 52]. However, cocaine abuse can also cause a number of psychological problems, which sometimes can worsen the symptoms of above-mentioned comorbidities. Schizophrenia patients, for example, have a higher suicide risk when they use cocaine [53]. Besides worsening the existing disorders, cocaine use can also cause psychological problems in healthy individuals.

Unwanted effects of cocaine use include panic attacks, paranoid ideation, agitation, anxiety, hallucinations, psychosis, and violence behavior [43, 45, 51, 54]. These effects can lead to dependence and subsequent dangerous behaviors and risky situations [47]. Epidemiological studies have shown that cocaine use is frequently associated with (car) accidents, homicides, and suicides (attempts) [43, 55].

In several studies cocaine has been shown to influence cognitive functioning, both negative and positive [56, 57]. The prefrontal cortex is the brain region which is most associated with affected cognitive functioning in cocaine users. Due to cocaine's effect on the mesolimbic dopamine pathway cocaine has a reducing metabolic effect on the prefrontal cortex, which among others can lead to some forms of cognitive impairment such as effects on speed of information processing and problem solving [17, 56, 58].

However, cocaine also has an effect on other brain regions. For example, cocaine affects verbal and visual memory functioning and impairment in verbal fluency and perceptual-sensory functions has been found [56, 58, 59].

Cocaine's negative effects are not limited to recent abusers. In the past cocaine users, cognitive impairment may persist [51, 58]. For example, Oliveira et al. [58] has found deficits in attentional and executive functioning in ex-users who were abstinent for at least 6 months.

Toxicity

Toxic effects have been described with a dose of approximately 1 mg/kg or a plasma concentration of 0.1 mg/l. However, this range can be large depending on the situation (purity, route of administration) and individual differences. There have been reports of lethal intravenous dosages of 20 mg, whereas an oral dose of 10 g administered to a chronic cocaine user was not fatal [60, 61].

Acute intoxication includes tremor, restlessness, irritability, emotional instability, panic, and paranoia. Higher dosages can cause hallucinations, paranoia, intense anxiety attacks, tachycardia, hypertension, ventricular irritability, respiratory depression, and hyperthermia. In case of an overdose, cocaine can cause serious problems like acute heart failure, stroke, seizures, and sudden death syndrome [25, 34, 43].

Interactions

Cocaine and Medication

Cocaine is metabolized by CYP3A4. Substances that effect CYP3A4 can affect the metabolism of cocaine and vice versa, which can lead to higher or lower plasma concentrations. Cocaine also inhibits CYP2D6 and can thereby decrease the metabolism of other substances [11].

Several medicinal drugs are known to interact with cocaine. For example, cocaine affects the same sodium channels as lidocaine. But lidocaine is able to displace cocaine from the sodium channels, and because of that able to reduce cocaine-induced QRS prolongation [12]. Phenothiazines and butyrophenones block potassium channels as well as sodium channels. In this way, they may enhance cocaine toxicity [41].

Use of cocaine and a beta-adrenergic antagonist at the same time leads to vasoconstriction, followed by hypertension, increased seizure frequency and coronary artery spasm, because of unopposed alpha-adrenergic effects as a result of blocking beta-adrenergic receptors [12, 42].

By interfering with cocaine metabolism by plasma cholinesterase, succinylcholine can cause higher plasma concentrations of cocaine, leading to subsequent increased toxicology. Monoamine oxidase inhibitors (MAOIs) are antidepressants with the same neurotransmitter systems as target as cocaine (dopamine, serotonin, norepinephrine). MAOIs decrease the metabolism of monoamines. The same applies for selective serotonin reuptake inhibitors (SSRIs) and drugs that inhibit the reuptake of dopamine-like bupropion [13]. This could lead to an increased or sustained effect of cocaine.

Cocaine and Alcohol

Cocaine is frequently used in combination with alcohol. People that used both cocaine and alcohol reported that this drug combination prolongs the high of cocaine and decrease the dysphoric feelings caused by alcohol. This can be explained by the formation of cocaethylene, which is formed out of cocaine by carboxyesterase in the presence of ethanol. Cocaethylene has a similar effect on heart rate and blood pressure and gives a euphoric feeling. Because of the longer half-life when compared to cocaine the euphoria is extended. Combining cocaine and alcohol also inhibits cocaine metabolism, which lead to higher blood concentrations of cocaine [14, 15, 41].

Cocaine, Marijuana, and/or Nicotine

The combination of cocaine and marijuana increases heart rate when compared to using these drugs individually [11, 62]. This effect may be a result of enhanced nasal absorption of cocaine caused by cannabinoid-induced vasodilatation [11].

Both cocaine and nicotine increase heart rate and coronary vasoconstriction, possibly increasing the risk for cardiovascular complications, especially when used in combination [5, 41].

Detection

Cocaine can be detected in urine, blood, perspiration, hair, saliva, and feces. Urine is most commonly used to detect cocaine, because it is easy to collect and it is a noninvasive method [60]. Usually urine is tested by enzyme-multiplied immunoassay, or less commonly by radioimmunoassay or thin-layer chromatography. Immunoassays are not very precise, so a positive result should be checked using chromatography [25]. Urine tests usually screen for the presence of its metabolite benzoylecgonine. Cocaine has a short elimination half-life (about 1 h), whereas benzoylecgonine has a half-life of 6 h. In contrast to cocaine, benzoylecgonine can still be detected 1 or 2 days after administration [63]. The detection of benzoylecgoine in urine does not necessarily prove cocaine abuse. A very high dose of prilocaine or coca tea (made of the leaves of the coca plant) can also give a positive result in urine immunoassays [64]. By adding bleach or sodium chloride to the urine, a false-negative result can be achieved. Other products that have been added to urine to prevent

detection of cocaine or its metabolite are vinegar, soap, or lemon juice [65]. Also, if the time between testing and cocaine use is too short, no benzoylecgonine is detected [5].

The benefit of testing in hair is the longer period that cocaine or its metabolite benzoylecgonine are detectable [66]. Hair analysis is also an easy and noninvasive method to test for cocaine use. Normally, 50–100 strands are enough for a good sample [67]. Because hair grows in a constant rate, it is also possible to say whether the use was chronic or episodic [33]. Detection of cocaine use in saliva is a less accurate method if exact concentrations are needed to be determined. In order to detect low concentrations, more sensitive methods are necessary [60].

Treatment of Cocaine Abuse

Currently, there is no specific effective pharmacological treatment available for cocaine addiction [68]. Based on general theories on brain mechanisms of addiction, several compounds have been studied. Xi and Gardner [69] recently reviewed several neurotransmitters and receptors that are involved in the reward pathway and the ways they can be targeted to develop pharmacological treatment (see Fig. 12.3).

Figure 12.3 represents a schematic presentation of the VTA–NAc–ventral pallidum (VP) reward pathway. Furthermore, it shows were psychostimulants affect this pathway and possible sites of actions for pharmacological treatment of cocaine addiction [69] (adapted with permission from Xi et al. 2008).

Activation of the ionotropic glutamate receptors (iGluR) leads to stimulation of the NAc medium-spiny GABAergic neurons, while activation of the D2 receptors leads to inhibition of these neurons. It seems that functional inhibition of the NAc-VP GABAergic pathway is essential in drug reward and addiction. Blocking or reversing of the DAT by psychostimulants leads to an increase of the extracellular dopamine concentration in the NAc dopamine axon terminals. This concentration rise leads to the release of endocannabinoids (eCBs) in the medium-spiny GABAergic neurons, eventually leading to reduction of glutamate in the NAc and GABA in the VP. Animal research has suggested seven possible points of pharmacological intervention, which can affect this mechanism of drug reward and addiction (1) blocking of the dopamine receptors (especially D_3) with dopamine antagonists, (2) inhibition of the DAT or other monoamine transporter with slow-onset long-acting inhibitors which substitute the cocaine, but have different pharmacokinetic properties, (3) affecting the GABAergic terminals in the VP (see Fig. 12.3) and VTA with GABAmimetic compounds, (4) acting on CB_1 receptors by cannabinoid CB_1 receptor antagonist, (5) modulating the release of presynaptic glutamate and/or neuronal activity of the postsynaptic NAc GABAergic

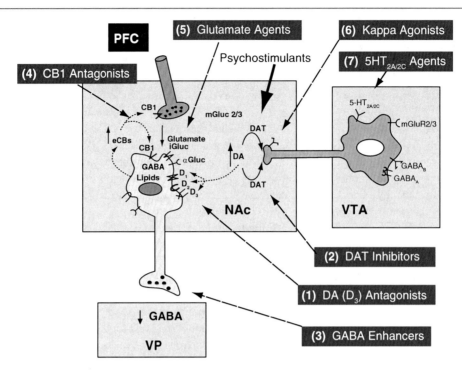

Fig. 12.3 Schematic presentation of the ventral tegmental area (VTA)–nucleus accumbens (NAc)–ventral pallidum (VP) reward pathway. Furthermore, it shows were psychostimulants affect this pathway and possible sites of actions for pharmacological treatment of cocaine addiction [69] (adapted with permission from Xi et al. 2008)

neurons by agents which act on the mGluRs, (6) decrease of the dopamine release in the NAc by κ-opioid agonists, and (7) modulating the dopamine neuron activity and dopamine release in the NAc by affecting the action of psychostimulants by the use of agents which act on 5-HT$_{2A}$ and/or 5$_{2C}$ receptors [69].

Human research has focused on points 1 to 3, 6, and 7. There are also some other forms of treatments which are currently applied or investigated in humans, e.g. vaccination and psychosocial interventions. However, none of these intervention options has a complete cure ratio, therefore more research is needed.

Dopamine-Related Treatment

The mesolimbic dopamine system has been a target for various compounds that aimed to modulate dopamine receptors or transporters [69]. The dopamine reuptake inhibitor bupropion [70, 71] showed no significant reduction in craving and self-administration of cocaine. Levodopa–carbidopa studies show conflicting outcomes, a study of Mooney et al. [72] shows no significant effect on cocaine addiction symptoms, whereas a study of Schmitz et al. [73] found contrasting detectable treatment effect for levodopa in comparison with placebo.

Antagonists acting at D$_1$ or D$_2$ receptors were not effective or produced unwanted adverse effects and are therefore not applicable in the treatment of cocaine dependence. However, D$_3$ receptor antagonists seem promising for the treatment of psychostimulant dependence [69]. Currently, several D$_3$ receptor antagonists are in development.

Replacement Therapy

Drugs that mimic cocaine's mechanism of action should be able to reduce craving, because they replace the effect of cocaine. This strategy has been successfully applied with methadone in heroin addicts and nicotine patches in smokers. Dopamine reuptake inhibitors and dopamine agonists are possible maintenance medications [74, 75]. Partial dopamine agonists are able to imitate some of cocaine's effects, without the particular toxic characteristics [76]. Several promising dopamine agonists have been studied.

For example, modafinil has been shown to significantly reduce cocaine use [77, 78]. Also, there is some evidence that disulfiram is effective in the treatment of cocaine dependence, but further research is needed [79]. Disulfiram is also used for the treatment of alcoholism. In patients with combined cocaine and alcohol use, disulfiram reduces both alcohol and cocaine use [80, 81].

Clinical trials have examined the effect of methylphenidate on cocaine addiction, but failed to show its clinical efficacy. Often these studies were performed in patients who also suffered from ADHD. Whereas methylphenidate was effective in the treatment of ADHD symptoms, no significant effects were reported on cocaine use outcomes [82].

GABA-Related Treatment

GABA also plays an important role in the mesolimbic dopamine reward system. Based on this knowledge, several potential treatments have been developed that aim to counteract inhibition of GABAergic neurons by cocaine. These include gabapentin, tiagabine, topiramate, vigabatrin, and baclofen. Baclofen decreased cocaine self-administration [83] and was especially effective in heavy cocaine users [84]. Vigabatrin also decreased cocaine use [85, 86]. The effect of treatment with tiagabine is not completely clarified, because Gonzalez et al. [87, 88] show a decrease in cocaine use after treatment, but Winhusen et al. [89] did not found a significant effect of tiagabine on drug usage.

In a pilot trial, after 3 weeks of treatment with topiramate 59% of cocaine addicts remained abstinent from the drug, twice as much as in the placebo-treated group [90]. Although not 100% effective, these drugs may help a substantial numbers of cocaine addicts in remaining abstinent.

Other Treatments

Other compounds that are currently under investigation are kappa opioid-receptor agonists such as nalfurafine. Kappa receptor agonists inhibit dopamine release and thus may antagonize cocaine's effects [69]. Also, $5HT_{2A}$ receptor antagonists and $5HT_{2C}$ agonists are in development, because serotonin receptors are present in the mesolimbic dopamine system as well. Ondansetron, a 5HT3 receptor antagonist, also produced a reduction in cocaine use [91].

N-acetylcysteine is a vaccine aiming to reduce craving and relapse by restoring glutamate levels in the NAc. Double-blind studies showed that the vaccine significantly reduced both craving for cocaine and the use of cocaine in addicted subjects [92, 93].

Psychosocial Interventions

A number of psychosocial interventions based on cognitive-behavioral approaches have received significant empirical attention in the literature on cocaine use disorders in the last two decades [94]. Approaches to increase coping skills and community reinforcement have been proven to be effective.

Psychosocial treatments may be useful in combination with pharmacotherapy for treating cocaine addiction. Several studies have proved to be effective; improving coping skills and motivation using psychosocial treatments on the one hand, while increasing abstinence from cocaine abstinence using pharmacological compounds on the other [75].

References

1. Monardes N. Joyfull Newes Out of the Newe Founde Worlde. New York, NY: Alfred Knopf; 1925.
2. Freud S. Uber coca. Centralblad fur die ges. Therapie. 1884;2:289–314.
3. Benson D. Coca kick in drinks spurs export fears. The Washington Times, April 20 2004
4. EM, Editors of Consumer Reports Magazine. The Consumers Union Report on licit and illicit drugs. Consumer Reports Magazine, 1972.
5. Goldstein R, DesLauriers C, Burda A. Cocaine history, social implications and toxicity a review. Dis Mon. 2009;55:6–38.
6. Kenyon SL, Ramsey JD, Lee T, Johnston A, Holt DW. Analysis for identification in amnesty bin samples from dance venues. Ther Drug Monit. 2005;27(6):793–8.
7. United Nations Office on Drugs and Crime (UNODC). World Drug Report 2008. Vienna: United Nations. http://www.unodc.org/documents/wdr/WDR_2008/WDR_2008_eng_web.pdf.
8. Moffat A. http://clarke.pharm.uu.nl:9876/. Accessed 27 Dec 2008.
9. Hardy J. http://ull.chemistry.uakron.edu/erd/. Accessed 27 Dec 2008.
10. Wishart D. http://www.drugbank.ca/. Accessed 27 Dec 2008.
11. Lexi-comp Online. Lexi-Interact. 1978–2008 Lexi-Comp, Inc. Retrieved June 2008.
12. Liu D, Hariman RJ, Bauman JL. Cocaine concentration-effect relationship in the presence and absence of lidocaine: evidence of competitive binding between cocaine and lidocaine. J Pharmacol Exp Ther. 1996;276(2):568–77.
13. O'Dell L, George FR, Ritz MC. Antidepressant drugs appear to enhance cocaine induced toxicity. Exp Clin Psychpharmacol. 2000;8(1):133–41.
14. Knuepfer M. Cardiovascular disorders associated with cocaine use: myths and truths. Pharmacol Ther. 2003;97(3):181–222.
15. Laizure SC, Mandrell T, Gades NM, et al. Cocaethylene metabolism and interaction with cocaine and ethanol: role of carboxylesterases. Drug Metab Dispos. 2003;31(1):16–20.
16. Stahl S (2008) Stahl's essential psychopharmacology; neuroscientific basis and practical applications, 3rd edition. Cambridge University Press, Cambridge
17. Dackis CA, O'Brien CP. Cocaine dependence: a disease of the brain's reward centers. J Subst Abuse Treat. 2001;21:111–7.
18. Filip M, Bubar MJ, Cunningham KA. Contribution of serotonin (5-HT) 5-HT2 receptor subtypes to the hyperlocomotor effects of cocaine: acute and chronic pharmacological analyses. J Pharmacol Exp Ther. 2004;310(3):1246–54.
19. Nestler E. The neurobiology of cocaine addiction. Sci Pract Perspect. 2005;3(1):4–10.
20. Narendran R, Martinez D. Cocaine abuse and sensitization of striatal dopamine transmission: a critical review of the preclinical and clinical imaging literature. Synapse. 2008;62(11):851–69.
21. Steketee JD. Cortical mechanisms of cocaine sensitization. Crit Rev Neurobiol. 2005;17(2):69–86.
22. Lu L, Hope BT, Dempsey J, Liu SY, Bossert JM, Shaham Y. Central amygdala ERK signaling pathway is critical to incubation of cocaine craving. Nat Neurosci. 2005;8(2):212–9.

23. Li YQ, Li FQ, Wang XY, Wu P, Zhao M, Xu CM, Shaham Y, Lu L. Central amygdala extracellular signal-regulated kinase signaling pathway is critical to incubation of opiate craving. J Neurosci. 2008;28(49):13248–57.

24. Fleming JA, Byck R, Barash PG. Pharmacology and therapeutic applications of cocaine. Anesthesiology. 1990;73:518–31.

25. Warner EA. Cocaine abuse. Ann Intern Med. 1993;119(3):226–35.

26. Hammer RP, Egilmez Y, Emmett-Oglesby MW. Neural mechanisms of tolerance to the effects of cocaine. Behav Brain Res. 1997;84:225–39.

27. Vanderschuren LJ, Everitt BJ. Behavioral and neural mechanisms of compulsive drug seeking. Eur J Pharmacol. 2005;526(1–3):77–88.

28. Childress AR, Mozley PD, McElgin W, Fitzgerald J, Reivich M, O'Brien CP. Limbic activation during cue-induced cocaine craving. Am J Psychiatry. 1999;156(1):11–8.

29. Kilts CD, Schweitzer JB, Quinn CK, Gross RE, Faber TL, Muhammad F. Neural activity related to drug craving in cocaine addiction. Arch Gen Psychiatry. 2001;58(4):334–41.

30. Volkow ND, Fowler JS, Wang G, Telang F, Logan J, Jayne M, et al. Cognitive control of drug craving inhibits brain reward regions in cocaine abusers. Neuroimage. 2010;49:2536–43.

31. Shannon M. Clinical toxicity of cocaine adulterants. Ann Emerg Med. 1988;17(11):1243–7.

32. Brunt TM, Rigter S, Hoek J, Vogels N, van Dijk P, Niesink RJ. An analysis of cocaine powder in the Netherlands: content and health hazards due to adulterants. Addiction. 2009;104(5):798–805.

33. Koren G, Klein J, Forman R, et al. Hair analysis of cocaine: differentiation between systemic exposure and external contamination. J Clin Pharmacol. 1992;32:671–5.

34. Boghdadi MS, Henning RJ. Cocaine: pathophysiology and clinical toxicology. Heart Lung. 1997;26(6):466–83.

35. Chychula NM, Okore C. The cocaine epidemic: a comprehensive review of use, abuse and dependence. Nurse Pract. 1990; 15(7):31–9.

36. Volkow ND, Wang GJ, Fischman MW, Foltin R, Fowler JS, Franceschi D. Effects of route of administration on cocaine induced dopamine transport blockade in the human brain. Life Sci. 2000;67:1507–15.

37. Fattinger K, Benowitz N, Jones R, Verotta D. Nasal mucosal versus gastrointestinal absorption of nasally administered cocaine. Eur J Clin Pharmacol. 2000;56:305–10.

38. Cone E. Recent discoveries in pharmacokinetics of drugs of abuse. Toxicol Lett. 1998;102–103:97–101.

39. Wilkinson P, van Dyke C, Jatlow P, Barash P, Byck R. Intranasal and oral cocaine kinetics. Clin Pharmacol Ther. 1980;27(3): 386–94.

40. Cone EJ. Pharmacokinetics and pharmacodynamics of cocaine. J Anal Toxicol. 1995;19:459–78.

41. Hoffman RS. Cocaine. In: Flomenbaum NE, Goldfrank LR, Hoffman RS, et al., editors. Goldfrank's toxicologic emergencies. 8th ed. New York, NY: McGraw Hill; 2006. p. 1133–46.

42. McCord J, Hani J, Hollander JE. Management of cocaine-associated chest pain and myocardial infarction: a scientific statement from the American Heart Association acute cardiac care committee of the council on clinical cardiology. Circulation. 2008;117(14): 1897–907.

43. Glauser J, Queen JR. An overview of non-cardiac cocaine toxicity. J Emerg Med. 2007;32(2):181–6.

44. Hagan I, Burney K. Radiology of recreational drug abuse. RadioGraphics. 2007;27:919–40.

45. Devlin R, Henry J. Clinical review: Major consequences of illicit drug consumption. Crit Care. 2008;12(1):202.

46. Restrepo CS, Carrillo JA, Martínez S, Ojeda P, Rivera AL, Hatta A. Pulmonary complications from cocaine and cocaine-based substances: imaging manifestations. Radiographics. 2007;27(4): 941–56.

47. Shanti CM, Lucas CE. Cocaine and the critical care challenge. Crit Care Med. 2003;31(6):1851–9.

48. Gitman M, Singhal P. Cocaine-induced renal disease. Expert Opin Drug Saf. 2004;3(5):441–8.

49. Linder JD, Monkemuller KE, Raijman I, et al. Cocaine-associated ischemic colitis. South Med J. 2000;93:909–13.

50. Thompson BL, Levitt P, Stanwood G. Prenatal exposure to drugs: effects on brain development and implications for policy and education. Neuroscience. 2009;10(4):303–12.

51. Nnadi CU, Olubansile AM, McCurtis HL, Cadet JL. Neuropsychiatric effects of cocaine use disorders. J Natl Med Assoc. 2005;197(11): 1504–15.

52. Rounsaville BJ. Treatment of cocaine dependence and depression. Biol Psychiatry. 2004;56(10):803–9.

53. Seibyl JP, Satel SL, Anthony D, Southwick SM, Krystal JH, Charney DS. Effects of cocaine on hospital course in schizophrenia. J Nerv Ment Dis. 1993;181(1):31–7.

54. Louwenstein DH, Massa SM, Rowbotham MC, Collins SD, McKinney HE, Simon RP. Acute neurologic and psychiatric complications associated with cocaine abuse. Am J Med. 1987;83:841–6.

55. Ryb GE, Cooper CC, Dischinger PC, Kufera JA, Auman KM, Soderstrom CA. Suicides, homicides, and unintentional injury deaths after trauma center discharge: cocaine use as a risk factor. J Trauma. 2009;67:409–97.

56. Jovanovski D, Erb S, Zakzanis KK. Neurocognitive deficits in cocaine users: a quantitative review of evidence. J Clin Exp Neuropsychol. 2005;27:189–204.

57. Goldstein RZ, Leskovjan AC, Hoff AL, Hitzemann R, Bashan F, Khalsa SS, et al. Severity of neuropsychological impairment in cocaine and alcohol addiction: association with metabolism in the prefrontal cortex. Neuropsycholgia. 2004;42:1447–58.

58. Oliveira LG, Barroso LP, Silveira CM, van der Meer Sanchez Z, Ponce JC, Vaz LJ, et al. Neuropsychological assesment of current and past crack cocaine users. Subst Use Misuse. 2009;44:1941–57.

59. Ardilla A, Rosselli M, Strumwasser S. Neuropsychological deficits in chronic cocaine abusers. Int J Neurosci. 1991;57:73–9.

60. Ursitti F, Klein J, Koren G. Confirmation of cocaine use during pregnancy: a critical review. Ther Drug Monit. 2001;23:347–53.

61. Meulenbelt J, de Vries I, Joore J. Behandeling van acute vergiftingen, Practische richtlijnen. 1997; Bohn Stafleu Van Loghum.

62. Foltin W, Fischman MW, Pedroso JJ, et al. Marijuana and cocaine interactions in humans: cardiovascular consequences. Pharmacol Biochem Behav. 1987;28(4):459–64.

63. Burke WM, Ravi NV, Dhopesh V, et al. Prolonged presence of metabolite in urine after compulsive cocaine use. J Clin Psychiatry. 1990;51(4):145–48.

64. Baselt RC, Baselt DR. Little cross-reactivity of local anesthetics with Abuscreen, EMIT d.a.u., and TDX immunoassays for cocaine metabolite (letter). Clin Chem. 1987;33(5):747.

65. Mikkelsen SL, Ash KO. Adulterants causing false negatives in illicit drug testing. Clin Chem. 1988;34(11):2233–6.

66. Gruszecki AC, Robinson CA, Embry JH, et al. Correlation of the incidence of cocaine and cocaethylene in hair and postmortem biologic samples. Am J Forensic Med Pathol. 2000;21(2):166–71.

67. Mazor SS, Mycyk MB, Wills BK, et al. Coca tea consumption causes positive urine cocaine assay. Eur J Emerg Med. 2006;13:340–1.

68. Karila L, Gorelick D, Wienstein A, Noble F, Benyamina A, Coscas S, et al. New treatments for cocaine dependence: a focused review. Int J Neuropsychopharmacol. 2008;11:425–38.

69. Xi Z-X, Gardner EL. Hypothesis-driven medication discovery for the treatment of psychostimulant addiction. Curr Drug Abuse Rev. 2008;1:303–27.

70. Margolin A, Kosten TR, Avants SK, Wilkins J, Ling W, Beckson M. A multicenter trial of bupropion for cocaine dependence in methadone-maintained patients. Drug Alcohol Depend. 1995;40: 125–31.

71. Shoptaw S, Heinzerling KG, Rotheram-Fuller E, Kao UH, Wang P, Bholat MA, et al. Bupropion hydrochloride versus placebo, in combination with cognitive behavioral therapy, for the treatment of cocaine abuse/dependence. J Addict Dis. 2008;27(1):13–23.

72. Mooney ME, Schmitz JM, Moeller FG, Grabowski J. Safety, tolerability and efficacy of levodopa-carbidopa treatment for cocaine dependence: two double-blind randomized, clinical trials. Drug Alcohol Depend. 2007;88:214–23.

73. Schmitz J, Mooney M, Moeller F, Stotts A, Green C, Grabowski J. Levodopa pharmacotherapy for cocaine dependence: choosing the optimal behavioral therapy platform. Drug Alcohol Depend. 2008;94(1–3):142–50.

74. Preti A. New developments in the pharmacotherapy of cocaine abuse. Addict Biol. 2007;12:133–51.

75. de Lima MS, de Oliveira Soares BG, Reisser AA, Farrell M. Pharmacological treatment of cocaine dependence: a systematic review. Addiction. 2002;97(8):931–49.

76. Platt DM, Rowlett JK, Spealman RD. Behavioral effects of cocaine and dopaminergic strategies for preclinical medication development. Psychopharmacology (Berl). 2002;163(3–4):265–82.

77. Dackis CA, Kampman KM, Lynch KG, Pettinati HM, O'Brien CP. A double-blind, placebo controlled trial of modafinil for cocaine dependence. Neuropsychopharmacology. 2005;30:205–11.

78. Anderson AL, Reid MS, Li S, Holmes T, Shemanski L, Slee A, Smith EV, et al. Modafinil for the treatment of cocaine dependence. Drug Alcohol Depend. 2009;104:133–9.

79. Pani P, Trogu E, Vacca R, Amato L, Vecchi S, Davoli M. Disulfiram for the treatment of cocaine dependence. Cochrane Database Syst Rev. 2010; 20(1):CD007024.

80. Carroll KM, Nich C, Ball SA, McCance E, Rounsaville BJ. Treatment of cocaine and alcohol dependence with psychotherapy and disulfram. Addiction. 1998;93:713–27.

81. Carroll KM, Nich C, Ball SA, McCance E, Frankforter TL, Rounsaville BJ. One year follow-up of disulfram and psychotherapy in cocaine-dependent outpatients: a randomized placebo-controlled trial. Addiction. 2000;95:1335–49.

82. Castells X, Casas M, Pérez-Mañá C, Roncero C, Vidal X, Capellà D. Efficacy of psychostimulant drugs for cocaine dependence. Cochrane Database Syst Rev. 2010;(2):CD007380.

83. Haney M, Hart CL, Foltin RW. Effects of baclofen on cocaine self-administration: opioid- and nonopioid-dependent volunteers. Neuropsychpharmacology. 2006;31:1814–21.

84. Shoptaw S, Yang X, Rotheram-Fuller E, Hsieh Y, Kintaudi P, Charuvastra V, Ling W. Randomized placebo-controlled trial of baclofen for cocaine dependence: preliminary effects for individuals with chronic patterns of cocaine use. J Clin Psychiatry. 2003;64(12):1440–8.

85. Brodie J, Figueroa E, Laska E, Dewey S. Safety and efficacy of gamma-vinyl GABA (GVG) for the treatment of methamphetamine and/or cocaine addiction. Synapse. 2005;55(2):122–5.

86. Fetchner R, Khouri A, Figueroa E, Ramirez M, Federico M, Dewey SM, et al. Short-treatment of cocaine and/or methamphetamine abuse with vigabatrin: occular safety pilot results. Arch Ophthalmol. 2006;124:1257–62.

87. Gonzalez G, Desai R, Sofuoglu M, Poling J, Oliveto A, Gonsar K, et al. Tiagebine increases cocaine-free urines in cocaine-dependent methadone treated patients: results of a randomized pilot study. Addiction. 2003;98:1625–32.

88. Gonzalez G, Desai R, Sofuoglu M, Poling J, Oliveto A, Gonsai K, et al. Clinical efficacy of gabapentin versus tiagebine for reducing cocaine use among cocaine-dependent methadone treated patients. Drug Alcohol Depend. 2006;87:1–9.

89. Winhusen T, Somoza E, Ciraulo DA, Harrer JM, Goldsmtih RJ, Grabowski J. A double-blind placebo controlled trial of tiagabine for the treatment of cocaine dependence. Drug Alcohol Depend. 2007;91:141–8.

90. Kampman KM, Pettinati H, Lynch KG, Dackis C, Sparkman T, Weigley C, et al. A pilot trial for the treatment of cocaine dependence. Drug Alcohol Depend. 2004;75:233–40.

91. Johnson BA, Roache JD, Ait-Daoud N, Javors MA, Harrison JM, Elkashef A, et al. A preliminary randomized, double-blind, placebo-controlled study of safety and efficacy of ondansetron in the treatment of cocaine dependence. Drug Alcohol Depend. 2006; 84:256–63.

92. LaRowe SD, Mardikian P, Malcolm R, et al. Safety and tolerability of N-acetylcysteine in cocaine-dependent individuals. Am J Addict. 2006;15:105–10.

93. Martell BA, Mitchell E, Poling J, Gonsai K, Kosten TR. Vaccine pharmacotherapy for the treatment of cocaine dependence. Biol Psychiatry. 2005;58(2):158–64.

94. Dutra L, Stathopoulou G, Basden SL, Leyro TM, Powers MB, Otto MW. A meta-analytic review of psychosocial interventions for substance use disorders. Am J Psychiatry. 2008;165(2): 179–87.

MDMA and LSD

13

A.C. Parrott

Abstract

MDMA is a methamphetamine derivative and powerful CNS stimulant, which is taken at dance clubs and parties under the street name of "ecstasy". MDMA or 3,4-methylene-dioxymethamphetamne is an indirect monoaminergic agonist, leading to increased levels of synaptic serotonin, dopamine, and other neurotransmitters. It also stimulates the hypothalamic–pituitary–adrenal (HPA) axis, increasing the release of many neurohormones. Recreational MDMA users at dance clubs demonstrate an 800% increase in the stress hormone cortisol. In acute terms, most ecstasy users are in a state of hyper-stimulation, and display elements of the serotonin syndrome. This is generally relieved by resting or "chilling out", although it can develop into severe hyperthermia. Medical treatment should focus on immediate rest and cooling. Blood tests are also needed to monitor potential hyponatraemia, when excessive fluid-intake dilutes sodium levels. In the absence of rapid medical intervention, fatalities may occur. Acute MDMA disrupts attention, impairs cognitive processing, and makes car driving hazardous. The period following recreational ecstasy/ MDMA is typified by neurochemical recovery, when feelings of lethargy, irritability, and depression predominate. Thermal stress and prolonged dancing when on-ecstasy can heighten the emergent neuropsychobiological problems. The dependence syndrome with MDMA has a two-factor structure, with compulsive usage and escalating doses/bingeing. Indeed chronic tolerance is almost universal amongst regular users (Table 13.1). Regular ecstasy users can display a range of neuropsychobiological problems, including memory deficits, impaired problem solving, reduced social intelligence, disrupted sleep architecture, sleep apnea, oxidative stress, and reduced immunocompetence (Table 13.2). Psychiatric symptom profiles are often raised. Interactive diathesis-stress models note that prior predisposition factors are exacerbated by repeated metabolic overstimulation. The psychedelic drug LSD is also associated with various psychiatric problems, including psychotic breakdown, paranoia, and perceptual flashbacks. These are most prevalent in regular LSD users. Medical problems with MDMA can include cardiac, renal, and hepatic damage. Neuroimaging indices often show a reduction in serotonin transporter density, consistent with the data on serotonergic neurotoxicity in laboratory animals. These multiple factors have been integrated into metabolic-distress model (Table 13.3). To summarise, MDMA is a powerful acute metabolic stressor, with a range of adverse acute effects, recovery problems, and long-term neuropsychobiological problems. The main problems with LSD are the risk of psychiatric breakdown, especially in susceptible individuals.

A.C. Parrott (✉)
Department of Psychology, Swansea University,
Swansea, SA2 8PPUK, Wales, UK
e-mail: a.c.parrott@swansea.ac.uk

J.C. Verster et al. (eds.), *Drug Abuse and Addiction in Medical Illness: Causes, Consequences and Treatment*,
DOI 10.1007/978-1-4614-3375-0_13, © Springer Science+Business Media, LLC 2012

Learning Objectives

- MDMA or ecstasy is a powerful CNS stimulant.
- It increases synaptic levels of serotonin, dopamine, noradrenaline, and other neurotransmitters.
- Recreational users show an 800% acute increase in the stress hormone cortisol.
- Acute MDMA boosts most mood states. Elation and euphoria generally predominate, although negative moods can also be intensified.
- MDMA impairs hypothalamic thermal control and increases body temperature.
- Medical emergencies need to be treated rapidly by rest and cooling, with blood tests for potential hyponatraemia.
- Car driving can be "extremely dangerous" in ecstasy/MDMA polydrug users.
- The days after ecstasy are typified by low moods, lethargy, tiredness, and depression.
- The dependence syndrome for MDMA is bi-factorial, with compulsive use, and escalating usage/bingeing.
- The long-term effects of regular usage can include memory deficits, higher cognitive deficits in reasoning, disturbed sleep architecture, sleep apnea, impaired sexual performance, reduced immunocompetence, and oxidative stress.
- Factors affecting these psychobiological changes include lifetime MDMA usage, intensive single session usage, thermal distress, and prolonged dancing when on-drug.
- Most ecstasy users are polydrug users, and these other drugs will contribute to the neuropsychobiological profiles.
- Psychiatric aspects may be interpreted via the diathesis-stress model, where predisposition factors interact with psychoactive drug use to heighten psychiatric distress.
- Metabolic distress provides an integrative factor for understanding the acute and chronic effects of MDMA [1].
- LSD causes perceptual distortions and can generate ideas of reference and paranoia.
- Diathesis-stress models may help to explain the increased risk of psychotic breakdown in susceptible LSD users.

Issues that Need to Be Addressed by Future Research

- The effect of MDMA on basic cell metabolism in humans.
- The long-term effects of regular MDMA use on basic cellular metabolic processes (viz. its potential for programmed cell death or apoptosis).
- The role of cumulative acute metabolic stress for the long-term neuropsychobiological problems of regular users.
- Plasma MDMA levels and psychobiological indices.
- Follow-up studies of medical emergency treatments for hyponatraemia and hyperthermia.
- The role of neurohormones (cortisol, oxytocin, others) in the acute, sub-acute, and chronic effects of MDMA.
- Closer integration between structural and functional MDMA studies.
- Dynamic models of psychoactive drug interactions.
- Contributory role of co-factors such as noise, dehydration, overcrowding, and physical exertion.
- Effects of MDMA on occupational skills and real world problem solving.
- Emotional information processing, interpersonal skills, and social intelligence, in drug-free recreational ecstasy users.
- Acute LSD effects on standard test batteries for mood and cognition.
- Long-term effects of regular LSD usage, on mood, cognition, health, and well-being.

MDMA Pharmacokinetics

Molecular structure of 3,4 Methylenedioxymethamphetamine (MDMA).

(continued)

(continued)

MDMA is normally taken as "ecstasy" pills or tablets, which typically contain around 75 mg. In recent years, ecstasy powders have also become popular, and they may be taken nasally. Some heavy users with chronic tolerance to MDMA [1] progress to MDMA injections. In a survey of 329 regular ecstasy users, 54 reported injecting MDMA [2]. One reason was the increased rush/high, although three-quarters had switched back to oral/intranasal route, as the feelings were too intense, the post-injection come-down was too rapid, stronger dependency, and increased health problems. MDMA is such a powerful CNS stimulant, that injecting only occurs in experienced users [3]. De la Torre et al. [4] administered single oral doses of 50 mg, 75 mg, 100 mg, 125 mg, 150 mg MDMA to human volunteers, and reported non-linear pharmacokinetics. They noted that a relatively small increase in MDMA could give rise to a disproportionate increase in drug plasma levels. The average t_{max} values were 1.5–3.0 h, and the half-life values ranged between 6 and 8 h. MDMA is metabolised, by n-demethylation, to 3,4-metheylene-dioxyamphetamine or MDA. This has similar psychoactive properties to MDMA [5], but has a slightly longer t_{max} and half-life. For fuller description of the metabolism of MDMA and MDA, see de la Torre et al. [3], or Green et al. [6]. The renal clearance of MDMA is relatively constant [3]. The hepatic breakdown of MDMA is via the CYP2D2 liver enzymes. Around 10% of the Caucasian population are deficient in CYP2D2, and this may make them more susceptible to adverse drug reactions [3, 5, 6]. In a field study of 12 dance clubbers [7], plasma levels were zero at predrug baseline, increased to 1,524 ng/dl (range 74–7,025) at 1 h, and 3,447 ng/dl (range 396–17,166) at 2.5 h. The wide variation in plasma levels was particularly noticeable. Future studies should investigate the relationship between plasma levels and psychobiological functioning.

Ecstasy/MDMA Usage

In the early 1980s MDMA was first used by Californians in search of pleasure and spiritual enlightenment [8–10]. Their weekend sessions in retreats have often been described as "psychotherapeutic", although this was of a very informal nature [8]. Most the participants at these weekend retreats were friends and acquaintances, and no formal measures of change were recorded. The on-drug experiences were often

extremely positive, although negative reactions also occurred, especially in those with previous psychiatric history. Greer and Tolbert [8] therefore warned against the use of MDMA with vulnerable individuals: "There is an indication that MDMA may predispose people to a recurrence of previous psychological disabilities" [10]. Laboratory research showed that MDA and MDMA were neurotoxic in animals, since they damage the distal axon terminals of serotonin neurons. The parent compound methamphetamine was an established neurotoxin, but MDA and MDMA were found to be much more damaging to the nerve terminals [11, 12].

During the middle years of the 1980s, the use of MDMA spread to youth culture, and the rave scene was born. All-night dance parties on the Balearic Island of Ibiza stimulated similar events in London and other European cities. In America the use of MDMA was mainly used at college campuses [13]. In those early days each "ecstasy" experience would be planned in advance. Most users would take a single tablet with their friends, then dance throughout the night before "crashing out" and sleeping. The inter-dosing interval trip was typically measured in weeks. In an interview survey of 100 MDMA users at an American college [14], most stated that waited 2–3 weeks between dosing, since "the good effects of the drug appear to diminish while the negative side-effects appear to increase if the drug is taken too frequently". During this period there was widespread recognition that MDMA was a very powerful stimulant, and it should not be mixed with other psychoactive drugs. The number of occasions it was being taken was also quite small. Peroutka et al. [13] noted that 66% of users in their survey had taken it between 1 and 5 occasions in total, and only 12% having taken MDMA more than 10 occasions. Solowij et al. [15] noted very similar findings in an Australian survey. Its popularity increased throughout the 1990s, so that demand often outstripped supply. This led to many "ecstasy" tablets not containing MDMA, and for several years tablet impurity was an issue, with various other chemicals being sold as ecstasy (see Table 13.2 in [16]). The impurity problem was eventually resolved, and by the end of the millennium most tablets sold as ecstasy contained MDMA. Since then purity rates have generally remained high at around 90–100%, although impure supplies still occur [16].

Acute Effects of Ecstasy/MDMA in Recreational Users

Ecstasy/MDMA is mostly taken at dance clubs and parties [17–19]. In surveys of young people around 5–15% report having taken it, whereas the equivalent percentage for dance clubbers is 80–90% [18, 20]. MDMA is a powerful indirect agonist for serotonin and dopamine [6]. In laboratory animals, the environmental conditions can also affect this neurotransmitter release. Temperature is particularly important, since MDMA impairs hypothalamic thermal control [21]. Hence laboratory rats overheat when given MDMA in a hot thermal environment [21]. The extent of MDMA-induced serotonergic neurotoxicity is also heightened by each 2°C increase in ambient temperature [22]. Hydration is another important factor, with water-deprivation increasing the hyperthermic response [23]. Social crowding in animals also increases the effects of CNS stimulant drugs such as methamphetamine, leading to "aggregate toxicity" [24].

These environmental co-factors can have important implications for recreational users. Dance clubs and raves are typified by loud music, bright light shows, dense crowds, and vigorous dancing. All these factors help to optimise environmental stimulation, Suy et al. [25] noted that at a Dutch rave of 14,000 dancers, the disc jockey employed massive auditory and visual sensory stimulation "to achieve a state of heightened arousal". An American ecstasy user recalled that felt they "had a stereo inside my body", while another commented that all their body sensations were "enhanced and pleasure filled" by ecstasy [26]. This sensory hyper-alertness is confirmed by the psychophysiological changes, with increased heart rate, heightened blood pressure, and faster breathing [27]. MDMA in the medical laboratory has clear stimulant effects [27], but at dance clubs and raves the overall stimulation seems to be much stronger, possibly because of the combined effects of drug and environmental factors [18].

Feeling hot is a typical experience for most ecstasy/MDMA users, along with excessive sweating, feelings of thirst, and dehydration [2, 7, 28]. One American dance clubber noted: "It feels like your blood is 115 degrees Fahrenheit" [26]. These subjective reports are confirmed by objective increase in body temperature, both in the laboratory [27, 29] and in dance clubbers [30]. Hot and cold flushes are also a typical experience for ecstasy using dance clubbers, although a minority may feel cold rather than hot [7]. Many thermally stressed dancers visit the "chill-out" room to rest and recover, although some continue dancing for prolonged periods. Some drink excessive amounts of water and develop hyponatraemia—the dilution of sodium electrolytes in the blood. Acute MDMA leads to mental confusion and poor memory [31], and this may impair the ability to monitor water intake. Rosenson et al. [32] reviewed 1,407 cases of MDMA-attributed hyponatraemia in California, and found a significant over-representation of females. There are several reports of stronger acute abreactions in females, presumably due to lower average body weight and higher plasma concentrations [1].

Sympathomimetic activation occurs with all the recreational stimulants such as amphetamine and cocaine [33]. With MDMA this is also accompanied by elements of the serotonin syndrome, since it causes a massive efflux (80%) of serotonin into the synaptic cleft [6]. In an earlier review [34] I noted: "Many ecstasy-using clubbers can be seen to display mild signs of the serotonin syndrome. Hyperactivity, mental confusion, hyperthermia, and trismus (jaw clenching) are typical on-drug experiences for most ecstasy users [28, 31] …. Ecstasy users sometimes develop stronger signs of serotonergic overactivity… Many inner-city hospitals report that the treatment of adverse drug reactions in clubbers has become part of the usual Saturday night routine". In most users overheating is treated effectively by rest, cooling down, and fluid replacement [25]. However, a minority need more urgent medical attention. White [35] recommended that acute methamphetamine and MDMA toxicity should be treated by aggressive cooling and sedation, with titratable agents being used for any cardiovascular abnormalities. Rusniak and Sprague [36] noted the need to clinically differentiate between hyperthermic syndromes induced by different drugs and toxins. With the serotonin syndrome induced by MDMA, a serotonergic antagonist such as cyproheptadine or chlorpromazine was recommended. This was contrasted with the Neuroleptic Malignant Syndrome, found in patients being treated with neuroleptics. Benzodiazepines were recommended as the safest option when these two syndromes could not be clinically differentiated (e.g. schizophrenics who have taken ecstasy). Hall and Henry [37] described the physiological abreactions to MDMA and outlined the best treatment options. They also noted: "Hyperpyrexia and multi-organ failure are now relatively well known, other serious effects have become apparent more recently. Patients with acute MDMA toxicity may present to doctors working in Anaesthesia, Intensive Care and Emergency Medicine. A broad knowledge of these pathologies and their treatment is necessary for those working in an acute medicine speciality".

Despite aggressive medical interventions, physical deterioration is sometime impossible to reverse, with fatal outcomes. Henry et al. [38] described MDMA-induced fatalities in seven young party-goers, whose body temperatures in the Intensive Care ward were all raised (range 40–43°C). Fantegrossi et al. [39] noted that with MDMA-related fatalities: "In almost every case, a recreational dose of the drug had been taken at a dance club or party where crowds danced vigorously". The causes of death can include various forms of organ failure. MDMA induces apoptosis or *programmed cell death* in cultured liver cells [40]. In some cases of liver failure the young person may require a liver transplant [41]. Other causes of rapid death include rhabdomyolysis (destruction of skeletal muscle tissue), disseminated intravascular coagulation (impaired blood clotting with bleeding though multiple sites), cardiac arrest, and brain seizure [6, 26, 37].

Acute MDMA can impair car driving and other psychomotor skills. Logan and Couper [42] reviewed the empirical literature in this area, but also described a number of case studies, often involving MDMA combined with other drugs. Six case studies involved drivers with blood samples positive

Table 13.1 Summary of the acute damaging effects of MDMA

Serotonin syndrome [34]
Metabolic stress [46]
Increased body temperature [29, 37]
Hyponatraemia [32]
Heightened cortisol release [7, 47, 48]
Mental confusion and poor attention [31]
Risky sexual behaviours [49]
Car driving impairments [42, 45]
Disrupted sleep [50–53]
Reduced appetite and food intake [54]
Mid-week depression and aggression [31, 55, 56]
Death [38, 57]

for MDMA alone: "Most subjects displayed muscle twitching and body tremors, dilated pupils, slow pupillary reaction to light, elevated pulse and blood pressure, lack of balance and coordination, and most were perspiring profusely"—despite their MDMA blood levels being described as not-excessive. On standard police sobriety tests they performed poorly, yet they were also described as being cooperative with the police. Logan and Couper [42] noted that in driving simulator studies, performance skills were sometimes only minimally impaired. Ramaekers et al. [43] also showed minimal performance changes, although "tracking accuracy" was improved (reflecting CNS alerting/stimulation), while "compensatory overshoot in braking" was impaired (reflecting poorer cognitive integration). Most simulator studies have involved low doses of MDMA. However, in applied human psychopharmacology, it is important to closely mimic the real world situation [44]. Brookhuis et al. [45] undertook such a hybrid study, with driving simulator performance being assessed under three real world scenarios: self-administered recreational ecstasy/MDMA, recreational MDMA-polydrug at a party, and drug-free control. Driving was significantly impaired by MDMA alone, and was further impaired after the MDMA-polydrug usage at the party. Brookhuis et al. [45] concluded that driving while on MDMA alone was "certainly not safe", whereas driving after partying on MDMA and other drugs was "extremely dangerous". Logan and Couper [42] similarly concluded that: "MDMA use is not consistent with safe driving", and that: "Impairments of various types may persist for a considerable time after last use" (Table 13.1).

Post-MDMA Recovery

Recreational ecstasy/MDMA is followed by low moods and feelings during the period of neurotransmitter depletion and recovery. Parrott and Lasky [31] prospectively monitored ecstasy users and non-users while at a Saturday night dance party, and during the days afterwards. The predominant post-MDMA feelings were of tiredness, lethargy, irritability, unpleasantness, and reduced sociability. Curran and Travill [58] noted that some users developed feelings of depression which occasionally reached clinical levels. Turner et al. [54] showed that another important psychobiological change during the post-MDMA recovery period was poor appetite, with reduced calorific intake for several days afterwards. Curran et al. [55] showed that subjective feelings of aggression were heightened mid-week, while behavioural measures of aggression were also increased. Hoshi et al. [56] confirmed this mid-week aggression occurred in both males and females.

Jones et al. [50] demonstrated that sleep was significantly impaired for several days after ecstasy. The reduction in total sleep time was accompanied by subjective complaints of decreased energy and other psychological impairments. The problems occurred on days 2–5 post-MDMA, and recovered to baseline by day 7. Indeed in all of the above studies, psychobiological functioning had returned to normal within the week (review: [1]). Since MDMA can also impair memory, it has been suggested that the memory deficits may be caused by poor sleep. However, Montgomery et al. [59] re-analysed their cognitive deficits in syllogistic reasoning, computational span, and paired associated learning, but when the sleep measures were included as covariates: "The effects of ecstasy on all cognitive measures remained significant". Blagrove et al. [60] investigated cognitive functioning and sleep in four groups of regular dance clubbers; again the memory impairments of the recent ecstasy users remained significant after controlling for sleep. Hence sleep and cognition are being impaired independently.

MDMA Dependence and Tolerance

It has taken many years for the dependency potential of MDMA to become recognised. In this respect MDMA is similar to every other CNS stimulant. When cocaine was first used in mid-Victorian era, it was initially thought to be non-problematic. Pope Leo XIII was very fond of Vin Mariani, an intoxicating mixture of cocaine and fortified wine. The Pope gave a gold medal to the originator of this powerful cocktail, citing Monsieur Mariani as a "benefactor for humanity". It took several decades for its addictiveness to become accepted. When amphetamine was first developed, it was initially marketed as a safe tonic and non-addictive stimulant; again it took many years for this belief to be reversed (Chap. 4 in [33]). In the early years of recreational ecstasy, there were few indications of drug dependence [9, 15]. This led to the erroneous belief that MDMA does not have an addiction potential. However in recent years, a number studies have demonstrated ecstasy tolerance, dependency, and cravings [61–65].

The first empirical demonstration of ecstasy dependence was published by Topp et al. in 1997 [61]. They interviewed 185 regular ecstasy users with the Composite International Diagnostic Interview (CIDI). Dependence on MDMA was apparent in 64% of the sample during their period of highest usage—generally one or two sessions per week. Dependence was linked with various indices of everyday distress, including interpersonal, financial, criminal, and occupational problems. These lifestyle problems were statistically associated with ecstasy/MDMA usage, rather than other recreational drugs. In an American study, Cottler et al. [62] interviewed 52 recent ecstasy users via the CIDI Substance Abuse Module. The most prevalent dependence indicator was "continuing to use despite knowledge of physical or psychological harm (64%), while ecstasy withdrawal symptoms (59%) were also noted". In overall terms, 43% of the sample met DSM-IV criteria for dependence, 34% met the DSM-IV criteria for abuse, and 23% met neither criterion for abuse or dependence. The assessment battery had high test–retest agreement, indicating that the MDMA dependence syndrome was reliable and robust.

Topp et al. [61] showed that MDMA dependence had a bifactorial structure, with two components, compulsive and escalating use. "Compulsive usage" loaded on questions such as continuing to use despite ecstasy-induced problems, unsuccessful attempts at cessation, and spending an excessive amount of time and effort in obtaining MDMA and using it. The "escalating usage" factor loaded on needing higher doses, taking it for longer than intended, and periods of bingeing. Most regular users take serial repeated doses, while some heavy users have continuous binges which last 48 h or more [2]. This is broadly similar to the 2–3 day binges of some heavy cocaine users. Bruno et al. [63] confirmed the same two-factor structure for MDMA dependency, in a large study of 1662 regular ecstasy users. The two assessment measures comprised the DSM-IV dependency scale and Severity of Dependence (SDS) scale. Amphetamine and cocaine generally demonstrate a unifactorial structure on the Severity of Dependence Scale [63]. Hence the ecstasy dependence syndrome differs from that found with other CNS stimulants [61–65].

Craving is a classic symptom of drug dependence [33, 66], although ecstasy cravings are limited to the periods when it is normally used. Hopper et al. [67] monitored a group of 22 regular ecstasy users over a 6 week period. A wrist actigraph allowed the times of drug taking to be recorded, while ecstasy cravings were completed at preset times. Cravings remained low over most days, but increased over the 24 h preceding MDMA usage. Hopper et al. [67] commented that cravings for the more traditional drugs of dependence (opiates, nicotine, cocaine) often remain low, only to increase under the appropriate environmental cues. Since MDMA is mostly taken only at weekends, this explains why cravings generally only occur then. However, a minority of heavy ecstasy users take it more frequently than once per week. Their intensive patterns of usage are accompanied by stronger ecstasy dependency, and multiple psychobiological problems [3]. One very heavy ecstasy/MDMA user: "Sold everything he owned so he could buy MDMA, alcohol and go clubbing. He sold his television, video and clothes. He would go without sleep for days, and would not eat" ([3]; see also [68]).

In 1986, Alexander Shulgin [9] suggested that: "MDMA does not lend itself to overuse because its most desirable effects diminish with frequency of use". Subsequent studies have confirmed the development of tolerance to MDMA, with Verheyden et al. [69] reporting that 90% of recreational users noted a decline in subjective efficacy. However, when chronic tolerance develops with other recreational stimulants, most users simply increase their self-dosing [33], and this also occurs with MDMA. Scholey et al. [70] noted that most novice ecstasy users took 1 or 2 tablets, whereas more experienced users sometimes took 10 or more tablets per session. Some very heavy users consume even more, with one of the problematic users in Janssen [3] "taking 25–30 tablets each weekend". Soar et al. [68] noted similar heavy usage. The hepatic, neuroadaptive, and neurotoxic changes, which underlie chronic tolerance to MDMA, in both animals and humans, are detailed elsewhere [71].

Psychobiological Problems in Regular Ecstasy/MDMA Users

Recreational ecstasy/MDMA users can display a range of neuropsychobiological problems. The first to be described were memory deficits [72], and these have been confirmed in numerous subsequent studies [1, 5, 73–75]. Retrospective memory is often impaired, with the Rivermead Paragraph Recall test, and Rey Auditory Verbal Learning task, showing deficits in numerous studies (review: [1]). Prospective memory, or remembering to do things in the future, is also often impaired in drug-free users [76–78]. This has practical implications for MDMA research. We now routinely phone participants to remind them of an impending test session, in order to minimise the frequent missed appointments we suffered in earlier studies. Spatial memory is also impaired in regular ecstasy/MDMA users [79], although we have not found it necessary to send out maps. In general, memory deficits are often demonstrable after 50 occasions of usage [1], although some studies have found deficits after just 10 occasions [31, 80]. In one prospective study, Schildt et al. [81] demonstrated significant deficits in immediate and delayed verbal recall and verbal recognition, after an average total consumption of 3.2 ecstasy tablets.

Table 13.2 Summary of the chronic damaging effects of MDMA

Memory problems [31, 60, 73–79, 81, 88, 89]
Impaired problem solving and other cognitive deficits [77, 79, 80, 82, 89, 90]
Social intelligence impaired [84]
Serotonergic neurotoxicity [80, 86, 87, 91]
Oxidative stress [92]
Neurohormonal changes [47, 48]
Immunocompetence reduced [93, 94]
Psychiatric problems [52, 64, 95, 96]
Substance abuse disorders [1, 97]
Sexual interest/ability reduced [98]
Increased risk of sexually transmitted diseases [99]
Sleep apnoea [100]
Interpersonal problems and occupational difficulties [2, 101]
Chronic tolerance to MDMA [9, 69, 71]
Ecstasy dependence and cravings [61, 63, 65, 102]
Food cravings [17]
Cardiac, hepatic, and renal damage [40, 41]

The other main area of cognitive deficits for ecstasy users is higher executive processing. The frontal cortex is important for many intellectual activities, such as organising complex material, decision taking, and integrating memory-related skills [76]. Montgomery and Fisk [82] showed that drug-free ecstasy users were significantly impaired on visual and verbal aspects of frontal information updating. Fox et al. [83] showed that ecstasy users displayed deficits on some difficult cognitive tasks, especially those with a temporal lobe component. Reay et al. [84] showed that ecstasy users were significantly impaired on various tasks of social intelligence. The authors suggested that these cognitive deficits may have reflected reduced serotonergic neurotransmission in the prefrontal cortex. This leads to the general topic of serotonergic neurotoxicity. In laboratory animals, MDMA selectively damages serotonin nerve terminals, but it is not straightforward to extrapolate the animal data to humans [85]. There have been a number of neuroimaging studies with humans, involving EEG, PET, MRI, and fMRI (reviews: [86, 87]). Significant deficits have been demonstrated in various brain regions, such as the hippocampus. Many of the findings are consistent with the notion of serotonergic neurotoxicity, although there is also considerable variance in the emergent data [86]. Nevertheless, Cowan et al. [87] noted in their most recent review: "Neuropsychological, neuroendocrine, and neuroimaging studies have all suggested that human MDMA users may have long-lasting changes in brain function consistent with 5-HT toxicity" (Table 13.2).

Serotonin is involved in a wide range of psychobiological functions, and many of these are also impaired in recreational MDMA users. In an overnight EEG study, Allen et al. [51] showed that drug-free MDMA users had significantly less stage-2 sleep than non-user controls. Parrott et al. [52] reported that heavy ecstasy users complained of more "restless sleep" than non-user controls. McCann et al. [53] reviewed the literature on MDMA and sleep, and debated their findings in relation to altered serotonin functioning. More recently, the Johns Hopkins group have reported that drug-free ecstasy users display a higher incidence of sleep apnoea, with the incidence of apnoea being significantly associated with lifetime MDMA usage [103]. This finding had not been predicted by the psychobiologists involved in the study, since their original concern had been changed in sleep architecture. However, the thoracic surgeons were not surprised, since serotonin is involved in breathing control.

Acute MDMA tends to delay ejaculation and orgasm, and hence it is sometimes used to prolong sexual intercourse and enhance sensory pleasures. However, when used for sex it is often accompanied by medically hazardous practices, such as multiple partners, and penetration without condoms [104]. This increases the risk of sexual transmitted diseases including HIV-AIDS. Theall et al. [99] reported that 79% of heavy ecstasy users had been tested for HIV, although a significant minority also stated that they had "no chance" of contacting the HIV virus. MDMA is often used within the gay community. Degenhardt [49] compared the patterns of ecstasy use amongst males and females grouped according to sexuality. The homosexual/bisexual men and women were more likely than the heterosexuals to use other recreational drugs such as crystal methamphetamine, to have multiple sexual partners, and to inject drugs. Finally, the regular use of MDMA to enhance sex can lead to more sexual problems in the longer term. Soar et al. [98] reported a higher incidence of "decrease in sexual desire, physical problems with sex, and difficulty in achieving orgasm", in a group of drug-free ecstasy users compared to polydrug user controls.

Any psychobiological function which is acutely enhanced by a psychoactive drug is likely to become more problematic in the longer term, due to adaptive neuropsychobiological processes [33]. This can explain the acute sexual changes, and the longer terms sexual problems of regular users noted above. It may also help to explain the similar data on neurohormonal functioning. Acute MDMA has a powerful stimulatory effect on neurohormones such as cortisol. In the medical laboratory, acute MDMA leads to an increase of around 100–150% in cortisol [47]. In dance clubbers, MDMA (biochemically confirmed) leads to a cortisol increase of around 800% [7]. In regular ecstasy uses, the repeated overstimulation of the HPA axis may be having long terms neuropsychobiological effects [1, 7]. For instance, Harris et al. [47] showed that drug free ecstasy users showed altered levels of cortisol functioning. Similar chronic changes may also occur with the other neurohormones [7, 105]. Regular users

Table 13.3 Bio-energetic stress in recreational ecstasy/MDMA users: main contributory factors and theoretical predictions (after [1])

Acute MDMA heightens neurotransmitter release for several hours, leading to acute metabolic distress in the serotonergic pre-synapse, greater oxidative stress, and impaired cellular recovery/repair. Hence intensive MDMA usage will be more damaging.

Chronic MDMA repeated sessions of acute metabolic stress lead to more chronic distress. Hence chronic use will lead to more neuropsychobiological problems over time.

MDMA tolerance will lead to increased self-dosing in parallel with reduced efficacy. This will contribute to more drug-related problems over time.

MDMA dependence and situational cravings will facilitate continued drug use, despite the emergence of further drug-related problems.

Other CNS stimulants such as amphetamine, cocaine, and nicotine, may heighten acute metabolic stress, and independently add to general neuropsychobiological distress.

Temperature. High temperature increase serotonergic neurotoxicity in rats. MDMA increases body temperature in animals and humans. The increase in acute metabolic distress will be greater when MDMA is taken under hot conditions.

Exercise/dancing will add to the metabolic stress of ecstasy/MDMA users and contribute to overheating and dehydration. It will exacerbate psychobiological/cognitive problems.

Nutrition. MDMA can reduce appetite and lead to weight loss. This may exacerbate the bio-energetic stressors of stimulant drugs such as MDMA.

Immunocompetence. MDMA can reduce immunocompetence. This may further impair the ability of the body to handle the repeated stress of stimulant drug usage.

of ecstasy also demonstrate reduced levels of immunocompetence [93, 94], and greater oxidative stress [92]. Darvesh and Gudelsky [46] noted that MDMA is an acute metabolic stressor. Indeed, the regular experience of acute metabolic stress will lead in a cumulative fashion to greater neuropsychobiological distress. This explanatory model is described more fully elsewhere [1, 48], but is summarised here (Table 13.3).

The metabolic stress model notes that the rate of development of psychobiological problems is dependent on several factors (Table 13.3). Two of the most important will be the intensity of ecstasy usage at each session, and cumulative or lifetime usage. MacInnes et al. [106] noted that scores on the Beck Depression Inventory (BDI) were significantly associated with the number of ecstasy tablets taken in a 12 h period. Thomasius et al. [107] found that psychopathology and structural aspects of serotonin integrity were "best predicted" by the number of ecstasy tablets generally taken. Topp et al. [2] reported that bingeing on ecstasy was statistically associated with more physical and psychological problems. Soar et al. [98] found a significant correlation between the average ecstasy dosage, and self-reported sexual dysfunctioning. Verheyden et al. [69] noted a positive correlation between the amount of MDMA normally taken, with Speilberger

anxiety and Hamilton depression scores. Zhou et al. [92] noted that various markers for oxidative stress, such as lipoperoxide levels, superoxide dismutase activity in erythrocytes, were significantly higher amongst drug-free MDMA users than healthy controls. Furthermore, the oxidative stress markers correlated both daily MDMA dosage, and with overall duration of usage.

Lifetime usage is also crucially important, with many studies demonstrating that heavy ecstasy users are significantly more impaired than light users. Fox et al. [79] found that spatial memory and logical problems solving were both significantly related to lifetime dosage. On the problem solving task (Tower of London), the illicit polydrug user controls took an average of 6.5 s, the low ecstasy user group took 8.9 s, the medium ecstasy user group took 9.8 s, while the heavy ecstasy users took an average of 15.3 s, to plan each solution. Fisk et al. [90] similarly found that logical reasoning impairments were correlated with lifetime ecstasy/MDMA usage; the authors also noted that heavy ecstasy users showed "qualitative changes" in their attempts at problem solving. In a psychophysiolgical study, Mejias et al. [108] noted that response latencies on a visual event-related-potential (ERP) task were significantly related to ecstasy usage. In an extensive review, Morgan [75] noted the crucial role of lifetime usage: "Chronic, heavy recreational use of ecstasy is associated with sleep disorders, depressed mood, persistent elevation of anxiety, impulsivity and hostility, and selective impairment of episodic memory, working memory and attention". The role of lifetime dosage is also apparent in the reports from users themselves, with far more problems being reported by the heavier users. In an Internet study [88] the following rates of ecstasy-attributed problems were noted by the experienced users: weight loss by 48%, poor sleep 52%, depression 65%, poor concentration 70%, poor memory 73%, and mood fluctuation by 80%.

Most ecstasy users are polydrug users, and these other psychoactive drugs will also affect neuropsychobiological functions [97]. Cannabis is taken by around 90–95% of ecstasy users [109]. Cannabis can cause memory problems, which raises the question of whether the memory deficits of ecstasy-cannabis polydrug users are due to MDMA, or cannabis, or both [77, 110–112]. These and many similar studies are reviewed in Parrott [1]. The main conclusion was that the lifetime usage of cannabis and ecstasy were the two crucial factors. For instance, in Croft et al. [110], the mean lifetime use of cannabis was 10,000 occasions, whereas the mean lifetime use of ecstasy was 40 occasions; this may help to explain why the observed cognitive deficits were associated with cannabis. In contrast, in Croft et al. [111] the average cannabis use was more modest at 2.3 joints per week, whereas the mean lifetime use of MDMA was far higher at 225 tablets; the psychobiological deficits were associated with

MDMA rather than cannabis. In many studies, cannabis and MDMA are *both* associated with neuropsychobiological problems—probably because each drug was being used regularly (review: [1]). However, the overall picture is even more complex, since cannabis and MDMA have opposing properties in three key areas: MDMA is a powerful CNS stimulant, whereas cannabis is a sedative/relaxant; MDMA is hyperthermic, whereas cannabis is hypothermic; MDMA increases oxidative stress, whereas cannabinoids are powerful antioxidants [109]. Hence MDMA and cannabis show some opposing/interactive properties [113]. In laboratory animals, cannabis can attenuate the acute effects of MDMA [114]. In recreational ecstasy users, light/moderate cannabis can ameliorate some indices of psychological distress, whereas heavy cannabis use can exacerbate psychopathological problems [64].

Scholey et al. [70] revealed that 69% of ecstasy users had also taken amphetamine, 60% had used LSD, while 56% had experience of psilocybin mushrooms; these rates were all far higher than with non-ecstasy users. Furthermore the use of cocaine, amphetamine, LSD, and magic mushrooms, was significantly higher amongst heavy compared to light MDMA users. Ecstasy users are also more likely to use legal psychoactive drugs such as alcohol and tobacco [95]; these other drugs will all contribute to the adverse neuropsychobiological profiles of ecstasy. Hence it is important to note that the deficits remain after statistically controlling for the influence of other drugs ([74, 79, 89, 90, 106, 115, 116], other studies). Although most ecstasy users take other drugs, there is an intriguing study by Halpern et al. [117], of sole ecstasy users from Salt Lake City in the USA. For religious reasons they avoided most psychoactive substances, including alcohol, nicotine, and cannabis, yet ecstasy/MDMA was sometimes used. Those with less than 50 ecstasy/MDMA experiences/lifetime displayed similar cognitive performance to the non-user controls. Whereas the more experienced ecstasy users (+50 occasions) demonstrated significant deficits on cognitive tasks involving working memory. In a study from China, Zhou et al. [92] investigated 120 young "self-confessed" MDMA users, where the exclusion criteria included cigarette smoking, drug, and alcohol abuse. Every marker for oxidative stress was significantly increased, with these biochemical stress markers correlating with lifetime MDMA usage. Finally, prolonged dancing while on MDMA, and extreme levels of thermal distress, can also affect the extent of psychobiological problems of recreational users [118].

Psychiatric Aspects of MDMA

Recreational ecstasy/MDMA is also associated with various forms of psychiatric distress. In a number of early reports, young recreational users complained of various clinical problems which were subsequently confirmed during formal psychiatric interviews [17, 119, 120]. In larger scale surveys, recreational ecstasy users also report significantly higher rates of psychiatric distress than non-user controls [52, 95, 106, 121]. The problems can include depression, anxiety, phobic anxiety, paranoia, bulimia, and impulsivity. In many of these surveys other types of illicit polydrug user also demonstrated raised psychiatric symptom profiles [95]. Various explanations have often been offered. The use of psychoactive drugs such as MDMA may directly cause psychopathological distress; for instance, Alati et al. [96] showed that MDMA was direly linked with the development of psychiatric problems. Susceptible individuals may also be overrepresented amongst ecstasy and other drug users; Lieb et al. [122] demonstrated this in a prospective study. Many cases will reflect a complex amalgam of both factors [1].

Diathesis-stress models [123] provide a theoretical framework for how internal predisposition factors interact with the biological stress of stimulant drug usage. It is important to note that every psychiatric concept is dimensional. Feelings of anxiety, irritability, impulsivity, stress, and depression are normal for everyone. The formal clinical diagnosis will depend on reaching a standard clinical criterion on a continuous scale (viz: an established clinical cut-off score). Hence everyone is potentially susceptible to a psychiatric drug abreaction—when the stressor is severe enough (viz: posttraumatic stress disorder in robust individuals). Interactive models note that a wide range of psychobiological outcomes can occur, depending on the complex interactions between numerous individual predisposition factors, and multiple drug stressors [123]. Individuals with high loadings on internal predisposition factors (genetic, biochemical, personality, psychiatric), will be at most risk of adverse drug sequelae [1]. Robust individuals will be more able to cope with the stress of repeated drug use, although they will develop problems if enough drug is taken; hence the crucial role of lifetime usage [2, 3, 88, 96, 120].

MacInnes et al. [106] debated their findings of increased depression in drug-free ecstasy users, using an interactive vulnerability model. Butler and Montgomery [124] reported that high ecstasy users displayed higher levels of impulsivity than light ecstasy users. They noted that impulsivity was a personality characteristic for all illicit drug users; they suggested that the repeated use of ecstasy/MDMA had intensified this inherent predisposition, possibly via serotonergic neurotoxicity. More examples of the interactive-stress model are summarised elsewhere [1]. Finally, diathesis-stress models also warn against the use of MDMA for "psychotherapeutic" purposes in clinically vulnerable individuals [10]. Vollenweider et al. [125] investigated the effects of acute MDMA in the laboratory, but excluded potential subjects with a psychiatric disorder (personal or family), and those with high "neuroticism" scores. The reason given was that those personality types were: "particularly liable to prolonged and severe responses to stimulant and hallucinogenic drugs

[126]". The primary concern is that those individuals with psychiatric vulnerability may be particularly prone to drug-induced abreactions [8, 10].

LSD

Lysergic Acid Diethylamide or LSD is one of the most powerful of all psychoactive drugs, since an extremely small dose can induce profound changes in thinking and perception. Its psychoactive properties were discovered accidentally by the research scientist Albert Hofmann, after he ingested a small amount of the drug and experienced: "An uninterrupted stream of fantastic pictures, extraordinary shapes with intense kaleidoscopic play of colours" [33, 127]. Like all good researchers he believed in scientific replication, and so a few days later he self-administered 0.25 mg LSD. He believed this would be a very small amount, but it is now known to be equivalent to *ten* doses. This caused the first "bad trip", with powerful perceptual distortions, paranoid and demonic feelings, and various aspects of ego disintegration. Its long duration of 14 h confirmed the very large dosage [127]. LSD was clinically tested in controlled trials during the 1950s, but no medical uses emerged [33]. In the mid-1960s, Timothy Leary and fellow hippies advocated the use of LSD to "turn-on … tune in … and drop out". Cannabis and LSD were the two main drugs used being during the classic 1960s hippie period. Since then, LSD has become one of the several compounds used by recreational drug users, typically in a polydrug context [33].

The brain areas affected by psychedelic drugs such as LSD include the locus coeruleus and raphe nuclei in the brain stem, which process incoming stimulus input. By enhancing initial stimulus reception, LSD intensifies the resulting perceptual experience. Synaesthesia, or the integration of information from different sense modalities, may also occur. For instance, colours and shapes may alter in time with the prevailing music. Cognitive processes, thoughts and ideas may also be boosted. Sometimes these cognitive insights may be enhancing and revelatory, whereas at other times they may be threatening and disturbing. One of the commonest side-effects of LSD is paranoia—when ideas of self-reference are boosted. Former friends may be misperceived as undercover police agents, and professional clinical support may be required [33, 128]. One of the main problems with LSD is its unpredictability, so that even experienced LSD users can have unpleasant trips. The uncontrolled pressure of new sensations and novel thoughts with LSD, may have similarities to the sensory and cognitive overload of acute schizophrenia.

Most individuals soon recover from any adverse experiences while on LSD, although they can occasionally develop into a more enduring psychotic breakdown. This may occur after a single LSD experience, but more typically they follow its regular usage [128]. In a clinical trial where LSD was given in a medically controlled setting as an "aid" for psychotherapy, around 1–4% of patients developed psychotic breakdowns afterwards [129]. The diathesis-stress model, as already described for MDMA, is again applicable here. This notes that individuals with prior susceptibility are most at risk from developing adverse sequelae, especially with cognitive distorting agents such as LSD. This has been confirmed by Shoval et al. [130], who prospectively monitored the use of recreational drugs in a cohort of young schizophrenic and schizoaffective patients, over 10 years. The recreational use of LSD and solvents were most strongly associated with suicide attempts, while MDMA and alcohol also showed a positive association. Flashbacks, or sudden LSD-like perceptual disturbances when drug-free, are another occupational hazard of users of psychedelic drugs. Batzer et al. [131] noted that the incidence of flashbacks was associated with the number of times LSD had been taken; they also suggested that unwanted flashbacks were a major reason for users ceasing to use it. The cognitive effects of LSD do not seem to have been empirically studied, although in mood terms, LSD can induce acute feelings of alertness, anxiety, and mental confusion [132]. Car driving will also be severely affected, since the profound perceptual distortions would seriously impair any skill requiring psychomotor integrity. However, formal car driving studies do not seem to have been undertaken. Ventegodt and Marrick [133] investigated the associations between various recreational drugs and the quality of life. The use of LSD was associated with a 10% reduction in the quality of life parameters, but more detailed studies are needed. One surprising aspect of LSD is the paucity of studies into its basic psychological and psychophysiological effects. One key are for future research is to assess the acute and chronic effects of LSD, using modern neuropsychobiological assessment batteries similar to those developed for recreational ecstasy/MDMA.

References

1. Parrott AC. MDMA in humans: factors which affect the neuropsychobiological profiles of recreational ecstasy users, the integrative role of bio-energetic stress. J Psychopharmacol. 2006;20:147–63.
2. Topp L, Hando J, Dillon P, Roche A, Solowij N. Ecstasy use in Australia: patterns of use and associated harm. Drug Alcohol Depend. 1999;55:105–15.
3. Jansen KLR. Ecstasy (MDMA) dependence. Drug Alcohol Depend. 1999;53:121–4.
4. De la Torre R, Farre M, Roset PN, Lopez CH, Mas M, Ortuno J, Menoyo E, Pizarro N, Segura J, Cami J. Pharmacology of MDMA in humans. Ann NY Acad Sci. 2000;914:225–37.
5. Parrott AC. Human psychopharmacology of ecstasy (MDMA): a review of fifteen years of empirical research. Hum Psychopharmacol. 2001;16:557–77.

6. Green AR, Mechan AO, Elliott JM, O'Shea E, Colado MI. The pharmacology and clinical pharmacology of 3,4-methylenedioxymethamphetamine (MDMA, "ecstasy"). Pharmacol Rev. 2003;55:463–508.

7. Parrott AC, Lock J, Conner AC, Kissling C, Thome J. Dance clubbing on MDMA and during abstinence from Ecstasy/MDMA: prospective neuroendocrine and psychobiological changes. Neuropsychobiology. 2008;57:165–80.

8. Greer G, Tolbert R. Subjective reports of the effects of MDMA in a clinical setting. J Psychoactive Drugs. 1986;18:319–27.

9. Shulgin AT. The background and chemistry of MDMA. J Psychoactive Drugs. 1986;18:291–304.

10. Parrott AC. The psychotherapeutic potential of MDMA (3,4-methylenedioxymethamphetamine): an evidence-based review. Psychopharmacology. 2007;191:181–93.

11. Ricaurte GA, Bryan G, Strauss L, Seiden LS, Schuster CR. Hallucinogenic amphetamine selectively destroys brain serotonin nerve terminals. Science. 1985;229:986–8.

12. Ricaurte GA, Yuan J, McCann UD. (+-) 3,4-methylenedioxymethamphetamine (MDMA, "Ecstasy")-induced serotonin neurotoxicity: studies in animals. Neuropsychobiology. 2000;42: 5–10.

13. Peroutka SJ, Newman H, Harris H. Subjective effects of 3,4-methylenedioxymethamphetamine in recreational users. Neuropsychopharmacology. 1988;1:273–7.

14. Peroutka SJ. 'Ecstasy': a human neurotoxin? Arch Gen Psychiatry. 1989;46:191.

15. Solowij N, Hall W, Lee N. Recreational MDMA use in Sydney: a profile of ecstasy users and their experiences with the drug. Br J Addict. 1992;87:1161–72.

16. Parrott AC. Is Ecstasy MDMA? A review of the proportion of ecstasy tablets containing MDMA, dosage levels, and the changing perceptions of purity. Psychopharmacology. 2004;173: 234–41.

17. Schifano F. Potential human neurotoxicity of MDMA ('Ecstasy') subjective self-reports, evidence form an Italian drug addiction centre and clinical case studies. Neuropsychobiology. 2000;42: 25–33.

18. Parrott AC. MDMA (3,4-methylenedioxymethamphetamine) or Ecstasy: the neuropsychobiological implications of taking it at dances and raves. Neuropsychobiology. 2004;50:329–35.

19. Leung KS, Cottler LB. Ecstasy and other club drugs: a review of recent epidemiologic studies. Curr Opin Psychiat. 2008;21:234–41.

20. Winstock AR, Griffiths P, Stewart D. Drugs and the dance music scene: a survey of current drug use patterns among a sample of dance music enthusiasts in the UK. Drug Alcohol Depend. 2001; 64:9–17.

21. Dafters RI, Lynch E. Persistent loss of thermoregulation in the rat induced by 3,4-methylenedioxymethamphetamine (MDMA or "ecstasy") but not by fenfluramine. Psychopharmacology. 1998; 138:207–12.

22. Malberg JE, Seiden LS. Small changes in ambient temperature cause large changes in 3,4-methylenedioxymethamphetamine (MDMA)- induced serotonin neurotoxicity and core body temperature in the rat. J Neurosci. 1998;18:5086–94.

23. Dafters R. Hyperthermia following MDMA administration in rats: effects of ambient temperature, water consumption, and chronic dosing. Physiol Behav. 1995;58:877–82.

24. Gunn J, Gurd M. The action of some amines related to adrenaline, Cyclohexylalkylamines. J Physiol. 1940;97:453–70.

25. Suy K, Gijsenbergh F, Baute L. Emergency medical assistance during a mass gathering. Eur J Emerg Med. 1999;6:249–54.

26. Cohen RS. The love drug: marching to the beat of ecstasy. New York: Haworth Medical Press; 1998.

27. Liechti ME, Gamma A, Vollenweider FX. Gender differences in the subjective effects of MDMA. Psychopharmacology. 2001;154: 161–8.

28. Davison D, Parrott AC. Ecstasy in recreational users: self-reported psychological and physiological effects. Hum Psychopharmacol. 1997;12:91–7.

29. Freedman RR, Johanson CE, Tancer ME. Thermoregulatory effects of 3,4-methylenedioxymethamphetamine (MDMA) in humans. Psychopharmacology. 2005;183:248–56.

30. Parrott AC, Young L. Increased body temperature in recreational Ecstasy/MDMA users out clubbing and dancing. J Psychopharmacol. 2005;19:a26.

31. Parrott AC, Lasky J. Ecstasy (MDMA) effects upon mood and cognition; before, during, and after a Saturday night dance. Psychopharmacology. 1998;139:261–8.

32. Rosenson J, Smollin C, Sporer KA, Blanc P, Olson KR. Patterns of ecstasy-associated hyponatremia in California. Ann Emerg Med. 2006;49:164–71.

33. Parrott A, Morinan A, Moss M, Scholey A. Understanding drugs and behaviour. Chichester: Wiley; 2004.

34. Parrott AC. Recreational Ecstasy/MDMA, the serotonin syndrome, and serotonergic neurotoxicity. Pharmacol Biochem Behav. 2002;71:837–44.

35. White SR. Amphetamine toxicity. Semin Respir Crit Care Med. 2002;23:27–36.

36. Rusyniak DE, Sprague JE. Toxin-induced hyperthermic syndromes. Med Clin North Am. 2005;89:1277–96.

37. Hall AP, Henry JA. Acute toxic effects of 'Ecstasy' (MDMA) and related compounds: overview of pathophysiology and clinical management. Br J Anaesth. 2006;96:678–85.

38. Henry JA, Jeffries KJ, Dawling S. Toxicity and deaths from 3,4-methylenedioxymethamphetamine ("Ecstasy"). Lancet. 1992;340:384–7.

39. Fantegrossi WE, Godlewski T, Karabenick RL, Stephens JM, Ullrich T, Rice KC, Woods JH. Pharmacological characterization of the effects of 3,4-methylenedioxymethamphetamine ("ecstasy") and its enantiomers on lethality, core temperature, and locomotor activity in singly housed and crowded mice. Psychopharmacology. 2003;166:202–11.

40. Montiel-Duarte C, Varela-Rey M, Oses-Prieto JA, Lopez-Zabalza MJ, Beitia G, Cenarruzabeitia E, Iraburu MJ. 3,4-Methylenedioxymethamphetamine ("Ecstasy") induces apoptosis of cultured rat liver cells. Biochim Biophys Acta. 2002;1588: 26–32.

41. Smith ID, Simpson KJ, Garden OJ, Wigmore SJ. Non-paracetamol drug-induced fulminant hepatic failure among adults in Scotland. Eur J Gastroenterol Hepatol. 2005;17:161–7.

42. Logan BK, Couper FJ. 3,4-Methylenedioxymethamphetamine (MDMA, ecstasy) and driving impairment. J Forensic Sci. 2001; 46:1426–33.

43. Ramaekers JG, Kuypers KP, Samyn N. Stimulant effects of 3,4-methylenedioxymethamphetamine (MDMA) 75 mg and methylphenidate 20 mg on actual driving during intoxication and withdrawal. Addiction. 2006;101:1614–21.

44. Parrott AC. Assessment of psychological performance in applied situations. In: Hindmarch I, Stonier PD, editors. Human psychopharmacology: methods and measurers, vol. 1. Chichester: Wiley; 1987.

45. Brookhuis KA, de Waard D, Samyn N. Effects of MDMA (ecstasy), and multiple drugs use on (simulated) driving performance and traffic safety. Psychopharmacology. 2004;173: 440–5.

46. Darvesh AS, Gudelsky GA. Evidence for a role of energy dysregulation in the MDMA-induced depletion of brain 5-HT. Brain Res. 2005;21:168–75.

47. Harris DS, Baggott M, Mendelson JH, Mendelson JE, Jones RT. Subjective and hormonal effects of 3,4-methylenedioxymethamphetamine (MDMA) in humans. Psychopharmacology. 2002;162:396–405.

48. Parrott AC. Cortisol and MDMA (3,4-methylenedioxymethamphetamine): neurohormonal aspects of bioenergetic stress in Ecstasy users. Neuropsychobiology. 2009;60:148–58.

49. Degenhardt L. Drug use and risk behaviour among regular ecstasy users: does sexuality make a difference? Cult Health Sex. 2005;7:599–614.

50. Jones KA, Callen F, Blagrove MT, Parrott AC. Sleep, energy and self rated cognition across 7 nights following recreational ecstasy/MDMA use. Sleep Hypn. 2008;10:16–28.

51. Allen RP, McCann UD, Ricaurte GA. Persistent effects of (+/-)3,4-methylenedioxymethamphetamine (MDMA, "ecstasy") on human sleep. Sleep. 1993;16:560–4.

52. Parrott AC, Sisk E, Turner J. Psychobiological problems in heavy 'ecstasy' (MDMA) polydrug users. Drug Alcohol Depend. 2000;60:105–10.

53. McCann UD, Ricaurte GA. Effects of (+/-) 3,4-methylenedioxymethamphetamine (MDMA) on sleep and circadian rhythms. Sci World J. 2007;7:231–8.

54. Turner JJD, Nicolas L, Parrott AC. Reduced calorie intake in the week following weekend MDMA (ecstasy) use. J Psychopharmacol. 1998;12:a43.

55. Curran HV, Rees H, Hoare T, Hoshi R, Bond A. Empathy and aggression: two faces of ecstasy? A study of interpretive cognitive bias and mood change in ecstasy users. Psychopharmacology. 2004;173:425–33.

56. Hoshi R, Pratt H, Mehta S, Bond AJ, Curran HV. An investigation into the sub-acute effects of ecstasy on aggressive interpretative bias and aggressive mood—are there gender differences? J Psychopharmacol. 2006;20:291–301.

57. Schifano F, Oyefeso A, Corkery J, Cobain K, Jambert-Gray R, Martinotti G, Ghodse AH. Death rates from ecstasy (MDMA, MDA) and polydrug use in England and Wales 1996-2002. Hum Psychopharmacol. 2003;18:519–24.

58. Curran HV, Travill RA. Mood and cognitive effects of 3,4-methylenedioxymethamphetamine (MDMA, "ecstasy"): weekend "high" followed by mid-week "low". Addiction. 1997;92:821–31.

59. Montgomery C, Fisk JE, Wareing M, Murphy P. Self reported sleep quality and cognitive performance in ecstasy users. Hum Psychopharmacol. 2007;22:537–48.

60. Blagrove M, Seddon J, George SA, Parrott AC, Morgan MJ, Stickgold R, Walker MP, Jones KA. Procedural and declarative memory task performance, and the memory consolidation function of sleep, in recent and abstinent ecstasy/MDMA users. J Psychopharmacol. 2011;25(4):465–77.

61. Topp L, Hall W, Hando J. Is there a dependence syndrome for ecstasy? Australian National Drug and Alcohol Research Centre Technical Report No. 51. NDARC, Sydney, Australia; 1997.

62. Cottler LB, Womack SB, Compton WM, Ben-Abdallah A. Ecstasy abuse and dependence: applicability and reliability of DSM-IV criteria among adolescents and young adults. Hum Psychopharmacol. 2001;16:599–606.

63. Bruno R, Matthews A, Degenhardt L, Topp L, Gomez R, Dunn M. Can the severity of dependence scale be usefully applied to 'Ecstasy'? Neuropsychobiology. 2008;60:137–47.

64. Milani RM, Parrott AC, Schifano F, Turner JJD. Patterns of cannabis use in ecstasy polydrug users: moderate cannabis use may compensate for self-rated aggression and somatic symptoms. Hum Psychopharmacol. 2005;20:1–13.

65. Milani RM. The nature of Ecstasy dependence. Neuropsychobiology. 2009;60:137–147.

66. Parrott AC. Nicotine psychobiology: how chronic-dose prospective studies can illuminate some of the theoretical issues from acute-dose research. Psychopharmacology. 2006;184:567–76.

67. Hopper JW, Su Z, Looby AR, Ryan ET, Penetar DM, Palmer CM, Lukas SE. Incidence and patterns of polydrug use and craving for ecstasy in regular ecstasy users: an ecological momentary assessment study. Drug Alcohol Depend. 2006;85:221–35.

68. Soar K, Parrott AC, Turner JJD. Persistent neuropsychological problems after seven years of abstinence from recreational Ecstasy (MDMA): a case study. Psychol Rep. 2004;95:192–6.

69. Verheyden SL, Henry JA, Curran HV. Acute, sub-acute and long-term subjective consequences of 'ecstasy' (MDMA) consumption in 430 regular users. Hum Psychopharmacol. 2003;18:507–17.

70. Scholey AB, Parrott AC, Buchanan T, Heffernan T, Ling J, Rodgers J. Increased intensity of Ecstasy and polydrug usage in the more experienced recreational Ecstasy/MDMA users: a www study. Addict Behav. 2004;29:743–52.

71. Parrott AC. Chronic tolerance to recreational MDMA (3,4-methylenedioxymethamphetamine) or Ecstasy. J Psychopharmacol. 2005;19:71–83.

72. Krystal JH, Price LH, Opsahl C, Ricaurte GA, Heninger GR. Chronic 3,4-methylenedioxymethamphetamine (MDMA) use: effects on mood and neuropsychological function? Am J Drug Alcohol Abuse. 1992;18:331–41.

73. Bolla KI, McCann UD, Ricaurte GA. Memory impairment in abstinent MDMA ("Ecstasy") users. Neurology. 1998;51:1532–7.

74. Morgan MJ. Memory deficits associated with recreational use of "ecstasy" (MDMA). Psychopharmacology. 1999;141:30–6.

75. Morgan MJ. Ecstasy (MDMA): a review of its possible persistent psychological effects. Psychopharmacology. 2000;152:230–48.

76. Heffernan TM, Ling J, Scholey AB. Subjective ratings of prospective memory deficits in MDMA ('ecstasy') users. Hum Psychopharmacol. 2001;16:339–44.

77. Rodgers J, Buchanan T, Scholey AB, Heffernan TM, Ling J, Parrott AC. Patterns of drug use and the influence of gender on self reports of memory ability in ecstasy users: a web based study. J Psychopharmacol. 2003;17:379–86.

78. Rendell PG, Gray TJ, Henry JD, Tolan A. Prospective memory impairment in "ecstasy" (MDMA) users. Psychopharmacology. 2007;194:497–504.

79. Fox H, Parrott AC, Turner JJD. Ecstasy/MDMA related cognitive deficits: a function of dosage rather than awareness of problems. J Psychopharmacol. 2001;15:273–81.

80. Jacobsen LK, Mencl WE, Pugh KR, Skudlarski P, Krystal JH. Preliminary evidence of hippocampal dysfunction in adolescent MDMA ("ecstasy") users: possible relationship to neurotoxic effects. Psychopharmacology. 2004;173:383–90.

81. Schilt T, de Win MM, Koeter M, Jager G, Korf DJ, van den Brink W, Schmand B. Cognition in novice ecstasy users with minimal exposure to other drugs: a prospective cohort study. Arch Gen Psychiatr. 2007;64:728–36.

82. Montgomery C, Fisk JE. Ecstasy-related deficits in the updating component of executive processes. Hum Psychopharmacol. 2008;23:495–511.

83. Fox HC, McLean A, Turner JJD, Parrott AC, Rogers R, Sahakian BJ. Neuropsychological evidence of a relatively selective profile of temporal dysfunction in drug-free MDMA ("ecstasy") polydrug users. Psychopharmacology. 2002;162:203–14.

84. Reay JL, Hamilton C, Kennedy DO, Scholey AB. MDMA polydrug users show process-specific central executive impairments coupled with impaired social and emotional judgment processes. J Psychopharmacol. 2006;20:385–8.

85. Eastern N, Marsden CA. Ecstasy: are animal data consistent between species and can they translate to humans? J Psychopharmacol. 2006;20:194–210.

86. Reneman L, de Win MM, van den Brink W, Booij J, den Heeten GJ. Neuroimaging findings with MDMA/ecstasy: technical aspects, conceptual issues and future prospects. J Psychopharmacol. 2006;20:164–75.

87. Cowan RL, Roberts DM, Joers JM. Neuroimaging in human MDMA (Ecstasy) users. Ann NY Acad Sci. 2008;1139:291–8.

88. Parrott AC, Buchanan T, Scholey AB, Heffernan TM, Ling J, Rodgers J. Ecstasy attributed problems reported by novice, moderate and heavy recreational users. Hum Psychopharmacol. 2002;17:309–12.

89. Wareing M, Murphy PN, Fisk JE. Visuospatial memory impairments in users of MDMA ('ecstasy'). Psychopharmacology. 2004; 173:391–7.

90. Fisk JE, Montgomery C, Wareing M, Murphy PN. Reasoning deficits in ecstasy (MDMA) polydrug users. Psychopharmacology. 2005;181:550–9.

91. Huether G, Zhou D, Ryuther E. Causes and consequences of the loss of serotonergic presynapses elicited by the consumption of 3,4-methylenedioxymethamphetamine (MDMA, "ecstasy") and its congeners. J Neural Transmiss. 1997;104:771–7941.

92. Zhou JF, Chen P, Zhou YH, Zhang L, Chen HH. 3,4-methylene-dioxymethamphetamine abuse may cause oxidative stress and potential free radical damage. Free Radic Res. 2003;37:491–7.

93. Pacifici R, Zuccaro P, Farre M, Pichini S, Di Carlo S, Roset PN, Palmi I, Ortuno J, Menoyo E, Segura J, de la Torre R. Cell-mediated immune response in MDMA users after repeated dose administration: studies in controlled versus non-controlled settings. Ann NY Acad Sci. 2002;965:421–33.

94. Connor TJ. Methylenedioxymethamphetamine (MDMA, 'Ecstasy'): a stressor on the immune system. Immunology. 2004;111:357–67.

95. Parrott AC, Milani R, Parmar R, Turner JJD. Ecstasy polydrug users and other recreational drug users in Britain and Italy: psychiatric symptoms and psychobiological problems. Psychopharmacology. 2001;159:77–82.

96. Alati R, Kinner SA, Hayatbakhsh MR, Mamun AA, Najman JM, Williams GM. Pathways to ecstasy use in young adults: anxiety, depression or behavioural deviance? Drug Alcohol Depend. 2008;92:108–15.

97. Wu LT, Parrott AC, Ringwalt CL, Patkar AA, Mannelli P, Blazer DG. The high prevalence of substance use disorders among adult MDMA users compared with former MDMA users and other drug users: implications for intervention. Addict Behav. 2009;34: 654–61.

98. Soar K, Parrott AC, Turner JJD. No more the "love drug": sexual behavior impairments in Ecstasy users. J Psychopharmacol. 2005;19:a25.

99. Theall KP, Elifson KW, Sterk CE. Sex, touch, and HIV risk among ecstasy users. AIDS Behav. 2006;10:169–78.

100. McCann UD, Sgambati FP, Schwartz AR, Ricaurte GA. Sleep apnea in young abstinent recreational MDMA ("ecstasy") consumers. Neurology. 2009;73:2011–7.

101. Parrott AC. Conscious awareness versus optimistic beliefs in recreational Ecstasy/MDMA users. In: Perry E, Collerton D, LeBeau F, Ashton HE, editors. New horizons in the neuroscience of consciousness. Amsterdam: John Benjamins; 2010.

102. Milani RM, Parrott AC. Psychological problems may be associated with Ecstasy dependence rather than Ecstasy lifetime dose. World J Biol Psychiatr. 2004;5:130.

103. McCann UD, Sgambati F, Ricaurte GA. Sleep disturbance in MDMA users. Neuropsychobiology. 2008;60:215.

104. McElrath K. MDMA and sexual behavior: ecstasy users' perceptions about sexuality and sexual risk. Subst Use Misuse. 2005;40: 1461–77.

105. McGregor IS, Callaghan PD, Hunt GE. From ultrasocial to antisocial: a role for oxytocin in the acute reinforcing effects and long-term adverse consequences of drug use? Br J Pharmacol. 2008; 154:358–68.

106. MacInnes N, Handley SL, Harding GFA. Former chronic methylenedioxymethamphetamine (MDMA or ecstasy) users report mild depressive symptoms. J Psychopharmacol. 2001;15:181–6.

107. Thomasius R, Petersen K, Buchert R, Andresen B, Zapletalova P, Wartberg L, Nebeling B, Schmoldt A. Mood, cognition and serotonin transporter availability in current and former ecstasy (MDMA) users. Psychopharmacology. 2003;167:85–96.

108. Mejias S, Rossignol M, Debatisse D, Streel E, Servais L, Guerit JM, Philippot P, Campanella S. Event-related potentials in ecstasy (MDMA) users during a visual oddball task. Biol Psychol. 2005;69:333–52.

109. Parrott AC, Milani RM, Gouzoulis-Mayfrank E, Daumann J. Cannabis and Ecstasy/MDMA (3,4-methylenedioxymethamphetamine): an analysis of their neuropsychobiological interactions in recreational users. J Neural Transmiss. 2007;114:959–68.

110. Croft RJ, Mackay AJ, Mills ATD, Gruzelier JGH. The relative contributions of ecstasy and cannabis to cognitive impairment. Psychopharmacology. 2001;153:373–9.

111. Croft RJ, Mackay AJ, Mills ATD, Gruzelier JGH. Electrophysiological evidence of serotonergic impairment in long-term MDMA ("Ecstasy") users. Am J Psychiatr. 2001;158: 1687–92.

112. Rodgers J. Cognitive performance amongst recreational users of "ecstasy". Psychopharmacology. 2000;151:19–24.

113. Sala M, Braida D. Endocannabinoids and 3,4-methylene-dioxymethamphetamine (MDMA) interaction. Pharmacol Biochem Behav. 2005;81:407–16.

114. Morley KC, Li KM, Hunt GE, Mallet PE, McGregor IS. Cannabinoids prevent the acute hyperthermia and partially protect against the 5-HT depleting effects of MDMA ("Ecstasy") in rats. Neuropharmacology. 2004;46:954–65.

115. Rizzo M, Lamers CTJ, Sauer CG, Ramaekers JG, Bechara A, Anderson GJ. Impaired perception of self-motion (heading) in abstinent ecstasy and marijuana users. Psychopharmacology. 2005;179:559–66.

116. Verkes RJ, Gigsman HJ, Pieters MSM, Schoemaker RC, de Visser S, Kuijpers M. Cognitive performance and serotonergic function in users of Ecstasy. Psychopharmacology. 2001;53: 196–202.

117. Halpern JH, Pope HG, Sherwood AR, Barry S, Hudson JI, Yurgelun-Todd D. Residual effects of illicit 3,4-methylene-dioxymethamphetamine in individuals with minimal exposure to other drugs. Drug Alcohol Depend. 2004;75:135–47.

118. Parrott AC, Rodgers J, Buchanan T, Ling J, Heffernan T, Scholey AB. Dancing hot on ecstasy: physical activity and thermal comfort ratings are associated with the memory and other psychobiological problems of recreational MDMA users. Hum Psychopharmacol. 2006;21:285–98.

119. McCann UD, Ricaurte GA. Lasting neuropsychiatric sequelae of (+-) Methylenedioxymethamphetamine ('Ecstasy') in recreational users. J Clin Psychopharmacol. 1991;11:302–5.

120. Soar K, Turner JJD, Parrott AC. Psychiatric disorders in recreational Ecstasy (MDMA) users: a literature review focusing upon personal predisposition factors and drug histories. Hum Psychopharmacol. 2001;16:641–6.

121. Roiser JP, Sahakian BJ. Relationship between ecstasy use and depression: a study controlling for poly-drug use. Psychopharmacology. 2004;173:411–7.

122. Lieb R, Schuetz CG, Pfister H, von Sydow K, Wittchen H-U. Mental disorders in ecstasy users: a prospective-longitudinal investigation. Drug Alcohol Depend. 2002;68:195–207.

123. Monroe SM, Simmons D. Diathesis-stress theories in the context of life stress research. Psychol Bull. 1991;110:406–25.

124. Butler GKL, Montgomery AMJ. Impulsivity, risk taking and recreational 'ecstasy' (MDMA) use. Drug Alcohol Depend. 2004; 76:55–62.

125. Vollenweider FX, Gamma A, Liechti M, Huber T. Psychological and cardiovascular effects and short-term sequelae of MDMA ("Ecstasy") in MDMA-naive healthy humans. Neuropsychopharmacology. 1998;19:241–51.

126. Dittrich A. Psychological aspects of altered states of consciousness of the LSD type. In: Pletscher A, Ladewig D, editors. Fifty years of LSD: current status and future perspectives of hallucinogens. New York: Parthenon; 1994.

127. Hofmann A. LSD: my problem child. New York: McGraw-Hill; 1980.

128. Boutros NN, Bowers MB. Chronic substance-induced psychotic disorders: state of the literature. J Neuropsychiat Clin Neurosci. 1996;8:262–9.

129. Abraham HD, Aldridge AM. Adverse consequences of lysergic acid diethylamide. Addiction. 1993;88:1327–34.

130. Shoval G, Sever J, Sher L, Diller R, Apter A, Weizman A, Zalsman G. Substance use, suicidality, and adolescent-onset schizophrenia: an Israeli 10-year retrospective study. J Child Adolesc Psychopharmacol. 2006;16:767–75.

131. Batzer W, Ditzler T, Brown C. LSD use and flashbacks in alcoholic patients. J Addict Dis. 1999;18:57–63.

132. Parrott AC, Stuart M. Ecstasy (MDMA), amphetamine, and LSD: comparative mood profiles in recreational polydrug users. Hum Psychopharmacol. 1997;12:501–4.

133. Ventegodt S, Merrick J. Psychoactive dugs and quality of life. Sci World J. 2003;3:694–706.

Inhalants Abuse: Status of Etiology and Intervention

14

Ty. A. Ridenour and Matthew O. Howard

Abstract

Inhalants differ from other psychoactive substances in that thousands of commercial products can produce intoxication and toxicity if inhaled, they are widely available, legal, inexpensive, and easily obtained. Moreover, relatively few parents, retailers, school personnel, law enforcement professionals, or human services workers are vigilant about inhalant use or inhalant-related health and social problems. Numerous medical, cognitive, emotional, and social consequences and correlates of inhalant use have been documented including abuse and dependence. Moreover, little research has tested prevention or treatment programs specifically for inhalant abuse. This chapter summarizes extant research on etiology and clinical practices pertaining to inhalant use and abuse.

Learning Objectives
- Psychopharmacological effects of inhalants appear to categorically differ between nitrites (smooth muscle relaxants) and other inhalants which act upon the central nervous system.
- Damage from inhalant exposure spans neurological, cognitive, affective, cardiovascular, immune, bone, social, and renal systems.
- Historically, research on inhalants has been scant, with such research rapidly increasing in recent years.
- Inhalant use and abuse generally goes undetected by health professionals.
- Although some efforts to curb inhalant use and abuse have been successful, no standardized intervention approach is available.

Ty.A. Ridenour, Ph.D. (✉)
Center for Education and Drug Abuse Research,
University of Pittsburgh, 3520 Forbes Ave., Rm 228,
Pittsburgh, PA 15213, USA
e-mail: tar27@pitt.edu

M.O. Howard
School of Social Work, The University of North Carolina
at Chapel Hill, Tate-Turner-Kuralt Building, Campus Box 3550,
Chapel Hill, NC 27599-3550, USA

Issues that Need to Be Addressed by Future Research
- The only areas of inhalant research characterized by conclusive evidence are prevalence estimates and gender comparisons.

J.C. Verster et al. (eds.), *Drug Abuse and Addiction in Medical Illness: Causes, Consequences and Treatment*,
DOI 10.1007/978-1-4614-3375-0_14, © Springer Science+Business Media, LLC 2012

Inhalant abuse has been researched much less than abuse of other psychoactive substances. Increasingly, inhalant use and abuse are recognized as dangerous and unique among addictive substances [1–3]. Between 2002 and 2004, about 600,000 youths between ages 12 and 17 initiated inhalant use annually in the USA [4]. This chapter summarizes the health risks, epidemiology, and emerging etiology of inhalant use and abuse as well as the tendency among U.S. health professionals to let inhalant use go undetected and untreated.

Heterogeneity of Inhalants

Classifications of inhalants have been proposed based on their delivery mechanisms and behavioral pharmacology. The National Institute on Drug Abuse proffers the most widely recognized categories: volatile solvents, aerosols, gases, and nitrites [5]. *Volatile solvents* vaporize upon opening and include adhesives, correction fluids, felt-tip markers, fuels, and paint thinners and removers. *Aerosols* are sprays that contain both propellants and solvents including personal hygiene products (e.g., deodorants and hair spray), spray paint, and household products (e.g., fabric protector or cooking oil). *Gases* include products that contain gases (butane lighters, propane tanks, refrigerants) and medical anesthetics such as ether, chloroform, halothane, and nitrous oxide. *Nitrites* ("poppers") consist of cyclohexyl nitrite, amyl (or isoamyl) nitrite, or butyl (or isobutyl) nitrite. Some products are sold primarily for recreational use of nitrites (e.g., Rush, Locker Room, and Climax).

Alternatively, DSM-IV nomenclature classifies aerosols and solvents as inhalants but gases and nitrites as "other substances" [6]. Balster suggested classifications based on pharmacological and behavioral effects: alkyl nitrites and nitrous oxide versus "volatile solvents" (solvents, fuels, and anesthetics) [7]. Nitrites are smooth muscle relaxants most frequently used to enhance sexual experience [5, 7]. Although the psychopharmacological profiles of Balster's volatile solvents vary, their effects appear to depend on similar molecular mechanisms in the central nervous system.

Bowen et al. [8] reviewed research on central nervous system mechanisms of inhalants. NMDA receptors are inhibited during acute solvent exposure (especially in the prefrontal cortex, nucleus accumbens, and hippocampus). Animal studies of chronic solvent exposure resembling binge usage in humans demonstrate a recovery of NMDA-evoked responses with a concurrent decrease in GABA-evoked responses, similar to processes that occur during alcohol tolerance and subsequent withdrawal [9]. Lopreato et al. reported that solvent exposure enhanced serotonin-3 receptor functioning, which also resembles alcohol exposure [10].

Animal research collectively suggests that solvent behavioral effects correlate strongly with their impact on $GABA_A$

receptors, with preliminary research implicating neurons in the medial prefrontal cortex, hippocampus, and substantia nigra. Also, resembling other abusable substances, repeated solvent exposure increases dopaminergic neuronal activity in the prefrontal cortex, ventral tegmental area, caudate, and nucleus accumbens. One hypothesis for this increased dopaminergic activity is that it results from changes in the GABA systems. With the relatively scant (but expanding) research on mechanisms underlying inhalant effects, Balster [7] and Paez-Martinez and colleagues [11] argued that further categorization of inhalants ought to be based on scientific evidence of distinct pharmacological and behavioral effects.

Why Be Concerned About Inhalant Use?

Acute Medical Effects

Symptoms of inhalant intoxication include dizziness, nystagmus, incoordination, slurred speech, ataxia, lethargy, depressed reflexes, psychomotor retardation, tremor, generalized muscle weakness, blurred vision, stupor or coma, euphoria, and other signs similar to alcohol intoxication [6]. Intoxication onset occurs rapidly following inhalation and lasts only minutes. Some users repeatedly self-administer inhalants to maintain a preferred level of intoxication [6]. Case reports and clinical studies have documented inhalant-related chemical and thermal burns [12–15], withdrawal symptoms [16], and persistent signs of psychosis [17] following discrete periods of solvent inhalation. Inhalant use can lead to disabling, life-threatening or fatal injuries (e.g., ventricular arrhythmias or "sudden sniffing death") [18–22]. "Sudden sniffing death" can occur when an intoxicated inhalant user is startled; the subsequent release of catecholamines can induce ventricular fibrillation leading to tissue and brain damage or even death.

Neurological and Cognitive Effects

Persistent neurological and cognitive impairments have been attributed to inhalant abuse [23–25]. Studies of occupationally exposed workers provide much of what is known about cognitive deficits due to inhalant exposure, although chemical exposures during recreational inhalant use surpass even toxic occupational exposures [26–29]. Morrow et al. reported significant impairments in learning and memory with slow recovery among journeyman painters [30–33].

Deficits in cognitive and sensory functions associated with occupational and recreational exposures to inhalants include impaired memory, vision, hearing, attention, recall, judgment, Parkinsonism, cerebellar ataxia, encephalopathy, trigeminal neuropathy, hepatotoxicity, and hepatorenal syndrome [34–47]. Neurological damage from inhalant use includes cerebral atrophy, thinning of the corpus collosum, lesions of the white matter with pyramidal tract/cranial nerve signs, and hypointensities of the thalamus/basal ganglia [48, 49]. SPECT findings indicate that inhalant abusers evidence hypoperfusion foci and nonhomogeneous uptake of radiopharmaceuticals [50]. Functional MRI studies indicate that decrements in cerebral blood flow occur after 1 year of inhalant use, whereas white matter changes may take more time to develop [51, 52]. Therefore, earlier identification of characteristic patterns of cognitive dysfunction in inhalant users may facilitate prevention and reduction of inhalant-related neuropsychological damage [26].

Other Chronic Health Consequences

Tenenbein reported a withdrawal syndrome occurs in neonates exposed to inhalants in utero that resembles fetal alcohol syndrome and includes craniofacial dysmorphologies, microencephalopathy, low birth weight, developmental delays, and other pregnancy and birth complications [53, 54]. Inhalants also exert pathophysiological effects across multiple organ systems [55]. Animal studies, case reports, and small clinical investigations implicate inhalant use in hepatotoxicity [56], cardiotoxicity [57], renal toxicity [58], bone demineralization [59], bone marrow suppression, reduced T cell responsivity, and diminished plasma and erythrocyte levels of selenium and zinc [60, 61]. The latter three conditions could predispose to serious infectious diseases. O'Brien et al. reported a case of hepatorenal failure in a 19-year-old who had sniffed glue for 3 years [62]. Wiseman et al. diagnosed irreversible congestive heart failure in a 15-year-old patient who had sniffed glue for 2 years [63]. Moreover, inhalant use increases risk for chronic pain, visual impairments from peripheral neuropathy or optic nerve damage, and other neuropathic conditions [64, 65]. Replicated studies suggest that nitrite use is associated with risk for HIV and HHV-8 and Kaposi's sarcoma [66–68], likely due to nitrite suppression of immune system responses to virus infections and tumor growth including HIV replication [69–71].

Focus groups recently conducted by Ridenour et al., provide case study evidence that even subjective experiences of neuropsychological deficits arise from binge usage of inhalants [3, 72]. Consider the following exchange between one group of participants.

#1: You just feel like out of it, like you can't think very quickly. Like, you've killed a lot of brain cells and you can feel it.
#3: It's like if you do heroin or crack or cocaine, the next day you feel stupid, like I regret I did that. But with [inhalants] you feel like you're kind of lost or something for a minute.
#4: [When doing poppers] we always made sure we were sitting down because I mean you would fall back and you can't stand up.

#6: Yeah, you could stand up and do one, but if you're going to do two cartridges, you're not going to be standing up. You're going down no matter what.

Psychosocial Dysfunction

Relatively little is known about psychosocial comorbidities associated with the natural history of inhalant use in the general population [73, 74]. Occupational exposure to inhalants evidences high post-exposure levels of depression and anxiety [75]. Condray et al. [76] found that journeyman painters were 3.5 times as likely as controls to have lifetime DSM-IV major depression. Virtually all of the painters who had a mood disorder experienced their first episode after starting their painting careers.

Several reports suggest that inhalants are among the first psychoactive substances used by youth and earlier onset of inhalant use presages later heroin use, intravenous drug use, and severity of substance use problems [77–81]. The notion that inhalants serve as gateway drugs has been rejected because noninhalant drug use generally precedes inhalant use within treated drug abusers; rather, inhalant use appears to reflect general deviancy proneness [82–85]. Howard et al. reported high rates of risky behavior during inhalant intoxication in a state population of antisocial youth [2]. Inhalant use in dangerous situations was often described during focus groups by Ridenour et al., illustrating poor judgment that can precede and accompany inhalant use [3, 72].

#8: We used to play a game by doing whip its while driving.
#10: I don't know what it is with the driving. Doing it you're obviously trying to get really messed up because it's not like smoking weed or something. You're completely out of your head when you do this stuff and I think the driving part of it is sort of an adventure. I've never gone out on a main road, but just driving down the street.

Clinical, criminological, and general population studies of youth have identified robust associations between lifetime inhalant use, other drug use, and psychiatric disorders [1, 2, 86–91]. In adults, inhalant use correlates with major depression, psychosis, suicidal ideation and attempts, anxiety disorders, personality disorders, and other substance use disorders [92]. Other psychosocial correlates of inhalant use include adverse life circumstances such as abuse, trauma, school drop out, job or school-related problems [93, 94], HIV/HCV infection [95], and arrest or incarceration [96–98].

Addiction

Although inhalant use has been regarded as an episodic behavior that is unlikely to develop into addiction [99], inhalant dependence, tolerance, and withdrawal have been reported [72, 88, 99, 100]. Lifetime prevalence of any substance use disorder among adult inhalant users was 96% in the *National Epidemiologic Survey on Alcohol and Related Conditions* (NESARC) [87]. Although 19% of NESARC adult inhalant users experienced inhalant use-related disorders, their prevalences were greater for disorders consequent to using alcohol (87%), marijuana (68%), nicotine (58%), cocaine (35%), hallucinogens (31%), and stimulants (28%). The reinforcing mechanisms of inhalant use also likely overlap with such mechanisms of other substances. Recent development of animal models for inhalants should lead to clarification of their reinforcing effects on the central nervous system as well as cellular-level effects [101–103].

Inhalant addiction can occur at relatively young ages. During the focus groups conducted by Ridenour et al. [3, 72], one adolescent recalled, "I ultimately stopped [using spray paint] because I could not keep from getting it all over myself. I heard my mother calling me and I passed out in my closet and the closet was painted. We had to throw away half of my clothes … I did it a lot when I was 13. I would do it every day and most of the time I could make myself stop after like 15 or 20 minutes. But then that one time my mother finally caught me, I thought hey, you lost like two hours there. I got really scared … I've done it since then when I was about 15 or 16. I had a group of friends that had never done it and I told them that I used to do it. So, they decided it was a good idea and they started doing it. I only did it with them once because doing it made me remember how scary it could be. To be that out of control and start spray painting things. Like I said, it happened to one of them and she had to go to the hospital."

Uniqueness of Inhalants as a Class of Substances

In the U.S., inhalant use first gained notoriety in the 1850s, but has since remained largely covert [104, 105]. Inhalant use and consequent disorders are more prevalent in isolated rural settings and geographic areas characterized by serious social disadvantage [106–113]. Perhaps, because inhalant use is so concealed, few interventions have been developed and tested specifically to curb inhalant involvement [114, 115].

Inhalant use differs from use of other psychoactive substances in additional respects. Over 3,400 commercial products contain agents that can produce intoxication (and toxicity) if inhaled [116]. Products containing inhalants are not only widely available, they also are legal, inexpensive, and easily obtained for free. Thus, children and adolescents, low income and unemployed adults, and persons living in isolated rural or institutional settings, such as prison or residential units, have greater access to inhalants than to other

psychoactive substances. Moreover, relatively few parents, retailers, school personnel, law enforcement professionals, or human services workers are vigilant about inhalant use or inhalant-related health and social problems. Detecting inhalant use can be difficult; to illustrate, youths with "white out" or nail polish can offer plausible explanations for possessing them other than for intoxication.

Most inhalant initiates appear to discontinue use. The 2006 MTF indicated that 44%, 52%, and 59% of lifetime inhalant users in 8th, 10th, and 12th grade, respectively, had not used inhalants in the prior 12 months [117]. However, youth at highest risk for continued use drop out of school at greater rates, potentially upwardly biasing estimates of discontinuance in the school-based MTF survey [118, 119]. Further, some studies suggest that substantial proportions of adolescent and young adult inhalant users do go on to develop inhalant use disorders [72].

Epidemiology

Prevalence

Lifetime inhalant use between ages 14 and 18 based on the MTF has remained near 15% since 1991 (Fig. 14.1) (monitoringthefuture.org/new.html). In the most comprehensive prevalence study to date, Wu et al. [120] reanalyzed the U.S. *National Survey on Drug Use and Health* (NSDUH) to estimate the prevalence of inhalant use and consequent disorders among 12–17-year-olds; their estimates of lifetime use, abuse, and dependence were 9.0%, 0.2%, and 0.2%, respectively. In adults of NSDUH, the prevalence of inhalant use, abuse, and dependence were 10%, 6.6%, and 1.1%, respectively [121]. These estimates resembled Anthony et al.'s (1994) findings from the National Comorbidity Study 15–24-year-olds of 8.1% for inhalant use and 0.6% for dependence [99]. Anthony et al. estimated the prevalence of inhalant use and dependence among U.S. adults as 6.8% and 0.3%, respectively [99].

Age Trends

Compared to illegal drugs, inhalant use is generally initiated at younger ages [122, 123]. In NSDUH, past-year inhalant use for ages 12–17, respectively, was 3.4%, 4.8%, 5.3%, 5.1%, 4.2%, and 3.9% [118]. Thus, although annual prevalence rates were similar from early to late adolescence, it peaked at age 14, a finding replicated in inhalant cases recorded in U.S. poison control centers from 1993 to 2008 [116]. Similarly, Siqueira et al. [119] found that lifetime inhalant use was most prevalent among 14-year-olds (16.5%) in their survey of 60,345 Floridian students in 6th to 12th

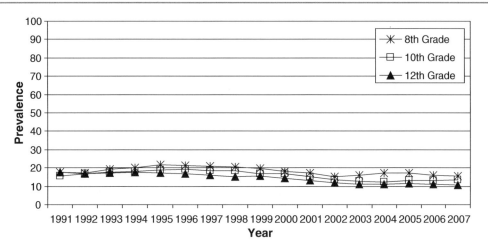

Fig. 14.1 Annual lifetime prevalence of inhalants use. *Note*: From monitoringthefuture.org/new.html

grades. Lubman et al. [9] argued these surveys may underestimate the prevalence of adolescent inhalant use, because "young people at high risk of becoming regular users (e.g., nonschool attendees) are unlikely to be included in such surveys. Epidemiological figures are also likely to be affected by the episodic and cyclical nature of inhalant abuse among youth populations, such that the brief periods of intensive use within distinct locations may not be accurately captured" (p. 317).

The prevalence of lifetime and past-year inhalant use is low among adults in the USA who are ages 50 and older. Moreover, there is a weak inverse relationship between ages 18 and 49 and lifetime or past-year history of inhalant use [121, 124]. Cohort effects many contribute to these trends as might homelessness or death among inhalant users in older generations because of the increased serious health risks resultant to inhalant use or associated risky behaviors later.

Gender Differences

Males and females differ in lifetime inhalant use according to age and sampling scheme [122]. Results of the 2006 MTF, suggest lifetime inhalant use was slightly greater in girls than boys in 8th (17.4% vs. 14.7%) and 10th (14.3% vs. 12.4%) grades, but less in 12th grade (10.3% vs. 12.0%) [117]. The paradoxical finding of lower lifetime prevalence rates for inhalant use in higher grades may be due to increased dropout rates among youth at highest risk for lifetime inhalant use [118, 119]. Likewise, the (small) reversal in gender prevalence of inhalant use may result from greater school dropout among female inhalant users. Similar gender differences occur in MTF prevalence of annual and 30-day inhalant use.

Conversely, 73.5% of the inhalant cases among 12- to 17-year-olds recorded by U.S. poison control centers from 1993 to 2008 were boys, suggesting genders differ considerably on riskier inhalant use [116].

Findings from the NSDUH replicated the similarity between genders in adolescent inhalant use; nearly 49% of the 2002–2004 overall samples, ages 12–17, were girls and 50.5% of past-year inhalant initiates were girls [118]. Similar results have been reported in other adolescent samples [125–127]. In contrast, Wu and Ringwalt [121] reported lower prevalence of lifetime and past-year inhalant use among adult women compared to men in the 2002–2003 administrations of the NSDUH. Recent NESARC findings demonstrated that adult women lifetime inhalant users had greater highest rates of co-occurring mood and anxiety disorders whereas adult men lifetime inhalant users had greater co-occurring polysubstance use disorders [87, 88].

Gender differences typically do not occur in criminal justice or clinical samples in the prevalence, age of onset, or lifetime frequency of inhalant use [126, 127]. The 1994 DSM-IV stated that inhalant use disorders were 3–4 times more prevalent among males than females [6]. In contrast, the 2000 text-revision of DSM-IV proffered no gender differences in inhalant use-related disorders [6].

Correlates of Inhalant Use

Others have reviewed research on correlates of inhalant use [9, 98, 123]. Compared to general populations, elevated prevalence of inhalant use occurs in U.S. and Canadian Native Indians, persons involved in the justice system, perpetrators of interpersonal violence, residents of isolated rural areas, and residents of Latin America, Asia, and Eastern Europe. Compared to nonusers, inhalant users experience greater rates of school dropout and discipline; poverty and social marginalization; intravenous and multiple drug use; suicidality; AD/HD, mood, anxiety, and personality disorders; dysfunctional family backgrounds including parental alcoholism and criminality, poor or absent parenting, and histories of physical or sexual abuse; socially deviant friends; and neuropsychological and learning disorders [77, 96, 98, 128].

Early-onset inhalant use is additionally associated with adverse outcomes. Wu et al. [120] reported that inhalant use prior to age 14 (versus initiation between ages 15 and 17) was associated with a five- to sixfold risk for past-year inhalant dependence. Early-onset inhalant use also presages later heroin and intravenous drug use [125, 126], antisocial behavior, and problematic use of other psychoactive drugs [127]. Perron et al. [129] reported that young adolescents who experienced inhalant-related problems and had a friend or sibling inhalant user were more likely than other inhalant users to intend to use inhalants in the future. This information may help to detect problematic inhalant use at an early stage to facilitate prevention of harmful outcomes.

Barriers to Inhalant Use

Compared to other substances, the barriers to using inhalants are few and consist mostly of naïveté about inhalants or a perception that they are harmful. More than one-third (35.8%) of U.S. 8th graders and 29.2% of 10th graders do not regard regular inhalant use as posing serious risk to their well-being. Declines occurred from the 2001 to 2006 MTF surveys in 8th and 10th graders' perceived risk of inhalant use. In response, MTF researchers suggested implementing public information campaigns and other interventions [117].

Care must be exercised when discussing inhalants with youth. Unfortunately, inhalant use demonstrations and information are widely accessible from internet sites such as *YouTube* and inhalant retailers. Merely providing information about inhalants, even accurate information, without strong warnings of their dangers can be harmful. This point may be best illustrated with an exchange during one of Ridenour et al.'s focus groups [3, 72]:

> #5: "I don't know if people realize how many kids get influenced into doing drugs because of the DARE program. You don't go searching out to do inhalants, you might know somebody who happened upon it. It's just something that you accidentally fall into. Like, 'hey, I can get high off of it!' "
> #11: "No. 11 agrees. The DARE program taught me that drugs are so good."

Prevention and Treatment of Inhalant Use Disorders and Associated Consequences

Little research has tested prevention or treatment programs specifically for inhalant abuse. Some insights may be gained from studies of programs for other substances that included inhalant use as a secondary outcome. For example, Caldwell et al. [130] reported that compared to a control group, inhalant use was lower in U.S. 9th grade boys (about age 15) enrolled in the *TimeWise* program. TimeWise is designed to promote youth's use of leisure time in goal-directed and constructive activities. In contrast, a similar-aged sample who at ages 5–7 had received a prevention program designed to improve classroom behavior had equivalent inhalant use as a control group [131]. These contrasting outcomes suggest inhalant use might be reduced more effectively by providing alternative leisure time activities or implementing interventions during the age at which inhalant initiation typically occurs.

In spite of the scant research on this topic, generalizing from studies of other substances and common sense may improve efforts to prevent inhalant use. Effective prevention and treatment of inhalant use problems and disorders requires increased awareness on the part of adolescents, adults, and professionals. Balster [105] referred to inhalant use as "the forgotten epidemic," reflecting the general tendency of health, education, and social service professionals to overlook inhalant use in their patients, students, and clients. Boylan et al. [132] documented deficits in practitioner knowledge about inhalant effects, appropriate treatments for inhalant users, and a lack of training opportunities to gain knowledge in these areas.

This general negligence of inhalant use and abuse among professionals is evidenced in a nosological study of inhalant use disorders [72]. Rates of detecting inhalant use disorders were compared between two assessment techniques: the layman-administered, structured interview, Substance Abuse Module (SAM) [133] versus the psychiatrist-administered, clinical interview style, Schedules for Clinical Assessment in Neuropsychiatry (SCAN) [134]. In a sample of adolescent and young adult inhalant users, only 57% of the SAM aerosol-related diagnoses were detected using the SCAN and only 36% of the SAM gases-related diagnoses were detected using the SCAN. Although notably fewer diagnoses were found related use of solvents and nitrites, nearly equal numbers of these disorders were detected by the SAM and SCAN techniques. Ongoing development of a laboratory test using gas chromatography and mass spectrometry to detect certain inhalants (dichloromethane, ethyl acetate, benzene, toluene, and xylene) in the blood stream may lead to improved screening for inhalant use and consequent disorders [135–137].

However, detection of inhalant use is of little utility without effective interventions to curb it.

Public Health

Efforts of mixed effectiveness have been implemented to reduce the availability or appeal of inhalants. In Australia, psychoactive components of gasoline have been replaced with more benign alternatives, chemicals such as oil of mustard have been added to certain inhalants (e.g., airplane glue and correction fluid), nozzles and other inhalant containers have been modified, and steps have been taken to restrict the sales of inhalants to minors [123]. Presently, however, inhalants remain the most unregulated of all abused psychoactive substances.

The minimal barriers to accessing inhalants require education to be a critical component in efforts to reduce inhalant use. Three simple steps can be taken within homes and organizations where youth are located. The first step is to reduce access to inhalants such as locking them in storage cabinets. Second, parents and professionals could be familiarized with the signs of inhalant use [129] and could help disperse information about the dangers of such toxins. A third step is to closely monitor youth's activities [138].

Medical Professionals

Several studies have examined inhalant-related deaths and calls to poison control centers [139, 140], yet whether inhalant use is associated with elevated rates of hospitalization or outpatient health care is unknown. Likewise, few concerted practice or research efforts have focused on intervention specifically for inhalant use, abuse, or dependence. Two exceptions exist in Canada and Australia. The Canadian Youth Solvent Addiction Committee oversees seven treatment agencies serving Native Indian youth with inhalant-related problems. This committee has delineated components needed for effective treatment of inhalant use disorders [141]. D'Abbs et al. [123] recently reviewed interventions for volatile solvent misuse in Australia including multi-level harm-reduction, prevention, and treatment approaches directed at environmental, social, and intrapersonal predictors of inhalant use problems.

Social Workers and Nurses

There are more social workers (595,000) and nurses (2.4 million) than any other U.S. physical or mental health profession and they work in any professional setting that involves youth. Given the frequency of their contacts with potential inhalant users, educating these professionals of the harmfulness and magnitude of inhalant use could greatly enhance efforts to screen, assess, prevent, and treat inhalant use and resultant disorders. For example, social workers often service disenfranchised and low-income clients and are trained to match clients with needed community services. Nurses work with persons having medical and mental health problems that correlate with inhalant use and abuse. Additionally, nurses come into contact with youth from all walks of life (e.g., schools and physician offices) and often easily establish caring and trusting rapport with them. Youth may disclose sensitive behavior such as inhalant use to nurses more readily than other professionals. Nurses educate patients about health concerns and can educate medical and school staff as to the prevalence, signs, and symptoms of inhalant use.

Juvenile Justice

High rates of inhalant use and associated problems occur in adjudicated youth [142–144]. Howard et al. [2, 145] found that 36.7% of 723 Missouri youths in juvenile justice residences and 34.3% of juveniles on probation had used inhalants. Inhalant users display greater frequency and earlier onset of illegal and antisocial behavior compared to nonusers [1, 146]. Given the well-documented association between adolescent inhalant use and antisocial behavior, screening and intervention for inhalants in juvenile justice facilities could be impactful because their clientele is at such elevated risk for inhalant use. Staff in these settings includes persons trained in health issues related to substance use and antisocial behavior who also often have extended contact with such youth and their families as well as contacts with community services where such youth and families may receive help. However, it may require the efforts of medical staff (e.g., psychiatrists and nurses) or social workers within justice settings to promote screening and intervention related to inhalants.

Conclusion

In sum, inhalants constitute a dangerous and unique class of abusable substances. Although there is much to learn about inhalant use, abuse, and underlying mechanisms of such behavior, accumulation of such research has accelerated in recent years. Ongoing inhalants research spans physiological and behavioral effects, international epidemiological studies, and prevention research. In terms of prevention and treatment, health professionals likely will have to provide the impetus for reducing inhalant use, abuse, and dependence including in nonmedical settings. Fortunately, the growing research literature should improve the information and tools available for screening and intervention specifically related to inhalant use.

Acknowledgement Funding for this research was provided by grants from the National Institute on Drug Abuse (R01 15984, P50 10075).

References

1. Howard MO, Walker RD, Walker PS, Cottler LB, Compton WM. Inhalant use among urban American Indian youth. Addiction. 1999;94:83–95.
2. Howard MO, Balster RL, Cottler LB, Wu LT, Vaughn MG. Inhalant use among incarcerated adolescents in the United States. Drug Alcohol Depend. 2008;93:197–209.
3. Ridenour TA. Inhalants: not to be taken lightly anymore. Curr Opin Psychiatry. 2005;18:243–7.
4. SAMHSA. Characteristics of recent adolescent inhalant initiates (issue 11). Washington, DC: Office of Applied Studies; 2006. p. 1–4.
5. National Institute on Drug Abuse. Inhalant abuse. Washington, DC: NIH; 2000. Pub No 00-3818.
6. American Psychiatric Association. Diagnostic and statistical manual of mental disorders. 4th ed. Washington, DC: American Psychiatric Association; 1994.
7. Balster RL. Neural basis of inhalant abuse. Drug Alcohol Depend. 1998;51:207–14.
8. Bowen SE, Batis JC, Paez-Martinez N, Cruz SL. The last decade of solvent research in animal models of abuse: mechanistic and behavioral studies. Neurotoxicol Teratol. 2006;28:636–47.
9. Lubman DI, Yucel M, Lawrence AJ. Inhalant abuse among adolescents: neurobiological considerations. Br J Pharmacol. 2008;154:316–26.
10. Lopreato GF, Phelan R, Borghese CM, Beckstead MJ, Mihic SJ. Inhaled drugs of abuse enhance serotonin-3-receptor function. Drug Alcohol Depend. 2003;70:11–5.
11. Paez-Martinez N, Cruz SL, Lopez-Rubalcava C. Comparative study of the effects of toluene, benzene, 1,1,1-trichloroethane, diethyl ether, and flurothyl on anxiety and nociception in mice. Toxicol Appl Pharmacol. 2003;193:9–16.
12. Kurbatt RS, Pollack CV. Facial injury and airway threat from inhalant abuse: a case report. J Emerg Med. 1998;16:167–9.
13. Cox MJ. Severe burn injury from recreational gasoline use. Am J Emerg Med. 1996;14:39–42.
14. Moreno C, Beierle EA. Hydrofluoric acid burn in a child from a compressed air duster. J Burn Care Res. 2007;28:909–12.
15. Foster KN, Jones L, Caruso DM. Hydrofluoric acid burns resulting from ignition of gas from a compressed air duster. J Burn Care Rehabil. 2003;24:234–7.
16. Keriotis AA, Upadhyaya HP. Inhalant dependence and withdrawal symptoms. J Am Acad Child Adolesc Psychiatry. 2000;39:679–80.
17. Jung I, Lee HJ, Cho BH. Persistent psychotic disorder in an adolescent with a past history of butane gas dependence. Eur Psychiatry. 2004;19:519–20.
18. Avella J, Wilson JC, Lehrer M. Fatal cardiac arrhythmia after repeated exposure to 1,1-difluoroethane. Am J Forensic Med Pathol. 2006;27:58–60.
19. Bowen CE, Daniel J, Balster RL. Deaths associated with inhalant abuse in Virginia from 1987 to 1996. Drug Alcohol Depend. 1999;53:239–45.
20. Esmail A, Warburton B, Bland JM, Anderson HR, Ramsey J. Regional variations in deaths from volatile solvent abuse in Great Britain. Addiction. 1977;92:1765–71.
21. Esmail A, Anderson JD, Ramsey JD, Taylor J, Pottier A. Controlling deaths from volatile substance use in under 18s: the effects of legislation. Br Med J. 1992;305:692.
22. Johns A. Volatile solvent use and 963 deaths. Br J Addict. 1991;86:1053–6.
23. Yamanouchi OS, Kodama K, Sakamoto T, Sekine H, Hirai S, Murkami A, Komatsu N, Sato T. Effects of MRI abnormalities on WAIS-R performance in solvent abusers. Acta Neurol Scand. 1997;96:34–9.
24. Tenbein M, Pillay N. Sensory evoked potential in inhalant (volatile solvent) abuse. J Paediatr Child Health. 1993;29:206–8.
25. Sharp CW, Rosenberg N. Inhalant-related disorders. In: Tasman A, Kay J, Lieberman JA, editors. Psychiatry, vol. 1. Philadelphia: Saunders; 1997.
26. Sharp CW, Rosenberg N. Inhalants. In: Lowinson JH, Ruiz P, Millman RB, Langrod JG, editors. Substance abuse: a comprehensive textbook. Baltimore: Williams & Wilkins; 1997.
27. Hoek JAF, Verberk MM, Hageman G. Criteria for solvent-induced chronic toxic encephalopathy: a systematic review. Int Arch Occup Environ Health. 2000;73:362–8.
28. Mikkelsen S. Epidemiological update on solvent neurotoxicity. Environ Res. 1997;73:101–12.
29. Soderkvist P, Ahnadi A, Akerback A, Axelson O, Flodin U. Glutathione S-transferase M1 null genotype as a risk modifier for solvent-induced chronic toxic encephalopathy. Scand J Work Environ Health. 1996;22:360–3.
30. Morrow LA, Stein L, Bagovich GR, Condray R. Neuropsychological assessment, depression, and past exposure to organic solvents. Appl Neuropsychol. 2001;8:65–73.
31. Morrow LA, Steinhauer SR, Condray R, Hodgson M. Neuropsychological performance of journeyman painters under acute solvent exposure and exposure-free conditions. J Int Neuropsychol Soc. 1997;3:269–75.
32. Morrow LA, Steinhauer SR, Condray R. Differential associations of P300 amplitude and latency with cognitive and psychiatric function in solvent-exposed adults. J Neuropsychiatry Clin Neurosci. 1996;8:446–9.
33. Morrow LA, Steinhauer SR, Condray R. Predictors of improvement in P300 latency in solvent-exposed adults. Neuropsychiatry Neuropsychol Behav Neurol. 1998;11:146–50.
34. Utti RJ, Snow BJ, Shinotoh H, Vingerhoets JG, Hayward M, Hashimoto S, Richmond J, Markey SP, Markey CJ, Calne DB. Parkinsonism induced by solvent abuse. Ann Neurol. 1994;35:616–9.
35. Brett A. Myeloneuropathy from whipped cream bulbs presenting as conversion disorder. Aust NZ J Psychiatry. 1997;31:131–2.
36. Weintraub E, Gandhi D, Robinson C. Medical complications due to mothball abuse. South Med J. 2000;93:427–9.
37. Meadows R, Verghese A. Medical complications of glue sniffing. South Med J. 1996;89:455–62.
38. Joe GW, Garriott JC, Simpson DD. Physical symptoms and psychological distress among inhalant users. Hisp J Behav Sci. 1991;13:297–314.
39. Matsuoka M. Neurotoxicity of organic solvents—recent findings. Brain Nerve. 2007;59:591–6.
40. Gautschi OP, Cadosch D, Zellweger R. Postural tremor induced by paint sniffing. Neurol India. 2007;55:393–5.
41. Valpey R, Sumi SM, Copass MK, Goble GJ. Acute and chronic progressive encephalopathy due to gasoline sniffing. Neurology. 1978;28:507–10.
42. Finch CK, Lobo BL. Acute inhalant-related neurotoxicity with delayed recovery. Ann Pharmacother. 2005;39:169–72.
43. Stolley BT. Long-term cognitive sequelae of solvent intoxication. Neurotoxicol Teratol. 1996;18:471–6.
44. Maruff P, Burns CB, Tyler P, Currie BJ, Currie J. Neurological and cognitive abnormalities associated with chronic petrol sniffing. Brain. 1998;121:1903–17.

45. Tenbein M, Pillay N. Sensory evoked potential in inhalant (volatile solvent) abuse. J Paediatr Child Health. 1993;29:206–8.

46. Hormes JT, Filley CM, Rosenberg NL. Neurologic sequelae of chronic solvent vapor abuse. Neurology. 1986;36:698–702.

47. Korman M, Trimboli F, Semler I. A comparative evaluation of 162 inhalant users. Addict Behav. 1980;5:143–52.

48. Yamanouchi N, Okada S, Kodama K, Hirai S, Sekine H, Murakami A, Komatsu N, Sakamoto T, Sato T. White matter changes caused by chronic solvent abuse. Am J Neuroradiol. 1995;16:1643–9.

49. Yamanouchi N, Okada S, Kodama K, Sakamoto T, Sekine H, Hirai S, Murakami A, Komatsu N, Sato T. Effects of MRI abnormalities on WAIS-R performance in solvent abusers. Acta Neurol Scand. 1997;96:34–9.

50. Kucuk NO, Kilic EO, Aysev A, Gencoglu EA, Aras G, Soylu A, Erbay G. Brain SPECT finding in long-term inhalant abuse. Nucl Med Commun. 2000;21:769–73.

51. Okada S, Yamanouchi N, Kodama K, Uchida Y, Hirai S, Sakamoto T, Noda S, Komatsu N, Sato T. Regional cerebral blood flow abnormalities in chronic solvent abusers. Psychiatry Clin Neurosci. 2000;53:351–6.

52. Yamanouchi N, Okada S, Kodama K, Sato T. Central nervous system impairment caused by chronic solvent abuse—a review of Japanese studies on the clinical and neuroimaging aspects. Addict Biol. 1998;3:15–27.

53. Tenebein M. Neonatal abstinence syndrome due to maternal inhalant abuse. Clin Res. 1993;41:298.

54. Tenenbein M, Casiro OG, Seshia MM, Debooy VD. Neonatal withdrawal from maternal volatile substance abuse. Arch Dis Child Fetal Neonatal Ed. 1996;74:F204–7.

55. Anderson CE, Loomis GA. Recognition and prevention of inhalant abuse. Am Fam Physician. 2003;68:869–74.

56. Kong JT, Schmiesing C. Concealed mothball abuse prior to anesthesia: mothballs, inhalants, and their management. Acta Anaesthesiol Scand. 2005;49:113–6.

57. Shepard RT. Mechanism of sudden death associate with volatile substance abuse. Hum Toxicol. 1989;8:287–92.

58. Marjot R, McLeod AA. Chronic non-neurological toxicity from volatile solvent abuse. Hum Toxicol. 1989;8:301–6.

59. Atay AA, Kismet E, Turkbay T, Kocaoglu M, Demirkaya E, Sarici SU, Congologlu A, Gokcay E. Bone mass toxicity associated with inhalation exposure to toluene. Bio Trace Elem Res. 2005;105:197–203.

60. Dundaroz MR, Turkbay T, Sarici SU, Akay C, Sayal A, Denli M. Selenium and zinc levels in volatile solvent abusers. Bio Trace Elem Res. 2002;88:119–23.

61. Guo GL, Rose D, Barnett JB, Soderberg LS. Acute exposure to the abused inhalant, isobutyl nitrite, reduced T cell responsiveness and spleen cellularity. Toxicol Lett. 2000;116:151–8.

62. O'Brien ET, Yeoman WB, Hobby JAE. Hepatorenal damage from toluene in a "glue sniffer". Br Med J. 1971;2:29–30.

63. Wiseman MN, Banim S. Glue-sniffers' heart? Br Med J. 1987;294:739.

64. Lorenc JD. Inhalant abuse in the pediatric population: a persistent challenge. Curr Opin Pediatr. 2003;15:204–9.

65. Dukanovic B. Consequences of abuse of inhalants. Med Arh. 1992;46:91–3.

66. Archibald CP, Schechter MT, Le TN, Craib KJ, Montaner JS, O'Shaughnessy MV. Evidence for a sexually transmitted cofactor for AIDS-related Kaposi's sarcoma in a cohort of homosexual men. Epidemiology. 1992;3:203–9.

67. Moss AR, Osmond D, Bacchetti P, Chermann JC, Barre-Sinoussi F, Carlson J. Risk factors for AIDS and HIV seropositivity in homosexual men. Am J Epdiemiol. 1987;125:1035–47.

68. Pauk J, Huang ML, Brodie SJ, Wald A, Koelle DM, Schacker T, Celum C, Selke S, Corey L. Mucosal shedding of human herpesvirus 8 in men. N Engl J Med. 2000;343:1369–77.

69. Soderberg LS, Ponnappan U, Roy A, Schafer R, Barnett JB. Production of macrophage IL-1B was inhibited both at the levels of transcription and maturation by caspase-1 following inhalation exposure to isobutyl nitrite. Toxicol Lett. 2004;152:47–56.

70. Soderberg LSF. T-cell functions are impaired by inhaled isobutyl nitrite through a T-independent mechanism. Toxicol Lett. 1994;70:319–29.

71. Soderberg LSF. Increased tumor growth in mice exposed to inhaled isobutyl nitrite. Toxicol Lett. 1999;104:35–41.

72. Ridenour TA, Bray BC, Cottler LB. Reliability of use, abuse, and dependence of four types of inhalants in adolescents and young adults. Drug Alcohol Depend. 2007;91:40–9.

73. Hansen WB, McNeal RB. Self-initiated cessation from substance use: a longitudinal study of the relationship between postulated mediators and quitting. J Drug Issues. 2001;31:957–75.

74. Smitham DM. Understanding inhalant abuse: an application of primary socialization theory. Diss Abstr Int. 2001;61:4430.

75. Morrow LA, Gibson C, Bagovich GR, Stein L, Condray R, Scott A. Increased incidence of anxiety and depressive disorders in persons with organic solvent exposure. Psychosom Med. 2000;62:746–50.

76. Condray R, Morrow LA, Steinhauer SR, Hodgson M, Kelley M. Mood and behavioral symptoms in individuals with chronic solvent exposure. Psychiatry Res. 2000;97:191–206.

77. Oetting ER, Edwards RW, Beauvais F. Social and psychological factors underlying inhalant abuse. In: Crider RA, Rouse CD, editors. Epidemiology of inhalant abuse: an update (NIDA Monograph No. 85, pp.172-203). Rockville, MD: U.S. Public Health Service; 1988.

78. Walker DD, Venner K, Hill DE, Meyers RJ, Miller WR. A comparison of alcohol and drug disorders: Is there evidence for a developmental sequence of drug abuse? Addict Behav. 2004;29:817–23.

79. Warner LA. Predictors of substance use, problems and dependence: results from the National Comorbidity Survey. Diss Abst Int. 1999;59:2722.

80. Matsumoto T, Kosaka K, Miyakawa T, Kamijo A, Endo K, Yabana T, Kishimoto H, Okudaira K. Clinical features of cigarette lighter fluid (butane gas) abusers. Clin Psychiatry. 2001;43:875–83.

81. Bennett ME, Walters ST, Miller JH, Woodall WG. Relationship of early inhalant use to substance use in college students. J Subst Abuse. 2000;12:227–40.

82. Ramirez JR, Crano WD, Quist R. Acculturation, familism, parental monitoring, and knowledge as predictors of marijuana and inhalant use in adolescents. Psychol Addict Behav. 2004;18:3–11.

83. Mosher C, Rotolo T, Phillips D, Krupski A, Stark K. Minority adolescents and substance use risk/protective factors: a focus on inhalant use. Adolescence. 2004;39:489–502.

84. Bonnheim ML, Korman M. Family interaction and acculturation in Mexican-American inhalant users. J Psychoactive Drugs. 1985;17:25–33.

85. Simpson DD, Joe GE, Barrett ME. Inhalant use by Mexican American youth: an introduction. Hisp J Behav Sci. 1991;13:246–55.

86. Howard MO, Jenson JM. Inhalant use among antisocial youth: prevalence and correlates. Addict Behav. 1999;41:59–74.

87. Wu T, Howard MO. Substance use disorders among inhalant users: findings from the National Epidemiologic Survey on Alcohol and Related Conditions. Addict Behav. 2008;33:968–73.

88. Wu LT, Howard MO. Psychiatric disorders among inhalant users: findings from the National Epidemiologic Survey on Alcohol and Related Conditions. Drug Alcohol Depend. 2007;88:146–55.

89. Freedenthal S, Vaughn MG, Jenson JM, Howard MO. Inhalant use and suicidality among incarcerated youth. Drug Alcohol Depend. 2007;90:129–33.

90. Jacobs AM, Ghodse AH. Delinquency and regular solvent abuse: an unfavorable combination? Br J Addict. 1988;83:965–8.

91. McGarvey EL, Canterbury RJ, Waite D. Delinquency and family problems in incarcerated adolescents with and without a history of inhalant use. Addict Behav. 1996;21:537–42.

92. Compton WM, Cottler LB, Dinwiddie SH, Spitznagel EL, Mager DE, Asmus G. Inhalant use: characteristics and predictors. Am J Addict. 1994;3:263–72.

93. Bates SC, Plemons BW, Jumper-Thurman P, Beauvais F. Volatile solvent abuse: patterns by gender and ethnicity among school attenders and dropouts. Drugs Soc. 1997;10:61–78.

94. Liu LY. Substance use among youths at high risk of dropping out: grades 7-12 in Texas, 1998. Texas Commission on Alcohol and Drug Abuse; 1998.

95. Wada K, Greberman SB, Konuma K, Hirai S. HIV and HCV infection among drug users in Japan. Addiction. 1999;94:1063–70.

96. Dinwiddie SH. Abuse of inhalants: a review. Addiction. 1994;89: 925–39.

97. Barnes GE. Solvent abuse: a review. Int J Addict. 1979;14:1–26.

98. Dinwiddie SH. Psychological and psychiatric consequences of inhalants. In: Tarter R, editor. Handbook of substance abuse: neurobehavioral pharmacology. New York: Plenum; 1998.

99. Anthony JC, Warner LA, Kessler RC. Comparative epidemiology of dependence on tobacco, alcohol, controlled substances, and inhalants: basic findings from the National Comorbidity Survey. Exp Clin Psychopharm. 1994;2:244–68.

100. Howard MO, Cottler LB, Compton WM, Ben-Abdallah A. Diagnostic concordance of DSM-III-R, DSM-IV, and ICD-10 inhalant use disorders. Drug Alcohol Depend. 2001;61:223–8.

101. Wiley JL, Bale AS, Balster RL. Evaluation of toluene dependence and cross-sensitization to diazepam. Life Sci. 2003;72:3023–33.

102. Blokhina EA, Dravolina OA, Bespalov AY, Balster RL, Zvartau EE. Intravenous self-administration of abused solvents and anesthetics in mice. Eur J Pharmacol. 2004;485:211–8.

103. Gerasimov MR, Collier L, Ferrieri A, Alexoff D, Lee D, Gifford AN, Balster RL. Toluene inhalation produces a conditioned place preference in rats. Eur J Pharmacol. 2003;477:45–52.

104. Howard MO, Cottler LB, Compton WM, Abdallah A. Diagnostic concordance of DSM-III-R, DSM-IV, and ICD-10 inhalant use disorders. Drug Alcohol Depend. 2001;61:223–8.

105. Balster RL. Inhalant abuse, a forgotten drug abuse problem. Proceedings of the College on Problems of Drug Dependence; 1996.

106. Committee on Substance Abuse and Committee on Native American Child Health. Am Acad Pediatr. Pediatrics. 1996;97: 420–3.

107. Smart RG. Inhalant abuse in Canada. Subst Use Misuse. 1997;32:1835–40.

108. Wingert JL, Fifield MG. Characteristics of Native American users of inhalants. Int J Addict. 1985;20:1575–82.

109. Burns CB, D'abbs P, Currie BJ. Patterns of petrol sniffing and other drug use in young men from an Australian Aboriginal community in Arnhem Land, Northern Territory. Drug Alcohol Rev. 1995;14:159–69.

110. Beauvais F, Oetting ER, Edwards RW. Trends in drug use of Indian adolescents living on reservations: 1975–1983. Am J Drug Alcohol Abuse. 1985;11:209–29.

111. Wittig MCW, Wright JD, Kaminsky DC. Substance use among street children in Honduras. Subst Use Misuse. 1997;32:805–27.

112. Smart RG. Inhalant use and abuse in Canada. In: Crider RA, Rouse BA, editors. Epidemiology of inhalant abuse: an update. NIDA Research Monograph 85, Rockville, MD; 1988.

113. Bachrach KM, Sandler IN. A retrospective assessment of inhalant use in the Barrio: implications for prevention. Int J Addict. 1985;20:1177–89.

114. Misa LK, Kofoed L, Fuller W. Treatment of inhalant abuse with risperidone. J Clin Psychiatry. 1999;60:620.

115. Lowenstein LF. Glue sniffing: background features and treatment by aversion methods and group therapy. Practitioner. 1982;226: 1113–6.

116. Marsolek MR, White NC, Litowitz TL. Inhalant abuse: monitoring trends by using poison control data, 1993-2008. Pediatrics. 2010;125:906–13.

117. Johnston LD, O'Malley PM, Bachman JG, Schulenberg JE. Monitoring the Future National Survey on Drug Use, 1975–2006. Vol I: Secondary Students. (NIH Pub. No. 07-6205); 2007.

118. Substance Abuse and Mental Health Administration, Office of Applied Studies. Inhalant use across the adolescent years. National Survey on Drug Use and Health, The NSDUH Report, March 13; 2008.

119. Siqueira LM, Crandall LA. Inhalant use in Florida youth. Subst Abuse. 2006;27:27–35.

120. Wu LT, Pilowsky DJ, Schlenger WE. Inhalant abuse and dependence among adolescents in the United States. J Am Acad Child Adolesc Psychiatry. 2004;43:1206–14.

121. Wu LT, Ringwalt CL. Inhalant use and disorders among adults in the United States. Drug Alcohol Depend. 2006;85:1–11.

122. Crocetti M. Inhalants. Pediatr Rev. 2008;29:33–4.

123. D'Abbs P, MacLean S. Volatile substance misuse: a review of interventions. Australian Department of Health and Aging, National Drug Strategy, Monograph Series No. 65; 2008.

124. Wu LT, Howard MO. Psychiatric disorders in inhalant users: results from the National Epidemiologic Survey on Alcohol and Related Conditions. Drug Alcohol Depend. 2007;88:146–55.

125. Wu L, Howard MO. Is inhalant use a risk factor for heroin and injection drug use among adolescents in the general population? Addict Behav. 2007;32:265–81.

126. Storr CL, Westergaard R, Anthony JC. Early onset inhalant use and risk for opiate addiction by young adulthood. Drug Alcohol Depend. 2005;78:253–61.

127. SAMHSA, Office of Applied Studies. Inhalant use and delinquent behaviors among young adolescents. National Survey on Drug Use and Health, NSDUH Report, March 17; 2007.

128. Williams JF, Storck M, Committee on Substance Abuse and Committee on Native American Child Youth. Inhalant abuse. Pediatrics. 2007;119:1009–17.

129. Perron BE, Howard MO. Perceived risk of harm and intentions of future inhalant use among adolescent inhalant users. Drug Alcohol Depend. 2008;97:185–9.

130. Caldwell LL, Ridenour TA, Smith EA, Maldonado-Molina M. Results from a three-year efficacy trial on the effects of a leisure-based intervention on substance use. (Under review).

131. Furr-Holden CDM, Ialongo NS, Anthony JC, Petras H, Kellam SG. Developmentally inspired drug prevention: middle school outcomes in a school-based randomized prevention trial. Drug Alcohol Depend. 2004;73:149–58.

132. Boylan J, Braye S, Worley C. Life's a gas? The training needs of practitioners and careers working with young people misusing volatile substances. Soc Work Educ. 2006;25:591–607.

133. Cottler LB, Robins LN, Helzer JE. The reliability of the CIDI-SAM: A comprehensive substance abuse interview. Br J Addict. 1989;84:801–14.

134. World Health Organization. Schedules for clinical assessment in neuropsychiatry. American Psychiatric Press, Washington, DC; 1993.

135. Wasfi IA, Al-Awadhi AH, Al-Hatali ZN, Al-Rayami FJ, Al Katheeri NA. Rapid and sensitive static headspace gas chromatography-mass spectrometry method for the analysis of ethanol and abused inhalants in blood. J Chromatogr B. 2004; 799:331–6.

136. Broussard LA, Broussard A, Pittman T, Lafferty D, Presley L. Headspace gas chromatographic method for the measurement of difluoroethane in blood. Clin Lab Sci. 2001;14:3–5.

137. Broussard LA. The role of the laboratory in detecting inhalant abuse. Clin Lab Sci. 2000;13:205–9.

138. Ramirez JR, Crano WD, Quist R, Burgoon M, Alvaro EM, Grandpre J. Acculturation, familism, parental monitoring, and knowledge as predictors of marijuana and inhalant use in adolescents. Psychol Addict Behav. 2004;18:3–11.

139. Spiller HA, Krenzelok EP. Epidemiology of inhalant abuse reported to two regional poison centers. J Toxicol Clin Toxicol. 1997;35:167–73.

140. Beasley M, Frampton L, Fountain J. Inhalant abuse in New Zealand. NZ Med J. 2006;119:1233.

141. Dell CA, Dell DE, Hopkins C. Resilience and holistic inhalant abuse treatment. J Aborig Health. 2005;2:4–12.

142. McGarvey EL, Canterbury RJ, Waite D. Delinquency and family problems in incarcerated adolescents with and without a history of inhalant use. Addict Behav. 1996;21: 537–42.

143. McGarvey EL, Clavet GJ, Mason W, Waite D. Adolescent inhalant abuse: environments of use. Am J Drug Alcohol Abuse. 1999;25:731–41.

144. Reed BJ, May PA. Inhalant abuse and juvenile delinquency: a control study in Albuquerque, New Mexico. Int J Addict. 1984;19:789–803.

145. Howard MO, Jenson JM. Inhalant use among antisocial youth: prevalence and correlates. Addict Behav. 1999;24:59–74.

146. Sakai JT, Hall SK, Mikulich-Gilbertson SK, Crowley TJ. Inhalant use, abuse, and dependence among adolescent patients: commonly comorbid problems. J Am Acad Child Adolesc Psychiatry. 2004;43:1080–8.

Ketamine

Kim Wolff

Abstract

Ketamine (2-(2-chlorophenyl)-2-(methylamino)-cyclohexanone), an anaesthetic derivative of phencyclidine (PCP) with analgesic, neuroprotective and psychedelic properties, is an unusual anaesthetic in its ability to produce a "dissociative" state. It is the action (antagonism) at NMDA (N-methyl aspartate) receptors that is thought to underlie ketamine's qualities. Whilst ketamine use in medicinal and veterinary settings is well documented and has a good safety record, the increase in its unregulated use outside of such controlled environments is a cause for concern. In non-medicinal use, the stereo-selective kinetics and the complex mechanism of action may lead to unpredictable effects. It is reported that the perceptual and mood changes observed in those who have consumed ketamine are highly sensitive to age, dose, route, previous experience and setting. At low doses stimulant effects predominate and environmental conditions are significant, but with higher doses psychedelic effects become the primary experience. When used recreationally in sub-therapeutic doses by inhalation (or insufflation) the alteration in perception of auditory, visual and painful stimuli result in a general "lack of responsive awareness" which puts the recreational user at risk of personal damage which can go unrecognized. The recreational use of this drug, the effects and potential risks associated with its unregulated use will be discussed.

Learning Objectives
- Ketamine (2-(2-chlorophenyl)-2-(methylamino)-cyclohexanone) is an anaesthetic derivative of phencyclidine developed by Parke Davis laboratories in 1962
- Ketamine is a dissociative anaesthetic with analgesic properties and has a wide range of clinical applications and a wide margin of safety in overdose
- Antagonism at NMDA (N-methyl aspartate) receptors underlies ketamine's analgesic, dissociative and neuroprotective qualities

- Complex in its pharmacology, the isomeric form of ketamine can exert a significant influence upon both monoaminergic and glutaminergic neurotransmission
- Ketamine, both acutely and chronically, may have specific and yet wide-ranging effects on memory systems
- Acute doses impair episodic memory (processes involved in retrieval and initial encoding of information)
- Ketamine has reinforcing properties when used chronically and sequential use may in susceptible individuals result in acute episodes of paranoia, panic and psychosis
- Recreational use of ketamine is now a global phenomenon

K. Wolff, Ph.D. (✉)
Addiction Science, Institute of Psychiatry, King's College London,
Addiction Sciences Building, 4 Windsor Walk, London SE5 8AF, UK
e-mail: kim.wolff@kcl.ac.uk

J.C. Verster et al. (eds.), *Drug Abuse and Addiction in Medical Illness: Causes, Consequences and Treatment*,
DOI 10.1007/978-1-4614-3375-0_15, © Springer Science+Business Media, LLC 2012

Issues that Need to Be Addressed by Future Research

- Investigations to explore acute cardio respiratory problems especially when combined with other (stimulant) drugs are necessary for prevention and harm reduction initiatives with recreational users
- Investigating some of the relatively unique effects of ketamine, for example on semantic memory, may provide clues as to the neurochemical basis of memory
- As a research probe in the study of schizophrenia, ketamine has given increasing prominence to the role of glutamate in the aetiology of this illness. Further research should seek to unravel this role
- In relation to the cognitive effects of chronic ketamine use, future work should address the neuroanatomical and neurochemical correlates of such impairments
- Future research into the long term consequences of misuse might need to include investigation of social–psychological as well as physiological parameters
- Ketamine can be subjectively reinforcing to both healthy volunteers and drug users. The addiction potential of ketamine needs to be further explored
- Knowledge of the chronic use of ketamine is a priority as the drug has become a preferred choice for many
- Systematic research is required to investigate animal evidence that indicates ketamine, as a NMDA antagonist, may be a potent neurotoxin [1]

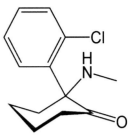

Fig. 15.1 Chemical structure of Ketamine (*RS*)-2-(2-chlorophenyl)-2-methylamino-cyclohexan-1-one)

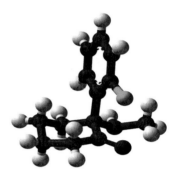

Fig. 15.2 Three dimentional structure of Ketamine (*RS*)-2-(2-chlorophenyl)-2-methylamino-cyclohexan-1-one); white balls-hydrogen atom; black balls-carbon atoms; red ball-oxygen atom; blue ball-nitrogen atom; green ball-chlorine atom

Clinical Disorders Research Use

The psychotogenic and cognitive effects of ketamine have led to the drug being used as a pharmacological model for studying transitory schizophrenic-thought disorder in normal subjects [7]. The state of dissociation achieved with ketamine are thought to mimic the phenomenology of schizophrenia [8] and reliably induce a psychosis like syndrome with cognitive, negative and positive features [9, 10] This has led to the so-called NMDA (*N*-methyl aspartate) hypothesis of schizophrenia [11] which has been the subject of debate for over 25 years [12]. Ketamine as with other drug models of clinical disorders only has partial validity, mimicking some but not other symptoms. For instance, acute ketamine administration is subjectively rewarding and produces euphoria, phenomena not often associated with the illness [13]. The similarity of the cognitive profile of an acute dose of ketamine with that observed in schizophrenia has been discussed in Fletcher and Honey's review [14]. According to the DSM-IV classification system a ketamine-induced psychosis would best fit the criteria for the disorganized or the undifferentiated subtype model of schizophrenia [15, 16].

Contemporary debate regarding the "ketamine (or NMDA-hypo function) model" of schizophrenia [17] has concerned itself with whether an acute dose of ketamine or chronic self-administration provides the better model of the cognitive deficits observed in schizophrenia in drug-naive volunteers.

Medicinal Use

Ketamine (2-(2-chlorophenyl)-2-(methylamino)-cyclohexanone) developed by Parke Davis laboratories in 1962 (Figs. 15.1 and 15.2) is an anaesthetic derivative of phencyclidine (PCP).

Manufactured as a hydrochloride, ketamine has been utilized effectively in several areas of medicine including paediatrics, anaesthesia (pre-operative, emergency and high altitude) [2], dentistry, obstetrics, battle-zones [3] and in the management of neuropathic and cancer pain. It is one of those rare anaesthetic agents that does not cause hypotension and this benefit is used to best advantage in treating patients with serious trauma and hypovolemic shock [4]. Ketamine is also widely used in veterinary practice, particularly to sedate large uncooperative animals at a distance, for example in the case of free-ranging giraffes and gorillas [5, 6].

There are evidence-based arguments for both models [18–20]. Although no work exists as yet to indicate whether NMDA-R up-regulation occurs in ketamine users, pre-clinical research seems to support this view [21] as do observations following repeated administration of the drug [22]. Meador-Woodruff and Healy [23] suggest that similar up-regulation occurs in schizophrenia. Thus, whilst not mimicking the aetiology or acute phases of the disorder, the ketamine-abusing population may still depict later functional changes.

Ketamine has been used as a probe to explore the potential clinical importance of NMDA receptor antagonism among the mechanisms underlying the subjective effects of ethanol in humans [24]. There is a growing body of research which indicates that alcohol acts in a similar way blocking glutamate effects at the NMDA receptor in a non-competitive and concentration dependent fashion at alcohol concentrations associated with alcohol intoxication (5–100 mmol/L) in man [25].

Ketamine has also been shown to attenuate the development of opioid tolerance and has been used as a research probe in studies of the modulation of opioid neurobiology [26]. Ketamine is thought to have a modulating effect on the analgesic (μ-opioid receptors) and dysphonic (kappa α-receptors) opioid receptors binding to these with one-tenth and one-fifth of its NMDA receptor affinity, respectively. The opioid antagonist Naloxone therefore has only a limited capacity to reverse the effects of ketamine and could not reverse key effects in vivo [27]. In animal models, ketamine and other NMDA antagonists such as methadone have been demonstrated to inhibit the development and acquisition of opioid dependence and tolerance [28], whilst small doses of ketamine have been shown to prevent tolerance developing acutely on repeated administration, of alfentanyl [29].

The use of ketamine as a research tool to study the pathophysiology of psychosis and as a screen to evaluate new drug action [29] has raised concerns in terms of the distress inflicted on patients. The potential for adverse events and the serious long-term effects that might be induced by the symptom-stimulating action of ketamine have led to the view that such use is unethical. Work to investigate the question of prolonged psychological effects as a result of the administration of ketamine in controlled experiments in the general population [30, 31] have however concluded that there was no evidence for long-lasting events nor increased distress [32, 33]. Safety aspects of the drug used in areas that do not permit these controls is, however, poorly researched.

Recreational Use

The recreational use of ketamine was first reported in 1971 in North America [34] linked by some to returning Vietnam veterans who may have been exposed to the drug on the battlefield [35, 36]. Intellectual hedonism popularized ketamine in the 1970s and 1980s, particularly in the United States and periodic reports of its misuse by healthcare professionals gradually appeared [37, 38]. This was followed by a growing number of reports of recreational use of the drug elsewhere, including in the United Kingdom [39, 40], Sweden [41] and Australia [42].

Ketamine use was linked to the gay dance scene during the early 1990s, with many users adhering to strict, carefully pre-planned, set and setting rituals [43, 44] emphasizing comfort and familiarity [45]. Its popularity as a recreational drug has continued to grow especially among UK dance and rave scene attendees. In a survey of club drug users in 1997, 32% reported having used ketamine [46]. A UK survey in 1999 reported a lifetime prevalence of use of 25% ($n = 1,100$), half of which used in combination with ecstasy. Prevalence had increased to 35% in a similar population 1 year later [47] and to 43% in 2004 [48]. Other surveys in Australia reported an increase in "ever use" of ketamine from 6 to 15% between 1997 and 2001 [49, 50] and surveys of year-on-year trends have reported similar findings [51]. Knowledge of the drug has also grown: 31% of young people surveyed aged 11–14 and 50% of 15 year olds reported knowledge of ketamine [45] and 0.8% of 16–24 year olds responding to the British Crime Survey had used the drug [51].

Seizures of ketamine intended for non-medical use have increased over the last decade: in the US (Drug Enforcement Administration 2001) by more than 500% [52], whilst in Hong Kong in 2002, of all reported drug users under the age of 21, 59% were using ketamine (greater numbers than ecstasy) [53]. The use of ketamine as a street drug has been recognized by the authorities and in 2006 ketamine was registered as a scheduled drug in the UK. In North America, possession of ketamine without a prescription had become illegal in 1997, and was listed as a controlled drug (Schedule III) in 1999. Ketamine use has grown exponentially during the first decade of the new millennium [54] recreational use of the drug is now a global phenomenon.

Ketamine: Sought After Effects

Ketamine is most frequently misused for its psychedelic properties sometimes as a dance drug and sometimes to "explore the mind" [55]. Used for recreational purposes ketamine has been reported to be a collection of "paradoxes" and has many effects that are associated with other substances: "cannabis-like imagery", "alcohol-like intoxication", cocaine-like stimulation and opiate-like calming [56].

Ketamine Preparations/Route of Administration

Ketamine can be purchased for recreational use in a number of preparations but is used mainly in powdered or liquid form or crystalline powder for intranasal use (Fig. 15.3).

Fig. 15.3 Solution of ketamine from a 10 ml ampoule drying into crystals (**a**) and dried and scraped onto a spoon for intranasal use (**b**). Doses of 100–400 mg of the drug are usual [54]

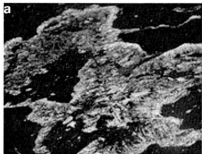
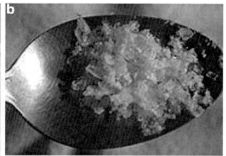

Ketamine for non-medical use may be smuggled into a country from China and India where it is legally manufactured [57], purchased entirely from legitimate medical supplies [58], such as in Holland, Germany, France and Mexico [40] or diverted directly from hospitals and vetinary clinics. The illicit manufacture of ketamine is almost unknown because it is very difficult to synthesize. Although those selling the drug for non-medical use reportedly add various adulterants to make the drug go further. The particular brand of pharmaceutical ketamine may make a difference to drug effects beyond anecdotal reports. Ketalar contains a preservative (benzthonium chloride, an anticholinergic agent) that has a significant effect upon the brain and Astrapin's ketamine-500 contains the toxic organic preservative chlorobutanol, which has shown harmful effects in some animal experiments [59].

In powdered form (Fig. 15.4), ketamine's appearance is similar to that of cocaine and the drug can be insufflated, injected, or dissolved in beverages. It is an inexpensive drug and can be purchased in the UK for between £6.00 and £10.00 a gramme. It is also possible to smoke the drug in a joint or pipe, usually mixed with marijuana and tobacco [60]. The smoke has a distinctive bitter taste but the onset of effects sought after occurs much faster than when insufflated, ingested or injected intramuscularly.

Oral use usually requires more drug, but results in prolonged effects due to the production of the inactive metabolite nor-ketamine (see box below), which possesses sedating effects; this route of administration is unlikely to produce a dissociative state unless very high doses (>500 mg) are ingested [61]. Ketamine has also appeared as a constituent of tablets purporting to be ecstasy (special K), often in combination with drugs such as ephedrine.

The nasal route of administration of ketamine tends to be favoured with users, snorting or inhaling lines (50–400 mg) of a powdered formulation although ketamine has also been produced as an intranasal spray (Fig. 15.3). There are some reports of "freebasing" ketamine, produced by the removal of benzthonimum chloride and salts from Ketalar to achieve fewer unwanted side-effects.

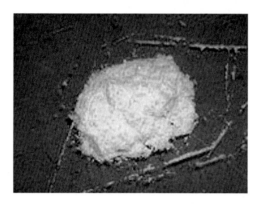

Fig. 15.4 Ketamine hydrochloride (500 mg) powder [54]

There is wide variation in consumption patterns among users with tolerant and experienced consumers reporting use of 1 g or more of ketamine over the course of an evening/weekend. A standard street dose of ketamine in a Scottish study was found to be much lower typically around 125 mg (⅛ g) [46], whilst recreational users with low tolerance will experience a mild "trippy" euphoria from a dose (a bump) of 10–30 mg.

Pharmacokinetics

Ketamine
- May be effectively administered medically by a number of routes (oral, intranasal, intravenous, intramuscular, intrathecal, intra-articular [62], transdermal [63], rectal [64] and subcutaneously) which all permit adequate absorption and excellent bioavailability [9].
- Intranasal use is common amongst recreational users, providing a rapid onset of action and an estimated duration of action of 2–3 h [65].
- Is rapidly distributed to highly perfused tissues (brain, heart and lungs).

(continued)

(continued)
- Doses for intravenous analgesia are <1 mg/kg with oral doses being much higher (100–500 mg).
- Has a short half-life and elimination is variable depending upon the route of administration, but is generally of the order of 1–3 h [66].
- Ketamine is metabolized and eliminated from the body within 24 h.
- Effects following oral administration may be prolonged due to the presence of the active metabolite—nor-ketamine, with anaesthetic potency approaching one-third, that of the parent compound [67].
- Ketamine is mainly eliminated by hydroxylation as conjugated metabolites, with <4% appearing in urine as the parent compound or as nor-ketamine.

Optical Isomers of Ketamine

Ketamine is manufactured as a racemic mixture of two optical isomers (enantiomers), $S(+)$-ketamine and $R(-)$-ketamine [68], with $S(+)$ ketamine being twice as potent an analgesic and a hypnotic as the racemic mixture (Fig. 15.5) [66].

The anaesthetic potency of $S(+)$-ketamine has been observed to be three times higher than $R(-)$-ketamine. Its higher anaesthetic potency and minor psychotomimetic side effects suggests $S(+)$-ketamine may have a better therapeutic efficacy when compared with the racemic form [68]. However, the likelihood of ketamine being formulated in its $S(+)$ form is unlikely due to cost and difficulty of production.

Pharmacological differences exist between the enantiomers of ketamine against several targets (transporter proteins) of the drug [69]. In particular, it was found that $S(+)$-ketamine binds with a 4–5 times higher affinity to the phencyclidine (PCP) binding site of the NMDA receptor complex in the human brain than $R(-)$-ketamine [70]. It was also found that at sub-anaesthetic (recreational) doses, racemic ketamine has a weak affinity for the sigma receptor sites, whereas $S(+)$-ketamine binds only negligibly [71]. It has been speculated that the occurrence of psychotomimetic effects results from the higher affinity of $R(-)$ ketamine to the sigma receptor site [72]. However, studies with $S(+)$-ketamine in healthy volunteers indicate that $S(+)$-ketamine is more likely to be associated with hallucinogenic effects than $R(-)$-Ketamine [73, 74]. This finding is conducive with the much higher affinity of $S(+)$-ketamine for the NMDA receptor.

Since psychotomimetic effects are generally considered to be caused by a relative excess of dopamine, it is possible to consider that stereo-selective inhibition of dopamine re-uptake might contribute to the ketamine-induced psychotomimetic effects. However, the inability of haloperidol to block these effects suggest other transmitters are involved [75] and would imply that nor-epinephrine and serotonergic systems are more strongly activated in those individuals who have greater $R(-)$ ketamine activity. The over stimulation of nor-epinephrinergic and serotonergic pathways by $R(-)$ ketamine may have a contributory role in the adverse effects observed in recreational users and in those who use the drug for non-medical purposes during ketamine-induced overdose. It has been postulated that the psychotomimetic and sympathomimetic effects of ketamine are thus mediated through this enhanced monoaminergic effect on the brain [25].

Neurochemical Effects

The activity of ketamine is complex with multiple actions at numerous receptor sites, particularly affecting glutaminergic and monoaminergic neurotransmission. The most significant pharmacological action of ketamine is the non-competitive antagonist binding at the cation channel of the NMDA receptor and consequent interference with excitatory amino acid transmitters—glutamate and aspartate [76, 77]. Not only thought to underlie its analgesic and dissociative effects, but action at the NMDA receptor is also thought to be important in its effects on memory. Antagonism at the NMDA receptor is thought to disrupt long-term potentiation and synaptic growth, which are crucial in the development of synaptic plasticity, learning and memory [78, 79]. Clinical studies also implicate glutamate in the mediation of the dissociative symptoms of ketamine with acute administration leading to a transient hyper-glutaminergic state [80]. Indeed the pre-administration of drugs that reduce glutamate release partly negate the perceptual disturbances seen with ketamine [81].

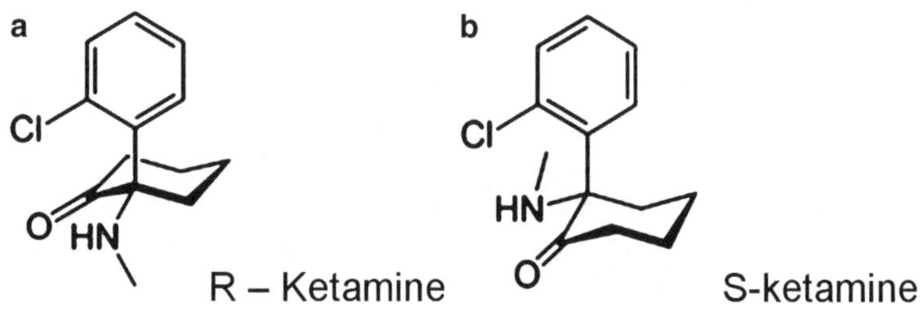

Fig. 15.5 Optical isomers of Ketamine [54] (**a**) R-Ketamine; (**b**) S-Ketamine

Research has begun to address the relationship between the modulation of other neurotransmitter systems by ketamine and its memory-impairing effects suggesting contributions of GABA-ergic and DA-ergic effects, in addition to the glutamatergic properties. Ketamine may then in part produce psychotomimetic effects through an increase in glutamate release that in turn acts on the AMPA subtype of glutamate receptor in the prefrontal cortex to induce a hyperdopaminergic state [82]. Ketamine can block excitotoxicity (brain damage due to low oxygen, low sugar, epilepsy, trauma, etc.) but it can also excite the brain at low doses by switching off the inhibitory system. Why this is not damaging in humans probably lies in the fact that ketamine binds to an increasingly wide range of different receptors: As the dose level rises some of these receptors act to shut down the excitement, by the time a potentially toxic dose is reached, the "excitement window" has been passed and the drug is starting to activate other systems that switch cells off again. Hence ketamine's promiscuity actually improves its safety [83].

Pharmacodynamics

Recreationally ketamine has been reported to have the advantage of being easy to administer: the clear dose response effect and relatively short half-life making the effects easier to titrate than LSD [36]. The spectrum of effects has been reported to be reflected in the different groups of users who choose ketamine for differing reasons. For instance, communal events where individual or small groups of users participate in sequential dosing over the evening are preferred by some and may well evoke different events to the over stimulation of a dance club venue [84].

Ketamine
- Produces anaesthesia at doses of 5–10 mg/kg (300–800 mg).
- With doses adequate to bring about anaesthesia, produces a *trance-like cataleptic state* with *amnesia*, without impairment of laryngeal and pharyngeal reflexes or depression of respiration or cardiac function [85].
- Is able to produce potent analgesia at sub-therapeutic concentrations.
- Produces dissociation at doses as low as 50–100 mg [2, 86] typically, eyes remain open with a disconnected stare: The recreational drug user may appear

to be awake but is dissociated from the environment, *immobile* and *unresponsive to pain* [87].
- Use may cause *Nystagmus* but this is not universally experienced [54].
- Induces with doses >150 mg a dissociation commonly referred to as the "*K hole*"—described as detachment from one's physical body (depersonalization) [83], the external world (derealization) [88] and from one's immediate surroundings.
- Insufflated or injected may cause hallucinations lasting about 1 h and up to 2 h when ingested [89].
- Hallucinations following a low dose are only experienced with closed eyes and in a darkened room [90] but distortion of time and space is achieved with mild dissociative effects.
- Has a wide margin of safety in overdose [2, 44].
- Is somewhat unusual, almost acting as a partial antagonist with regard to brain reward enhancements; being stimulatory at low doses and inhibiting brain reward centres at higher doses.
- May produce problematic emergence phenomena and other unpleasant experiences. These appear maximal in early adolescence.

The characteristic most commonly associated with ketamine is the cerebral "dissociative" state following anaesthesia [86, 88]. It is the action at NMDA receptors that underlies these qualities inducing a functional and electrophysiological dissociation between the thalamoneocortical and limbic systems [75, 76]. This is potentially hazardous outside clinical settings with great risk of injuries being masked and the risk of accidents increased.

Low Dose Administration

Ketamine may initially be thought of as an odd choice of drug given its dissociating and immobilizing effects; however, the drug in fact produces a syndrome of effects in individuals who take sub-therapeutic doses in a recreational manner. Reactions to low sub-anaesthetic doses illustrated in a number of texts [91] describe disoriented perceptions and the total loss of an observer consciousness. However, immobility has been reported to be reduced by the concurrent use of amphetamine, or cocaine. The symptoms of low dose ketamine intoxication appear to be short-lived and in line with the pharmacokinetics of the drug. In a case series study of North American ketamine users, 18 of 20 patients were discharged from the Emergency Department within 5 h of presentation [69]. The commonest complaints in these were symptoms of a stimulatory event (anxiety, chest pain and palpitations) with tachycardia being the most common finding following physical examination [92, 93].

The short duration of effect and rapid onset of action when taken by intranasal or intravenous routes often leads recreational users to administer repeated doses in order to maintain a desired psychoactive effect. The amnesic properties of the drug may make it difficult to remember the total number of doses consumed, increasing the likelihood of prolonged intoxication. Indeed the acute amnesic effects have been reported to be marked and subjects given ketamine under experimental conditions have struggled to describe their experience to researchers attempting to record the episode [94]. Johnston [95], who self-administered ketamine, reported "cycling into and out of awareness—a frightening experience".

In laboratory settings one-off sub-anaesthetic doses of ketamine have led to transient disruption of attentional performance, impaired performance on tests of vigilance, recognition memory, verbal fluency, working, and episodic memory. On tests of higher executive function such as the Wisconsin Card Sorting Test, ketamine use led to an increase in perseverative errors and preferentially disrupts delayed word recall, sparing immediate recall and post-distraction recall [10, 26, 96]. Dysfunction seen in episodic memory (personal life event) is of particular note, since this highly correlated with everyday memory difficulties [9, 97, 98].

Ketamine can leave the user in a confused state, since the principal physical dangers of most non-medical use are believed to arise mainly from the setting, or an interaction between the user and the setting [37, 40, 55]. This can result in falls (sometimes fatal), drowning, road traffic accidents and becoming a victim of crimes such as sexual assault [68, 99]. The likelihood of such incidences is enhanced when the drug is consumed unwittingly when it has been marketed under the guise of another drug such as ecstasy [100, 101] or as a spike in a beverage.

High Dose Administration

The perceptual and mood changes observed in those who have consumed ketamine are, as with other effects, highly sensitive to age, dose, route, previous experience (expectations, personality, motivation and mood) and setting (social, physical and emotional environment) [101–104]. The collective term for the myriad of experiences associated with the use of higher doses of ketamine is known as the "K hole" [105]. Users may feel as though their perceptions are located so deep inside the mind that the real world seems distant (hence the use of the word "hole" to describe the experience). Reported experiences are wide ranging and have included emergence and toxic effects such as out-of-body experi-

ences, temporal and spatial distortion, a sense of floating, rebirthing and experiencing evolution, and sudden insights into the meaning of existence, as well as tactile and visual distortions and hallucinations [40, 55].

Sometimes the "K hole" can reproduce the features of a "near-death" experience, including buzzing/ringing/whistling sounds at the beginning, travel through a dark tunnel into light, at a high speed, with intense visions [106]. Users may experience worlds or dimensions that are ineffable, all the while being completely unaware of their individual identities or the external world [56, 87, 107]. Some users may not remember the "K-hole" experience after regaining consciousness, in the same way that a person may forget a dream. The "re-integration" process following intoxication is slow, and the user gradually becomes aware of surroundings. At first, users may not remember their own names, or even know that they are human, or what that means. Movement is extremely difficult, and a user may not be aware that he or she has a body at all.

Ketamine Dependence

Ketamine demonstrates reinforcing efficacy in animal self-administration models and is found to be a discriminative stimuli in operant tasks [108, 109], with the ability to release dopamine within the reward pathway [110]. Heavy habitual use has been described [111], and cases of dependence have been reported among anaesthetic staff [112, 113]. Heavy users report a rapid increase in tolerance with extended use and "a line" (when snorted) which might leave a naive user passed out may have no effect on a more experienced user. It is not known how long it takes to become dependent, or the risk factors that influence this eventuality.

Historical data on the long-term consequences of ketamine use has been difficult to collect due to limited access to those using ketamine as a drug of choice. Early reports in social users of ketamine record prolonged "psychic" phenomena occurring for periods of up to 1 year [1, 114] including "flashbacks", attentional dysfunction, anxiety, and decreased sociability following nasal, intravenous or intramuscular use of the drug [115]. However, flashbacks reported following repetitive use [65], may only be "a graininess of vision" under anxiety provoking circumstances [116]. Long-term users also reportedly experience stimulant-like weight loss and loss of appetite during periods of heavy use.

Chronic intravenous use by the American psychiatrist Lilly [117] led to several admissions for paranoid psychosis; self-reported attentional difficulties and social withdrawal. Employment problems have also been reported in survey respondents, linked to vagueness affecting work performance [48, 49]. Conversely, however, some report positive long-term effects such as chronic elevation in mood, and deeper insights into one self and others [65]. Long-term users report "K-Pains" or "Ketamine cramps" the exact cause of these are unknown but seem to relate to extreme pain in the lower abdomen. Symptoms include an increased need to urinate, passing blood in urine, leakage of urine and pain on urination [118]. In a case study, Colebunders [119] found cystitis following recreational use of ketamine, and more recently abdominal pain and lower urinary tract symptoms were reported as common in ketamine users presenting at emergency departments in Hong Kong [120].

Overdose

The most frequent complications reported following ketamine overdose were severe agitation and rhabdomyolysis. In an Australian study, which surveyed 100 lifetime ketamine users, many reported regularly experiencing an inability to speak, blurred vision, lack of co-ordination and increased body temperature [48, 49]. It is reported that sequential dosing, variations in purity, intravenous route, tolerance and the amnesic effects of the drug (which may impair recall of total dose consumed) could result in acute episodes of paranoia, panic and psychosis [121]. A study of ketamine anaesthesia in over 300 subjects identified premorbid anosognosia and paranoia (as assessed with MMPI) as risk factors for experiencing psychotic disorders after ketamine administration [122].

Summary

Ketamine is a dissociative anaesthetic with a wide range of clinical applications and a wide margin of safety in overdose. The marked perceptual and cognitive psychedelic effects of ketamine have led to a global rise in prominence in the recreational drug scene. Somewhat complex in its pharmacology, ketamine effects are dose dependent and somewhat unusual, almost acting as a partial antagonist with regard to brain reward enhancements; being stimulatory at low doses and inhibiting brain reward centres at higher doses [1]. Acutely there is significant disturbance in semantic and episodic memory as well as in attention and higher executive functioning. Acute adverse psychological reactions may also occur and many regular users report "grainy" flashbacks following consumption of ketamine. Chronic use has been associated with acute cardio respiratory problems especially when combined with other (stimulant) drugs and may lead to accidental injury. Numbers involved in habitual use have grown significantly during recent years. Its future as a novel clinical and research tool is matched; it would appear, by its abuse potential outside medical settings.

References

1. Gardner EL. Brain reward mechanisms. In: Lowinson H, Ruiz P, Millman RB, Langrod JG, editors. Substance abuse: a comprehensive textbook. 3rd ed. Baltimore: Williams and Wilkins; 1996. p. 51–85.
2. Bishop RA, Litch JA, Stanton JM. Ketamine anesthesia at high altitude. High Alt Med Biol. 2000;1(2):111–4.
3. Cottingham R, Thomson K. Use of ketamine in prolonged entrapment. J Accid Emerg Med. 1994;11(3):189–91.
4. White PF, Way WL, Trevor AJ. Ketamine: its pharmacology and therapeutic uses. Anaesthesiology. 1982;56:1.
5. Bush M, Grobler DG, Raath JP, Phillips Jr LG, Stamper MA, Lance WR. Use of medetomidine and ketamine for immobilization of free-ranging giraffes. J Am Vet Med Assoc. 2001;218(2):245–9.
6. Vercruysse Jr J, Mortelmans J. The chemical restraint of apes and monkeys by means of phencyclidine or ketamine. Acta Zool Pathol Antverpiensia. 1978;70:211–20.
7. Hetem LA, Danion JM, Diemunsch P, Brandt C. Effect of a subanesthetic dose of ketamine on memory and conscious awareness in healthy volunteers. Psychopharmacology. 2001;22:59–72.
8. Giannini AJ. Drugs of abuse. 2nd ed. Los Angeles: Practice Management Information Company; 1997. ISBN 1-57066-053-0.
9. Newcomber JW, Farber NB, Jevtovic-Todorovic V, Selke G, Melson AK, Hershey T, Craft S, Olney JW. Ketamine induced NMDA receptor hypofunction as a model of memory impairment and psychosis. Neuropsychopharmacology. 1999;20:106–18.
10. Krystal JH, Karper LP, Seibyl JP, Freeman GK, Delaney R, Bremner JD, Heninger GR, Bowers MB, Charney DS. Subanaesthetic effects of the noncompetitive NMDA antagonist, ketamine, in humans: psychotomimetic, perceptual, cognitive, and neuroendocrine responses. Arch Gen Psychiatry. 1994;51(3):199–214.
11. Abi-Saab WM, D'Souza DC, Moghaddam B, Krystal JH. The NMDA antagonist model for schizophrenia: promise and pitfalls. Pharmacopsychiatry. 1998;31:104–9.
12. Carpenter WT. The schizophrenia ketamine challenge study debate. Biol Psychiatry. 1999;46(8):1081–91.
13. Morgan CAJ, Curran HJ. Acute and chronic effects of ketamine upon human memory: a review. Psychopharmacology. 2006;188:408–24.
14. Fletcher PC, Honey GD. Schizophrenia, ketamine and cannabis: evidence of overlapping memory deficits. Trends Cogn Sci. 2006;10:167–74.
15. Green MF. What are the functional consequences of neurocognitive deficits in schizophrenia? Am J Psychiatry. 1996;153:321–30.
16. Malhotra AK, Pinals DA, Caleb MA, Elman I, Clifton A, Pickar D, Breier A. Ketamine-induced exacerbation of psychotic symptoms and cognitive impairment in neuroleptic-free schizophrenics. Neuropsychopharmacology. 1997;17:141–50.
17. Olney J, Labruyere J, Wang G, Wozniak D, Price MT, Sesma M. NMDA antagonist neurotoxicity: mechanism and prevention. Science. 1991;254:1515–8.
18. Harvey PD, Green MF, McGurk SR, Meltzer HY. Changes in cognitive functioning with risperidone and olanzapine treatment: a large-scale, double-blind, randomized study. Psychopharmacology. 2003;169:404–11.
19. Tamlyn D, McKenna PJ, Mortimer AM, Lund CE, Hammond S, Baddeley AD. Memory impairment in schizophrenia: its extent, affiliations and neuropsychological character. Psychol Med. 1992;22:101–15.

20. Saykin AJ, Gur RC, Gur RE, Mozeley PD, Mozeley LH, Resnick SM, Kester DB, Stafiniak P. Neuropsychological function in schizophrenia: selective impairment in memory and learning. Arch Gen Psychiatry. 1991;48:618–24.

21. Keilhoff G, Bernstein HG, Becker A, Grecksch G, Wolf G. Increased neurogenesis in a rat ketamine model of schizophrenia. Biol Psychiatry. 2004;56:317–22.

22. Feldman RS, Meyer JS, Quenzer LF. Principles of neuropsychopharmacology. Sunderland, MA: Sinauer; 1997.

23. Meador-Woodruff JH, Healy DJ. Glutamate receptor expression in schizophrenic brain. Brain Res Rev. 2000;31:288–94.

24. Rothman SM, Thurston JB, Hauhart RE, Clark GD, Soloman JS. Ketamine protects hippocampal neurons from anoxia in vitro. Neuroscience. 1987;21:673–8.

25. Meldrum B. Possible therapeutic applications for antagonists of excitatory amino acid neurotransmitters. Clin Sci. 1985;68: 113–22.

26. Sonsalla PK, Nicklas WJ, Heikkila RE. Role for excitatory amino acids in methamphetamine-induced nigrostriatal dopaminergic toxicity. Science. 1989;243(4889):398–400.

27. Krystal JH, Petrakis IL, Webb E, Cooney NL, Karper LP, Namanworth S, Stetson P, Trevisan LA, Charney DS. Dose-related ethanol-like effects of the NMDA antagonist, ketamine, in recently detoxified alcoholics. Arch Gen Psychiatry. 1998;55(4): 354–60.

28. Trujillo KA. The effects of non-competitive N-methyl-D-aspartate receptor antagonists on opiate tolerance and physical dependence. Neuropsychopharmacology. 1995;13(4):301–7.

29. Byrd LD, Standish LJ, Howell LL. Behavioral effects of phencyclidine and ketamine alone and in combination with other drugs. Eur J Pharmacol. 1987;144(3):331–41.

30. Kissin I, Bright CA, Bradley Jr EL. The effect of ketamine on opioid-induced acute tolerance: can it explain reduction of opioid consumption with ketamine-opioid analgesic combinations? Anaesth Analg. 2000;91(6):1483–8.

31. Lahti AC, Warfel D, Michaelidis T, Weiler MA, Frey K, Tamminga CA. Long-term outcome of patients who receive ketamine during research. Biol Psychiatry. 2001;49:869–75.

32. Hersack RA. Ketamine's psychological effects do not contraindicate its use based on a patient's occupation. Aviat Space Environ Med. 1994;65:1041–6.

33. Ishihara H, Kudo H, Murakawa T, Kudo A, Takahashi S, Matsuki A. Uneventful total intravenous anaesthesia with ketamine for schizophrenic surgical patients. Eur J Anaesthesiol. 1997;14: 47–51.

34. Carpenter WT. The schizophrenia ketamine challenge study debate. Biol Psychiatry. 1999;46:1081–91.

35. Lahti AC, Warfel D, Michaelidis T, Weiler MA, Frey K, Tamminga CA. Outcome of patients who receive ketamine. Biol Psychiatry. 2001;49:869–75.

36. Gboniem MM, Hinricks JV, Mewaldt SP, Peterson RC. Ketamine: behavioural effects of subanaesthetic doses. J Clin Psychopharmacol. 1985;5:70–7.

37. Dillon P, Copeland J, Jansen K. Patterns of use and harms associated with non-medical ketamine use. Drug Alcohol Depend. 2003;69:23–8.

38. Dotson JW, Ackerman DL, West LJ. Ketamine abuse. J Drug Issues. 1995;25:751–7.

39. Zinberg NE. The basis for controlled intoxicant use. New Haven: Yale University Press; 1984.

40. Jansen KL. Non medical use of ketamine. BMJ. 1993;306(6878): 601–2.

41. Jansen KLR. Ketamine: dreams and realities. Santa Cruz: Multi disciplinary Association for Psychedelic Studies; 2000.

42. Release. Release drugs and dance survey: an insight into the culture. London: Release; 1997 (Contact: Release, 388 Old Street, London EC1V 9LT, UK).

43. Skovmand K. Swedes alarmed at ketamine misuse. Lancet. 1996;348(9020):122.

44. White JM, Ryan CF. Pharmacological properties of ketamine. Drug Alcohol Rev. 1996;15(2):145–55.

45. Shapiro H. Ketamine fact sheet. London: Institute for the Study of Drug Dependence (ISDD); 1991.

46. Winstock AR, Griffiths P, Stewart D. Drugs and the dance music scene: a survey of current drug use patterns among a sample of dance music enthusiasts in the UK. Drug Alcohol Depend. 2001;64(1):9–17.

47. Mixmag. The Mixmag drug survey 2004: the world's biggest drug survey. London: Emap; 2004. p. 30–51.

48. Topp L, Hando J, Degenhardt L, Dillon P, Roche A, Solowiji N. Ecstasy use in Australia, Monograph Number 39. Sydney: National Drug and Alcohol Research Centre; 1998.

49. Topp L, Breen C, Kaye S, Darke S, NSW Party Drug Trends. Findings from the Illicit Drug Reporting System (IDRS), Technical Report Number 136. Sydney: National Drug and Alcohol Research Centre; 2001.

50. McCambridge J, Winstock A, Hunt N, Mitcheson L. 5-Year trends in use of hallucinogens and other adjunct drugs among UK dance drug users. Eur Addict Res. 2007;13(1):57–64.

51. Murphy R, Roe S. Drug misuse declared: findings from the 2006/2007 British Crime Survey. 2007. ISBN: 978-1-84726-541-8. http://www.homeoffice.gov.uk/rds/pdfs07/hosb1807.pdf.

52. Drug Enforcement Agency, Ketamine abuse increasing, February 4, 1997.

53. Gough N. Ketamine: China's other white powder. Time Asia. com. 2003. http://www.time.com/time/asia/covers/1101020520/ketamine.html.

54. Hansen G, Jenson SB, Chandresh L, Hilden T. The psychotropic effect of ketamine. J Psychoactive Drugs. 1988;20(4):419–25.

55. Jansen KL. A review of the nonmedical use of ketamine: use, users and consequences. Psychoactive Drugs. 2000; 32(4):419–33.

56. Tori SP. Ketamine abuse "Special K". Pennsylvania: Middle Atlantic-Great Lakes Organized Crime Law Enforcement Network (MAGLO-CLEN); 1996.

57. Winstock AR, Wolff K, Ramsey J. Ecstasy pill testing: harm minimisation gone too far? Addiction. 2001;96(8):1139–48.

58. Bohr N. On atoms and human knowledge. Daedalus. 1958;87(2): 53–61.

59. Muetzelfeldt L, Kamboj SK, Rees H, Taylor J, Morgan CJA, Curran HV. Journey through the K-hole: phenomenological aspects of ketamine use. Drug Alcohol Depend. 2008;95:219–29.

60. http://en.wikipedia.org/wiki/Ketamine. Wikipedia, the free encyclopedia. Accessed 23 April 2009.

61. Dalgarno PJ, Shewan D. Illicit use of ketamine in Scotland. J Psychoactive Drugs. 1996;28(2):191–9.

62. Huang GS, Yeh CC, Kong SS, Lin TC, Ho ST. Wong Intra-articular ketamine for pain control following arthroscopic knee surgery. Acta Anaesthesiol. 2000;152(3):283–8.

63. Azevedo VM, Lauretti GR, Pereira NL, Reiss MP. Transdermal ketamine as an adjuvant for post operative analgesia after abdominal gynecological surgery using lidocaine epidural blockade. Anesth Analg. 2000;91(6):1479–82.

64. Marhofer P, Freitag H, Hochtl A, Greher M, Erlacher W, Semsroth M. S(+)-Ketamine for rectal premedication in children. Anesth Analg. 2001;92(1):62–5.

65. Siegel RK. Phencyclidine and ketamine intoxication: a study of four populations of recreational users. In: Peterson RC, Stillman RC, editors. Phencyclidine abuse: an appraisal. Rockville: National Institute on Drug Abuse; 1978.

66. Kienbaum P, Heuter T, Pavlakovic G, Michel MC, Peters J. S(+)-ketamine increases muscle sympathetic activity and maintains the neural response to hypotensive challenges in humans. Anesthesiology. 2001;94(2):252–8.

67. Grant IS, Nimmo WS, Clements JA. Pharmacokinetics and analgesic effects of MI and oral ketamine. Br J Anaesth. 1981;53: 805–10.

68. Reich DL, Silvay G. Ketamine: an update on the first twenty-five years of clinical experience. Can J Anesth. 1989;36(2):186–97.

69. Weiner AL, Vieria L, McKay CA, Bayer MJ. Ketamine abusers presenting to the Emergency Department: a case series. J Emerg Med. 2000;18(4):447–51.

70. Doenicke A, Kugler J, Mayer M, Angster R, Hoffman P. Influence of racemic ketamine and S-(+) – ketamine on vigilance, performance and wellbeing. Anaesthestist. 1992;41:610–8.

71. Oye I, Paulsen O, Maurset A. Effects of ketamine on sensory perception: evidence for a role of N-methyl-D-aspartate receptors. J Pharmacol Exp Ther. 1992;260(3):1209–13.

72. Zeilhofer HU, Swandulla D, Geisslinger G, Brune K. Differential effects of ketamine enantiomers on NMDA receptor currents in cultured neurons. Eur J Pharmacol. 1992;213:155–8.

73. Engelhardt W. Recovery and psychic emergence reactions after S-(+)-ketamine. Anaesthesist. 1997(Suppl 1);46:538–42.

74. Vollenweider FX, Leenders KL, Oye I, Hell D, Angst J. Differential psychopathology and patterns of cerebral glucose utilization produced by (s)- and (R) – ketamine in healthy volunteers using positron emission tomography (PET). Eur Neuropsychopharmacol. 1997;7:25–38.

75. Øye I, Hustveit O, Maurset A, Ratti Moberg E, Paulsen O, Skoglund LA. The chiral forms of ketamine as probes for NMDA-receptor function in humans. In: Kameyama T, Nabeshima T, Domino EF, editors. NMDA receptor related agents: biochemistry, pharmacology and behavior. Ann Arbor: NPP Books; 1991. p. 381–9.

76. Fagg GE. Phencyclidine and related drugs bind to the activated NMDA receptor channel complex in rat brain membranes. Neurosci Lett. 1987;76:221–9.

77. Anis NA, Berry SC, Burton NR, Lodge D. The dissociative anaesthetics ketamine and phencyclidine selectively reduce excitation of central mammalian neurons by N-methyl-D-Aspartate. Br J Pharmacol. 1983;79:565–75.

78. Morris RGM, Anderson E, Lynch GS, Baudry M. Selective impairment of learning and blockade of long-term potentiation by an N-methyl-D-aspartate receptor antagonist. AP5. Nature. 1986;319:774–6.

79. Lynch G, Baudry M. The biochemistry of memory: a new and specific hypothesis. Science. 1984;224:1057–63.

80. Cotman CW, Monaghan DT. Excitatory amino acid neurotransmission: NMDA receptors and Hebb-type synaptic plasticity. Annu Rev Neurosci. 1988;11:60–80.

81. Chambers RA, Bremner JD, Moghaddam B, Southwick SM, Charney DS, Krystal JH. Glutamate and post-traumatic stress disorder: toward a psychobiology of dissociation. Semin Clin Neuropsychiatry. 1999;4(4):274–81.

82. Anand A, Charney DS, Oren DA, Berman RM, Hu XS, Cappiello A, Krystal JH. Attenuation of the neuropsychiatric effects of ketamine with lamotrigine: support for hyperglutamatergic effects of N-methyl-D- aspartate receptor antagonists. Arch Gen Psychiatry. 2000;57(3):270–6.

83. Moghaddam B, Adams B, Verma A, Daly A. Activation of glutaminergic neurotransmission by ketamine: a novel step in the pathway from NMDA receptor blockade to doperminergic and cognitive disruptions associations with the prefrontal cortex. J Neurosci. 1997;17:2921–7.

84. Stone JM, Erlandsson K, Arstad E, Bressan RA, Squassante L, Teneggi V, Ell PJ, Pilowsky LS. Ketamine displaces the novel NMDA receptor SPET probe [(123)I]CNS-1261 in humans in vivo. Nucl Med Biol. 2006;33:239–43.

85. Wolff K, Winstock. Ketamine: from medicine to misuse. Rev CNS Drugs. 2006;20:199–218.

86. Dillon P, Copeland J, Jansen K. Patterns of use and harms associated with non-medical ketamine use. Drug Alcohol Depend. 2003;69:23–8.

87. Leary T, Sirius RU. Design for dying. London: Thorsons/Harper Collins; 1997.

88. Adams HA, Thiel A, Jung A, Fengler G, Hempelman G. Effects of S-(=)-ketamine on the endocrine and cardiovascular parameters. Recovery and psychomimetic reactions in volunteers. Anaesthesist. 1992;41:558–96.

89. Jevtovic-Todorovic V, Todorovic SM, Mennerick S, Powell S, Dikranian K, Benshoff N, Zorumsk CF, Olney JW. Nitrous Oxide (laughing gas) is an NMDA antagonist, neuroprotectant and neurotoxin. Nat Med. 1998;4:460–3.

90. Grinspoon L, Bakalar JB. The major psychedelic drugs: sources and effects. Chap 2. New York: Basic Books; 1981. p. 32–6.

91. Giannini AJ, Loiselle RH, Giannini MC, Price WA. Phencyclidine and the dissociatives. Med Psychiatry. 1987;3(3):197–204.

92. Stafford P. Contrasting profiles. In: Stafford P, editor. Psychedelics encyclopedia. 3rd ed. Berkeley, CA: Ronin; 1991. p. 392–5.

93. Gill JR, Stajic M. Ketamine in non-hospital and hospital deaths in New York City. J Forensic Sci. 2000;45(3):655 8.

94. Baer G, Parkas P. Ketamine-induced psychopathological changes in normal volunteers during conditions used for experimental psychoses (author's transl). Anaesthesist. 1981;30(5):251–6.

95. Johnston REA. Ketamine trip. Anaesthesiology. 1973;39:460–1 (Clinical workshop, Letter to Editor).

96. Malhotra AK, Pinals DA, Weingartner H, Sirocco K, Missar CD, Pickar D, Breier A. NMDA receptor function and human cognition: the effects of ketamine in healthy volunteers. Neuropsychopharmacology. 1996;16:120–25.

97. Green SM, Johnson NE. Ketamine sedation for pediatric procedures: part 2, review and implications. Ann Emerg Med. 1990;19:1033–46.

98. Ghonheim MM, Hinrichs JV, Mewaldt SP, Peterson RC. Ketamine: behavioural effects of subanaesthetic doses. J Clin Psychopharmacol. 1985;5:70–7.

99. Merle R. "Special-K" is latest US drug fad. The Seattle Times, 1997, June 20.

100. Hansen G, Jenson SB, Chandresh L, Hilden T. The psychotropic effect of ketamine. J Psychoactive Drugs. 1988;20(4):419–25.

101. Wolff K, Hay AWM, Sherlock K, Conner M. Contents of Ecstasy. Lancet. 1996;346:1100–1.

102. Ahmed SN, Petchkovsky L. Abuse of ketamine. Br J Psychiatry. 1980;137:303.

103. Curran HV, Morgan C. Cognitive dissociative and psychogenic effects of ketamine in recreational users on the night of drug use and 3 days later. Addiction. 2000;95(4):575–90.

104. Curran HV, Monaghan L. In and out of the K-hole: a comparison of the acute and residual effects of ketamine in frequent and infrequent ketamine users. Addiction. 2001;96(5):749–60.

105. Smith GS, Schloesser R, Brodie JD, Dewey SL, Logan J, Vitkuns SA, Simkovitz P, Hurley A, Cooper T, Volkow ND, Cancro R. Glutamate modulation of dopamine measured in vivo with positron emission tomography (PET) and 11-raclopride in normal human subjects. Neuropsychopharmacology. 1998;18:18–25.

106. Klein M, Calderon S, Hayes B. Abuse liability assessment of neuro-protectants. Ann NY Acad Sci. 1999;890:515–2.

107. Beardsley PM, Balster RL. Behavioral dependence upon phencyclidine and ketamine in the rat. J Pharmacol Exp Ther. 1987;242(1):203–112.

108. Jansen KL. Ketamine–can chronic use impair memory? Int J Addict. 1990;25(2):133–9.

109. Kamaya H, Krishna PR. Ketamine addiction. Anesthesiology. 1987;67(5):861–2.

110. Hurt PH, Ritchie EC. A case of ketamine dependence. Am J Psychiatry. 1994;151(5):779.

111. Moore NN, Bostwick JM. Ketamine dependence in anesthesia providers. Psychosomatics. 1999;40(4):356–9.
112. Steen PA, Michenfelder JD. Neurotoxicity of anesthetics. Anesthesiology. 1997;50:437.
113. Schorn TOF, Whitwam JG. Are there long term effects of ketamine on the central nervous system? Br J Anaesth. 1980;52:967–8.
114. Siegal RK. Phenocyclidine and ketamine intoxication a study of 4 populations of recreational users. Natl Inst Drug Abuse Res Monogr Ser. 1978;21:110–9.
115. Lilly JC. The scientist: a novel autobiography. New York: J.B. Lippincott; 1978.
116. Adler CM, Goldbert TE, Malhotra AU, Pickar D, Breir A. Effects of ketamine on thought disorder, working memory and semantic memory in healthy volunteers. Biol Psychiatry. 1998;43:811–6.
117. Albin M, Dresner J, Paolin A, Sweet R, Virtue R, Miller G. Long-term personality evaluation in patients subjected to ketamine hydrochloride and other anaesthetic agents. Pharmacology: Abstracts of Scientific Papers. American Society of Anesthesiologists Annual Meeting, 1970. p. 166.
118. Cottrell AM, Athreeres R, Weinstock P, Warren K, Gillatt D. An emerging problem: urinary tract disease associated with chronic ketamine use. BMJ. 2008;336(7651):973. doi:10.1136/bmj.39562.711713.80.
119. Colebunders B, Van Erps P. Cystitis due to the use of ketamine as a recreational drug: a case report. J Med Case Rep. 2008;2:219. doi:10.1186/1752-1947-2-219.
120. Ng SH, Tse ML, Ng HW, Lau FL. Emergency department presentation of ketamine abusers in Honmg Kong: a review of 233 cases. Hong Kong Med J. 2010;16:6–11.
121. Lily JC. The scientist: a novel autobiography. New York: J.B Lippincott; 1978.
122. Melkonian DL, Meschcheriakov AV. Possibility of predicting and preventing psychotic disorders during ketamine anesthesia. Anesteziol Reanimatol. 1989;3:15–8.

Prescription Drug Misuse Across the Lifespan: A Developmental Perspective

16

Megan E. McLarnon, Sean P. Barrett, Tracy L. Monaghan, and Sherry H. Stewart

Abstract

The misuse of psychoactive prescription drugs, including opioids, sedatives, anxiolytics, and stimulants, is an issue of growing concern. Factors contributing to the increasing prevalence of prescription drug misuse are thought to include rising prescription rates, social acceptability of use, and lack of perceived harm from use. Prescription drug misuse is associated with a number of direct and indirect costs. Risks to the user include development of substance use disorders, overdose, and other adverse medical consequences. Medication misuse is also responsible for a sizable burden on the health care system. Despite the indications of a growing trend, the literature is far from conclusive regarding the correlates of prescription drug misuse. Existing research is characterized by inconsistency in how prescription drug misuse is operationalized. Depending on how *misuse* is defined, it may encompass a heterogeneous group of motivations for use with varying associated behavioral patterns. Another impediment to understanding prescription drug misuse is the tendency for this phenomenon to manifest in different ways across the lifespan. Studies have documented patterns of misuse in young people that differ strikingly from those in older adults. This chapter considers the misuse of psychoactive prescription medications using a developmental framework, focusing separately on adolescence and early, middle, and late adulthood. The implications for detection, prevention, and treatment of prescription drug misuse are discussed for each age group.

Learning Objectives
- Inconsistencies in the operational definition of prescription drug misuse employed in the research literature have made it difficult to compare findings across studies.
- Age-specific patterns and correlates of prescription drug misuse can be identified by focusing separately on adolescence, young adulthood, middle adulthood, and later adulthood.
- Treatment and prevention implications differ by age group.

M.E. McLarnon • T.L. Monaghan
Department of Psychology, Dalhousie University,
Halifax, Nova Scotia, B3H 4R2 Canada

S.P. Barrett
Departments of Psychology and Psychiatry, Dalhousie University,
Halifax, Nova Scotia, B3H 4R2 Canada

S.H. Stewart (✉)
Departments of Psychiatry, Psychology, and Community
Health and Epidemiology, Dalhousie University, Halifax,
Nova Scotia, B3H 4R2 Canada
e-mail: sherry.stewart@dal.ca

J.C. Verster et al. (eds.), *Drug Abuse and Addiction in Medical Illness: Causes, Consequences and Treatment*,
DOI 10.1007/978-1-4614-3375-0_16, © Springer Science+Business Media, LLC 2012

> **Issues that Need to Be Addressed by Future Research**
> - Standardized terminology for describing and referring to the various forms of prescription drug misuse will facilitate cross-study comparisons.
> - Future inquiries will benefit from examining individuals' contexts of use and motivations for misuse of prescription medications.
> - Researchers should increase their focus on middle adulthood, a demographic group that has received little attention in the literature on prescription drug misuse.

Prescription Drug Misuse Across the Lifespan: A Developmental Perspective

Psychoactive prescription medications, including opioid analgesics, anxiolytics, sedatives, and stimulants, have important therapeutic applications in pain management, relief from insomnia, and the treatment of psychiatric conditions, such as attention-deficit hyperactivity disorder (ADHD) and anxiety disorders [1–4]. Although medications from these four classes play a crucial role in alleviating distress and discomfort in those who suffer from these conditions, many also have psychoactive effects that render them liable to be misused. In recent years, the misuse of prescription medications has garnered a substantial amount of attention in the scientific literature and the popular media. A growing body of research has documented increases in the prevalence of prescription drug misuse [3, 5, 6]. Epidemiological data collected in the USA indicate that of all individuals initiating use of an intoxicating substance illicitly in the past year, nearly one-third reported nonmedical use of a prescription psychotherapeutic medication [7]. Rates of substance use disorders involving psychoactive prescription drugs, as categorized according to *Diagnostic and Statistical Manual of Mental Disorders* (DSM-IV) [8] criteria have also shown an increase [9]. Correspondingly, concern over nonmedical use of prescription medications has grown, with the issue being labeled an "epidemic" and a problem of "staggering" proportions [10].

The rising popularity of these types of prescription medications for nonmedical reasons has been linked both to an increase in their availability and to a general perception that they are relatively less harmful than illicit drugs [10, 11]. Pharmaceuticals may be misused for a multitude of reasons, including enhancing the effects of other drugs, achieving an intoxicating effect, and managing symptoms of withdrawal. They may also be used with the intent of self-medicating psychiatric or medical symptoms [12–14]. The potential for abuse of and dependence on each of these classes of substances has been noted as a major focus of concern [4, 10, 15, 16]. Although much of the epidemiological data concerning prescription drug misuse has been collected in the USA [7] emerging data suggest that this phenomenon is increasing worldwide [17, 18]. Expenditures for psychoactive prescription drugs continue to increase [19], and despite concerns about their misuse, opioid analgesics, anxiolytics, sedatives, and stimulants remain among the most frequently prescribed classes of prescription medications [20].

What Do Researchers Mean by "Misuse"?

A major problem in the existing prescription drug literature is a lack of a universally accepted definition of misuse [21], an issue that has long been identified as a major impediment to making cross-study comparisons [22]. This issue impedes conducting comprehensive evaluations of the literature, including those related to the epidemiology of prescription drug misuse, the factors associated with misuse, and the possible negative consequences of misuse. Unfortunately, a wide range of operational criteria continues to persist in this field, resulting in the grouping of a heterogeneous collection of behaviors and motivations under the same descriptive term [21, 23].

One common way of characterizing prescription drug misuse is on the basis of prescription status. Numerous existing studies have defined misuse as any prescription drug use without a physician's prescription [24–31]. By definition, all forms of nonprescribed use may be considered to be misuse, as they take place without a physician's oversight and are inherently risky. These individuals do not receive clinical assessments, follow-up, or medical information from a health care provider [29]. However, equating misuse with nonprescribed use fails to take into account individuals' motives for use of prescription drugs [21]. Understanding motives for substance use is crucial for predicting risk for problematic consequences [32]. Griffiths and Johnson describe two forms of prescription drug self-administration that differ in motive and associated patterns of use [33]. Recreational use, or use for the purposes of experimentation or intoxication, is thought to be distinct from self-administration with quasi-therapeutic intent, which is generally an attempt to self-medicate undiagnosed or undertreated physical (e.g., pain) or psychiatric (e.g., anxiety) symptoms [33, 34].

Another limitation to this definition of misuse is that it excludes individuals who possess a valid prescription but use their medication in unsanctioned ways. Examples include increasing the dosage or frequency of administration, coadministering with other substances (licit and illicit), and altering the route of administration by injecting, smoking, or inhaling the prescription drug [21]. Furthermore, defining misuse as use without a prescription does not take into account individuals who procure prescriptions for unsanctioned reasons; for example, with the intent of using them recreationally or diverting to others.

Characterizing prescription drug misuse by evaluating symptoms of problematic prescription drug use based on formal DSM-IV [8] diagnostic criteria is another method which has been employed [9, 15, 35, 36]. Although this approach may yield information that aids in treatment planning for some individuals [35], it is problematic for several reasons. Hazardous use of prescription drugs may occur even when diagnostic criteria for a substance use disorder are not met. Conversely, symptoms of dependence, such as physiological tolerance to a drug's effects and symptoms of withdrawal following its cessation, have long been observed to develop as a consequence of long-term use of certain medications, even when used according to a physician's instructions [15]. In this situation, the patient and physician may decide that the risk of this occurrence is outweighed by the benefit that the medication provides in controlling the symptoms for which it was prescribed. Studies that classify prescription drug misuse based on symptoms of substance use disorders may describe a heterogeneous group of individuals and therefore be of limited predictive value [21].

Several large-scale epidemiological studies have been conducted in the USA examining patterns of substance use, including misuse of prescription drugs, at a population-based level. The National Survey on Drug Use and Health (NSDUH) is one such ongoing investigation [7]. The NSDUH assesses nonmedical use of prescription psychotherapeutics, defined as use without a prescription, for the experience, or for the feeling that the substance caused [7]. This definition of prescription drug misuse is congruent with the definition currently recommended by Canada's national public health agency [37]. As this characterization has been adopted by numerous recent studies focusing on prescription drug misuse [9, 16, 38–44], the term "misuse" in the current chapter will be employed to correspond with this definition.

It should be noted that the NSDUH definition presents some inherent limitations. By capturing a wide range of behaviors, respondents may potentially be required to recall multiple instances of substance use in order to provide an accurate response to a single survey item [23]. For researchers, it is impossible to tease apart the specific factors associated with risk for different forms of prescription misuse; for instance, that engaged by prescribed users versus nonprescribed users. Despite the inclusiveness of the NSDUH definition, some forms of misuse may nevertheless be underreported. For example, using a prescribed sedative to minimize the negative side effects of stimulant drugs [45] corresponds to none of the behaviors described in the definition.

Numerous researchers have identified the need to adopt a standard definition of prescription drug misuse in order to coordinate the efforts to better understand the nature, extent, and complexity of this issue [10, 21]. This avenue of research represents an important area for future investigations.

Risks and Consequences Associated with Prescription Drug Misuse

There are a number of reasons why prescription drug misuse is of critical concern to health care professionals, policymakers, and the general public [9]. Misuse of prescription drugs may reportedly transition to use of illicit drugs over time [46]. Misuse has also been reported as a risk factor for subsequent onset of prescription drug abuse and dependence [47] and may also play a role in exacerbating existing substance use disorders involving other substances [48]. This may result in direct costs to the user, such as poor health and diminished quality of life, as well as indirect societal costs, such as lost productivity and increased demands upon the health care and criminal justice systems [49]. In addition to increased risk of developing a prescription drug use disorder, adverse medical sequelae of misuse can include cardiac arrhythmia, respiratory depression, and overdose [3, 33]. Use of prescription medications in ways that are not in accordance with physician recommendations has also been associated with a host of other factors, including psychiatric symptoms [15, 16] and risk for accidents and injury [33].

Prescription Drug Misuse Across the Lifespan

The use and misuse of psychoactive substances are closely related to age, developing and varying in correspondence with the life cycle [50]. Forms of prescription medication misuse have been reported in all age groups from early adolescence [42, 51] to late adulthood [52–54]. Epidemiological data indicate that prevalence rates tend to vary by age, with the highest rates reported in the late teens and early twenties [7]. Other studies have found that older adults are also at elevated risk for prescription drug misuse [53, 54]. Despite the indications of a growing trend of misuse, existing research is far from conclusive as to the demographic features or other characteristics associated with increased risk for misuse of prescription drugs [10].

Another rarely acknowledged issue in the literature is that prescription drug misuse appears to manifest in different ways across development, suggesting that studies that investigate misuse in a given age group are unlikely to generalize to other populations. The remainder of this chapter will employ a developmental framework to describe the heterogeneity of prescription drug misuse across the lifespan. Specifically, patterns of use, correlates, and treatment considerations will be examined in various age groups, including adolescents, young adults, middle age, and older adults.

Prescription Drug Misuse in Adolescence

Adolescence, defined chronologically as the period between approximately age 12 and 17 and socially as a transitional period between childhood and adulthood [55], is a time of rapid development, growth, and change—physically, emotionally, and intellectually. For many adolescents, it is also a time of experimentation with substance use. Initiation of the use of many types of substances, including alcohol, tobacco, and illicit drugs, is commonly documented to occur in the teen years [43, 56]. Prevention and treatment initiatives have long been employed to educate teens about the harms associated with substance use, and encouragingly, rates of tobacco and alcohol use in teens are at historically low levels [51]. However, the issue of prescription drug misuse in adolescent populations has increasingly drawn the attention of health professionals, educators, policymakers, and the general public [57]. The alarm this issue has prompted is exemplified by phrases such as "Generation Rx," coined to refer to teenagers in North America in the twenty-first century [58].

Although research documenting prescription drug misuse in adolescent populations suggests that there is cause for concern, researchers are far from reaching a consensus about the nature and extent of this issue [57]. Results from several large-scale epidemiological surveys have detailed widespread misuse of prescription psychoactive medications among teens [7, 51]. However, as described previously, comparisons between different studies are complicated by varying operational definitions of "misuse" employed by different researchers [21, 42]. Considerable variation is evident even in the findings of studies purporting to study the same phenomenon [59]. For example, depending on the definition used, prevalence estimates among adolescents for having engaged in misuse use of any of the most commonly misused psychoactive prescription drug classes, including sedatives, tranquilizers, stimulants, and opioids, range from 1.1% [59] to 20% [60, 61]. Although specific prevalence estimates are difficult to agree upon, there are a number of trends indicative of a growing problem. In contrast to the declining prevalence of alcohol and illicit drug use documented among adolescents in recent years, most studies indicate that rates of misuse of prescription medications have grown [51, 55]. Recent reports from the USA indicate that in relation to other drug use, the prevalence of prescription drug misuse among teens is second only to that of marijuana. Teens represent the fastest-growing segment of new misusers of prescription drugs [7]. Though diagnosable prescription medication-related substance use disorders were thought to manifest infrequently during adolescence as recently as a decade ago

[59], more current data suggest that symptoms of prescription medication abuse and dependence may also be increasing [40]. One large, population-based study found that over 17% of adolescents who reported misusing a prescription medication in the previous year met diagnostic criteria for substance abuse or dependence, with nearly two-thirds of those cases relating solely to opioid analgesics [41].

In addition to signs that adolescent prescription medication misuse is becoming more widespread, a number of other considerations make this a particularly vital issue. Adolescent substance use is associated with increased likelihood of injury, fights, declining school performance, unwanted sexual activity, peer conflict, property damage, and trouble with police [55]. The risk of accident or injury may be particularly heightened with the use of sedatives and opioids, which can affect cognition and motor skills even at low doses [62]. Another reason for the concern surrounding adolescent prescription drug misuse is that brain development progresses through critical stages during the teenage years. In fact, changing connectivity, neurotransmitter activity, and neurocognitive function are thought to be some of the factors underlying the increase in high-risk and disinhibitory behavior seen in adolescents [63]. Exposure to psychoactive prescription drugs at this time has the potential to induce lasting neurobiological changes in the brain [10, 62]. Although the behavioral consequences are unknown, research does indicate that early onset of prescription misuse also appears to be associated with increased risk of substance use disorders in adulthood [64]. McCabe et al. found that for each year prescription drug misuse was delayed, risk for subsequent abuse of or dependence on a prescription medication declined by 5% [47]. With a growing body of evidence documenting the potential for negative outcomes of prescription drug misuse in adolescence, it is critical that more efforts be directed to increasing our understanding of this phenomenon, to developing ways to prevent its occurrence, and to providing appropriate intervention when problems are identified.

Patterns of Prescription Drug Misuse in Adolescence

Although the media has often portrayed adolescent prescription drug misuse as a unitary construct, a review of the existing literature suggests that the nature of the issue is far more complex. Although misuse of all forms of psychoactive prescription medications has been documented in adolescents, the highest rates have been found for opioid painkillers, followed, in decreasing order of prevalence, by sleeping, sedative/anxiety, and stimulant medications [13, 61, 65, 66]. Patterns of use are thought to vary by class of medication used [13, 42, 61].

Further complicating these investigations is the diversity of pharmaceutical products and drug formulations within a given class of medications [57]. For example, misuse of stimulant medications, such as methylphenidate and dextroamphetamine, is well documented [27, 40, 67]. However, this class of medications includes a number of substances that are chemically distinct from one another, have different functions in the brain, and that are produced in a variety of formulations. Some of the sustained-release formulations are specifically designed to decrease the likelihood of their being administered through an altered route of administration [68]. Patterns of misuse observed with short-acting stimulant medications may not generalize to the extended-release formulations; unfortunately, existing studies often fail to make this distinction [69].

As noted, increases in prescription drug misuse have been partially attributed to availability of abusable prescription drugs [13, 51]. Children and adolescents under the age of 19 receive, per capita, the highest proportion of stimulant medications for treatment of Attention-Deficit Hyperactivity Disorder (ADHD) of any age group [20]. These drugs may be misused by the individuals they were intended to treat or diverted to users without a prescription [60]. Indeed, diversion, including "borrowing" or "sharing" of all types of prescription drugs, is particularly prevalent among teens [60, 70]. Several North American studies report that between one-quarter and one-third of middle- and high-school students with prescriptions for stimulant medications have been approached to sell, trade, or give away their prescription [27, 71, 72]. Additionally, adolescents have ready access to prescription drugs in their own homes, often attaining prescription painkillers and anti-anxiety medications from family members or friends, both with their permission and via theft [60].

Although friends and family with prescriptions appear to be the primary sources from which adolescents obtain diverted prescription medications [7, 40, 60, 73], the recent proliferation of online pharmacies has raised the concern that teens may be illicitly obtaining prescription drugs over the Internet [18, 74]. As yet, data do not support Internet pharmacies as a major source, perhaps due to the ready availability of medications from other sources [60, 70]. One large survey asked American teens to estimate the time it would take them to attain prescription drugs for the purposes of intoxication. More than one-third of these participants reported being able to attain illicit prescription drugs within a day's time, with the vast majority listing parents, other family members, and friends as the sources of these drugs [75].

Coupled with easier access to prescription medications is the issue of lower perceived harm, which is also thought to be a major contributing factor to this growing problem [62]. One study found that 40% of teens believed prescription drugs to be "much safer" than illegal drugs, while 25% believed that painkillers were not addictive [76]. Societal shifts in attitudes toward medications and drugs and their perceived negative effects may be reflected in changing patterns of substance use [51]. In the context of widespread medical use and direct-to-consumer advertising, it is not surprising to find that many adolescents perceive prescription drug use to be acceptable and consider the hazards associated with their use to be minimal compared to the use of illicit street drugs [10, 51, 62].

In addition to the influences of society, community, and culture on teens' substance use, when exploring how prescription drug misuse in adolescence may be differentiated from other age groups, it is also important to take into account more proximal environments and contexts in which the misuse takes place [42]. The attitudes, beliefs, and customs of adolescents' peer groups are thought to have a profound effect on teens' patterns of substance use. Peer group approval has been shown to be associated with increased misuse of medications [51], and having friends who use illicit drugs is associated with increased risk for prescription drug misuse in teens [66, 77]. Parental expectations and modeling are also important predictors of substance use [10]. Permissive attitudes toward the use of alcohol and marijuana among parents are associated with greater use of these substances by teens; although not yet evaluated empirically, this relationship may also apply to prescription drugs [75].

Intrinsic to the current review is the idea that considering motives for use of prescription medications is crucial to making sense of the heterogeneity within the group of behaviors broadly classified as prescription medication misuse. Contrary to representations in the popular media which suggest that most adolescents using prescription drugs nonmedically are doing so for recreational purposes, empirical results suggest that adolescent prescription drug misuse is more frequently in keeping with the accepted therapeutic purpose of the medications [13, 62]. For instance, teens have reported self-medication with tranquilizers to help with sleep or decrease stress, with stimulants to enhance their level of concentration while studying, and with analgesics to manage pain [13, 60]. As these individuals may be unaware of the side effects or drug interactions, this is far from being a risk-free activity; yet, the potential harms associated with this type of therapeutically motivated misuse are likely to differ from purely recreational use. Boyd et al. examined motives for use of prescription sedatives, anxiolytics, stimulants, and painkillers in an adolescent student sample and found that motives varied by substance used [13]. While three-quarters of nonmedical sedative use was reported as being solely for the purpose of helping with sleep, motives for use of analgesic and stimulant medications were much more diverse, with many students reporting multiple concurrent motives. These researchers found that as the number of motives for use of prescription drugs increased, so too did the risk for other substance use problems [13]. Adolescents reporting purely self-medication motives for prescription drug misuse demonstrated no increased risk of other substance problems.

Correlates of Prescription Drug Misuse in Adolescent Populations

Investigations of prescription drug misuse in adolescence have emphasized quantifying the extent of the problem, rather than characterizing it. Existing research has tended to focus on misuse of opioid analgesics and stimulants, with sedatives and tranquilizers receiving relatively less attention [41]. Although evidence for correlates of prescription misuse in adolescents is just beginning to accumulate, these studies have identified a number of factors associated with the misuse of prescription medications in this age group. The most commonly replicated finding is a strong association between prescription drug misuse and increased likelihood of engaging in all other forms of substance use, including alcohol, tobacco, and illicit drugs [27, 41, 43, 60, 66, 67, 72, 77]. For instance, one study found that adolescent non-medical prescription drug users were seven times more likely to smoke cigarettes, five times more likely to drink alcohol and smoke marijuana, almost four times more likely to binge drink, and eight times more likely to have used several other illicit drugs [60]. This association holds across the various categories of abusable prescription drugs. Additionally, adolescent prescription drug misuse appears to often take place in a polysubstance context [41]. Teens who misuse prescription stimulants [43] and analgesics [77] have reported a high level of coadministration with other drugs, putting them at risk for adverse consequences from drug interactions.

A general tendency toward risk-taking behavior among adolescents has also been found to be predictive of misuse of all categories of commonly misused prescription drugs [41]. For example, teens who reported stimulant misuse were more likely to have been a passenger in a car driven by someone who had consumed alcohol [27]. McCabe, Boyd, and Teter found that opioid painkiller misuse was associated with a range of "problem behaviors," including having been suspended or expelled from school, skipping school in the past month, buying illegal drugs at school, and frequently using drugs to get high [77].

Several studies have examined relationships between demographic variables and prescription drug misuse. Rates of prescription drug misuse have been shown to increase consistently from early to late adolescence [27, 51, 60, 67]. The association between gender and medication misuse appears to vary between drug classes. Studies of prescription stimulant misuse typically report similar rates in adolescent males and females [40, 43], or slightly higher rates in males [27, 72]. In contrast, females appear to be more likely than males to misuse opioids and tranquilizers [13, 60, 66]. This may reflect either the higher frequency with which females receive prescriptions for these medications and/or self-medication of disorders such as depression or anxiety, which occur more often in females. Prescription misuse also appears to differ across racial and ethnic groups. Most studies report the highest prevalence of misuse among Caucasian adolescents [27, 40, 67]. However, Boyd and colleagues found equal rates of prescription opioid misuse among Caucasian and African-American students in an ethnically diverse school district in the USA [13], and Sung et al. found that African-American teens were actually at higher risk for opioid misuse compared to other racial groups [66].

The likelihood of methylphenidate misuse appears to be greater among students with poorer academic performance [41, 66, 67, 72]. Adolescent stimulant misuse has also been found to be more common in low-income families and families receiving government assistance [40, 66].

Only a few studies have looked at the relationship between mental health and prescription misuse in adolescents. Poulin found that high school students with elevated levels of depressive symptoms, as well as those screening positive for ADHD, had a higher likelihood of having used stimulant medication without a prescription [72]. Schepis and Krishnan-Sarin reported a positive association between misuse of any prescription drug and experiencing a major depressive episode or receiving mental health treatment in the preceding year [41]. Further examining these relationships, as well as identifying associations with any other psychiatric conditions (e.g., anxiety disorders), represents an important area for future investigations.

Implications for Prevention and Treatment in Adolescents

The recent escalation in prescription medication misuse among adolescents and the increasingly well-documented risks of such misuse make it essential to develop initiatives to minimize the negative effects to teens. The body of literature described above indicates that adolescents involved in prescription drug misuse are a heterogeneous group. Individual differences in the particular prescription medications used, patterns of use, and motives for use, are all essential to consider when developing prevention or treatment interventions [37].

As mentioned, motivations for prescription drug misuse are commonly reported to be therapeutic; thus, traditional anti-drug campaigns may be inappropriate for addressing prescription misuse in teens [13]. Effective treatment programs will need to consider the motivations and perceptions that may have encouraged adolescents to initially misuse medications [40, 42]. One of the most important prevention strategies may be education programs targeted at adolescents that highlight the dangers and risks of misusing prescription medications [60] while at the same time taking care not to downplay their legitimate use [42].

Considering the frequency of self-medication motives for prescription drug misuse, it is also important that adolescents receive appropriate treatment for relevant psychological conditions [13]. Poulin found that less than 10% of those with symptoms of ADHD or depression were actually receiving appropriate medication; the presence of these psychiatric symptoms was linked to taking stimulant medications illicitly [72]. Better screening programs are needed to detect and address adolescent mental health conditions that may be linked to prescription drug misuse [72].

For adolescents, family involvement may prove to be a key to prevention in a number of important ways. Parents can limit their teens' access to abusable prescription drugs in the home by monitoring and securing any medications that are present, as well as appropriately disposing of expired or unused medications. Schinke et al. found that female teens in families with better parent–child communication and clear anti-drug views were less likely to have misused prescription drugs [78]. Higher parental involvement in teens' lives has also been associated with lower rates of opioid misuse [66]. More favorable outcomes may be achieved if parents participate in prevention programs along with their children [42].

Other potential targets for intervention programs to reduce prescription drug misuse in adolescents include schools and the health care system. Educators can discuss potential harms of prescription misuse and diversion with teens, focusing on the specific hazards of each drug class [51, 62]. Because of the high occurrence of polysubstance use among adolescents misusing prescription drugs, preventative efforts should educate adolescents about the risks for adverse drug interactions [77]. Given the frequency of diversion from peer sources [60] especially in schools [73], strict school policy and monitoring of legitimate prescription drug use is also crucial.

Clinicians and service providers who work with adolescents, including doctors, nurses, social workers, and pharmacists, can act as "gatekeepers," monitoring teens' prescription use in order to detect signs of diversion and being mindful of the risk factors for misuse, particularly given the relationship with other substance use [27, 41]. Although it is important to be able to identify specific risk factors to minimize access to medications that may be harmful if used inappropriately, clinicians face a challenge in balancing the effective delivery of care with the risk for misuse of certain medications.

Prescription Drug Misuse in Young Adults

Like adolescence, early adulthood is a time of transition. During this period of life, defined approximately as ages 18 to 25 [79], individuals begin to assume adult responsibilities and pursue new educational and vocational goals [79]. This age group comprises the largest proportion of students at postsecondary educational institutions in North America [80, 81]. Enrollment in colleges and universities has grown over recent decades, with current data indicating that nearly 40% of 18- to 25-year-olds are current postsecondary students [82]. This population has been the recipient of much attention in the literature, due to the prevalence of substance use among college and university students [51, 79] as well as their proximity to academic researchers. Accordingly, this section on prescription drug misuse in young adults will focus primarily on postsecondary students.

Culturally, the college years are perceived as a time of experimentation and risk taking [83], in which substance use is often viewed as normative [79, 84]. In addition to reporting the highest rates of illicit drug use of any age group, 18- to 25-year-olds in North America report the highest rates of prescription drug misuse [7], with evidence suggesting that prevalence rates are increasing [85]. Although representing only 13% of the US population [7], recent epidemiological investigations found that this age group accounted for 32% of all opioid pain reliever misuse [86], 35% of prescription stimulant misuse [40], and 21% of prescription tranquilizer misuse [7]. Although much of the existing research has been conducted in the US and Canada, worldwide data appear to corroborate this trend [59, 87].

As with other age groups, methodological differences between studies and variations in the operationalization of misuse make it difficult to determine definitive estimates of the extent of prescription drug misuse in college- and university-age populations. However, particular attention has been paid to the misuse of stimulant medications [32, 57, 88–92]. The lifetime prevalence of prescription stimulant misuse in college and university students has been reported to range from 7% [88] to 43% [93], greatly exceeding the lifetime prevalence of between 2 and 5% reported in the general population [3, 40]. Hall et al. found the rate of nonprescribed use of prescription stimulants in a college sample to be second only to marijuana, with nearly half of the respondents stating that they knew a fellow student who had misused these drugs [90]. Far fewer studies have been conducted examining rates of opioid, anxiolytic, and sedative medication misuse in postsecondary students, but preliminary data have reported prevalence rates of approximately 15% for opioids [38, 94, 95] and 8% for anxiolytics and sedatives [25].

There are a number of reasons why prescription medication misuse in young adult populations is of particular concern. Misuse is frequently reported to occur in the context of simultaneous polysubstance use [92, 95–98], putting users at risk for adverse drug interactions. Co-administration of stimulants [92, 96], opioids [83], and tranquilizers [83] with alcohol has been reported among university students. In a study focusing on prescription stimulants, Barrett et al. found that co-administration of other substances was common even when students reported using stimulants exclusively when studying [97].

One study that examined students' perceptions of nonprescribed stimulant use found that 79% of the students who engaged in this behavior reported no concerns about potential negative consequences, suggesting many may underestimate the potency and adverse health effects of stimulant misuse [91]. Quintero, Peterson, and Young found that college students tended to describe the use of prescription drugs as more socially and legally acceptable and less hazardous than illicit drugs [83]. Many college students do not appear aware that one of the risks of prescription drug misuse is the development of medication-related substance abuse or dependence [47]. In fact, one large population-based study found that the mean age of onset for medication-related substance use disorders was in the early 20s [3]. Kroutil et al. reported that young adults who had misused prescription drugs in the past year were at higher risk for dependence on and abuse of prescription medications, as compared to older age groups [40].

Patterns of Prescription Drug Misuse in Young Adult Populations

As with adolescents, young adults' motives for misuse of prescription medications are essential to consider [14]. Within individual classes of medication, multiple motives for use have been reported. The majority of research on prescription drug misuse in young adult populations has focused on the misuse of stimulant medications, including various forms of methylphenidate (Ritalin, Concerta), dextroamphetamine (Dexedrine), and mixed-salts amphetamine (Adderall). Given the high level of demands in college environments, students may seek out stimulant medications to assist in staying awake and focused while studying [32, 57, 90], a form of misuse which is somewhat congruent with these medications' intended therapeutic purpose [14]. This supposition is borne out by a series of studies reporting that students' primary motives for taking a stimulant medication without a prescription were to concentrate and increase alertness [32, 38, 92, 93, 99, 100]. Judson and Langdon also found that individuals who had self-diagnosed themselves as having ADHD were more likely to use stimulant medications without a prescription [100]. Although some reports suggest that many students believe that stimulant medications will improve their academic performance [93, 100], interestingly, one study found that only 14% of nonprescribed stimulant users agreed that using these drugs had had a positive long-term effect on their academic achievements [90].

Given that stimulant medications act in similar ways in the brain to illicit stimulant drugs, they may also be used for recreational purposes [101]. Although recreational use of prescription stimulants has been found to be prevalent, evidence suggests that it is less commonly students' primary motive for use [92, 99, 100]. Emerging evidence suggests that these two motives, self-medication and recreation, may describe distinct subtypes of prescription drug misuse among college students [14].

Less evidence has documented differing motives for use in other prescription drug classes in university and college students. One study found that the primary purpose for non-prescribed use of opioids was to relieve pain, with 63% of students endorsing this motive. However, other motives were common, with 32% reporting having taken prescription opioids to get high and 29% reporting use for experimentation [94]. Although engaging in prescription drug misuse for any reason has the potential to escalate into problematic patterns of use [101], gaining a better understanding of young adults' motives for use will help provide insights into the potential short- and long-term consequences of this behavior [32].

Another important avenue of investigation concerns misuse among individuals with prescriptions for psychoactive drugs. Several studies have examined prescription drug misuse in college students with prescriptions to treat ADHD [90, 91, 99]. Arria et al. found that 27% of the students reported overuse of their own medication and 16% reported nonprescribed stimulant use [99]. Teter et al. found similar rates of stimulant misuse in students with and without past prescriptions for stimulant medications [32], while Judson and Langdon found that students with current prescriptions for stimulants were more likely to report misuse [100]. These results suggest that medication misuse among students with prescriptions is also a concern.

Studies assessing patterns of diversion among prescribed young adult users of psychoactive medications are equally important. The literature indicates that most nonprescribed medication administered by individuals in this age range originates from peers with prescriptions [11, 86, 91, 94, 95, 99, 102]. In a sample of students with prescriptions for stimulant medications to treat ADHD, Advokat et al. found that 83% had been asked to give their medications away and 54% had been asked to sell their medications [93]. Undergraduate men have been found to be more likely than women to have been approached to divert their opioid medication [95]. As compared to other sources, students who obtained prescription drugs from peers reported more frequent heavy episodic alcohol use, higher rates of drug use, and a greater tendency to engage in polysubstance use [102]. These students were also more likely to report symptoms of drug and alcohol use disorders [94]. One study reported that opioids diverted from peers were commonly co-administered with alcohol, while those diverted from family members were exclusively used for pain management [95]. Several studies have found gender differences in sources for diverted prescription drugs, with females more likely than males to have received sedative, anxiolytic, and pain medications from familial sources [94, 95, 102]. Obtaining medications using methods such as pharmacy theft, prescription fraud, online pharmacies, or seeking prescriptions from multiple doctors is thought to be rare among young adults [11, 86, 94, 99].

A further consideration when examining patterns of misuse of prescription drugs in young adult populations is the drug formulation and route of administration used. Extended-release formulations appear to have lower misuse liability; however, tampering with medications may allow faster drug delivery, alternate routes of administration, and separation and purification of active drug ingredients [68]. Not surprisingly, most stimulant medication misuse appears to involve short-acting methylphenidate and dextroamphetamine, but misuse of long-acting forms has also been reported [40].

The most common route of administration for misused prescription stimulants among young adults appears to be oral, followed by intranasal [91, 97]. Likewise, the most common route of administration for opioids appears to be oral [94], with other routes reported much less frequently. Interestingly, the route of administration for opioids has been shown to vary depending on prescription source and motive for use. McCabe et al. found that less than 1% of the students reporting pain management as their motive for opioid misuse reported intranasal use [94]. No student who obtained prescription opioids from a parent reported intranasal administration, while more than 16% of the students obtaining these drugs from non-parent sources (predominantly friends) reported intranasal use [94], Eighty percent of the group of intranasal users was composed of students who reported using the medications to get high [94]. Overall, those students reporting non-oral routes of administration had increased odds of experiencing drug-related problems [94].

Correlates of Prescription Drug Misuse in Young Adult Populations

As with adolescent populations, studies focusing on young adults have consistently found a relationship between prescription drug misuse and increased prevalence and frequency of other substance use [11, 32, 93, 102], as well as problems associated with alcohol and other drugs [28, 30, 103]. These studies have overwhelmingly concentrated on nonprescribed stimulant use, which has been associated with higher rates of binge drinking [26, 32, 88, 89, 104, 105], tobacco use [32, 88, 104], marijuana use [88, 89, 97, 105], ecstasy use [26, 88, 89, 97], cocaine use [26, 88, 97], and other illicit drug use [26, 97, 105]. Nonprescribed stimulant medication users are more likely to report adverse consequences related to substance use, including missing classes, developing a hangover, and being injured while under the influence of alcohol or drugs [89]; risky activities such as having unplanned sex and driving while intoxicated [88, 89]; and antisocial behaviors such as being arrested, stealing, and selling drugs [105]. Interestingly, some studies have found that compared to nonusers, college students who had engaged in nonprescribed stimulant use reported more

extensive alcohol and other drug use histories regardless of whether their primary motive for using the medication was to help concentrate or for recreation [32, 97]. Teter et al. argue that this finding runs contrary to the notion that students who use stimulant medications without a prescription to study are engaging in relatively less hazardous behaviors [32]. Although most studies have investigated the correlates of nonprescribed stimulant use, higher rates of substance use, as well as increased risk for alcohol and marijuana dependence, have also been observed in prescribed stimulant users who report overuse of their own medications [99].

As noted, considerably fewer studies have examined opioid, sedative, and anxiolytic misuse in young adult populations. Existing evidence supports a link between misuse of these medications and other substance use in this age range [11]; however, the patterns appear to differ somewhat from those observed with young adults' stimulant misuse. For instance, other substance use has been found to differ among nonprescribed opioid users depending on their motives for use [94] and on the source of the medication [95]. Students who reported using opioids exclusively to manage pain did not differ from nonusers in terms of binge drinking and alcohol use disorders, while those reporting nontherapeutic motives for use had elevated rates of these problems [94]. As compared to nonusers, higher rates of tobacco use, illicit drug use, and binge drinking were observed in nonprescribed opioid users who obtained the medication from their peers, while no such elevations were found among those who obtained opioids from familial sources [95].

Multiple studies have examined demographic correlates of prescription drug misuse in an attempt to better understand the risk factors for misuse [16]. Findings relating to gender are inconsistent across studies. Several investigations have demonstrated similar overall prevalence of prescription drug misuse in male and female young adults [89, 91, 105, 106], while others have found higher rates in males [11, 26, 32, 90, 92, 95]. Less commonly, higher rates in females have also been reported [59]. The reason for this lack of clarity may stem from variations between studies in how prescription misuse was operationalized. Some evidence suggests that an interaction between gender and motives for use may be present, such that young women may be more likely to misuse prescription drugs for medical reasons, while young men may be more likely to report nonmedical motives [77, 94]. One study [11] found that although young women were prescribed anti-anxiety and pain medications at higher rates than young men, men reported more misuse of these substances, defined in this study as use without a prescription.

Studies analyzing use in different racial or ethnic groups have found the highest rates of misuse of prescription stimulants, opioids, and anxiolytics among Caucasian postsecondary students [11, 25, 26, 94, 105, 107]. One study [32], however, reported similarly high levels of stimulant misuse among Hispanic students. Typically, African-American and Asian young adults have been reported to be at lower risk.

A number of other socio-demographic factors appear to be correlated with prescription drug misuse in young adults. Having a higher family income [89] and having attended a private high school [91] have been associated with increased use of stimulant medications without a prescription, suggesting a relationship between higher socio-economic status (SES) and stimulant misuse in postsecondary students, a pattern which differs from that observed in high school students. Interestingly, colleges with more competitive entrance requirements have been found to have higher rates of stimulant misuse [88]. The authors of this study suggest that competitive entrance requirements may be serving as a proxy for SES. In addition, although this study did not measure students' motivations for prescription stimulant misuse, it suggests that misuse of these medications may be more common in environments that place a high degree of emphasis on academic achievement. More research is needed to examine this pattern and explore the potential reasons (developmental and otherwise) for the differing relationships between stimulant misuse observed in adolescent and young adult populations.

Several studies have found that postsecondary students with lower grade point averages are more likely to report prescription drug misuse [107]. In particular, this relationship has been noted for both opioids [95] and stimulants [26, 88]. Arria et al. found that nonmedical users of stimulants and analgesics skipped more classes, spent more time socializing and less time studying, and had lower GPAs. These authors suggest that students engaging in prescription drug misuse represent a high-risk group for academic problems in college [38].

Further investigations of individual differences in this area have suggested relationships between misuse of prescription drugs and physical health, mental health, and personality. Poorer health has been found to be correlated with increased risk for misuse [107], while involvement in athletics appears to be a protective factor for sedative, anxiolytic, and painkiller misuse, especially among females [108]. Surprisingly, few studies have examined the role of mental health in young adults' prescription drug misuse. Herman-Stahl et al. found that higher scores on a broad measure of psychological distress were associated with vulnerability to engage in prescription misuse [105]. Consistent with past studies finding a robust association between sensation seeking and drinking behavior in postsecondary students [79], high sensation seeking appears to be associated with greater risk for stimulant medication misuse [92, 109]. This relationship was found to be especially pronounced among students with high perfectionism scores, leading the authors to speculate that perfectionism appears to function synergistically with sensation seeking to predict misuse of prescription stimulants [92].

Implications for Prevention and Treatment in Young Adults

College and university environments present unique challenges to implementing intervention strategies to minimize the diversion and misuse of prescription medications [88]. Institutions need to act proactively to address substance-related problems experienced by their students [110], which may include developing educational initiatives targeted at students, their parents, and health care providers. Treatment programs could be designed to address the specific demands intrinsic to college life, especially regarding the intensity of the social environment and academic pressures [110].

At the health care provider level, clinicians may be able to make use of some of the demonstrated correlates of prescription drug misuse, particularly the strong relationship between alcohol and illicit drug use and prescription drug misuse. In all cases, there is a need to strike a balance between the delivery of essential medications and the need to reduce misuse of these drugs [95]. As evidence suggests that malingering of symptoms of ADHD in order to obtain medications for misuse is becoming more common [111], it is essential that patients be given a thorough and comprehensive assessment before medications with known misuse liability are prescribed. Because most college students who misuse prescription medications obtain them from their peers, clinicians need to appropriately monitor students with prescriptions for abusable prescription drugs, not only to improve clinical outcomes, but also to help prevent the misuse of these medications [40]. When treating students with ADHD who may be at risk for misuse or diversion, physicians may wish to consider nonstimulant alternatives [112] or pharmaceutical delivery systems that are less prone to misuse [88].

Assessing young adults' motives for use of prescription drugs is critical, as the correlates of different motives appear to vary by drug class. As noted, studies indicate that for those endorsing pain relief as the sole reason for nonprescribed opioid use, there was no increase in risk for substance use problems [94], while both academic and recreational stimulant misusers reported higher rates of such problems. Health care professionals should also inquire about the routes of administration used and the sources of medications, as the associated risks also appear to vary considerably depending on these factors.

Prescription Drug Misuse in Middle Adulthood

The period of life defined herein as middle adulthood extends roughly from the early 30s to the early 60s. Some of the key developmental challenges encountered by individuals in this age group involve establishing a career, maintaining stable marital and family relationships, and parenting [113]. Despite comprising the largest proportion of the population, research examining prescription drug misuse in middle adulthood is by far the sparsest. The investigations of adolescents and postsecondary students described previously in this review portray distinct patterns of use (e.g., stimulant misuse in academic contexts) that are unlikely to generalize to individuals in middle adulthood. Perhaps in recognition of the unique characteristics of adolescent and college-age populations, epidemiological studies often report prevalence rates and demographic correlates of prescription drug misuse in adults separately from those in younger groups [35, 40]. However, grouping individuals in middle adulthood together with older adults fails to take into account that patterns and correlates of prescription drug misuse are dynamic and likely to continue changing over the lifespan. In addition, many of the studies that do include participants in this age range focus on specific subpopulations, such as street drug users [114], hospital inpatients [115], military veterans [116], and chronic pain patients [117, 118], precluding extrapolation of their findings to the broader adult population.

Patterns of Prescription Drug Misuse in Middle Adulthood

After peaking in late adolescence and early adulthood, the evidence suggests that prescription drug misuse in the general population begins to decline steadily [7]. In a large population-based study, Blanco et al. found past-year prevalence of prescription drug misuse and prescription drug use disorders in middle adulthood were intermediate between young adults and those over age 55 [9]. In another epidemiological study, the prevalence of prescription drug misuse in adults aged 30–64 was found to be similar to those aged 18–29, but significantly more frequent than in those aged 65 and above [3]. No significant differences were found in the prevalence of misuse between sedatives, tranquilizers, opioids, and stimulants. Using the nationally representative NSDUH dataset, Blazer and Wu found that the rates of opioid pain reliever misuse were significantly greater in middle-aged adults as compared to those over age 65 [39]. Interestingly, the majority of opioid misusers in this study reported that they initiated misuse in adulthood, with more than 20% of these individuals reporting initiation at age 50 or above.

Anxiolytics, sedatives, and opioid painkillers are prescribed more frequently for adults in middle age as compared to younger age groups [20]. As noted previously, symptoms of substance dependence, particularly physiological dependence, tolerance, and withdrawal, are known to occur routinely following long-term use of these medications, even when used according to a physician's prescription [45]. Many of these users may be unaware of this dependence until they attempt to discontinue taking the medication [15].

Although this form of prescription drug use is not encompassed by the definition of prescription drug misuse employed by many studies, it represents a problematic consequence of medication use that is nevertheless an important target for research and clinical attention.

Correlates of Prescription Drug Misuse in Middle Adulthood

Studies examining prescription drug misuse in middle adulthood have focused on a disparate set of subpopulations. Although the findings from these investigations cannot be extrapolated directly to the general population, they provide important contributions to our understanding of the heterogeneity and diversity of individuals engaging in misuse of prescription drugs.

Among an urban sample of street drug users, prescription opioid misuse was most commonly reported for the purposes of pain reduction and withdrawal management [114]. Only 37% of this sample reported misuse of opioids for their euphoric effects; these individuals were more likely to report administering the drugs intranasally or by injecting. Conversely, in a study of rural illicit stimulant users, prescription opioid misuse was associated with comorbid anxiety and illicit drug use, but not with higher levels of chronic pain [119]. Although these samples differ considerably, self-medication of physical or psychological symptoms may have contributed to opioid misuse in both cases.

Studies in the alcohol literature have suggested that failure to master the typical developmental goals of adulthood is associated with increased risk for alcohol use problems [113]. Although research in the prescription drug misuse literature has yet to address this topic directly, some evidence suggests a similar association with prescription drug use problems. An association between prescription drug misuse and unemployment has been reported in studies involving participants ranging from US military veterans, hospital inpatients [115], and a general community-based sample [120]. In a large sample of military veterans in the USA, Becker et al. found that prescription drug misuse was associated with being unmarried and experiencing financial difficulties [116]. In this study, misuse of prescription drugs was also associated with smoking, illicit drug use, chronic pain, and depression.

The role of gender in prescription drug misuse and dependence has long been a focus of attention. Women receive prescriptions for psychotropic medications at higher rates than men, particularly those with the potential for misuse [121]. Several factors have been proposed to contribute to this difference, including higher rates of mood, anxiety, and pain-related problems, an increased willingness to seek treatment, and a tendency of physicians to interpret symptoms as indicative of psychiatric complaints [122]. Green et al. reported that the strongest risk factor for opioid misuse was recent use of prescribed opioid medication; unsurprisingly, they also found that women were 50% more likely to report recent opioid misuse [123]. Simoni-Wastila, Ritter, and Strickler found that being female increased the odds of reporting problem use of opioid analgesics, including symptoms of dependence [124]. In a sample of general hospital patients, prescription drug dependence was more prevalent in females, and was found to be commonly associated with comorbid mood, anxiety, and other substance use disorders [115].

Implications for Prevention and Treatment in Middle Adulthood

Although onset of prescription drug misuse typically occurs during adolescence or early adulthood, a substantial number of older adults have reported engaging in misuse for the first time after age 50 [39], indicating that prevention efforts for this age group are still warranted. One investigation found that patients with comorbid substance use disorders actually had an increased likelihood of receiving a prescription medication with misuse potential as compared to those with no comorbid substance use disorder [125]. Primary care physicians can play an important role in minimizing psychoactive prescription drug misuse in adults by recognizing factors associated with risk for misuse, such as a history of alcohol or illicit drug problems. However, as demonstrated with gender, it is important to be aware that the relationships between prescription drug misuse and factors correlating with misuse may be indirect or moderated by other variables, such as prescription rates.

Physicians have an ethical responsibility to balance the provision of safe and effective care with the risks associated with various prescription drugs [125]. Based on the potential for abuse of and dependence on opioid analgesics and benzodiazepine anxiolytics, many researchers have argued that the use of these medications should be restricted as much as possible to the treatment of short-term pain, anxiety, and insomnia [20, 45]. If the symptoms are likely to persist for a longer duration, an alternative treatment may be indicated. In cases where no viable alternative is available, more careful monitoring by health care providers is warranted.

Prescription Drug Misuse in Older Adults

As described previously, the highest prevalence of substance use across the lifespan has been reported to occur in late adolescence and early adulthood. Correspondingly, clinical and research attention has focused primarily on these younger populations, with relatively less attention paid to examining substance use and misuse in older adults [50]. Illicit drug use

in adults over age 60 is relatively rare, yet the misuse of alcohol and prescription drugs among this population has been identified as a substantial public health concern [54, 126, 127]. Prescription medication misuse has been described as the most widespread pattern of problematic substance use among senior populations [50]. Although the epidemiology and treatment of alcohol abuse in older adults has been relatively well described, comparable data on prescription drug misuse are lacking [54]. Investigations into the causes, correlates, and sequelae of prescription misuse in this population are few [128], and, surprisingly, no validated screening or assessment tools for identifying this phenomenon among older adults have been developed [129].

Adults over 60 years of age are the fastest growing segment of the population. As life expectancy continues to rise and the average overall age of the population increases, the consumption of psychoactive prescription medications has been predicted to grow [50]. This has the potential to profoundly affect all sectors of the health care system, including addiction-related services [130]. Compared to younger individuals, seniors are prescribed more medications and tend to take them more frequently [50]. It is estimated that in the USA, at least one in four older adults has a prescription for a psychoactive medication with the potential for misuse [54]. In North America, adults over 60 years of age represent just 13% of the population, yet they are the consumers of an estimated 50% of all psychoactive prescription medications [130, 131]. This disproportionate share is thought to occur, at least in part, because older individuals tend to experience a relatively greater number of illnesses for which these medications are typically prescribed [50]. Some of the most commonly reported health issues in old age are insomnia and mental health issues; correspondingly, the medications most frequently prescribed to this population include sedatives and anxiolytics [132]. Older adults are also more likely to continue use of these psychoactive medications for longer periods of time than younger individuals [126]. In particular, benzodiazepine anxiolytics and opioid analgesics are prescribed on a long-term basis more frequently for elderly patients than for any other age group [128].

Despite data indicating a growing population of older individuals with exposure to prescription medications with misuse potential, there is considerably less information available about the actual prevalence rates of medication misuse in this age group. In the general population, researchers have argued that observed increases in the rates of prescription drug misuse may be attributed to increased medication availability and social acceptance surrounding the use of sedatives, anxiolytics, and analgesics [6, 53]. The lack of empirical data specific to older adults is thought to be related to a number of issues, including undersampling of older adults in population-based studies, inconsistent definitions of substance abuse and dependence, and prevalence estimates based on subpopulations such as emergency department patients and residents of long-term care facilities that may not accurately represent older prescribed medication users in general [54, 133, 134].

Patterns of Prescription Drug Misuse in Older Adult Populations

Researchers have reported a number of ways in which prescription drug misuse may differ qualitatively and quantitatively in older adults as compared to those earlier in life [129]. Older adults use fewer classes of prescription drugs, most commonly sedatives, opioids, and anxiolytics [133]. Most older adults obtain medications from a physician by means of a legitimate prescription [128]. Use of medications obtained from illicit sources is thought to be much rarer than in younger populations, although risky behaviors such as seeking prescriptions from multiple doctors, taking pills from family or friends, or stockpiling medications over time have been reported in older prescription drug users [129]. Existing research suggests that the use of prescription medications for recreational purposes or in the context of polysubstance use occurs less frequently in older adults than their younger counterparts [129]. More typically, the motivation for use of prescription medications is therapeutic. As mentioned previously, however, problems with psychoactive prescription drug use can manifest even when medications are used with therapeutic intent. For instance, Busto et al. reported that older adults tended to take benzodiazepines for longer periods of time and have more problems with withdrawal than younger adults, both signs of physiological dependence [135].

Raffoul described several different patterns of medication misuse in older adult populations [136]. One form of misuse may result from the use of medications following incorrect instructions or from misunderstanding the directions for appropriate medication administration. Older individuals with cognitive impairments may be particularly at risk for adverse consequences resulting from this type of unintended noncompliance with prescription regimens. Another form of unintentional misuse may result from the simultaneous use of multiple medications. For many older adults, polypharmacy is the norm. In a sample of older adults accessing a community-based mental health clinic, Jinks and Raschko found that 92% of these participants had current prescriptions for three or more medications [134]. Finlayson and Davis reported an average of approximately 2.9 psychoactive drugs per person administered concurrently within a geriatric inpatient population, in addition to an average of 2.8 nonpsychoactive medications per person [133]. Older adults may also supplement prescribed medications with over-the-counter preparations, which have the potential to interact and produce harmful side effects [137].

Although use of prescription medications for recreational purposes in older adults is thought to be rare, different forms of intentional misuse of prescription medications have been reported, ranging from deficient to excessive use [50]. Medication noncompliance and underutilization may be associated with health risks, such as failure to adequately treat a health condition. Overuse of medications such as anxiolytics and opioid analgesics can increase the risk for accidents (e.g., falls), injury, or overdose, particularly if used in combination with alcohol or other drugs [33].

Correlates of Prescription Drug Misuse in Older Adult Populations

Problematic substance use in older adults has been described as a "hidden epidemic" [138]. One reason that this population has received less attention than younger individuals may be due to the differing manifestations of prescription drug misuse in older adults. Zimberg noted that family members or friends often do not identify alcohol problems in seniors, as there may be fewer consequences in social, legal, occupational, and interpersonal domains in older people [137]. Prescription drug misuse in older adults may be underreported for similar reasons.

Another important consideration in older adult populations is the role of biological factors. Physiological sensitivity to some medications increases with age, which can result in negative side effects even at previously tolerated dosages [50]. For example, benzodiazepine anxiolytics, which are widely prescribed in older adults, may cause multiple cognitive side effects, including sedation, memory problems, and attentional impairments [139]. Changes in body composition, including less body water, more fat stores, and changes in organ function may also affect how a given medication acts in older adults [138].

Researchers have suggested a wide variety of factors that may increase vulnerability for prescription drug misuse in seniors. Despite the widespread utilization of medications with misuse potential in older adults, intentional misuse in those without a history of other substance use problems is relatively uncommon [54, 129]. High rates of psychiatric comorbidity are common in elderly patients with prescription drug dependence [133]. In one investigation of individuals with prescription drug dependence, a diagnosable psychiatric illness was present in 85% of elderly patients but in only 36% of younger patients [140]. In this sample, older patients were more likely to have a history of memory loss, sleep disturbance, irritability, delusions, and inability to conduct daily activities without assistance. Younger patients, in contrast, were more likely to have experienced blackouts and to report that prescription medication misuse had negatively affected their relationships and careers. Unintentional misuse in older adults may be more likely to occur when individuals suffer from more health problems, lack knowledge about the medications and their effects, visit a greater number of physicians and pharmacists, and live further from the medical clinic at which treatment is received [141].

A number of psychosocial factors unique to older populations have been associated with the risk for prescription drug misuse [50]. Elderly individuals are likely to encounter a range of difficult life circumstances, including loss of status following retirement, diminished social support and self-esteem, financial hardship, reduced mobility and social isolation, compromised physical health, or loneliness following the death of a spouse or close friends [138]. The use of psychoactive prescription medications has been suggested as a means of coping with these difficulties [50]. Of these negative factors, depression and social isolation are thought to be some of the most potent risk factors for prescription medication misuse [138]. For individuals with a history of using substances to cope with negative life events, the stresses associated with aging may be compounded by an exacerbation of existing substance-related problems [142].

Implications for Prevention and Treatment in Older Adults

A number of barriers have been identified that may impede the detection of problematic prescription drug use in older adults [128]. In addition to the lack of formal diagnostic tools [129], the negative consequences of misuse may be subtle and thus more difficult for health care providers to discern [138]. Potential warning signs of prescription misuse, such as concurrent alcohol or illicit drug use, prescription forgery, acquisition from nonmedical sources, or dose escalation may be less commonly observed in older adults as compared to their younger counterparts [128]. Consequences of misuse, including cognitive or psychomotor impairment or exacerbation of depression or anxiety, may be overlooked or attributed to the effects of aging. It may be difficult to determine whether an individual's difficulties are due to the effects of a medication, related withdrawal symptoms, the underlying condition the medication is prescribed to treat, or an interaction of these and other factors [128]. Complicating matters further, evidence suggests that elderly patients may underreport their medication usage [143] and that health care workers tend to display a low index of suspicion regarding substance misuse in older patients [137].

Access to appropriate treatment services presents another important consideration regarding older prescription drug misusers. Increased awareness of the problem of prescription drug misuse in older adults has provided some impetus for the development of intervention programs [50]. Zimberg argues for an aging-specific approach to treatment that aims to decrease problem substance use in the context of the other stresses associated with aging [137]. Treatments aimed at increasing social support and self-esteem may be more acceptable for older adults than interventions aimed solely at decreasing problem prescription drug use. Additionally, promoting the involvement of family members in the treatment process may produce better outcomes [50].

General Conclusions

Although the many definitions of prescription drug misuse used within the literature make it difficult to arrive at specific estimates of prevalence, existing research portrays a growing problem which, thus far, has been inadequately characterized and addressed [42, 66]. Distinct patterns of prescription drug misuse are evident in the various age groups covered in this review.

Patterns of prescription drug misuse are strikingly different across developmental stages and demographic classifications. More research is needed on socio-cultural factors relating to prescription drug misuse, as well as personality correlates and psychiatric comorbidities [83]. One consistent finding across age groups is the association between prescription drug misuse and increased use of alcohol and illicit drugs, a finding that has implications for the detection, assessment, and treatment of prescription drug misuse, abuse, and dependence. It is essential that prevention and intervention efforts take into account individual differences in motivations for misuse of prescription drugs, as the patterns and correlates of use tend to vary depending on whether a medication is self-administered for therapeutic or nontherapeutic reasons.

The body of research examining prescription drug misuse focuses on the extremities of the age continuum, a problem that is shared with the alcohol use literature [113]. Although many studies have examined the patterns and predictors of prescription drug misuse in young adulthood and older age, information about the intervening period is scarce and little is known about transitions between developmental stages.

Methodological considerations for future research include employing standardized definitions of prescription drug misuse, abuse, and dependence. Additionally, agreement on standard age ranges would facilitate comparisons across studies [113]. It should be noted that most existing research in this area is cross-sectional and should not be interpreted as implying causal relationships. For example, young adults may engage in prescription drug misuse to cope with negative feelings associated with poor academic performance. Alternately, prescription misuse may impair functioning, resulting in poorer grades. Either, or both, of these relationships may be true. The cross-sectional nature of these data also renders it difficult to track trends in prescription drug misuse over time [86]. Cohort differences could imply that as these individuals age, higher rates of misuse now observed in younger age groups will manifest as increased prevalence in older age groups in the future. It is also possible that the findings reported here demonstrate age-specific correlates of prescription drug misuse that reflect changing life circumstances [86], suggesting that the observed patterns of prescription drug misuse should remain relatively constant over time. Further longitudinal investigations are needed to clarify these relationships.

References

1. Augustin SG. Anxiety disorders. In: Koda-Kimble MA, Young LY, Kradjan WA, Guglielmo BJ, editors. Applied therapeutics: the clinical use of drugs. 7th ed. Philadelphia, PA: Lippincott Williams & Wilkins; 2001. p. 74.1–8.
2. Greenhill LL, Pliszka S, Dulcan MK, Bernet W, Arnold V, Beitchman J, et al. Practice parameters for the use of stimulant medications in the treatment of children, adolescents, and adults. J Am Acad Child Adolesc Psychiatry. 2002;41 Suppl 2: 26S–49S.
3. Huang B, Dawson DA, Stinson FS, Hasin DS, Ruan WJ, Saha TD, et al. Prevalence, correlates, and comorbidity of nonmedical prescription drug use and drug use disorders in the United States: results of the National Epidemiologic Survey on Alcohol and Related Conditions. J Clin Psychiatry. 2006;67:1062–73.
4. Zacny J, Bigelow G, Compton P, Foley F, Iguchi M, Sannerud C. College on problems of drug dependence taskforce on prescription opioid non-medical use and abuse. Drug Alcohol Depend. 2003;69:215–32.
5. Hertz JA, Knight JR. Prescription drug misuse: a growing national problem. Adolesc Med. 2006;17:751–69.
6. McCarthy M. Prescription drug abuse up sharply in the USA. Lancet. 2007;369:1505–6.
7. Substance Abuse and Mental Health Services Administration. Results from the 2007 National Survey on Drug Use and Health: National findings [Online]. Rockville (MD): Substance Abuse and Mental Health Services Administration, Office of Applied Studies, NSDUH Series H-34, DHHS Publication No. SMA 08-4343. Sept, 2008. http://www.oas.samhsa.gov/nsduh/2k7nsduh/2k7Results.pdf.
8. American Psychiatric Association. Diagnostic and statistical manual of mental disorders (Text Revision) (DSM-IV-TR). 4th ed. Washington, DC: American Psychiatric Association; 2000.
9. Blanco C, Alderson D, Ogburn E, Grant BF, Nunes EV, Hatzenbuehler ML, et al. Changes in the prevalence of non-medical prescription drug use and drug use disorders in the United States: 1991-1992 and 2001-2002. Drug Alcohol Depend. 2007;90:252–60.
10. Compton WM, Volkow ND. Abuse of prescription drugs and the risk of addiction. Drug Alcohol Depend. 2006;83S:S4–7.
11. McCabe SE, Teter CJ, Boyd CJ. Medical use, illicit use, and diversion of abusable prescription drugs. J Am Coll Health. 2006;54: 269–78.
12. Australian Crime Commission. Australian Crime Commission illicit drug data report, 2007-08. [Online]. Canberra City (Australia): Australian Crime Commission. Jun, 2009. http://www.crimecommission.gov.au/publications/iddr/_files/2007_08/IDDR%202007-08%20FINAL%20030609.pdf.
13. Boyd CJ, McCabe SE, Cranford JA, Young A. Adolescents' motivations to abuse prescription medications. Pediatrics. 2006;118: 2472–80.
14. McCabe SE, Boyd CJ, Teter CJ. Subtypes of nonmedical prescription drug misuse. Drug Alcohol Depend. 2009;102:63–70.
15. O'Brien CP. Benzodiazepine use, abuse, and dependence. J Clin Psychiatry. 2005;66 Suppl 2:28–33.
16. Becker WC, Fiellin DA, Desai RA. Non-medical use, abuse and dependence on sedatives and tranquilizers among U.S. adults: psychiatric and socio-demographic correlates. Drug Alcohol Depend. 2007;90:280–87.
17. Zarocostas J. Abuse of prescription drugs is second only to abuse of cannabis in US, UN drugs panel says. Br Med J. 2009;338:b684.
18. International Narcotics Control Board. Report of the International Narcotics Control Board for 2008. [Online]. New York, NY: United Nations. 2009. http://www.incb.org/incb/annual-report-2008.html.
19. Canadian Community Epidemiology Network on Drug Use. 2002 National Report: Drug trends and the CCENDU network. [Online]. Ottawa, ON: Canadian Centre on Substance Abuse. 2003. http://www.ccsa.ca/2003%20and%20earlier%20CCSA%20Documents/CCENDU-National-2002-e.pdf.
20. Morgan SG, Raymond C, Mooney D, Martin D. The Canadian Rx atlas, 2nd Ed. [Online]. Vancouver, BC: UBC Centre for Health Services and Policy Research. 2008. http://www.chspr.ubc.ca.
21. Barrett SP, Meisner JR, Stewart SH. What constitutes prescription drug misuse? Problems and pitfalls of current conceptualizations. Curr Drug Abuse Rev. 2008;1:255–62.
22. Shader RI, Greenblatt DJ. Use of benzodiazepines in anxiety disorders. N Engl J Med. 1993;328:1398–405.
23. Boyd CJ, McCabe SE. Coming to terms with nonmedical use of prescription medications. Subst Abuse Treat Prev Policy. 2008;3: 22–5.
24. Kelly B, Parsons J. Prescription drug misuse among club drug-using young adults. Am J Drug Alcohol Abuse. 2007;33:875–84.
25. McCabe SE. Correlates of nonmedical use of prescription benzodiazepine anxiolytics: results from a national survey of U.S. college students. Drug Alcohol Depend. 2005;79:53–62.
26. McCabe SE, Teter CJ, Boyd CJ. Medical use, illicit use and diversion of prescription stimulant medication. J Psychoactive Drugs. 2006;38:43–56.
27. McCabe SE, Teter CJ, Boyd CJ. The use, misuse and diversion of prescription stimulants among middle and high school students. Subst Use Misuse. 2004;39:1095–116.
28. McCabe SE. Screening for drug abuse among medical and nonmedical users of prescription drugs in a probability sample of college students. Arch Pediatr Adolesc Med. 2008;162:225–31.
29. McCabe SE, Cranford JA, Boyd CJ, Morales M. In pursuit of a more complex understanding of non-medical use of prescription drugs: broadening perspective by sharpening our tools. Addiction. 2008;103:1051–2.
30. McCabe SE, Teter CJ. Drug use related problems among nonmedical users of prescription stimulants: a web-based survey of college students from a midwestern university. Drug Alcohol Depend. 2007;91:69–76.
31. McCabe SE, West B, Wechsler H. Alcohol-use disorders and nonmedical use of prescription drugs among U.S. college students. J Stud Alcohol Drugs. 2007;68:543–7.
32. Teter CJ, McCabe SE, Cranford JA, Boyd CJ, Guthrie SK. Prevalence and motives for illicit use of prescription stimulants in an undergraduate student sample. J Am Coll Health. 2005;53: 253–62.
33. Griffiths RR, Johnson MW. Relative abuse liability of hypnotic drugs: a conceptual framework and algorithm for differentiating among compounds. J Clin Psychiatry. 2005;66 Suppl 9:31–41.
34. Fischer B, Rehm J. Understanding the parameters of non-medical use of prescription drugs: moving beyond mere numbers. Addiction. 2007;102:1931–2.

35. McCabe SE, Cranford JA, West BT. Trends in prescription drug abuse and dependence, co-occurrence with other substance use disorders, and treatment utilization: results from two national surveys. Addict Behav. 2008;33:1297–305.

36. Simoni-Wastila L, Strickler G. Risk factors associated with problem use of prescription drugs. Am J Public Health. 2004;94:266–8.

37. Weekes J, Rehm J, Mugford R. Prescription drug abuse FAQs. [Online]. Ottawa, ON: Canadian Centre on Substance Abuse. Jun, 2007. http://www.ccsa.ca/2007%20CCSA%20Documents/ccsa-011519-2007.pdf.

38. Arria AM, O'Grady KE, Caldeira KM, Vincent KB, Wish ED. Nonmedical use of prescription stimulants and analgesics: associations with social and academic behaviors among college students. J Drug Issues. 2008;38:1045–60.

39. Blazer DG, Wu LT. Nonprescription use of pain relievers by middle-aged and elderly community-living adults: National Survey on Drug Use and Health. J Am Geriatr Soc. 2009;57:1252–7.

40. Kroutil LA, Van Brunt DL, Herman-Stahl MA, Heller DC, Bray RM, Penne MA. Nonmedical use of prescription stimulants in the United States. Drug Alcohol Depend. 2006;84:135–43.

41. Schepis TS, Krishnan-Sarin S. Characterizing adolescent prescription misusers: a population-based study. J Am Acad Child Adolesc Psychiatry. 2008;47:745–54.

42. Twombly EC, Holtz KD. Teens and the misuse of prescription drugs: evidence-based recommendations to curb a growing societal problem. J Prim Prev. 2008;29:503–16.

43. Wu L-T, Pilowsky DJ, Schlenger WE, Galvin DM. Misuse of methamphetamine and prescription stimulants among youths and young adults in the community. Drug Alcohol Depend. 2007;89:195–205.

44. Wu L-T, Pilowsky DJ, Patkar AA. Non-prescribed use of pain relievers among adolescents in the United States. Drug Alcohol Depend. 2008;94:1–11.

45. O'Brien CP. Drug abuse and drug addiction. In: Brunton LL, editor. Goodman & Gilman's the pharmacological basis of therapeutics. 11th ed. New York, NY: McGraw-Hill, Medical Publishing Division; 2006. p. 607–28.

46. Inciardi JA, Surratt HL, Cicero TJ, Beard RA. Prescription opioid abuse and diversion in an urban community: the results of an ultra-rapid assessment. Pain Med. 2009;10:537–48.

47. McCabe SE, West BT, Morales M, Cranford JA, Boyd CJ. Does early onset of non-medical use of prescription drugs predict subsequent prescription drug abuse and dependence? Addiction. 2007;102:1920–30.

48. Roache JD, Meisch RA, Henningfield JE, Jaffe JH, Klein S, Sampson A. Reinforcing effects of triazolam in sedative abusers: correlation of drug liking and self-administration measures. Pharmacol Biochem Behav. 1995;50:171–9.

49. Becker WC, Sullivan LE, Tetrault JM, Desai RA, Fiellin DA. Non-medical use, abuse and dependence on prescription opioids among U.S. adults: psychiatric, medical and substance use correlates. Drug Alcohol Depend. 2008;94:38–47.

50. Barnea Z, Teichman M. Substance misuse and abuse among the elderly: implications for social work intervention. J Gerontol Social Work. 1994;21(3):133–48.

51. Johnston LD, O'Malley PM, Bachman JG, Schulenberg JE. Monitoring the Future national results on adolescent drug use: Overview of key findings, 2006. [Online]. Bethesda, MD: National Institute on Drug Abuse. 2007. http://www.monitoringthefuture.org/pubs.html.

52. Bodigger D. Drug abuse in older US adults worries experts. Lancet. 2008;372:1622.

53. Riggs P. Non-medical use and abuse of commonly prescribed medications. Curr Med Res Opin. 2008;24:869–77.

54. Simoni-Wastila L, Yang HK. Psychoactive drug abuse in older adults. Am J Geriatr Pharmacother. 2006;4:380–94.

55. Smith A, Stewart D, Peled M, Poon C, Saewyc E. A picture of health: Highlights from the 2008 BC Adolescent Health Survey. [Online]. Vancouver, BC: McCreary Centre Society. 2009. http://www.mcs.bc.ca/pdf/AHS%20IV%20March%2030%20Final.pdf.

56. Kandel DB, Logan JA. Patterns of drug use from adolescence to young adulthood. I: periods of risk for initiation, continued use, and discontinuation. Am J Public Health. 1984;74:660–6.

57. Arria AM, Wish ED. Nonmedical use of prescription stimulants among students. Pediatr Ann. 2006;35:565–71.

58. Partnership for a Drug-Free America. Generation Rx: National study reveals new category of substance abuse emerging: Teens abusing Rx and OTC medications intentionally to get high. [Online]. Nov 2005. http://www.drugfree.org/General/Articles/article.aspx?id=df07cc48-88e2-4fc5-abdf-c83c0e22e943&Site=Print&PrintPage=true.

59. Lieb R, Pfister H, Wittchen H. Use, abuse and dependence of prescription drugs in adolescents and young adults. Eur Addict Res. 1998;4:67–74.

60. Boyd CJ, McCabe SE, Teter CJ. Medical and nonmedical use of prescription pain medication by youth in a Detroit-area public school district. Drug Alcohol Depend. 2006;81:37–45.

61. McCabe SE, Boyd CJ, Young A. Medical and nonmedical use of prescription drugs among secondary school students. J Adolesc Health. 2007;40:76–83.

62. Friedman RA. The changing face of teenage drug abuse—the trend toward prescription drugs. N Engl J Med. 2006;354:1448–50.

63. Schepis TS, Adinoff B, Rao U. Neurobiological processes in adolescent addictive disorders. Am J Addict. 2008;17:6–23.

64. Colliver JD, Kroutil LA, Dai L, Gfroerer JC. Misuse of prescription drugs: Data from the 2002, 2003, and 2004 National Surveys on Drug Use and Health. [Online]. Rockville, MD: Substance Abuse and Mental Health Services Administration, Office of Applied Studies. DHHS Publication No. SMA 06-4192, Analytic Series A-28. Sept, 2006. http://www.oas.samhsa.gov/prescription/toc.htm.

65. Boyd CJ, McCabe SE, Cranford JA, Young A. Prescription drug abuse and diversion among adolescents in a southeast Michigan school district. Arch Pediatr Adolesc Med. 2007;161:276–81.

66. Sung H, Richter L, Vaughan R, Johnson PB, Thom B. Nonmedical use of prescription opioids among teenagers in the United States: trends and correlates. J Adolesc Health. 2005;37:44–51.

67. McCabe SE, Teter CJ, Boyd CJ, Guthrie SK. Prevalence and correlates of illicit methylphenidate use among 8th, 10th, and 12th grade students in the United States, 2001. J Adolesc Health. 2004;35:501–4.

68. Cone EJ. Ephemeral profiles of prescription drug and formulation tampering: evolving pseudoscience on the Internet. Drug Alcohol Depend. 2006;83S:S31–9.

69. Meisner JR, Darredeau C, McLarnon ME, Barrett SP. Extended release stimulant medication misuse with alcohol co-administration. J Can Acad Child Adolesc Psychiatry. 2008;17:181–2.

70. Daniel KL, Honein MA, Moore CA. Sharing prescription medication among teenage girls: potential danger to unplanned/undiagnosed pregnancies. Pediatrics. 2003;111(Suppl):1167–70.

71. Moline S, Frankenberger W. Use of stimulant medication for treatment of Attention-Deficit/Hyperactivity Disorder: a survey of middle and high school students' attitudes. Psychol Sch. 2001;38:569–84.

72. Poulin C. Medical and nonmedical stimulant use among adolescents: from sanctioned to unsanctioned use. CMAJ. 2001;165:1039–44.

73. Poulin C. From attention-deficit/hyperactivity disorder to medical stimulant use to the diversion of prescribed stimulants to

non-medical stimulant use: connecting the dots. Addiction. 2007;102:740–51.

74. Califano J. You've got drugs! V: Prescription drug pushers on the Internet. [Online]. New York, NY: The National Center on Addiction and Substance Abuse, Columbia University. 2008. http://www.casacolumbia.org/templates/publications_reports. aspx.

75. The National Center on Addiction and Substance Use at Columbia University (CASA). National survey of American attitudes on substance abuse XIV: teens and parents. [Online]. New York, NY: The National Center on Addiction and Substance Abuse, Columbia University. Aug, 2009. http://www.casacolumbia.org/templates/ publications_reports.aspx.

76. The Partnership for a Drug-Free America. The Partnership Attitude Tracking Study (PATS): teens in grades 7 through 12. [Online]. May, 2006. http://www.drugfree.org/files/full_teen_report.

77. McCabe SE, Boyd CJ, Teter CJ. Illicit use of opioid analgesics by high school seniors. J Subst Abuse Treat. 2005;28:225–30.

78. Schinke SP, Fang L, Cole KCA. Substance use among early adolescent girls: risk and protective factors. J Adolesc Health. 2008;43:191–4.

79. Prendergast M. Substance use and abuse among college students: a review of recent literature. J Am Coll Health. 1994;43:99–113.

80. The Association of Universities and Colleges of Canada. Trends in higher education. Vol 1: Enrolment. [Online]. Ottawa, ON: The Association of Universities and Colleges of Canada; 2007. http://www.aucc.ca/_pdf/english/publications/trends_2007_ vol1_e.pdf.

81. U.S. Census Bureau. School enrollment: Social and economic characteristics of students. [Online]. Oct, 2007. http://www. census.gov/population/www/socdemo/school/cps2007.html.

82. Snyder TD, Dillow SA, Hoffman CM. Digest of education statistics, 2008 (NCES 2009-020), Chap. 3. [Online]. Washington, DC: National Center for Education Statistics, U.S. Department of Education; 2009. http://nces.ed.gov/pubsearch/pubsinfo. asp?pubid=2009020.

83. Quintero G, Peterson J, Young B. An exploratory study of sociocultural factors contributing to prescription drug misuse among college students. J Drug Issues. 2006;36:903–32.

84. Quintero G. Controlled release: a cultural analysis of collegiate polydrug use. J Psychoactive Drugs. 2009;41:39–47.

85. McCabe SE, West B, Wechsler H. Trends and college-level characteristics associated with the non-medical use of prescription drugs among US college students from 1993 to 2001. Addiction. 2007;102:455–65.

86. Hurwitz W. The challenge of prescription drug misuse: a review and commentary. Pain Med. 2005;6:152–61.

87. Australian Institute of Health and Welfare. 2007 National Drug Strategy Household Survey: Detailed findings. [Online]. Canberra: AIHW; 2008. http://www.aihw.gov.au/publications/phe/ndshs07-df/ndshs07-df.pdf.

88. McCabe SE, Knight JR, Teter CJ, Wechsler H. Non-medical use of prescription stimulants among US college students: prevalence and correlates from a national survey. Addiction. 2005;99: 96–106.

89. Teter CJ, McCabe SE, Boyd CJ, Guthrie SK. Illicit methylphenidate use in an undergraduate student sample: prevalence and risk factors. Pharmacotherapy. 2003;23:609–17.

90. Hall K, Irwin M, Bowman K, Frankenberger W, Jewett D. Illicit use of prescribed stimulant medication among college students. J Am Coll Health. 2005;53:167–74.

91. Prudhomme White B, Becker-Blease KA, Grace-Bishop K. Stimulant medication use, misuse, and abuse in an undergraduate and graduate student sample. J Am Coll Health 2006;54:261–8.

92. Graff Low K, Gendaszek AE. Illicit use of psychostimulants among college students: a preliminary study. Psychol Health Med 2002;7:283–7.

93. Advokat CD, Guidry D, Martino L. Licit and illicit use of medications for Attention-Deficit Hyperactivity Disorder in undergraduate college students. J Am Coll Health. 2008;56:601–6.

94. McCabe SE, Cranford JA, Boyd CJ, Teter CJ. Motives, diversion and routes of administration associated with nonmedical use of prescription opioids. Addict Behav. 2007;32:562–75.

95. McCabe SE, Teter CJ, Boyd CJ. Illicit use of prescription pain medication among college students. Drug Alcohol Depend. 2005;77:37–47.

96. Barrett SP, Pihl RO. Oral methylphenidate-alcohol co-abuse. J Clin Psychopharmacol. 2002;22:633–4.

97. Barrett SP, Darredeau C, Bordy L, Pihl RO. Characteristics of methylphenidate misuse in a university student sample. Can J Psychiatry. 2005;50(8):457–61.

98. McCabe SE, Cranford JA, Morales M, Young A. Simultaneous and concurrent polydrug use of alcohol and prescription drugs: prevalence, correlates, and consequences. J Stud Alcohol. 2006;67: 529–37.

99. Arria AM, Caldeira KM, O'Grady KE, Vincent KB, Johnson EP, Wish ED. Nonmedical use of prescription stimulants among college students: associations with ADHD and polydrug use. Pharmacotherapy. 2008;28:156–69.

100. Judson R, Langdon S. Illicit use of prescription stimulants among college students: prescription status, motives, theory of planned behaviour, knowledge and self-diagnostic tendencies. Psychol Health Med. 2009;14:97–104.

101. Swanson JM, Volkow ND. Increasing use of stimulants warns of potential abuse. Nature. 2008;454:586.

102. McCabe SE, Boyd CJ. Sources of prescription drugs for illicit use. Addict Behav. 2005;30:1342–50.

103. McCabe SE, Cranford JA, Boyd CJ. The relationship between past-year drinking behaviors and nonmedical use of prescription drugs: prevalence of co-occurrence in a national sample. Drug Alcohol Depend. 2006;84:281–8.

104. Scotter E, Meaux J. Prescription stimulant misuse among college students. J Pediatr Nurs. 2008;23:e21.

105. Herman-Stahl M, Krebs C, Kroutil L, Heller D. Risk and protective factors for methamphetamine use and nonmedical use of prescription stimulants among young adults aged 18 to 25. Addict Behav. 2007;32:1003–15.

106. Sharp J, Rosén L. Recreational stimulant use among college students. J Subst. 2007;12:71–82.

107. Ford J, Arrastia M. Pill-poppers and dopers: a comparison of non-medical prescription drug use and illicit/street drug use among college students. Addict Behav. 2008;33:934–41.

108. Ford J. Nonmedical prescription drug use among college students: a comparison between athletes and nonathletes. J Am Coll Health. 2008;57:211–9.

109. Arria AM, Caldeira KM, Vincent KB, O'Grady KE, Wish ED. Perceived harmfulness predicts nonmedical use of prescription drugs among college students: interactions with sensation-seeking. Prev Sci. 2008;9:191–201.

110. Arria AM, Caldeira KM, O'Grady KE, Vincent KB, Fitzelle DB, Johnson EP, Wish ED. Drug exposure opportunities and use patterns among college students: results of a longitudinal prospective cohort study. Subst Abus. 2008;29:19–38.

111. Harrison AG. Adults faking ADHD: you must be kidding! ADHD Rep. 2006;14:1–7.

112. Kollins SH. Abuse liability of medications used to treat Attention-Deficit/Hyperactivity Disorder (ADHD). Am J Addict. 2007;16: 35–44.

113. Handley SM, Ward-Smith P. Alcohol misuse, abuse, and addiction in young and middle adulthood. Annu Rev Nurs Res. 2005;23: 213–44.

114. Davis WR. Prescription opioid use, misuse, and diversion among street drug users in New York City. Drug Alcohol Depend. 2008;92:267–76.

115. Fach M, Bischof G, Schmidt C, Rumpf H. Prevalence of dependence on prescription drugs and associated mental disorders in a representative sample of general hospital patients. Gen Hosp Psychiatry. 2007;29:257–63.

116. Becker WC, Fiellin DA, Gallagher RM, Barth KS, Ross JT, Oslin DW. The association between chronic pain and prescription drug abuse in veterans. Pain Med. 2009;10:531–6.

117. Manchikanti L, Giordano J, Boswell MV, Fellows B, Manchukonda R, Pampati V. Psychological factors as predictors of opioid abuse and illicit drug use in chronic pain patients. J Opioid Manag. 2007;3:89–100.

118. Morasco BJ, Dobscha SK. Prescription medication misuse and substance use disorder in VA primary care patients with chronic pain. Gen Hosp Psychiatry. 2008;30:93–9.

119. Havens JR, Stoops WW, Leukefeld CG, Garrity TF, Carlson RG, Falck R, et al. Prescription opiate misuse among rural stimulant users in a multistate community-based study. Am J Drug Alcohol Abuse. 2009;35:18–23.

120. Merline AC, O'Malley PM, Schulenberg JE, Bachman JG, Johnston LD. Substance use among adults 35 years of age: prevalence, adulthood predictors, and impact of adolescent substance use. Am J Public Health. 2004;94:96–102.

121. Rasu RS, Shenolikar RA, Nahata MC, Balkrishnan R. Physician and patient factors associated with the prescribing of medications for sleep difficulties that are associated with high abuse potential or are expensive: an analysis of data from the National Ambulatory Medical Care Survey for 1996-2001. Clin Ther. 2005;27:1970–9.

122. Cooperstock R. Sex differences in psychotropic drug use. Soc Sci Med Med Anthropol. 1978;12:179–86.

123. Green TC, Grimes Serrano JM, Licari A, Budman SH, Butler SF. Women who abuse prescription opioids: findings from the Addiction Severity Index-Multimedia Version® Connect prescription opioid database. Drug Alcohol Depend. 2009;103:65–73.

124. Simoni-Wastila L, Ritter G, Strickler G. Gender and other factors associated with the nonmedical use of abusable prescription drugs. Subst Use Misuse. 2004;39:1–23.

125. Clark RE, Xie H, Brunette MF. Benzodiazepine prescription practices and substance abuse in persons with severe mental illness. J Clin Psychiatry. 2004;65:151–5.

126. Blow FC. Substance abuse among older adults (Treatment Improvement Protocol (TIP) Series No. 26). Rockville, MD: U.S. Department of Health and Human Services, Public Health Service, Substance Abuse and Mental Health Services Administration, Center for Substance Abuse Treatment, 1998.

127. Reid MC, Anderson PA. Geriatric substance use disorders. Med Clin North Am. 1997;81:999–1016.

128. Juergens SM. Prescription drug dependence among elderly persons. Mayo Clin Proc. 1994;69:1215–7.

129. Culberson JW, Ziska M. Prescription drug misuse/abuse in the elderly. Geriatrics. 2008;63:22–31.

130. Canadian Centre for Substance Abuse (CCSA). The essentials of seniors and substance abuse. [Online]. Ottawa, ON: Canadian Centre on Substance Abuse, 2007. http://www.cnsaap.ca/SiteCollectionDocuments/PT-Essentials%20of%20Seniors%20and%20Substance%20Abuse-20071101-e.pdf.

131. National Institute on Drug Abuse. Prescription drugs: Abuse and addiction. [Online]. U.S. Department of Health and Human Services, National Institutes of Health, 2005. http://www.nida.nih.gov/PDF/RRPrescription.pdf.

132. Prinz PN, Vitiello MV, Raskind MA, Thorpy MJ. Geriatrics: sleep disorders and aging. N Engl J Med. 1990;323:520–6.

133. Finlayson RE, Davis Jr LJ. Prescription drug dependence in the elderly population: demographic and clinical features of 100 inpatients. Mayo Clin Proc. 1994;69:1137–45.

134. Jinks MJ, Raschko RR. A profile of alcohol and prescription drug abuse in a high-risk community-based elderly population. DICP. 1990;24:971–5.

135. Busto U, Sellers EM, Naranjo CA, Cappell HD, Sanchez-Craig M, Simpkins J. Patterns of benzodiazepine abuse and dependence. Br J Addict. 1986;81:87–94.

136. Raffoul PR. Drug misuse among older people: focus for interdisciplinary efforts. Health Soc Work. 1986;11:197–203.

137. Zimberg S. Alcoholism and substance abuse in older adults. In: Frances RJ, Miller SI, Mack AH, editors. Clinical textbook of addictive disorders. 3rd ed. New York, NY: Guilford; 2005. p. 396–410.

138. Center for Substance Abuse Treatment. Substance abuse relapse prevention for older adults: a group treatment approach. [Online]. Rockville, MD: Substance Abuse and Mental Health Services Administration, 2005. http://www.kap.samhsa.gov/products/manuals/pdfs/substanceabuserelapse.pdf.

139. Buffett-Jerrott SE, Stewart SH. Cognitive and sedative effects of benzodiazepine use. Curr Pharm Des. 2002;8:45–58.

140. Solomon K, Stark S. Comparison of older and younger alcoholics and prescription drug abusers: history and clinical presentation. Clin Gerontol. 1993;12:41–56.

141. Fincham JE. The aging of America: how to deal with the geriatric patient in the community pharmacy. J Geriatr Drug Ther. 1989;4:33–49.

142. Levenson MR, Aldwin CM. A Generation at risk… Applying prevention concepts to the elderly. [Online]. Folsom, CA: EMT Group. 2001. http://www.ca-cpi.org/Publications/Prevention_Tactics/Archive_tactics/elderly.pdf.

143. Ready LB, Sarkis E, Turner JA. Self-reported vs. actual use of medications in chronic pain patients. Pain 1982;12:285–94.

Anxiolytics and Sedatives

17

Alyson Bond and Malcolm Lader

Abstract

Benzodiazepines are classified as anxiolytics or hypnotics, but the term "sedative" describes a group of drugs, including barbiturates and tricyclic antidepressants as well as benzodiazepines, which are abused. These drugs have different pharmacokinetic characteristics. Patients prescribed benzodiazepines seldom escalate their doses, and primary benzodiazepine abuse is rare. However, secondary abuse of all sedative drugs is common, and high doses are frequently consumed by patients dependent on opiates or alcohol to enhance the effects and by stimulant users to alleviate offset effects after a binge. Benzodiazepines cause dependence on prescribed doses with a clear withdrawal syndrome lasting a few weeks evident in 20–30% patients. The consumption of high doses can result in more severe withdrawal symptoms. Benzodiazepines should never be withdrawn abruptly because of the risk of fits or paranoid psychosis. A stepped care approach to reduction is recommended. All sedative drugs have characteristic pharmacodynamic effects, causing sedation, psychomotor slowing and memory impairment. They increase the risk of accidents and injuries and contribute to specific drug-related harms in abusers. Tolerance develops to some effects but long-term users are impaired compared with non-users. However, gradually stopping the drugs, even after several years of use, results in improvement in functioning, and there is no evidence of lasting impairment or cognitive decline. Newer anxiolytics and SSRIs appear to cause less impairment and have lower abuse potential.

Learning Objectives
- This class of drug includes a range of compounds with differing pharmacokinetics.
- The field is dominated by the benzodiazepines which have a characteristic pharmacodynamic profile and high abuse liability among polydrug users.
- SSRIs provide a better risk/benefit ratio.

Issues that Need to Be Addressed by Future Research
- Can we identify who is likely to become dependent on BZDs?
- Can we identify who is likely to abuse BZDs?
- The natural history of sedative abuse with opioids.

A. Bond (✉)
Department of Addiction, Institute of Psychiatry,
King's College London, London, SE5 8AF, UK
e-mail: alyson.bond@kcl.ac.uk

M. Lader
Institute of Psychiatry, Kings College,
London, UK

Introduction and Definition of Anxiolytics and Sedatives

Some characteristic benzodiazepines are listed in Tables 17.1 and 17.2. These groups of drugs are discussed together as their use is dictated by custom rather than by their

J.C. Verster et al. (eds.), *Drug Abuse and Addiction in Medical Illness: Causes, Consequences and Treatment*,
DOI 10.1007/978-1-4614-3375-0_17, © Springer Science+Business Media, LLC 2012

Table 17.1 Some benzodiazepine anxiolytics

Drug	Trade name in the UK	Half-life
Alprazolam	Xanax (not available in the UK)	12–15 h
Chlordiazepoxide	None—used to be Librium	6–30 h
Diazepam	None—used to be Valium	1–4 days
Lorazepam	None—used to be Ativan	12–16 h
Oxazepam	None—used to be Serenid	7–20 h

Table 17.2 Benzodiazepine and related drugs used as hypnotics

Drug	Trade name in the UK	Half-life
Flurazepam	Dalmane (not available in the UK)	1–4 days
Loprazolam	None	12–16 h
Lormetazepam	None	8–12 h
Nitrazepam	Mogadon	18–24 h
Temazepam	None	7–11 h
Triazolam	(Not available in the UK)	2–4 h
Zaleplon	Sonata	1–2 h
Zolpidem	Stilnoct	2–4 h
Zopiclone	Zimovane	4–8 h
Eszopiclone	(Not available in the UK)	4–8 h

pharmacology. However, differences in pharmacokinetic properties do play some part.

The term "sedative" originally meant allaying anxiety, but it now has the connotation of causing unwanted drowsiness. Instead the term "anxiolytic" or (minor) "tranquilliser" is used to describe drugs that lessen anxiety. The term "hypnotic" is applied to medications taken at night to induce sleep. A range of substances including alcohol, bromides, chloral and paraldehyde were used in the nineteenth century as both sedatives and hypnotics but were supplanted by a range of barbiturates in the twentieth century. These were effective but caused over-sedation and confusion, were prone to be abused and were dangerous in over dosage. In turn they were replaced by first meprobamate and then by numerous benzodiazepines from the 1960s onwards. However, in the drug abuse field, the term sedative is still used to describe a group of drugs that are often used to induce soporific feelings of relaxation. This term includes not only benzodiazepines but also barbiturates and tricyclic antidepressants such as amitriptyline.

The *benzodiazepines* (hereafter abbreviated to BZD) group of drugs is characterised by an ability to bind to specific benzodiazepine-type receptors on the GABA chloride ion channel complex. Included in the class are the so-called "Z-drug" hypnotics—zopiclone, eszopiclone, zolpidem and zaleplon. Although these drugs are chemically dissimilar to the BZDs, they bind to varying degrees to the same receptors.

The mode of action of the benzodiazepines is to potentiate the inhibitory neurotransmitter GABA by binding to specific receptors [1]. This can reduce the turnover of several neurotransmitters such as norepinephrine and serotonin. The main sites of action of the BZDs are in the spinal cord where they mediate muscle relaxation, the brain stem, the cerebellum, causing ataxia, and the limbic and cortical areas involved in emotional experience and behaviour [2]. The BZDs vary in their profile and activity, for example, clonazepam has more anticonvulsant properties than most of the others.

A BZD antagonist, flumazenil, is available. It binds to BZD receptors and prevents the actions of BZDs. It can be used to reverse BZD over dosage. Finally, BZD inverse agonists have been described that have the opposite effects to BZDs, being proconvulsant and anxiogenic.

Pharmacokinetics

The chemical formulae of some BZDs are shown in Fig. 17.1. Chemically, they are 1:4 or 1:5 benzodiazepines. Well over 1,000 have been synthesised.

- They are generally well absorbed by mouth but vary in their rate of absorption after being injected intramuscularly. Diazepam in particular is absorbed erratically by this modality. Intravenous preparations are available but can result in local irritation. A special formulation, diazemuls, is better tolerated than simple solutions.
- Some BZDs have a pronounced redistribution alpha phase, diazepam being a case in point.
- The metabolic half-lives of the BZDs vary greatly (Fig. 17.2). The key compound is the desmethylated

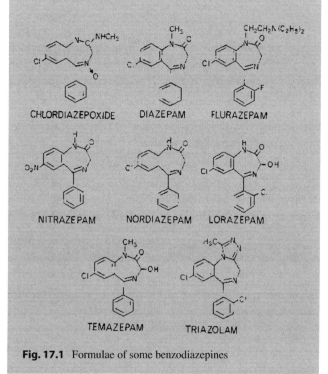

Fig. 17.1 Formulae of some benzodiazepines

(continued)

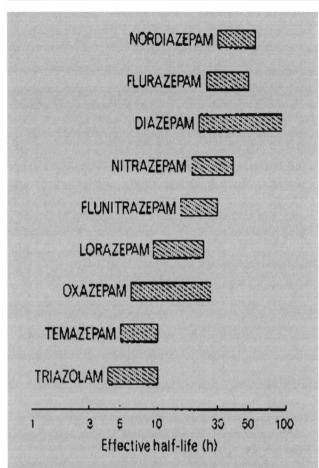

Fig. 17.2 Elimination half-lives of some benzodiazepines

derivative desmethyldiazepam. This has a very long half-life. Metabolism is slower in the elderly and in patients with liver impairment. Clobazam also has a long-acting metabolite. By contrast, lorazepam, oxazepam and temazepam have half-lives averaging less than 12 h. The Z-drugs used as hypnotics are appropriate as very short-acting hypnotics. The half-life of zopiclone is around 5 h, zolpidem 3 h and zaleplon as short as 1 h. Elimination of diazepam, chlordiazepoxide and clobazam is by Phase I processes, followed by Phase II glucuronide conjugation. Lorazepam, oxazepam and temazepam are mainly conjugated.

- BZDs do not induce microsomal enzymes, and pharmacokinetic interactions are uncommon. An exception is a potential interaction with methadone in the form of QT interval prolongation on the electrocardiogram. Most BZDs are metabolised by the CYP3A4 enzyme system. Pharmacodynamic interactions are more of a problem, particularly the interaction with alcohol.
- Overdosage, accidental or deliberate, is common but not usually dangerous. However, it can potentiate alcohol and the combination can be lethal.

Clinical Pharmacology

It would seem logical to use long-acting BZDs as anxiolytics, reserving shorter-acting ones for hypnotic use. For complex historical reasons this is not so, and anxiolytic BZDs vary greatly in their duration of action. In the clinic, BZDs reduce generalised anxiety and muscle tension and induce sleep. They also cause detectible cognitive and psychomotor impairment and subjective sedation. Careful testing shows that, although the subjective sedation subsides as tolerance sets in after a few days, the objective impairments may persist into the longer-term, showing that tolerance is system-specific. In parallel, the EEG fast beta activity which is increased by BZDs persists. An additional complexity is that anxious and insomniac patients tend to perform poorly anyway. Anxiolytic/hypnotic treatment will improve that performance, so the depressant effects of the BZDs will tend to be obscured by their beneficial effects. As the beneficial effects wane when tolerance sets in, only the impairments remain. However, when treatment is stopped, functioning gradually improves and there is no evidence of lasting anatomical or functional changes in the brain.

Clinical Uses

BZDs, as adumbrated before, are mainly used to treat anxiety and insomnia. Other uses include the management of some forms of epilepsy, severe muscle spasm and contractions, and as pre-medication before surgical procedures. BZDs also have an important role in the management of severely disturbed psychotic patients, the so-called "rapid tranquillisation". Other adjunctive uses are to allay anxiety in depressed patients and those suffering from schizophrenic illnesses. BZDs such as lorazepam are used in conjunction with antipsychotic medication to sedate the acutely disturbed psychotic patient, and appear to have a potentiating action. Longer-term usage in psychotic disorders is not established.

The target symptoms in the use of BZDs as *anxiolytics* are pathological ("free-floating", generalised) anxiety, tension and agitation. It is generally thought that psychological processes such as a bereavement reaction can be impaired by BZDs but there is no convincing evidence supporting this contention. Nor is there any firm evidence that they can impede cognitive behavioural therapy (CBT).

Because of the risks of tolerance and dependence, it is widely recommended that the use of anxiolytic BZDs be restricted to 4 weeks and 2 weeks as hypnotics. These injunctions are largely ignored by some prescribers who inadvertently or deliberately allow the usage to become chronic with the risk of withdrawal and dependence problems.

According to the UK Government advisory body, the National Institute for Clinical Excellence, BZDs do not have antidepressant properties [3]. Even the adjunctive use along with antidepressants early in treatment was regarded as unnecessary. Concern that they may even induce depression is probably misplaced. However, as they lessen anxious symptoms in patients with both anxiety and depression, the depressive symptoms may come to the fore. NICE [4] recommends that the BZDs should not be used in Panic Disorder as CBT is superior.

When administered as *hypnotics*, BZDs lessen REM sleep; when they are discontinued, REM rebound occurs. They are effective but their mode of action is as general depressants lowering arousal rather than having any specific effects on sleep mechanisms. A range of hypnotics are available (Table 17.2). Usage is still widespread especially in patients admitted to hospital [5]. Before treating insomnia with BZDs and related drugs, it is necessary to consider the possibility of any underlying causes such as depression, mania, anxiety, respiratory complaints, urinary frequency and, in particular, pain. Substance misuse particularly of stimulants and alcohol may be a problem. Simple "sleep hygiene" measures should first be instituted.

Abuse of Benzodiazepines

Prevalence of sedative misuse has been calculated from data from the National Comorbidity Study in the US [6]. The lifetime prevalence of non-prescribed sedative use was found to be 7.1% among adults. However, the type of sedative was not specified in this study and other similar surveys suffer from the same drawback. In fact abuse of benzodiazepines, in particular, is likely to be higher in countries where they are easily obtainable and there are fewer controls, e.g. parts of Asia and South America. However, much of the literature relates to the US and European nations where misuse often results from diverted prescriptions.

Patients who are prescribed benzodiazepines for problems with anxiety or sleep rarely escalate their doses even over a lengthy period of use. However, high-dose benzodiazepine mono-dependence has been reported [7, 8] with doses ranging up to 95 mg/day lorazepam. Laboratory studies of abuse liability show that although benzodiazepines have the potential for abuse, this is at a much lower level than for heroin, cocaine or the barbiturates [9]. Primary benzodiazepine abuse is therefore rare, but secondary abuse with alcohol or other drugs is much more common. It usually involves high doses as part of a pattern of polydrug abuse [10]. Patients with problems with alcohol abuse or dependence are more likely to use higher doses of benzodiazepines [11]. Initially, patients with drug or alcohol abuse may be prescribed higher-than-average doses by GPs or other medical specialists for problems with anxiety or insomnia, but they may then exceed the prescribed dose, obtain prescriptions from different sources or buy them on the illicit market. Sometimes they are taken regularly, but they are also taken in an intermittent binge pattern. They are frequently taken with alcohol because the combination results in increased feelings of intoxication [12] or with other sedative drugs such as tricyclic antidepressants or opiates [13]. They are used by heroin-dependent individuals [14] and by patients in opioid substitution treatment [15] to prolong and enhance the opiate effects. Benzodiazepines can also be used when preferred drugs are scarce. They are used by stimulant users to alleviate the increased jitteriness and anxiety after a binge and to induce sleep. They are usually taken orally, but both intranasal [16] and intravenous abuse [17] does occur, the pattern of use varying according to compound, formulation and country. Snorted flunitrazepam has high abuse liability [18], and this type of abuse is popular in Chile. Other benzodiazepines have been abused intravenously. For example, the intravenous abuse of temazepam liquid-filled capsules, in particular, spread rapidly among opiate users in the UK, causing the drug company to alter the filling to a hard gel but this, in turn, led to serious physical complications [19] and so now temazepam is only available in a tablet formulation in the UK. The abuse of high doses of benzodiazepines in combination with opiates is implicated in potentially fatal overdoses [20, 21].

Dependence and Withdrawal

It is important to emphasise that most of these patients, who show clear signs of dependence as evidenced by a characteristic syndrome on attempted withdrawal, are still taking the original prescribed dose. Only a minority escalate their dosage above recommended therapeutic levels. Those who do attain high doses usually have a more severe form of dependence than those patients keeping to the therapeutic dosage range. The high-dose users usually indulge in a form of BZD misuse (see above).

Withdrawal symptoms from the BZDs can ensue after 4–6 weeks of use, but only in about 20–30% of patients [22]. The reasons why some can withdraw with impunity after even years of continuous use while others undergo agonies remains unclear. Dosage reduction as well as complete withdrawal can result in withdrawal symptoms. These include physical symptoms such as muscle tension and spasm, or weakness; pins and needles and flu-like symptoms. Perceptual hypersensitivity and depersonalisation are common. Anxiety/insomnia may increase, nightmares may wake the patient, memory and concentration are impaired and depressive symptoms may ensue. Occasionally, fits or a paranoid psychosis may occur. The symptoms come on within 2–3 half-lives of the particular BZD and subside within a few weeks [23]. Some patients claim that their symptoms have persisted for months or indefinitely [24].

Minimal interventions are often helpful. Simple advice given by the GP can be quite effective [25]. Withdrawal schedules are widely available and involve tapering usually after substituting diazepam [26]. However, such substitution has little evidence to support it [27]. Equivalent dosages for such switching schedules are set out in Table 17.3. The rate of taper is not based on good evidence but the clinical experience of the prescriber. A typical reducing schedule is set out in Table 17.4. An important observation is that the early stages of withdrawal are easier to tolerate than the later and last stages. For example, a person may reduce quite quickly from 15 mg of diazepam a day to 5 mg, and then stall as the symptoms increase from 5 downwards. Therefore, a regular reduction may not be the most appropriate. It is usual to start fairly briskly and then slow down.

The prognosis is often poor with a high rate of relapse. Predictive factors include previous failed attempts, lack of family or social support, an unsympathetic general practitioner, a history of alcohol-related problems, older age, co morbid depression or physical problems or a personality problem. A careful appraisal may conclude that long-term maintenance is the best option, but the patient must be monitored to prevent accumulation with toxicity such as cognitive impairment.

Adjunctive treatments include antidepressant medication. Carbamazepine has also some evidence supporting its use [28]. However, psychological therapies or support groups should be used during the period of withdrawal. Group therapy may instil the patient with confidence that as others can withdraw, so can she. Once a patient has experienced withdrawal problems, they should not be prescribed a BZD again.

Withdrawal from high doses of benzodiazepines is conducted in a similar way, although supervision of doses may be necessary in polydrug abusers, diazepam being administered alongside methadone in specialist drug services, to avoid diversion of the medicine. A different approach using the BZD antagonist and partial agonist, flumazenil, has been tried with some success [29]. This procedure involved stabilising the patients on high doses of oxazepam (120 mg/day) for a week. The experimental group were then treated with gradual infusion of flumazenil 1.0 mg for 4 h in the morning and then 4 h in the afternoon for 8 days with low doses of oxazepam for the first 3 nights. This was compared with tapering of the oxazepam doses with a placebo infusion and placebo tablets and infusion. Treatment with flumazenil was found to be more effective than tapering or placebo. It reversed BZD effects without precipitating severe withdrawal symptoms and also reduced craving. This procedure involves inpatient treatment and is likely to be suitable only

Table 17.3 Switching to diazepam: equivalent doses to 10 mg/day

	Milligrams per day
Chlordiazepoxide	25
Clonazepam	1–2
(Diazepam	10)
Lorazepam	1
Lormetazepam	1
Nitrazepam	10
Oxazepam	30
Temazepam	20

Table 17.4 An example of a fairly rapid discontinuation schedule

Week	
0	Starting dose, again, as an example, 15 mg/day
2	15 mg/day down to 10 mg/day
4	10 mg/day down to 5 mg/day
6	5 mg/day down to 2.5 mg/day
8	2.5 mg/day down to 0—stop

for a small number of severely dependent patients with a history of prolonged BZD abuse.

Short- and Long-Term Effects on Brain and Behaviour

Subjective Sedation

Sedation is the most common subjective effect of this group of drugs. Despite improved specificity of action compared with barbiturates, drowsiness and tiredness are still the most common unwanted effects of benzodiazepines at recommended therapeutic doses. Increased sedation can also be detected after each dose even after a week of treatment in healthy volunteers [30]. Although tolerance does appear to develop after a few weeks' treatment, some residual effects may remain as increased alertness is reported by patients on stopping treatment with benzodiazepines [31]. Sedation is not always an unwelcome effect as high doses of benzodiazepines are commonly abused with alcohol or tricyclic antidepressants to deliberately increase sedation by polydrug users. Amitriptyline was taken by 26% of opiate users in one study [32].

Objective Sedation and Psychomotor Effects

Barbiturates produce a characteristic pattern of sedation in high doses. They produce unsteadiness, poor coordination, slurred speech and disorientation. Benzodiazepines do not produce as much sedation but nevertheless effects such as poor coordination are related to dose, compound and individual vulnerability. Both benzodiazepines and other sedative drugs have been shown consistently to have effects on psychomotor performance both in acute and repeated doses [33]. They impair the ability to perform simple repetitive tasks both when these are performed on their own and as a component of more complex tasks. The effect is related to speed of execution, participants slowing down to maintain accuracy of performance. They also impair simple attentional tasks. A positive relationship was found between size of effect and dose level several years ago [34].

Although tolerance has been found to develop to some measures of sedation and psychomotor performance [35, 36], impaired performance on simple repetitive tasks has been shown to persist after 1 year [37] and on tests of attention after several years of treatment [38] in long-term benzodiazepine users compared with control groups.

Cognitive Effects

Higher functions such as learning and memory have been shown to be impaired by acute and short-term administration of benzodiazepines in many studies [33, 39]. Memory for information acquired pre-drug administration (retrograde memory) is not impaired and may even be improved acutely, but acquisition of new material post-drug (anterograde memory) is consistently impaired by benzodiazepines. The more demands that are made on memory, e.g. increased task complexity and delay in recall, the greater the effect [40]. There are also differences between benzodiazepine compounds. The majority of compounds do not affect implicit memory or priming but lorazepam has been found to impair this aspect of memory as well [41].

The characteristic effects of benzodiazepines on episodic memory can still be found after months or even years of treatment [26, 42, 43] and was not reversed by flumazenil [43]. In a recent meta-analysis of 13 studies Barker et al. [44] found that benzodiazepine users performed worse on the majority of cognitive tasks used, in particular verbal memory, compared with controls or test norms. It should be noted that the studies were very diverse in variables such as length of use, dose and diagnosis. This has sparked a debate on whether sedative drugs including benzodiazepines cause lasting cognitive impairment or decline.

Cognitive Decline

Sedative drugs can produce cognitive disorders such as delirium at any age. This is often associated with different drug combinations. In the young, these effects can be associated with problematic alcohol use and in the elderly they can occur because of age-related altered pharmacokinetics

and polypharmacy [45]. Drug-induced cognitive impairment in older adults can be a confounding factor in dementia, in some cases leading to the apparent worsening of cognitive decline and pseudo-dementia [46]. In a further meta-analysis of 12 of the same studies, Barker et al. [47] found that although there was improvement in all areas of cognitive function up to 6 months after withdrawal, former benzodiazepine users performed worse on the majority of cognitive tasks used, in particular verbal memory, compared with controls or test norms. Verdoux et al. [48] investigated this issue further by reviewing six prospective studies carried out in older adults. Of these, two studies reported a lower risk of cognitive decline in former or ever users, two found no association and three found an increased risk of cognitive decline in users. However, withdrawal of the medication generally leads to steady, if gradual, resolution of the effects and improvement on both psychomotor tasks and tests of working and episodic memory has been found in two studies comparing patients who have discontinued compared with those who have continued with benzodiazepine medication [31, 49]. It is likely that effects are related to both dose and task complexity, those on higher doses taking longer to recover on more complex functions and so testing should be carried out at longer follow-up times. In illustration, Tata et al. [50] found impairment did not remit a relatively short time (6 months) after withdrawal of high doses of a benzodiazepine (diazepam 48 mg) but a follow-up study of patients showing impairment of episodic memory while being treated with alprazolam [42] showed no impairment 3.5 years later [51].

Accidents and Injuries

The risk of accidents, injuries and cognitive failures (problems of memory, attention or action) is increased by sedative drugs. In a postal questionnaire survey, completed by a community sample of approximately 8,000 people in two districts of Wales, benzodiazepine use was associated with injuries outside work and tricyclic antidepressant use both with injuries inside and outside work and cognitive failures [52]. These relationships were stronger in those with other risk factors and continuing mental health problems. The association between accidents and sedative drug use is even more apparent in the elderly [53, 54] who are more likely to experience falls and hip fractures while taking both benzodiazepines and tricyclic antidepressants [55, 56]. The risk of hip fractures in older adults can be increased by as much as 50% [57]. However, it is important to recognise that polypharmacy is common among this population and side effects of other drugs, e.g. postural hypotension, may also increase the risk of falls and accidents.

Complex Skills and Driving

Increased sedation and impaired psychomotor skills have implications for complex skills such as operating machinery or driving. Sedative drugs have been shown to impair both simulated driving performance and actual driving ability [58]. They have also been shown to be associated with accidents in both pepetrators and victims [59]. Epidemiological studies have confirmed that road traffic accidents involving injury or death are associated with sedative drug use [33, 60–62]. This relationship has been found to be related to dose, and the risk is increased by the presence of alcohol [62] and age [63, 64].

Forensic or Behavioural Problems

Paradoxical excitement is another unwanted effect which also has possible legal complications [65]. This disinhibitory effect of the BZDs can cause increased anxiety, acute excitement and hyperactivity. Aggressive impulses maybe released with hostility and rage; criminal acts such as assault and rape have been documented. Depending on the patient sample, estimates of incidence range from less than 1% to at least 20%. High-risk patients include borderline personality disorders, impulse control disorder and those with alcohol problems. The combination of a BZD and alcohol is particularly prone to lead to paradoxical reactions. The patient may have complete or partial amnesia for the event such as an episode of "air-rage". Disinhibitory reactions to sedative drugs are related to dose and mode of administration [66]. Therefore, intravenous administration of high doses of high potency BZDs poses an enhanced risk.

Effects in Drug Abusers

The effects of benzodiazepines and other sedative drugs are increased by their combination with alcohol. There has been relatively a little research examining the effects of BZDs in opioid-dependent individuals, but clear acute effects have been found in the few studies that have been done, which parallel the acute effects of benzodiazepines alone described above. Diazepam, flunitrazepam and triazolam in combination with methadone produced increased sedation [67–70], decreased psychomotor performance and attention [68–70] and impaired episodic memory [69]. Diazepam in combination with buprenorphine produced similar but less significant effects [69, 70]. Impairment increased with higher doses, simulating abuse conditions.

These impairments not only increase the risks already mentioned above, but are likely to contribute to specific drug-related harms involved in the preparing and injecting of drugs, increasing the risk of transmission of blood borne viruses such as HIV and Hepatitis C and of missing veins, causing abscesses. Polydrug misuse involving sedatives has also been associated with criminal activity and increased risk of overdose in both heroin users and those on opioid maintenance programmes [20, 21].

Other Anxiolytics and Sedatives

Buspirone is the only available member of the azapirone compounds and is a partial 5-HT$_{1A}$ agonist. It is a reasonably effective anxiolytic in general [71], but its onset of action is delayed. It is not as effective in patients with extensive prior experience of BZD treatment. Side effects include headache, dizziness and nausea. It is not associated with sedation, tolerance or withdrawal problems and has a low abuse liability.

Hydroxyzine is an antihistamine/anticholinergic drug with some anxiolytic properties [72]. Some antihistamines have been found to be liable to abuse.

A recent introduction is pregabalin. This compound was already licenced to treat neuropathic pain and some forms of epilepsy. It binds to the alpha-2-lambda subunit of voltage-gated calcium channels in the CNS. It reduces neurotransmitter release. It has proven efficacy in GAD in clinical trials [73]. It has a low incidence of side effects such as dizziness, somnolence and dry mouth. Tolerance, dependence and addiction potentials are low.

The drug treatment of choice in the anxiety disorders is the SSRI/SNRI group of drugs [4]. These drugs appear to have a much lower abuse liability than benzodiazepines or sedative tricyclic antidepressants. Antipsychotic drugs are favoured by some but no firm evidence backs their use and olanzapine has shown some abuse potential. Some primary care practitioners still use beta-blockers, but this use is not evidence-based.

Other Hypnotics

A range of hynotic BZDs are available. Barbiturates are still occasionally used in severe and intractable insomniacs with a history of persistent use. They are dependence inducing, dangerous in over dosage, and interact with a range of other medications. Barbiturates were extensively abused prior to the introduction of benzodiazepines. They were abused on their own for their positive effects but also as part of polydrug abuse. This has declined as availability is now much more restricted.

The Z-drugs—zopiclone, zolpidem and zaleplon—are essentially short- or very short-acting BZD-like drugs [74]. The short duration of action confers advantages such as lack of daytime sedation, but they are inappropriate for patients with early-morning awakening [75]. They probably have less propensity to rebound and withdrawal problems than BZDs of equivalent duration of action. These drugs appear to have similar abuse liability as the benzodiazepines, but as they are not yet tested for on routine drug urine screens, the evidence is based on case reports at present.

Whatever hypnotic is chosen, it should be given at the lowest effective dose for no more than 2 weeks. Usage on an intermittent basis is desirable. Withdrawal should be slow. It is doubtful if the risk/benefit ratio is favourable in the elderly [76].

Melatonin has a long tradition of being used to induce sleep. A sustained release preparation (Circadin) is licenced for use in Europe for insomniacs aged over 55 [77].

Sedative antidepressants such as amitriptyline and trazodone are prescribed to help induce sleep [78]. However, it is these very qualities that make these drugs prone to abuse in polydrug users [13]. Sedative antihistamines are also available over-the-counter but can cause troublesome residual sedation the next morning. Other over-the-counter herbal remedies include valerian and hops [79].

Finally, as with treatment of anxiety, CBT has been adapted to treat insomnia but is not widely available. Therefore, anxiolytic and hypnotic drugs are only recommended for short-term use. Newer compounds may cause less impairment and have lower abuse potential. SSRIs are licenced for some anxiety disorders.

References

1. Kerr DI, Ong J. GABA-B receptors. Pharmacol Ther. 1995;67:187–246.
2. Nutt DJ. New insights into the role of the GABA(A)-benzodiazepine receptor in psychiatric disorder. Br J Psychiatry. 2001;179:390–6.
3. National Institute for Clinical Excellence. Depression: management of depression in primary and secondary care—Clinical guidance. http://www.nice.org.uk. 2004.
4. National Institute for Clinical Excellence. Anxiety: management of anxiety (panic disorder, with or without agoraphobia, and generalised anxiety disorder) in adults in primary, secondary and community care. Clinical Guidance 22. http://www.nice.org.uk. 2004.
5. Mahomed R, et al. Prescribing hypnotics in a mental health trust: what consultants say and what they do. Pharm J. 2002;268:657–9.
6. Goodwin RD, Hasin DS. Sedative use and misuse in the United States. Addiction. 2001;97:555–62.
7. Hallstrom C, Lader MH. Benzodiazepine withdrawal phenomena. Int Pharmacopsychiatry. 1981;16:235–44.
8. Martinez-Cano H, Vela-Bueno A, De Iceta M, Pomalima R, Martinez-Gras I, Sobrino MP. Benzodiazepine types in high versus therapeutic dose dependence. Addiction. 1996;91:1179–86.
9. De Wit H, Griffiths RR. Testing the abuse liability of anxiolytic and hypnotic drugs in humans. Drug Alcohol Depend. 1991;28:83–111.
10. Seivewright NA, Dougal W. Benzodiazepine misuse. Curr Opin Psychiatry. 1992;5:408–11.
11. Wolf B, Grohmann R, Biber D, Brenner PM, Ruther E. Benzodiazepine abuse and dependence in psychiatric inpatients. Pharmacopsychiatry. 1989;22:54–60.
12. Bond AJ, Silveira JC, Lader MH. Effects of single doses of alprazolam alone and alcohol alone and in combination on psychological performance. Hum Psychopharmacol. 1991;6:219–28.
13. Peles E, Schreiber S, Adelson M. Tricyclic antidepressants abuse, with or without benzodiazepines abuse, in former heroin addicts currently in methadone maintenance treatment (MMT). Eur Neuropsychopharmacol. 2007;18:188–93.
14. Darke S. Benzodiazepine use among injecting drug users: problems and implications. Addiction. 1994;89:379–82.
15. Stitzer M, Griffiths R, McLellan A, Grabowski J, Hawthorne J. Diazepam use among methadone maintenance patients: patterns and dosages. Drug Alcohol Depend. 1981;8:189–99.
16. Sheehan MF, Sheehan DV, Torres A, Coppola A, Francis E. Snorting benzodiazepines. Am J Drug Alcohol Abuse. 1991;17:457–68.
17. Strang J, Griffiths P, Abbey J, Gossop M. Survey of injected benzodiazepines among drug users in Britain. BMJ. 1994;308:1082.
18. Bond AJ, Seijas D, Dawling S, Lader MH. Systematic absorption and abuse liability of snorted flunitrazepam. Addiction. 1994;89:821–30.
19. Launchbury AP, Drake J, Seager H. Misuse of temazepam. BMJ. 1992;305:252–3.
20. Oliver P, Keen J. Concomitant drugs of misuse and drug using behaviours associated with fatal opiate-related poisonings in Sheffield, UK, 1997-2000. Addiction. 2003;98(2):191–7.
21. Pirnay S, Borron S, Giudicelli C, Tourneau J, Baud F, Ricordel I. A critical review of the causes of death among post-mortem toxicological investigations: analysis of 34 buprenorphine-associated and 35 methadone-associated deaths. Addiction. 2004;99:978–88.
22. Lader M. Withdrawal reactions after stopping hypnotics in patients with insomnia. CNS Drugs. 1998;10:425–40.
23. Schweitzer E, et al. Benzodiazepine dependence and withdrawal: a review of the syndrome and its clinical management. Acta Psychiatrica Scand. 1998;393:95–101.
24. Royal College of Psychiatrists. Benzodiazepines: risks, benefits and dependence: a re-evaluation. Council Report 59. 1997. http://www.rcpsych.ac.uk/(London).
25. Lader M, Tylee A, Donoghue J. Withdrawing benzodiazepines in primary care. CNS Drugs. 2009;23(1):19–34.
26. Voshaar RCO, Couvee JE, Van Balkom AJLM, et al. Strategies for discontinuing long-term benzodiazepine use: meta-analysis. Br J Psychiatry. 2006;189:213–20.
27. Denis C, et al. Pharmacological interventions for mono-dependence benzodiazepine management in outpatient settings. Cochrane Database Syst Rev. 2006;CD005194.
28. Schweitzer E, et al. Carbamazepine treatment in patients discontinuing long-term benzodiazepine therapy. Effects on withdrawal severity and outcome. Arch Gen Psychiatry. 1991;48:448–52.
29. Gerra G, Zaimovic A, Giusti F, Moi G, Brewer C. Intravenous flumazenil versus oxazepam tapering in the treatment of benzodiazepine withdrawal: a randomised, placebo-controlled study. Addict Biol. 2002;7:385–95.
30. Bond AJ, Lader MH, Shotriya R. Comparative effects of a repeated dose regime of diazepam and buspirone on subjective ratings, psychological tests and the EEG. Eur J Clin Pharm. 1983;24:463–7.
31. Curran HV, Collins R, Fletcher S, Kee SCY, Woods B, Iliffe S. Older adults and withdrawal from benzodiazepine hypnotics in general practice: effects on cognitive function, sleep, mood and quality of life. Psychol Med. 2003;33:1223–37.
32. Darke S, Ross J. The use of antidepressants among injecting drug users in Sydney, Australia. Addiction. 2000;95:407–17.
33. Woods JH, Katz JL, Winger G. Benzodiazepine use, abuse and consequences. Pharmacol Rev. 1992;44:151–347.
34. Wittenborn JR, Flaherty CF, McGough WE, Nash RJ. Psychomotor changes during initial day of benzodiazepine medication. Br J Clin Pharmacol. 1979;7:69S–76S.

35. Buffet-Jerrott SE, Stewart SH. Cognitive and sedative effects of benzodiazepine use. Curr Pharm Des. 2002;8:45–58.

36. Lucki I, Rickels K, Geller AM. Chronic use of benzodiazepines and psychomotor and cognitive test performance. Psychopharmacology. 1986;88:426–33.

37. Golombok S, Moodley P, Lader M. Cognitive impairment in long-term benzodiazepines users. Psychol Med. 1988;18:365–74.

38. Petursson H, Gudjonsson G, Lader M. Psychiatric performance during withdrawal form long-term benzodiazepine treatment. Psychopharmacology. 1983;81:345–9.

39. Curran HV. Benzodiazepines, memory and mood: a review. Psychopharmacology. 1991;105:1–8.

40. Curran H. Tranquillising memories: a review of the effects of benzodiazepines on human memory. Biol Psychol. 1986;23:179–213.

41. Curran HV, Gorenstein C. Differential effects of lorazepam and oxazepam on priming. Int Clin Psychopharmacol. 1993;8:37–42.

42. Curran HV, Bond A, O'Sullivan G, Bruce M, Marks I, Lelliot P, Shine P, Lader M. Memory functions, alprazolam and exposure therapy: a controlled longitudinal trial of agoraphobia with panic disorder. Psychol Med. 1994;24:969–76.

43. Gorenstein C, Bernik MA, Pompeia S. Differential acute psychomotor and cognitive effects of diazepam on long-term benzodiazepine users. Int Clin Psychopharmacol. 1994;9:145–53.

44. Barker MJ, Greenwood KM, Jackson M, Crowe SF. Cognitive effects of long-term benzodiazepine use: a meta-analysis. CNS Drugs. 2004;18:37–48.

45. Gray S, Lai KV, Larson EB. Drug-induced cognition disorders in the elderly: incidence, prevention and management. Drug Saf. 1999;21:101–22.

46. Paterniti S, Dufouil C, Alperovitch A. Long-term benzodiazepine use and cognitive decline in the elderly: the Epidemiology of Vascular Aging Study. J Clin Psychopharmacol. 2002;22:285–93.

47. Barker MJ, Greenwood KM, Jackson M, et al. Persistence of cognitive effects after withdrawal from long-term benzodiazepine use: a meta-analysis. Arch Clin Neuropsychol. 2004;19:437–54.

48. Verdoux H, Lagnaoui R, Begaud B. Is benzodiazepine use a risk factor for cognitive decline and dementia? A literature review of epidemiological studies. Psychol Med. 2005;35:307–15.

49. Salzman C, Fisher J, Nobel K, Glassman R, Wolfson A, Kelley M. Cognitive improvement following benzodiazepine discontinuation in elderly nursing home residents. Int J Geriatr Psychiatry. 1992;7:89–93.

50. Tata PR, Rollings J, Collins M, Pickering A, Jacobson RR. Lack of cognitive recovery following withdrawal from long-term benzodiazepine use. Psychol Med. 1994;24:203–13.

51. Kilic C, Curran HV, Noshirvani H, Marks IM, Basoglu M. Long-term effects of alprazolam on memory: a 3.5 year follow-up of agoraphobial panic patients. Psychol Med. 1999;29:225–31.

52. Wadsworth EJK, Moss SC, Simpson SA, Smith AP. Psychotropic medication use and accidents, injuries and cognitive failures. Hum Psychopharmacol. 2005;20:391–400.

53. Kallin K, Lundin-Olsson L, Jensen J, Nyberg L, Gustafson Y. Predisposing and precipiataing factors for falls among older people in residential care. Public Health. 2002;116:263–71.

54. Taylor S, McCracken CF, Wilson KC, et al. Extent and appropriateness of benzodiazepine use. Results from an elderly urban community. Br J Psychiatry. 1998;173:433–8.

55. Ray WA, Griffin MR, Schaffner W, Baugh DK, Melton 3rd LJ. Psychotropic drug use and the risk of hip fracture. New Engl J Med. 1987;316:363–9.

56. Sternbacka M, Jansson B, Leufman A, Romelsjo A. Association between use of sedatives or hypnotics, alcohol consumption, or other risk factors and single injurious fall or multiple injurious falls: a longitudinal general population study. Alcohol. 2002;28:9–16.

57. Cumming RG, Le Couteur DG. Benzodiazepines and risk of hip fractures in older people: a review of the evidence. CNS Drugs. 2003;17:825–37.

58. O'Hanlon JF, de Gier JJ. Drugs and driving (Taylor and Francis, London, 1986). Addiction. 2003; 98:191–7.

59. Currie D, Hashemi K, Fothergill J, Findlay A, Harris A, Hindmarch I. The use of antidepressants and benzodiazepines in the perpetrators and victims of accidents. Occup Med. 1995;45:323–5.

60. Skegg DCC, Richards SM, Doll R. Minor tranquillisers and road accidents. BMJ. 1979;1:917–9.

61. Thomas RE. Benzodiazepine use and motor vehicle accidents. Systematic review of reported association. Can Fam Physician. 1998;44:799–808.

62. Barbone F, McMahon AD, Davey PG, et al. Association of road-traffic accidents with benzodiazepine use. Lancet. 1998;352:1331–6.

63. Hemmelgarn B, Suissa S, Huang A, Boivin JF, Pinard G. Benzodiazepine use and the risk of motor vehicle crash in the elderly. JAMA. 1997;278:27–31.

64. Ray WA, Fought RL, Decker MD. Psychoactive drugs and the risk of injurious motor vehicle crashes in elderly drivers. Am J Epidemiol. 1992;136:873–83.

65. Paton C. Benzodiazepines and disinhibition: a review. Psychiatr Bull. 2002;26:460–2.

66. Bond AJ. Drug-induced behavioural disinhibition. Incidence, mechanisms and therapeutic implications. CNS Drugs. 1998;9:41–57.

67. Preston K, Griffiths R, Cone E, Darwin W, Gorodetzky C. Diazepam and methadone blood levels following concurrent administration of diazepam and methadone. Drug Alcohol Depend. 1986;18:195–202.

68. Farre M, Teran M, Roset P, Mas M. Abuse liability of flunitrazepam among methadone-maintained patients. Psychopharmacology. 1998;140:486–95.

69. Lintzeris N, Mitchell TB, Bond AJ, Nestor L, Strang J. Interactions on mixing diazepam with methadone or buprenorphine in maintenance patients. J Clin Psychopharmacol. 2006;26:274–83.

70. Lintzeris N, Mitchell TB, Bond AJ, Nestor L, Strang J. Pharmacodynamics of diazepam co-administered with methadone or buprenorphine under high dose conditions in opioid dependent patients. Drug Alcohol Depend. 2007;91:187–94.

71. Sramek JJ, Tansman M, Suri A, et al. Efficacy of buspirone in generalized anxiety disorder with coexisting mild depressive symptoms. J Clin Psychiatry. 1996;57:287–91.

72. Lader M. Anxiolytic effect of hydroxyzine: a double-blind trial versus placebo and buspirone. Hum Psychopharmacol. 1999;14 Suppl 1:S94–S102.

73. Montgomery SA. Pregabalin for the treatment of generalised anxiety disorder. Expert Opin Pharmacother. 2006;7:2139–54.

74. National Institute for Clinical Excellence. Insomnia—newer hypnotic drugs. Zaleplon, zolpidem and zopiclone for the management of insomnia. Technology Appraisal 77. http://www.nice.org.uk. 2004.

75. Benca RM. Diagnosis and treatment of chronic insomnia: a review. Psychiatr Serv. 2005;56:332–43.

76. Glass J, Lanctot KL, Herrmann N, et al. Sedative hypnotics in older people with insomnia: meta-analysis of risks and benefits. BMJ. 2005;331:1169.

77. Zisapel N. Development of a melatonin-based formulation for the treatment of insomnia in the elderly. Drug Dev Res. 2000;50:226–34.

78. James SP, Mendelson WB. The use of trazodone as a hypnotic: a critical review. J Clin Psychiatry. 2004;65:752–5.

79. Morin CM, Koetter U, Bastien C, et al. Valerian-hops combination and diphenhydramine for treating insomnia: a randomized placebo-controlled clinical trial. Sleep. 2005;28:1465–71.

Opioids and Other Analgesics

18

Jane C. Ballantyne

Abstract

The opioids hold a unique place amongst addictive substances in that they have a critical and indispensable role in medical treatment. This is as true today as it was in ancient times, for despite medical advances, palliation is still needed, and there are no better drugs than the opioids for treating severe pain and suffering. Recreational use of opioids, once as opium, has an established place in human history and is more prevalent today than ever because of a number of geopolitical and societal factors (Administration USDE. Automation of Reports and Consolidated Orders System (ARCOS), Retail Drug Summary Report; http://www.deadiversion.usdoj.gov/arcos/retail_drug_summary/index.html; Associated Press Analysis. http://wwwihtcom/articles/ap/2007/08/20/america/NA-FEA-GEN-US-World-of-Painphp). That these two often conflicting roles for opioids exist presents real difficulty in terms of how these drugs should be used and controlled so as to help patients and not harm them. This chapter will explore some of the issues surrounding opioid pain therapy, and how opioid addiction impacts this.

Role of Opioids in Pain Management

Despite monumental efforts to find alternatives to opioids for treating pain, or to modify opioid drugs to make them more durable or less addictive, we are still left with classic opioids (Table 18.1) as the only systemically administered drugs capable of relieving severe pain. Whereas before the twentieth century, cure was rare, and opioids and palliation were central to the physician's craft, recent medical advances have made early death and rapidly progressive illness unusual, and chronic disease more prominent. At the same time, opioid regulations, introduced in the USA and Europe at the beginning of the twentieth century, have stigmatized addiction and opioids (because they are addictive), making patients and prescribers fearful of using opioids to treat either pain or opioid addiction [1]. All in all, we are confused about the proper role for opioids in pain management, and our practices are

now driven by conflicting regulations, guidelines, and mandates [2–7]. For example, in the USA, hospitals must show that pain evaluation and treatment (often necessitating opioids) are part of their standard of care, yet the US Drug Enforcement Agency (DEA) comes down heavily on misguided opioid prescribing [8, 9].

Acute Pain

Despite these difficulties, there are areas of pain practice where opioid use is established as effective, necessary, and virtually free from addiction risk. The first of these is the treatment of acute pain. Acute pain is predominantly nociceptive, that is produced by injury and carried by nociceptors, which is a type of pain particularly sensitive to opioids. Moreover, acute pain is short lived, so its treatment with opioids tends not to be complicated by the several factors that can ultimately result in deterioration of efficacy: tolerance, sensitization (hyperalgesia), and psychological factors such as loss of placebo effect [10]. Acute opioid pain treatment is remarkably effective as long as the dose is adequate (the dose

J.C. Ballantyne (✉)
Penn Pain Medicine Center, 2nd floor Tuttleman Building,
1840 South Street, Philadelphia, PA 19146, USA
e-mail: jane.ballantyne@uphs.upenn.edu

J.C. Verster et al. (eds.), *Drug Abuse and Addiction in Medical Illness: Causes, Consequences and Treatment*,
DOI 10.1007/978-1-4614-3375-0_18, © Springer Science+Business Media, LLC 2012

Table 18.1 Classification of opioids

Naturally occurring
  Morphine
  Papaverine
  Codeine
  Thebaine

Semisynthetic
  Heroin
  Hydromorphone
  Hydrocodone
  Buprenorphine
  Oxycodone

Synthetic
  Morphinan series (levophanol, butorphanol)
  Diphenylpropylamine series (methadone)
  Benzomorphinan series (pentazocine)
  Phenylpiperidine series (meperidine, fentanyl, sufentanil, alfentanil)

needed being extremely variable between individuals), and success is generally limited only by side effects. Early opioid side effects include nausea, somnolence, euphoria or dysphoria, bowel slowing, pruritus, and urinary retention. In some cases, opioid side effects are undesirable because they delay mobilization and recovery, in other cases because they are intolerable to the patient. Development of addiction is virtually unheard of in the setting of acute pain treatment, although established addicts may be difficult to control during an acute pain episode, and addicts in remission may be fearful of triggering a relapse by accepting opioid pain treatment [11]. Despite the long history of success for opioid treatment of acute pain, more recently, a limitation on this success has been produced by widespread chronic opioid use which may induce a state of opioid refractoriness [12–14]. The mechanisms for this effect are currently under intense study, but appear to involve complex adaptations that produce the clinical picture of insurmountable tolerance with or without hyperalgesia [15]. The clinical picture is one of a high opioid dose requirement, inadequate pain relief despite high doses, disconnected side effect risk, especially respiratory depression which may occur even in the presence of severe pain (unlike the picture in opioid naïve individuals who generally exhibit pain relief before respiratory depression).

Pain During Terminal Illness

The second area of established and successful opioid pain therapy is the treatment of pain and suffering during terminal illness. Again, though, this success is partly related to the fact that the course of treatment has tended to be short. But recently there have been changes in medical treatment, notably in the treatment of cancer, that have extended both the course of diseases and their terminal phase. Cancer, and indeed many other diseases, no longer progress rapidly

towards death. In fact, cancer could now be termed a chronic relapsing and remitting disease. Pain can be a prominent factor during treatment phases, and even during remission, cancer treatment and the disease itself can leave patients with pain. It may be that by the time a patient reaches the terminal phase of a disease, a chronic opioid regime has been established, and the success of opioid treatment for end of life palliation can be compromised. Whereas we could once be confident that the opioid option was available for relief of terminal suffering, we must now reevaluate the role of opioids during chronic disease management and continue the quest to unravel mechanisms of opioid refractoriness to preserve this invaluable option for terminal care. Addiction risk is not considered important during the management of terminal illness. However, even during terminal illness, it is possible for patients to exhibit opioid seeking behavior. Yet there are many reasons for terminally ill patients to seek opioids, including inadequate control of pain, helplessness, anxiety and grief, and most people would be reluctant to label this type of opioid seeking as addiction. Considering addiction an irreversible neurobiological state produced by repeated drug procurement, de novo opioid seeking during terminal illness would rarely meet the criteria for addiction [16]. This does not mean that addiction does not arise during a prolonged course of cancer or any other chronic life-threatening disease. The risk of iatrogenic addiction must be the same during any long-term course of opioid treatment, regardless of underlying diagnosis, and it is time to start treating prolonged cancer pain much as any other chronic pain state with a goal of maintaining function, preserving efficacy, and minimizing addiction risk.

Chronic Pain

It seems inherently appealing to use opioids to treat chronic pain. After all, if opioids can relieve the suffering associated with surgery and trauma and other acute pain states, and relieve suffering during terminal illness, why should patients with chronic pain not be treated the same way. In fact there has not been a tradition of treating chronic pain with opioids, partly because of fear of addiction, partly because chronic pain was previously less prevalent or at least less overt, and partly because chronic pain states (typically neuropathic pain, i.e., pain associated with a diseased or altered nervous system) were not considered sensitive to opioids. The recent popularization of opioids for treating chronic pain must be regarded as an experiment, and the treatment remains under considerable scrutiny, with many diverse opinions about the wisdom of using opioids to treat chronic pain. Many questions remain unanswered, but most important: is analgesic efficacy maintained, is future analgesic efficacy compromised, and how does dependence interfere?

There are now multiple randomized controlled trials (RCTs) that confirm the efficacy of opioids in treating chronic pain states, and these convincingly refute earlier concerns that chronic pain states are not responsive to opioids [10, 17, 18]. However, being RCTs, they are only conducted over a limited time frame (up to 8 months) and they do not inform about longer-term use. Observational studies produce a conflicting picture about long-term opioid effectiveness and efficacy with some case series suggesting good effectiveness [19], while epidemiological studies often suggest the opposite [20, 21]. There are several putative mechanisms for a decline in opioid analgesic efficacy over time, and these include pharmacological tolerance, sensitization (hyperalgesia and withdrawal), and psychological factors including loss of placebo and associative tolerance [10].

Perhaps of even greater concern than loss of analgesic efficacy over the course of chronic pain treatment is the issue of opioid refractoriness whereby new onset pain cannot be treated effectively with opioids in a patient who is opioid tolerant. This phenomenon is seen increasingly in operating rooms, recovery settings and during the treatment of terminal illness, as chronic opioid treatment is used more widely and for longer. The mechanisms for this effect may be similar or the same as those that produce the clinical picture of loss of analgesic efficacy, although it is likely that cellular and molecular adaptations play a more prominent and psychological factors a less prominent role. In any case, opioid refractoriness is becoming a concerning clinical occurrence that interferes with pain management, and there is an urgent need to understand the mechanisms for this effect so that it can be avoided, treated, or reversed [14].

Concerns about addiction arising in patients treated with opioid analgesics are multiple, and arise chiefly during chronic pain treatment precisely because it is conducted over prolonged periods of time, and conducted out of hospital. Can opioid-treated pain patients develop addiction as a direct consequence of their treatment (this being termed "iatrogenic opioid addiction" [15])? Do patients come to pain clinics or to doctors' surgeries to satisfy a preexisting addiction? Do prescription analgesics get diverted to addicts in the community? Do the many comorbidities shared by chronic pain patients and addicts increase the risk of addiction arising in chronic pain patients treated with opioids? [22] None of these questions has a clear answer, but let us focus here on the first question, whether iatrogenic opioid addiction interferes with successful opioid treatment of chronic pain. Efforts to quantify the risk of iatrogenic opioid addiction have been greatly hampered by lack of consensus over exactly what addiction looks like when it arises in patients who are prescribed opioids. All patients on a steady, continuous dose of opioids will become dependent, that is they will exhibit some form of withdrawal upon dose reduction or cessation of opioid treatment. Many will exhibit problematic opioid seeking behaviors that could be related to poor pain relief, chemical coping (i.e., using medications to reduce life stresses) or dependence; behaviors that disappear either when pain and distress are adequately controlled, or once the opioids are discontinued. Largely because of their reversibility, these behaviors do not constitute addiction, although they do interfere with the success of the pain treatment. At some point, though, a line might be crossed and the behaviors, their motivators, and the patients' ability to control the behaviors might reach criteria for true addiction. There are some opioid-treated pain patients whose behavior is exemplary; there are some who are clearly out of control and should receive an addiction diagnosis so that they can be appropriately treated. But most patients lie between these two extremes and receive an addiction diagnosis according to the opinion of the treating clinician, which varies greatly between clinicians. It is not surprising then that published estimates of addiction arising in opioid-treated chronic pain patients range widely from 5 % [19] up to 50 % [23–25].[1] We do not really understand the extent to which true iatrogenic opioid addiction develops, and to some extent it might be avoidable with careful screening both in and out of treatment [26–30]. Nevertheless, when true addiction does arise it has a devastating effect on the effort to improve a patient's life through pain treatment, and a careful approach to opioid treatment of chronic pain is always warranted [1].

Alternatives to Opioids

Although much of this chapter is devoted to opioids, justifiably given their key role in pain treatment and addiction, it should be remembered that there are many alternatives to opioids for managing pain. In fact, because of the many problems associated with opioid therapy, and despite the fact that opioids are the strongest analgesics available, the thrust of pain management, whether acute, terminal, or chronic, is to minimize opioid usage. This means using every available alternative to reduce reliance on opioids.

For acute pain management, local anesthetic blocks are extremely useful because they will last long enough to get patients over the initial severe postoperative pain period, or can be prolonged using catheters. Neuraxial and regional techniques are widely used to reduce opioid requirements after surgery. Non-steroidal anti-inflammatory drugs (NSAIDs) and acetaminophen are also useful and used for their opioid-sparing effect. A variety of other adjuncts are used less commonly including ketamine, clonidine, local anesthetics, and anticonvulsants. For opioid-dependent and

---

[1] May include concomitant substance use disorders as well as iatrogenic opioid addiction (addiction arising directly out of opioid pain treatment), since in several studies there is no distinction made.

addicted patients, these options are indispensable since without them patients who have become opioid refractory may not get any effective analgesia.

For terminal pain relief, which was traditionally treated successfully with opioids alone, it has become necessary to think about alternatives because opioid refractoriness can become a problem during a prolonged course of treatment. Since much cancer pain is neuropathic (due to changes in peripheral or central nervous system), it makes sense to treat with the neuropathic pain medications (anticonvulsants such as gabapentin and pregabalin or antidepressants such as amitryptilline), as tolerated. The benzodiazepines have a dual role as anxiolytics and muscle relaxants and are often useful. Terminally ill patients suffer much inner turmoil for which they need support, whether in the form of family or professional counseling, or in the form of medications. Either way, optimizing their psychological status will greatly reduce pain and analgesic requirements, and is an invaluable adjunct to opioid pain management. For opioid refractoriness that cannot be overcome by opioid rotation (switching to a different opioid that may reduce opioid dose requirement) [31, 32], treatment with an N-methyl-D-aspartate receptor antagonist, typically ketamine, may help. Steroids are useful analgesics at the end of life. Cannabinoid treatment, or allowing patients to use marijuana, may also be useful during terminal illness to improve pain relief and reduce nausea and distress.

Given the high degree of uncertainty about whether chronic opioid therapy is a good idea, when managing chronic pain few would disagree that opioids are a last resort. The first option must always be to change lifestyle if necessary, and optimally treat the underlying cause of pain. Patients who are willing can help themselves with the aid of self-help books, videos, or face-to-face counseling. Pain related to the spine might be helped by spine injections or other minimally invasive interventions before the surgical option is pursued. Surgery and other interventions can completely reverse pain when carefully applied, or make things worse when not. Alternative approaches such as acupuncture and massage are useful. Physical, behavioral, and occupational therapy can be tried, and are particularly helpful in a rehabilitation setting as part of comprehensive approach to teaching patients to cope with pain. Medications are helpful to some extent, especially in the short term, when they can help patients get over periods in their lives when pain is particularly troublesome. However, for nearly all the medications used to treat pain, many patients abandon their therapy after several months of treatment, or seek alternatives, when they begin to feel that the medication is no longer helping. The more commonly used chronic pain medications are the anticonvulsants, antidepressants, and NSAIDs. Opioids, of course, are not so easily abandoned, even when they stop providing good analgesia, because of dependence. This is one of many reasons to be highly selective about opioid treatment for chronic pain, and to regard it as a last resort.

Opioids and Addiction

Addiction Mechanisms in Opioid-Treated Pain Patients

A key difference between opioid-treated pain patients and illicit opioid addicts is the way in which dependence is manifest. Dependence and addiction definitions have produced a great deal of confusion in the pain field, especially after chronic opioid pain treatment was popularized and it become obvious that all patients treated continuously and long term with opioids develop dependence, but few manifest "substance dependence" as identified by DSM-IV criteria [16]. The word "dependence" was commandeered into addiction definitions partly to medicalize addiction and remove the stigma associated with the word "addiction," and partly because physical dependence often characterizes drug addiction. Yet opioid-treated pain patients may become dependent and tolerant without developing any of the compulsive behaviors that comprise the other addiction criteria [16, 33, 34]. One of the difficulties we face in understanding dependence during opioid treatment of pain is that while the manifestations of dependence in pain patients may include some of the same characteristics and those in addicts, they present differently. Thus, opioid addicts in withdrawal exhibit a characteristic withdrawal syndrome with central neurologic arousal and sleeplessness, irritability, psychomotor agitation, diarrhea, rhinorrhea, and piloerection. The pain patient, on the other hand, is more likely to simply experience a general feeling of malaise or being let down (withdrawal anhedonia) [35–38], possibly a worsening of pain, or an increase in pain sensitivity (withdrawal hyperalgesia) [39], and no overt physical symptoms. This state in pain patients could be thought of as a sub-threshold withdrawal. The difference between withdrawal states in addicts and pain patients can be explained partly by the fact that doses and dose fluctuations in pain patients are typically much smaller than in addicts. In addition, associative tolerance (learned tolerance) [37, 40, 41], thus dose effect, may fluctuate even during the course of a day, with consequent subtle withdrawal effects. In pain patients, withdrawal anhedonia and hyperalgesia are likely to play an important role in the common clinical scenario where opioid-treated pain patients are not experiencing good pain relief, yet discontinuing treatment or dose reduction makes things worse and is not acceptable to them. Dependence understood in this way first differs markedly from the "substance dependence" described by DSM criteria, and second characterizes the state that is reached by many opioid-treated pain patients of poor analgesia and mood in the face of immediate worsening of pain and mood upon opioid withdrawal.

Regulations and Guidelines in Pain Management

Whatever one thinks of opioid regulations in terms of their effect on recreational opioid use in society, the effect of regulations on the medical use of opioids has been substantial, and in many ways has compromised physicians' ability to provide pain management. What is seen throughout history and across cultures is that the more draconian the regulations, the greater the effect on medical use. In the USA, for example, where the regulations introduced at the beginning of the twentieth century made it illegal for physicians to prescribe opioids for addiction [42], prescribing for both pain and addiction virtually stopped because physicians were afraid of losing their medical licenses. It took the pioneering work of addiction researchers in Lexington, Kentucky, to establish a role for opioid maintenance for the treatment of opioid addiction, culminating in a change in the regulations to allow such prescribing, but not until 1974 (Narcotic Addict Treatment Act, 1974) [43, 44]. A parallel effort was underway in the pain field, and pain advocacy first reestablished the rightful role of opioids in cancer pain treatment, and later evidence-based guidelines were produced by US government agencies to encourage opioid prescribing for acute and cancer pain on the basis of proven improvements in outcome related to better pain control [45, 46]. Unfortunately, though, it is always difficult to achieve a balance, and despite the efforts of both the detractors and the advocates, there continue to be abuses on both sides, all be they rare, that encourage the growth of even more draconian regulations on the one side [9, 47], and unreasonable pain mandates on the other [7, 48, 49]. What has become clear, however, as the two parallel fields (pain and addiction) have developed, is that guidelines for controlling use during opioid maintenance treatment of addiction [50, 51] have become remarkably similar to those for controlling use during opioid treatment of pain [2–7]. This suggests that expert opinion recognizes that opioid maintenance, whether for the treatment of addiction or the treatment of pain, needs careful monitoring and a willingness to stop the treatment if it is not achieving its stated goals. It is not a coincidence, either, that the drugs used conventionally for opioid maintenance (methadone and buprenorphine) are used increasingly for the treatment of chronic pain.

Pain and Addiction Comorbidities

Chronic pain patients commonly present with psychiatric comorbidities, the most frequent being depression, anxiety, substance use disorders, somatization, and personality disorders [52–56]. For example, between 18% and 32% of chronic low back pain patients are found to have major depression during the course of their treatment [55] compared with 5%

point prevalence in the general US population [56–59]. Rates of substance use disorders in chronic pain patients, estimated at between 5% and 50% [19, 23–25, 53], may also be markedly greater than in the general population (estimated at a point prevalence of 16.7%) [53]. Whether the comorbidity is depression, anxiety, substance use disorder, somatization, or personality disorder, high rates of concurrence with chronic pain are well documented. It is less clear, however, which comes first, the pain or the psychopathology [22]. Although the high incidence of psychiatric comorbidity in both chronic pain patients and addicted individuals is well documented, the processes by which comorbidities alter the initiation and development of pain and addiction remain elusive. The diathesis-stress model, in which genetic and biological vulnerability (diathesis) interacts with life experiences (stress), is a useful construct on which to base studies that attempt to elucidate the interplay between chronic pain, addiction, and their shared comorbidities [60]. On the basis of this construct, it is reasonable to suppose that chronic pain patients, having a high rate of shared psychiatric comorbidities with addiction, might be at increased risk of developing iatrogenic opioid addiction. Maladaptive responses of the hypothalamic–pituitary–adrenal axis arising through disruption of normal responses by chronic stressors, including chronic pain, may be important common mechanisms in pain chronicity, addiction, and other psychiatric comorbidities, especially depression [61, 62].

Prescription Drug (Opioid) Abuse

Drug abuse has grown to be a societal problem of enormous proportions, influenced by globalization, lucrative trading, and the availability of increasingly refined and therefore increasingly addictive substances [63, 64]. Prescription drugs are affected by the same factors that have produced marked growth in illicit drug abuse. In fact, in the USA, rates of prescription drug abuse may have overtaken those of illicit drug abuse as prescription drugs become increasingly favored by addicts because of their purity, relative safety, and easy availability [65–68]. The result is an alarming increase in prescription drug abuse. Opioids, prevalent both in medical usage as analgesics, and in illicit usage (heroin and prescription opioids), are the prescription drugs of greatest concern because opioid use is medically necessary and widespread. Physicians are faced with an ethical dilemma: can they deny patients relief of chronic pain, or should they offer long-term opioid treatment and risk opioid abuse. If the latter, do they need to select patients for this treatment, and on what grounds can they ever deny patients opioids. Full discussion of these issues is beyond the scope of this review, nevertheless there are important issues at stake, with protection of patients and the community being the end goal for all clinicians providing opioids and guiding practice.

The question facing us now is can we realistically make a complicated treatment widely available and unfettered, and if not, what is the best way to control it.

Conclusion

It is easy to dismiss addiction as something that arises only rarely during opioid treatment of pain, yet prescription opioid abuse is growing [65–68] and clinicians providing opioids are increasingly troubled by the failure of their patients to meet the promise of good pain control and a better quality of life. This may have as much to do with failing to understand the complexity of long-term opioid pain management, as with the failure of the treatment per se. It may be, for example, that more patients would be helped and fewer harmed if a more careful treatment approach were adopted, with stricter selection criteria, and more time spent with fewer carefully selected patients. We need to find out. What we know already, though, is that the careless use of opioids is never successful, and leaves patients and those around them open to the risk of opioid abuse.

Opioids can be classified as naturally occurring, semisynthetic and synthetic (Table 18.1). Morphine, codeine, papaverine, and thebaine are naturally occurring constituents of opium. The semisynthetic drugs are derived from morphine, codeine, and thebaine. The synthetic drugs structurally resemble morphine but do not occur in nature. They are produced by gradually reducing the number of rings from the 5-ring structure of morphine, through the 4-ring "morphinans," the 3-ring "benzomorphinans" to the 2-ring "phenylpiperidines" (Fig. 18.1). There are alternative classifications of opioids: the drugs may be grouped according to the specific receptors on which they act, or according to whether they are agonist, antagonists, or some combination of the two (Table 18.2, Fig. 18.2).

Absorption: The opioids vary in their absorption according to their molecular size and shape, lipophilicity, first-pass effect, and the compartment into which they are delivered. The hepatic first-pass effect is significant for many of the commonly prescribed opioids, including morphine, oxycodone, and dilaudid, with an oral:parenteral ratio of 3:1. After neuraxial administration (intrathecal

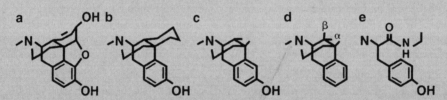

Fig. 18.1 Structure of morphine-like opioids. (**a**) Morphine, (**b**) morphinan, (**c**) benzomorphan, (**d**) phenylpiperidine, and (**e**) tyramine moiety of endogenous opioids. Note the progressive removal of ring structures from five-ring morphine to two-ring phenylpiperidine (Reproduced with permission from Carr DB. Opioids. *Int Anesthesiol Clin* 1988; 26:273.)

Table 18.2 Alternative classification of opioids

Class	Definition	Example
Agonist	A drug which, when bound to the receptor, stimulates the receptor to the maximum level; by definition, the intrinsic activity of a full agonist is unity	Morphine
Antagonist	A drug which, when bound to the receptor, fails completely to produce any stimulation of that receptor; by definition, the intrinsic activity of a pure antagonist is zero	Naloxone
Partial agonist	A drug which, when bound to the receptor, stimulates the receptor to a level below the maximum level; by definition, the intrinsic activity of a partial agonist lies between zero and unity	Buprenorphine (partial mu agonist)
Mixed agonist–antagonist	A drug which acts simultaneously on different subtypes, with the potential for agonist action on one or more subtypes and antagonist action on one or more subtypes	Nalbuphine (partial mu agonist, kappa agonist, delta antagonist)

From Textbook of Pain, Melzack and Wall, 1994, Chap. 49, table 49.1

Fig. 18.2 Examples of opioid receptor antagonists and agonists

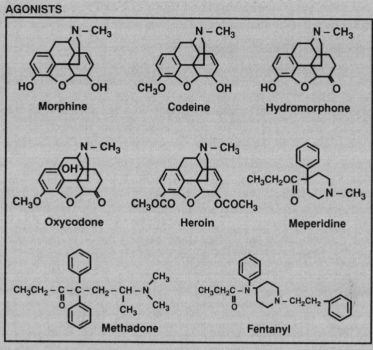

and epidural), both lipophilicity and molecular shape influence absorption into cerebrospinal fluid (CSF) and subsequently onto spinal receptor sites. The globular shape and extreme hydrophilicity of morphine delay its absorption and favor its passage in CSF to higher centers.

Distribution: Most opioid drugs are rapidly distributed throughout the body, and reach their central nervous system (CNS) target sites within 5–20 min. The physical characteristics of opioids that determine distribution are protein binding, ionization, and lipophilicity. The extreme hypdrophilicity of morphine slows its passage across the blood–brain barrier, so compared with the more lipophilic opioids, its onset is slow and its action prolonged.

Actions: Opioids act via specific receptors on cell membranes. There are three well-defined "classical" opioid receptors (mu, delta, and kappa). The more recently identified "orphan" receptor has a high degree of similarity to the "classical" opioid receptors and has been named *opioid receptor-like* (ORL). There is also pharmacological evidence for subtypes of each known receptor, and for other, less well-characterized opioid receptors, including epsilon and gamma. Opioid receptors exist largely in the

CNS, although there are opioid receptors importantly in the bowel (bowel slowing), on immune cells (immune suppression), in endocrine tissue (pituitary–adrenal and –gonadal suppression), and in other peripheral locations (sparsely, role unknown).

Opioid receptors are coupled to G-proteins, and are thus able to affect protein phosphorylation via second messenger systems, thereby altering ion channel conductance. Opioids act both presynaptically and postsynaptically on C and Aδ nerves. Presynaptically they inhibit the release of neurotransmitters, including substance P and glutamate. Postsynaptically they can inhibit neurons by opening potassium channels that hyperpolarize the cell. They also activate presynaptic receptors on GABA neurons which inhibit the release of GABA in the ventral tegmental area, thus allowing vigorous firing of dopaminergic neurons in the nucleus accumbens, which is intensely pleasurable. Ultimately these cellular processes can result in gene regulation with potential long-term effects.

Some opioid actions are mediated by non-opioid receptors. N-methyl-D-aspartate (NMDA)-sensitive glutamate receptors are involved in nociceptive transmission in the spinal dorsal horn. Norepinephrine, serotonin, and sodium channels are also involved, and it is possible that a central nitric oxide–cyclic guanosine monophosphate signaling pathway may help mediate nociception. These pathways may be important in opioid-induced hyperalgesia, and in top-down regulation of opioid analgesia.

Elimination: The metabolism of opioids is thought to occur predominantly in the liver. Most opioids are metabolized by glucuronidation or by the cytochrome P450 system. The basal rate of metabolism is determined by genetics, gender, age, environmental factors including diet, state of health, and concurrent medications. Several opioids, notably morphine and meperidine, have active and potentially toxic metabolites, and these metabolites can accumulate when renal function is impaired. Methadone metabolism is highly variable and this drug can accumulate due to its long half-life, variable metabolism, and potential for drug interactions [1–5].

References

References to Chapter

1. Ballantyne JC, Mao J. Opioid therapy for chronic pain. N Engl J Med. 2003;349:1943–53.
2. Haddox JD, Joranson D, Angarola RT, et al. The use of opioids for the treatment of chronic pain. A consensus statement from the American Academy of Pain Medicine and the American Pain Society. Clin J Pain. 1997;13:6–8.
3. West JE, Aronoff G, Dahl J, et al. Model guidelines for the use of controlled substances for the treatment of pain. A policy document of the Federation of State Medical Boards of the United States Inc. Euless, TX: Federation of State Medical Boards of the United States Inc; 1998.
4. Evidence-based recommendations for medical management of chronic non-malignant pain. Reference guide for clinicians. The College of Physicians and Surgeons of Ontario 2000.
5. Jovey R, Ennis J, Gardner-Nix J, et al. Use of opioid analgesics for the treatment of chronic noncancer pain–a consensus statement and guidelines from the Canadian Pain Society, 2002. Pain Res Manag. 2003;8(Suppl A):3A–28A.
6. Recommendations for the appropriate use of opioids for persistent non-cancer pain. A consensus statement prepared on behalf of the British Pain Society, the Royal College of Anaesthetists, the Royal College of General Practitioners and the Royal College of Psychiatrists. London: The British Pain Society, ISBN 0-9546703-5-3; 2005.
7. Organizations JCoAoH. Pain management standards. Effective January 1, 2001. http://www.jcaho.org/standard/.
8. Drug Enforcement Administration, 21 Health Care Organizations News Release, October 23, 2001. http://www.lastacts.org.
9. Department of Justice DEA. Issuance of multiple prescriptions for schedule II controlled substances. Notice of proposed rulemaking.

21 CFR Part 1306, RIN 1117-AB01. Fed Regist. 2006;71:52724–6.
10. Ballantyne JC, Shin NS. Efficacy of opioids for chronic pain: a review of the evidence. Clin J Pain. 2008;24:469–78.
11. Porter J, Jick H. Addiction rare in patients treated with narcotics (letter). N Engl J Med. 1980;302:123.
12. Mao J. Opioid induced abnormal pain sensitivity: implications in clinical opioid therapy. Pain. 2002;100:213–7.
13. Angst MS, Clark JD. Opioid-induced hyperalgesia: a qualitative systematic review. Anesthesiology. 2006;104:570–87.
14. Chu LF, Angst MS, Clark D. Opioid-induced hyperalgesia in humans: molecular mechanisms and clinical considerations. Clin J Pain. 2008;24:479–96.
15. Ballantyne JC, LaForge SL. Opioid dependence and addiction in opioid treated pain patients. Pain. 2007;129:235–55.
16. American Psychiatric Association. Diagnostic and statistical manual of mental disorders. 4th ed. Washington, DC: American Psychiatric Association; 1994.
17. Kalso E, Edwards J, Moore R, McQuay H. Opioids in chronic non-cancer pain: systematic review of efficacy and safety. Pain. 2004;112:372–80.
18. Eisenberg E, McNicol ED, Carr DB. Efficacy and safety of opioid agonists in the treatment of neuropathic pain of non-malignant origin: systematic review and meta-analysis of randomized controlled trials. JAMA. 2005;293:3043–52.
19. Portenoy RK, Foley KM. Chronic use of opioid analgesics in non-malignant pain: report of 38 cases. Pain. 1986;25:171–86.
20. Eriksen J, Sjogren P, Bruera E, Ekholm O, Rasmussen NK. Critical issues on opioids in chronic non-cancer pain. An epidemiological study. Pain. 2006;125:172–9.
21. Ballantyne JC. Opioids for chronic pain: taking stock. Pain. 2006;125:3–4.
22. Fishbain D, Cutler R, Rosomoff HL, Rosomoff RL. Chronic pain-associated depression: antecedent or consequence of chronic pain? A review. Clin J Pain. 1997;113:116–37.

23. Hojsted J, Sjogren P. Addiction to opioids in chronic pain patients: a literature review. Eur J Pain. 2007;11(5):490–518.

24. Fishbain DA, Rosomoff HL, Rosomoff RS. Drug abuse, dependence and addiction in chronic pain patients. Clin J Pain. 1992;8:77–85.

25. Martell BA, O'Connor PG, Kerns RD, et al. Systematic review: opioid treatment for chronic back pain: prevalence, efficacy, and association with addiction. Ann Intern Med. 2007;146:116–27.

26. Belgrade MJ, Schamber CD, Lindgren BR. The DIRE score: predicting outcomes of opioid prescribing for chronic pain. J Pain. 2006;7:671–81.

27. Akbik H, Butler SF, Budman SH, Fernandez K, Katz NP, Jamison RN. Validation and clinical application of the Screener and Opioid Assessment for Patients with Pain (SOAPP). J Pain Symptom Manage. 2006;32:287–93.

28. Butler SF, Budman SH, Fernandez KC, et al. Development and validation of the current opioid misuse measure. Pain. 2007;130:144–56.

29. Passik SD, Kirsh KL, Whitcomb L, et al. A new tool to assess and document pain outcomes in chronic pain patients receiving opioid therapy. Clin Ther. 2004;26:552–61.

30. Passik SD, Kirsh KL, Whitcomb L, et al. Monitoring outcomes during long-term opioid therapy for noncancer pain: results with the Pain Assessment and Documentation Tool. J Opioid Manag. 2005;1:257–66.

31. Indelicato RA, Portenoy RK. Opioid rotation in the management of refractory cancer pain. J Clin Oncol. 2002;20:348–52.

32. Vorobeychik Y, Chen L, Bush MC, Mao J. Improved opioid analgesic effect following opioid dose reduction. Pain Med. 2008;9:724–7.

33. 30th report. WHO Expert Committee on drug dependence. Geneva: WHO; 1998.

34. World Health Organization. The ICD-10 classification of mental and behavioral disorders: clinical descriptions and diagnostic guidelines. Geneva: WHO; 1992.

35. Koob GF, Le Moal M. Drug abuse: hedonic homeostatic dysregulation. Science. 1997;278:52–8.

36. Koob GF, Le Moal M. Drug addiction, dysregulation of reward, and allostasis. Neuropsychopharmacology. 2001;24:97–129.

37. Koob GF, Maldonado R, Stinus L. Neural substrates of opiate withdrawal. Trends Neurosci. 1992;15:186–91.

38. Hyman SE, Malenka RC, Nestler EJ. Neural mechanisms of addiction: the role of reward-related learning and memory. Annu Rev Neurosci. 2006;29:565–98.

39. Compton P, Athanasos P, Elashoff D. Withdrawal hyperalgesia after acute opioid physical dependence in nonaddicted humans: a preliminary study. J Pain. 2003;4:511–9.

40. South SM, Smith MT. Analgesic tolerance to opioids. Pain Clin Updates. 2001;9:1–4.

41. von Zastrow M. A cell biologist's perspective on physiological adaptation to opiate drugs. Neuropharmacology. 2004;47 Suppl 1:286–92.

42. U.S. Supreme Court, WEBB, et al. v. United States, 249 U.S. 96 (1919), No. 370., Argued Jan. 16, 1919., Decided March 3, 1919.

43. Dole VP. What we have learned from three decades of methadone maintenance treatment. Drug Alcohol Rev. 1994;13:3–4.

44. Dole VP, Nyswander M, Kreek MJ. Narcotic blockade. Arch Intern Med. 1966;188:304–9.

45. Jacox A, Carr DB, Payne R, et al. Management of cancer pain: clinical practice guideline. Washington, DC: US Department of Health and Human Services, AHCPR Publication No 94-0592; March 1994.

46. Carr DB. Acute pain management: operative or medical procedures and trauma. In: Clinical practice guideline. Rockville, MD: Agency for Health Care Policy and Research, Public Health Service, US Department of Health and Human Services, AHCPR Pub No 92-0032; 1992.

47. Department of Justice DEA. Dispensing of controlled substances for the treatment of pain. Interim policy statement. Docket No DEA-258S 2004.

48. Frasco PE, Sprung J, Trentman TL. The impact of the joint commission for accreditation of healthcare organizations pain initiative on perioperative opiate consumption and recovery room length of stay. Anesth Analg. 2005;100:162–8.

49. Overdyk F, Carter R, Maddox R. New JCAHO pain standard bigger threat to patient safety than envisioned. Anesth Analg. 2006;102:1596; author reply -7.

50. Fiellin DA, O'Connor PG. Office-based treatment of opioid-dependent patients. N Engl J Med. 2002;347:817–23.

51. Krantz M, Mehler P. Treating opioid dependence. Growing implications for primary care. Arch Intern Med. 2004;164:277–88.

52. Webster L, Webster R. Predicting aberrant behaviors in opioid-treated patients: preliminary validation of the Opioid Risk Tool. Pain Med. 2005;6:432–42.

53. Dersh J, Polatin PB, Gatchell RJ. Chronic pain and psychopathology: research finding and theoretical considerations. Psychom Med. 2002;64:773–86.

54. Fishbain DA, Goldberg M, Labbe E, Steele R, Rosomoff HL. Compensation and non-compensation chronic pain patients compared for DSM-III operational diagnoses. Pain. 1988;32:197–06.

55. Katon W, Egan K, Miller D. Chronic pain: lifetime psychiatric diagnoses and family history. Am J Psychiatry. 1985;142:1156–60.

56. McWilliams L, Goodwin R, Cox B. Depression and anxiety associated with three pain conditions: results from a nationally representative sample. Pain. 2004;111:77–83.

57. Magni G, Caldieron C, Rigatti-Luchini S, Merskey H. Chronic musculoskeletal pain and depressive symptoms in the general population. An analysis of the 1st National Health and Nutrition Examination Survey data. Pain. 1990;43:299–307.

58. Wasan AD, Davar G, Jamison R. The association between negative affect and opioid analgesia in patients with discogenic low back pain. Pain. 2005;117:450–61.

59. Blazer D, Kessler R, McGonagle K, Swartz M. The prevalence of major depression in a national community sample: the national comorbidity survey. Am J Psychiatry. 1994;151:979–86.

60. Banks S, Kerns R. Explaining high rates of depression in chronic pain: a diathesis-stress framework. Psychol Bull. 1996;119:95–110.

61. Blackburn-Munro G, Blackburn-Munro R. Chronic pain, chronic stress and depression: coincidence or consequence? J Neuroendocrinol. 2001;13:1009–23.

62. Kreek MJ, Nielsen DA, LaForge KS. Genes associated with addiction: alcoholism, opiate, and cocaine addiction. Neuromol Med. 2004;5:85–108.

63. Administration USDE. Automation of Reports and Consolidated Orders System (ARCOS), Retail Drug Summary Report; http://www.deadiversion.usdoj.gov/arcos/retail_drug_summary/index.html.

64. Associated Press Analysis. http://wwwihtcom/articles/ap/2007/08/20/america/NA-FEA-GEN-US-World-of-Painphp.

65. Year-end 2000 emergency department data from the Drug Abuse Warning Network. DAWN series D-18. Rockville, MD: Substance Abuse and Mental Health Services Administration, 2001 (DHHS publication no (SMA) 01-3532) http://wwwsamhsagov/oas/dawn/200yrendpdf.

66. DHHS, SAMHSA: National Household Survey on Drug Abuse Main Findings. Series H-11. 1998.

67. DHHS, SAMHSA: National Survey on Drug Use and Health http://www.oas.samha.gov. 2003.

68. Compton WM, Volkow ND. Major increases in opioid analgesic abuse in the United States: concerns and strategies. Drug Alcohol Depend. 2006;81:103–7.

References to Box

1. Nestler EJ. Molecular mechanisms of drug addiction. Neuropharmacology. 2004;47 Suppl 1:24–32.
2. Ballantyne JC, LaForge SL. Opioid dependence and addiction in opioid treated pain patients. Pain. 2007;129:235–55.
3. Inturrisi CE. Clinical pharmacology of opioids for pain. Clin J Pain. 2002;18:S3–13.
4. Trescot AM, Datta S, Lee M, Hansen H. Opioid pharmacology. Pain Physician. 2008;11:S133–53.
5. Uppington J. Opioids. In: Ballantyne JC, editor. The Massachusetts General Hospital handbook of pain management. 3rd ed. Philadelphia: Lippincott Williams & Wilkins; 2005.

Anabolic–Androgenic Steroids

19

Harrison G. Pope Jr. and Gen Kanayama

Abstract

The anabolic–androgenic steroids (AAS) are a family of hormones that includes the natural male hormone, testosterone, together with a group of synthetic derivatives of testosterone. These drugs are widely abused by men (and rarely, women) to gain muscle mass and lose body fat. Prior to about 1980, abuse of AAS was confined largely to elite competitive athletes, but in recent decades, AAS abuse has broken out of the athletic community and into the general population. Many modern AAS users have no specific athletic aspirations at all, but simply want to become bigger and more muscular. About 2–6% of men in many Western industrialized countries have used AAS, but AAS use is rare in Asian societies. Individuals with body image concerns, such as "muscle dysmorphia," appear more prone to abuse AAS. Male muscularity is more strongly emphasized and rewarded in industrialized Western cultures than in Asia, and this difference likely explains the geographic distribution of AAS abuse. AAS cause few serious short-term medical effects, but over the long term may cause suppression of hypothalamic–pituitary–gonadal function, adverse effects on serum lipids, and cardiomyopathy. The most common psychiatric effects of AAS are mood disorders (typically hypomanic or manic syndromes during AAS exposure and depressive symptoms during AAS withdrawal); these are idiosyncratic, affecting a minority of AAS users, but are occasionally severe. A growing literature describes syndromes of AAS dependence, where individuals use AAS almost continuously despite adverse medical or psychiatric effects. Individuals displaying AAS abuse or dependence may also exhibit other forms of substance dependence. Unfortunately, AAS users rarely seek treatment, but this situation may change as the first large wave of illicit AAS users—those who first began AAS as youths in the 1980s—now reaches middle age and enters the age of risk for long-term cardiac, neuroendocrine, and psychiatric complications from these drugs.

Learning Objectives
- Anabolic–androgenic steroid (AAS) abuse is no longer restricted to competitive athletes; many AAS abusers are men with no athletic aspirations who simply want to become more muscular.
- AAS abuse is widespread in Western industrialized countries, but rare in Asia, probably because of the greater emphasis on male muscularity in western cultural traditions.

H.G. Pope Jr., M.D. (✉)
Biological Psychiatry Laboratory, McLean Hospital,
Belmont, MA 02178, USA
e-mail: hpope@mclean.harvard.edu

G. Kanayama, M.D., Ph.D.
Department of Psychiatry, Harvard Medical School, Boston, MA, USA

(continued)

J.C. Verster et al. (eds.), *Drug Abuse and Addiction in Medical Illness: Causes, Consequences and Treatment*,
DOI 10.1007/978-1-4614-3375-0_19, © Springer Science+Business Media, LLC 2012

(continued)

- The psychiatric effects of AAS are idiosyncratic, with many users exhibiting few psychiatric symptoms, but occasional individuals developing marked hypomanic or manic symptoms, sometimes associated with aggression and violence, while taking AAS.
- AAS withdrawal is often characterized by depression, fatigue, and loss of libido, partially mediated by suppression of the hypothalamic–pituitary–gonadal axis. These dysphoric symptoms may cause some individuals to quickly resume AAS use and eventually to go on to develop a syndrome of AAS dependence.
- Individuals exhibiting AAS abuse and dependence often display a history of other forms of classical substance abuse and dependence.
- AAS users rarely seek treatment, but this situation may change in the near future as increasing numbers of AAS users reach middle age.

Issues that Need to Be Addressed by Future Research
- The phenomenon of AAS dependence should be further characterized, and risk factors for development of AAS dependence should be assessed.
- Little is known about treatment of AAS abuse and dependence, and future studies should focus on the unique features of this class of substance abusers.
- The long-term psychiatric and medical effects of AAS must be better studied, now that substantial numbers of former illicit AAS users are moving into middle age, and entering the age of risk for some of these possible effects.

The anabolic–androgenic steroids (AAS) are a family of hormones comprising the natural male hormone, testosterone, together with numerous synthetic derivatives of testosterone developed over the last 70 years [1, 2]. Testosterone itself was first isolated in the 1930s [3, 4] and synthetic derivatives quickly followed [5]. All AAS have both *anabolic* ("muscle building") effects and *androgenic* ("masculinizing") effects; no compound has been created that produces one effect without the other. AAS have become widespread drugs of abuse because they allow users to gain large amounts of muscle mass and to lose body fat—often well beyond the limits of what would naturally be possible without drugs [6].

Throughout the following discussion of AAS, it is important to note that AAS should be distinguished from other types of steroid hormones. Many individuals, especially those without medical training, are misled by the generic term "steroids" and fail to recognize that the vast majority of "steroids" prescribed by doctors are not AAS, but instead corticosteroids, which have no anabolic properties and no abuse potential [7]. This confusion has likely led to inflated estimates of the prevalence of AAS use among students receiving anonymous survey instruments, because many students likely responded that they had used "steroids" when in fact they had been prescribed corticosteroids (see below) [8]. Therefore, throughout the following discussion, we will use the term "AAS" to indicate that we are talking specifically about testosterone and its synthetic relatives, and not about other types of "steroids."

Pharmacology

Testosterone is synthesized in the body from cholesterol; like cholesterol, it has a four-ring structure containing 19 carbon atoms. Most synthetic AAS represent slight variations on this molecule, particularly variations created by addition of an alkyl group to the C-17 alpha position, which allows the compounds to survive first-pass metabolism and become orally active [5, 9].

Testosterone is rapidly metabolized in the body, and thus synthetic testosterone preparations are generally produced as injectable esters, such as testosterone decanoate, testosterone cypionate, testosterone propionate, testosterone enanthate, and various blends of these esters. These esters are gradually hydrolyzed to testosterone after they are absorbed and produce a plateau of testosterone levels lasting for a few days to several weeks. Thus, when testosterone is used in the treatment of hypogonadal men, injections can be administered at weekly or longer intervals [10]. By contrast, orally active AAS are metabolized fairly quickly, and thus are generally administered on a daily basis [10].

AAS bind to intracellular receptors, and this AAS–receptor complex then enters the nucleus of the cell, where it stimulates gene transcription, leading eventually to new protein synthesis [9]. It is this effect that leads to the muscle gains for which AAS are illicitly used [7, 11]. The mechanism of the mood-altering effects of AAS (discussed below) is less well understood and may involve actions at various androgen receptors, together with the formation of psychoactive metabolites of the parent AAS [12–14]. Animal studies suggest that AAS modulate a number of neurotransmitter systems, including the GABA [13], opioid [13–20], dopamine [13, 21–23], and serotonin [24–27] systems—and these effects may contribute both to the psychoactive effects of AAS and to the evolution of AAS dependence and withdrawal (see below) [14, 16, 20].

Therapeutic Use of AAS

By far the most important legitimate use of AAS is in the treatment of male hypogonadism [9, 10, 28–30]. Healthy men normally display plasma testosterone concentrations of 300–1,000 ng/dL; men who fail to achieve this range can usually be restored to normal physiological levels by administration of testosterone esters in the range of 100 mg per week or by use of transdermal testosterone preparations such as patches or gels [30–33]. There is rarely any basis for the use of synthetic AAS in the treatment of male hypogonadism, given the availability of testosterone itself. Testosterone and other AAS may rarely be used for a handful of other medical disorders, such as certain types of anemia, hereditary angioedema, and occasionally breast cancer in women [10]. Testosterone has also been found effective for the wasting syndrome associated with HIV infection [34, 35], and two controlled studies [36, 37]—but not one other [38]—have indicated that testosterone may also have antidepressant properties in this population. Several recent studies, extrapolating from this experience, have attempted to use testosterone, either alone [39, 40] or as an augmentation strategy [41–44] in men with a poor response to conventional antidepressant treatment, but experience in this area remains inconclusive [30]. A large controlled trial of testosterone as an augmentation strategy in depressed men incompletely responsive to serotonergic antidepressants has recently been completed [45]; this study failed to find a significant difference between testosterone and placebo in the degree of improvement of depressive symptoms.

Nontherapeutic AAS Use

Initially, during the decades after AAS were first synthesized, nontherapeutic use of these drugs was confined largely to elite athletes [46]. However, by about 1980, bodybuilding and the cult of muscularity had begun to spread through Western societies [47]—a phenomenon evident in movies, magazines [48], and even in children's action toys [49]. In this climate, AAS use began to spread out from the athletic world and into the general population, abetted by various underground guides offering advice on how to self-administer the drugs by mouth or by injection [50–53]. By 1990, concern about illicit AAS use in the United States reached the point where the American government enacted the Steroid Trafficking Act [54], which defined AAS as federally controlled substances, under the jurisdiction of the Drug Enforcement Administration.

Despite more aggressive attempts at enforcement, however, AAS remain readily available to illicit users throughout Western countries. Today, a majority of these illicit AAS users are not competitive athletes at all, but simply men who want to become leaner and more muscular [55–57]. Contrary to some popular beliefs, illicit AAS use is often not associated with a health-conscious "bodybuilding lifestyle," but instead may be only one form of substance abuse in individuals who use a wide variety of illicit drugs [58–63].

AAS Usage Patterns

As noted earlier, many AAS, including testosterone itself, are ineffective when taken orally, and are usually administered by injection; others can survive first-pass metabolism and are effective when taken in oral form [2, 61]. Illicit AAS users often take a combination of both injectable and oral agents simultaneously, a practice colloquially called "stacking" [64]. Characteristically, AAS are taken for courses of time, colloquially called "cycles," typically ranging from 4 to 16 weeks, interspersed with off-drug periods [65]. One rationale for using AAS in cycles is that exogenous AAS will suppress the hypothalamic–pituitary–testicular axis (HPT axis), thus suppressing endogenous testosterone production [2, 61, 66, 67]. By using the drugs in cycles, therefore, a user can allow his own HPT axis to rebound to normal function during the drug-free intervals.

AAS users typically use doses far above the normal physiologic range. A normal man produces about 35–70 mg of endogenous testosterone per week [67], whereas AAS users may often use doses equivalent to more than 1,000 mg of testosterone per week [65], and sometimes even the equivalent of 3,000–5,000 mg [64, 65, 68, 69]. As will be discussed below, the psychiatric effects of AAS appear to be much more prominent in individuals who take doses in these higher ranges [70].

Epidemiology of AAS Use

As mentioned earlier, anonymous surveys of illicit AAS use have often been compromised by the fact that respondents answered that they had used "steroids" when in fact they had not used actual AAS, but merely had been prescribed corticosteroids, or had used over-the-counter supplements that they believed to be AAS. As a result, anonymous surveys have often generated substantial numbers of "false positive" responses, leading to inflated estimates of the true prevalence of AAS use—especially among female respondents [8]. Nevertheless, even correcting for these possible sources of error, it seems likely that at least 2–6% of men have used AAS at some time in their lives in many Western countries, including the United States [71–73], British Commonwealth countries [74, 75], Scandinavia [76–78], Brazil [79], and elsewhere [80, 81]. However, AAS use is uncommon in

Asian countries, probably because these cultures place less value on muscularity [82]. AAS use in women is rare, since women are less likely to want to become very muscular, and also because women are vulnerable to the masculinizing effects of AAS, such as beard growth, deepening of the voice, and masculinized sexual characteristics [8]. Indeed, we are aware of only one published study in the last 15 years where the investigators succeeded in recruiting and evaluating a group of actual women who had used AAS [83, 84]—and even this investigation located only 25 women with a history of AAS use, despite a 2-year period of advertising in three metropolitan areas of the United States.

Adverse Medical Effects of AAS

AAS produce several short-term adverse medical effects, such as acne, gynecomastia, hypertension, and adverse effects on lipid profiles [46, 85]. However, these effects are generally modest (or detectable only on clinical evaluation) and rarely dissuade young men from using AAS [47]. Very rarely, orally active AAS can cause hepatotoxicity, including peliosis hepatis [86] and even liver cancer [87–90], but the risk of these phenomena has often been overstated [91]. AAS may also contribute to a focal segmental glomerulonephritis, although the magnitude of this risk remains uncertain [92].

Probably the greatest long-term risk of AAS is on the cardiovascular system. AAS may produce a range of adverse cardiovascular effects, including myocardial damage [93–97] sometimes leading to dilated cardiomyopathy [98–101]. One recent report of cardiac function in American AAS users has suggested that the extent of myocardial pathology may be greater than previously anticipated, potentially placing long-term AAS users at significant risk for heart failure [102]. AAS also increase low-density lipoprotein cholesterol and decrease high-density lipoprotein cholesterol [103–105] and may affect blood coagulation, leading to an increased risk of thrombus formation [106–108]. These effects may have been responsible for many reported myocardial infarctions and cerebrovascular accidents in AAS users under age 40 [109–119]; as AAS users age, the risk of such events likely rises. One recent study found cardiac abnormalities on the autopsies of 12 out of 34 deceased AAS users [120].

AAS may also sometimes cause persistent HPT axis suppression, especially if these drugs are self-administered for prolonged periods. The authors have encountered several individuals who displayed hypogonadism for more than 6 months after discontinuing AAS and cases lasting more than a year have been reported in the literature [121–123]. Persistent hypogonadism has important psychiatric consequences, including depressive syndromes [64, 65, 70, 124–129] and potentiation of AAS dependence syndromes [16, 126, 130–132] as will be discussed below.

Adverse Psychiatric Effects of AAS Use

There are four general categories of AAS-associated psychiatric effects: (1) major mood syndromes (typically manic or hypomanic symptoms during AAS exposure and depressive symptoms during AAS withdrawal); (2) violent or aggressive behavior; (3) AAS dependence syndromes; and (4) progression to other forms of substance misuse, especially opioid dependence.

Mood Syndromes

Hypomanic and manic reactions to AAS, in rare cases associated with psychotic symptoms, have been reported anecdotally as far back as the early 1980s [133, 134]. In the late 1980s, the first psychiatric case series appeared, describing 39 male AAS users who were administered systematic psychiatric interviews [64, 135]. Five of these men reported a manic syndrome while using the drugs; none reported a manic or hypomanic episode when not taking AAS. Three of the men with manic syndromes, plus two others not meeting criteria for mania, reported psychotic symptoms (delusions or hallucinations) while using AAS; none reported psychotic symptoms of AAS. Five also reported depressive symptoms after stopping an AAS "cycle," but two of these men had also displayed major depression at times unrelated to AAS use.

The last two decades have produced numerous additional naturalistic studies describing apparent hypomanic or manic symptoms associated with AAS use. These studies have used varying assessment methods, including both personal interviews and various psychological rating scales to measure indices such as mood, hostility, and aggression. Study designs have included case reports or small case series [136–138]; longitudinal assessment of users before, during, and after AAS use [68, 139–141]; retrospective comparisons of AAS users on-drug vs. off-drug [64, 69, 142]; comparisons of AAS users on- and off-drug with matched nonusers [65, 128, 142–150]; and even a longitudinal evaluation of two pairs of monozygotic twins where one used AAS and the other did not [151]. Two other retrospective accounts have also described pairs of monozygotic twins where one used AAS and the other did not; in both cases, the AAS-using twin exhibited severe psychopathology associated with AAS use—suicide in one case [129] and extreme violence in the other [152]—whereas the non-AAS-using twin exhibited no psychiatric problems. Details of these various studies are provided in several recent review articles [70, 153–156].

However, the findings of the above studies vary considerably, with some describing very pronounced effects of irritability, aggressiveness, grandiosity, and even occasional psychotic symptoms during AAS use [64], others describing only infrequent or modest effects, and at least one study finding no effects at all [143]. Upon inspection, however, the differences among studies may be partially related to differences in the doses of AAS used by the men in the different studies. For example, one study compared 12 low-dose AAS users (defined as less than 300 mg of testosterone or equivalent per week), 51 medium-dose users (300–1,000 mg per week), and 25 high-dose users (greater than 1,000 mg per week). Only one (8.3%) of the low-dose users and 5 (9.8%) of the medium-dose users reported that they had ever experienced an AAS-associated mood syndrome, as compared to 7 (28%) of the high-dose users. Similarly, high rates of psychopathology were reported in the 1988 Pope and Katz study described earlier in this section [64]; the 8 men reporting manic and/or psychotic symptoms in this study were ingesting a mean weekly dose of 900 mg. At the other end of the spectrum are the subjects of Bahrke and colleagues [143], who exhibited virtually no psychiatric symptoms; these men were using a mean of only 318 mg per week, with none higher than 620 mg per week. Studies of users taking intermediate doses of AAS have tended to show intermediate levels of psychiatric symptoms. Taken collectively, then, naturalistic studies suggest that psychiatric symptoms associated with AAS are rare up to AAS doses of 300 mg per week, somewhat more frequent (though still uncommon) at 300–1,000 mg per week, and much more common above 1,000 mg per week.

The above naturalistic observations, however, do not establish that AAS actually *caused* the symptoms observed. For example, it might be argued that mood symptoms in AAS users are not attributable to AAS per se, but instead are attributable to premorbid psychological traits of the users themselves [68, 146, 149], or to expectational factors, or to psychosocial influences of the weightlifting culture, as some have speculated [157–160]. The only good way to resolve these questions is with randomized controlled trials where volunteers are administered AAS vs. placebo under blinded conditions.

Of course, one cannot ethically administer grossly supraphysiologic doses of AAS, comparable to the doses taken by illicit users, to normal volunteers—but there are published studies using more modest supraphysiologic doses. Several studies have used doses up to a maximum of 300 mg of testosterone equivalent per week and found very few psychiatric effects [159, 161–166]. However, these studies are not very useful for our purposes, because a dose of 300 mg per week is much lower than the doses used by most illicit AAS users. Thus, it is inappropriate to extrapolate from these results to the case of illicit users.

There are four laboratory studies, however, that have used doses of 500 mg per week or more, and which therefore come a little closer to approximating the doses used by illicit AAS users [167–171]. We have described these studies in detail in previous reviews [2, 70, 168]. In these studies collectively, 109 men received testosterone or other AAS under double-blind conditions; 5 (4.6%) of these men developed hypomanic or manic syndromes on AAS, but none exhibited such syndromes on placebo. This rate is almost certainly an underestimate of the true rate of such reactions among illicit users in the field, for several reasons: (1) illicit users may take much larger doses of AAS, and for much longer periods, than was the case in any of these studies; (2) users may ingest ("stack") multiple AAS simultaneously, with possible augmentation of psychiatric effects; and (3) the laboratory studies recruited participants screened to eliminate cases with a history of psychopathology or substance use, whereas actual AAS users do not screen themselves with such care. Finally, AAS effects may be further potentiated by external influences, such as provocative psychosocial influences or simultaneous use of other drugs (such as alcohol) in conjunction with AAS.

Laboratory studies have not documented depressive symptoms associated with AAS use, largely because it would be unethical to deliberately administer AAS for prolonged periods to intentionally suppress the HPT axis or otherwise attempt to induce depression. However, several field studies have described depressive syndromes associated with AAS use, especially during the period of potential HPT suppression after discontinuing a lengthy "cycle" [65, 85, 127, 128]. Among these reports are several cases of suicides [124, 126, 129, 138, 172]. Like manic and hypomanic symptoms, AAS-associated depressive symptoms may be highly variable, with most individuals showing few symptoms during AAS withdrawal and occasional individuals showing severe symptoms [12]. This idiosyncratic pattern has been replicated in the laboratory, where it has been shown that pharmacologically induced hypogonadism precipitates pronounced depression in a small minority of men, but not in the majority, for reasons that remain incompletely understood [173].

In conclusion, an important observation in both laboratory studies and naturalistic studies is that the psychological effects of AAS are idiosyncratic: a majority of users, even at high doses, exhibit little or no psychopathology, whereas an occasional user exhibits severe effects. Interestingly, the same idiosyncratic pattern is observed in nonhuman mammals; most hamsters administered AAS display pronounced aggressiveness, whereas some show little behavioral change [17, 174, 175]. Similarly, the hypogonadism induced during AAS withdrawal may also produce idiosyncratic responses; as just mentioned, some hypogonadal men show marked depressive symptoms, while most show none [173]. Clearly, this variability in response cannot be ascribed purely to psychological or expectational factors, since it has been documented under double-blind conditions in both humans and animals. Although the nonuniform pattern of response has long been recognized [176], its mechanism is still not understood, and available findings in animals [17, 175, 177, 178] and humans [24, 179, 180] are still preliminary.

Aggression and Violence

A growing scientific literature has described unusually violent or criminal behaviors, including many cases of murder or attempted murder, apparently associated with AAS use. Most of these reports have described individual cases or small case series. In most instances, the individual had displayed no history of comparable aggression or violence prior to AAS exposure. For example, Conacher and Workman described a 32-year-old bodybuilder who beat his wife to death while he was taking AAS [181]. Choi and colleagues [139] described longitudinal observations of a 22-year-old bodybuilder who attempted to kill his girlfriend while he was on AAS. Pope and Katz described three men who developed grandiosity, aggressiveness, and violence while taking AAS [152]. One man abducted a woman and shot her in the spine when she tried to escape; the second murdered a hitchhiker; and the third planted an explosive device in the car of his ex-fiancée and detonated it by remote control. None of these three men had any prior criminal record, nor had any of them displayed a major psychiatric disorder or violence prior to AAS use. Several other recent case reports have described comparable cases [137, 182–184]. Thiblin and colleagues [185] described 14 violent offenders who were evaluated for current or past AAS use. These cases included six individuals with apparent AAS-related violence, which the authors said was "characterized by minimal provocation, great intensity and long duration" (p. 305). These authors caution that one cannot be certain that AAS played an etiologic role in each case, but suggest that collectively, the 14 case reports provide additional evidence that AAS may lead to violent behavior and other mental disturbances, including psychotic symptoms. Subsequently, Thiblin and colleagues [186] described five additional young AAS users who became involved in criminal activities, including violent offenses. One of these showed evidence of conduct disorder prior to AAS use, but the others were not known to have acted out during early adolescence before AAS exposure. A recent review [153] mentions six cases of AAS-induced criminal behavior seen by the authors, including three homicides and three violent assaults. The men in these cases apparently experienced psychotic symptoms, with "stereotypic qualities of irritability, aggressiveness, and grandiosity" (p. 287). The authors report that "the mental status of all six perpetrators cleared within weeks to 2 months, and they had specific memory of the act and of their delusional thinking at the time the act was committed" (p. 287).

Clearly, it is difficult to draw causal inferences from AAS use to violence in all of the cases described above. However, as noted earlier, many of the cases involved individuals with no evidence of psychiatric disorder, violence, or criminality when not using AAS—suggesting that AAS was likely a necessary causal factor in the behavior. Many of the cases also share very similar symptomatic features—what Hall and colleagues have referred to as the "stereotypic qualities of irritability, aggressiveness, and grandiosity"—again suggesting that they do not represent chance phenomena, but are indeed attributable to AAS intoxication.

A Swedish forensic research group has recently used epidemiological techniques to assess possible links between AAS use and violent crimes. For example, one study of prisoners (using an analysis that excluded cases referred from substance abuse centers) found that individuals testing positive for AAS were significantly less likely to have been convicted of a crime against property, but significantly more likely to have been convicted of a weapons offense, as compared to AAS-negative prisoners [187]. Another study examined the criminal history of deceased individuals testing positive for AAS, other drugs of abuse, or both categories; the findings suggested that criminal violence observed among AAS users was not confounded in any systematic way by the abuse of other drugs [188]. An earlier study from the same group found that deceased AAS users were significantly more likely to have died from homicide or suicide than a comparison group of deceased amphetamine and/or heroin users [189]. Although these findings do not permit causal inferences in specific cases, they all appear consistent with the findings described earlier in this section.

AAS Dependence

A growing literature has shown that individuals can develop a syndrome of AAS dependence, in which they progress from using AAS in individual "cycles" and go on to use AAS on an almost continuous basis, with little or no time between cycles of use [190]. AAS-dependent individuals may continue usage despite significant adverse medical and psychiatric effects, and they frequently describe withdrawal symptoms when they attempt to stop AAS. These withdrawal symptoms typically include decreased libido, depressed mood, sleep disorder, loss of appetite, and fatigue; AAS-dependent individuals will frequently resume use of the drugs to avoid these symptoms.

In addition, a substantial animal literature has shown that AAS can produce dependence syndromes. For example, rats and mice will selectively spend time in environments where they have received AAS [191, 192], and hamsters will self-administer testosterone, even to the point of death [193]. Interestingly, these hamsters will develop a syndrome of testosterone intoxication that has opioid-like features [193]. This syndrome can be antagonized by naltrexone, and indeed pretreatment with naltrexone will block testosterone self-administration [15]. These and other animal data, recently comprehensively reviewed by Wood [14], provide strong evidence that AAS can produce a biological dependence syndrome, mediated in particular by neuroendocrine and opioidergic mechanisms [14, 16, 20], and likely also modulated by input from various other neurotransmitter systems [13, 21–27].

Over the past 20 years, eight field studies of human AAS users, to our knowledge, have attempted to apply the criteria for substance dependence from various editions of the American Psychiatric Association's *Diagnostic and Statistical Manual of Mental Disorders* [194–196] to these individuals [65, 128, 130, 197–201]. These eight studies have collectively diagnosed AAS dependence in 197 (30.2%) of 653 AAS users, suggesting that AAS dependence is a relatively common outcome of AAS use, likely afflicting millions of individuals worldwide. Although the *DSM* diagnostic criteria are not ideally suited for diagnosing AAS dependence, recent diagnostic criteria modeled on DSM-IV and specifically adapted to AAS have been proposed [201]. A recent pilot study, using a structured diagnostic interview based on these criteria, has shown that these criteria can yield good interrater reliability and evidence of construct and discriminant validity [202]. Nevertheless, the true prevalence of AAS dependence in the overall population of illicit users remains difficult to estimate because of the difficulty of obtaining a representative sample of these individuals. In any event, it seems likely that the prevalence of AAS dependence may be increasing, because widespread illicit AAS use did not appear until approximately the 1980s, as discussed earlier. Thus, many users are only now becoming old enough to have established a dependence pattern.

Concomitant Substance Use Disorders

Several studies suggest that AAS use and dependence are associated with other forms of substance dependence, especially opioids. For example, two reports have described abuse of nalbuphine, an opioid agonist–antagonist, among AAS-using weightlifters [203, 204]. In another study at a substance abuse clinic in New Jersey, the authors found that 21 (9%) of 227 sequential male heroin addicts appeared to have been first introduced to opioids through their use of AAS [205]. Yet another study evaluated 223 consecutive male inpatients at a substance abuse treatment center [62]. Among 88 men with a primary diagnosis of opioid dependence in this study, 22 (25%) reported a past history of AAS use, as compared to only 7 (5%) of 135 men with a primary diagnosis of other forms of substance dependence ($p < 0.001$). Although these data are preliminary, they appear consistent with animal observations summarized earlier, suggesting possible common mechanisms in the effects of AAS and of opioids.

Treatment Implications

Despite the various adverse medical and psychiatric effects enumerated earlier, AAS users rarely seek treatment. Often, they view their drug use positively and are apprehensive about stopping AAS for fear that they will lose muscular size. Thus, they often do not present in the clinic unless they develop a serious mood disorder (e.g., depression with suicidal ideation or a suicide attempt); aggressive behavior leading to a forensic evaluation (e.g., being arrested for violent behavior); or some other form of substance abuse that drives them to treatment (e.g., opioid dependence). Even in situations where AAS users do present in clinical settings, treatment may be difficult, since they often do not trust medical personnel. For example, one recent study found that among a group of 43 AAS users recruited in the field, 40% reported that they would trust their drug dealer as much as they would trust any physician that they had seen, and 56% reported that they had never disclosed their AAS use to any physician [206].

Because of these considerations, the treatment options for AAS dependence are still incompletely understood. One recent review article suggests that AAS dependence may arise via any or all of three separate pathways: (1) an *anabolic* pathway, where individuals with body-image concerns might become dependent on AAS for their muscle-building effects; (2) an *androgenic* pathway, where men might repeatedly use AAS to self-treat hypogonadism from AAS withdrawal; and (3) a *hedonic* pathway, where AAS dependence may arise via mechanisms shared with classical addictive drugs. Each pathway, if supported, would suggest specific clinical treatments.

Looking first at the anabolic pathway, individuals with "muscle dysmorphia," a form of body dysmorphic disorder characterized by an exaggerated preoccupation with muscularity [207], may become dependent on AAS because they are pathologically afraid that they will lose muscular size if they discontinue these drugs [208, 209]. Thus, treatment of the underlying pathology of muscle dysmorphia may be beneficial. Although to our knowledge there are no specific studies of treatment of muscle dysmorphia, a substantial literature has shown that other forms of body dysmorphic disorder respond to cognitive behavioral therapies [210–213] or to serotonergic antidepressants [214–216]. Thus, these modalities may also be effective for underlying muscle dysmorphia in some individuals with AAS dependence.

Looking at the androgenic pathway, a growing literature has suggested that it is important to identify and treat hypogonadism associated with AAS withdrawal, lest the individual be tempted to resume AAS in an attempt to self-treat these symptoms [61, 217]. Treatment of hypogonadism may involve administration of human chorionic gonadotropin to stimulate testicular testosterone production [122, 218, 219] and clomiphene to stimulate pituitary function [220–222]. Sexual dysfunction associated with AAS withdrawal may be ameliorated by phosphodiesterase inhibitors such as sildenafil. Finally, AAS withdrawal may be associated with marked symptoms of depression in susceptible individuals, as discussed earlier. Case reports have described successful treatment of such symptoms with fluoxetine [127] and with electroconvulsive therapy [124], but these data remain limited. It seems likely that depression associated with AAS withdrawal should be treated with the same medications and psychosocial therapies used for ordinary biological depressions, but the clinician should be particularly careful to treat the endocrine component [12].

Finally, looking at the hedonic pathway, it seems likely that AAS dependence shares brain mechanisms with classical substance dependence, as discussed earlier, and thus may respond to both psychosocial and pharmacological interventions known to be effective in classical substance dependence. Many psychosocial treatments have been shown to be effective across a range of different drugs of abuse [223–225], and thus might well be effective for AAS dependence as well, especially in situations where AAS dependence occurs comorbidly with other forms of substance dependence, as is often the case [59, 60]. Also, given evidence for the apparent overlap between the mechanisms of AAS dependence and opioid dependence, described earlier, it seems possible that AAS dependence might be effectively treated in selected cases with naltrexone [12], although to our knowledge this possibility has not been described in the literature to date.

Conclusions

Illicit AAS use and AAS dependence represent a major public health in many Western industrialized societies, but the full public health implications of AAS abuse remain incompletely understood. Our understanding of this form of substance abuse is limited by the fact that AAS use is often highly surreptitious—and indeed, in the authors' experience, perhaps more covert than any other form of illicit substance abuse [206]. As a result, fewer investigators have "penetrated" the AAS subculture to perform field studies of these individuals, and the literature hence remains limited. Understanding of AAS is further compromised by the fact that widespread illicit AAS use in the general population did not arise until the early 1980s, as discussed earlier. As a result, it is only now that large numbers of former (and sometimes still current) AAS users are reaching middle age. Thus, the full magnitude of long-term AAS effects, both psychiatric and medical, may still not be fully appreciated, because only now are sufficient numbers of individuals entering the

age of risk for some of these conditions. As these aging AAS users develop adverse effects from long-term AAS exposure, such as cardiomyopathy, atherosclerotic disease, persistent hypogonadism, major mood disorders, and other forms of substance dependence, it seems likely that increasing numbers will present for treatment, which must be performed with recognition for the multiple pathways by which AAS dependence may arise, as discussed earlier.

Acknowledgment This study was supported in part by United States National Institutes on Drug Abuse Grant DA016744 and DA029141.

References

1. Kanayama G, Hudson JI, Pope HG. Illicit anabolic-androgenic steroid use. Horm Behav. 2010;58(1):111–21.
2. Pope HG, Brower KJ. Anabolic-androgenic steroid-related disorders. In: Sadock B, Sadock V, editors. Comprehensive textbook of psychiatry. 9th ed. Philadelphia, PA: Lippincott Williams & Wilkins; 2009. p. 1419–31.
3. David K, Dingemanse E, Freud J, Laquer E. Uber Krystallinisches mannliches Hormon Hoden (Testosteron), wirksamer als aus Harn oder aus Cholesterin Bereitetes Androsteron. Zeit Physiol Chem. 1935;233:281–2.
4. Wettstein A. Uber die kunstliche Herstellung des Testikelhormons Testosteron. Schweiz Med Wochenschr. 1935;16:912.
5. Kopera H. The history of anabolic steroids and a review of clinical experience with anabolic steroids. Acta Endocrinol. 1985; 271:11–8.
6. Kouri EM, Pope Jr HG, Katz DL, Oliva P. Fat-free mass index in users and nonusers of anabolic-androgenic steroids. Clin J Sports Med. 1995;5(4):223–8.
7. Sheffield-Moore M, Urban RJ. An overview of the endocrinology of skeletal muscle. Trends Endocrinol Metab. 2004;15(3): 110–5.
8. Kanayama G, Boynes M, Hudson JI, Field AE, Pope HG, Jr. Anabolic steroid abuse among teenage girls: an illusory problem? Drug Alcohol Depend. 2007;88(2–3):156–62.
9. Shahidi NT. A review of the chemistry, biological action, and clinical applications of anabolic-androgenic steroids. Clin Ther. 2001;23(9):1355–90.
10. Basaria S, Wahlstrom JT, Dobs AS. Clinical review 138: Anabolic-androgenic steroid therapy in the treatment of chronic diseases. J Clin Endocrinol Metab. 2001;86(11):5108–17.
11. Wu FC. Endocrine aspects of anabolic steroids. Clin Chem. 1997;43(7):1289–92.
12. Kanayama G, Brower KJ, Wood RI, Hudson JI, Pope HG. Treatment of anabolic-androgenic steroid dependence: emerging evidence and its implications. Drug Alcohol Depend. 2010; 109(1–3):6–13.
13. Frye CA. Some rewarding effects of androgens may be mediated by actions of its 5alpha-reduced metabolite 3alpha-androstanediol. Pharmacol Biochem Behav. 2007;86(2):354–67.
14. Wood RI. Anabolic-androgenic steroid dependence? Insights from animals and humans. Front Neuroendocrinol. 2008;29(4): 490–506.
15. Peters KD, Wood RI. Androgen dependence in hamsters: overdose, tolerance, and potential opioidergic mechanisms. Neuroscience. 2005;130(4):971–81.
16. Kashkin KB, Kleber HD. Hooked on hormones? An anabolic steroid addiction hypothesis. JAMA. 1989;262(22):3166–70.

17. Clark AS, Henderson LP. Behavioral and physiological responses to anabolic-androgenic steroids. Neurosci Biobehav Rev. 2003;27(5):413–36.

18. Celerier E, Yazdi MT, Castane A, Ghozland S, Nyberg F, Maldonado R. Effects of nandrolone on acute morphine responses, tolerance and dependence in mice. Eur J Pharmacol. 2003;465(1–2):69–81.

19. Johansson P, Ray A, Zhou Q, Huang W, Karlsson K, Nyberg F. Anabolic androgenic steroids increase beta-endorphin levels in the ventral tegmental area in the male rat brain. Neurosci Res. 1997;27(2):185–9.

20. Hochberg Z, Pacak K, Chrousos GP. Endocrine withdrawal syndromes. Endocr Rev. 2003;24(4):523–38.

21. Kindlundh AM, Lindblom J, Bergstrom L, Nyberg F. The anabolic-androgenic steroid nandrolone induces alterations in the density of serotonergic 5HT1B and 5HT2 receptors in the male rat brain. Neuroscience. 2003;119(1):113–20.

22. Kindlundh AM, Rahman S, Lindblom J, Nyberg F. Increased dopamine transporter density in the male rat brain following chronic nandrolone decanoate administration. Neurosci Lett. 2004;356(2):131–4.

23. Schroeder JP, Packard MG. Role of dopamine receptor subtypes in the acquisition of a testosterone conditioned place preference in rats. Neurosci Lett. 2000;282(1–2):17–20.

24. Daly RC, Su TP, Schmidt PJ, Pickar D, Murphy DL, Rubinow DR. Cerebrospinal fluid and behavioral changes after methyltestosterone administration: preliminary findings. Arch Gen Psychiatry. 2001;58(2):172–7.

25. Lindqvist AS, Johansson-Steensland P, Nyberg F, Fahlke C. Anabolic androgenic steroid affects competitive behaviour, behavioural response to ethanol and brain serotonin levels. Behav Brain Res. 2002;133(1):21–9.

26. Ricci LA, Rasakham K, Grimes JM, Melloni Jr RH. Serotonin-1A receptor activity and expression modulate adolescent anabolic/androgenic steroid-induced aggression in hamsters. Pharmacol Biochem Behav. 2006;85(1):1–11.

27. Tamaki T, Shiraishi T, Takeda H, Matsumiya T, Roy RR, Edgerton VR. Nandrolone decanoate enhances hypothalamic biogenic amines in rats. Med Sci Sports Exerc. 2003;35(1):32–8.

28. Sih R, Morley JE, Kaiser FE, Perry 3rd HM, Patrick P, Ross C. Testosterone replacement in older hypogonadal men: a 12-month randomized controlled trial. J Clin Endocrinol Metab. 1997;82(6):1661–7.

29. Wang C, Alexander G, Berman N, Salehian B, Davidson T, McDonald V, et al. Testosterone replacement therapy improves mood in hypogonadal men–a clinical research center study. J Clin Endocrinol Metab. 1996;81(10):3578–83.

30. Kanayama G, Amiaz R, Seidman S, Pope Jr HG. Testosterone supplementation for depressed men: current research and suggested treatment guidelines. Exp Clin Psychopharmacol. 2007;15(6):529–38.

31. Dobs AS, Meikle AW, Arver S, Sanders SW, Caramelli KE, Mazer NA. Pharmacokinetics, efficacy, and safety of a permeation-enhanced testosterone transdermal system in comparison with bi-weekly injections of testosterone enanthate for the treatment of hypogonadal men. J Clin Endocrinol Metab. 1999;84(10):3469–78.

32. Steidle C, Schwartz S, Jacoby K, Sebree T, Smith T, Bachand R. AA2500 testosterone gel normalizes androgen levels in aging males with improvements in body composition and sexual function. J Clin Endocrinol Metab. 2003;88(6):2673–81.

33. Wang C, Swerdloff RS, Iranmanesh A, Dobs A, Snyder PJ, Cunningham G, et al. Transdermal testosterone gel improves sexual function, mood, muscle strength, and body composition parameters in hypogonadal men. J Clin Endocrinol Metab. 2000;85(8):2839–53.

34. Newshan G, Leon W. The use of anabolic agents in HIV disease. Int J STD AIDS. 2001;12(3):141–4.

35. Johns K, Beddall MJ, Corrin RC. Anabolic steroids for the treatment of weight loss in HIV-infected individuals. Cochrane Database Syst Rev (Online). 2005;(4):CD005483.

36. Grinspoon S, Corcoran C, Stanley T, Baaj A, Basgoz N, Klibanski A. Effects of hypogonadism and testosterone administration on depression indices in HIV-infected men. J Clin Endocrinol Metab. 2000;85(1):60–5.

37. Rabkin JG, Wagner GJ, Rabkin R. A double-blind, placebo-controlled trial of testosterone therapy for HIV-positive men with hypogonadal symptoms. Arch Gen Psychiatry. 2000;57(2):141–7; discussion 55–6.

38. Rabkin JG, Wagner GJ, McElhiney MC, Rabkin R, Lin SH. Testosterone versus fluoxetine for depression and fatigue in HIV/AIDS: a placebo-controlled trial. J Clin Psychopharmacol. 2004;24(4):379–85.

39. Seidman SN, Spatz E, Rizzo C, Roose SP. Testosterone replacement therapy for hypogonadal men with major depressive disorder: a randomized, placebo-controlled clinical trial. J Clin Psychiatry. 2001;62(6):406–12.

40. Perry PJ, Yates WR, Williams RD, Andersen AE, MacIndoe JH, Lund BC, et al. Testosterone therapy in late-life major depression in males. J Clin Psychiatry. 2002;63(12):1096–101.

41. Seidman SN, Rabkin JG. Testosterone replacement therapy for hypogonadal men with SSRI-refractory depression. J Affect Disord. 1998;48(2–3):157–61.

42. Seidman SN, Miyazaki M, Roose SP. Intramuscular testosterone supplementation to selective serotonin reuptake inhibitor in treatment-resistant depressed men: randomized placebo-controlled clinical trial. J Clin Psychopharmacol. 2005;25(6):584–8.

43. Pope Jr HG, Cohane GH, Kanayama G, Siegel AJ, Hudson JI. Testosterone gel supplementation for men with refractory depression: a randomized, placebo-controlled trial. Am J Psychiatry. 2003;160(1):105–11.

44. Orengo CA, Fullerton L, Kunik ME. Safety and efficacy of testosterone gel 1% augmentation in depressed men with partial response to antidepressant therapy. J Geriatr Psychiatry Neurol. 2005;18(1):20–4.

45. Pope H, Amiaz R, Brennan B, Orr G, Weiser M, Kelly JF, et al. A parallel-group placebo-controlled trial of testosterone gel in men with major depressive disorder displaying an incomplete response to standard antidepressant treatment. J Clin Psychopharmacol. 2010;30(2):126–34.

46. Kanayama G, Hudson JI, Pope Jr HG. Long-term psychiatric and medical consequences of anabolic-androgenic steroid abuse: a looming public health concern? Drug Alcohol Depend. 2008;98(1–2):1–12.

47. Pope H, Phillips K, Olivardia R. The Adonis complex: the secret crisis of male body obsession. New York: Simon & Schuster; 2000.

48. Pope Jr HG, Olivardia R, Borowiecki 3rd JJ, Cohane GH. The growing commercial value of the male body: a longitudinal survey of advertising in women's magazines. Psychother Psychosom. 2001;70(4):189–92.

49. Pope Jr HG, Olivardia R, Gruber A, Borowiecki J. Evolving ideals of male body image as seen through action toys. Int J Eat Disord. 1999;26(1):65–72.

50. Phillips W. Anabolic reference guide. Golden, CO: Mile High; 1985.

51. Phillips W. Anabolic reference update. Golden, CO: Mile High; 1991.

52. Duchaine D. The original underground steroid handbook. Santa Monica, CA: OEM; 1981.

53. Duchaine D. Underground steroid handbook II. Los Angeles, CA: HLR Technical Books; 1988.

54. One Hundred First United States Congress. The Steroid Trafficking Act of 1990. Washington: U.S. Government Printing Office; 1990.

55. Kanayama G, Pope Jr HG, Hudson JI. "Body image" drugs: a growing psychosomatic problem. Psychother Psychosom. 2001;70(2):61–5.

56. Parkinson AB, Evans NA. Anabolic androgenic steroids: a survey of 500 users. Med Sci Sports Exerc. 2006;38(4):644–51.

57. Evans NA. Current concepts in anabolic-androgenic steroids. Am J Sports Med. 2004;32(2):534–42.

58. Brennan BP, Kanayama G, Hudson JI, Pope HG. Illicit human growth hormone abuse in male weightlifters. Addict Behav. 2011; 20(1):9–13.

59. Skarberg K, Nyberg F, Engstrom I. Multisubstance use as a feature of addiction to anabolic-androgenic steroids. Eur Addict Res. 2009;15(2):99–106.

60. Kanayama G, Hudson JI, Pope Jr HG. Features of men with anabolic-androgenic steroid dependence: a comparison with nondependent AAS users and with AAS nonusers. Drug Alcohol Depend. 2009;102(1–3):130–7.

61. Brower KJ. Anabolic steroid abuse and dependence in clinical practice. Phys Sportsmed. 2009;37:1–11.

62. Kanayama G, Cohane GH, Weiss RD, Pope HG. Past anabolic-androgenic steroid use among men admitted for substance abuse treatment: an underrecognized problem? J Clin Psychiatry. 2003;64(2):156–60.

63. Kanayama G, Pope HG, Cohane G, Hudson JI. Risk factors for anabolic-androgenic steroid use among weightlifters: a case-control study. Drug Alcohol Depend. 2003;71(1):77–86.

64. Pope Jr HG, Katz DL. Affective and psychotic symptoms associated with anabolic steroid use. Am J Psychiatry. 1988;145(4): 487–90.

65. Pope Jr HG, Katz DL. Psychiatric and medical effects of anabolic-androgenic steroid use. A controlled study of 160 athletes. Arch Gen Psychiatry. 1994;51(5):375–82.

66. Reyes-Fuentes A, Veldhuis JD. Neuroendocrine physiology of the normal male gonadal axis. Endocrinol Metab Clin North Am. 1993;22(1):93–124.

67. Swerdloff RS, Wang C, Hikim APS. Hypothalamic-pituitary-gonadal axis in men. In: Pfaff D, Arnold A, Etgen A, Fahrbach S, Rubin R, editors. Hormones, brain and behavior. San Diego: Elsevier; 2002. p. 1–36.

68. Fudala PJ, Weinrieb RM, Calarco JS, Kampman KM, Boardman C. An evaluation of anabolic-androgenic steroid abusers over a period of 1 year: seven case studies. Annu Clin Psychiatry. 2003;15(2):121–30.

69. Parrott AC, Choi PY, Davies M. Anabolic steroid use by amateur athletes: effects upon psychological mood states. J Sports Med Phys Fitness. 1994;34(3):292–8.

70. Pope HG, Katz DL. Psychiatric effects of exogenous anabolic-androgenic steroids. In: Wolkowitz OM, Rothschild AJ, editors. Psychoneuroendocrinology: the scientific basis of clinical practice. Washington, DC: American Psychiatric Press; 2003. p. 331–58.

71. Kanayama G, Gruber AJ, Pope Jr HG, Borowiecki JJ, Hudson JI. Over-the-counter drug use in gymnasiums: an underrecognized substance abuse problem? Psychother Psychosom. 2001;70(3): 137–40.

72. Buckley WE, Yesalis 3rd CE, Friedl KE, Anderson WA, Streit AL, Wright JE. Estimated prevalence of anabolic steroid use among male high school seniors. JAMA. 1988;260(23):3441–5.

73. McCabe SE, Brower KJ, West BT, Nelson TF, Wechsler H. Trends in non-medical use of anabolic steroids by U.S. college students: results from four national surveys. Drug Alcohol Depend. 2007; 90(2–3):243–51.

74. Handelsman DJ, Gupta L. Prevalence and risk factors for anabolic-androgenic steroid abuse in Australian high school students. Int J Androl. 1997;20(3):159–64.

75. Melia P, Pipe A, Greenberg L. The use of anabolic-androgenic steroids by Canadian students. Clin J Sports Med. 1996;6(1):9–14.

76. Nilsson S, Baigi A, Marklund B, Fridlund B. The prevalence of the use of androgenic anabolic steroids by adolescents in a county of Sweden. Eur J Public Health. 2001;11(2):195–7.

77. Thiblin I, Petersson A. Pharmacoepidemiology of anabolic androgenic steroids: a review. Fundam Clin Pharmacol. 2005;19(1): 27–44.

78. Pallesen S, Josendal O, Johnsen BH, Larsen S, Molde H. Anabolic steroid use in high school students. Subst Use Misuse. 2006;41(13):1705–17.

79. Galduróz JC, Noto AR, Nappo SA, Carlini EA. Household survey on drug abuse in Brazil: study involving the 107 major cities of the country–2001. Addict Behav. 2005;30(3):545–56.

80. Rachon D, Pokrywka L, Suchecka-Rachon K. Prevalence and risk factors of anabolic-androgenic steroids (AAS) abuse among adolescents and young adults in Poland. Sozial- und Praventivmedizin. 2006;51(6):392–8.

81. Wanjek B, Rosendahl J, Strauss B, Gabriel HH. Doping, drugs and drug abuse among adolescents in the State of Thuringia (Germany): prevalence, knowledge and attitudes. Int J Sports Med. 2007; 28(4):346–53.

82. Yang CF, Gray P, Pope Jr HG. Male body image in Taiwan versus the West: Yanggang Zhiqi meets the Adonis complex. Am J Psychiatry. 2005;162(2):263–9.

83. Gruber AJ, Pope Jr HG. Compulsive weight lifting and anabolic drug abuse among women rape victims. Compr Psychiatry. 1999; 40(4):273–7.

84. Gruber AJ, Pope Jr HG. Psychiatric and medical effects of anabolic-androgenic steroid use in women. Psychother Psychosom. 2000;69(1):19–26.

85. Brower KJ. Anabolic steroid abuse and dependence. Curr Psychiatry Rep. 2002;4(5):377–87.

86. Karasawa T, Shikata T, Smith RD. Peliosis hepatis. Report of nine cases. Acta Pathol Jpn. 1979;29(3):457–69.

87. Schumacher J, Muller G, Klotz KF. Large hepatic hematoma and intraabdominal hemorrhage associated with abuse of anabolic steroids. New Engl J Med. 1999;340(14):1123–4.

88. Bagia S, Hewitt PM, Morris DL. Anabolic steroid-induced hepatic adenomas with spontaneous haemorrhage in a bodybuilder. Aust NZ J Surg. 2000;70(9):686–7.

89. Socas L, Zumbado M, Perez-Luzardo O, Ramos A, Perez C, Hernandez JR, et al. Hepatocellular adenomas associated with anabolic androgenic steroid abuse in bodybuilders: a report of two cases and a review of the literature. Br J Sports Med. 2005; 39(5):e27.

90. Patil JJ, O'Donohoe B, Loyden CF, Shanahan D. Near-fatal spontaneous hepatic rupture associated with anabolic androgenic steroid use: a case report. Br J Sports Med. 2007;41(7):462–3.

91. Dickerman RD, Pertusi RM, Zachariah NY, Dufour DR, McConathy WJ. Anabolic steroid-induced hepatotoxicity: is it overstated? Clin J Sports Med. 1999;9(1):34–9.

92. Herlitz LC, Markowitz GS, Farris AB, Schwimmer JA, Stokes MB, Kunis C, et al. Development of focal segmental glomerulosclerosis after anabolic steroid abuse. J Am Soc Nephrol. 2010;21(1):163–72.

93. Nottin S, Nguyen LD, Terbah M, Obert P. Cardiovascular effects of androgenic anabolic steroids in male bodybuilders determined by tissue Doppler imaging. Am J Cardiol. 2006;97(6):912–5.

94. Sullivan ML, Martinez CM, Gennis P, Gallagher EJ. The cardiac toxicity of anabolic steroids. Prog Cardiovasc Dis. 1998;41(1): 1–15.

95. Di Bello V, Giorgi D, Bianchi M, Bertini A, Caputo MT, Valenti G, et al. Effects of anabolic-androgenic steroids on weight-lifters' myocardium: an ultrasonic videodensitometric study. Med Sci Sports Exerc. 1999;31(4):514–21.

96. D'Andrea A, Caso P, Salerno G, Scarafile R, De Corato G, Mita C, et al. Left ventricular early myocardial dysfunction after chronic misuse of anabolic androgenic steroids: a Doppler myocardial and strain imaging analysis (Commentary). Br J Sports Med. 2007; 41(3):149–55.

97. Kasikcioglu E, Oflaz H, Umman B, Bugra Z. Androgenic anabolic steroids also impair right ventricular function. Int J Cardiol. 2009;134(1):123–5.

98. Ferenchick GS. Association of steroid abuse with cardiomyopathy in athletes. Am J Med. 1991;91(5):562.

99. Stolt A, Karila T, Viitasalo M, Mantysaari M, Kujala UM, Karjalainen J. QT interval and QT dispersion in endurance athletes and in power athletes using large doses of anabolic steroids. Am J Cardiol. 1999;84(3):364–6. A9.

100. Sullivan ML, Martinez CM, Gallagher EJ. Atrial fibrillation and anabolic steroids. J Emerg Med. 1999;17(5):851–7.

101. Vogt AM, Geyer H, Jahn L, Schanzer W, Kubler W. Cardiomyopathy associated with uncontrolled self medication of anabolic steroids. Zeitschrift fur Kardiologie. 2002;91(4):357–62.

102. Baggish AL, Weiner RB, Kanayama G, Hudson JI, Picard MH, Hutter AM, et al. Long-term anabolic-androgenic steroid use is associated with left ventricular dysfunction. Circ Heart Fail. 2010;3:472–6.

103. Kuipers H, Wijnen JA, Hartgens F, Willems SM. Influence of anabolic steroids on body composition, blood pressure, lipid profile and liver functions in body builders. Int J Sports Med. 1991;12(4):413–8.

104. Kouri EM, Pope Jr HG, Oliva PS. Changes in lipoprotein-lipid levels in normal men following administration of increasing doses of testosterone cypionate. Clin J Sports Med. 1996;6(3):152–7.

105. Lajarin F, Zaragoza R, Tovar I, Martinez-Hernandez P. Evolution of serum lipids in two male bodybuilders using anabolic steroids. Clin Chem. 1996;42(6 Pt 1):970–2.

106. Ferenchick GS. Anabolic/androgenic steroid abuse and thrombosis: is there a connection? Med Hypoth. 1991;35(1):27–31.

107. Ferenchick G, Schwartz D, Ball M, Schwartz K. Androgenic-anabolic steroid abuse and platelet aggregation: a pilot study in weight lifters. Am J Med Sci. 1992;303(2):78–82.

108. McCarthy K, Tang AT, Dalrymple-Hay MJ, Haw MP. Ventricular thrombosis and systemic embolism in bodybuilders: etiology and management. Annu Thoracic Surg. 2000;70(2):658–60.

109. McNutt RA, Ferenchick GS, Kirlin PC, Hamlin NJ. Acute myocardial infarction in a 22-year-old world class weight lifter using anabolic steroids. Am J Cardiol. 1988;62(1):164.

110. Ferenchick GS, Adelman S. Myocardial infarction associated with anabolic steroid use in a previously healthy 37-year-old weight lifter. Am Heart J. 1992;124(2):507–8.

111. Kennedy C. Myocardial infarction in association with misuse of anabolic steroids. Ulster Med J. 1993;62(2):174–6.

112. Kennedy MC, Corrigan AB, Pilbeam ST. Myocardial infarction and cerebral haemorrhage in a young body builder taking anabolic steroids. Aust NZ J Med. 1993;23(6):713.

113. Kennedy MC, Lawrence C. Anabolic steroid abuse and cardiac death. Med J Aust. 1993;158(5):346–8.

114. Dickerman RD, Schaller F, Prather I, McConathy WJ. Sudden cardiac death in a 20-year-old bodybuilder using anabolic steroids. Cardiology. 1995;86(2):172–3.

115. Fisher M, Appleby M, Rittoo D, Cotter L. Myocardial infarction with extensive intracoronary thrombus induced by anabolic steroids. Br J Clin Pract. 1996;50(4):222–3.

116. Hausmann R, Hammer S, Betz P. Performance enhancing drugs (doping agents) and sudden death–a case report and review of the literature. Int J Legal Med. 1998;111(5):261–4.

117. Godon P, Bonnefoy E, Guerard S, Munet M, Velon S, Brion R, et al. Myocardial infarction and anabolic steroid use. A case report. Arch Mal Coeur Vaiss. 2000;93(7):879–83.

118. Tischer KH, Heyny-von Haussen R, Mall G, Doenecke P. [Coronary thrombosis and ectasia of coronary arteries after long-term use of anabolic steroids]. Zeitschrift fur Kardiologie. 2003;92(4):326–31.

119. Halvorsen S, Thorsby PM, Haug E. Acute myocardial infarction in a young man who had been using androgenic anabolic steroids. Tidsskr Nor Laegeforen. 2004;124(2):170–2.

120. Thiblin I, Lindquist O, Rajs J. Cause and manner of death among users of anabolic androgenic steroids. J Forensic Sci. 2000;45(1): 16–23.

121. Boyadjiev NP, Georgieva KN, Massaldjieva RI, Gueorguiev SI. Reversible hypogonadism and azoospermia as a result of anabolic-androgenic steroid use in a bodybuilder with personality disorder. A case report. J Sports Med Phys Fitness. 2000;40(3):271–4.

122. Menon DK. Successful treatment of anabolic steroid-induced azoospermia with human chorionic gonadotropin and human menopausal gonadotropin. Fertil Steril. 2003;79 Suppl 3: 1659–61.

123. van Breda E, Keizer HA, Kuipers H, Wolffenbuttel BH. Androgenic anabolic steroid use and severe hypothalamic-pituitary dysfunction: a case study. Int J Sports Med. 2003;24(3):195–6.

124. Allnutt S, Chaimowitz G. Anabolic steroid withdrawal depression: a case report. Can J Psychiatry. 1994;39(5):317–8.

125. Brower KJ. Withdrawal from anabolic steroids. Curr Ther Endocrinol Metab. 1997;6:338–43.

126. Brower KJ, Blow FC, Beresford TP, Fuelling C. Anabolic-androgenic steroid dependence. J Clin Psychiatry. 1989;50(1): 31–3.

127. Malone Jr DA, Dimeff RJ. The use of fluoxetine in depression associated with anabolic steroid withdrawal: a case series. J Clin Psychiatry. 1992;53(4):130–2.

128. Malone Jr DA, Dimeff RJ, Lombardo JA, Sample RH. Psychiatric effects and psychoactive substance use in anabolic-androgenic steroid users. Clin J Sport Med. 1995;5(1):25–31.

129. Thiblin I, Runeson B, Rajs J. Anabolic androgenic steroids and suicide. Annu Clin Psychiatry. 1999;11(4):223–31.

130. Brower KJ, Blow FC, Young JP, Hill EM. Symptoms and correlates of anabolic-androgenic steroid dependence. Br J Addict. 1991;86(6):759–68.

131. Brower KJ, Catlin DH, Blow FC, Eliopulos GA, Beresford TP. Clinical assessment and urine testing for anabolic-androgenic steroid abuse and dependence. Am J Drug Alcohol Abuse. 1991; 17(2):161–71.

132. Cole JC, Smith R, Halford JC, Wagstaff GF. A preliminary investigation into the relationship between anabolic-androgenic steroid use and the symptoms of reverse anorexia in both current and ex-users. Psychopharmacology. 2003;166(4):424–9.

133. Freinhar JP, Alvarez W. Androgen-induced hypomania. J Clin Psychiatry. 1985;46(8):354–5.

134. Annitto WJ, Layman WA. Anabolic steroids and acute schizophrenic episode. J Clin Psychiatry. 1980;41(4):143–4.

135. Pope Jr HG, Katz DL. Bodybuilder's psychosis. Lancet. 1987;1(8537):863.

136. Cooper CJ, Noakes TD. Psychiatric disturbances in users of anabolic steroids. S Afr Med J. 1994;84:509–12.

137. Stanley A, Ward M. Anabolic steroids–the drugs that give and take away manhood. A case with an unusual physical sign. Med Sci Law. 1994;34(1):82–3.

138. Papazisis G, Kouvelas D, Mastrogianni A, Karastergiou A. Anabolic androgenic steroid abuse and mood disorder: a case report. Int J Neuropsychopharmacol. 2007;10(2):291–3.

139. Choi PY, Parrott AC, Cowan D. High-dose anabolic steroids in strength athletes: effects upon hostility and aggression. Hum Psychopharmacol. 1990;5:349–56.

140. Pagonis TA, Angelopoulos NV, Koukoulis GN, Hadjichristodoulou CS. Psychiatric side effects induced by supraphysiological doses

of combinations of anabolic steroids correlate to the severity of abuse. Eur Psychiatry. 2006;21(8):551–62.

141. Wilson-Fearon C, Parrott AC. Multiple drug use and dietary restraint in a Mr. Universe competitor: psychobiological effects. Percept Motor Skills. 1999;88(2):579–80.

142. Cooper CJ, Noakes TD, Dunne T, Lambert MI, Rochford K. A high prevalence of abnormal personality traits in chronic users of anabolic-androgenic steroids. Br J Sports Med. 1996;30(3): 246–50.

143. Bahrke MS, Wright JE, Strauss RH, Catlin DH. Psychological moods and subjectively perceived behavioral and somatic changes accompanying anabolic-androgenic steroid use. Am J Sports Med. 1992;20(6):717–24.

144. Choi PY, Pope Jr HG. Violence toward women and illicit androgenic-anabolic steroid use. Ann Clin Psychiatry. 1994;6(1):21–5.

145. Lefavi R, Reeve T, Newland M. Relationship between anabolic steroid use and selected psychological parameters in male bodybuilders. J Sports Behav. 1990;13:157–66.

146. Midgley SJ, Heather N, Davies JB. Levels of aggression among a group of anabolic-androgenic steroid users. Med Sci Law. 2001;41(4):309–14.

147. Moss H, Panzak G, Tarter R. Personality, mood, and psychiatric symptoms among anabolic steroid users. Am J Addict. 1992; 1:315–24.

148. Perry PJ, Andersen KH, Yates WR. Illicit anabolic steroid use in athletes. A case series analysis. Am J Sports Med. 1990; 18(4):422–8.

149. Perry PJ, Kutscher EC, Lund BC, Yates WR, Holman TL, Demers L. Measures of aggression and mood changes in male weightlifters with and without androgenic anabolic steroid use. J Forensic Sci. 2003;48(3):646–51.

150. Yates WR, Perry P, Murray S. Aggression and hostility in anabolic steroid users. Biol Psychiatry. 1992;31(12):1232–4.

151. Pagonis TA, Angelopoulos NV, Koukoulis GN, Hadjichristodoulou CS, Toli PN. Psychiatric and hostility factors related to use of anabolic steroids in monozygotic twins. Eur Psychiatry. 2006; 21(8):563–9.

152. Pope Jr HG, Katz DL. Homicide and near-homicide by anabolic steroid users. J Clin Psychiatry. 1990;51(1):28–31.

153. Hall RC, Hall RC, Chapman MJ. Psychiatric complications of anabolic steroid abuse. Psychosomatics. 2005;46(4):285–90.

154. Talih F, Fattal O, Malone D Jr. Anabolic steroid abuse: psychiatric and physical costs. Cleve Clin J Med 2007;74(5):341–4, 346, 349–52.

155. Trenton AJ, Currier GW. Behavioural manifestations of anabolic steroid use. CNS Drugs. 2005;19(7):571–95.

156. Hartgens F, Kuipers H. Effects of androgenic-anabolic steroids in athletes. Sports Med. 2004;34(8):513–54.

157. Bahrke MS, Yesalis 3rd CE. Weight training. A potential confounding factor in examining the psychological and behavioural effects of anabolic-androgenic steroids. Sports Med. 1994; 18(5):309–18.

158. Bahrke MS, Yesalis 3rd CE, Wright JE. Psychological and behavioural effects of endogenous testosterone and anabolic-androgenic steroids. An update. Sports Med. 1996;22(6):367–90.

159. Björkqvist K, Nygren T, Björklund A-C, Björkqvist S-E. Testosterone intake and aggressiveness: real effect or anticipation? Aggress Behav. 1994;20(1):17–26.

160. Riem K, Hursey K. Using anabolic-androgenic steroids to enhance physique and performance: effects on moods and behavior. Clin Psychol Rev. 1995;15:235–56.

161. Friedl KE, Dettori JR, Hannan Jr CJ, Patience TH, Plymate SR. Comparison of the effects of high dose testosterone and 19-nortestosterone to a replacement dose of testosterone on strength and body composition in normal men. J Steroid Biochem Mol Biol. 1991;40(4–6):607–12.

162. Friedl KE, Jones RE, Hannan Jr CJ, Plymate SR. The administration of pharmacological doses of testosterone or 19-nortestosterone to normal men is not associated with increased insulin secretion or impaired glucose tolerance. J Clin Endocrinol Metab. 1989; 68(5):971–5.

163. Hannan Jr CJ, Friedl KE, Zold A, Kettler TM, Plymate SR. Psychological and serum homovanillic acid changes in men administered androgenic steroids. Psychoneuroendocrinology. 1991;16(4):335–43.

164. Matsumoto AM. Effects of chronic testosterone administration in normal men: safety and efficacy of high dosage testosterone and parallel dose-dependent suppression of luteinizing hormone, follicle-stimulating hormone, and sperm production. J Clin Endocrinol Metab. 1990;70(1):282–7.

165. Forbes GB, Porta CR, Herr BE, Griggs RC. Sequence of changes in body composition induced by testosterone and reversal of changes after drug is stopped. JAMA. 1992;267(3):397–9.

166. Bagatell CJ, Heiman JR, Matsumoto AM, Rivier JE, Bremner WJ. Metabolic and behavioral effects of high-dose, exogenous testosterone in healthy men. J Clin Endocrinol Metab. 1994;79(2): 561–7.

167. Bhasin S, Storer TW, Berman N, Callegari C, Clevenger B, Phillips J, et al. The effects of supraphysiologic doses of testosterone on muscle size and strength in normal men. New Engl J Med. 1996;335(1):1–7.

168. Pope HG Jr, Kouri EM, Hudson JI. Effects of supraphysiologic doses of testosterone on mood and aggression in normal men: a randomized controlled trial. Arch Gen Psychiatry 2000;57(2):133–40; discussion 55–6.

169. Su TP, Pagliaro M, Schmidt PJ, Pickar D, Wolkowitz O, Rubinow DR. Neuropsychiatric effects of anabolic steroids in male normal volunteers. JAMA. 1993;269(21):2760–4.

170. Tricker R, Casaburi R, Storer TW, Clevenger B, Berman N, Shirazi A, et al. The effects of supraphysiological doses of testosterone on angry behavior in healthy eugonadal men–a clinical research center study. J Clin Endocrinol Metab. 1996;81(10): 3754–8.

171. Yates WR, Perry PJ, MacIndoe J, Holman T, Ellingrod V. Psychosexual effects of three doses of testosterone cycling in normal men. Biol Psychiatry. 1999;45(3):254–60.

172. Agren G, Thiblin I, Tirassa P, Lundeberg T, Stenfors C. Behavioural anxiolytic effects of low-dose anabolic androgenic steroid treatment in rats. Physiol Behav. 1999;66(3):503–9.

173. Schmidt PJ, Berlin KL, Danaceau MA, Neeren A, Haq NA, Roca CA, et al. The effects of pharmacologically induced hypogonadism on mood in healthy men. Arch Gen Psychiatry. 2004;61(10): 997–1004.

174. Melloni Jr RH, Connor DF, Hang PT, Harrison RJ, Ferris CF. Anabolic-androgenic steroid exposure during adolescence and aggressive behavior in golden hamsters. Physiol Behav. 1997; 61(3):359–64.

175. DeLeon KR, Grimes JM, Melloni Jr RH. Repeated anabolic-androgenic steroid treatment during adolescence increases vasopressin V(1A) receptor binding in Syrian hamsters: correlation with offensive aggression. Horm Behav. 2002;42(2):182–91.

176. Rubinow DR, Schmidt PJ. Androgens, brain, and behavior. Am J Psychiatry. 1996;153(8):974–84.

177. Fischer SG, Ricci LA, Melloni Jr RH. Repeated anabolic/androgenic steroid exposure during adolescence alters phosphate-activated glutaminase and glutamate receptor 1 (GluR1) subunit immunoreactivity in Hamster brain: correlation with offensive aggression. Behav Brain Res. 2007;180(1):77–85.

178. Grimes JM, Melloni Jr RH. Prolonged alterations in the serotonin neural system following the cessation of adolescent anabolic-androgenic steroid exposure in hamsters (Mesocricetus auratus). Behav Neurosci. 2006;120(6):1242–51.

179. Daly RC. Anabolic steroids, brain and behaviour. Irish Med J. 2001;94(4):102.
180. Daly RC, Su TP, Schmidt PJ, Pagliaro M, Pickar D, Rubinow DR. Neuroendocrine and behavioral effects of high-dose anabolic steroid administration in male normal volunteers. Psychoneuroendocrinology. 2003;28(3):317–31.
181. Conacher GN, Workman DG. Violent crime possibly associated with anabolic steroid use. Am J Psychiatry. 1989;146(5):679.
182. Dalby JT. Brief anabolic steroid use and sustained behavioral reaction. Am J Psychiatry. 1992;149(2):271–2.
183. Schulte HM, Hall MJ, Boyer M. Domestic violence associated with anabolic steroid abuse. Am J Psychiatry. 1993;150(2):348.
184. Pope Jr HG, Kouri EM, Powell KF, Campbell C, Katz DL. Anabolic-androgenic steroid use among 133 prisoners. Compr Psychiatry. 1996;37(5):322–7.
185. Thiblin I, Kristiansson M, Rajs J. Anabolic androgenic steroids and behavioural patterns among violent offenders. J Forensic Psychiatry Psychol. 1997;8:299–310.
186. Thiblin I, Parlklo T. Anabolic androgenic steroids and violence. Acta Psychiatr Scand Suppl. 2002;412:125–8.
187. Klotz F, Garle M, Granath F, Thiblin I. Criminality among individuals testing positive for the presence of anabolic androgenic steroids. Arch Gen Psychiatry. 2006;63(11):1274–9.
188. Klotz F, Petersson A, Isacson D, Thiblin I. Violent crime and substance abuse: a medico-legal comparison between deceased users of anabolic androgenic steroids and abusers of illicit drugs. Forensic Sci Int. 2007;173(1):57–63.
189. Petersson A, Garle M, Holmgren P, Druid H, Krantz P, Thiblin I. Toxicological findings and manner of death in autopsied users of anabolic androgenic steroids. Drug Alcohol Depend. 2006;81(3):241–9.
190. Kanayama G, Brower KJ, Wood RI, Hudson JI, Pope HG. Anabolic-androgenic steroid dependence: an emerging disorder. Addiction. 2009;104:1966–78.
191. Alexander GM, Packard MG, Hines M. Testosterone has rewarding affective properties in male rats: implications for the biological basis of sexual motivation. Behav Neurosci. 1994;108(2):424–8.
192. Arnedo MT, Salvador A, Martinez-Sanchis S, Gonzalez-Bono E. Rewarding properties of testosterone in intact male mice: a pilot study. Pharmacol Biochem Behav. 2000;65(2):327–32.
193. Wood RI. Anabolic steroids: a fatal attraction? J Neuroendocrinol. 2006;18(3):227–8.
194. American Psychiatric Association. Diagnostic and statistical manual of mental disorders (revised edition). 3rd ed. Washington, DC: American Psychiatric Association; 1987.
195. American Psychiatric Association. Diagnostic and statistical manual of mental disorders (DSM-IV). 4th ed. Washington, DC: American Psychiatric Association; 1994.
196. American Psychiatric Association. Diagnostic and statistical manual of mental disorders (Text Revision) (DSM-IV-TR). 4th ed. Washington: American Psychiatric Association; 2000.
197. Copeland J, Peters R, Dillon P. Anabolic-androgenic steroid use disorders among a sample of Australian competitive and recreational users. Drug Alcohol Depend. 2000;60(1):91–6.
198. Midgley SJ, Heather N, Davies JB. Dependence-producing potential of anabolic-androgenic steroids. Addict Res. 1999;7:539–50.
199. Gridley DW, Hanrahan SJ. Anabolic-androgenic steroid use among male gymnasium participants: knowledge and motives. Sports Health. 1994;12:11–4.
200. Perry PJ, Lund BC, Deninger MJ, Kutscher EC, Schneider J. Anabolic steroid use in weightlifters and bodybuilders: an internet survey of drug utilization. Clin J Sports Med. 2005;15(5):326–30.
201. Kanayama G, Brower KJ, Wood RI, Hudson JI, Pope Jr HG. Issues for DSM-V: clarifying the diagnostic criteria for anabolic-androgenic steroid dependence. Am J Psychiatry. 2009;166(6):642–5.
202. Pope HG, Kean J, Nash A, Kanayama G, Samuel DB, Bickel WK, et al. A diagnostic interview module for anabolic-androgenic steroid dependence: preliminary evidence of reliability and validity. Exp Clin Psychopharmacol. 2010;18:203–13.
203. McBride AJ, Williamson K, Petersen T. Three cases of nalbuphine hydrochloride dependence associated with anabolic steroid use. Br J Sports Med. 1996;30(1):69–70.
204. Wines Jr JD, Gruber AJ, Pope Jr HG, Lukas SE. Nalbuphine hydrochloride dependence in anabolic steroid users. Am J Addict. 1999;8(2):161–4.
205. Arvary D, Pope Jr HG. Anabolic-androgenic steroids as a gateway to opioid dependence. N Engl J Med. 2000;342(20):1532.
206. Pope HG, Kanayama G, Ionescu-Pioggia M, Hudson JI. Anabolic steroid users' attitudes towards physicians. Addiction. 2004;99(9):1189–94.
207. Pope Jr HG, Gruber AJ, Choi P, Olivardia R, Phillips KA. Muscle dysmorphia. An underrecognized form of body dysmorphic disorder. Psychosomatics. 1997;38(6):548–57.
208. Choi PY, Pope HG, Jr., Olivardia R. Muscle dysmorphia: a new syndrome in weightlifters. Br J Sports Med. 2002;36(5):375–6; discussion 377.
209. Kanayama G, Barry S, Hudson JI, Pope Jr HG. Body image and attitudes toward male roles in anabolic-androgenic steroid users. Am J Psychiatry. 2006;163(4):697–703.
210. McKay D. Two-year follow-up of behavioral treatment and maintenance for body dysmorphic disorder. Behav Modif. 1999;23(4):620–9.
211. McKay D, Todaro J, Neziroglu F, Campisi T, Moritz EK, Yaryura-Tobias JA. Body dysmorphic disorder: a preliminary evaluation of treatment and maintenance using exposure with response prevention. Behav Res Ther. 1997;35(1):67–70.
212. Rosen JC, Reiter J, Orosan P. Cognitive-behavioral body image therapy for body dysmorphic disorder. J Consult Clin Psychol. 1995;63(2):263–9.
213. Veale D, Gournay K, Dryden W, Boocock A, Shah F, Willson R, et al. Body dysmorphic disorder: a cognitive behavioural model and pilot randomised controlled trial. Behav Res Ther. 1996;34(9):717–29.
214. Phillips KA, Rasmussen SA. Change in psychosocial functioning and quality of life of patients with body dysmorphic disorder treated with fluoxetine: a placebo-controlled study. Psychosomatics. 2004;45(5):438–44.
215. Phillips KA, Albertini RS, Rasmussen SA. A randomized placebo-controlled trial of fluoxetine in body dysmorphic disorder. Arch Gen Psychiatry. 2002;59(4):381–8.
216. Hollander E, Allen A, Kwon J, Aronowitz B, Schmeidler J, Wong C, et al. Clomipramine vs desipramine crossover trial in body dysmorphic disorder: selective efficacy of a serotonin reuptake inhibitor in imagined ugliness. Arch Gen Psychiatry. 1999;56(11):1033–9.
217. Tan RS, Scally MC. Anabolic steroid-induced hypogonadism–towards a unified hypothesis of anabolic steroid action. Med Hypotheses. 2009;72(6):723–8.
218. Medras M, Tworowska U. Treatment strategies of withdrawal from long-term use of anabolic-androgenic steroids. Pol Merkur Lekarski. 2001;11(66):535–8.
219. Turek PJ, Williams RH, Gilbaugh 3rd JH, Lipshultz LI. The reversibility of anabolic steroid-induced azoospermia. J Urol. 1995;153(5):1628–30.
220. Guay AT, Jacobson J, Perez JB, Hodge MB, Velasquez E. Clomiphene increases free testosterone levels in men with both secondary hypogonadism and erectile dysfunction: who does and does not benefit? Int J Impot Res. 2003;15(3):156–65.

221. Tan RS, Carrejo MH, Chen D. An unusual case of vascular hypogonadism treated with clomiphene citrate and testosterone replacement. Andrologia. 2009;41(1):63–5.
222. Tan RS, Vasudevan D. Use of clomiphene citrate to reverse premature andropause secondary to steroid abuse. Fertil Steril. 2003; 79(1):203–5.
223. Carroll KM, Onken LS. Behavioral therapies for drug abuse. Am J Psychiatry. 2005;162(8):1452–60.
224. Stitzer ML, Vandrey R. Contingency management: utility in the treatment of drug abuse disorders. Clin Pharmacol Ther. 2008; 83(4):644–7.
225. Woody GE. Research findings on psychotherapy of addictive disorders. Am J Addict. 2003;12 Suppl 2:S19–26.

Comorbid Anxiety and Substance Use Disorders

Kathleen Brady

Abstract

The relationship between symptoms of anxiety, anxiety disorders and substance use, abuse and dependence is complex. Converging evidence from epidemiologic studies as well as studies of treatment-seeking individuals indicates that anxiety disorders, symptoms of anxiety, and substance use disorders (SUDs) commonly co-occur, and the interaction is not unidirectional, but multifaceted and variable. Anxiety symptoms often emerge during the course of chronic intoxication and withdrawal. Anxiety disorders may be a risk factor for the development of SUDs. Anxiety disorders modify the presentation and treatment outcome for SUDs. Substance use, abuse and SUDs modify the presentation and treatment outcome for anxiety disorders. In this chapter, recent findings on co-occurring SUDs and anxiety disorders will be reviewed including prevalence, diagnostic, and treatment issues.

Prevalence

General Population

A number of epidemiologic studies conducted over the past 20 years consistently indicate that anxiety disorders and SUDs co-occur more commonly than would be expected by chance alone [1–3]. The National Epidemiological Survey on Alcohol and Related Conditions (NESARC) surveyed more than 43,000 adults and is the most recent and largest survey study focused on psychiatric and SUDs to date [4]. Approximately, 15% of those with any anxiety disorder in the past 12 months had at least one co-occurring SUD and 17.7% of respondents with a SUD in the past 12 months also met criteria for an independent (i.e., not attributed to withdrawal or intoxication) anxiety disorder. The relationship between anxiety disorders and drug use disorders (OR = 2.8) was stronger than the relationship between anxiety and

alcohol use disorders (OR = 1.7). Associations between SUDs and specific anxiety disorders were virtually all significantly positive ($p < 0.05$) with the odds ratios for abuse more positive than those for dependence and the ORs for women more positive than those for men. Among individuals with anxiety disorders, marijuana use disorders were the most common drug use disorder (15.1%) followed by cocaine (5.4%), amphetamine (4.8%), hallucinogen (3.7%), and sedative (2.6%) use disorder [5].

Addiction and Psychiatric Treatment Populations

Because the relationship between anxiety and SUDs is fraught with symptom overlap and diagnostic difficulties, estimates of co-occurring disorders in treatment settings are variable and depend upon the diagnostic techniques used and the specific disorder being assessed. Specific prevalence estimates will be addressed in more detail in sections focused on individual anxiety disorders. In one study of a large sample of SUD treatment clinics, 80% of individuals in treatment had at least one co-occurring anxiety disorder and comorbidity had a significant relationship to mental distress at initial interview and 6 years later [6].

K. Brady, M.D., Ph.D. (✉)
Department of Psychiatry and Behavioral Sciences,
Medical University of South Carolina, 67 President St,
Box 250861, Charleston, SC 29425, USA
e-mail: bradyk@musc.edu

J.C. Verster et al. (eds.), *Drug Abuse and Addiction in Medical Illness: Causes, Consequences and Treatment*,
DOI 10.1007/978-1-4614-3375-0_20, © Springer Science+Business Media, LLC 2012

Screening and Differential Diagnosis

One of the most challenging areas when addressing co-occurring anxiety and SUDs is diagnosis. Anxiety is a common symptom during withdrawal from substances of abuse and symptoms associated with substance use and withdrawal can mimic most anxiety disorders. Substances of abuse also have profound effects on neurotransmitter systems involved in the pathophysiology of anxiety disorders and may unmask vulnerability or lead to neurobiological changes that manifest as an anxiety disorder. The best way to differentiate substance-induced, transient symptoms of anxiety from anxiety disorders that warrant treatment is through observation of symptoms during abstinence, as transient substance-related symptoms will improve with time. The duration of abstinence necessary for accurate diagnosis remains controversial and is likely to be influenced by the specific anxiety disorder being assessed and the substance of abuse. For example, long half-life drugs (e.g., some benzodiazepines, methadone) may require several weeks of abstinence for withdrawal symptoms to subside, but shorter acting substances (e.g., alcohol, cocaine, short half-life benzodiazepines) require shorter periods of abstinence to make valid diagnoses. The onset of anxiety symptoms before the onset of SUD, a family history of anxiety disorder, and/or sustained anxiety symptoms during lengthy periods of abstinence all suggest an anxiety disorder that will warrant treatment.

Because of the high rate of co-occurrence of anxiety and SUDs, screening patients presenting at primary care, substance use, or psychiatric treatment settings is critical. This is especially important because early diagnosis and treatment can improve treatment outcomes. Screening tools can help to identify high-risk individuals, but because of symptom overlap and diagnostic difficulties, a detailed interview is likely to be necessary to fully differentiate substance-induced symptoms, which should resolve with abstinence from primary anxiety disorders that warrant treatment.

General Treatment Considerations

In general, treatment efforts addressing SUDs and psychiatric disorders have developed in parallel. The integration of services and efficacious treatments from both fields is critical to the optimal treatment of individuals with co-occurring disorders. Maximizing the use of nonpharmacologic treatment strategies is also important. Learning strategies to self-regulate anxiety symptoms and alternative coping strategies can interrupt the cycle of using alcohol and drugs of abuse to combat intolerable subjective states. Among psychosocial treatments, cognitive behavioral therapies (CBT) are among

the most effective for both anxiety disorders and SUDs. Promising pilot work investigating the integration of treatments to develop therapies specifically targeting co-occurring anxiety and SUDs will be discussed in the sections below, but there is much work to be done.

The investigation of pharmacotherapeutic treatments for both anxiety disorders and SUDs is progressing rapidly. The pharmacotherapeutic treatment of specific anxiety disorders will be discussed in detail below, but there are some general principles that apply across disorders. In some SUD treatment settings, the use of psychotropic medications is sometimes discouraged and this can undermine treatment [7–9]. In addition, individuals in recovery often have complex and conflicting feelings and attitudes about medications and may see the need for medications as a sign of defectiveness or failure. It is important to address feelings and attitudes about the use of medications and to develop a therapeutic partnership focused on medication adherence in a proactive manner in cases where medications are an important part of optimal treatment.

When the relationship between psychiatric symptoms and substance use is unclear, the risks and benefits of using medications must be carefully considered. If medications are used, treatment should generally follow routine clinical practice for the anxiety disorder with some specific issues taken into consideration. Potential toxic interactions between the prescription medications and illicit drugs and alcohol must be carefully assessed and reviewed with the patient. The abuse potential of therapeutic agents should be considered and an efficacious agent with the least abuse potential should be used. In particular, the use of benzodiazepines in the treatment of co-occurring anxiety disorders and SUDs is a controversial issue. Despite their effectiveness in immediate relief of panic and other anxiety symptoms, these agents are generally avoided in substance-using populations because of abuse potential. However, during the early treatment phase when activation or latency of onset of antidepressant/anxiolytic is an issue with some medications, benzodiazepines may be a reasonable adjunctive medication. When benzodiazepines are prescribed to patients with co-occurring SUDs, limited amounts of medication should be given and patients should be monitored closely for relapse. As a rule, benzodiazepines should be avoided in patients with a current SUD and used with caution in those with a history of SUDs. Benzodiazepines should be considered for chronic treatment only when other pharmacological and nonpharmacological treatment options have been exhausted.

The use of agents targeting SUDs specifically, such as naltrexone or disulfiram, as add-on treatment for individuals with comorbid anxiety disorders and SUDs is underexplored. In one study of 254 outpatients with alcohol dependence and a variety of comorbid psychiatric disorders, Petrakis and colleagues [10] investigated the efficacy of disulfiram and naltrexone alone and in combination in a 12-week trial. Participants treated with either active agent, as compared to placebo, had significantly more consecutive weeks of abstinence and fewer drinking days per week. Disulfiram-treated participants reported less craving from pre- to posttreatment as compared to the naltrexone or placebo-treated groups. The effects of the medications by specific comorbid psychiatric disorder were not discussed, but active medication was associated with improvement in anxiety symptoms. There was no advantage of combining medications. This study argues for the use of adjunctive pharmacotherapeutic treatment targeting SUDs in individuals co-occurring anxiety disorders and SUDs. Hopefully this area will be further investigated and these treatments will become integrated into routine clinical practice.

In the sections that follow, prevalence rates, differential diagnosis, and treatment of posttraumatic stress disorder (PTSD), panic disorder, social anxiety disorder (SAD), generalized anxiety disorder (GAD), and obsessive compulsive disorder (OCD) will be reviewed. Simple phobia will not be covered because most evidence suggests that this disorder has no specific relationship with SUDs.

Posttraumatic Stress Disorder

Data from a number of studies over the last 20 years have emphasized the high co-occurrence of PTSD with SUDs. For example, a recent multisite longitudinal study of almost 1,000 individuals demonstrated that a history of PTSD predisposes individuals to elevated rates of drug abuse and dependence [11]. In the National Comorbidity Study, the odds ratio for SUDs was 2–3 for men and 2.5–4.5 for women with PTSD [12]. In one study using data from the ECA study [13], the assault history and PTSD prevalence in individuals with SUDs were compared to the assault history and PTSD prevalence in those without SUDs. Of all subgroups studied, cocaine/opiate users were most likely to report a PTSD-qualifying traumatic event (43%), and the overall rate of PTSD was 10 times higher among these individuals compared with individuals without a SUD. Among treatment-seeking individuals with SUDs, the prevalence of lifetime PTSD has been reported as high as 50% or greater [14]. In the majority of cases, the development of PTSD precedes the development of the SUD [15].

While the treatment of PTSD is generally multimodal, pharmacotherapy is playing an increasingly important role. Literature on the use of the selective serotonin reuptake inhibitors (SSRIs) in the treatment of PTSD is the most extensive. A number of SSRIs (sertraline, paroxetine, fluoxetine) have received FDA approval for the treatment of PTSD. There is one, double-blind, placebo-controlled study of sertraline in the treatment of PTSD in men and women

with comorbid alcohol dependence [16]. Sertraline treatment was more efficacious than placebo in the treatment of PTSD symptoms, but there were no overall differences between groups in alcohol consumption. However, post hoc analysis revealed that treatment with sertraline significantly decreased alcohol consumption in a subgroup of individuals with early onset PTSD (before age 18), and later onset, less severe alcohol dependence.

Several other classes of compounds are of particular interest in the treatment of co-occurring PTSD and SUDs. A number of case series, open-label and small placebo-controlled trials suggest that anticonvulsant agents may be useful in the treatment of PTSD [17]. Of particular interest, Topiramate demonstrated efficacy in secondary measures of PTSD symptoms in one small placebo controlled trial [18]. Topiramate has also demonstrated efficacy in one placebo-controlled trial and one open-label study [19]. Positive results have been reported in case series and open label studies for both gabapentin and vigabatrin in the treatment of PTSD [20]. These agents also show promise in alcohol and cocaine dependence [21]. Also, there is evidence that adjunctive treatment with atypical antipsychotic agents, including risperidone and quetiapine, can provide therapeutic benefit in the treatment of PTSD [22, 23]. A recent preliminary study ($N=61$) demonstrated decreased alcohol consumption in a subgroup of individuals treated with quetiapine as compared to placebo [24]. Because of potential efficacy in treating PTSD and SUDs, select anticonvulsant and antipsychotic agents warrant further exploration in the treatment of individuals with co-occurring PTSD/SUDs.

There are a number of investigations suggesting that integrative psychotherapies addressing trauma/PTSD among SUD patients are beneficial and typically leads to significant reductions in both PTSD and SUD symptoms. The most widely studied integrated therapy to date is Seeking Safety (SS), a 25-session, manualized treatment that provides psychoeducation and teaches coping skills [25].

In a recent controlled trial comparing SS to a health education group in 353 women, both groups demonstrated significant improvement in substance use and PTSD-related outcomes, but there was no significant difference in improvement between groups [26]. Of interest, improvement in PTSD symptoms was associated with improvement in substance use outcomes, arguing for aggressive treatment of PTSD symptoms in individuals with co-occurring PTSD/SUD (NIH/NIDA CTN-0015, Women's Treatment for Trauma and Substance Use Disorders).

Several small studies have systematically examined the integration of exposure-based treatment for PTSD with empirically validated treatments for SUDs. Triffleman and colleagues developed a manualized treatment combining RP, coping skills, psychoeducation, and in vivo exposure. In a small ($N=19$) pilot trial it was shown to be as effective as, but not superior to, Twelve-Step Facilitation Therapy with regard to PTSD symptoms and drug use [27]. In another uncontrolled trial, Brady and colleagues [28] developed a 16-session, manualized treatment consisting of combined *imaginal* and in vivo exposure therapy for PTSD, and cognitive-behavioral RP techniques for cocaine dependence. Among treatment completers ($N=39$), the intervention was associated with significant reductions in all three clusters of PTSD symptoms and cocaine use. Preliminary data ($N=20$) from an ongoing RCT show substantial reductions in both PTSD symptoms and substance use severity in subjects receiving COPE vs. treatment as usual for substance use [29].

Several other studies have preliminarily explored the use of psychosocial treatments among PTSD/SUD patients with favorable results [30, 31]. While more randomized, controlled trials in this area are needed, the studies to date demonstrate that for the majority of PTSD/SUD patients, addressing PTSD confers substantial therapeutic benefit.

Panic Disorder

In the NESARC study, lifetime prevalence of panic disorder (with or without agoraphobia) was 5.1% and was twice as common in women as compared to men [32] and lifetime risk of both alcohol and drug dependence was increased in individuals with panic disorder [33]. In a recent review of the literature, the risk of panic disorder in the presence of alcohol use disorders was 2–4 times higher than in the absence of an alcohol use disorder [34]. In the Collaborative Study on the Genetics of Alcoholism, lifetime risk for panic disorder was increased in individuals with alcohol use disorders (4.2% vs. 1.0%, respectively).

Alcohol withdrawal can cause panic attacks. However, as compared to individuals with panic disorder, withdrawal-precipitated panic attacks generally markedly improve during the first several weeks of abstinence [35]. Alternatively, individuals with panic attacks may use alcohol to decrease panic symptoms and, consequently, develop an alcohol use disorder [34]. Panic attacks early in recovery that decrease in frequency may respond to support and reassurance. However, if the panic attacks continue or increase over several weeks of abstinence, the diagnosis of panic disorder should be made. Without treatment, the risk of relapse to alcohol use is increased [36]. In one prospective study of alcoholics recruited from acute treatment, panic disorder was the most common diagnosis and was predictive of relapse. After 4 months, approximately 50% of those who had initially met criteria for an anxiety disorder no longer met diagnostic criteria [37]. This finding emphasizes the need to carefully track anxiety symptoms early in recovery and to provide normalizing information to patients about common withdrawal symptoms and the typical course of recovery.

The relationship between panic disorder and smoking is well studied and of interest. In the NESARC study, individuals with panic disorder had elevated 12-month prevalence rates of nicotine dependence [38]. Daily smoking is associated with an increased risk for the first occurrence of a panic attack or panic disorder and the risk is higher in active smokers than past smokers [39]. Early smoking increases the risk of panic disorder [40], and the initiation of smoking may precede the onset of panic disorder by many years (median = 12 years) [41]. In addition, individuals with panic disorder who smoke regularly report more severe anxiety symptoms and social impairment as compared to nonsmokers [42].

According to current guidelines, four classes of medications—SSRIs, TCAs, benzodiazepines, and MAOIs—have approximately comparable efficacy in the treatment of panic disorder [37]. As previously discussed, benzodiazepines are generally avoided in individuals with SUDs. The SSRIs fluoxetine, sertraline, paroxetine, and fluvoxamine have all demonstrated effectiveness in clinical trials, have no abuse potential, and are the best choice for individuals with co-occurring panic disorder and SUD [37].

There is an extensive body of literature supporting the efficacy of CBT in the treatment of panic disorder [37]. In one controlled trial of standard alcohol treatment vs. combined CBT for panic disorder plus alcohol use disorder [43], improvement of panic symptoms and relapse rates did not differ between the two groups. The authors hypothesized that typical strategies for managing anxiety such as stress management, relaxation training, and relapse prevention present in standard alcohol treatment programs may have made it difficult to detect between-group differences [43].

Social Anxiety Disorder

The lifetime prevalence of SAD ranges from 3 to 13% [44]. Approximately, 20% of individuals with SAD also suffer from a drug or alcohol use disorder and the lifetime prevalence of an alcohol use disorder with SAD (48%) is more than double that of individuals without lifetime SAD (29%) [45]. As the average onset of social phobia is before adolescence, symptoms of social anxiety typically precede the initiation of alcohol or drug use [46]. In one study, SAD was diagnosed in 24.7% of 300 patients hospitalized for AUD and preceded AUD in 90.2% of cases.

The current treatment recommendations for SAD include SSRIs or beta blockers in combination with integrated psychosocial treatment. There are a few studies examining treatment options in comorbid populations. Schade and colleagues randomized 96 alcohol-dependent patients with comorbid anxiety disorders, including SAD ($N=87$) to CBT plus optional fluvoxamine (150 mg per day) versus treatment as usual. There was greater improvement in the combined treatment group in anxiety outcomes. Fluvoxamine was not associated with better outcomes [47].

Two small placebo-controlled studies of paroxetine in co-occurring AUD and SAD have demonstrated significant improvement in social anxiety with paroxetine treatment but no significant group differences in alcohol use in either study [48, 49]. Gabapentin is an anticonvulsant agent with demonstrated efficacy in the treatment of social phobia [50]. This is of particular interest because gabapentin has also demonstrated efficacy in the treatment of alcohol withdrawal [51]; and unlike benzodiazepines, gabapentin has no abuse potential. One case report of a polysubstance-dependent individual with comorbid SAD who was treated with gabapentin documented significant improvement in craving and substance use [52], but there are currently no controlled trials examining the efficacy of gabapentin in co-occurring SAD and SUDs.

In a study of individual CBT for alcohol use disorders versus concurrent alcohol use/SAD therapy, individuals who received concurrent treatment had worse alcohol outcomes [53]. The authors hypothesized that exposure to anxiety-provoking social situations in concurrent treatment may have increased drinking to cope [53]. Terra and colleagues followed 300 detoxified alcohol-dependent patients with and without SAD following standard treatment and found no difference in treatment adherence and outcomes, individuals with SAD chaired AA meetings less often, were more ashamed of attendance, felt less integrated into the group, and were less likely to feel better after a meeting [54]. Individuals with SAD may need treatment targeting their social anxiety before being able to benefit from group interventions. Individual therapy may be better tolerated than group therapy and a period of sobriety and skills training may be important before increasing exposure to social situations.

Generalized Anxiety Disorder

SUDs are one of the most common comorbid psychiatric disorders among individuals with GAD [55]. In the NESARC study, approximately 90% of individuals with GAD had at least one other co-occurring disorder and GAD was strongly associated with alcohol use disorders [56]. Another epidemiologic study of 5,877 adults found that GAD was the anxiety disorder most often associated with using alcohol or drugs to self-medicate symptoms [57]. In adolescents, the presence of GAD is associated with a more rapid progression from age of first drink to alcohol dependence [58]. GAD follows a chronic course with low rates of remission and frequent relapses/recurrences. Comorbid SUD decreases the likelihood of recovery from GAD and increases the risk of exacerbation [59, 60].

As GAD symptoms can be mimicked by substance use or withdrawal, diagnostic complications can arise. Assessment of GAD should be delayed until intoxication or withdrawal has terminated. For short-acting drugs (e.g., cocaine) it may be possible to assess GAD after 1 week of abstinence, but longer periods of time (e.g., 4–8 weeks) may be required for longer acting drugs (e.g., methadone, valium) [61]. Patients should also be assessed for use of over-the-counter substances that can induce anxiety (e.g., caffeine, diet pills). DSM-IV requires that a core number of anxiety symptoms be present for at least 6 months in order to meet diagnostic criteria for GAD. Substance use during those 6 months needs to be considered, and symptoms of GAD must have been present during times other than when the patient was using or recovering from alcohol or drugs. This can be challenging to assess because many SUD patients presenting for treatment and complaining of anxiety will not have had 6 months of abstinence.

The treatment of GAD in the context of addiction can also be challenging. The most current guidelines for the pharmacotherapeutic treatment of GAD are from the Canadian Psychiatric Association [62]. First-line medications include: paroxetine, escitalopram, sertraline, and venlafaxine XR. While controlled trials support the use of SRIs and NSRIs in GAD, no clinical trials of these agents have been conducted in individuals with comorbid GAD/SUD. Second-line agents include: alprazolam, bromazepam (not available in the United States), lorazepam, diazepam, buspirone, imipramine, pregabalin, and buproprion XL. Third-line medications to be considered are mirtazapine, citalopram, trazodone, hydroxyzine, and adjunctive olanzapine or risperidone. While affective for some individuals, controlled trials do not support the use of B-blockers. Paroxetine, escitalopram, and venlafaxine have demonstrated long-term efficacy with increasing response rates over 6 months. Because approximately 20–40% of patients with GAD relapse within 6–12 months after the discontinuation of pharmacotherapy, long-term treatment may be needed [62].

While benzodiazepines are effective in the treatment of GAD, their use in individuals with current or former SUDs is controversial because of their abuse liability. Some authors posit, however, that the empirical evidence regarding these concerns is lacking and suggests that benzodiazepines may be safely used to treat anxiety disorders in some SUD patients [63]. Buspirone, a partial 5-hydroxytryptamine [5-HT]1A agonist with low abuse potential, has been shown to be efficacious in some studies in anxious alcoholics [61, 64, 65], but the results are mixed [66, 67] and more evidence supporting the use of buspirone in SUD patients with GAD is needed.

Among psychosocial treatments, CBT may help decrease both anxiety symptoms and risk of relapse. Patients with both GAD and SUDs may benefit from the education of relaxation techniques, coping skills, cognitive restructuring, behavioral activation, problem solving, and sleep hygiene

[61]. Nutritional counseling and regular exercise may also prove beneficial for GAD/SUD patients, although empirical trials are lacking.

Obsessive Compulsive Disorder

In comparison to other anxiety disorders, the association between OCD and SUDs is less robust [68]. For example, in a clinical sample of 254 individuals, approximately 4% of OCD patients met criteria for a lifetime SUD [69]. In the National Comorbidity Survey Replication study, OCD was negatively correlated with SUDs [68]. The Collaborative Study on the Genetics of Alcoholism found no significant increase in rates of OCD in individuals with alcohol use disorders [35]. The lower rates of OCD among SUD patients may be due, in part, to the generally low levels of impulsive or spontaneous behaviors and high levels of harm avoidance exhibited by individuals with OCD. When OCD patients do use substances, they typically choose sedating agents (e.g., alcohol, marijuana).

Some substances of abuse (e.g., alcohol, stimulants) and medications (e.g., benzodiazepines) can produce obsessive-compulsive behaviors [61, 70]. This potential confound should be ruled out when diagnosing OCD among SUD patients. In general, the differential diagnosis of OCD in individuals with SUDs is not as difficult as that of some of the other anxiety disorders because there is less symptom overlap. For SUD patients, the content of obsessions and compulsions is restricted to alcohol or drug use. Obsessions and compulsions focused on procuring and using drugs alone or that occur only during intoxication do not meet diagnostic criteria for OCD.

Little research on the treatment of co-occurring OCD and SUDs has been conducted to date, and there are no randomized controlled trials examining the use of a pharmacologic treatment for this patient population. First-line medications for OCD are clomipramine, fluoxetine, fluvoxamine, paroxetine, and sertraline. In individuals with SUDs, SSRIs are preferable to clomipramine because of more favorable side effect profiles [71]. Fals-Stewart and Schafer randomly assigned 60 substance abusers with OCD in a drug-free therapeutic community to combined OCD and SUD treatment, SUD treatment alone, or SUD treatment plus progressive muscle relaxation. At 12 months, the group receiving combined treatment had higher abstinence, longer duration in treatment, and a greater reduction in OCD symptoms [72].

Nicotine and Anxiety Disorders

In the NESARC study, 28% of the participants used tobacco products and 25% were current cigarette smokers [38]. The 12-month prevalence rate of nicotine dependence was 13% in the general population and 25% among individuals with anxiety disorders. The risk of anxiety disorder among individuals with nicotine dependence was more than twice that of any other psychiatric disorder. Conversely, the prevalence rates of nicotine dependence were also increased in individuals with anxiety disorders (panic disorder 40%, SAD 27%, and GAD 33%) [38]. Despite the strong associations between smoking, nicotine dependence, and anxiety disorders, there has been relatively little investigation of causal connections or treatment. A recent review suggested that smoking, and nicotine in particular, can alleviate anxiety, but other studies indicate that nicotine use and withdrawal can cause anxiety [40]. The Development and Assessment of Nicotine Dependence in Youth (DANDY) study followed a cohort of seventh graders for 3.5 years and found a strong association between trait anxiety and all measures of tobacco use and nicotine dependence. A relaxing effect from initial exposure to nicotine, distinct from relief of withdrawal symptoms, was predictive of a sixfold increase in risk for nicotine dependence [73]. Smokers with a history of panic attacks have significantly more anxiety-related withdrawal symptoms and shorter quit attempts compared to those without panic attacks [74]. Models currently being used to explain the relationship between nicotine dependence and anxiety disorders include conditioning theory, cognitive theory and anxiety.

Conclusions

Because of the high co-occurrence of anxiety and SUDs and their prevalence in the population, primary care and mental health providers will encounter these conditions frequently in the course of their work. It is essential that providers address anxiety symptoms in individuals with SUDs as a routine part of treatment. This requires careful differential diagnosis, which usually requires at least a brief period of sustained abstinence. It also requires providers to consider the mechanism of action of different medications and to choose those with the lowest risk for abuse. Psychosocial treatments for anxiety and substance use are excellent primary and adjunct treatments for these co-occurring disorders and referrals should be made as necessary.

References

1. Kessler RC, Crum RM, Warner LA, Nelson CB, Schulenberg J, Anthony JC. Lifetime co-occurrence of DSM-III-R alcohol abuse and dependence with other psychiatric disorders in the National Comorbidity Survey. Arch Gen Psychiatry. 1997;54(4):313–21.
2. Kessler RC, McGonagle KA, Zhao S, Nelson CB, Hughes M, Eshleman S, et al. Lifetime and 12-month prevalence of DSM-III-R psychiatric disorders in the United States. Results from the National Comorbidity Survey. Arch Gen Psychiatry. 1994;51(1):8–19.
3. Regier DA, Farmer ME, Rae DS, Locke BZ, Keith SJ, Judd LL, et al. Comorbidity of mental disorders with alcohol and other drug

abuse. Results from the Epidemiologic Catchment Area (ECA) Study [see comments]. JAMA. 1990;264(19):2511–8.

4. Grant BF, Stinson FS, Dawson DA, Chou SP, Dufour MC, Compton W, et al. Prevalence and co-occurrence of substance use disorders and independent mood and anxiety disorders: results from the National Epidemiologic Survey on Alcohol and Related Conditions. Arch Gen Psychiatry. 2004;61(8):807–16.

5. Conway KP, Compton W, Stinson FS, Grant BF. Lifetime comorbidity of DSM-IV mood and anxiety disorders and specific drug use disorders: results from the National Epidemiologic Survey on Alcohol and Related Conditions. J Clin Psychiatry. 2006;67(2):247–57.

6. Bakken K, Landheim AS, Vaglum P. Axis I and II disorders as long-term predictors of mental distress: a six-year prospective follow-up of substance-dependent patients. BMC Psychiatry. 2007;7:29.

7. Aagaard J, Vestergaard P, Maarbjerg K. Adherence to lithium prophylaxis: II. Multivariate analysis of clinical, social, and psychosocial predictors of nonadherence. Pharmacopsychiatry. 1988;21(4):166–70.

8. Danion JM, Neunreuther C, Krieger-Finance F, Imbs JL, Singer L. Compliance with long-term lithium treatment in major affective disorders. Pharmacopsychiatry. 1987;20(5):230–1.

9. Keck Jr PE, McElroy SL, Strakowski SM, Stanton SP, Kizer DL, Balistreri TM, et al. Factors associated with pharmacologic noncompliance in patients with mania. J Clin Psychiatry. 1996;57(7):292–7.

10. Petrakis IL, Poling J, Levinson C, Nich C, Carroll K, Rounsaville B. Naltrexone and disulfiram in patients with alcohol dependence and comorbid psychiatric disorders. Biol Psychiatry. 2005;57(10):1128–37.

11. Reed PL, Anthony JC, Breslau N. Incidence of drug problems in young adults exposed to trauma and posttraumatic stress disorder: do early life experiences and predispositions matter? Arch Gen Psychiatry. 2007;64(12):1435–42.

12. Kessler RC, Sonnega A, Bromet E, Hughes M, Nelson CB. Posttraumatic stress disorder in the National Comorbidity Survey. Arch Gen Psychiatry. 1995;52(12):1048–60.

13. Cottler LB, Compton 3rd WM, Mager D, Spitznagel EL, Janca A. Posttraumatic stress disorder among substance users from the general population. Am J Psychiatry. 1992;149(5):664–70.

14. Dansky BS, Brady KT, Roberts JT. Post-traumatic stress disorder and substance abuse: empirical findings and clinical issues. Subst Abuse. 1994;15(4):247–57.

15. Jacobsen LK, Southwick SM, Kosten TR. Substance use disorders in patients with posttraumatic stress disorder: a review of the literature. Am J Psychiatry. 2001;158(8):1184–90.

16. Brady KT, Sonne S, Anton RF, Randall CL, Back SE, Simpson K. Sertraline in the treatment of co-occurring alcohol dependence and posttraumatic stress disorder. Alcohol Clin Exp Res. 2005;29(3):395–401.

17. Van Ameringen M, Mancini C, Pipe B, Bennett M. Antiepileptic drugs in the treatment of anxiety disorders: role in therapy. Drugs. 2004;64(19):2199–220.

18. Tucker P, Trautman RP, Wyatt DB, Thompson J, Wu SC, Capece JA, et al. Efficacy and safety of topiramate monotherapy in civilian posttraumatic stress disorder: a randomized, double-blind, placebo-controlled study. J Clin Psychiatry. 2007;68(2):201–6.

19. Johnson DR, Rosenheck R, Fontana A, Lubin H, Charney D, Southwick S. Outcome of intensive inpatient treatment for combat-related posttraumatic stress disorder. Am J Psychiatry. 1996;153(6):771–7.

20. Zvolensky MJ, Bernstein A, Sachs-Ericsson N, Schmidt NB, Buckner JD, Bonn-Miller MO. Lifetime associations between cannabis, use, abuse, and dependence and panic attacks in a representative sample. J Psychiatr Res. 2006;40(6):477–86.

21. Bonn-Miller MO, Zvolensky MJ, Bernstein A. Marijuana use motives: concurrent relations to frequency of past 30-day use and anxiety sensitivity among young adult marijuana smokers. Addict Behav. 2007;32(1):49–62.

22. Bartzokis G, Lu PH, Turner J, Mintz J, Saunders CS. Adjunctive risperidone in the treatment of chronic combat-related posttraumatic stress disorder. Biol Psychiatry. 2005;57(5):474–9.

23. Reich DB, Winternitz S, Hennen J, Watts T, Stanculescu C. A preliminary study of risperidone in the treatment of posttraumatic stress disorder related to childhood abuse in women. J Clin Psychiatry. 2004;65(12):1601–6.

24. Kampman KM, Pettinati HM, Lynch KG, Whittingham T, Macfadden W, Dackis C, et al. A double-blind, placebo-controlled pilot trial of quetiapine for the treatment of Type A and Type B alcoholism. J Clin Psychopharmacol. 2007;27(4):344–51.

25. Najavits LM. Seeking safety: a treatment manual for PTSD and substance abuse. New York: Guilford; 2002.

26. Hien DA, Wells EA, Jiang H, Suarez-Morales L, Campbell AN, Cohen LR, et al. Multisite randomized trial of behavioral interventions for women with co-occurring PTSD and substance use disorders. J Consult Clin Psychol. 2009;77(4):607–19.

27. Triffleman E. Gender differences in a controlled pilot study of psychosocial treatments in substance dependent patients with posttraumatic stress disorder: design considerations and outcomes. Alcohol Treat Q. 2000;18(3):113–26.

28. Brady KT, Dansky BS, Back SE, Foa EB, Carroll KM. Exposure therapy in the treatment of PTSD among cocaine-dependent individuals: preliminary findings. J Subst Abuse Treat. 2001;21(1):47–54.

29. Mills KL, Teesson M, Back SE, Hopwood S, Brady KT. Integrated treatment for substance use and PTSD using exposure therapy: preliminary findings. Paper presented at the College on Problems of Drug Dependence, San Juan, Puerto Rico, 2008.

30. Donovan B, Padin-Rivera E, Kowaliw S. "Transcend": initial outcomes from a posttraumatic stress disorder/substance abuse treatment program. J Trauma Stress. 2001;14(4):757–72.

31. Harris M. Trauma recovery and empowerment: a clinician's guide for working with women in groups. New York: Free; 1998.

32. Grant BF, Hasin DS, Stinson FS, Dawson DA, Goldstein RB, Smith S, et al. The epidemiology of DSM-IV panic disorder and agoraphobia in the United States: results from the National Epidemiologic Survey on Alcohol and Related Conditions. J Clin Psychiatry. 2006;67(3):363–74.

33. Ormel J, VonKorff M, Ustun TB, Pini S, Korten A, Oldehinkel T. Common mental disorders and disability across cultures. Results from the WHO Collaborative Study on Psychological Problems in General Health Care. JAMA. 1994;272(22):1741–8.

34. Cosci F, Schruers KR, Abrams K, Griez EJ. Alcohol use disorders and panic disorder: a review of the evidence of a direct relationship. J Clin Psychiatry. 2007;68(6):874–80.

35. Schuckit MA, Tipp JE, Bucholz KK, Nurnberger Jr JI, Hesselbrock VM, Crowe RR, et al. The life-time rates of three major mood disorders and four major anxiety disorders in alcoholics and controls. Addiction. 1997;92(10):1289–304.

36. American Psychiatric Association. Practice guideline for the treatment of patients with panic disorder. Work Group on Panic Disorder. Am J Psychiatry. 1998;155:1–34.

37. Kushner MG, Abrams K, Thuras P, Hanson KL, Brekke M, Sletten S. Follow-up study of anxiety disorder and alcohol dependence in comorbid alcoholism treatment patients. Alcohol Clin Exp Res. 2005;29(8):1432–43.

38. Grant BF, Hasin DS, Chou SP, Stinson FS, Dawson DA. Nicotine dependence and psychiatric disorders in the United States: results from the national epidemiologic survey on alcohol and related conditions. Arch Gen Psychiatry. 2004;61(11):1107–15.

39. Breslau N, Klein DF. Smoking and panic attacks: an epidemiologic investigation. Arch Gen Psychiatry. 1999;56(12):1141–7.

40. Morissette SB, Tull MT, Gulliver SB, Kamholz BW, Zimering RT. Anxiety, anxiety disorders, tobacco use, and nicotine: a critical review of interrelationships. Psychol Bull. 2007;133(2):245–72.

41. Amering M, Bankier B, Berger P, Griengl H, Windhaber J, Katschnig H. Panic disorder and cigarette smoking behavior. Compr Psychiatry. 1999;40(1):35–8.

42. Zvolensky MJ, Schmidt NB, McCreary BT. The impact of smoking on panic disorder: an initial investigation of a pathoplastic relationship. J Anxiety Disord. 2003;17(4):447–60.

43. Bowen RC, D'Arcy C, Keegan D, Senthilselvan A. A controlled trial of cognitive behavioral treatment of panic in alcoholic inpatients with comorbid panic disorder. Addict Behav. 2000;25(4):593–7.

44. American Psychiatric Association. Diagnostic and statistical manual of mental disorders (4th text revision). Washington, DC: American Psychiatric Press; 2000.

45. Grant BF, Hasin DS, Blanco C, Stinson FS, Chou SP, Goldstein RB, et al. The epidemiology of social anxiety disorder in the United States: results from the National Epidemiologic Survey on Alcohol and Related Conditions. J Clin Psychiatry. 2005;66(11):1351–61.

46. Sareen J, Chartier M, Kjernisted KD, Stein MB. Comorbidity of phobic disorders with alcoholism in a Canadian community sample. Can J Psychiatry. 2001;46(8):733–40.

47. Schade A, Marquenie LA, van Balkom AJ, Koeter MW, de Beurs E, van den Brink W, et al. The effectiveness of anxiety treatment on alcohol-dependent patients with a comorbid phobic disorder: a randomized controlled trial. Alcohol Clin Exp Res. 2005;29(5): 794–800.

48. Book SW, Thomas SE, Randall PK, Randall CL. Paroxetine reduces social anxiety in individuals with a co-occurring alcohol use disorder. J Anxiety Disord. 2008;22(2):310–8.

49. Randall CL, Johnson MR, Thevos AK, Sonne SC, Thomas SE, Willard SL, et al. Paroxetine for social anxiety and alcohol use in dual-diagnosed patients. Depress Anxiety. 2001;14(4):255–62.

50. Pande AC, Davidson JR, Jefferson JW, Janney CA, Katzelnick DJ, Weisler RH, et al. Treatment of social phobia with gabapentin: a placebo-controlled study. J Clin Psychopharmacol. 1999;19(4):341–8.

51. Malcolm R, Myrick H, Brady KT, Ballenger JC. Update on anticonvulsants for the treatment of alcohol withdrawal. Am J Addict. 2001;10(Suppl):16–23.

52. Verduin ML, McKay S, Brady KT. Gabapentin in comorbid anxiety and substance use. Am J Addict. 2007;16(2):142–3.

53. Randall CL, Thomas S, Thevos AK. Concurrent alcoholism and social anxiety disorder: a first step toward developing effective treatments. Alcohol Clin Exp Res. 2001;25(2):210–20.

54. Terra MB, Barros HM, Stein AT, Figueira I, Athayde LD, Spanemberg L, et al. Does co-occurring social phobia interfere with alcoholism treatment adherence and relapse? J Subst Abuse Treat. 2006;31(4):403–9.

55. Wittchen HU, Zhao S, Kessler RC, Eaton WW. DSM-III-R generalized anxiety disorder in the National Comorbidity Survey. Arch Gen Psychiatry. 1994;51(5):355–64.

56. Grant BF, Hasin DS, Stinson FS, Dawson DA, June Ruan W, Goldstein RB, et al. Prevalence, correlates, co-morbidity, and comparative disability of DSM-IV generalized anxiety disorder in the USA: results from the National Epidemiologic Survey on Alcohol and Related Conditions. Psychol Med. 2005;35(12):1747–59.

57. Bolton JM, Sareen J. Lifetime mood, anxiety, and drug use disorders are common in the United States population. Evid Based Ment Health. 2006;9(4):113.

58. Sartor CE, Lynskey MT, Heath AC, Jacob T, True W. The role of childhood risk factors in initiation of alcohol use and progression to alcohol dependence. Addiction. 2007;102(2):216–25.

59. Bruce SE, Yonkers KA, Otto MW, Eisen JL, Weisberg RB, Pagano M, et al. Influence of psychiatric comorbidity on recovery and recurrence in generalized anxiety disorder, social phobia, and panic disorder: a 12-year prospective study. Am J Psychiatry. 2005;162(6):1179–87.

60. Compton 3rd WM, Cottler LB, Jacobs JL, Ben-Abdallah A, Spitznagel EL. The role of psychiatric disorders in predicting drug dependence treatment outcomes. Am J Psychiatry. 2003;160(5): 890–5.

61. McKeehan MB, Martin D. Assessment and treatment of anxiety disorders and co-morbid alcohol/other drug dependency. Alcohol Treat Q. 2002;20:45–59.

62. Clinical practice guidelines: management of anxiety disorders. Can J Psychiatry. 2006;51.

63. Posternak MA, Mueller TI. Assessing the risks and benefits of benzodiazepines for anxiety disorders in patients with a history of substance abuse or dependence. Am J Addict. 2001;10(1):48–68.

64. Kranzler HR, Burleson JA, Del Boca FK, Babor TF, Korner P, Brown J, et al. Buspirone treatment of anxious alcoholics. A placebo-controlled trial. Arch Gen Psychiatry. 1994;51(9): 720–31.

65. Malec E, Malec T, Gagne MA, Dongier M. Buspirone in the treatment of alcohol dependence: a placebo-controlled trial. Alcohol Clin Exp Res. 1996;20(2):307–12.

66. Malcolm R, Anton RF, Randall CL, Johnston A, Brady K, Thevos A. A placebo-controlled trial of buspirone in anxious inpatient alcoholics. Alcohol Clin Exp Res. 1992;16(6):1007–13.

67. Tollefson GD, Montague-Clouse J, Tollefson SL. Treatment of comorbid generalized anxiety in a recently detoxified alcoholic population with a selective serotonergic drug (buspirone). J Clin Psychopharmacol. 1992;12(1):19–26.

68. Kessler RC, Chiu WT, Demler O, Merikangas KR, Walters EE. Prevalence, severity, and comorbidity of 12-month DSM-IV disorders in the National Comorbidity Survey Replication. Arch Gen Psychiatry. 2005;62(6):617–27.

69. Sbrana A, Bizzarri JV, Rucci P, Gonnelli C, Doria MR, Spagnolli S, et al. The spectrum of substance use in mood and anxiety disorders. Compr Psychiatry. 2005;46(1):6–13.

70. Satel SL, McDougle CJ. Obsessions and compulsions associated with cocaine abuse. Am J Psychiatry. 1991;148(7):947.

71. Koran LM, Hanna GL, Hollander E, Nestadt G, Simpson HB. Practice guideline for the treatment of patients with obsessive-compulsive disorder. Am J Psychiatry. 2007;164(7 Suppl):5–53.

72. Chatterjee CR, Ringold AL. A case report of reduction in alcohol craving and protection against alcohol withdrawal by gabapentin. J Clin Psychiatry. 1999;60(9):617.

73. DiFranza JR, Savageau JA, Rigotti NA, Ockene JK, McNeill AD, Coleman M, et al. Trait anxiety and nicotine dependence in adolescents: a report from the DANDY study. Addict Behav. 2004;29(5):911–9.

74. Zvolensky MJ, Lejuez CW, Kahler CW, Brown RA. Nonclinical panic attack history and smoking cessation: an initial examination. Addict Behav. 2004;29(4):825–30.

Depression and Substance Use

21

Clare J. Mackie, Patricia Conrod, and Kathleen Brady

Abstract

Depression and substance use disorders (SUD) commonly co-occur in adult [10, 13, 97] and adolescent samples [98, 99]. Epidemiological studies that have begun in childhood and adolescence and followed cohorts over time have provided valuable information on changes in prevalence, trajectories of comorbid associations, and in highlighting key issues about their underlying causal mechanisms. This chapter draws together recent findings in this area, using examples from a wide range of sources to highlight key themes emerging from both adult and adolescent research. We begin with an overview of the concurrent prevalence of depression and SUD in adult and adolescent samples. We then explore longitudinal patterns of depression and SUD comorbidity from adolescence to adulthood to illustrate the varying mechanisms now thought to contribute to this comorbidity. Finally, we consider the implications of these findings for clinical practice.

Learning Objectives
- Clinical and epidemiological studies demonstrate elevated prevalence rates of depression and SUD.
- Conflicting findings exist concerning the causal association of depression and SUD.
- Antecedents such as personality characteristics, genetic and environmental factors contribute to both depression and SUD.

Issues that Need to Be Addressed by Future Research
- Knowledge of antecedents would enable an identification of adolescents at risk for depression and SUD.
- This would lead to the development of preventative interventions that address both depression and SUD.
- How developmental change underpins the co-occurrence of depression and SUD should be examined.

C.J. Mackie (✉) • P. Conrod
National Addiction Centre, Institute of Psychiatry,
King's College London, 4 Windsor Walk, Denmark Hill,
London SE5 8AF, UK
e-mail: clare.mackie@kcl.ac.uk

K. Brady, M.D., Ph.D.
Department of Psychiatry and Behavioral Sciences, Clinical
Neurosciences Division, Medical University of South Carolina,
67 President St, PO Box 250861, Charleston, SC 29425, USA
e-mail: bradyk@musc.edu

Prevalence

Before establishing the concurrent prevalence rates of depression and SUD, there are a number of considerations on which the evidence of a co-occurrence of depression and SUD might be differentiated. For instance, differences in the prevalence rates of depression and SUD across studies might reflect variations in the measurement of both disorders. Some studies examine major depression as defined by the Diagnostic and Statistical Manual of mental disorders (DSM-IV) [1], while others have examined measures of symptom severity. Studies that utilize a higher cutoff for clinically defined depression might indicate lower levels of prevalence than studies which encompass a range of depression symptoms. With regard to substance use, some studies group different types of substances together, often including alcohol, cigarettes, and illicit drug use, so it is not clear what the independent contribution of each makes to the co-occurrence of depression. Investigators have also examined problematic use of substances in terms of "abuse" and/or "dependence." However, it is not unreasonable to expect that low levels of substance use can be associated with depression in individuals who are susceptible to the development of both problems. Measurement issues such as the ones outlined earlier might account for differences in prevalence of concurrent comorbidity and in its predictive course.

The concurrent prevalence of SUD among adults receiving treatment for major depression is between 8% and 25%, and the lifetime prevalence of SUD is even higher (30–42%) [2, 3]. Similar prevalence rates have been reported in adolescent clinical samples [2–4]. In an adolescent sample (13–19 years of age) with a diagnosis of depressive disorders, 16% of participants reported a current comorbid SUD compared to only 2% of the comparison group with no depressive disorder [4]. High rates of depression are also shown in adults and adolescents seeking treatment for SUD [5–7].

Several epidemiological studies have shown that depression and SUD co-occur in the general population [8–12]. In adults, the prevalence rates for the co-occurrence of depression with any substance use disorder in the previous 12 months range from 5% to 19.2% [11], with lifetime prevalence rates ranging from 9.1% to 32% [9]. Aside from confirming these basic associations, research has shown that depression is more often associated with substance dependence than substance abuse. An examination of the co-occurrence of alcohol dependence and abuse with other mental health disorders in the general population showed that women were more likely to show a co-occurrence of major depression and alcohol dependence than men [13]. The Odds Ratio (OR), which compares the observed co-occurrence of the two disorders with their expected co-occurrence, considering their prevalence in the general population, was reported to be 4.05 for women and 2.95 for men, meaning that for women with alcohol dependence they were 4 times more likely to have a diagnosis of major depression compared to 2.9 times more likely for men with alcohol dependence.

Several studies have reported the co-occurrence of depression and SUD in adolescent samples [14–21]. An increase in the prevalence of mood disorders from 5% in adolescents

who had never consumed alcohol to 23.8% in adolescents who reported consuming alcohol almost weekly has been shown [12]. Similar results were also shown for frequency of cigarette and illicit drug use. Concurrent comorbidity between SUD and depression has been estimated to range from 11% to 32% across studies [22]. Examining the Odds Ratios showed a range from 1.1 for comorbid depression and cannabis use to 8.0 for any concurrent SUD [8, 22].

Individual Differences in Age and Gender

An upsurge in the rate of depression often accompanies the onset of puberty, at which point the female predominance of mood disorders first emerges [23]. Differences exist between prepuberal depression with its onset in childhood and adolescent onset depression. Twin studies suggest a greater genetic component for adolescent rather than childhood onset depression [24, 25] supporting the view that childhood and adolescent onset depression differs in etiology. Research has often reported that in clinical samples, SUD is more associated with adolescent onset depression than childhood onset depression [26].

Gender-specific relationships are also shown to occur between depression and SUD [14, 18]. Even though depression is more common in females than males, the presence of depression prior to 13 years of age increased the risk for SUD between 13 and 16 years more for boys than for girls [18]. This can be an example of the often stated gender paradox [27] in that disorders might be more severe in the gender in which they are less common. Until recently, SUD demonstrated a higher prevalence in adolescent males than in females; currently, girls are shown to be increasing in their quantity and frequency of alcohol use, particularly in the UK [28]. Early onset alcohol and substance use (prior to age 15) is associated with an increased risk for adult mental health disorders [29], particularly depression and suicidal behavior [30, 31]. These findings thus raise the question of whether an earlier age of onset per se contributes to these effects or whether it functions as a marker for more severe, or a more generalized liability, to subsequent difficulties [32].

Causal Models

For the purpose of understanding the nature of this comorbidity, it is important to consider the causal relationships between these two sets of symptoms. In this case, the diagnosis of a disorder may be of less interest, but rather its timing or onset may be of greater importance. Therefore, longitudinal data are important for examining causal mechanisms and risk factors. Prospective studies of clinical and epidemiological samples have the benefit of a longitudinal design in that they involve multiple waves of assessment and allow for tests of the timing and patterning of symptoms. Moreover, they allow for opportunities to examine focused hypotheses about causal mechanisms. Epidemiological samples provide a number of advantages over clinical samples in that they can examine behaviors that fall short of a clinical diagnosis. However, one known disadvantage is that epidemiological studies are based on large samples which may only include a small number of participants who show high levels of symptom prevalence. An alternative is to identify high-risk participants with known risk factors for the development of both disorders, which allows for greater variability and frequency of symptoms that would not be available in a community sample. The major limitation of this design, however, lies in uncertainties over the extent to which findings are specific to that selected group or generalizable to the broader population.

A number of theoretical models have been posited in an attempt to explain comorbid psychopathology and substance use [33–35]. Causal models would suggest that either psychopathology can increase an individual's potential vulnerability to develop an SUD or that substance use may trigger psychopathological symptoms. The common factor or correlated liabilities model would posit that high rates of comorbidity are the result of a shared vulnerability to both disorders (e.g., genetic risk, personality, or temperament). An alternative model would highlight bidirectional effects between symptoms, in that each disorder has independent origins but its course and severity is exacerbated by the other disorder over time. Research has provided support for all models of comorbidity with the causation [36, 37] and common factor model [34, 38] receiving the most attention. However, caution is needed before assuming that earlier behaviors necessarily cause later ones. It is possible that at some stage this temporal sequence is simply a function of maturational processes, whereby the earlier disorder manifests itself earlier in time than the other.

Depression Causes an Increase in the Vulnerability for Substance Use

Theories that have been presented to support the idea that psychopathology can precipitate an increase in substance use include the self-medication model [39], the tension reduction [40], and the stress–response dampening model [41] all of which would suggest that depressed individuals would use substances to reduce feelings of negative effect. The majority of studies that provide support for self-medication models of comorbidity tend to include adolescents or young adults who are at the onset of substance use. Elevated depression symptoms in adolescence often predict future alcohol use [42, 43], alcohol use problems, particularly in males [44], and alcohol

abuse/dependence [21]. In a sample of 1,545 Finnish twins, early onset depressive disorder at 14 years was shown to predict frequent alcohol use and recurrent intoxication at 17.5 years, even after controlling for other psychiatric disorders and other substance use [43]. Depression symptoms and depressive disorder are also shown to be a risk factor for cigarette use and dependence [15, 17, 42, 45]. For instance, major depression assessed at 16 and 18 years increased the risk for daily cigarette smoking at 21 years by 19% compared to adolescents without such a diagnosis [17]. Less support has been shown for a predictive relationship between depression and cannabis use [46]. Although, one recent study did demonstrate a predictive relationship between major depression at 14 years and subsequent cannabis onset and cannabis use disorder at 17 years after controlling for externalizing behavior [47].

Substance-Induced Depression

Substance use may predispose individuals to the development of depression, either through the physiological effects of heavy substance use [48] or due to the consequences of heavy use (e.g., family problems, occupational, school). The majority of evidence that supports this causation model is often found in adults or college students where substance use has reached relatively elevated levels [49–52]. Binge drinking and alcohol dependence are found to increase the odds of reporting depression [12], with 11.3% of adults with an alcohol dependence diagnosis reporting an episode of depression in the previous 12 months [9]. In a prospective longitudinal study, it was reported that tobacco and illicit drug use in adolescence were predictive of major depression in early adulthood [53]. In an examination of the cumulative affect of substance use in the same sample, it was demonstrated that heavy alcohol use, cannabis use, and more frequent illicit drug use in childhood, adolescence, and young adulthood predicted major depression in late adulthood [36]. More recently, the predictive association between drinking patterns and depression in a nationally representative sample of Finnish adults was examined [52]. The authors demonstrated that binge drinking predicted symptoms of depression 5 years later, over and above potential confounders such as average alcohol use, and preexisting alcohol dependence. In fact, the frequency of a hangover was the best predictor of later depression, suggesting that the link between alcohol use and depression in adults is limited to the effects of heavy drinking.

Concerns about the impact of cannabis use on depression are often related to the effects of THC on serotonin and other neurotransmitters in a way that can produce depression-like symptoms. A prospective study examined the relationship between cannabis use and depression in adulthood.

This study used data from the Epidemiological Catchment Area study in which a subsample of 1,920 individuals were followed-up 14–16 years later. Respondents who reported cannabis use and at least one symptom of either cannabis use dependence or abuse at baseline were 4.5 times more likely to report depressive symptoms in the follow-up period than individuals who were none users [50]. This association remained even after controlling for confounders and baseline depression. An Australian cohort of adolescents was followed-up into adulthood to examine the link between early onset regular cannabis use and early adulthood depression. It was found that among females only, weekly cannabis use in adolescence predicted a twofold increase in rates of depression at 20–21 years, and daily use predicted a fourfold increase in depression risk [54].

Reciprocal Associations

There is the possibility that depression and substance use are reciprocally related to each other, in which the onset of depression can increase substance use and subsequently the consumption of substances can increase the risk for depression. Studies that employ structural equation models can estimate simultaneous directional effects. Five such studies have utilized these techniques to examine sequential effects while estimating the reverse association [37, 55–58]. In young adults, one study showed that heavy weekend drinking predicted later weekday negative affect [55], while another study demonstrated the reverse association, from alcohol dependence at 17 years to major depression at 25 years [37]. However, in adults directional effects might have already been established earlier in development. One study examined the reciprocal relationships between depression and three separate substance use outcomes (frequency of alcohol, cigarette, and cannabis use) in 951 adolescents (12–14 years). Positive relationships were shown between change in one construct and change in the other reflecting that both domains increase (or decrease) in parallel, but predictive relationships from one disorder to the other were not demonstrated [57]. In a UK sample of adolescents (mean age 13; 9 years), elevated initial levels in depression predicted growth in quantity and frequency of alcohol use over an 18-month period [58].

Summary

The previous review demonstrated conflicting findings with regard to the causal relationship between depression and SUD, and there are a number of potential factors that might account for this discrepancy in findings. Firstly, it is possible that significant directional effects are demonstrated at

short-term intervals rather than yearly spaced assessments. Secondly, studies demonstrate stronger predictive associations between early onset depression and later substance use in adolescence. Whether this is due to the age of onset of depression occurring prior to the onset of SUD is unclear. Thirdly, differences may occur according to gender. Cross-sectional associations between depression and SUD are stronger in females than males, while longitudinal associations are stronger in males than females [14, 18]. Fourthly, associations can differ according to the substance assessed. Limited evidence has shown that depression is a stronger predictor of later alcohol use/dependence [42, 43, 58], while cannabis use is a stronger predictor of later depression [50, 54].

Common Factors

A third possible model that might explain the high rates of comorbidity of depression and substance use is that a third factor or a common underlying vulnerability contributes to the association between the two domains. Possible candidates for a third factor are certain personality characteristics, a genetic vulnerability, or common environmental factors.

Personality Characteristics

Separate lines of research have shown that broad indices of personality traits, such as neuroticism and lower order facets, such as hopelessness, are associated with alcohol and substance use and abuse [59–61] and depression [62, 63]. Neuroticism refers to a broad temperamental sensitivity to negative stimuli and a tendency to experience negative emotional states [64, 65], and forms the cornerstone of the tripartite model of personality in depression and anxiety [66].

A number of prospective studies have examined how neuroticism or negative emotionality impacts on substance misuse and depression. In a sample of 378 college students, neuroticism accounted for a significant proportion of the variance in the association between alcohol use disorders and psychological distress [56]. Initial associations between major depression in mid-adolescence and alcohol abuse/dependence and nicotine dependence in young adulthood were shown prior to controlling for additional variables [67]. After controlling for neuroticism these associations were not maintained, suggesting that neuroticism is not only associated with an increased risk of depression and SUD, but can account for the association between adolescent depression and later adult SUD.

It has been posited that hopelessness, a lower order trait of neuroticism would be associated with a specific pattern of substance misuse. Specifically, in a sample of substance abusing women, hopelessness was associated with major and recurrent depression, and a threefold increased risk for opioid dependence, indicating that hopelessness might predispose individuals to depressed feelings and thus encourage the use of analgesics to reduce feelings of negative affect [68]. Furthermore, in college students, the same measure of hopelessness was associated with depressive symptoms, alcohol and sedative drug use, and coping with depression [69], providing further support that individuals who score high in hopelessness are using substance to self-medicate painful depressive feelings. The idea that poor problem-solving skills might mediate the relationship between hopelessness and substance misuse was explored in an adolescent sample (mean age 16.9 years). The authors posited that individuals high in hopelessness when encountering problematic events might not engage in rational problem solving due their personality style as characterized by a belief that negative events will occur. It was demonstrated that poor rational problem solving mediated the predictive association between depression and lifetime alcohol and cannabis use [70]. Research has also examined the association between the personality impulsivity, heavy alcohol use, and depression. A recent study demonstrated that adolescents who scored high in impulsivity and were consuming elevated levels of alcohol use did not demonstrate a developmental decrease in depression over time [58]. Research that has focused on depression and impulsivity at the biological levels has examined decreased serotonin levels in adolescents with alcohol use disorders, and in turn might lead to depression [71]. In addition, interactions with the environment need to be considered as impulsive individuals might be at risk of stressful or negative life events as a consequence of their risky behavior (alcohol/drug use, antisocial behavior) and due to their poor decision making/poor planning.

Genetic Risk Factors

Depression and SUD might share an underlying genetic etiology that increases the likelihood of their co-occurrence. However, the evidence for a shared familial relationship of alcohol disorder and depression is ambiguous. If such a relationship exists, family studies should demonstrate higher rates of alcoholism in first-degree relatives of depressed probands and/or higher rates of depression in first-degree relatives of alcoholic probands. In support of a genetic etiology, studies have reported higher rates of alcoholism among relatives of depressed adults [72, 73], suggesting a familial vulnerability that is common to both disorders. Twin studies, which examine if this familial vulnerability is related to genetic or environmental factors, have demonstrated that both genetic and specific environmental sources of vulnerability to depression overlap with those of alcohol dependence in adults [74]. However, no evidence has been shown for a

causal effect model, in that the genetic risk for one disorder predicts the genetic risk for the other [75, 76]. Instead, research has shown that within an individual, a person's susceptibility for depression and alcohol dependence was correlated. For instance, if relative 1 has depression, then the risk for relative 2 for alcohol dependence is increased, this would occur regardless if relative 2 had depression.

Sex differences are also demonstrated in the genetic and environmental contributions to depression and alcohol dependence comorbidity. For females half the risk for depression and alcohol dependence was due to genetic and specific environmental factors, whereas for males it was due largely to genetic factors. These findings suggest that genetics play a role in the vulnerability to both alcohol risk and depression, and that specific environmental stresses are associated with this comorbidity.

Although twin studies do not provide information on the specific genes that might contribute to both disorders, studies by other research groups might shed light on this issue. For example, studies have found that a polymorphism in the serotonin transporter gene (5-HTTLPR) was associated with greater alcohol use and dependence (see [77] for a review). It has also been examined in relation to depression [78], neuroticism [79], and using alcohol to cope with stress [80].

Environmental Risk Factors

In addition to genetic risk factors, studies have examined the long-term effects of early environmental risk on subsequent depression and SUD. Several studies have confirmed associations between early adversity and an increased risk for SUD and internalizing disorders. Collectively this work has focused on adverse rearing environments such as high conflict, parental divorce, low parental monitoring and harsh parenting, and at the extreme end physical and sexual abuse on both adolescent alcohol use and depression [81, 82]. In addition, a growing interest in the role of prenatal exposures, such as maternal smoking in pregnancy, has attracted interest in early onset substance use [83], evidence for maternal stress in pregnancy on later emotional and behavioral disorders [84], and links between prematurity/low birth weight and subsequent depression [85]. Genetically informative studies are also utilized to establish to what extent environmental risk factors are in fact truly, "environmental" in nature. For instance, having substance-using peers are shown to be highly predictive of both the initiation of alcohol use in adolescence as well as its continuation [86] with perceived peers' attitudes towards alcohol use and number of alcohol-using peers as important factors contributing to adolescents' problem alcohol and drug use [87]. Therefore, peer relationships are argued to be a form of environmental mediated risk for the development of SUD. However, evidence points to other possibilities, for instance the genetically influenced child characteristics can evoke responses from peers. Evidence suggests that adolescents who demonstrate impulsive personality characteristics are more likely to select substance-using peers [88], highlighting the interplay between genetic risk and susceptibility to risk environments in predicting SUD.

Moderating Mechanisms

The previous review demonstrated that environmental risk mediated the link between personality characteristics and SUD. There is consistent evidence that early adolescent depression interacts with conduct disorder to predict SUD [21, 89, 90]. For instance, elevated rates of depression early in adolescence is associated with higher rates of alcohol use disorder, but only in boys with high levels of conduct disorder [21]. Recently, it was hypothesized that adolescents with both high rates of depression and conduct disorder were more likely to use substances to elevate negative affective states because they were relatively unconcerned about violating social norms [90].

Treatment Studies

Well-controlled treatment studies can also provide an opportunity to understand mechanisms maintaining comorbidity. If an evidence-based intervention for a particular set of symptoms, e.g., relapse prevention for alcohol dependence, is shown to reduce the other set of symptoms, then findings might have implications for how we understand causal relationships between the two sets of symptoms. However, before we review the literature examining these very findings, it is worth mentioning some methodological issues pertaining to this type of investigation. First, while certain evidence-based interventions might be originally conceptualized as targeting a specific set of problems, e.g., relapse prevention for alcohol dependence, the therapy might also contain some generic treatment effects, which would broadly impact on a variety of symptoms and problems. This such a case, the intervention might be shown to have an impact on the other comorbid disorder, i.e., depression, but this effect is achieved independent of any effect on drinking behavior. Therefore, when reviewing the treatment literature for this purpose, it is not only important to examine the dual effects of the treatment on each set of problems, but to also examine the extent to which specific components of the treatment might impact each set of symptoms. Well-conceptualized research designs, particularly those that include relevant control conditions, can be more helpful in this regard.

Two previous reviews of outcome studies for behavior therapies for co-occurring substance use and mood disorders [35, 91] have concluded that a number of evidence-based therapies for substance use disorders, particularly, cognitive-behavioral or relapse prevention therapies, not only impact on substance use, but also have been shown to have broad effects on physical, social, and mental health. What is unclear is whether these secondary outcomes are the result of exposure to generic therapeutic principles that might also have beneficial effects in other domains of life, whether they are real secondary outcomes of reduction in substance use, or they are necessary outcomes for effective substance use treatment, thus suggesting that substance use might be consequential to these other changes.

With respect to substance dependence and depression more specifically, three well-controlled randomized trials involving substance using patients with elevated levels of depression shed some light on this issue. In one study, alcohol-dependent patients with elevated depressive symptom profiles received either an eight-session CBT for depression (CBT-D) or a relaxation training control in addition to their attendance at a partial-day hospitalization program for alcohol dependence [92]. This study showed that over and above traditional addiction treatment and the relaxation control, the CBT-D condition was associated with more enhanced and sustained recovery from depressive symptoms, as well as reductions in drinking. Similarly, a re-analysis of a randomized controlled trial of CBT and desipramine for cocaine-dependent individuals showed that in those patients with elevated levels of depression, CBT was associated with longer periods of abstinence and improved treatment retention [93]. Finally, a CBT that included mood management strategies was significantly more effective than a 12-step treatment approach for cocaine-dependent patients with a history of major depression [94]. The findings from these three well-controlled randomized trials suggest that some of the variance in substance-related behavior in patients with comorbid substance dependence and depressive symptoms is consequential to the depressive symptoms.

Summary and Conclusions

Multiple findings have documented the importance of examining comorbid depression and SUD. These include their increased prevalence, associated impairment, and the increased risk for social and occupational impairment later in adulthood. Clinical studies have generated lifetime co-occurrence rates between 8 and 25% of SUD and depressive disorders, with females overrepresented [95, 96]. Epidemiological samples highlight similar associations albeit at slightly lower prevalence rates [11]. Prospective studies allow for opportunities to examine whether one domain is a causal risk factor of the other. However, there are conflicting findings with regard to the causal relationship of depression and SUD, with predictive associations varying according to gender, type of substance assessed, and age of onset of disorder. Knowledge of antecedents would enable identification of adolescents at risk and provide information for the development of preventative interventions. Personality risk factors such as neuroticism and impulsivity are often associated with both depression and SUD [56, 58, 67]. A modest influence for genetic transmission has been found, with males showing a larger genetic influence than females [74]. Environmental risk factors contribute to both depression and SUD independently, but research is lacking in the consideration of genetic influences on the susceptibility to environmental risks in relation to comorbid depression and SUD. Treatment of depression and SUD encompasses psychotherapeutic and psychopharmological interventions. Most behavioral treatment studies involving substance-using patients show evidence of desistence of depressive symptoms as well reductions in alcohol and drug use [92, 93]. The field has now moved beyond examining the extent of the co-occurrence of depression and SUD to asking questions about the nature of these associations and their etiological links. Future research investigating the underlying mechanisms of influence will necessarily involve integrating a range of interdisciplinary approaches. Furthermore, these integrative studies should be considered within the context of developmental change.

References

1. American Psychiatric Association. Diagnostic and statistical manual of mental health disorders. 4th ed. Washington DC: Author; 1994.
2. Libby AM, Orton HD, Stover SK, Riggs PD. What came first, major depression or substance use disorder? Clinical characteristics and substance use comparing teens in a treatment cohort. Addict Behav. 2005;30:1649–62.
3. Becker DF, Grilo CM. Prediction of drug and alcohol abuse in hospitalized adolescents: comparisons by gender and substance type. Behav Res Ther. 2006;44:1431–40.
4. Karlsson L, Pelkonen M, Ruuttu T, Kiviruusu O, Heilä H, Holi M, Kettunen K, Tuisku V, Tuulio-Henriksson A, Törrönen J, Marttunen M. Current comorbidity among consecutive adolescent psychiatric outpatients with DSM-IV mood disorders. Eur Child Adolesc Psychiatry. 2006;15:220–31.
5. Clark DB, Pollock N, Bukstein OG, Mezzich AC, Bromberger JT, Donovan JE. Gender and comorbid psychopathology in adolescents with alcohol dependence. J Am Acad Child Adolesc Psychiatry. 1997;36:1195–203.
6. Chinet L, Plancherel B, Bolognini M, Bernard M, Laget J, Daniele G, Halfon O. Substance use and depression. Comparative course in adolescents. Eur Child Adolesc Psychiatry. 2006;15:149–55.
7. Merikangas K, Gelernter C. Comorbidity for alcoholism and depression. Psychiatr Clin North Am. 1990;13:613–32.
8. Rohde P, Lewinsohn PM, Seeley JR. Comorbidity of unipolar depression: II. Comorbidity with other mental disorders in adolescents and adults. J Abnorm Psychol. 1991;100:214–22.
9. Kessler RC, Nelson CB, McGonagle KA, Edlund MJ, Frank RG, Leaf PJ. The epidemiology of co-occurring addictive and mental disorders. Am J Orthopsychiatry. 1996;66:17–31.
10. Reiger DA, Farmer ME, Rae DS, Locke BZ, Keith SJ, Judd LL, Goodwin FK. Comorbidity of mental disorders with alcohol and other drug abuse: results from the Epidemiologic Catchment area (ECA) study. JAMA. 2000;264:2511–8.
11. Grant BF, Stinson FS, Dawson DA, Chou P, Dufour MC, Compton W, Pickering RP, Kaplan K. Prevalence and co-occurrence of substance use disorders and independent mood and anxiety disorders. Arch Gen Psychiatry. 2004;61:807–16.
12. Haynes JC, Farrell M, Singleton N, Meltzer H, Araya R, Lewis G, Wiles NJ. Alcohol consumption as a risk factor for anxiety and depression: results from the longitudinal follow-up of the National Psychiatric Morbidity Survey. Br J Psychiatry. 2005;187:544–51.
13. Kessler RC, Crum RM, Warner LA, Nelson CB, Schulenberg J, Anthony JC. The lifetime co-occurrence of DSM-III-R alcohol abuse and dependence with other psychiatric disorders in the National Comorbidity Survey. Arch Gen Psychiatry. 1997;54: 313–21.
14. Costello JE, Erkanli A, Federman E, Angold A. Development of Psychiatric comorbidity with substance abuse in adolescents: effects of timing and sex. J Clin Child Psychol. 1999;28: 298–311.
15. Dierker LC, Avenevoli SA, Merikangas KR, Flaherty BP, Stolar M. Association between psychiatric disorders and the progression of tobacco use behaviors. J Am Acad Child Adolesc Psychiatry. 2001;40:1159–67.
16. Costello JE, Mustillo S, Erkanli A, Keeler G, Angold A. Prevalence and development of psychiatric disorders in childhood and adolescence. Arch Gen Psychiatry. 2003;60:837–44.
17. Fergusson DM, Goodwin RD, Horwood LJ. Major depression and cigarette smoking: results of a 21-year longitudinal study. Psychol Med. 2003;33:1357–67.
18. Sung M, Erkanli A, Angold A, Costello EJ. Effects of age at first substance use and psychiatric comorbidity on the development of substance use disorders. Drug Alcohol Depend. 2004;75:287–99.
19. Measelle JR, Stice E, Hogansen JM. Developmental trajectories of co-occurring depressive, eating, anti-social and substance abuse problems in female adolescents. J Abnorm Psychol. 2006;115: 524–38.
20. Hayatbakhsh MR, Najman JM, Jamrozik K, Mumun AA, Alati R, Bor W. Cannabis and anxiety and depression in young adults: a large prospective study. J Am Acad Child Adolesc Psychiatry. 2007;46:408–17.
21. Pardini D, Raskin White H, Stouthamer-Loeber M. Early adolescent psychopathology as a predictor of alcohol use disorders by young adulthood. Drug Alcohol Depend. 2007;88S:S38–49.
22. Boyle MH, Offord DR. Psychiatric disorder and substance use in adolescence. Can J Psychiatry. 1991;36:699–705.
23. Angold A, Costello EJ, Erkanli A, Worthman CM. Pubertal changes in hormonal levels and depression in girls. Psychol Med. 1999;29:1043–53.
24. Eley TC, Stevenson J. Using genetic analyses to clarify the distinction between depressive and anxious symptoms in children and adolescents. J Abnorm Child Psychol. 1999;27:105–14.
25. Scourfield J, Rice F, Thapar A, Harold GT, Martin N, McGuffin P. Depressive symptoms in children and adolescents: changing aetiological influences with development. J Child Psychol Psychiatry. 2003;44:968–76.
26. Yorbik O, Birmaher B, Axelson D, Williamson DE, Ryan ND. Clinical characteristics of depressive symptoms in children and adolescents with major depressive disorder. J Clin Psychiatry. 2004;65:1654–9.
27. Keenan K, Loeber R, Green S. Conduct disorder in girls: a review of the literature. Clin Child Fam Psychol Rev. 1999;2:3–19.

28. Smith LA, Foxcroft DR. Drinking in the UK: an exploration of trends. York: Joseph Rowntree Foundation; 2009.

29. McGue M, Slutske W, Iacono WG. Personality and substance use disorders: II. Alcoholism versus drug use disorders. J Consult Clin Psychol. 1999;67:394–404.

30. Landheim AS, Bakken K, Vaglum P. Impact of comorbid psychiatric disorders on the outcome of substance abusers: a six year prospective follow-up in two Norwegian counties. BMC Psychiatry. 2006;6:44.

31. Swahn MH, Bossarte RM, Sullivent EE. Age of alcohol use initiation, suicidal behavior, and peer and dating violence victimization and perpetration among high-risk, seventh-grade adolescents. Pediatrics. 2008;121:297–305.

32. McGue M, Iacono WG. The association of early adolescent problem behavior with adult psychopathology. Am J Psychiatry. 2005;162:1118–24.

33. Mueser KT, Drake RE, Wallach MA. Dual diagnosis: a review of etiological theories. Addict Behav. 1998;23:717–34.

34. Krueger RF, Hicks BM, Patrick CJ, Carlson SR, Iacono WG, McGue M. Etiological connections among substance dependence, antisocial behavior and personality: modeling the externalizing spectrum. J Abnorm Psychol. 2002;111:411–24.

35. Conrod PJ, Stewart S. A critical look at dual-focused cognitive-behavioral treatments for comorbid substance use and psychiatric disorders: strengths, limitations, and future directions. J Cogn Psychother. 2005;19:261–84.

36. Brook DW, Brook J, Zhang C, Cohen P, Whiteman M. Drug use and the risk of major depressive disorder, alcohol dependence, and substance use disorders. Arch Gen Psychiatry. 2002;59:1039–44.

37. Fergusson DM, Boden JM, Horwood LJ. Test of causal links between alcohol abuse or dependence and major depression. Arch Gen Psychiatry. 2009;66:260–6.

38. Kendler KS, Prescott CA, Myers J, Neale MC. The structure of genetic and environmental risk factors for common psychiatric and substance use disorders in men and women. Arch Gen Psychiatry. 2003;60:929–37.

39. Khantzian EJ. The self-medication hypothesis of addictive disorders: focus on heroin and cocaine dependence. Am J Psychiatry. 1985;142:1259–64.

40. Greeley J, Oei T. Alcohol and tension reduction. In: Leonard KE, Blane HT, editors. Psychological theories of drinking and alcoholism. New York: Guilford; 1999. p. 14–53.

41. Sher K, Levenson R. Risk for alcoholism and individual differences in the stress-response-dampening effect of alcohol. J Abnorm Psychol. 1982;91:350–67.

42. King SM, Iacono WG, McGue M. Childhood internalizing and internalizing psychopathology in the prediction of early substance use. Addiction. 2004;99:1548–9.

43. Sihvola E, Rose RJ, Dick DM, Pulkkinen L, Marttunen M, Kaprio J. Early onset depressive disorders predict the use of addictive substances in adolescence: a prospective study of adolescent Finnish twins. Addiction. 2008;103:2045–53.

44. Marmorstein NR. Longitudinal associations between alcohol problems and depressive symptoms: early adolescence through early adulthood. Alcohol Clin Exp Res. 2009;33:49–59.

45. Loeber R, Stouthamer-Loeber M, Raskin-White. Developmental aspects of delinquency and internalizing problems and their association with persistent juvenile substance use between ages 7 and 18. J Clin Child Psychol. 1999;28:322–32.

46. Degenhault L, Hall W, Lynskey M. Exploring the association between cannabis use and depression. Addiction. 2003;98: 1493–504.

47. Wittchen HU, Frohlich C, Behrendt S, Gunther A, Rehm J, Zimmermann P, Lieb R, Perkonigg A. Cannabis use and cannabis use disorders and their relationship to mental disorders: a 10-year prospective longitudinal community study in adolescents. Drug Alcohol Depend. 2007;88S:S60–70.

48. Schuckit MA. Comorbidity between substance use disorders and psychiatric conditions. Addiction. 2006;101:76–88.

49. Brown SA, Inaba RK, Gillin JC, Schuckit MA, Stewart MA, Irwin MR. Alcoholism and affective disorder: clinical course of depressive symptoms. Am J Psychiatry. 1995;152:45–52.

50. Bovasso GB. Cannabis abuse as a risk factor for depressive symptoms. Am J Psychiatry. 2001;158:2033–7.

51. Agosti V, Levin F. The effects of alcohol and drug dependence on the course of depression. Am J Addict. 2006;15:71–5.

52. Paljärvi T, Koskenvuo M, Poikolainen K, Kauhanen J, Sillanmäki L, Mäkelä P. Binge drinking and depressive symptoms: a 5-year population-based cohort study. Addiction. 2009;104:1168–78.

53. Brook JS, Cohen P, Brook DW. Longitudinal study of co-occurring psychiatric disorders and substance use. J Am Acad Child Adolesc Psychiatry. 1998;37:322–30.

54. Patton GC, Coffey C, Carlin JB, Degenhardt L, Lynskey M, Hall W. Cannabis use and mental health in young people: cohort study. Br Med J. 2002;325:1195–8.

55. Hussong AM, Hicks RE, Levy SA, Curran PJ. Specifying the relations between affect and heavy alcohol use among young adults. J Abnorm Psychol. 2001;110:449–61.

56. Jackson KM, Sher KJ. Alcohol use disorder and psychological distress: a prospective state-trait analysis. J Abnorm Psychol. 2003;112:599–613.

57. Fleming CB, Masan WA, Mazza JJ, Abott RD, Catalano RF. Latent growth internal of the relationship between depressive symptoms and substance use during adolescence. Psychol Addict Behav. 2008;22:186–97.

58. Mackie CJ, Castellanos-Ryan N, Conrod PJ. Personality moderates the longitudinal relationship between psychological symptoms and alcohol use in adolescents. Alcohol Clin Exp Res. 2011;35(4):703–16.

59. Wills TA, Sandy JM, Shinar O, Yaeger A. Contributions of positive and negative affect to adolescent substance use: test of a bidimensional model in a longitudinal study. Psychol Addict Behav. 1999;13:327–38.

60. Krueger RF, Caspi A, Moffitt TE. Epidemiological personology: the unifying role of personality in population-based research on problem behaviors. J Pers. 2000;68:967–98.

61. Elkins IJ, McGue M, Malone S, Iacono WG. The effect of parental alcohol and drug disorders on adolescent personality. Am J Psychiatry. 2004;161:670–76.

62. Caspi A, Moffitt TE, Newman DL, Silva PA. Behavioural observations at the age of 3 years predict adults psychiatric disorders: longitudinal evidence from a birth cohort. Arch Gen Psychiatry. 1996;53:1033–9.

63. Cox BJ, McWilliams LA, Enns MW, Clara IP. Broad and specific personality dimensions associated with major depression in a nationally representative sample. Compr Psychiatry. 2004;45: 246–53.

64. Eysenck BG, Eysenck HJ. Personality differences between prisoners and controls. Psychol Rep. 1977;40:1023–8.

65. Costa PT, McCrae RR. Normal personality assessment in clinical practice: the NEO Personality Inventory. Psychol Assess. 1992; 4:5–13.

66. Clark LA, Watson D. Tripartite model of anxiety and depression: psychometric evidence and taxonomic implications. J Abnorm Psychol. 1991;100:316–36.

67. Fergusson DM, Woodward LJ. Mental health, educational and social role outcomes of depressed adolescents. Arch Gen Psychiatry. 2002;59:225–31.

68. Conrod PJ, Pihl RO, Stewart SH, Dongier M. Validation of a system of classifying female substance abusers on the basis of personality

and motivational risk factors for substance abuse. Psychol Addict Behav. 2000;14:243–56.

69. Woicik PA, Stewart SH, Pihl RO, Conrod PJ. The Substance Use Risk Profile Scale: a scale measuring traits linked to reinforcement-specific substance use profiles. Addict Behav. 2009;34:1042–55.

70. Jaffee WB, D'Zurilla TJ. Personality, problem solving, and adolescent substance use. Behav Ther. 2009;40:93–101.

71. Clark DB. Serum tryptophan ratio and suicidal behavior in adolescents: a prospective study. Psychol Res. 2003;119:199–204.

72. Winokur G, Coryell W. Familial alcoholism in primary unipolar major depressive disorder. Am J Psychiatry. 1991;148:184–8.

73. Kendler KS, Neale MC, Kessler RC, Heath AC, Eaves LJ. A longitudinal twin study of personality and major depression in women. Arch Gen Psychiatry. 1993;50:853–62.

74. Prescott CA, Aggen SH, Kendler KS. Sex-specific genetic influences on the comorbidity of alcoholism and major depression in a population-based sample of US twins. Arch Gen Psychiatry. 2000;57:803–11.

75. Kendler KS, Prescott CA. Genes, environment, and psychopathology: understanding the causes of psychiatric and substance use disorders. New York: Guilford; 2006.

76. Lyons MJ, Schultz M, Neale M, Brady K, Eisen S, Toomey R, Rhein A, Faraone S, Tsuang M. Specificity of familial vulnerability for alcoholism versus major depression in men. J Nerv Ment Dis. 2006;194:809–17.

77. Dick DM, Foroud T. Candidate genes for alcohol dependence: a review of genetic evidence from human studies. Alcohol Clin Exp Res. 2003;27:868–79.

78. Enoch M. Genetic and environmental influences on the development of alcoholism. Resilience vs. risk. Ann NY Acad Sci. 2006;1094:193–201.

79. Greenberg BD, Li Q, Lucas FR, Hu S, Sirota LA, Benjamin J, Lesch K-P, Hamer D, Murphy DL. Association between the serotonin transporter promoter polymorphism and personality traits in a primarily female population sample. Am J Med Genet. 2000;96:202–16.

80. Armeli S, Connor TS, Covault J, Tennen H, Kranzler HR. A serotonin transporter gene polymorphism (5-HTTLPR), drinking to cope motivation, and negative life events among college students. J Stud Alcohol Drugs. 2008;69:814–26.

81. Clark DB, de Bellis MD, Lynch KG, Cornelius JR, Martin CS. Physical and sexual abuse, depression and alcohol use disorders in adolescents: onsets and outcomes. Drug Alcohol Depend. 2005;69:51–60.

82. Sartor CE, Lynskey MT, Heath AC, Jacob T, True W. The role of childhood risk factors in initiation of alcohol use and progression to alcohol dependence. Addiction. 2007;102:216–25.

83. Wakschlag L, Pickett K, Cook E, Benowitz N, Leventhal B. Maternal smoking during pregnancy and severe antisocial behavior in offspring: a review. Am J Public Health. 2002;92:966–74.

84. O'Connor TG, Ben-Shlomo Y, Heron J, Golding J, Adams D, Glover V. Prenatal anxiety predicts individual differences in cortisol in pre-adolescent children. Biol Psychiatry. 2005;58:211–7.

85. Patton GC, McMorris BJ, Toumbourou JW, Hemphill SA, Donath S, Catalano RF. Puberty and the onset of substance use and abuse. Pediatrics. 2004;114:e300–6.

86. Walden B, McGue M, Iacono WG, Burt SA, Elkins I. Identifying shared environmental contributions to early substance use: the respective roles of peers and parents. J Abnorm Psychol. 2004;113:440–50.

87. Curran PJ, Stice E, Chassin L. The relation between adolescent alcohol use and peer alcohol use: a longitudinal random coefficients model. J Consult Clin Psychol. 1997;65:130–40.

88. Feske U, Tarter RE, Kirisci L, Gao Z, Reynolds M, Vanyukov M. Peer environment mediates parental history and individual risk in the etiology of cannabis use disorders in boys: a 10-year prospective study. Am J Drug Alcohol Abuse. 2008;34:307–20.

89. Miller-Johnson S, Lochman JE, Coie JD, Terry R, Hyman C. Comorbidity of conduct and depressive problems at sixth grade: substance use outcomes across adolescence. J Abnorm Child Psychol. 1998;26:221–32.

90. Marmorstein NR, Icono WG. Major depression and conduct disorder in a twin sample: gender, functioning, and risk for future psychopathology. J Am Acad Child Adolesc Psychiatry. 2003;42:225–33.

91. Carroll KM. Behavioural therapies for co-occurring substance use and mood disorders. Biol Disord. 2004;56:778–84.

92. Brown RA, Evans DM, Miller IW, Burgess ES, Mueller TI. Cognitive-behavioural treatment for depression in alcoholism. J Consult Clin Psychol. 1997;65:715–26.

93. Carroll KM, Nich C, Rounsaville BJ. Differential symptom reduction in depressed cocaine abusers treated with psychotherapy and pharmacotherapy. J Nerv Ment Dis. 1995;183:251–9.

94. Maude-Griffin PM, Hohenstein JM, Humfleet GL, Reilly PM, Tusel DJ, Hall SM. Superior efficacy of cognitive-behavioural therapy for urban crack cocaine abusers: main and matching effects. J Consult Clin Psychol. 1998;66:832–7.

95. Melartin TK, Rytsälä HJ, Leskelä US, Lestelä-Mielonen PS, Sokero TS, Isometsä ET. Current comorbidity of psychiatric disorders among DSM-IV major depressive disorder patients in psychiatric care in the Vantaa Depression Study. J Clin Psychiatry. 2002;63:126–34.

96. Grant BF, Harford TC. Comorbidity between DSM-IV alcohol use disorders and major depression: results of a national survey. Drug Alcohol Depend. 1995;39:197–206.

97. Swendsen JD, Merikangas KR. The comorbidity of depression and substance use disorder. Clin Psychol Rev. 2000;20:173–89.

98. Armstrong TD, Costello EJ. Community studies on adolescent substance use, abuse, or dependence and psychiatric comorbidity. J Consult Clin Psychol. 2002;70:1224–39.

99. Cerdá M, Sagdeo A, Galea S. Comorbid forms of psychopathology: key patterns and future research directions. Epidemiol Rev. 2008;30:155–77.

ADHD

Pieter-Jan Carpentier

Abstract

Attention deficit/hyperactivity disorder (ADHD) is a chronic illness that begins in childhood and is characterized by inattention, hyperactivity, and impulsivity. In adulthood, ADHD is an invalidating illness, often with psychiatric comorbidity, including substance abuse and addiction. In children and adults, ADHD is very treatable. Medication forms the basis of treatment, with psychostimulants as the first choice. Additional cognitive therapy and coaching are necessary to help patients improve their functioning and organizational skills.

The high prevalence of ADHD in adults with substance use disorders (SUDs) points to the causal role of the disorder in the development of addiction. Many patients with ADHD and SUDs have a history of childhood behavioral problems, with early initiation of drug use and a more severe addiction course. ADHD has a negative influence on the course of SUDs. Until now, the diagnosis and treatment of ADHD has received too little attention in this patient group. The limited number of controlled trials showed that ADHD in combination with SUDs is more difficult to treat with medication and that treatment for the ADHD hardly has any influence on the course of addiction. However, there is evidence that early treatment of ADHD has a preventive effect on the development of addiction.

When treating this patient group with psychostimulants, it is important to bear in mind the risk of abuse of the medication. Further research is necessary to optimize the treatment of ADHD and comorbid SUDs.

Learning Objectives
- ADHD is a common and highly treatable disorder in children and adults, typically presenting with psychiatric comorbidity
- ADHD is a risk factor in the development of addiction; treatment for ADHD in childhood might have a preventive effect
- ADHD is common in adults with SUDs, and has a negative influence on the course of the addiction
- Treatment with psychostimulants involves the risk of misuse that should preferably be avoided by prescribing modern drug formulations or curtailed by making strict agreements
- Pharmacotherapy for ADHD is less effective in adults with SUDs

P.-J. Carpentier (✉)
Reinier van Arkel groep,
PO Box 70058, 5201DZ's Hertogenbosch
e-mail: P.carpentier@rvagroep.nl

J.C. Verster et al. (eds.), *Drug Abuse and Addiction in Medical Illness: Causes, Consequences and Treatment,*
DOI 10.1007/978-1-4614-3375-0_22, © Springer Science+Business Media, LLC 2012

Issues that Need to Be Addressed for Future Research

- Firstly, more studies should confirm that ADHD in patients with various SUDs can be treated effectively
- More extensive research is also necessary to identify the reasons why pharmacotherapy for ADHD is less effective in addicted patients (e.g. clarify the influence of long-term substance use)
- Additional knowledge can provide important indications to optimize the treatment of ADHD (e.g. the relevance of tailored psychosocial interventions)
- More systematic studies are needed on the influence of effective treatment of ADHD on addiction, in order to identify significant prognostic factors

Introduction

Attention deficit/hyperactivity disorder (ADHD) in children was first described at the beginning of the twentieth century. The positive effect of psychostimulants was discovered as early as in 1937, and these drugs have been used to treat children for almost half a century [1]. In contrast, the adult manifestations of ADHD have only been receiving attention over the past 20 years. ADHD in adulthood is an invalidating but quite treatable condition that in conformity with childhood ADHD is often accompanied by other psychiatric disorders. This chapter mainly describes the association with substance use disorders (SUDs) and the consequences of this association on the treatment of the two disorders.

ADHD in Adults

Definition

The disorder characterized by the chronic presence of concentration problems, restlessness, and/or impulsiveness in children has been described under various names in the medical literature and is presently defined as ADHD in the DSM-IV-TR [2]. This internationally accepted definition denotes that the symptoms are present from a young age and cause problems in two or more settings. The disorder has a chronic course. In 30–60% of the cases, the complaints and symptoms remain problematic into adulthood. However, it appears that hyperactivity and impulsivity are remitting sooner with age than the concentration problems [3].

Prevalence

ADHD has been diagnosed in children and adults in all racial groups that have been studied. In children, ADHD is the most common psychiatric illness, with a prevalence of between 3% and 12% [4, 5]. The illness is diagnosed two to four times more often in boys than in girls. In adults, the worldwide prevalence has recently been estimated to be 3.4% (range 1.2–7.3%) on the basis of an overview of international publications [6]. Higher prevalences have been found in specific populations, for example, detainees, psychiatric patients, and patients with addiction problems [7–10].

Clinical Characteristics

A striking characteristic of ADHD in adults is that in the majority of cases, the illness has not been previously diagnosed or treated. Patients tend to underreport their complaints. Owing to the chronic course of the illness, patients become used to the symptoms and have learned to compensate for them. In many cases, the illness is not immediately apparent, because the most obvious symptom, motor restlessness, is the first to remit [3, 11]. More characteristic is the underachievement that marks the lives of the majority of patients [12]. Adults with ADHD are commonly unable to perform at the level of their (intellectual) abilities, while failures in different fields are typical in their life stories [13]. Although patients do attribute these features to themselves, the chronic dysfunction is often not the primary reason to seek psychiatric help.

The clinical symptoms in adults are varied (see Table 22.1) and changeable: it is distinctive that these patients do not function at a constant level. ADHD is a disorder of performance, not of skill; it is not a disorder of knowing what to do, but of doing what one knows [15]. Patients have great difficulty with organizing and structuring their activities. They appear to function better in a structured environment, but also have great difficulty with routine and monotonous tasks. The concentration problems (such as easily becoming distracted, forgetfulness) occur particularly during monotonous, time-consuming (i.e. mentally frustrating) tasks. The motor unrest usually changes with age into inner restlessness and rapid boredom [16].

Comorbidity is a marked clinical feature of childhood and adult ADHD [17]. It has been estimated that up to 87% of adults with ADHD have one or more comorbid psychiatric disorders [18]. The most frequent disorders include: mood disturbances (depressive disorder, seasonal affective disorder, and bipolar disorder), anxiety disorders, addictions, and personality disorders. Many patients with an autistic spectrum disorder also have ADHD characteristics [19].

Table 22.1 Proposed age-specific diagnostic criteria for ADHD in adults[a]

1. Is often easily distracted by extraneous stimuli
2. Often make decisions impulsively
3. Often has difficulty stopping activities or behavior when he/she should
4. Often starts a project or task without carefully reading or listening to directions
5. Often shows poor follow-through on promises or commitments made to others
6. Often has trouble doing things in their proper order or sequence
7. Is often more likely to drive a motor vehicle much faster than others (excessive speeding)
   [For nondrivers, substitute this item:
   "Often has difficulty engaging in leisure activities or doing fun things quietly."]
8. Often has difficulty sustaining attention in tasks or play activities (optional)
9. Often has difficulty organizing tasks and activities (optional)

[a]Complaints and symptoms that were most specific to adults with ADHD identified on the basis of a comparative study on ADHD patients ($N = 142$), psychiatric patients, ($N = 97$), and a control group ($N = 109$) [14]

Table 22.2 Diagnosis of ADHD in adults according to the DSM-IV-TR criteria

1. Symptoms beginning in childhood (before the age of 7 years)
2. As a child:
   – A minimum of 6/9 DSM-IV-TR criteria of attention deficit and/or hyperactivity/impulsivity
   – Leading to significant dysfunctioning in different settings (home, school)
3. Continuous presence of the symptoms over the course of time, with persistent dysfunctioning
4. At the time of testing:
   – A minimum of 5/9 DSM-IV-TR criteria of attention deficit and/or hyperactivity/impulsiveness
   – With significant dysfunction

Etiology

ADHD is a neurobehavioral disorder with genetic, environmental, and biological etiologies. Primarily, ADHD is a multifactorially determined hereditary disorder. In monozygotic twins, concordance is 60–80%, while in heterozygotic twins, concordance is 30% [20]. Between 10% and 35% of the immediate family members of children with ADHD are also likely to have the disorder. When one of the parents has ADHD, the chance of ADHD in the children is up to 57% [21]. Until now, molecular genetic studies have only revealed a limited number of candidate genes, each of which makes no more than a small contribution to the development of the disorder. A number of these genes are involved in dopamine and serotonin neurotransmission [20]. Recent genome-wide association studies has also identified genes that are involved in neural cell growth and metabolism [22].

Presently, little is known about how these genes interact with each other and with environmental factors in the development of the disorder. It is also unclear which environmental factors play a protective role or aggregative role. Although it has been established that ADHD is not caused by negative circumstances in the upbringing or traumatization, these factors are expected to have a negative influence on existing vulnerability. This also applies to neurotoxic influences (lead poisoning) and other forms of brain damage (perinatal brain damage, traumatic brain injury) [23].

Imaging techniques in ADHD patients have chiefly revealed abnormalities in the frontal, prefrontal, and subcortical parts of the brain [24]. Currently, it is impossible to capture the clinical entity of ADHD in a single neuropsychological model. The most widely accepted neuropsychological explanation model for ADHD focuses on disruption of the executive functions, which can be demonstrated in many of the patients. The executive functions of the brain are responsible for planning and organization of purposeful behavior in response to incoming stimuli. As a result of too little inhibition of unimportant stimuli, problems arise in the regulation and control of planned behavior [15]. Another current theory (delay aversion) focuses on the difficulty ADHD patients have with maintaining long-term goals and postponing rewards. They are far more likely to target immediate gratification than delayed rewards [25].

Prognosis

If left untreated, adult ADHD is characterized by chronic dysfunctioning and can cause significant personal, social, and economic problems that negatively influence overall quality of life [13]. Owing to the often thoughtless, irresponsible, and unhealthy behavior, this group is at greater risk of material problems (unemployment, poor finances) and health problems [26]. Additional dilemmas are caused by the comorbid psychiatric disorders that are commonly present.

Diagnostic Assessment

The basis of the diagnosis of ADHD in adulthood is to establish the lifelong presence of distressing concentration problems, restlessness, and/or impulsivity (Table 22.2). This means that the diagnosis is not so much determined by the clinical symptoms, but by anamnestic information that should preferably be obtained from multiple sources. As has already been stated earlier, the patient is not always the best informant. More clarity about the severity of the disturbance can be obtained from the partner, while the parents or family members can provide more information about the presence of symptoms in childhood [11, 27]. The lack of validated age-specific criteria for adults is an important obstacle in the rapid recognition of the illness (also see Table 22.1) [14].

Table 22.3 Medication choice in the treatment of ADHD in adults

Order of precedence	Name	Usual dosage range	N daily doses	References
1	Methylphenidate	0.5–1.0 mg/kg/day	4–5 (IR)	[34–37]
	Dextroamphetamine	0.25–0.50 mg/kg/day	3–4 (IR)	[38–41]
2	Atomoxetine	80–100 mg/day	1–2	[42, 43]
3	Bupropion	300–450 mg/day	1–2	[44]
4	TCA: desipramine	100–200 mg/day	1–2	[45]
	imipramine	50–150 mg/day		
5	Venlafaxine	75–225 mg/day	1–2	[46]
	Modafinil	200–400 mg/day	1	[38]
	Moclobemide	300–600 mg/day	3	[47]

IR immediate release

Consequently, the clinical diagnosis is still being based on DSM-IV-TR criteria that were developed for children (Table 22.2). A number of screening and diagnostic instruments have been developed, including the well-known Conners rating scale [28]. Lacking in specificity and sensitivity for diagnostic purposes, neuropsychological testing offers little additional value [11]. Lastly, assessing psychiatric comorbidity is an integral and indispensable part of the diagnostic procedure [12].

Treatment

ADHD is quite treatable in children and good results have also been reported in adults (without comorbid psychiatric problems) [29, 30]. Extensive patient education about the illness, the causes and consequences is a fixed component of successful treatment [27, 31]. As is also the case in children, medication forms the basis of the treatment [32]; in many cases medication will lead to stabilization of the ADHD symptoms. Essentially, adults receive the same types of medication as children. The activity of these drugs has not been studied as extensively as in children but guidelines are starting to emerge [27, 33]. Two specific psychostimulants, methylphenidate (MPH) and dextroamphetamine (or dexamphetamine), are still the first choice (Table 22.3) [48]. Their effectivity in children and adults has been documented in several controlled trials [49, 50]. Although less effective in adults than in children, they can decrease the hyperactivity and impulsivity as well as improve the concentration problems. Small differences in working mechanism of these drugs in improving dopamine neurotransmission can explain why some patients do not respond to one drug, but experience great benefit from the other [48, 51]. The side effects are actually fairly mild (anorexia, palpitations, headaches) without long-term toxicity. The short duration of effectiveness of the two drugs (MPH: 3–4 h, dextroamphetamine: 4–5 h) places high demands on the therapy compliance of the patient. Their immediate but short effect is also the foundation of their abuse potential; therapeutic use of psychostimulants is subject to controlling laws in most countries. To a large extent it is possible to solve both problems of lack of compliance and risk of misuse by using reliable MPH slow-release formulations (Concerta, with a duration of action of up to 12 h, Equasym and Medikinet working up to 8 h). Long-action dexamphetamine formulations are not available in Europe. However, lisdexamfetamine, currently in use in the USA, will shortly be released on the European market. It is a prodrug that comprises dexamphetamine conjugated to the amino acid lysine. After oral administration, the prodrug is activated in the gastrointestinal tract by splitting off lysine and releasing the active substance dexamphetamine. Because of the need for metabolic activation, this product has a reduced potential for parenteral abuse [52].

Alternatives to these drugs are atomoxetine that chiefly acts on noradrenergic neurotransmission [42] and bupropion that also acts dopaminergically [44]. The clinical impression is that these substances are less effective than the stimulants [43], particularly with regard to the concentration problems. Further options for pharmacological treatment are limited. Double-blind studies have documented a positive effect of tricyclic antidepressants (particularly desipramine) [45], but these medications often have to be discontinued owing to bothersome side effects. The positive effect of modafinil in one smaller controlled study [38] has not yet been replicated. Efficacy of venlafaxine [46] and moclobemide [47] has only been reported in case reports or open studies. Monoamine oxidase inhibitors (MAOI) have hardly been studied in adult ADHD [53] and are seldom used because of their potential for serious adverse reactions and drug interactions. In the past, clonidine was prescribed for children with ADHD, but this drug has become less popular due to limited effectiveness and negative side effects. Another current medication strategy is to combine drugs with different mechanisms of action [48].

In the majority of patients, pharmacotherapy alone is insufficient; they derive great benefit from additional cognitive therapy or psychosocial interventions (especially in the form of coaching), aimed at helping them to cope with their ADHD and learn skills in the fields of planning and organization [54–57]. Coaching is a collaborative relationship between the patient and a professional to develop strategies for managing problems such as procrastination, time management, and organization. These therapies also have scope for emotional themes, such as coping with the disappointments and failures that result from the disorder [31, 58]. Offering these treatments in group form enables mutual recognition and the exchange of experiences. It is also recommended to involve the patient's partner in the treatment.

ADHD and Addiction

Prevalence

In adult as well as in childhood ADHD, psychiatric comorbidity determines clinical presentation and treatment strategy to a large extent. The SUDs belong to the most frequently occurring problems in adults with ADHD: in some studies, the life-time prevalence rates of substance abuse and dependence were as high as 52% [59]. ADHD has consistently been found in a substantial minority of addicted patients. Although higher rates were found in the early studies [60] (probably as a result of less strict criteria), more recent research (based on DSM-IV criteria) has revealed a prevalence in SUD patients of between 10% and 24% [61–64]. A trend seems visible in which the prevalence of the combination increases with the severity of the disorders: the more severe the ADHD, the greater the chance of addiction and vice versa.

Clinical Characteristics

In the majority of addicted patients, the diagnosis of ADHD has never been made previously; thus, they have never received treatment for ADHD. Contrary to what has often been assumed, SUD patients with ADHD do not seem to have a selective preference for stimulants (cocaine, amphetamines); they also use sedatives (soft drugs, alcohol and heroine) [63]. It is common to encounter polydrug abuse. Some patients reported paradoxical effects of stimulant use (amphetamines, cocaine): they became calm and bright instead of driven and agitated. These findings are a strong indication of ADHD, but do not form proof of the diagnosis: not all patients with ADHD react to psychostimulants in this way and in addition, the higher dosages have a predominantly stimulant effect.

Many patients with ADHD and SUDs have a history of serious behavioral problems in childhood: 40% to even 93% of these patients conformed with the diagnosis of the

oppositional defiant disorder (ODD) and/or conduct disorder (CD) in their youth [64, 65]. In addition, many of them have an antisocial personality disorder (ASP): research showed a prevalence of 50% [64], compared to 25% in SUD patients without ADHD. Another characteristic of this patient population is early initiation of substance use, most often before the age of 20 years and not unusually before the age of 15 years [66]. There are indications that the presence of ADHD accelerates the transitions from use to abuse to dependence and the progression to hard drugs [67].

Etiology

The elevated association between ADHD and SUDs can be seen as the product of developmental interactions with ADHD symptoms (e.g. impulsivity or behavioral dysregulation) and the consequences of ADHD (e.g. poor academic achievement), which increase the opportunity for the development of SUDs. Genetic factors have a strong influence in these interactions. ADHD and addiction are to a large extent genetically determined. Moreover, ADHD seems to occur more frequently in the families of addicted patients, while SUDs occur more frequently in the families of ADHD patients [60]. Patterns revealed by familial risk analyses suggested that the association between ADHD and alcohol dependence is most consistent with the hypothesis of independent genetic transmission of these disorders, whereas the association between ADHD and drug dependence is best explained by the hypothesis of variable expressivity of a common risk factor [68]. This seems to indicate a common genetic basis for ADHD and addiction, in which dopamine neurotransmission most springs to mind, because it plays a role in both ADHD and SUDs [20, 69, 70].

Behavioral problems in childhood (ODD and CD), which are often combined with ADHD, have an even stronger influence: it has been known for some time that these disorders strongly increase the risk of addiction problems in adulthood [71]. Some authors hold the view that this is the principal (if not the only) explanation for the association between ADHD and addiction; it is not the ADHD that plays a causal role in the development of the addiction, but the serious behavioral problems which are often accompanied by ADHD [72]. This might also explain the negative influence of ADHD on the prognosis of addiction. In practice, the combination of ADHD and CD is chiefly found in patients with severe SUDs (particularly hard-drug addiction): many of them also have an antisocial personality disorder (ASP) [64, 65, 73].

Other research has shown sufficient evidence that ADHD alone is a risk factor for the development of addiction. It is likely that the more severe forms of the disorder involve greater risk; this is in agreement with the finding that persistent ADHD in adulthood is more commonly combined with addiction problems than ADHD in childhood alone [74]. In addition, the risk seems to be more closely associated with the hyperactive/impulsive symptoms than with the concentration problems [75]. The self-medication hypothesis has often been cited in this connection [76, 77]. According to this explanation model, patients with a psychiatric disorder use substances in an attempt to influence their psychiatric symptoms and control them. In practice, many ADHD patients will mention this type of experience, even spontaneously: particularly the fact that substance use makes them feel calmer is given as the reason for (continued) substance use. This working mechanism, which has not yet been studied systematically, might play a prominent role in the development of problematic substance use.

Secondary problems that often occur in ADHD (such as frequent failure and demoralization) and other comorbid disorders (such as depression and anxiety disorders) can increase the vulnerability towards addiction even further [60]. In summary, ADHD can be considered as a moderately serious risk factor for the development of addiction, with the possibility of early recognition and good treatability as important advantages.

Prognosis

Studies have shown that in patients with untreated ADHD, the course of addiction is more difficult; these patients seem to derive less benefit from treatment, show poorer treatment compliance, and have greater difficulty with achieving and maintaining abstinence [78, 79]. It is possible that the instability caused by the ADHD symptoms contributes to earlier substance use relapse. In addition, the ADHD cannot be treated adequately until the addiction has been stabilized. Therefore, the two disorders need to be treated together, preferably in an integrated approach.

Diagnosis

A careful diagnostic assessment is certainly recommended in addicted ADHD patients. The psychiatric comorbidity that is to be expected in these patients can also give rise to differential diagnostic problems. Another diagnostic issue is that the ADHD symptomatology can be masked or even mimicked by symptoms of intoxication or withdrawal [80]. Although abstinence at the time of assessment is clearly preferable, it is still possible to reliably diagnose ADHD in nonabstinent patients. As mentioned earlier, the diagnosis is not based primarily on clinical findings, but chiefly on anamnestic information that supports the lifelong presence of concentration problems, restlessness, and impulsivity. Special attention

must therefore be focused on the presence of ADHD symptoms in childhood (before the initiation of drug use) and in periods of abstinence and/or periods of relatively stable substance use [81]. Bringing in other informants (partner, parents, family) can help to clarify the picture [11]. To accurately judge the severity of the ADHD symptomatology (and in the case of persistent diagnostic uncertainty) it is recommended to repeat the evaluation after stable abstinence has been achieved [60].

Treatment

Treatment Planning

As patients with ADHD and SUDs have multiple problems that are complicated by further comorbidity (mood disturbances, anxiety disorders, personality disorders), it is important to draw up a detailed treatment plan in advance in order to approach these complex problems in a systematic and integrated manner. In the majority of cases, abstinence will be the first step in the treatment. Subsequent treatment aims at stabilization of the psychiatric situation, usually by means of symptomatic treatment of the psychiatric comorbidity, mostly by using medication. ADHD medication can be considered at this point. When patients are sufficiently stable, a start can be made on the more extensive treatment of the addiction (relapse prevention) and psychiatric comorbidity (e.g. treatment for the personality disorder or anxiety disorder). In this phase, the psychotherapeutic and psychosocial treatment of ADHD can be initiated.

The Importance of Abstinence

In principle, abstinence is a necessary precondition for the treatment of ADHD. Persistent substance use will have a negative effect on the medication, either directly through interference on neurotransmitter level or indirectly due to reduced treatment compliance and irregular medication intake. In addition, possible positive effects of the medication might be masked by substance use [58]. Another problem is the risk of dangerous interactions between medication and psychoactive drugs (although this does not seem to be too detrimental in the case of psychostimulants) [82]. If the patient is unable to remain abstinent with outpatient support, inpatient detoxification should be considered.

In the past, medication was not started until after long-term abstinence, in order to totally exclude interference from the addiction. The disadvantage of this approach is that after detoxification, many patients experience more trouble from their ADHD symptoms, which makes it difficult for them to remain abstinent and engage in therapy. Particularly on the basis of clinical experience, it is now advised to start ADHD medication shortly after detoxification [60, 81]. This approach can also be applied to outpatient patients who are not too

Table 22.4 Randomized controlled trials of ADHD medication in SUD patients

Study, year (ref)	Sample size	SUD type	Medication (dose)	Effect on ADHD[a]	Effect on SUD[a]
Schubiner et al., 2002 [84]	48	Cocaine	Methylphenidate 3×30 mg	+	0
Riggs et al., 2004 [85]	69	Various	Pemolide 75–112.5 mg	+	0
Carpentier et.al., 2005 [86]	25	Various	Methylphenidate 3×15 mg	0	
Levin et al., 2006 [87]	98	Opioid (MMT)	Methylphenidate 2×20–40 mg SR	0	0
Levin et al., 2007 [88]	106	Cocaine	Methylphenidate 40+20 mg SR	0	0 (+)
Wilens et al., 2008 [89]	72+75	Alcohol	Atomoxetine 25–100 mg	++	+
Thurstone, 2010 [90]	70	Various	Atomoxetine 25–100 mg	0	0
Konstenius, 2010 [91]	24	Amfetamine	Methylphenidate (OROS) 72 mg	0	0

[a]Symbols used to indicate effectiveness

MMT methadone maintenance treatment, *SR* slow release formulation (duration of action 4–6 h)

0—no significant difference

+/++/+++—strength of the difference (when positive effect of active treatment)

severely addicted and who are motivated to stop their substance use; in these cases, the attempts to achieve abstinence and medication intake can be launched simultaneously.

Efficacy of Medication

There are still no widely accepted guidelines for the appropriate pharmacological treatment of ADHD in the presence of SUDs [83]. In principle, the same medication is prescribed as that for ADHD adults without SUDs [58]. Although positive results have been published in case reports and open studies, convincing scientific evidence of the effectiveness of these types of medication in this patient group is still lacking [50]. Over the years only a limited number of placebo-controlled trials have been conducted and they were hardly able to demonstrate any positive effect (Table 22.4). Only one recent study on atomoxetine in patients with alcohol addiction has produced more positive results [89]. These negative results are surprising, because, as highlighted before, ADHD is considered to be eminently treatable, both in children and in adults, with robust effectiveness of pharmacotherapy in placebo-controlled trials [30].

More research is necessary to confirm the assumed causes of these negative results. Firstly, there is the influence of the psychiatric comorbidity; the best results have always been achieved in patients with a definite diagnosis of (genetically determined) ADHD without comorbidity; patients with addiction problems are usually excluded from controlled trials [34, 42]. In patients with more complex problems, diagnostic inaccuracy is more likely to occur. The ADHD symptoms can be caused or aggravated by other disorders

(e.g. traumatic brain injury), which would explain a decreased effectiveness of the medication. In addition, it is quite plausible that the long-term use of psychoactive substances reduces the effectiveness of the medication due to constant interaction with the same neurotransmitter systems [92]. In most of the outpatient studies mentioned earlier, abstinence was not maintained [84, 87, 88]. The studies on stimulants were conducted with older formulations that were less reliable [87, 88]. Furthermore, inadequate dosages of the medication played a role [86]. On the basis of case reports, there is evidence that (some) ADHD patients with addiction need a higher dosage as a result of their substance use. The type of addiction may play a role: there is speculation that ADHD in patients with alcohol use disorders responds better to medication [89]. The placebo response in ADHD medication trials is usually limited (to about 25% of the participants) [48] and is lower than in mood disturbances or anxiety disorders. However, when the effectiveness of the active drug is fairly low, even a limited placebo response will make it more difficult to demonstrate a significant difference.

Based on these considerations, the best results of pharmacotherapy will be seen in patients with a clear ADHD diagnosis with limited or stable comorbidity, during stable abstinence and using modern formulations: hardly the conditions one expects when treating complex patients with chronic addictions. The combination of ADHD and addiction is frequently a complex constellation, so it is hardly surprising that a single therapeutic factor (in this case, medication) is unable to have a significant impact.

Psychostimulant Diversion and Abuse

The risk of diversion and abuse of psychostimulants in the treatment of ADHD forms an important consideration in SUD patients. When prescribing psychostimulants, the treating physician must be prepared for abuse by the patient and/ or others nearby. In animal experiments, methylphenidate showed characteristics similar to cocaine [93]. Although it has euphoric activity, this effect does not occur when therapeutic dosages are taken orally; higher dosages are necessary with faster absorption by the body via the intranasal or intravenous route. Regular use of therapeutic dosages does not lead to misuse or addiction [94].

It is possible to avoid the risk of diversion and abuse in various ways. Abuse potential is significantly lower (and therapy compliance is clearly better) when longer acting psychostimulant formulations are prescribed. However, these longer acting formulations are yet not widely available. The same applies for lisdexamfetamine and for atomoxetine, which lacks abuse potential [95]. As the other pharmacological alternatives (mentioned previously) are seldom as effective, it may be necessary to prescribe the traditional short-acting psychostimulant formulations. A safe strategy is to prescribe these medications under strict conditions only and to discontinue prescription when these conditions are not met. A central issue is a reliable working alliance with the patient: the patient must be informed about the risks of the medication and agree to the conditions of its use. Obviously, there must be no doubt about the diagnosis of ADHD. Continued prescription of the medication should only take place after a trial period with convincing effectiveness of the medication. In cooperation with the pharmacy, the medication is dispensed in small quantities. It is recommended to involve a person who is close to the patient, in order to supervise the correct and regular intake of the medication. Abstinence during treatment is not only a precondition for optimal effectiveness, but also provides a means to measure the commitment of the patient to the therapy. The same applies to meeting appointments and participating in treatment. Under these circumstances, psychostimulants can be used fairly safely by this patient group. Moreover, the above-mentioned controlled studies have demonstrated that psychostimulant use does not lead to an increase in substance use [96]. However, it is also important to be aware of the poor therapy compliance associated with multiple dosages per day to be taken at fixed times [97].

Although the psychostimulants methylphenidate and dexamphetamine have documented abuse potential, there is very little evidence that these drugs, in the formulations prescribed to treat ADHD, are abused in any widespread manner. According to the literature and clinical experience, it is comparatively rare for the psychostimulants prescribed for ADHD to lead to clinically significant levels of abuse or dependence [98]. However, more large-scale problems seem to be related to the misuse and diversion of these drugs to individuals who do not have ADHD. This diversion is usually associated with efforts to increase concentration and attention, often times in competitive academic environments [99, 100].

Choice of Medication

The choice of medication not only depends on the characteristics and circumstances of the patient, but also on the pharmacotherapeutics available. In conformity with adult ADHD patients without addiction, psychostimulants still are the medication of first choice, despite the lack of hard evidence about their effectiveness. As mentioned earlier, the modern long-action formulations take clear preference, whereas the short-action formulations should only be prescribed under the above-described conditions. If the conditions are not met, other choices are atomoxetine (if available) or bupropion. Further alternatives (with decreasing efficacy) are the tricyclic antidepressants or venlafaxine.

Owing to the limited effectiveness of the medication, it is important to closely monitor the treatment and to optimize the treatment circumstances. Frequent checkups are necessary to strengthen the working alliance as well as to safeguard abstinence and correct medication intake. Good integration of the pharmacotherapy in the overall treatment strategy will be advantageous to compliance.

Other Treatment

Besides medication treatment, further psychotherapy and psychosocial support are certainly indicated in patients with ADHD and SUDs to preserve the prospect of stabilizing the two disorders [58]. Appropriate treatment, such as relapse prevention, is necessary to maintain abstinence. Preferably, the cognitive treatment and coaching of ADHD should be tailored to the unhealthy aspects of the patient's life style, with extensive attention to the role of substance use. This kind of specific treatment for the combination of ADHD and addiction has not yet been developed for general use and will be scarcely available.

The Influence of ADHD Treatment on the Addiction

In principle, effective treatment of the ADHD can be expected to have a positive effect on the prognosis of the addiction: patients are more stable and controlled, which should help them to engage in treatment and maintain abstinence. A number of case reports illustrated the impressive progress made by some addicted patients after effective treatment of their ADHD [101–103]. However, very little research has been conducted into the effect of treatment for ADHD on the prognosis of the addiction. In as far as the controlled trials addressed this topic, they hardly showed any positive influence on the course of the addiction [84, 87–89] (Table 22.4).

A more realistic view holds that effective treatment of ADHD will be feasible in many addicted patients, without having any direct positive influence on the addiction. Such an assumption is based on the results achieved in other addicted patients with different comorbid psychiatric disorders (such as mood disturbances and anxiety disorders) [104, 105]. Active treatment alleviates the comorbid disorder, but does not directly influence the SUD [106]. This classic pattern in dual diagnosis treatment can also be expected to apply to ADHD.

In spite of these limited expectations, there are enough convincing arguments to continue to actively identify and treat ADHD in SUD patients. Addiction is a multicausal disorder that has many more influencing factors, but in which improvement of ADHD can help to tip the balance in a positive direction.

Prevention

In the majority of cases, ADHD precedes the addiction. Therefore, the question arises as to whether effective treatment of the ADHD in childhood influences the increased risk of SUDs in these patients. At the same time, there is concern about the late effects of the use of psychostimulants in childhood. Animal studies drew attention to the potentially increased risk of psychoactive drug use as a result of exposure to psychostimulants in childhood through the mechanism of sensitization that increases the reinforcing effects of the drug [107]. Fortunately, scientific research has not found any evidence of this. Moreover, a meta-analysis on several follow-up studies gave clear indications that pharmacotherapy of ADHD in childhood (i.e. with psychostimulants) reduced the risk of addiction in adulthood [108]. These important findings were not confirmed in longer term follow-up [109]; however, it should be emphasized that in this naturalistic study after 10 years only 22% of the original patient group were still actively receiving treatment, which is not an optimal situation to demonstrate the protective effect of treatment. In all these longitudinal studies, there were hardly ever indications that treatment of ADHD with psychostimulants in childhood increased the risk of addiction [96]. All these findings link up well with the important role that ADHD seems to play in the initiation of substance use and the development of addiction. This might explain why treatment of ADHD appears to have less influence on an existing SUD; the greatest benefit would be achieved though prevention, before the addiction has fully developed. The possible preventive influence of ADHD treatment on the addiction risk is another reason to identify and treat ADHD at a young age.

Conclusion

In research as well as in clinical practice, ADHD in SUD patients is still an underexposed diagnosis. Despite the fact that this condition is very treatable in children and adults, until now it has not been possible to sufficiently demonstrate the effectiveness of treatment in this adult patient group by means of controlled studies. Furthermore, the expected positive (albeit limited) effect on the course of the addiction still needs to be confirmed. In anticipation of further research, more attention to this disorder in clinical practice may provide indications for the improvement of treatment and for clearer determination of the importance of ADHD in the diagnosis and treatment of addicted patients.

References

1. Bradley C. The behavior of children receiving benzedrine. Am J Psychiatry. 1937;94:577–85.
2. Barkley RA. Primary symptoms, diagnostic criteria, prevalence and gender differences. In: Barkley RA, editor. Attention-deficit hyperactivity disorder: a handbook for diagnosis and treatment. New York: Guilford; 2006. p. 76–121.
3. Mick E, Faraone SV, Biederman J. Age-dependent expression of attention-deficit/hyperactivity disorder symptoms. Psychiatr Clin North Am. 2004;27(2):215–24.
4. Faraone SV, Sergeant J, Gillberg C, Biederman J. The worldwide prevalence of ADHD: is it an American condition? World Psychiatry. 2003;2(2):104–13.
5. Polanczyk G, de Lima MS, Horta BL, Biederman J, Rohde LA. The worldwide prevalence of ADHD: a systematic review and metaregression analysis. Am J Psychiatry. 2007;164(6):942–8.
6. Fayyad J, de GR, Kessler R, Alonso J, Angermeyer M, Demyttenaere K, de GG, Haro JM, Karam EG, Lara C, Lepine JP, Ormel J, Posada-Villa J, Zaslavsky AM, Jin R. Cross-national prevalence and correlates of adult attention-deficit hyperactivity disorder. Br J Psychiatry. 2007;190:402–9.
7. Rosler M, Retz W, Retz-Junginger P, Hengesch G, Schneider M, Supprian T, Schwitzgebel P, Pinhard K, Dovi-Akue N, Wender P, Thome J. Prevalence of attention deficit-/hyperactivity disorder (ADHD) and comorbid disorders in young male prison inmates. Eur Arch Psychiatry Clin Neurosci. 2004;254(6):365–71.
8. Rosler M, Retz W, Yaqoobi K, Burg E, Retz-Junginger P. Attention deficit/hyperactivity disorder in female offenders: prevalence, psychiatric comorbidity and psychosocial implications. Eur Arch Psychiatry Clin Neurosci. 2008;259(2):98–105.
9. Almeida Montes LG, Hernandez Garcia AO, Ricardo-Garcell J. ADHD prevalence in adult outpatients with nonpsychotic psychiatric illnesses. J Atten Disord. 2007;11(2):150–6
10. Nylander L, Holmqvist M, Gustafson L, Gillberg C. ADHD in adult psychiatry. Minimum rates and clinical presentation in general psychiatry outpatients. Nord J Psychiatry. 2008;1–8
11. Murphy KR, Gordon M. Assessment of adults with ADHD. In: Barkley RA, editor. Attention-deficit hyperactivity disorder: a handbook for diagnosis and treatment. New York: Guilford; 2006. p. 425–52.

12. Adler L, Cohen J. Diagnosis and evaluation of adults with attention-deficit/hyperactivity disorder. Psychiatr Clin North Am. 2004;27(2):187–201.

13. Biederman J, Petty CR, Fried R, Kaiser R, Dolan CR, Schoenfeld S, Doyle AE, Seidman LJ, Faraone SV. Educational and occupational underattainment in adults with attention-deficit/hyperactivity disorder: a controlled study. J Clin Psychiatry. 2008;69(8):1217–22.

14. Barkley RA, Murphy KR, Fischer M. ADHD in adults: what the science says. New York: Guilford; 2008.

15. Barkley RA. A theory of ADHD. In: Barkley RA, editor. Attention-deficit hyperactivity disorder: a handbook for diagnosis and treatment. New York: Guilford; 2006. p. 297–336.

16. Barkley RA. ADHD in adults: developmental course and outcome of children withADHD, and ADHD in clinic-referred adults. In: Barklay RA, editor. Attention-deficit hyperactivity disorder: a handbook for diagnosis and treatment. New York: Guilford; 2006. p. 248–96.

17. Spencer TJ, Biederman J, Mick E. Attention-deficit/hyperactivity disorder: diagnosis, lifespan, comorbidities, and neurobiology. Ambul Pediatr. 2007;7(1 Suppl):73–81.

18. McGough JJ, Smalley SL, McCracken JT, Yang M, Del'Homme M, Lynn DE, Loo S. Psychiatric comorbidity in adult attention deficit hyperactivity disorder: findings from multiplex families. Am J Psychiatry. 2005;162(9):1621–7.

19. Holtmann M, Bolte S, Poustka F. Attention deficit hyperactivity disorder symptoms in pervasive developmental disorders: association with autistic behavior domains and coexisting psychopathology. Psychopathology. 2007;40(3):172–7.

20. Faraone SV, Perlis RH, Doyle AE, Smoller JW, Goralnick JJ, Holmgren MA, Sklar P. Molecular genetics of attention-deficit/hyperactivity disorder. Biol Psychiatry. 2005;57(11):1313–23.

21. Biederman J, Faraone SV, Mick E, Spencer T, Wilens T, Kiely K, Guite J, Ablon JS, Reed E, Warburton R. High risk for attention deficit hyperactivity disorder among children of parents with childhood onset of the disorder: a pilot study. Am J Psychiatry. 1995;152(3):431–5.

22. Lasky-Su J, Neale BM, Franke B, Anney RJ, Zhou K, Maller JB, Vasquez AA, Chen W, Asherson P, Buitelaar J, Banaschewski T, Ebstein R, Gill M, Miranda A, Mulas F, Oades RD, Roeyers H, Rothenberger A, Sergeant J, Sonuga-Barke E, Steinhausen HC, Taylor E, Daly M, Laird N, Lange C, Faraone SV. Genome-wide association scan of quantitative traits for attention deficit hyperactivity disorder identifies novel associations and confirms candidate gene associations. Am J Med Genet B Neuropsychiatr Genet. 2008;147(8):1345–54.

23. Barkley RA. Etiologies. In: Barkley RA, editor. Attention-deficit hyperactivity disorder: a handbook for diagnosis and treatment. New York: Guilford; 2006. p. 219–47.

24. Bush G, Valera EM, Seidman LJ. Functional neuroimaging of attention-deficit/hyperactivity disorder: a review and suggested future directions. Biol Psychiatry. 2005;57(11):1273–84.

25. Sonuga-Barke EJ, Sergeant JA, Nigg J, Willcutt E. Executive dysfunction and delay aversion in attention deficit hyperactivity disorder: nosologic and diagnostic implications. Child Adolesc Psychiatr Clin N Am. 2008;17(2):367–84, ix.

26. Goodman DW. The consequences of attention-deficit/hyperactivity disorder in adults. J Psychiatr Pract. 2007;13(5):318–27.

27. Gibbins C, Weiss M. Clinical recommendations in current practice guidelines for diagnosis and treatment of ADHD in adults. Curr Psychiatry Rep. 2007;9(5):420–6.

28. Conners CK. Clinical use of rating scales in diagnosis and treatment of attention-deficit/hyperactivity disorder. Pediatr Clin North Am 1999;46(5):857–70, vi.

29. Spencer TJ. ADHD treatment across the life cycle. J Clin Psychiatry 2004; 65 Suppl:322–6.

30. Biederman J, Faraone SV. Attention-deficit hyperactivity disorder. Lancet. 2005;366(9481):237–48.

31. Murphy K. Psychosocial treatments for ADHD in teens and adults: a practice-friendly review. J Clin Psychol. 2005;61(5):607–19.

32. A 14-month randomized clinical trial of treatment strategies for attention-deficit/hyperactivity disorder. The MTA Cooperative Group. Multimodal Treatment Study of Children with ADHD. Arch Gen Psychiatry. 1999;56(12):1073–86.

33. Attention deficit hyperactivity disorder; diagnosis and management of ADHD in children, young people and adults. National clinical practice guideline (NICE) 72. London, Royal College of Psychiatrists, 2009.

34. Spencer T, Wilens T, Biederman J, Faraone SV, Ablon JS, Lapey K. A double-blind, crossover comparison of methylphenidate and placebo in adults with childhood-onset attention-deficit hyperactivity disorder. Arch Gen Psychiatry. 1995;52(6):434–43.

35. Kooij JJ, Burger H, Boonstra AM, Van der Linden PD, Kalma LE, Buitelaar JK. Efficacy and safety of methylphenidate in 45 adults with attention-deficit/hyperactivity disorder. A randomized placebo-controlled double-blind cross-over trial. Psychol Med. 2004;34(6):973–82.

36. Spencer T, Biederman J, Wilens T, Doyle R, Surman C, Prince J, Mick E, Aleardi M, Herzig K, Faraone S. A large, double-blind, randomized clinical trial of methylphenidate in the treatment of adults with attention-deficit/hyperactivity disorder. Biol Psychiatry. 2005;57(5):456–63.

37. Biederman J, Mick E, Surman C, Doyle R, Hammerness P, Harpold T, Dunkel S, Dougherty M, Aleardi M, Spencer T. A randomized, placebo-controlled trial of OROS methylphenidate in adults with attention-deficit/hyperactivity disorder. Biol Psychiatry. 2006;59(9):829–35.

38. Taylor FB, Russo J. Efficacy of modafinil compared to dextroamphetamine for the treatment of attention deficit hyperactivity disorder in adults. J Child Adolesc Psychopharmacol. 2000;10(4):311–20.

39. Paterson R, Douglas C, Hallmayer J, Hagan M, Krupenia Z. A randomised, double-blind, placebo-controlled trial of dexamphetamine in adults with attention deficit hyperactivity disorder. Aust NZ J Psychiatry. 1999;33(4):494–502.

40. Spencer T, Biederman J, Wilens T, Faraone S, Prince J, Gerard K, Doyle R, Parekh A, Kagan J, Bearman SK. Efficacy of a mixed amphetamine salts compound in adults with attention-deficit/hyperactivity disorder. Arch Gen Psychiatry. 2001;58(8):775–82.

41. Taylor FB, Russo J. Comparing guanfacine and dextroamphetamine for the treatment of adult attention-deficit/hyperactivity disorder. J Clin Psychopharmacol. 2001;21(2):223–8.

42. Michelson D, Adler L, Spencer T, Reimherr FW, West SA, Allen AJ, Kelsey D, Wernicke J, Dietrich A, Milton D. Atomoxetine in adults with ADHD: two randomized, placebo-controlled studies. Biol Psychiatry. 2003;53(2):112–20.

43. Newcorn JH, Kratochvil CJ, Allen AJ, Casat CD, Ruff DD, Moore RJ, Michelson D. Atomoxetine and osmotically released methylphenidate for the treatment of attention deficit hyperactivity disorder: acute comparison and differential response. Am J Psychiatry. 2008;165(6):721–30.

44. Wilens TE, Spencer TJ, Biederman J, Girard K, Doyle R, Prince J, Polisner D, Solhkhah R, Comeau S, Monuteaux MC, Parekh A. A controlled clinical trial of bupropion for attention deficit hyperactivity disorder in adults. Am J Psychiatry. 2001;158(2):282–8.

45. Wilens TE, Biederman J, Prince J, Spencer TJ, Faraone SV, Warburton R, Schleifer D, Harding M, Linehan C, Geller D. Six-week, double-blind, placebo-controlled study of desipramine for adult attention deficit hyperactivity disorder. Am J Psychiatry. 1996;153(9):1147–53.

46. Findling RL, Schwartz MA, Flannery DJ, Manos MJ. Venlafaxine in adults with attention-deficit/hyperactivity disorder: an open clinical trial. J Clin Psychiatry. 1996;57(5):184–9.

47. Vaiva G, De Lenclave MB, Bailly D. Treatment of comorbid opiate addiction and attention-deficit hyperactivity disorder (residual type) with moclobemide: a case report. Prog Neuropsychopharmacol Biol Psychiatry. 2002;26(3):609–11.

48. Prince JB, Wilens TE, Spencer TJ, Biederman J. Pharmacotherapy of ADHD in adults. In: Barkley RA, editor. Attention-deficit hyperactivity disorder: a handbook for diagnosis and treatment. New York: Guilford; 2006. p. 704–36.

49. Faraone SV, Spencer T, Aleardi M, Pagano C, Biederman J. Meta-analysis of the efficacy of methylphenidate for treating adult attention-deficit/hyperactivity disorder. J Clin Psychopharmacol. 2004;24(1):24–9.

50. Koesters M, Becker T, Kilian R, Fegert JM. Weinmann S (2008) Limits of meta-analysis: methylphenidate in the treatment of adult attention-deficit hyperactivity disorder. J Psychopharmacol. 2008;23(7):733–44.

51. Pliszka SR, Browne RG, Olvera RL, Wynne SK. A double-blind, placebo-controlled study of Adderall and methylphenidate in the treatment of attention-deficit/hyperactivity disorder. J Am Acad Child Adolesc Psychiatry. 2000;39(5):619–26.

52. Faraone SV. Lisdexamfetamine dimesylate: the first long-acting prodrug stimulant treatment for attention deficit/hyperactivity disorder. Expert Opin Pharmacother. 2008;9(9):1565–74.

53. Ernst M, Liebenauer LL, Jons PH, Tebeka D, Cohen RM, Zametkin AJ. Selegiline in adults with attention deficit hyperactivity disorder: clinical efficacy and safety. Psychopharmacol Bull. 1996;32(3):327–34.

54. Safren SA, Sprich S, Chulvick S, Otto MW. Psychosocial treatments for adults with attention-deficit/hyperactivity disorder. Psychiatr Clin North Am. 2004;27(2):349–60.

55. Safren SA, Sprich S, Mimiaga MJ, Surman C, Knouse L, Groves M, Otto MW. Cognitive behavioral therapy vs relaxation with educational support for medication-treated adults with ADHD and persistent symptoms: a randomized controlled trial. JAMA. 2010;304(8):875–80.

56. Knouse LE, Cooper-Vince C, Sprich S, Safren SA. Recent developments in the psychosocial treatment of adult ADHD. Expert Rev Neurother. 2008;8(10):1537–48.

57. Solanto MV, Marks DJ, Wasserstein J, Mitchell K, Abikoff H, Alvir JM, Kofman MD. Efficacy of meta-cognitive therapy for adult ADHD. Am J Psychiatry. 2010;167(8):958–68.

58. Mariani JJ, Levin FR. Treatment strategies for co-occurring ADHD and substance use disorders. Am J Addict. 2007;16 Suppl:145–54.

59. Biederman J, Wilens T, Mick E, Milberger S, Spencer TJ, Faraone SV. Psychoactive substance use disorders in adults with attention deficit hyperactivity disorder (ADHD): effects of ADHD and psychiatric comorbidity. Am J Psychiatry. 1995;152(11):1652–8.

60. Wilens TE. Attention-deficit/hyperactivity disorder and the substance use disorders: the nature of the relationship, subtypes at risk, and treatment issues. Psychiatr Clin North Am. 2004;27(2):283–301.

61. Levin FR, Evans SM, Kleber HD. Prevalence of adult attention-deficit hyperactivity disorder among cocaine abusers seeking treatment. Drug Alcohol Depend. 1998;52(1):15–25.

62. King VL, Brooner RK, Kidorf MS, Stoller KB, Mirsky AF. Attention deficit hyperactivity disorder and treatment outcome in opioid abusers entering treatment. J Nerv Ment Dis. 1999;187(8):487–95.

63. Clure C, Brady KT, Saladin ME, Johnson D, Waid R, Rittenbury M. Attention-deficit/hyperactivity disorder and substance use: symptom pattern and drug choice. Am J Drug Alcohol Abuse. 1999;25(3):441–8.

64. Schubiner H, Tzelepis A, Milberger S, Lockhart N, Kruger M, Kelley BJ, Schoener EP. Prevalence of attention-deficit/hyperactivity disorder and conduct disorder among substance abusers. J Clin Psychiatry. 2000;61(4):244–51.

65. Carroll KM, Rounsaville BJ. History and significance of childhood attention deficit disorder in treatment-seeking cocaine abusers. Compr Psychiatry. 1993;34(2):75–82.

66. Wilens TE, Biederman J, Mick E, Faraone SV, Spencer T. Attention deficit hyperactivity disorder (ADHD) is associated with early onset substance use disorders. J Nerv Ment Dis. 1997;185(8):475–82.

67. Biederman J, Wilens TE, Mick E, Faraone SV, Spencer T. Does attention-deficit hyperactivity disorder impact the developmental course of drug and alcohol abuse and dependence? Biol Psychiatry. 1998;44(4):269–73.

68. Biederman J, Petty CR, Wilens TE, Fraire MG, Purcell CA, Mick E, Monuteaux MC, Faraone SV. Familial risk analyses of attention deficit hyperactivity disorder and substance use disorders. Am J Psychiatry. 2008;165(1):107–15.

69. Kalivas PW, Volkow ND. The neural basis of addiction: a pathology of motivation and choice. Am J Psychiatry. 2005;162(8): 1403–13.

70. Volkow ND, Wang GJ, Kollins SH, Wigal TL, Newcorn JH, Telang F, Fowler JS, Zhu W, Logan J, Ma Y, Pradhan K, Wong C, Swanson JM. Evaluating dopamine reward pathway in ADHD: clinical implications. JAMA. 2009;302(10):1084–91.

71. Kim-Cohen J, Caspi A, Moffitt TE, Harrington H, Milne BJ, Poulton R. Prior juvenile diagnoses in adults with mental disorder: developmental follow-back of a prospective-longitudinal cohort. Arch Gen Psychiatry. 2003;60(7):709–17.

72. Lynskey MT, Hall W. Attention deficit hyperactivity disorder and substance use disorders: is there a causal link? Addiction. 2001;96(6):815–22.

73. Carpentier PJ, van Gogh MT, Knapen LMJ, Buitelaar J, De Jong CA. Influence of ADHD and Conduct Disorder on opioid dependence severity and psychiatric comorbidity in chronic methadone maintained patients. Eur Addict Res. 2011;17(1):10–20.

74. Wilens TE, Biederman J. Alcohol, drugs, and attention-deficit/hyperactivity disorder: a model for the study of addictions in youth. J Psychopharmacol. 2006;20(4):580–8.

75. Elkins IJ, McGue M, Iacono WG. Prospective effects of attention-deficit/hyperactivity disorder, conduct disorder, and sex on adolescent substance use and abuse. Arch Gen Psychiatry. 2007;64(10):1145–52.

76. Khantzian EJ. The self-medication hypothesis of addictive disorders: focus on heroin and cocaine dependence. Am J Psychiatry. 1985;142(11):1259–64.

77. Khantzian EJ. The self-medication hypothesis of substance use disorders: a reconsideration and recent applications. Harv Rev Psychiatry. 1997;4(5):231–44.

78. Levin FR, Evans SM, Vosburg SK, Horton T, Brooks D, Ng J. Impact of attention-deficit hyperactivity disorder and other psychopathology on treatment retention among cocaine abusers in a therapeutic community. Addict Behav. 2004;29(9):1875–82.

79. Wilens TE, Biederman J, Mick E. Does ADHD affect the course of substance abuse? Findings from a sample of adults with and without ADHD. Am J Addict. 1998;7(2):156–63.

80. Levin FR. Diagnosing attention-deficit/hyperactivity disorder in patients with substance use disorder. J Clin Psychiatry. 2007;68(Suppl):119–14.

81. Schubiner H. Substance abuse in patients with attention-deficit hyperactivity disorder: therapeutic implications. CNS Drugs. 2005;19(8):643–55.

82. Winhusen T, Somoza E, Singal BM, Harrer J, Apparaju S, Mezinskis J, Desai P, Elkashef A, Chiang CN, Horn P. Methylphenidate and cocaine: a placebo-controlled drug interaction study. Pharmacol Biochem Behav. 2006;85(1):29–38.

83. Wilson JJ, Levin FR. Attention deficit hyperactivity disorder (ADHD) and substance use disorders. Curr Psychiatry Rep. 2001;3(6):497–506.

84. Schubiner H, Saules KK, Arfken CL, Johanson CE, Schuster CR, Lockhart N, Edwards A, Donlin J, Pihlgren E. Double-blind placebo-controlled trial of methylphenidate in the treatment of adult ADHD patients with comorbid cocaine dependence. Exp Clin Psychopharmacol. 2002;10(3):286–94.

85. Riggs PD, Hall SK, Mikulich-Gilbertson SK, Lohman M, Kayser A. A randomized controlled trial of pemoline for attention-deficit/hyperactivity disorder in substance-abusing adolescents. J Am Acad Child Adolesc Psychiatry. 2004;43(4):420–9.

86. Carpentier PJ, de Jong CA, Dijkstra BA, Verbrugge CA, Krabbe PF. A controlled trial of methylphenidate in adults with attention deficit/hyperactivity disorder and substance use disorders. Addiction. 2005;100(12):1868–74.

87. Levin FR, Evans SM, Brooks DJ, Kalbag AS, Garawi F, Nunes EV. Treatment of methadone-maintained patients with adult ADHD: double-blind comparison of methylphenidate, bupropion and placebo. Drug Alcohol Depend. 2006;81(2):137–48.

88. Levin FR, Evans SM, Brooks DJ, Garawi F. Treatment of cocaine dependent treatment seekers with adult ADHD: double-blind comparison of methylphenidate and placebo. Drug Alcohol Depend. 2007;87(1):20–9.

89. Wilens TE, Adler LA, Weiss MD, Michelson D, Ramsey JL, Moore RJ, Renard D, Brady KT, Trzepacz PT, Schuh LM, Ahrbecker LM, Levine LR. Atomoxetine treatment of adults with ADHD and comorbid alcohol use disorders. Drug Alcohol Depend. 2008;96(1–2):145–54.

90. Thurstone C, Riggs PD, Salomonsen-Sautel S, Mikulich-Gilbertson SK. Randomized, controlled trial of atomoxetine for attention-deficit/hyperactivity disorder in adolescents with substance use disorder. J Am Acad Child Adolesc Psychiatry. 2010;49(6):573–82.

91. Konstenius M, Jayaram-Lindstrom N, Beck O, Franck J. Sustained release methylphenidate for the treatment of ADHD in amphetamine abusers: a pilot study. Drug Alcohol Depend. 2010;108(1–2):130–3.

92. Thomas MJ, Kalivas PW, Shaham Y. Neuroplasticity in the mesolimbic dopamine system and cocaine addiction. Br J Pharmacol. 2008;154(2):327–42.

93. Kollins SH. A qualitative review of issues arising in the use of psycho-stimulant medications in patients with ADHD and co-morbid substance use disorders. Curr Med Res Opin. 2008;24(5):1345–57.

94. Volkow ND, Swanson JM. Variables that affect the clinical use and abuse of methylphenidate in the treatment of ADHD. Am J Psychiatry. 2003;160(11):1909–18.

95. Jasinski DR, Faries DE, Moore RJ, Schuh LM, Allen AJ. Abuse liability assessment of atomoxetine in a drug-abusing population. Drug Alcohol Depend. 2008;95(1–2):140–6.

96. Wilens TE, Monuteaux MC, Snyder LE, Moore H, Whitley J, Gignac M. The clinical dilemma of using medications in substance-abusing adolescents and adults with attention-deficit/hyperactivity disorder: what does the literature tell us? J Child Adolesc Psychopharmacol. 2005;15(5):787–98.

97. Swanson J. Compliance with stimulants for attention-deficit/hyperactivity disorder: issues and approaches for improvement. CNS Drugs. 2003;17(2):117–31.

98. Kollins SH. ADHD, substance use disorders, and psychostimulant treatment: current literature and treatment guidelines. J Atten Disord. 2008;12(2):115–25.

99. Wilens TE, Adler LA, Adams J, Sgambati S, Rotrosen J, Sawtelle R, Utzinger L, Fusillo S. Misuse and diversion of stimulants prescribed for ADHD: a systematic review of the literature. J Am Acad Child Adolesc Psychiatry. 2008;47(1):21–31.

100. Teter CJ, McCabe SE, LaGrange K, Cranford JA, Boyd CJ. Illicit use of specific prescription stimulants among college students: prevalence, motives, and routes of administration. Pharmacotherapy. 2006;26(10):1501–10.

101. Khantzian EJ, Gawin F, Kleber HD, Riordan CE. Methylphenidate (Ritalin) treatment of cocaine dependence–a preliminary report. J Subst Abuse Treat. 1984;1(2):107–12.

102. Schubiner H, Tzelepis A, Isaacson JH, Warbasse III LH, Zacharek M, Musial J. The dual diagnosis of attention-deficit/hyperactivity disorder and substance abuse: case reports and literature review. J Clin Psychiatry. 1995;56(4):146–50.

103. Levin FR, Evans SM, McDowell DM, Kleber HD. Methylphenidate treatment for cocaine abusers with adult attention-deficit/hyperactivity disorder: a pilot study. J Clin Psychiatry. 1998;59(6):300–5.

104. Schade A, Marquenie LA, van Balkom AJ, Koeter MW, et al. The effectiveness of anxiety treatment on alcohol-dependent patients with a comorbid phobic disorder: a randomized controlled trial. Alcohol Clin Exp Res. 2005;29(5):794–800.

105. Ostacher MJ. Comorbid alcohol and substance abuse dependence in depression: impact on the outcome of antidepressant treatment. Psychiatr Clin North Am. 2007;30(1):69–76.

106. Tiet QQ, Mausbach B. Treatments for patients with dual diagnosis: a review. Alcohol Clin Exp Res. 2007;31(4):513–36.

107. Robbins TW. ADHD and addiction. Nat Med. 2002;8(1):24–5.

108. Wilens TE, Faraone SV, Biederman J, Gunawardene S. Does stimulant therapy of attention-deficit/hyperactivity disorder beget later substance abuse? A meta-analytic review of the literature. Pediatrics. 2003;111(1):179–85.

109. Biederman J, Monuteaux MC, Spencer T, Wilens TE, Macpherson HA, Faraone SV. Stimulant therapy and risk for subsequent substance use disorders in male adults with ADHD: a naturalistic controlled 10-year follow-up study. Am J Psychiatry. 2008;165(5):597–603.

Judith H. Miles and Denis M. McCarthy

Abstract

Autism and alcoholism are common behavioral disorders with no phenotypic similarities to suggest underlying biological or etiologic connections. However, a number of studies have reported family overlaps which suggest these two behavioral disorders may have underlying associations. Our analysis of 167 families ascertained through an autistic child found that 39% of families had a significant family history of alcoholism; the remainder reported scattered individuals with alcoholism in unrelated branches of the family. High alcoholism families differed from low alcoholism families in multiple measures including an 18-fold increase in alcoholism in females and more than twice the percentage of relatives with affective disorders. Children with autism from high and low alcoholism families differed in the clinical course of their disorder and head size. Children from high alcoholism families were 1.5 times more apt to present with a regressive onset and 2.8 times less likely to have macrocephaly, a common feature of autism. In contrast, families ascertained through a proband with alcoholism have not been noted to have an increased incidence of autism. This disparity can be understood by comparing the very different prevalence rates. We postulate that subsets of these two clearly heterogeneous behavioral disorders have a genetic overlap, such that families identified with genetic loading for both disorders may have a common cause(s). This subset of families is expected to be more homogeneous and therefore a valuable resource for investigation of candidate genes and pathways common to autism and alcoholism.

Learning Objectives

- Families ascertained through a child with autism cleanly separate into those with high and low incidences of alcoholism.
- Thirty-nine percent of autism ascertained families have a high family history of alcoholism, defined by alcoholism in either a parent or multiple family members in an apparent Mendelian pattern.
- High and low alcoholism families differ in both the characteristics of the alcoholism and the autism.
- Autism and alcoholism are clinically distinct with no overlapping symptoms.
- The family overlap appears to identify a more homogeneous subset of both disorders which should provide a resource for the investigation of candidate genes and pathways common to both disorders.

J.H. Miles, M.D., Ph.D. (✉)
Thompson Center for Autism and Neurodevelopmental Disorders,
University of Missouri, 205 Portland Street, Columbia,
MO 65211, USA
e-mail: milesjh@missouri.edu

D.M. McCarthy, Ph.D.
Department of Psychological Sciences, University of Missouri, 213
McAlester Hall, Columbia, MO 65211, USA
e-mail: mccarthydm@missouri.edu

J.C. Verster et al. (eds.), *Drug Abuse and Addiction in Medical Illness: Causes, Consequences and Treatment*,
DOI 10.1007/978-1-4614-3375-0_23, © Springer Science+Business Media, LLC 2012

Issues that Need to Be Addressed by Future Research
- Identify more homogeneous subsets of both alcoholism and autism.
- Identify candidate genes with evidence of involvement in both disorders.
- Identify research populations ascertained with autism plus apparent familial alcoholism and vice versa.
- Test candidate genes in these more homogeneous populations.

Autism, or what is more appropriately called the Autism Spectrum Disorders (ASD) [1], is a neurodevelopmental disorder defined completely on the basis of persistent impairments in social interaction, impairments in communication, and repetitive and stereotypic behaviors. For most children, the development of autism symptoms is gradual; however, approximately 30% have a "regressive" onset usually between 18 and 24 months [2–4]. Fifty to seventy percent of children with autism are defined as mentally retarded by nonverbal IQ testing. Seizures develop in approximately 25% of children with autism. About 25% of children who fit the diagnostic criteria for autism at age 2 or 3 years subsequently begin to talk and communicate, and by age 6 or 7 years blend to varying degrees into the regular school population. The remaining 75% continue to have a lifelong disability requiring intensive parental, school, and societal support [5–7].

An increase in the prevalence of all the ASD has been reported worldwide. Prior to 1990, most studies estimated a general population prevalence for autism of 4–5 per 10,000 (1/2,000–1/2,500) [8]. During the 1990s, studies of preschool children in Japan, England, and Sweden reported prevalence rates for autism of 21–31 per 10,000 (1/476–1/323) [9, 10]. A CDC case-finding study in Brick Township, New Jersey, reported prevalence at 40 per 10,000 (1/250) for autism and 67 per 10,000 (1/149) for all PDDs [11]. An important epidemiologic study from the United Kingdom utilizing specialized visiting nurses who monitored child health and development at ages 7 months, 18–24 months, and 3 years reported a prevalence rate of 16.8 per 10,000 (1/595) for autism and 63 per 10,000 (1/159) for all PDDs in children younger than age 5 years [12]. Those rates were recently confirmed, reporting a prevalence rate of 22 per 10,000 (1/455) for autism and 59 per 10,000 (1/169) for all PDDs in children younger than age 6 years [13]. The most recent United States study identified 1/152 eight year old children across 14 sites diagnosed with an ASD [14].

Epidemiologic evidence, however, indicates that the "autism epidemic" is not a reflection of an increased incidence of ASDs, but rather is attributable to a gradual broadening of the diagnostic criteria plus increased autism awareness by both the public and professionals, which has led to more complete case finding [15–18]. Studies that find the greatest increase in the non-autism PDDs are also recording lower rates of mental retardation in these children. Only 30% of children with PDDs ascertained by Chakrabarti and Fombonne [13] were mentally retarded compared with 70% of children in earlier studies. This suggests that many high functioning children with milder autistic symptoms had not been counted in past epidemiologic surveys. A recent update from the California Autism Surveillance Project shows that the increase of autism in California shows no sign of plateauing and though the earlier age at diagnosis and inclusion of milder cases account for more than two thirds of the change, they cannot rule out that the remainder does not represent a true increase in the occurrence of autism [19].

Establishing the Diagnosis

The behavioral criteria, compiled by the American Psychiatric Association Manual of Psychiatric Diseases, 4th edition (DSM-IV-TR) [20], remain the standard for making an ASD diagnosis in the United States. The 2000 update of the 1994 DSM-IV included changes in accompanying text but did not change actual diagnostic criteria.

DSM-IV Diagnostic Criteria for 299.00 Autistic Disorder

I. A total of six (or more) items from A, B, and C, with at least two from A, and one each from B and C:
   A. Qualitative impairment in social interaction, as manifested by at least two of the following:
      1. Marked impairment in the use of multiple nonverbal behaviors such as eye-to-eye gaze, facial expression, body postures, and gestures to regulate social interaction
      2. Failure to develop peer relationships appropriate to developmental level
      3. A lack of spontaneous seeking to share enjoyment, interests, or achievements with other people (e.g., by a lack of showing, bringing, or pointing out objects of interest)
      4. Lack of social or emotional reciprocity
   B. Qualitative impairments in communication as manifested by at least one of the following:
      1. Delay in, or total lack of, the development of spoken language (not accompanied by an attempt to compensate through alternative modes of communication such as gesture or mime)

2. In individuals with adequate speech, marked impairment in the ability to initiate or sustain a conversation with others

3. Stereotyped and repetitive use of language or idiosyncratic language

4. Lack of varied, spontaneous make-believe play or social imitative play appropriate to developmental level

C. Restricted repetitive and stereotyped patterns of behavior, interests, and activities, as manifested by at least one of the following:

1. Encompassing preoccupation with one or more stereotyped and restricted patterns of interest that is abnormal either in intensity or focus

2. Apparently inflexible adherence to specific, non-functional routines or rituals

3. Stereotyped and repetitive motor mannerisms (e.g., hand or finger flapping or twisting or complex whole-body movements)

4. Persistent preoccupation with parts of objects

II. Delays or abnormal functioning in at least one of the following areas, with onset prior to age 3 years (1) social interaction, (2) language as used in social communication, or (3) symbolic or imaginative play

III. The disturbance is not better accounted for by Rett syndrome or childhood disintegrative disorder

If a child does not meet all the criteria, he or she may be given a diagnosis of Asperger syndrome (AS) or Pervasive Developmental Disorder-Not Otherwise Specified (PDD-NOS). These three diagnoses comprise the ASD. Diagnosis of an ASD does not imply etiology; rather autism is an umbrella diagnosis with many etiologic subsets.

Diagnostic Tools

To diagnose autism, one must precisely enumerate the autism symptoms and their age of occurrence. This can be done by using a copy of the *DSM-IV-TR* or a number of checklists. The most commonly used is the CARS (Childhood Autism Rating Scale) [21], which consists of 15 questions scored by the parent and the tester. The CARS is a reliable, well-verified measure, which is relatively fast and easy to administer. A score of 30–35 indicates mild autism and 36 or higher moderate-to-severe autism. Similar checklists, including the ABC (Autism Behavior Checklist) [22] and the GARS (Gilliam Autism Rating Scale) [23], are frequently used. The most commonly used screening tool is the M-CHAT (Checklist for Autism in Toddlers-modified) [24]. This 23 item checklist is designed as a screening tool for primary care providers to identify at-risk toddlers at the 18-month visit, can be filled out by parents in the waiting room, and is available in Spanish and English [25]. A recent replication

study [26] confirmed the validity in detecting possible ASD in both low and high risk groups aged 16–30 months.

In North America, research criteria for autism depend primarily on the ADI-R (Autism Diagnostic Interview-Revised) [27], which is a detailed parent interview, which takes between 2 and 3 h to administer and the shorter ADOS (Autism Diagnostic Observation Schedule) [28]. Both scales follow the DSM-IV criteria and were developed in an attempt to sort autism by its behavioral symptoms to permit identification of homogeneous ASD populations. Although required for research studies, these scales are not widely used in clinical practice because of the time and expense to administer them; the shorter ADOS is used in an increasing number of clinics.

Autism Heritability and Etiologies

Twin and family studies indicate that autism is fundamentally a genetic disorder with the highest heritability index (>0.90) of the behavioral diagnoses. Monozygotic twins are concordant for autism 60–92% of the time, compared with 0–10% concordance for dizygotic twins [29–31]. Family studies provide an average sib recurrence risk of 4% for classical autism and an additional 4% for milder symptoms of the disorder [12]. These numbers however are somewhat misleading since recurrence risks for different autism subgroups vary from minimal to around 20%, depending on the underlying etiology [32, 33]. Moreover, more than 60 specific genetic disorders are known to cause an autism behavioral phenotype [34–37]. Routine karyotype analysis reveals chromosome aneuploidy in ~5% of children with ASD [38, 39]. About half are maternally derived duplications of 15q11-q13, including both supernumerary isodicentric 15q chromosomes detectable by routine cytogenetic studies and small interstitial duplications which can only be detected by aCGH (array comparative genomic hybridization) or interphase FISH of the *SNRPN* gene [40, 41]. Other commonly reported chromosome abnormalities include deletions of 2q,18q, 22q13, Xp, trisomy 21, and the sex chromosome aneuploidies, 47,XYY and 45,X [42, 43]. aCGH, which is quickly replacing routine chromosome analysis for evaluation of children with ASDs, identifies another 5–10% of children with other copy number variations. These numbers are expected to increase as more dense microarrays become clinically available [44–47]. Finally, autism is also a prominent phenotype in a large number of single gene disorders including Fragile X syndrome (FMR1 trinucleotide repeat expansion), Tuberous Sclerosis (TSC1 and TSC2 gene mutations), Sotos syndrome (mutation or deletion of *NSD1*), Rett syndrome (MECP2 gene mutations), Timothy syndrome (*CACNA1C* gene), PTEN mutations, and a variety of mitochondrial respiratory chain disorders [37].

Neurodevelopmental Foundation

There is abundant evidence that autism is predominantly neurodevelopmental in origin. Abnormalities in brain size and structure are common. Macrocephaly defined as occipital frontal circumference ≥2SD above the mean reflects brain size [48, 49] and occurs in 20–30% of ASD children and 37–45% of their non-autistic parents [50–52]. Courchesne et al. [53, 54] found that 90% of children with autism between 2 and 4 years of age have a brain volume larger than the normal average. Hazlett et al. [55] observed similar cerebral volume enlargement. The significance of macrocephaly was underscored by Bolton's report [56] that infantile macrocephaly was a significant predictor (OR = 5.44) for the development of autism. Recent studies find that head circumference at birth may actually be within the normal range or even reduced [57–59] and move postnatally into the macrocephalic range. Our studies indicate that head growth surges throughout childhood is more consistent with autism than ultimate head size. This may explain why macrocephaly by itself has not been found to be a strong predictor of outcome or other phenotypic traits in autism [60, 61]. Understanding brain overgrowth in autism is incomplete with some conflicting data which undoubtedly reflects both the paucity of longitudinal studies and autism's inherent heterogeneity. Genes involved in brain overgrowth have been reviewed by McCaffery and Deutsch [57].

In addition to brain size differences, between 10% and 40% of children with autism have abnormal brain structure by MRI. A recent study of 77 children with idiopathic autistic disorder, uncomplicated by seizures, severe mental retardation, major anomalies, or focal neurologic signs found that in 40% of the children the MRI was read as abnormal by neuroradiologists with white matter signal abnormalities, severely dilated Virchow–Robin spaces and temporal lobe structural abnormalities being the most common [62]. This level of pathology in children with non-syndromic autism lends support to the controversial recommendation to obtain brain MRIs as a standard diagnostic test in autism. Structural imaging studies in autism have reported abnormalities in multiple structures, including the brainstem [63], cerebellum [50, 53], thalamus [64], corpus callosum [65–68], amygdala [69], hippocampus [70, 71], and cortical sulcal patterns [72, 73]. Unfortunately the results are generally inconclusive, and sometimes even contradictory. These inconsistencies are most likely a consequence of heterogeneity. A unifying theory, proposed by Minshew and Williams [74], is that autism is a primarily a disorder of abnormal neuronal connectivity.

Physical anomalies are observed in a significant proportion of children with autism [30, 75–77]. Their presence or absence at birth can be used as an indirect measure of perturbations during embryonic and fetal development. Early studies reported that children with behavioral disorders including autism have a higher risk of physical anomalies [78–85]. Walker, for example, studied 74 autistic and non-autistic children matched for age, sex, and socioeconomic group, using the Waldrop weighted scoring scale [86] for 16 anomalies. This study found that the mean minor anomaly score of 5.76 for the autistic children was significantly higher than the control group score of 3.53. He concluded this shift to a greater number of anomalies in the autistic children proved organicity in autism. Links et al. [82] recognized that autistic children had more anomalies than their sibs and that the autistic children with the higher anomaly scores had lower IQs, spent more time in the hospital, and had less frequent family histories of psychiatric illness or of drug or alcohol abuse. They concluded that the anomalies were the result of some unknown organic factor that played a role in the etiology of autism. Rodier et al. [76, 87] proposed that physical phenotypic features could be used to pick out the children whose autism was due to mutations in the embryologically important homeobox genes that model the development of the brain stem and face. She also demonstrated how environmental teratogens, such as valproic acid and thalidomide, may produce teratogenic phenocopies by influencing the same early developmental pathways.

In 2000, we proposed that physical dysmorphology can be used to identify a subset of children whose development was marred by abnormal processes during embryogenesis [88]. Subsequently, we defined complex autism as the ASD subset who displayed either significant dysmorphology or microcephaly [89]. The complex autism subgroup comprises about 20% of the total poulation studied, and individuals with complex autism have poorer outcomes with lower IQs, more seizures, more abnormal EEGs (46% vs. 30%) and more brain abnormalities on MRI (28% vs. 13%). The remainder have essential autism, which is more heritable, with a higher sib recurrence (4% vs. 0%), more relatives with autism (20% vs. 9%) and a higher male to female ratio (6.5:1 vs. 3.2:1). These group differences between individuals with complex and essential autism are predicated on the developmental principle that individuals for whom there is evidence of an insult to morphogenesis will be etiologically distinct from those whose development proceeded normally and who will almost certainly differ in outcome and response to therapies.

Currently, a specific etiology can be identified for 15–20% of children with autism; the rest remain idiopathic. Just as mental retardation and cerebral palsy have moved from the status of distinct disorders to clinical symptom complexes, autism is being documented in hundreds of neurologically based syndromes with various causes, outcomes and treatment responses [36, 90, 91]. This suggests that the brain, when perturbed, has a limited number of responses of which autism is one, a point of view which has been amplified by the paucity of autism specific genes identified in the last decade despite autism's high heritability index [29]. The general consensus is that the failure to find major autism genes is primarily a reflection of etiologic heterogeneity [42, 92–98].

Comparing and Contrasting Autism and Alcoholism

Alcoholism, or more specifically the alcohol use disorders of alcohol abuse and alcohol dependence, are very common, with a lifetime prevalence rate of >12% for alcohol dependence [99]. Although there are criteria with physiological components (tolerance, withdrawal), alcohol abuse and dependence are diagnosed on the basis of their behavioral phenotype. Comparing alcohol dependence and autism, there are many more differences than similarities in the clinical phenotypes of the two disorders. Perhaps the most striking difference is their developmental course. While the age of onset of autism is in early childhood, the peak age of onset for an alcohol dependence diagnosis is in young adulthood [100]. So while there is clearly a strong genetic basis for alcohol use disorder, with heritability estimates of 40–70% [101], the course of the disorder is such that a broad range of environmental factors (e.g., family/peer modeling, psychosocial stressors, personality development) are also important contributors to its development and can exert a significant moderating influence on any genetic etiologic factors.

There are a number of other phenotypic differences between the two disorders. For example, alcoholism is not associated with seizures, mental retardation, physical anomalies or abnormalities in brain structure or size. There is also no evidence for comorbidity between the two disorders. Although people with ASD certainly could develop alcohol dependence, there are no reports that they do so at higher rates than the general population [102–105]. In fact, Santosh and Mijovic reported significantly lower drug and alcohol use in adolescents with PDDs and IQs >70 compared to those with other psychiatric disorders (3% versus 17%) [105]. A recent report by Sizoo et al. found that of 68 high functioning (IQ ≥80) adults with ASD, recruited from adult diagnostic centers, 19% could be classified with alcohol abuse or dependence and an additional 9% reported past alcoholism [106]. Risk factors for alcoholism included parental alcoholism, early smoking, and higher adverse family events. These results were similar to a comparison group of adults with ADHD. Although this observed rate of alcohol use disorder is fairly high, the authors point out that their data are based on adults referred to specialized centers, and that the availability of addiction treatment facilities might have led to a relatively high prevalence of substance abuse comorbidity in their population.

When queried on overlap between autism and alcoholism, many clinicians recall reports attributing autism to maternal alcohol use in pregnancy [107–109]. Whether there was a causal relationship was initially unclear. We know that a number of teratogens will cause the autism phenotype, including thalidomide, valproic acid, and Misoprostol, an abortifactant commonly used in South America [110]. And children with Fetal Alcohol Syndrome (FAS) do have a number of overlapping behavioral issues that are also seen in autism including social problems, hyperactivity, impulsivity, irritability, tantrums, cognitive delays, and sensory aversions [111, 112]. However, re-examination of these early studies makes a causal association doubtful, as none were based on currently available standardized autism diagnostic measures and in the series taken from FAS registries only 1–2% of the children were considered autistic. A recent behavioral study of autism symptoms based on the gold standard autism diagnostic measures (ADI-R, Autism Diagnostic Observation Scale) showed that the children with autism and PDD-NOS were clearly distinguishable from children with FAS [113]. In our experience providing comprehensive genetic and dysmorphology evaluations in a dedicated autism clinic, FAS is rarely identified and we have never made a dual diagnosis of the two disorders. This is consistent with the experience of a number of other centers [36, 37]. Thus, we conclude that prenatal alcohol exposure does not cause autism and is not the explanation for the family history association between the two disorders.

Evidence of an etiologic connection between autism and alcoholism is based almost completely on the finding that families of children with autism have higher that expected alcoholism histories. In addition to alcoholism, numerous autism family studies show significant clustering of other neuropsychiatric disorders including depression, manic depression, obsessive compulsive disorder, social phobia, anxiety disorders, substance abuse, and motor tics in relatives of autism probands. This apparent genetic overlap between autism and other neuropsychiatric disorders has suggested that at least for certain types of autism there are common biochemical and genetic aberrations. Lobascher et al. [114] compared the family histories of 23 autistic children with normal controls and found a greater incidence of alcoholism (35%), psychiatric illness (35%), and mental retardation (26%) in the parents of autistic children. DeLong and Dwyer [115] reported that 55% of their 51 autism families had a first or second degree relative with alcoholism though the overall incidence rate of alcoholism among all 929 first and second degree relatives was only 6.5%. Piven et al. [116] reported that 12.3% of 81 parents of autistic children were alcoholic compared with 0% of 34 Down syndrome parents; the difference was not statistically significant. In a study of 36 autism families, Smalley et al. [117] compared the lifetime rates of psychopathology based on direct

SADS-LA interviews of parents and adult siblings of autism probands versus controls who had either tuberous sclerosis or an unspecified seizure disorder. They found that 47% (17/36) of the autism families had a first degree relative with substance abuse, including alcoholism, versus none in the 21 control families. And 22% of first degree relatives reported substance abuse compared to none in the controls ($p=0.002$). They also found increased rates of depression (32.3% vs. 11.1%; $p=0.013$) and social phobia (20.2% vs. 2.4%; $p=0.016$). Not all family studies have reported increased rates of alcoholism. Bolton et al. [118] using direct SADS-L interviews to assess the lifetime prevalence rates of psychopathology found a significant increase in major depression in first degree relatives of individuals with autism but no significant increase in other psychiatric disorders including alcoholism and drug abuse.

In 2003 we reported family history analyses of 167 autism families [119]. Families were ascertained through an autistic child and queried using the family history method [120–125] to determine the prevalence and pedigree configuration of alcoholism and related neuropsychiatric disorders and to determine whether a family history of alcoholism correlated with any identifiable subset of individuals with autism. Looking at the population as a whole, we found 13.5% of the first degree relatives and 13.6% of second degree adults were reported to have alcoholism including, 6.6% of mothers, 20.4% of fathers, 8.4% of grandmothers, and 27.5% of grandfathers. As expected, men were significantly more likely to have a history of alcoholism than women (20.3% vs. 6.6%) $\chi^2(1)=74.1, p<0.0001$. Alcoholism rates in the autism ascertained families were compared to a control population of 22 families ascertained through a child with Down syndrome and to lifetime alcohol prevalence data reported by three large United States alcoholism epidemiological studies, including a Missouri rural and suburban cohort [126–129]. The Down syndrome families reported significantly less alcoholism in all family members ($p<0.0001$), comprising 0% (0/44) of first degree relatives and 0.4% (1/234) of second degree relatives, 0% (0/22) of mothers, 0% (0/22) of fathers, 0% (0/44) of grandmothers, and 2.3% (1/44) of grandfathers. Compared to the 15.2% lifetime prevalence of alcoholism reported for suburban, small town and rural Missouri [127], the overall 13.7% rate of alcoholism reported by the autism families was similar, $\chi^2(1)=1.7, p=0.19$. The women in our population, however, were significantly more likely to report alcoholism than all women in Missouri (6.6% vs. 4.3%); $\chi^2(1)=7.1, p=0.008$.

Since alcoholism, like autism, is a heterogeneous disorder [130–136], we wanted to distinguish families with strongly genetic alcoholism from those with only sporadic or occasional cases that might be more environmentally induced. Using strict criteria to pick out the families with clusters of alcoholism, we classified 39% (65/167) of the families as

having probable genetic alcoholism. A family history was rated as significant or "probably genetic" for alcoholism if the proband had (1) a first degree relative with alcoholism (manifesting prior to concerns about the health of the proband), (2) a second degree relative plus at least two additional individuals in the same family branch in a pattern suggesting Mendelian inheritance, or (3) alcoholism in at least four individuals all in the same branch of the family. The high alcoholism families had an elevated percentage of affected relatives in all categories, with 17% of mothers, 52% of fathers, 14% of maternal grandmothers, 41% of maternal grandfathers, 21% of paternal grandmothers, and 45% of paternal grandfathers reported as alcoholic. The remaining 102 families reported scattered individuals with alcoholism in unrelated branches of the family (less than 1% of females and less than 10% males).

Families and children whose pedigrees revealed an apparent genetic distribution of alcoholism (designated high alcoholism families) were compared with those that did not (low alcoholism families). The family histories differed in two ways. First, the high alcoholism families had a significantly higher proportion of affected (alcoholic) females. In the high alcoholism families, the number of female alcoholics was 18 times the number in the low alcoholism families, whereas males were only 4 times more likely to be alcoholic (15.9% vs. 0.9% females; 38.2% vs. 8.7% males). The ratio of female to male alcoholics was significantly higher in the high alcoholism families compared to the low (0.46 vs. 0.052, $p=0.0001$). And compared with unselected Missouri families [125], the females in our high alcohol families were 3.7 times more apt to be alcoholic. Secondly, high alcoholism families had more relatives with affective disorders, also distributed in a familial pattern (50.8% vs. 24%), $\chi^2(1)=11.93$, $p=0.0006$. This is consistent with previous studies of alcoholism which report an association between alcoholism and affective disorders in families [137–140]. A significant family history of alcoholism did not associate preferentially with any other family history categories (cognitive, language, dyslexia, ADHD, or seizures). It is important to note that children from the high affective disorder families did not differ in any of the ways described in the next paragraph.

Evaluation of the autism probands from the high and low alcoholism groups differed in two important autism phenotypes, macrocephaly, and type of autism onset. Children from the high alcoholism families were 2.8 times *less likely* to be macrocephalic (14.7% vs. 40.6%) $\chi^2(1)=11.76$, $p=0.0006$. We had noted this inverse relationship between macrocephaly and alcohol family histories in our previous study of head circumference and autism [50]. In that study we found that only 20.7% of macrocephalic probands had strong histories of addictive disorders, compared with 37.2% of the normocephalic probands. In addition, we observed that macrocephaly in autism was highly familial with 45% of the macrocephalic autistic children having at least one macrocephalic parent, which suggests that there must be gene(s) which cause macrocephaly and also predispose to autism, and that non-autistic macrocephalic parents may be carrying gene(s) that put them at risk for having a child with autism. The very significant inverse relationship between high alcoholism family histories and macrocephaly suggest that whatever the genes are that predispose to both autism and macrocephaly are different and operate independently from gene(s) that predispose to alcoholism and autism.

The second difference between the autism probands from high versus low alcohol families was the clinical course of their autistic disorder. Children from high alcoholism families were 1.5 times more apt to present with a regressive onset (52.5% vs. 35.8%) $\chi^2(1)=4.19$, $p=0.04$. This was found predominately in families where the mother was alcoholic (80% vs. 40%) $\chi^2(1)=5.36$, $p=0.05$. There was no correlation with paternal alcoholism. This raised the question of a direct teratogenic effect of alcohol on the developing fetus. However, only one mother with a history of alcoholism reported drinking during the pregnancy. And in all of the children, FAS was ruled out by careful physical examinations. We believe that the connection between autism and familial alcoholism is consistent with the idea that there is an alcoholism subtype that is genetically mediated, highly penetrant, and predisposes to the development of autism.

It is tempting to look for evidence of some shared biochemical pathways or genes. Theoretically, a maternal factor is of interest since recent studies have reported that autism is associated with the maternal dopamine β-hydroxylase alleles and that there is sib concordance for maternal, but not paternal alleles, linked to dopamine, serotonin, and norepinephrine transmitters [141]. Clarification of our association between regressive autism and maternal alcoholism will depend on replication of the studies in a larger sample of families. Nevertheless, it does recommend that for autism, like other complex disorders [142] parental genotypes should be considered as possible risk factors.

Future Directions: Examining Autism in Studies of Alcoholism and Potential Common Genetic Pathways

With this clear observation of alcoholism in autism families, there is, to our knowledge, no mention in the alcohol literature of an association with autism. In this section, we will discuss what we think are the primary reasons for this disparity, as well as potential directions for future research to understand the potential overlap between alcoholism and autism.

The first and possibly most important reason that the alcohol literature does not report any overlap with autism is that there is no evidence for an increased rate of alcoholism in

individuals with autism [102–105]. In fact, anecdotal evidence would suggest that the rate of alcoholism is lower in autistic individuals than in the general population, most likely due to the fact that initiation of alcohol use is typically in early adolescence and is almost always in social contexts. The observed overlap between the two disorders we review here is at the level of the family, rather than the individual. This means that in order to detect this overlap, alcoholism researchers need to examine rates of autism in alcoholic families. As there is no evidence for high rates of autism in alcoholics themselves, there has previously not been a clear reason to examine rates of autism in alcoholic families.

An additional reason why alcohol researchers may not have observed an overlap with autism is the large difference in prevalence rates between the two disorders. Any overlap between autism and alcoholism families would be reflected in larger increases in family history of alcoholism within autistic families than the corresponding increases in autism in families with a history of alcoholism. In other words, the rate of positive family histories of alcoholism in families ascertained based on the presence of autism is expected to be higher than the rate of autism in families ascertained based on the presence of alcoholism. These rates differ to the extent that the base rates of the two disorders differ. This lack of symmetry between two apparently similar conditional probabilities is well known in the literature on assessment and probability.

The probability of having alcoholism in the family, given that there is autism in the family, is indicated by the joint probability of the disorders divided by the rate of autism. The probability of having autism in the family, given that there is alcoholism in the family, is indicated by the joint probability of the disorders divided by the rate of alcoholism. These two formulas diverge to the extent that their denominators, the base rate of the two disorders, differ. To illustrate, consider a conservative example, assuming a rate of 12% for family history of alcohol dependence and a 0.66% prevalence rate for autism, we would expect an 18-fold difference between the two calculations. This makes it much easier to detect an increased rate of alcoholism in autism families than the converse. If the overlap in family history of the two disorders was as high as 50%, we would expect the rate of alcoholism in autistic families to be 18%, while the rate of autism in families with alcoholism would only be 0.99%. In this example, a study of autism families looking at the probability of alcoholism would need a sample size sufficient to detect that the rate (18%) is higher than that of the general population (12%). On the other hand, a study of families with a positive family history of alcoholism would need to be of sufficient size to detect that the rate of autism (0.99%) is higher than that of the general population (0.66%). A similar phenomenon in the literature is the overlap between nicotine use and schizophrenia. The base rates of cigarette smoking (about 25% of the general population) and schizophrenia (approximately 1%) also differ markedly. Studies of those with schizophrenia easily detect a higher rate of cigarette use (upwards of 50%) [143] than in the general population, and this increased rate of smoking in those with schizophrenia is well known. However, it would be quite difficult for a study of cigarette smokers to detect a rate of schizophrenia in their sample that significantly exceeded 1%. Both the overlap between smoking and schizophrenia and our hypothetical numbers for autism/alcoholism overlap likely understate the difficulty in detecting higher rates of autism in families of alcoholics. The overlap between autism and alcoholism is in reality probably much lower than the overlap between schizophrenia and smoking and lower than the 50% estimate we used above. Estimates of the rate of having a positive family history of alcoholism are typically much higher [144]. Given the difficulty in detecting an increased rate of autism in alcoholic families, one direction for future research is for large scale epidemiologic studies to examine potential overlap between these two disorders in families.

Further complicating the picture is the potential that only a subgroup of alcoholism is linked to genes which also contribute to autism. While alcohol dependence is undoubtedly etiologically heterogeneous, there is no fully accepted system of subtyping alcohol dependence. There have been a broad range of approaches to subtyping alcoholism [129, 134, 145]. Subtypes have been identified by etiologic, phenotypic or developmental differences, as well as through comorbid conditions and combinations of these criteria. In a recent review, Hesselbrock and Hesselbrock [134] noted that despite the various approaches to alcoholism subtyping, there is remarkable agreement about classifying subtypes by severity (chronic/severe vs. mild) and by personality/psychopathology (depressed/anxious vs. antisocial). As noted, our prior study of autistic families found a higher rate of affective disorders in those classified as having strong family history of alcoholism [117]. This may suggest that the observed overlap between alcoholism and autism in families may be specific to a depressed/anxious subtype of alcoholism. In a recent study of adults with ASD [146] a higher level of harm avoidance associated with type 1 alcoholism [129] was observed in those with ASD compared to general population norms. However, harm avoidance did not differentiate ASD participants with and without substance use disorder. Describing the phenotypic details of alcoholism in autism ascertained families would make a significant contribution to our current knowledge.

An essential approach to discovering genetic causes of heterogeneous disorders is to meticulously describe the phenotype and on that basis identify homogeneous subgroups which have the likelihood of being etiologically discrete. The most accepted method has been to define biomarkers/endophenotypes. This has been easier in autism which is associated with its many structural, functional, and bio-physiologic variants than for alcoholism where the phenotype is almost completely behavioral. However, both autism and alcoholism do provide researchers a number of "genetics related" markers, including the high male prevalence, recurrence risk variations, and family histories loaded for specific psychiatric diagnoses. We suggest that identifying families who overlap for autism and alcoholism may identify a subgroup with a likelihood of carrying a limited number of genes which influence the development of both disorders [147]. As discussed above, identifying the smaller number of alcohol ascertained families which have individuals with autism will require a larger population. There is, however, ample evidence that the family history method is a specific and sensitive tool for both autism and alcoholism as family members are likely to know which family members are affected [120–123, 148]. Cooperative studies to identify familial alcoholism through autism probands could provide large enough populations for molecular analyses. Autism research is blessed with families who are advocates and willing to participate in research studies. One excellent resource is IAN, the Interactive Autism Network [149], a national registry which currently has collected comprehensive data on more than 25,000 autism families. Researchers are able to post requests for research participants and also to analyze the database.

Candidate gene searches are becoming more and more productive for both autism and alcoholism. More than 100 genes and multiple copy number variants have been identified for autism [37, 90, 150–152], the majority of which do not overlap with biochemical pathways or genes implicated in alcoholism. Neurodevelopmental genes, for instance, are commonly implicated in autism, but not alcoholism. Nevertheless, there are areas of overlap. Dysregulation of the major neurotransmitter systems for GABA and serotonin occur in autism and in alcoholism (Table 23.1). And recently genes that encode structural cell adhesion molecule subfamilies which specify brain connectivity during development and in adulthood have been linked to both autism and alcoholism. Autism is now considered a disorder of connectivity [95, 176, 177] and is linked to numerous genes involved in neural cell adhesion (Neuroligin 3 and 4, Neurexin 1, SH3 and multiple ankyrin repeat domains, Contactin-associated protein-like 2, Contactin 4 and Contactin 3, Protocadherin 1). Recently, addiction researchers have also queried relationships with neural adhesion related genes. Uhl et al. [171] analyzed convergence data from genome wide association studies identifying 27 candidate genes that link addiction and co-occurring brain disorders ranging from smoking to Alzheimer's disease; three cell adhesion genes (Neurexin 1, Contactin-associated protein-like 2, and Contactin 4) previously linked to autism were identified in addictive disorder populations. Moreover, addiction and autism share associations with a number of cell adhesion gene subfamilies.

Table 23.1 Genes implicated in both autism and alcoholism susceptibility

	Gene symbol and location	Autism	Alcoholism
Neurotransmitter genes			
GABA receptor subunits (major inhibitory transmitter receptors in the brain)	GABRG3 15q11.2-q12	Cook et al. [153] Martin et al. [154] Collins et al. [155] Buxbaum et al. [156] Menold et al. [157]	Dick et al. [158] Namkoong et al. [159]
Serotonin transporter gene 5-HTT	SLC6A4 17q11.1-q12	Sutcliffe et al. [160] McCauley et al. [161] Wassink et al. [162]	Hammoumi et al. [163] Feinn et al. [164] Seneviratne et al. [165]
Cell adhesion related genes			
Neurexin 1 (trans-synaptic binding partner for neuroligins; involved in development and function of glutamatergic and GABAergic synapses)	NRXN1 2p16.3	Szatmari et al. [166] Lise and El-Husseini [167] Feng et al. [168] Kim et al. [169] Yan et al. [170]	Uhl et al. [171]
Contactin-associated protein-like 2 (synaptic binding partner for contactin molecules involved in neuronal migration)	CNTNAP2 7q35-q36 7q36SCN7A	Alarcón et al. [172] Arking et al. [173] Bakkaloglu et al. [174]	Uhl et al. [171]
Contactin 4 (neuronally expressed adhesion molecules)	CNTN4 3p26-p25	Bakkaloglu et al. [174] Roohi et al. [175]	Uhl et al. [171]

For instance, nicotine dependence as well as autism has been associated with Neurexin 1 [178], alcoholism with Neurexin 3 [179]. These data support the concept that the same genetic variants can have overlapping or pleiotropic influences on more than one brain-based disorder.

Summary

Though autism and alcoholism are very different disorders, one with onset prior to age three and the other a disorder of adolescence and adulthood, we see evidence of shared familial predispositions and overlapping candidate genes and neurologic processes. The notion of different disorders sharing defects in the same genes and pathways has been explored best in addictive disorders where twin studies identify overlapping genetic predispositions to dependence to most substance classes. And molecular genome wide association studies as well as meta-analyses are beginning to pick out candidate genes associated with more neurologic diseases than multiple addictions [171, 180]. These types of analysis have not been extended to autism, though Uhl et al. [171] do suggest autism as a strong contender to share connectivity gene dysfunction with addictive disorders. These cross disorder comparisons are in their infancy and in most cases might best be considered hypotheses. We do not have the biological explanation for our observation that alcoholism is a significant trait in 39% of families identified through a child with an ASD. But it does indicate that when looking for autism gene associations, groups with and without high alcoholism family loading should be analyzed separately. The association between a maternal family history of alcoholism and regressive onset autism raises questions of possible imprinting or even the presence of genes active in adulthood that function as fetal morphogens. Both possibilities are open to currently accessible investigative approaches. Success in the study of these complex disorders will require that we identify and systematically address subtypes both within the confines of each disorder and more broadly across disorders that overlap in family pedigrees. Simultaneously, the study of biological pathways and neurological systems within these subtypes should accelerate identification of specific genetic etiologies.

References

1. National Institute of Mental Health. National Institute of Mental Health. 3-31-2009. 4-17-0009.
2. Chawarska K, Klin A, Paul R, Volkmar F. Autism spectrum disorder in the second year: stability and change in syndrome expression. J Child Psychol Psychiatry. 2007;48(2):128–38.
3. Rogers SJ, Young GS, Cook I, Giolzetti A, Ozonoff S, Rogers SJ, et al. Deferred and immediate imitation in regressive and early onset autism. J Child Psychol Psychiatry. 2008;49(4):449–57.
4. Ozonoff S, Heung K, Byrd R, Hansen R, Hertz-Picciotto I. The onset of autism: patterns of symptom emergence in the first years of life. Autism Res. 2008;1(6):320–8.
5. Bailey A, Luthert P, Dean A, Harding B, Janota I, Montgomery M, et al. A clinicopathological study of autism. Brain. 1998;121 (Pt 5):889–905.
6. Silverman JM, Smith CJ, Schmeidler J, Hollander E, Lawlor BA, Fitzgerald M, et al. Symptom domains in autism and related conditions: evidence for familiality. Am J Med Genet. 2002;114(1): 64–73.

7. Spence MA. The genetics of autism. Curr Opin Pediatr. 2001;13(6):561–5.

8. Fombonne E. Is there an epidemic of autism? Pediatrics. 2001;107(2):411–2.

9. Arvidsson T, Danielsson B, Forsberg P, Gillberg C, Johansson M, Kjellgren G. Autism in 3–6-year-old children in a suburb of Goteborg, Sweden. Autism. 1997;1:163–73.

10. Baird G, Charman T, Baron-Cohen S, Cox A, Swettenham J, Wheelwright S, et al. A screening instrument for autism at 18 months of age: a 6-year follow-up study. J Am Acad Child Adolesc Psychiatry. 2000;39(6):694–702.

11. Centers for Disease Control and Prevention. Prevalence of Autism and Brick Township, New Jersey, 1998: community report. Atlanta, GA: Department of Health and Human Services; 2000.

12. Chakrabarti S, Fombonne E. Pervasive developmental disorders in preschool children. JAMA. 2001;285(24):3093–9.

13. Chakrabarti S, Fombonne E. Pervasive developmental disorders in preschool children: confirmation of high prevalence. Am J Psychiatry. 2005;162(6):1133–41.

14. Centers for Disease Control and Prevention. Prevalence of Autism Spectrum Disorders—Autism and Developmental Disabilities Monitoring Network, Six Sites, United States, 2000. MMWR Morb Mortal Wkly Rep. 2007;56:1–11.

15. Atladottir HO, Parner ET, Schendel D, Dalsgaard S, Thomsen PH, Thorsen P. Time trends in reported diagnoses of childhood neuropsychiatric disorders: a Danish cohort study. Arch Pediatr Adolesc Med. 2007;161(2):193–8.

16. Shattuck PT. Diagnostic substitution and changing autism prevalence. Pediatrics. 2006;117(4):1438–9.

17. Gernsbacher M, Dawson M, Goldsmith H. Three reasons not to believe and autism epidemic. Curr Dir Psychol Sci. 2005;14(2):55–8.

18. Fombonne E, Zakarian R, Bennett A, Meng L, McLean-Heywood D. Pervasive developmental disorders in Montreal, Quebec, Canada: prevalence and links with immunizations. Pediatrics. 2006;118(1):e139–50.

19. Hertz-Picciotto I, Delwiche L. The rise in autism and the role of age at diagnosis. Epidemiology. 2009;20(1):84–90.

20. American Psychiatric Association. Diagnostic and Statistical Manual of Mental Disorders. 4th Edition, text revised ed. Washington DC: APA; 2000.

21. Schopler E, Reichler RJ, Renner BR. The Childhood Autism Rating Scale (CARS) for diagnostic screening and classification of autism. New York: Irvington; 1986.

22. Aman MG, Singh NN, Stewart AW, Field CJ. The aberrant behavior checklist: a behavior rating scale for the assessment of treatment effects. Am J Ment Defic. 1985;89(5):485–91.

23. Gilliam JE. Gilliam Autism Rating Scale (GARS). Austin, TX: Pro Ed; 1995.

24. Robins DL, Fein D, Barton ML, Green JA. The modified checklist for autism in toddlers: an initial study investigating the early detection of autism and pervasive developmental disorders. J Autism Dev Disord. 2001;31(2):131–44.

25. California Department of Developmental Services. Autistic spectrum disorders changes in the California caseload an update: 1999–2002. Sacramento, CA: California Health and Human Services Agency; 2002.

26. Kleinman JM, Robins DL, Ventola PE, Pandey J, Boorstein HC, Esser EL, et al. The modified checklist for autism in toddlers: a follow-up study investigating the early detection of autism spectrum disorders. J Autism Dev Disord. 2008;38(5):827–39.

27. Lord C, Rutter M, Le Couteur A. Autism Diagnostic Interview-Revised: a revised version of a diagnostic interview for caregivers of individuals with possible pervasive developmental disorders. J Autism Dev Disord. 1994;24(5):659–85.

28. Lord C, Rutter M, Goode S, Heemsbergen J, Jordan H, Mawhood L, et al. Autism diagnostic observation schedule: a standardized observation of communicative and social behavior. J Autism Dev Disord. 1989;19(2):185–212.

29. Bailey A, Le Couteur A, Gottesman I, Bolton P, Simonoff E, Yuzda E, et al. Autism as a strongly genetic disorder: evidence from a British twin study. Psychol Med. 1995;25(1):63–77.

30. Smalley SL, Asarnow RF, Spence MA. Autism and genetics. A decade of research. Arch Gen Psychiatry. 1988;45(10):953–61.

31. Le Couteur A, Bailey A, Goode S, Pickles A, Robertson S, Gottesman I, et al. A broader phenotype of autism: the clinical spectrum in twins. J Child Psychol Psychiatry. 1996;37(7):785–801.

32. Miles JH, McCathren RB. Autism Overview. GenesReviews. 12-1-2009. University of Washington, Seattle. GeneTests: Medical Genetics Information Resource (database online).

33. Sumi S, Taniai H, Miyachi T, Tanemura M. Sibling risk of pervasive developmental disorder estimated by means of an epidemiologic survey in Nagoya, Japan. J Hum Genet. 2006;51(6):518–22.

34. Coleman M. Advances in autism research. Dev Med Child Neurol. 2005;47(3):148.

35. Herman GE, Henninger N, Ratliff-Schaub K, Pastore M, Fitzgerald S, McBride KL. Genetic testing in autism: how much is enough? Genet Med. 2007;9(5):268–74.

36. Schaefer GB, Mendelsohn NJ. Clinical genetics evaluation in identifying the etiology of autism spectrum disorders. Genet Med. 2008;10(4):301–5.

37. Smith M, Spence MA, Flodman P. Nuclear and mitochondrial genome defects in autisms. Ann NY Acad Sci. 2009;1151:102–32.

38. Wassink TH, Piven J, Patil SR. Chromosomal abnormalities in a clinic sample of individuals with autistic disorder. Psychiatr Genet. 2001;11(2):57–63.

39. Reddy KS. Cytogenetic abnormalities and fragile-X syndrome in Autism Spectrum Disorder. BMC Med Genet. 2005;6:3.

40. Borgatti R, Piccinelli P, Passoni D, Dalpra L, Miozzo M, Micheli R, et al. Relationship between clinical and genetic features in "inverted duplicated chromosome 15" patients. Pediatr Neurol. 2001;24(2):111–6.

41. Dykens EM, Sutcliffe JS, Levitt P. Autism and 15q11-q13 disorders: behavioral, genetic, and pathophysiological issues. Ment Retard Dev Disabil Res Rev. 2004;10(4):284–91.

42. Gillberg C. Chromosomal disorders and autism. J Autism Dev Disord. 1998;28(5):415–25.

43. Manning MA, Cassidy SB, Clericuzio C, Cherry AM, Schwartz S, Hudgins L, et al. Terminal 22q deletion syndrome: a newly recognized cause of speech and language disability in the autism spectrum. Pediatrics. 2004;114(2):451–7.

44. Beaudet AL. Autism: highly heritable but not inherited. Nat Med. 2007;13(5):534–6.

45. Marshall CR, Noor A, Vincent JB, Lionel AC, Feuk L, Skaug J, et al. Structural variation of chromosomes in autism spectrum disorder. Am J Hum Genet. 2008;82(2):477–88.

46. Christian SL, Brune CW, Sudi J, Kumar RA, Liu S, Karamohamed S, et al. Novel submicroscopic chromosomal abnormalities detected in autism spectrum disorder. Biol Psychiatry. 2008;63(12):1111–7.

47. Weiss LA, Shen Y, Korn JM, Arking DE, Miller DT, Fossdal R, et al. Association between microdeletion and microduplication at 16p11.2 and autism. N Engl J Med. 2008;358(7):667–75.

48. Stanfield AC, McIntosh AM, Spencer MD, Philip R, Gaur S, Lawrie SM. Towards a neuroanatomy of autism: a systematic review and meta-analysis of structural magnetic resonance imaging studies. Eur Psychiatry. 2007;23(4):289–99.

49. Casanova MF. The neuropathology of autism. Brain Pathol. 2007;17(4):422–33.

50. Miles JH, Hadden L, Takahashi TN, Hillman RE. Head circumference is an independent clinical finding associated with autism. Am J Med Genet. 2000;95:339–50.

51. Fombonne E, Roge B, Claverie J, Courty S, Fremolle J. Microcephaly and macrocephaly in autism [In Process Citation]. J Autism Dev Disord. 1999;29(2):113–9.

52. Lainhart JE, Piven J, Wzorek M, Landa R, Santangelo SL, Coon H, et al. Macrocephaly in children and adults with autism. J Am Acad Child Adolesc Psychiatry. 1997;36(2):282–90.

53. Courchesne E, Karns CM, Davis HR, Ziccardi R, Carper RA, Tigue ZD, et al. Unusual brain growth patterns in early life in patients with autistic disorder: an MRI study. Neurology. 2001;57(2):245–54.

54. Courchesne E, Carper R, Akshoomoff N. Evidence of brain overgrowth in the first year of life in autism. JAMA. 2003;290(3):337–44.

55. Hazlett HC, Poe M, Gerig G, Smith RG, Provenzale J, Ross A, et al. Magnetic resonance imaging and head circumference study of brain size in autism: birth through age 2 years. Arch Gen Psychiatry. 2005;62(12):1366–76.

56. Bolton PF, Roobol M, Allsopp L, Pickles A. Association between idiopathic infantile macrocephaly and autism spectrum disorders. Lancet. 2001;358(9283):726–7.

57. McCaffery P, Deutsch CK. Macrocephaly and the control of brain growth in autistic disorders. Prog Neurobiol. 2005;77(1–2):38–56.

58. Courchesne E, Pierce K. Brain overgrowth in autism during a critical time in development: implications for frontal pyramidal neuron and interneuron development and connectivity. Int J Dev Neurosci. 2005;23(2–3):153–70.

59. Pardo CA, Eberhart CG. The neurobiology of autism. Brain Pathol. 2007;17(4):434–47.

60. Stoelb M, Yarnal R, Miles JH, Takahashi TN, Farmer J, McCathren R. Predicting responsiveness to treatment of children with autism: the importance of physical dysmorphology. Focus on Autism and Other Developmental Disabilities 2004;19(2):66–77.

61. Keegan MM, Takahashi TN, Miles JH. Macrocephaly in autism is not a homogeneous marker phenotype. American Society of Human Genetics Annual Meeting, San Diego, A755, 2007.

62. Boddaert N, Zilbovicius M, Philipe A, Robel L, Bourgeois M, Barthelemy C, et al. MRI findings in 77 children with non-syndromic autistic disorder. PLoS ONE. 2009;4(2):e4415.

63. Hashimoto T, Tayama M, Miyazaki M, Murakawa K, Shimakawa S, Yoneda Y, et al. Brainstem involvement in high functioning autistic children. Acta Neurol Scand. 1993;88(2):123–8.

64. Tsatsanis KD. Outcome research in Asperger syndrome and autism. Child Adolesc Psychiatr Clin N Am. 2003;12(1):47–63, vi.

65. Boger-Megiddo I, Shaw DW, Friedman SD, Sparks BF, Artru AA, Giedd JN, et al. Corpus callosum morphometrics in young children with autism spectrum disorder. J Autism Dev Disord. 2006;36(6):733–9.

66. Egaas B, Courchesne E, Saitoh O. Reduced size of corpus callosum in autism. Arch Neurol. 1995;52(8):794–801.

67. Piven J, Bailey J, Ranson BJ, Arndt S. An MRI study of the corpus callosum in autism. Am J Psychiatry. 1997;154(8):1051–6.

68. Vidal CN, Nicolson R, DeVito TJ, Hayashi KM, Geaga JA, Drost DJ, et al. Mapping corpus callosum deficits in autism: an index of aberrant cortical connectivity. Biol Psychiatry. 2006; 60(3):218–25.

69. Nacewicz BM, Dalton KM, Johnstone T, Long MT, McAuliff EM, Oakes TR, et al. Amygdala volume and nonverbal social impairment in adolescent and adult males with autism. Arch Gen Psychiatry. 2006;63(12):1417–28.

70. Dager SR, Wang L, Friedman SD, Shaw DW, Constantino JN, Artru AA, et al. Shape mapping of the hippocampus in young children with autism spectrum disorder. Am J Neuroradiol. 2007;28(4):672–7.

71. Nicolson R, DeVito TJ, Vidal CN, Sui Y, Hayashi KM, Drost DJ, et al. Detection and mapping of hippocampal abnormalities in autism. Psychiatry Res. 2006;148(1):11–21.

72. Levitt JG, O'Neill J, Blanton RE, Smalley S, Fadale D, McCracken JT, et al. Proton magnetic resonance spectroscopic imaging of the brain in childhood autism. Biol Psychiatry. 2003; 54(12):1355–66.

73. Hadjikhani N, Joseph RM, Snyder J, Chabris CF, Clark J, Steele S, et al. Activation of the fusiform gyrus when individuals with autism spectrum disorder view faces. Neuroimage. 2004; 22(3):1141–50.

74. Minshew NJ, Williams DL. The new neurobiology of autism: cortex, connectivity, and neuronal organization. Arch Neurol. 2007;64(7):945–50.

75. Jones KL. Smith's recognizable patterns of human malformation. 6th ed. Philadelphia: Elsevier Saunders; 2006.

76. Rodier PM, Ingram JL, Tisdale B, Nelson S, Romano J. Embryological origin for autism: developmental anomalies of the cranial nerve motor nuclei. J Comp Neurol. 1996;370(2): 247–61.

77. Rodier PM. 2003 Warkany Lecture: autism as a birth defect. Birth Defects Res A Clin Mol Teratol. 2004;70(1):1–6.

78. Waldrop MF, Halverson CF. Minor physical anomalies: their incidence and relation to behavior in a normal and deviant sample. In: Smart RC, Smart MS, editors. Readings in development and relationships. New York: Macmillan; 1971.

79. Mnukhin SS, Isaev DN. On the organic nature of some forms of schizoid or autistic psychopathy. J Autism Child Schizophr. 1975; 5(2):99–108.

80. Campbell M, Geller B, Small AM, Petti TA, Ferris SH. Minor physical anomalies in young psychotic children. Am J Psychiatry. 1978;135(5):573–5.

81. Walker HA. Incidence of minor physical anomaly in autism. J Autism Child Schizophr. 1977;7(2):165–76.

82. Links PS, Stockwell M, Abichandani F, Simeon J. Minor physical anomalies in childhood autism. Part I. Their relationship to pre- and perinatal complications. J Autism Dev Disord. 1980;10(3): 273–85.

83. Links PS. Minor physical anomalies in childhood autism. Part II. Their relationship to maternal age. J Autism Dev Disord. 1980; 10(3):287–92.

84. Steg JP, Rapoport JL. Minor physical anomalies in normal, neurotic, learning disabled, and severely disturbed children. J Autism Child Schizophr. 1975;5(4):299–307.

85. Gualtieri CT, Adams A, Shen CD, Loiselle D. Minor physical anomalies in alcoholic and schizophrenic adults and hyperactive and autistic children. Am J Psychiatry. 1982;139(5):640–3.

86. Waldrop MF, Halverson CF. Minor physical anomalies and hyperactive behavior in young children. In: Hellmuth J, editor. Exceptional infant: studies in abnormalities. New York: Brunner/ Mazel; 1971. p. 343–81.

87. Rodier PM. Converging evidence for brain stem injury in autism. Dev Psychopathol. 2002;14(3):537–57.

88. Miles JH, Hillman RE. Value of a clinical morphology examination in autism. Am J Med Genet. 2000;91(4):245–53.

89. Miles JH, Takahashi TN, Bagby S, Sahota PK, Vaslow DF, Wang CH, et al. Essential versus complex autism: definition of fundamental prognostic subtypes. Am J Med Genet A. 2005;135(2): 171–80.

90. O'Roak BJ, State MW. Autism genetics: strategies, challenges, and opportunities. Autism Res. 2008;1(1):4–17.

91. Rapin I, Tuchman RF, Rapin I, Tuchman RF. What is new in autism? Curr Opin Neurol. 2008;21(2):143–9.

92. Folstein SE, Rosen-Sheidley B. Genetics of autism: complex aetiology for a heterogeneous disorder. Nat Rev Genet. 2001;2(12): 943–55.

93. Arndt TL, Stodgell CJ, Rodier PM. The teratology of autism. Int J Dev Neurosci. 2005;23(2–3):189–99.

94. Freitag CM. The genetics of autistic disorders and its clinical relevance: a review of the literature. Mol Psychiatry. 2007; 12(1):2–22.

95. Geschwind DH, Levitt P. Autism spectrum disorders: developmental disconnection syndromes. Curr Opin Neurobiol. 2007;17(1):103–11.

96. Spence SJ. The genetics of autism. Semin Pediatr Neurol. 2004; 11(3):196–204.

97. Wassink TH, Brzustowicz LM, Bartlett CW, Szatmari P. The search for autism disease genes. Ment Retard Dev Disabil Res Rev. 2004;10(4):272–83.

98. Coon H. Current perspectives on the genetic analysis of autism. Am J Med Genet C Semin Med Genet. 2006;142(1):24–32.

99. Hasin DS, Grant BF. The co-occurrence of DSM-IV alcohol abuse in DSM-IV alcohol dependence: results of the National Epidemiologic Survey on Alcohol and Related Conditions on heterogeneity that differ by population subgroup. Arch Gen Psychiatry. 2004;61(9):891–6.

100. Li J, Nguyen L, Gleason C, Lotspeich L, Spiker D, Risch N, et al. Lack of evidence for an association between WNT2 and RELN polymorphisms and autism. Am J Med Genet B Neuropsychiatr Genet. 2004;126(1):51–7.

101. Agrawal A, Pergadia ML, Saccone SF, Lynskey MT, Wang JC, Martin NG, et al. An autosomal linkage scan for cannabis use disorders in the nicotine addiction genetics project. Arch Gen Psychiatry. 2008;65(6):713–21.

102. Howlin P, Goode S, Hutton J, Rutter M. Adult outcome for children with autism. J Child Psychol Psychiatry. 2004;45(2): 212–29.

103. Szatmari P, Bremner R, Nagy J. Asperger's syndrome: a review of clinical features. Can J Psychiatry. 1989;34(6):554–60.

104. Venter A, Lord C, Schopler E. A follow-up study of high-functioning autistic children. J Child Psychol Psychiatry. 1992;33(3): 489–507.

105. Santosh PJ, Mijovic A. Does pervasive developmental disorder protect children and adolescents against drug and alcohol use? Eur Child Adolesc Psychiatry. 2009;15:183–8.

106. Sizoo B, Brink W, Koeter M, Eenige MG, Wijngaarden-Cremers P, Gaag RJ. Treatment seeking adults with autism or ADHD and co-morbid substance use disorder: prevalence, risk factors and functional disability. Drug Alcohol Depend. 2010;107(1):44–50. doi:10.1016/j.drugalcdep.2009.09.003.

107. Aronson M, Hagberg B, Gillberg C. Attention deficits and autistic spectrum problems in children exposed to alcohol during gestation: a follow-up study. Dev Med Child Neurol. 1997;39(9): 583–7.

108. Harris SR, MacKay LL, Osborn JA. Autistic behaviors in offspring of mothers abusing alcohol and other drugs: a series of case reports. Alcohol Clin Exp Res. 1995;19(3):660–5.

109. Nanson JL. Autism in fetal alcohol syndrome: a report of six cases [see comments]. Alcohol Clin Exp Res. 1992;16(3):558–65.

110. Miller MT, Stromland K, Ventura L, Johansson M, Bandim JM, Gillberg C. Autism with ophthalmologic malformations: the plot thickens. Trans Am Ophthalmol Soc. 2004;102:107–20.

111. Steinhausen HC, Willms J, Metzke CW, Spohr HL. Behavioural phenotype in foetal alcohol syndrome and foetal alcohol effects. Dev Med Child Neurol. 2003;45(3):179–82.

112. Burd L, Klug MG, Martsolf JT, Kerbeshian J. Fetal alcohol syndrome: neuropsychiatric phenomics. Neurotoxicol Teratol. 2003;25(6):697–705.

113. Bishop S, Gahagan S, Lord C. Re-examining the core features of autism: a comparison of autism spectrum disorder and fetal alcohol spectrum disorder. J Child Psychol Psychiatry. 2007;48(11): 1111–21.

114. Lobascher ME, Kingerlee PE, Gubbay SS. Childhood autism: an investigation of aetiological factors in twenty-five cases. Br J Psychiatry. 1970;117(540):525–9.

115. DeLong GR, Dwyer JT. Correlation of family history with specific autistic subgroups: Asperger's syndrome and bipolar affective disease. J Autism Dev Disord. 1988;18(4):593–600.

116. Piven J, Chase GA, Landa R, Wzorek M, Gayle J, Cloud D, et al. Psychiatric disorders in the parents of autistic individuals. J Am Acad Child Adolesc Psychiatry. 1991;30(3):471–8.

117. Smalley SL, McCracken J, Tanguay P. Autism, affective disorders, and social phobia. Am J Hum Genet. 1995;60(1): 19–26.

118. Bolton PF, Pickles A, Murphy M, Rutter M. Autism, affective and other psychiatric disorders: patterns of familial aggregation. Psychol Med. 1998;28(2):385–95.

119. Miles JH, Takahashi TN, Haber A, Hadden L. Autism families with a high incidence of alcoholism. J Autism Dev Disord. 2003;33(4):403–15.

120. Andreasen NC, Rice J, Endicott J, Reich T, Coryell W. The family history approach to diagnosis. How useful is it? Arch Gen Psychiatry. 1986;43(5):421–9.

121. Orvaschel H, Thompson WD, Belanger A, Prusoff BA, Kidd KK. Comparison of the family history method to direct interview. Factors affecting the diagnosis of depression. J Affect Disord. 1982;4(1):49–59.

122. Yuan H, Marazita ML, Hill SY. Segregation analysis of alcoholism in high density families: a replication. Am J Med Genet. 1996;67(1):71–6.

123. Thompson WD, Orvaschel H, Prusoff BA, Kidd KK. An evaluation of the family history method for ascertaining psychiatric disorders. Arch Gen Psychiatry. 1982;39(1):53–8.

124. Rice JP, Reich T, Bucholz KK, Neuman RJ, Fishman R, Rochberg N, et al. Comparison of direct interview and family history diagnoses of alcohol dependence. Alcohol Clin Exp Res. 1995;19(4):1018–23.

125. Davies NJ, Sham PC, Gilvarry C, Jones PB, Murray RM. Comparison of the family history with the family study method: report from the Camberwell Collaborative Psychosis Study. Am J Hum Genet. 1997;74(1):12–7.

126. Eaton WW, Kramer M, Anthony JC, Dryman A, Shapiro S, Locke BZ. The incidence of specific DIS/DSM-III mental disorders: data from the NIMH Epidemiologic Catchment Area Program. Acta Psychiatr Scand. 1989;79(2):163–78.

127. Robins LN, Helzer JE, Weissman MM, Orvaschel H, Gruenberg E, Burke Jr JD, et al. Lifetime prevalence of specific psychiatric disorders in three sites. Arch Gen Psychiatry. 1984;41(10): 949–58.

128. Kessler RC, McGonagle KA, Zhao S, Nelson CB, Hughes M, Eshleman S, et al. Lifetime and 12-month prevalence of DSM-III-R psychiatric disorders in the United States. Results from the National Comorbidity Survey. Arch Gen Psychiatry. 1994;51(1):8–19.

129. Grant BF. Prevalence and correlates of alcohol use and DSM-IV alcohol dependence in the United States: results of the National Longitudinal Alcohol Epidemiologic Survey. J Stud Alcohol. 1997;58(5):464–73.

130. Johnson BA, Roache JD, Javors MA, DiClemente CC, Cloninger CR, Prihoda TJ, et al. Ondansetron for reduction of drinking among biologically predisposed alcoholic patients: a randomized controlled trial. JAMA. 2000;284(8):963–71.

131. Cloninger CR. Neurogenetic adaptive mechanisms in alcoholism. Science. 1987;236(4800):410–6.

132. Brown TG, Seraganian P, Tremblay J. Alcoholics also dependent on cocaine in treatment: do they differ from "pure" alcoholics? Addict Behav. 1994;19(1):105–12.

133. Litt MD, Babor TF, DelBoca FK, Kadden RM, Cooney NL. Types of alcoholics. II. Application of an empirically derived typology to treatment matching. Arch Gen Psychiatry. 1992;49(8): 609–14.

134. Hesselbrock VM, Hesselbrock MN. Are there empirically supported and clinically useful subtypes of alcohol dependence? Addiction. 2006;101 Suppl 1:97–103.

135. Edenberg HJ, Foroud T. The genetics of alcoholism: identifying specific genes through family studies. Addict Biol. 2006;11(3–4): 386–96.

136. Zucker RA, Ellis DA, Bingham CR, Fitzgerald HE. The development of alcoholic subtypes: risk variation among alcoholic families during the early childhood years. Alcohol Health Res World. 1996;20:46–55.

137. Kendler KS, Heath AC, Neale MC, Kessler RC, Eaves LJ. Alcoholism and major depression in women. A twin study of the causes of comorbidity. Arch Gen Psychiatry. 1993;50(9):690–8.

138. Bierut LJ, Dinwiddie SH, Begleiter H, Crowe RR, Hesselbrock V, Nurnberger Jr JI, et al. Familial transmission of substance dependence: alcohol, marijuana, cocaine, and habitual smoking: a report from the Collaborative Study on the Genetics of Alcoholism. Arch Gen Psychiatry. 1998;55(11):982–8.

139. Tsuang MT, Lyons MJ, Meyer JM, Doyle T, Eisen SA, Goldberg J, et al. Co-occurrence of abuse of different drugs in men: the role of drug-specific and shared vulnerabilities. Arch Gen Psychiatry. 1998;55(11):967–72.

140. Nurnberger Jr JI, Wiegand R, Bucholz K, O'Connor S, Meyer ET, Reich T, et al. A family study of alcohol dependence: coaggregation of multiple disorders in relatives of alcohol-dependent probands. Arch Gen Psychiatry. 2004;61(12):1246–56.

141. Robinson PD, Schutz CK, Macciardi F, White BN, Holden JJ. Genetically determined low maternal serum dopamine beta-hydroxylase levels and the etiology of autism spectrum disorders. Am J Med Genet. 2001;100(1):30–6.

142. Labuda D, Krajinovic M, Sabbagh A, Infante-Rivard C, Sinnett D. Parental genotypes in the risk of a complex disease. Am J Hum Genet. 2002;71(1):193–7.

143. Lasser K, Boyd JW, Woolhandler S, Himmelstein DU, McCormick D, Bor DH. Smoking and mental illness: a population-based prevalence study. JAMA. 2000;284(20):2606–10.

144. Dawson DA, Grant BF. Family history of alcoholism and gender: their combined effects on DSM-IV alcohol dependence and major depression. J Stud Alcohol. 1998;59(1):97–106.

145. Babor TF, Hofmann M, DelBoca FK, Hesselbrock V, Meyer RE, Dolinsky ZS, et al. Types of alcoholics. I. Evidence for an empirically derived typology based on indicators of vulnerability and severity. Arch Gen Psychiatry. 1992;49(8):599–608.

146. Sizoo B, Brink W, Eenige MG, Gaag RJ. Personality characteristics of adults with autism spectrum disorders of attention deficit hyperactivity disorder with and without substance use disorders. J Nerv Ment Dis. 2009;197(6):450–4.

147. Sauer CD, Takahashi TN, Miles JH. Autism and alcoholism: quest for genetic linkage. Am J Hum Genet. 2005;A127.

148. Vandeleur CL, Rothen S, Jeanpretre N, Lustenberger Y, Gamma F, Ayer E, et al. Inter-informant agreement and prevalence estimates for substance use disorders: direct interview versus family history method. Drug Alcohol Depend. 2008;92(1–3):9–19.

149. Interactive Autism Network. Baltimore, MD: Kennedy Krieger Institute. http://www.ianproject.org/. Accessed 17 Apr 2007.

150. Grice DE, Buxbaum JD. The genetics of autism spectrum disorders. Neuromol Med. 2006;8(4):451–60.

151. Lintas C, Persico AM. Autistic phenotypes and genetic testing: state-of-the-art for the clinical geneticist. J Med Genet. 2009; 46(1):1–8.

152. Losh M, Sullivan PF, Trembath D, Piven J. Current developments in the genetics of autism: from phenome to genome. J Neuropathol Exp Neurol. 2008;67(9):829–37.

153. Cook EHJ, Courchesne RY, Cox NJ, Lord C, Gonen D, Guter SJ, et al. Linkage-disequilibrium mapping of autistic disorder, with 15q11-13 markers. Am J Hum Genet. 1998;62(5):1077–83.

154. Martin ER, Menold MM, Wolpert CM, Bass MP, Donnelly SL, Ravan SA, et al. Analysis of linkage disequilibrium in gamma-aminobutyric acid receptor subunit genes in autistic disorder. Am J Med Genet. 2000;96(1):43–8.

155. Collins AL, Ma D, Whitehead PL, Martin ER, Wright HH, Abramson RK, et al. Investigation of autism and GABA receptor subunit genes in multiple ethnic groups. Neurogenetics. 2006; 7(3):167–74.

156. Buxbaum JD, Silverman JM, Smith CJ, Greenberg DA, Kilifarski M, Reichert J, et al. Association between a GABRB3 polymorphism and autism. Mol Psychiatry. 2002;7(3):311–6.

157. Menold MM, Shao Y, Wolpert CM, Donnelly SL, Raiford KL, Martin ER, et al. Association analysis of chromosome 15 gabaa receptor subunit genes in autistic disorder. J Neurogenet. 2001; 15(3–4):245–59.

158. Dick DM, Edenberg HJ, Xuei X, Goate A, Kuperman S, Schuckit M, et al. Association of GABRG3 with alcohol dependence. Alcohol Clin Exp Res. 2004;28(1):4–9.

159. Namkoong K, Cheon KA, Kim JW, Jun JY, Lee JY. Association study of dopamine D2, D4 receptor gene, GABAA receptor beta subunit gene, serotonin transporter gene polymorphism with children of alcoholics in Korea: a preliminary study. Alcohol. 2008;42(2):77–81.

160. Sutcliffe JS, Delahanty RJ, Prasad HC, McCauley JL, Han Q, Jiang L, et al. Allelic heterogeneity at the Serotonin Transporter Locus (SLC6A4) confers susceptibility to autism and rigid-compulsive behaviors. Am J Hum Genet. 2005;77(2):265–79.

161. McCauley JL, Olson LM, Dowd M, Amin T, Steele A, Blakely RD, et al. Linkage and association analysis at the serotonin transporter (SLC6A4) locus in a rigid-compulsive subset of autism. Am J Med Genet B Neuropsychiatr Genet. 2004;127(1):104–12.

162. Wassink TH, Losh M, Piven J, Sheffield VC, Ashley E, Westin ER, et al. Systematic screening for subtelomeric anomalies in a clinical sample of autism. J Autism Dev Disord. 2007;37(4):703–8.

163. Hammoumi S, Payen A, Favre JD, Balmes JL, Benard JY, Husson M, et al. Does the short variant of the serotonin transporter linked polymorphic region constitute a marker of alcohol dependence? Alcohol. 1999;17(2):107–12.

164. Feinn R, Nellissery M, Kranzler HR. Meta-analysis of the association of a functional serotonin transporter promoter polymorphism with alcohol dependence. Am J Med Genet B Neuropsychiatr Genet. 2005;133B(1):79–84.

165. Seneviratne C, Huang W, Ait-Daoud N, Li MD, Johnson BA. Characterization of a functional polymorphism in the 3′ UTR of SLC6A4 and its association with drinking intensity. Alcohol Clin Exp Res. 2009;33(2):332–9.

166. Szatmari P, Paterson AD, Zwaigenbaum L, Roberts W, Brian J, Liu XQ, et al. Mapping autism risk loci using genetic linkage and chromosomal rearrangements. Nat Genet. 2007;39(3):319–28.

167. Lise MF, El Husseini A. The neuroligin and neurexin families: from structure to function at the synapse. Cell Mol Life Sci. 2006;63(16):1833–49.

168. Feng J, Schroer R, Yan J, Song W, Yang C, Bockholt A, et al. High frequency of neurexin 1beta signal peptide structural variants in patients with autism. Neurosci Lett. 2006;409(1):10–3.

169. Kim HG, Kishikawa S, Higgins AW, Seong IS, Donovan DJ, Shen Y, et al. Disruption of neurexin 1 associated with autism spectrum disorder. Am J Hum Genet. 2008;82(1):199–207.

170. Yan J, Noltner K, Feng J, Li W, Schroer R, Skinner C, et al. Neurexin 1alpha structural variants associated with autism. Neurosci Lett. 2008;438(3):368–70.

171. Uhl GR, Drgon T, Johnson C, Li CY, Contoreggi C, Hess J, et al. Molecular genetics of addiction and related heritable phenotypes: genome-wide association approaches identify "connectivity constellation" and drug target genes with pleiotropic effects. Ann NY Acad Sci. 2008;1141:318–81.

172. Alarcon M, Abrahams BS, Stone JL, Duvall JA, Perederiy JV, Bomar JM, et al. Linkage, association, and gene-expression analyses identify CNTNAP2 as an autism-susceptibility gene. Am J Hum Genet. 2008;82(1):150–9.

173. Arking DE, Cutler DJ, Brune CW, Teslovich TM, West K, Ikeda M, et al. A common genetic variant in the neurexin superfamily member CNTNAP2 increases familial risk of autism. Am J Hum Genet. 2008;82(1):160–4.

174. Bakkaloglu B, O'Roak BJ, Louvi A, Gupta AR, Abelson JF, Morgan TM, et al. Molecular cytogenetic analysis and resequencing of contactin associated protein-like 2 in autism spectrum disorders. Am J Hum Genet. 2008;82(1):165–73.

175. Roohi J, Montagna C, Tegay DH, Palmer LE, DeVincent C, Pomeroy JC, et al. Disruption of contactin 4 in three subjects with autism spectrum disorder. J Med Genet. 2009;46(3):176–82.

176. Garber K. Neuroscience. Autism's cause may reside in abnormalities at the synapse. Science. 2007;317(5835):190–1.

177. Persico AM, Bourgeron T. Searching for ways out of the autism maze: genetic, epigenetic and environmental clues. Trends Neurosci. 2006;29(7):349–58.

178. Nussbaum J, Xu Q, Payne TJ, Ma JZ, Huang W, Gelernter J, et al. Significant association of the neurexin-1 gene (NRXN1) with nicotine dependence in European- and African-American smokers. Hum Mol Genet. 2008;17(11):1569–77.

179. Hishimoto A, Liu QR, Drgon T, Pletnikova O, Walther D, Zhu XG, et al. Neurexin 3 polymorphisms are associated with alcohol dependence and altered expression of specific isoforms. Hum Mol Genet. 2007;16(23):2880–91.

180. Li MD, Burmeister M. New insights into the genetics of addiction. Nat Rev Genet. 2009;10(4):225–31.

Personality Disorders

24

Louisa M.C. van den Bosch and Roel Verheul

Abstract

Subject of this chapter is the often found combination of personality disorders and substance abuse disorders. The serious nature of this comorbidity is shown through the discussion of prevalence and epidemiological data. Literature shows that the comorbidity, hampering the diagnostic process, is seen as complicating for treatment planning. Therefore, etiological models that explain the co-occurrence of both disorders are helpful. Several models, among them the Behavioral Disinhibition Pathway, the Stress Reduction Pathway, and the Reward Sensitivity Pathway are described. Next, treatment programs, focusing on one or on both disorders are described, and research results are shown. Finally, clinical implications are described. The most important conclusion drawn is that treatment of dually diagnosed patients with severe problems needs to include both foci, and because of that conclusion, therapists need to be trained to address a range of symptomatic manifestations of personality pathology in the impulse control spectrum.

Learning Objectives
- High joint comorbidity is evident for ASPD/BPD and substance use disorder.
- Assessment and diagnosis require careful attention to disentangling substance-related and independent personality pathology.
- Several causal pathways can be distinguished, that can have important consequences for planning treatment.
- Contrary to expectations, recent evidence has convincingly demonstrated that comorbid patients usually benefit from addiction treatments, but they often only improve to a level of problem severity that leaves them at considerable risk for relapse.
- Some evidence suggests that comorbid patients benefit from treatments focusing on the personality disorder as much as do those without substance use disorder.
- Results show that treatment of dually diagnosed patients with severe problems needs to include both foci (substance use disorder and personality disorder), because of the enormous gain for patients when personality disorders are addressed too.
- Therapists need to be trained to address a range of symptomatic manifestations of personality pathology in the impulse control spectrum.

L.M.C. van den Bosch, Ph.D. (✉)
Psychiatric Hospital de Gelderse Roos,
Wagnerlaan 2, 6815 AG Arnhem, The Netherlands

Centre of Specific Psychotherapy, Rhijngeesterstraatweg 13c,
2342 AN Oegstgeest, The Netherlands
e-mail: wiesvdbosch@planet.nl

R. Verheul, Ph.D.
Department of Clinical Psychology, University of Amsterdam,
Roetersstraat 15, 1018 WB Amsterdam, The Netherlands

Viersprong Institute for Studies on Personality Disorders (VISPD),
Center of Psychotherapy De, Viersprong, Post Box 7,
4660 AA Halsteren, The Netherlands

Issues that Need to Be Addressed by Future Research

- More research focusing on the effectivity of DFST, especially: what elements work.
- Research on the effectivity of DBT for, other than BPD, personality disorders in dually focused treatment programs.
- Research on the question whether treatment for Drug or Alcohol abuse needs to be different, what creates the differences and why.
- Examining effectivity of programs aimed at training therapist in multiple problem targeting.
- Research in which the effectivity of a chain of interconnected, and theory consistent, treatment modalities (like day treatment, long-term after care, outpatient treatment) is examined.

Introduction

Literature searches show that the evaluation of co-occurring personality disorders has been the subject of countless studies by addiction researchers. Interestingly, very little attention is paid by personality disorder researchers to the co-occurrence of substance abuse. This state of affairs is difficult to understand since prevalence rates show that comorbidity of substance abuse and personality disorders is the most common form of dual diagnosis to be found. Still, the topic of substance abuse is covered in only a very limited way in most personality disorder books and in the education of psychotherapists. A number of reasons might account for this: (1) the field of personality disorder research is relatively young, whereas the field of addiction has a long history; (2) the mental health field is, except for some addiction programs that have been adapted for treatment of personality disorders—particularly therapeutic communities—segregated in treatment for mental health that excludes substance use disorders (SUD), and centers for treatment of SUD; (3) there is a differentiation in treatment programs for personality disorders and addiction problems, focusing on one kind of disorder only; (4) funding for personality disorder research has been more limited than funding for research on Axis I disorders. Finally, patients with addictive behaviors are often excluded from treatment programs and studies of personality disorders, because substance abuse patients are considered to have little potential for change, are a strain to the therapist, and are at high risk for dropout. Thus, most research on patients with co-occurring personality disorders have been conducted in patients referred for treatment of substance abuse.

This chapter aims to review the empirical and scientific literature on the occurrence and treatment implications of comorbid substance use and personality disorders, based mostly on studies of substance use populations. *Prevalence and Epidemiology* provides an overview of empirical studies of comorbidity, and covers factors that affect prevalence estimates. *Assessment and diagnosis* discusses probable reasons for the differences found in prevalence and epidemiological studies, and aims to advice clinicians on how to deal with diagnostic problems. In *Etiology* we examine the direction of the relationship between personality disorders and substance use disorders. *Treatment* builds on the etiological models that have been shown to have important implications for treatment planning and clinical management. Finally, *Clinical implications* will be discussed and some *conclusions* are drawn.

Prevalence and Epidemiology

Prevalence Studies of Comorbidity Among Individuals with Personality Disorders

Reported prevalence rates of personality disorders (PD) in non-patient samples of individuals with substance use disorder are at least three times higher than in normal individuals (i.e., those without mental disorders including substance use disorder), ranging from 43% to 77% among patients with various personality disorders [1, 2]. In a sample of more than 500 psychiatric patients, Zanarini et al. [3] found substance use disorders in 64% of patients with borderline personality disorder (BPD) and in 54% of patients with other personality disorders. Toner et al. [4] found a prevalence rate of substance use disorder of 100% among patients with cluster B personality disorders and no substance use disorders in cluster A or C.

Prevalence Studies of Comorbidity Among Individuals with Substance Use Disorders

Numerous studies have shown that DSM-IV personality disorders are highly prevalent among individuals with substance use disorders, particularly antisocial, borderline, avoidant, and paranoid personality disorders. Prevalence rates of personality disorders have ranged widely from 30% to 75% in those with alcohol use disorders and from 30% to 90% in those with drug addiction [1, 5, 6]. The estimate of personality disorder prevalence ranged from 44% among alcoholic patients to 79% among opiate abusers. The two most prevalent personality disorders among patients with substance use disorder are antisocial personality disorder (ASPD) and BPD, with reported estimates of 22% for ASPD and 18% for BPD. Reported estimates for paranoid and avoidant personality disorders are 11% and 10%, respectively [7]. The other personality disorders are found in less than 10% of patients with substance use disorder (range 1–9%).

Epidemiological Studies

Many studies have stressed the negative effect of the combination of personality disorders and substance use disorder (SUD), as a strong predictor of relapse in addictive behavior [8–10]. The combination of *ASPD* and SUD is particularly negative one, not only in a prognostic sense [11–14]. Costs and duration of treatment are higher (i.e., [15]), as well as the risk of somatic illness [16, 17] and premature mortality [18]. ASPD/SUD patients also create a strain to therapists because they show more aggressive and impulsive behaviors compared to others [18]. The combination of *BPD* and SUD has proved to be a significant predictor of a lifetime diagnosis of SUD, even when the effects of other cluster B and all cluster C PDs are statistically controlled for [19]. Risks for and rates of suicide and suicide attempts, already high among individuals with BPD or substance abuse are even higher for individuals with both disorders [20–22]. Among the other effects of the combination of BPD and SUD, unemployment is found [23], as well as sexually promiscuous behavior [24].

Although the evidence seems overwhelming, the conclusion about the negative effect of combined SUD and PD needs to be called inconclusive. A number of studies have pointed out that the combined PD/SUD does not inevitably lead to negative prognostic consequences (i.e., [25–29]). For example, the combination of ASPD/SUD and a comorbid affective disorder seems to influence the prognosis in a beneficial way [30, 31].

The differences found in epidemiological studies can be accounted for by the many methodological and interpretative problems faced by researchers of these populations: for example, differences in substances used, setting, differences in the diagnostic criteria employed (classification system, criteria for excluding substance-related pathology, timeframe criteria), assessment procedures (time of measurement, method), and sampling factors (gender, age). For example, alcohol use is less destructive when compared to heroin and cocaine use [28, 32–34]. Adult ASPD has a much better prognosis compared to ASPD diagnosed before adulthood [35, 36]. The number of BPD criteria met appears critical [37]. Males and females differ in their patterns of comorbid personality and substance use disorders [30, 38–40]. And, finally, the assessment method employed seems to affect the observed prevalence to a great extent [41]. It can be expected that recent developments in psychiatric diagnostic modules will contribute to the validity of conclusions drawn in future research of substance use and psychiatric disorder epidemiology [42].

Assessment and Diagnosis

According to DSM-IV-TR, it is only when the consequences of substance abuse persist beyond the period of alcohol and/or drug consumption that these features constitute personality pathology. There is some consensus that self-reports overdiagnose personality disorders, especially in patients with substance use disorder [41]. Diagnostic (semi-structured) interviews may have greater specificity because questions and answers can clarify if a symptom is chronic and pervasive, more situation-specific, or related to substance abuse [9, 43]. Further clinical inquiry can also determine whether other behavioral examples of the trait exist that are not specifically related to substance abuse. An interview also provides important behavioral observations of the patient's interpersonal style that may inform clinical judgment [44].

In treatment planning, one of the most problematic diagnostic questions for clinicians seems to be which personality disorder symptoms that may be substance related need to be included or excluded. It is important to realize that excluding all symptoms that have ever been related to substance use will probably exclude all secondary personality pathology and may even exclude primary personality pathology. This could lead to an extremely restricted, and perhaps ineffective, treatment plan, especially in clinical situations with comorbid patients where their problems are directly related to intoxication and/or withdrawal. A correct answer to these questions, however, seems to be nearly impossible. This task becomes almost impossible when the patient's entire adolescent and adult life is characterized by chronic substance abuse. A further problem is created because of the inability of most addicted patients to distinguish between behaviors that are related to substance intoxication, substance withdrawal, or obtaining drugs and non-substance use-related behavior. This requires an empathic awareness of the impact of one's behavior on self and others and a willingness to accept responsibility for one's actions [44]. A high level of introspection and cognitive competence is, therefore, required and such qualities are often impaired in these patients. Patients have difficulties distinguishing what behavior is connected to drug use, and what behavior that was part of their not-using history, will stay when they no longer have a substance use disorder. In particular, distinguishing the antisocial activities, like lying and cheating that may be related to obtaining substances, from non-substance-related behaviors, plays an important role. These behaviors are often seen as sign of personality disturbance but can in fact be a consequence of the drug use. Also, these behaviors are often interpreted as signs of an ASPD (lying, aggression/assault, breaking the law), often a criterion that leads to exclusion from treatment. Consistent with this view, Rounsaville et al. [45] found that excluding substance-related symptoms reduced the reliability of ASPD diagnoses (but not of BPD diagnoses).

In general, a PD diagnosis should be kept "in store," until at least 2 weeks of abstinence has passed. Or, when time is too short, a collateral informant should be interviewed to gain valid information for diagnosis. In clinical practice it is probably more reliable to determine whether a symptom should be considered substance related on an item-by-item basis and not wait until the end of the interview or until all items relating to a specific disorder are administered. Also, DSM criteria in which substance dependence is an inherent part should be scored as due to substance abuse unless non-substance-related behavioral indicators of the trait (e.g., impulsivity, unlawful behaviors) are also present. In our experience it is important that the clinician should periodically remind patients that questions refer to the way they usually are. All studies on the subject of comorbidity of PDs and SUD agree that a careful diagnostic process should be undertaken, but they emphasize that it is a prerequisite when the patient shows life-threatening behavior or risky behavior, such as exchanging used needles [13, 46].

Etiology

It is now widely agreed in the literature that the addictive personality does not exist, and that no particular personality type is predisposed to addiction. But how do we account then for the common comorbidity of SUD and personality disorders? Evidence for causal relationships between SUD and personality disorders can be derived from the fact that the rate of co-occurrence exceeds that by chance alone, as evidenced by familial aggregation studies, epidemiological findings, genetic epidemiology, long-term longitudinal studies, and retrospective studies that account for the order of onset of each disorder. The available evidence suggests at least three different possible developmental pathways to comorbidity: the primary substance use disorder model, the primary personality disorder model, and the common factor model. It is important to note that the different models are not necessarily mutually exclusive. In any individual case, more than one model may have explanatory value. Furthermore, it is possible that one model best describes the initiation of a comorbid disorder, whereas another describes long-term maintenance of the comorbid association.

Primary Substance Use Disorder Model

The primary substance use disorder model in which substance abuse contributes to the development of personality pathology has received relatively little empirical attention. Three mechanisms are proposed [47]: (1) substance abuse often occurs within the context of a deviant peer group, and antisocial behaviors might be shaped and reinforced by social group norms (social learning hypothesis); (2) some Cluster A traits (e.g., suspiciousness, eccentric behaviors, magical thinking), Cluster B traits (e.g., egocentrism, manipulativeness), and Cluster C traits (e.g., passivity, social avoidance) may be shaped and maintained by the reinforcing and conditioning properties of psychoactive substances (behaviorist learning hypothesis); and (3) chronic substance abuse or withdrawal may alter personality through neuro-adaptive changes or a direct effect on brain chemistry (neuro-pharmacological hypothesis).

To the best of our knowledge, there are no studies that empirically support the primary substance use disorder model. The possibility that some symptoms in some individual patients with substance use disorder are shaped and maintained by the reinforcing and conditioning properties of social group norms or psychoactive substances, however, should not be rejected. For example, with comorbid patients that stay in high-security hospitals for a very long period, it can be expected that the effect of the reinforcement contingencies and the need to cope with the environment may lead to permanent changes in personality patterns.

Primary Personality Disorder Model

The primary personality disorder model describes comorbid relationships in which (pathological) personality traits contribute to the development of substance use disorder. Since the 1990s, many studies have yielded empirical support for a more dimensional adaptation of this model (i.e., [48]). The available evidence suggests at least three different developmental pathways from personality to addiction, associated with the clusters of personality disorder [9, 49, 50]. These pathways were defined as the behavioral disinhibition pathway, the stress reduction pathway, and the reward sensitivity pathway.

Behavioral Disinhibition Pathway
Individuals scoring high on antisocial traits like deceitfulness, or failure to conform to social norms, and impulsivity and low on constraint or conscientiousness have lower thresholds for deviant behaviors, and thus, they can easily become engaged in alcohol and drug abuse, especially when the circumstances in which they live are favorable [51, 52]. This model might account for the often found association of ASPD and, to some extent, BPD, with substance abuse. This model is the best documented one of the three. Firstly, as already pointed out, high comorbidity is observed between substance use disorder and Axis I and personality disorders from the impulse control spectrum [2, 53, 54]. Secondly, in addition to several longitudinal studies [48, 55, 56], more direct evidence can be derived from Cohen et al. [57] who found personality disorders, especially from cluster B, diagnosed on average at age thirteen to be highly predictive of diagnoses and symptoms of SUDs. Thirdly, based on a nationally representative epidemiologic sample ($N=43,093$), Goldstein et al. [58] concluded that onset of conduct disorder (CD) in childhood before age ten results in significantly elevated odds of drug dependence.

Stress Reduction Pathway

The stress reduction pathway (the affect-regulation model) to substance abuse argues that individuals scoring high on traits such as stress reactivity, anxiety sensitivity, and neuroticism (sometimes associated with stressful childhood experiences) are vulnerable to stressful life events, and thus to the way of coping that includes drug and alcohol use. This pathway might account for the comorbidity with BPD, avoidant, dependent, and obsessive-compulsive personality disorder. Substances can be either used to enhance positive affect or for symptom relief. These individuals typically respond to stress with anxiety and mood instability, which in turn can become a motive for substance use as self-medication. Longitudinal studies have shown that teachers' ratings of negative emotionality, stress reactivity, and low harm avoidance in children predicted substance abuse in adolescence and young adulthood [48, 52, 55]. James [59] showed the importance of negative emotionality in 617 university students with self-reported substance use problems and Cluster B PD symptoms. Furthermore, Conrod et al. [60] showed that coping motives for drinking as well as the fear-dampening properties of alcohol were far more pronounced among men scoring high on anxiety-sensitivity than among their low-scoring counterparts. Finally, individuals who score high on measures reflecting impulsivity/disinhibition seem to experience pronounced alcohol effects and may be more sensitive to alcohol [61]. The self-medication pathway, which has most frequently been investigated for alcoholism, typically accounts for late-onset alcohol use disorders and is more prevalent among women than among men. Finally, indirect support for this pathway is found in a study in which 58 female BPD patients were treated with standard Dialectical Behavior Therapy (DBT) [62]. Results showed that with the reduction of the impulsive self-destructive behavior, alcohol use was significantly reduced too.

Reward Sensitivity Pathway

It can be predicted that individuals scoring high on traits such as novelty seeking, reward seeking, and extraversion, will be motivated to use substances for their positive reinforcing properties. This pathway might account for the comorbidity of substance use disorder with antisocial, histrionic, and narcissistic personality disorders. Consistent with this hypothesis, some longitudinal studies [48, 52, 56] have shown that novelty seeking as a temperamental trait in childhood predicts later substance use problems. Also, hyperresponsiveness or hypersensitivity to the rewarding effects of substances, which in itself can be the result of repetitive use of the substances themselves, might develop most strongly among individuals characterized by a more general sensitivity to positive reinforcements [63, 64]. Furthermore, some evidence suggests that scores of extraversion, predict alcohol and drug dependence [65, 66]. Finally, Conrod et al. [60]

demonstrated that men with multigenerational family histories of alcoholism demonstrated elevated resting heart rates (index of psychostimulation) in response to alcohol intake, suggesting that this pathway partly mediates the role of genetic vulnerability in the etiology of alcoholism.

Common Factor Model

The common factor model assumes that both personality pathology and substance abuse are linked to an independent third factor that contributes to the development of both disorders. This model is more likely for personality disorders that show relatively high joint comorbidity, such as ASPD and BPD [67]. This hypothesis is consistent with a psychobiological perspective on personality disorders suggesting that BPD and ASPD are phenomenologically, genetically, and/or biologically related to Axis I impulse disorders such as substance abuse [68, 69].

Family, twin, and adoption studies are generally considered most appropriate to evaluate whether a common risk factor is transmitted genetically or otherwise. Until now, no evidence for cross-transmission of pure forms and no support for the shared-etiology model have been found. Behavior genetic studies need to avoid biases in estimates of genetic and environmental effects, like the possibility of substantial non-random mating with regard to ASPD and substance use [70].

Another approach in the search for common factors has relied on high-risk strategies, with the aim of identifying markers of biological vulnerability for both conditions. Justus et al. [71] found that a reduced amplitude of the P300 component of the scalp-recorded event-related brain potential in men is strongly associated with a general tendency toward antisocial, defiant, and impulsive traits, which in turn increase the risk for alcohol abuse [71]. Furthermore, some reviewers [47, 68] have concluded that abnormalities in serotonergic function may form a biological substrate underlying both substance abuse and impulsive/aggressive behavior.

Treatment

Outcomes of Treatments Focusing on Substance Abuse

Several studies published recently have showed convincingly that personality pathology, although associated with pre- and post-treatment problem severity, is not a robust predictor of the amount of improvement, which is in sharp contrast to clinical experiences and knowledge (e.g., [28, 72]). Furthermore, some studies showed that PD comorbidity is not associated with premature dropout or a shorter time-in-program [73, 74], or outcomes in pharmacotherapy [75].

Most studies have focused on cluster B disorders. Some factors seem to influence compliance to treatment, such as case management. Havens et al. [76] showed that injection drug users with and without comorbid ASPD, who spent 25 or more minutes with their case manager prior to their treatment entry date, were 3.51 times more likely to enter treatment than those who received less than 5 min. Ball et al. [73] found that lost motivation or hope for change appeared to be associated with dropout reasons. One study supported this finding. Carroll et al. [74], in a study focused on motivation, found that participants assigned to motivational interviewing had significantly better retention rates, but there were no significant effects on substance use outcomes. The question whether staff functioning or attitude contributes to early dropout is still left unanswered, although several authors have suggested that these factors play a significant motivational role [73, 77, 78]. Also mandatory treatment can have beneficial effects [79, 80], giving a whole new meaning to the concept "motivation."

In a prospective 4-year study, Krampe et al. [81] found that chronicity and the presence of a personality disorder were independently associated with decrease of cumulative 4-year abstinence probability. Thus, it seems that "an equal amount of improvement" does not resemble a similar risk of relapse. A possible explanation for this apparent discrepancy is that patients without personality pathology improve to a level of problem severity that no longer leaves them at risk for relapse, whereas patients with personality pathology are at risk for relapse despite their improvement. One study suggested that the level of emotional reactivity is lower among antisocial comorbid patients, compared to "normal" SUD patients, thereby hampering treatment [82]. Verheul, van den Bosch, and Ball [41] show that it is important to differentiate between individuals with only antisocial behaviors and individuals with ASPD, including traits such as shallow affect, grandiosity, and lack of empathy and remorse. The latter group might be more at risk for poor treatment response and outcome as Marmorstein and colleagues [83] show. This study also illustrates how significant the impact of gender is in the treatment of patients with comorbid problems. In a population-based sample of twins, the course of antisocial behavior with persisting (beginning by early adolescence and continuing through late adolescence) and desisting (stopping by mid-adolescence) antisocial behavior in terms of risk for later substance dependence and background risk factors was examined. Late-onset antisocial behavior has many of the same negative correlates of persisting antisocial behavior but occurs in significantly more females. Although they are excluded from the diagnosis of ASPD, these youths have clinically significant problems similar to those adults with this diagnosis. In this respect it creates hope that there is a growing body of studies on the adequate detection of comorbidity among adolescents and young adults aimed at the development of early specific interventions [84–86].

Consistently, several studies stress the importance of diagnosing and treating both substance use disorder and personality disorders in the same program [87, 88], because patients continued to exhibit high levels of risk and mental distress, long after treatment for SUD. Furthermore, Fridell and Hesse [89] showed that even if treating psychiatric problems has modest effects on abstinence, effective treatment of psychiatric symptoms in substance abusers might be life saving, because it decreases mortality.

Outcomes of Treatments Focusing on Personality Disorder

Little is known about the impact of substance abuse on treatment outcome of patients in treatment for their personality problems. Patients with comorbid SUD are often excluded from studies examining the efficacy of treatments designed to target personality disorder symptoms, although several studies have shown a lack of differences in clinical characteristics and/or etiological background between patients with and without SUD [14, 90].

To the best of our knowledge there is only one study that has investigated the impact of substance abuse on the outcome of a treatment focusing on PDs. In their randomized trial of DBT among Dutch borderline women, Verheul et al. [91] and van den Bosch et al. [62] found no differences in effectiveness for patients with and without substance use problems. However, studies of the efficacy of Mentalization Based Treatment (MBT) for severe BPD have typically included a large number of comorbid substance use disorders, and have showed extremely favorable outcomes [92], also in the long run [93].

Outcomes of Dual Focus Treatments

Only two psychotherapies have been developed for dual treatment, i.e., Schema Focused Therapy and DBT.

The only documented integrated dual focus treatment for the broad range of personality disorders is dual focus schema therapy (DFST), developed by Ball and Young [94, 95]. DFST is a 24-week, manual-guided individual therapy including both symptom-focused relapse prevention and coping skills techniques and schema-focused techniques for maladaptive schemas and coping styles.

Ball and colleagues [96] examined the treatment retention and utilization of DFST for a sample of 52 predominantly homeless men within a homeless drop-in center. The subjects could be characterized as a group with all the persistent and pervasive deficits that define personality disorder in combination with substance abuse. Superior utilization of DFST over Drug Counseling (DC) for participants was found, although further analyses of separate Cluster A,

Cluster B, and Cluster C symptoms scores favored DC over DFST for therapy utilization by more severe Cluster A and C clients. In a second randomized pilot study among 30 methadone-maintenance patients comparing DFST to 12-Step Facilitation Therapy (12FT), Ball [97] found some preliminary empirical support. Patients met criteria for an average of 3.3 personality disorders per patient, with ASPD present in over 70% and BPD and avoidant personality disorder present in over 50% of the cases. There were no significant differences between the two therapies for retention, utilization, or reductions in psychiatric symptoms or psychosocial impairment. Both therapy conditions demonstrated significant reductions in various severity indicators. DFST participants, however, demonstrated more rapid decreases in the frequency of their substance use over 6 months of DFST in comparison to 12FT. However, DFST patients and therapists reported an increase from a good early therapeutic alliance to a very strong alliance.

The two published randomized trials of DFST suggest this is a promising approach, but further research is necessary.

The second dual focus treatment involves a modified version of DBT known as DBT-S. This program includes all of the components of standard DBT (i.e., weekly individual cognitive-behavioral psychotherapy sessions with the primary therapist, weekly skills training groups lasting 2–2.5 h per session, weekly supervision and consultation meetings for the therapists, and phone consultation) plus application of dialectics to abstinence issues, application of a specific pharmacotherapy module, a treatment target hierarchy relevant to substance abuse, new strategies to keep difficult-to-engage and easily lost patients, the addition of six new and modified skills, an individual skills consultation mode, and increased emphasis on using natural and arbitrary reinforcers for maintenance of abstinence.

In a randomized trial, Linehan et al. [98] compared DBT-S to Treatment as Usual (TAU). Subjects assigned to DBT-S had significantly lower dropout rates and significantly greater reductions in substance-related outcomes and psychiatric functioning (although not parasuicidality) throughout the treatment year and at 16-month follow-up compared to control subjects. A second randomized trial [99] showed somewhat mixed results. DBT-S and comprehensive validation therapy incorporating 12-step facilitation (CVT + 12 S) both effectively reduced opiate use and level of psychopathology, when combined with LAAM replacement medication. DBT participants maintained reductions in mean opiate use through 12 months of active treatment while CVT + 12 S participants significantly increased opiate use during the last 4 months. CVT + 12 S, however, was remarkably effective in retaining patients (100% vs. 64% DBT-S).

The efficacy of DBT-S has been clearly established in a subgroup of substance abuse patients with BPD, but not with the wide range of other personality disorders found in substance abusers. Further research is necessary.

Outcomes of Treatments Focusing on Pharmacotherapy

Pharmacotherapy may have an important role in the treatment of dual diagnosis patients. Medications may ameliorate some personality disorder symptoms while simultaneously improving the outcome of SUD. It should be noted, however, that the co-occurrence of these disorders is also associated with high rates of non-compliance and an increased risk of lethal overdose, as well as the potential for dependence on medication.

Surprisingly, the number of studies focusing on pharmacotherapy in dual diagnosis patients is very limited. In the last 2 years, only one study was published. In a study on buprenorphine treatment outcome in heroin-dependent patients with personality disorders, Gerra et al. [100] showed that high doses of buprenorphine predict a better outcome as measured by negative urines, but not as measured by retention.

Clinical Implications

In general, clinical guidelines for the treatment of personality disorder recommend psychotherapy whenever possible, complemented by symptom-targeted pharmacotherapy whenever necessary or useful.

The authors wish to mention some essential ingredients of effective treatment of patients with both SUD and personality disorders.

- In treatment of comorbid patients, risk assessment always needs to take place and should be a critical focus of treatment efforts [101–105].
- The treatment requires special and professional attention to both foci (substance use disorder and personality disorders) from the very beginning, i.e., the program should consist of an integrated package of these elements, with a particular emphasis on motivational interviewing and validation throughout the entire treatment process [73, 74, 106].
- In addition to the regular program modules, intensive individual counseling, with therapeutic contact for extended periods of time, is recommended to establish a working alliance and to prevent these patients from leaving treatment early [107]. Treatment programs should integrate targeted behavior therapy interventions with empirical support for their use with specific disorders found in substance abusers, particularly antisocial [108] and borderline [109, 110]. But psychotherapy with

patients with both SUD and personality disorder is likely to have greater success if it is provided in the context of a relatively long-term treatment program that provides sufficient structure and safety (e.g., day hospital, residential treatment, or methadone maintenance program), and is combined with a skill training or relapse prevention program.

– Patients with SUD and severe personality disorders consume a disproportionate amount of staff time. They tend to be admitted into treatment repeatedly and exhaust the resources of one counselor after the next. Therapists treating these dual disorders should be professional or highly skilled therapists with extensive education and training in psychotherapy, psychopathology, personality disorders, and addiction. Given the challenges of treating this population, all therapists should be obliged to take part in some forum for supervision or consultation.

– Finally, participation in an appropriate aftercare program is highly recommended.

Conclusions

We have seen that (1) high joint comorbidity is evident for ASPD/BPD and substance use disorder, (2) assessment and diagnosis require careful attention to disentangling substance-related and independent personality pathology, (3) several causal pathways can be distinguished, that can have important consequences for planning treatment, (4) contrary to expectations, recent evidence has convincingly demonstrated that comorbid patients usually benefit from addiction treatments, but they often only improve to a level of problem severity that leaves them at considerable risk for relapse, (5) some evidence suggests that comorbid patients benefit from treatments focusing on the personality disorder as much as do those without substance use disorder, (6) results show that treatment of dually diagnosed patients with severe problems needs to include both foci, because of the enormous gain for patients when personality disorders are addressed too, and (7) therapists need to be trained to address a range of symptomatic manifestations of personality pathology in the impulse control spectrum.

The lack of more significant progress in treatment for comorbid disorders has been attributed to stigma, clinical lack of knowledge, uncertainty regarding assessment, and insufficient organizational support. Dissemination of information on recent advancements in the treatment of comorbidity, including manual-driven, empirically validated treatment approaches (e.g., motivational enhancement, 12-step and/or cognitive-behavioral therapies) is required.

Acknowledgments Special thanks to Rebecca Dulitt and Lisa Davies.

References

1. Verheul R, van den Brink W, Hartgers C. Personality disorders predict relapse in alcoholic patients. Addict Behav. 1998; 23:869–82.
2. Zimmerman M, Coryell WH. DSM-III personality disorder diagnoses in a nonpatient sample: demographic correlates and comorbidity. Arch Gen Psychiatry. 1989;46:682–9.
3. Zanarini MC, Frankenburg FR, Dubo ED. Axis I comorbidity of borderline personality disorder. Am J Psychiatry. 1998;155: 1733–9.
4. Toner BB, Gillies LA, Prendergast P, Cote FH, Browne C. Substance use disorders in a sample of Canadian patients with chronic mental illness. Hosp Commun Psychiatry. 1992;43(3): 251–4.
5. Grant BF, Stinson FS, Dawson DA, Chou SP, Ruan WJ, Pickering RP. Co-occurrence of 12-month alcohol and drug use disorders and personality disorders in the United States. Arch Gen Psychiatry. 2004;61:361–7.
6. Verheul R, Kranzler HR, Poling J. Axis I and Axis II disorders in substance abusers: fact or artifact? J Stud Alcohol. 2000;61: 101–10.
7. Ministry of Health, the Netherlands. Multidisciplinary guideline personality disorders. Utrecht, the Netherlands: Trimbos Instituut; 2008.
8. Ross S, Dermatis H, Levounis P, Galanter M. A comparison between dually diagnosed inpatients with and without Axis II comorbidity and the relationship to treatment outcome. Am J Drug Alcohol Abuse. 2003;29(2):263–79.
9. Verheul R, van den Brink W. Substance abuse and personality disorders. In: Kranzler HR, Rounsaville BJ, editors. Dual diagnosis and treatment. New York: Marcel Dekker; 2000.
10. Pettinati HM, Pierce JD, Belden PP. The relationship of Axis II personality disorders to other known predictors of addiction treatment outcome. Am J Addict. 1999;8:136–47.
11. Goldstein RB, Compton WM, Pulay AJ, Ruan WJ, Pickering RP, Stinson FS, Grant BF. Antisocial behavioral syndromes and DSM-IV drug use disorders in the United States: results from the National Epidemiologic Survey on Alcohol and Related Conditions. Drug Alcohol Depend. 2007;90(2–3):145–58.
12. Fridell M, Hesse M, Billsten J. Criminal behavior in antisocial substance abusers between five and fifteen years follow-up. Am J Addict. 2007;16(1):10–4.
13. Fridell M, Hesse M. Psychiatric severity and mortality in substance abusers: a 15-year follow-up of drug users. Addict Behav. 2006;31(4):559–65.
14. Westermeyer J, Thuras P, Carlson G. Association of antisocial personality disorder with psychiatric morbidity among patients with substance use disorder. Subst Abus. 2005;26(2):15–24.
15. Murray MG, Anthenelli RM, Maxwell RA. Use of health services by men with and without antisocial personality disorder who are alcohol dependent. Psychiatr Serv. 2000;51(3):380–2.
16. Ladd GT, Petry NM. Antisocial personality in treatment-seeking cocaine abusers: psychosocial functioning and HIV risk. J Subst Abuse Treat. 2003;24(4):323–30.
17. Kelley JL, Petry NM. HIV risk behaviors in male substance abusers with and without antisocial personality disorder. J Subst Abuse Treat. 2000;19(1):59–66.
18. Cornelius JR, Reynolds M, Martz BM, Clark DB, Kirisci L, Tarter R. Premature mortality among males with substance use disorders. Addict Behav. 2008;33(1):156–60.
19. Moeller FG, Dougherty DM, Barratt ES, Oderinde V, Mathias CW, Harper RA, Swann AC. Increased impulsivity in cocaine dependent subjects independent of antisocial personality disorder and aggression. Drug Alcohol Depend. 2002;68(1):105–11.

20. Feske U, Tarter RE, Kirisci L, Pilkonis PA. Borderline personality and substance use in women. Am J Addict. 2006;15(2):131–7.

21. Darke S, Williamson A, Ross J, Teesson M, Lynskey M. Borderline personality disorder, antisocial personality disorder and risk-taking among heroin users: findings from the Australian Treatment Outcome Study (ATOS). Drug Alcohol Depend. 2004;74(1): 77–83.

22. Welch SS, Linehan MM. High-risk situations associated with parasuicide and drug use in borderline personality disorder. J Pers Disord. 2002;16(6):561–9.

23. Links PS, Heslegrave RJ, Mitton JE, van Reekum R, Patrick J. Borderline personality disorder and substance abuse: consequences of comorbidity. Can J Psychiatry. 1995;40(1):9–14.

24. Miller FT, Abrams T, Dulit R, Fyer M. Substance abuse in borderline personality disorder. Am J Drug Alcohol Abuse. 1993; 19(4):491–7.

25. Morgenstern J, Langenbucher J, Labouvie E, Miller KJ. The comorbidity of alcoholism and personality disorders in a clinical population: prevalence rates and relation to alcohol typology variables. J Abnorm Psychol. 1997;106(1):74–84.

26. Neufeld KJ, Kidorf MS, Kolodner K, van King L, Clark M, Brooner RK. Behavioral treatment for opioid-dependent patients with antisocial personality. J Subst Abuse. 2008;34(1):101–11.

27. Messina NP, Wish ED, Hoffman JA, Nemes S. Antisocial personality disorder and TC treatment outcomes. Am J Drug Alcohol Abuse. 2002;28(2):197–212.

28. Verheul R, van den Brink W, Koeter MWJ. Antisocial alcoholics show as much improvement at 14-month follow-up as non-antisocial alcoholics. Am J Addict. 1999;8:24–33.

29. Goldstein RB, Powers SI, McCusker J, Lewis BF, Bigelow C, Mundt KA. Antisocial behavioral syndromes among residential drug abuse treatment clients. Drug Alcohol Depend. 1999; 53(2):171–87.

30. Grella CE, Joshi V, Hser YI. Followup of cocaine-dependent men and women with antisocial personality disorder. J Subst Abuse Treat. 2003;25(3):155–64.

31. Compton WM, Cottler LB, Ben-Abdallah A, Cunningham-Williams R, Spitznagel EL. The effects of psychiatric comorbidity on response to an HIV prevention intervention. Drug Alcohol Depend. 2000;58(3):247–57.

32. Penick EC, Powell BJ, Campbell J, Liskow BI, Nickel EJ, Dale TM, Thomas HM, Laster LJ, Noble E. Pharmacological treatment for antisocial personality disorder alcoholics: a preliminary study. Alcohol Clin Exp Res. 1996;20(3):477–84.

33. Cecero JJ, Ball SA, Tennen H, Kranzler HR, Rounsaville BJ. Concurrent and predictive validity of antisocial personality disorder subtyping among substance abusers. J Nerv Ment Dis. 1999;187(8):478–86.

34. Cacciola JS, Rutherford MJ, Alterman AI, McKay JR, Snider EC. Personality disorders and treatment outcome in methadone maintenance patients. J Nerv Ment Dis. 1996;184(4):234–9.

35. Cacciola JS, Rutherford MJ, Alterman AI, Snider EC. An examination of the diagnostic criteria for antisocial personality disorder in substance abusers. J Nerv Ment Dis. 1994;182(9):517–23.

36. Goldstein RB, Bigelow C, McCusker J, Lewis BF, Mundt KA, Powers SI. Antisocial behavioral syndromes and return to drug use following residential relapse prevention/health education treatment. Am J Drug Alcohol Abuse. 2001;27(3):453–82.

37. Asnaani A, Chelminski I, Young D, Zimmerman M. Heterogeneity of borderline personality disorder: do the number of criteria met make a difference? J Pers Disord. 2007;21(6):615–25.

38. Verona E, Sachs-Ericsson N, Joiner Jr TE. Suicide attempts associated with externalizing psychopathology in an epidemiological sample. Am J Psychiatry. 2004;161(3):444–51.

39. Landheim AS, Bakken K, Vaglum P. Gender differences in the prevalence of symptom disorders and personality disorders among poly-substance abusers and pure alcoholics. Substance abusers

40. Pelissier BM, O'Neil JA. Antisocial personality and depression among incarcerated drug treatment participants. J Subst Abuse. 2000;11(4):379–93.

41. Verheul R, van den Bosch LMC, Ball SA. Substance abus. In: Oldham J, Skodol AE, Bender DS, editors. Textbook of personality disorders. Washington DC: American Psychiatric Publishing; 2005. p. 463–76.

42. Ruan WJ, Goldstein RB, Chou SP, Smith SM, Saha TD, Pickering RP, Dawson DA, Huang B, Stinson FS, Grant BF. The alcohol use disorder and associated disabilities interview schedule-IV (AUDADIS-IV): reliability of new psychiatric diagnostic modules and risk factors in a general population sample. Drug Alcohol Depend. 2008;92(1–3):27–36.

43. Skodol AE, Oldham JM, Gallaher PE. Axis II comorbidity of substance use disorders among patients referred for treatment of personality disorders. Am J Psychiatry. 1999;156:733–8.

44. Zimmerman M. Diagnosing personality disorders: a review of issues and research methods. Arch Gen Psychiatry. 1994;51: 225–45.

45. Rounsaville BJ, Kranzler HR, Ball S. Personality disorders in substance abusers: relation to substance use. J Nerv Ment Dis. 1998;186:87–95.

46. Schuckit MA. The clinical implications of primary diagnostic groups among alcoholics. Arch Gen Psychiatry. 1985;42(11): 1043–9.

47. Bernstein DP, Handelsman L. The neurobiology of substance abuse and personality disorders. In: Ratey J, editor. Neuropsychiatry of personality disorders. Cambridge: Blackwell Science; 1995.

48. Cloninger CR, Sigvardsson S, Bohman M. Childhood personality predicts alcohol abuse in young adults. Alcohol Clin Exp Res. 1988;12:494–505.

49. Damen KF, DeJong CA, Nass GC, VanderStaak CP, Breteler MH. Interpersonal aspects of personality disorders in opioid-dependent patients: the convergence of the ICL-R and the SIDP-IV. Eur Addict Res. 2005;11(3):107–14.

50. Finn PR, Sharkansky EJ, Brandt KM. The effects of familial risk, personality, and expectancies on alcohol use and abuse. J Abnorm Psychol. 2000;109:122–33.

51. Tarter RE, Vanyukov M. Alcoholism: a developmental disorder. J Consult Clin Psychol. 1994;62:1096–107.

52. Wills TA, Windle M, Cleary SD. Temperament and novelty seeking in adolescent substance use: convergence of dimensions of temperament with constructs from Cloninger's theory. J Pers Soc Psychol. 1998;74:387–406.

53. Patrick CJ. Antisocial personality disorder and psychopathy. In: Lilienfeld SO, O'Donohue W, Fowler KA, editors. Personality disorders: toward the DSM-V. Thousand Oaks, CA: Sage; 2007.

54. Taylor J. Substance use disorders and Cluster B personality disorders: physiological, cognitive, and environmental correlates in a college sample. Am J Drug Alcohol Abuse. 2005;31(3):515–35.

55. Caspi A, Begg D, Dickson N. Personality differences predict health-risk behaviors in young adulthood: evidence from a longitudinal study. J Pers Soc Psychol. 1997;73:1052–63.

56. Masse LC, Tremblay RE. Behavior of boys in kindergarten and the onset of substance use during adolescence. Arch Gen Psychiatry. 1997;54:62–8.

57. Cohen P, Chen H, Crawford TN, Brook JS, Gordon K. Personality disorders in early adolescence and the development of later substance use disorders in the general population. Drug Alcohol Depend. 2007;88 suppl 1:S71–84.

58. Goldstein RB, Grant BF, Ruan WJ, Smith SM, Saha TD. Antisocial personality disorder with childhood- vs. adolescence-onset conduct disorder: results from the National Epidemiologic Survey on Alcohol and Related Conditions. J Nerv Ment Dis. 2006; 194(9):667–75.

treated in two counties in Norway. Eur Addict Res. 2003; 9(1):8–17.

59. James LM, Taylor J. Impulsivity and negative emotionality associated with substance use problems and Cluster B personality in college students. Addict Behav. 2007;32(4):714–27.

60. Conrod PJ, Pihl RO, Vassileva J. Differential sensitivity to alcohol reinforcement in groups of men at risk for distinct alcoholism subtypes. Alcohol Clin Exp Res. 1998;22:585–97.

61. Levenson RW, Oyama ON, Meek PS. Greater reinforcement from alcohol for those at risk: parental risk, personality risk, and sex. J Abnorm Psychol. 1987;96(3):242–53.

62. van den Bosch LMC, Koeter M, Stijnen T, Verheul R, van den Brink W. Sustained efficacy of dialectical behavior therapy for borderline personality disorder. Behav Res Ther. 2005;43:1231–41.

63. Robinson TE, Berridge KC. The neural basis of craving: an incentive-sensitization theory of addiction. Brain Res Rev. 1993; 18:247–91.

64. Zuckerman M. Vulnerability to psychopathology: a biosocial model. Washington, DC: American Psychological Association; 1999. p. 255–317.

65. Khan AA, Jacobson KC, Gardner CO, Prescott CA, Kendler KS. Personality and comorbidity of common psychiatric disorders. Br J Psychiatry. 2005;186:190–6.

66. Schuckit MA, Klein J, Twitchell G. Personality test scores as predictors of alcoholism almost a decade later. Am J Psychiatry. 1994;151:1038–43.

67. Compton WM, Thomas YF, Stinson FS, Grant BF. Prevalence, correlates, disability, and comorbidity of DSM-IV drug abuse and dependence in the United States: results from the national epidemiologic survey on alcohol and related conditions. Arch Gen Psychiatry. 2007;64(5):566–76.

68. Siever LJ, Davis KL. A psychological perspective on the personality disorders. Am J Psychiatry. 1991;148:1647–58.

69. Zanarini MC. Borderline personality disorder as an impulse spectrum disorder. In: Paris J, editor. Borderline personality disorder: etiology and treatment. Washington, DC: American Psychiatric Press; 1993. p. 67–86.

70. Sakai JT, Stallings MC, Mikulich-Gilbertson SK, Corley RP, Young SE, Hopfer CJ, Crowley TJ. Mate similarity for substance dependence and antisocial personality disorder symptoms among parents of patients and controls. Drug Alcohol Depend. 2004;75(2): 165–75.

71. Justus AN, Finn PR, Steinmetz JE. P300, disinhibited personality, and early-onset alcohol problems. Clin Exp Res. 2001;25: 1457–66.

72. Cacciola JS, Alterman AI, Rutherford MJ, McKay JR, Mulvaney FD. The relationship of psychiatric comorbidity to treatment outcomes in methadone maintained patients. Drug Alcohol Depend. 2001;61(3):271–80.

73. Ball SA, Carroll KM, Canning-Ball M, Rounsaville BJ. Reasons for dropout from drug abuse treatment: symptoms, personality, and motivation. Addict Behav. 2006;31(2):320–30.

74. Carroll KM, Ball SA, Nich C, Martino S, Frankforter TL, Farentinos C, Kunkel LE, Mikulich-Gilbertson SK, Morgenstern J, Obert JL. Motivational interviewing to improve treatment engagement and outcome in individuals seeking treatment for substance abuse: a multisite effectiveness study. Drug Alcohol Depend. 2006;81(3):301–12.

75. Ralevski E, Ball S, Nich C, Limoncelli D, Petrakis I. The impact of personality disorders on alcohol-use outcomes in a pharmacotherapy trial for alcohol dependence and comorbid Axis I disorders. Am J Addict. 2007;16:443–9.

76. Havens JR, Cornelius LJ, Ricketts EP, Latkin CA, Bishai D, Lloyd JJ, Huettner S, Strathdee SA. The effect of a case management intervention on drug treatment entry among treatment-seeking injection drug users with and without comorbid antisocial personality disorder. J Urban Health. 2007;84(2):267–71.

77. Claus RE, Kindleberger LR. Engaging substance abusers after centralized assessment: predictors of treatment entry and dropout. J Psychoactive Drugs. 2002;34:25–31.

78. Blondelle GCJ, Williams GL, van den Bosch LMC. 'OPERANT MILIEU' in een TBS-kliniek. MGv 2007;7/8(62):634–9.

79. Daughters SB, Stipleman BA, Sargeant MN, Schuster R, Bornovalova MA, Lejuez CW. The interactive effects of antisocial personality disorder and court-mandated status on substance abuse treatment dropout. J Subst Abuse Treat. 2008;34(2):157–64.

80. Hesse M. Antisocial personality disorder and retention: a systematic review. Int J Ther Support Org. 2006;27(4):495–504.

81. Krampe H, Wagner T, Stawicki S, Bartels C, Aust C, Kroener-Herwig B, Kuefner H, Ehrenreich H. Personality disorder and chronicity of addiction as independent outcome predictors in alcoholism treatment. Psychiatr Serv. 2006;57(5):708–12.

82. Miranda Jr R, Meyerson LA, Myers RR, Lovallo WR. Altered affective modulation of the startle reflex in alcoholics with antisocial personality disorder. Alcohol Clin Exp Res. 2003;27(12): 1901–11.

83. Marmorstein NR, Iacono WG. Longitudinal follow-up of adolescents with late-onset antisocial behavior: a pathological yet overlooked group. J Am Acad Child Adolescent Psychiatry. 2005; 44(12):1284–91.

84. Carballo JJ, Oqendo MA, Giner L, Zalsman G, Roche AM, Sher L. Impulsive-aggressive traits and suicidal adolescents and young adults with alcoholism. Int J Adolesc Med Health. 2006; 18(1):15–9.

85. Carballo JJ, Oqendo MA, Garcia-Moreno M, Poza B, Giner L, Baca E, Zalsman G, Roche AM, Sher L. Demographic and clinical features of adolescents and young adults with alcohol-related disorders admitted to the psychiatric emergency room. Int J Adolesc Med Health. 2006;18(1):87–96.

86. Stepp SD, Trull TJ, Sher KJ. Borderline personality features predict alcohol use problems. J Pers Disord. 2005;19(6):711–22.

87. Bakken K, Landheim AS, Vaglum P. Axis I and II disorders as long-term predictors of mental distress: a six-year prospective follow-up of substance-dependent patients. BMC Psychiatry. 2007;7:29.

88. Darke S, Ross J, Williamson A, Teesson M. The impact of borderline personality disorder on 12-month outcomes for the treatment of heroin dependence. Addiction. 2005;100(8):1121–30.

89. Fridell M, Hesse M, Johnson E. High prognostic specificity of antisocial personality disorder in patients with drug dependence: results from a five-year follow-up. Am J Addict. 2006;15(3): 227–32.

90. van den Bosch LMC, Verheul R, van den Brink W. Substance abuse in borderline personality disorder: clinical and etiological correlates. J Pers Disord. 2001;15(5):416–24.

91. Verheul R, van den Bosch LMC, Koeter MWJ, de Ridder MAJ, Stijnen T, van den Brink W. Efficacy of dialectical behavior therapy: a Dutch randomized controlled trial. Br J Psychiatry. 2003;182:135–40.

92. Bateman A, Fonagy P. Treatment of borderline personality disorder with psychoanalytically oriented partial hospitalization: an 18-month follow-up. Am J Psychiatry. 2001;158:36–42.

93. Bateman A, Fonagy P. 8-year follow-up of patients treated for borderline personality disorder: mentalization-based treatment versus treatment as usual. Am J Psychiatry. 2008;165:556–9.

94. Ball SA. Manualized treatment for substance abusers with personality disorders: dual focus schema therapy. Addict Behav. 1998;23:883–91.

95. Ball SA, Young JE, Rounsaville BJ. Dual focus schema therapy vs. 12-step drug counseling for personality disorders and addiction: randomized pilot study. Paper presented at the ISSPD 6th International Congress of the Disorders of Personality, Geneva, Switzerland; 2000.

96. Ball SA, Cobb-Richardson P, Connolly AJ, Bujosa CT, O'Neall TW. Substance abuse and personality disorders in homeless drop-in centre clients: symptom severity and psychotherapy retention in a randomized clinical trial. Compr Psychiatry. 2005;46:371–9.

97. Ball SA. Comparing individual therapies for personality disordered opioid dependent patients. J Pers Disord. 2007;21:305–21.

98. Linehan MM, Schmidt H, Dimeff LA. Dialectical behaviour therapy for patients with borderline personality disorder and drug-dependence. Am J Addict. 1999;8:279–92.

99. Linehan MM, Dimeff LA, Reynolds SK, Comtois KA, Welch SS, Heagerty P, Kivlahan DR. Dialectical behavior therapy versus comprehensive validation therapy plus 12-step for the treatment of opioid dependent women meeting criteria for borderline personality disorder. Drug Alcohol Depend. 2002;67:13–26.

100. Gerra G, Leonardi C, D'Amore A, Strepparola G, Fagetti R, Assi C, Zaimovic A, Lucchini A. Buprenorphine treatment outcome in dually diagnosed heroin dependent patients: a retrospective study. Prog Neuropsychopharmacol Biol Psychiatry. 2006;30(2):265–72.

101. Preuss UW, Koller G, Barnow S, Eikmeier M, Soyka M. Suicidal behavior in alcohol- dependent subjects: the role of personality disorders. Alcohol Clin Exp Res. 2006;30(5):866–77.

102. Sher KJ, Trull TJ. Personality and disinhibitory psychopathology: alcoholism and antisocial personality disorder. J Abnorm Psychol. 1994;103:92–102.

103. Cottler LB, Campbell W, Krishna VA, Cunningham-Williams RM, Abdallah AB. Predictors of high rates of suicidal ideation among drug users. J Nerv Ment Dis. 2005;193(7):431–7.

104. Zanarini MC, Frankenburg FR, Hennen J, Reich DB, Silk KR. Axis I comorbidity in patients with borderline personality disorder: 6-year follow-up and prediction of time to remission. Am J Psychiatry. 2004;161:2108–14.

105. Tidemalm D, Elofsson S, Stefansson CG, Waern M, Runeson B. Predictors of suicide in a community-based cohort of individuals with severe mental disorder. Soc Psychiatry Psychiatr Epidemiol. 2005;40(8):595–600.

106. Martino S, Carroll K, Kostas D, Perkins J, Rounsaville B. Dual diagnosis motivational interviewing: a modification of motivational interviewing for substance-abusing patients with psychotic disorders. J Subst Abuse Treat. 2002;23(4):297–308.

107. McKay JR. Is there a case for extended interventions for alcohol and drug use disorders? Addiction. 2005;100:1594–610.

108. Messina N, Farabee D, Rawson R. Treatment responsivity of cocaine-dependent patients with antisocial personality disorder to cognitive-behavioral and contingency management interventions. J Consult Clin Psychol. 2003;71(2):320–9.

109. Linehan MM. Cognitive behavioral therapy of borderline personality disorder. New York: Guilford; 1993.

110. Young JE. Cognitive therapy for personality disorders: a schema-focused approach (Revised edition). Sarasota: Professional Resource Press; 1994.

Schizophrenia and Other Psychotic Disorders

L. Gregg

Abstract

Around half of all people with psychosis have a co-occurring substance use problem, a much higher prevalence rate than that found in the general population. Alcohol and cannabis are the most frequently used substances, and multiple substance use is common. This comorbidity has profound implications for the course and treatment of psychotic disorders. People with psychosis who use drugs and alcohol have been reported to have poorer symptomatic and functional outcomes than their non-substance using counterparts: they experience more symptoms, are less likely to be compliant with medication, are at greater risk of relapse and hospitalisation and as a consequence make greater use of mental health services. The causes of this increased comorbidity are not yet fully understood. There is evidence that cannabis may act as a specific trigger for psychosis in some vulnerable individuals but simple broad models of either substance use causing schizophrenia or schizophrenia causing substance use have largely been discredited. Multiple risk factor models of comorbidity have not been adequately tested. Research on treatment development is limited and the findings contradictory: there is preliminary evidence for Clozapine but no evidence to support any one atypical antipsychotic over another. Likewise, despite promising findings for a combination of motivational interviewing and cognitive behavioural therapy there is little evidence for its superiority when compared to other psychosocial interventions. More good-quality longitudinal research is needed.

Learning Objectives
- Large numbers of people with schizophrenia and other psychotic disorders use drugs and alcohol.
- Drug and alcohol use results in poorer symptomatic and functional outcomes for many people with psychosis, even at relatively low levels of use.
- Clozapine may be effective at decreasing substance use but the evidence for other atypical antipsychotics is either insubstantial or conflicting.
- There is currently little evidence to support any one psychosocial intervention over another.

Issues that Need to Be Addressed by Future Research
- Comorbidity models require further investigation.
- More randomised controlled trials are needed to identify effective pharmacological and psychosocial treatments.

Psychotic disorders are estimated to affect around 3% of the population [1]. Schizophrenia is the most common of these. Characterised by both positive and negative symptoms such as disturbed perception (in the form of auditory, visual, olfactory or tactile hallucinations), disturbances of thought (in the form of delusions), cognitive impairment (in the areas of attention, memory and problem solving) and apathy and avolition [2], schizophrenia is a severe and generally debilitating

L. Gregg (✉)
Division of Clinical Psychology, School of Psychological Sciences, University of Manchester, Brunswick Street, Manchester, UK
e-mail: lynsey.gregg@manchester.ac.uk

J.C. Verster et al. (eds.), *Drug Abuse and Addiction in Medical Illness: Causes, Consequences and Treatment*,
DOI 10.1007/978-1-4614-3375-0_25, © Springer Science+Business Media, LLC 2012

disorder with an often poor prognosis. Behavioural disturbance is common and the major areas of functioning such as work, interpersonal relations and self-care are usually adversely affected. People with schizophrenia and other psychotic disorders may also experience elevated levels of anxiety and depression and be affected by distress; feelings of stigmatisation and social exclusion as a result of their illness.

Substance Use Prevalence

Research shows that large numbers of people diagnosed with schizophrenia or other psychotic disorders use drugs or alcohol. Estimates of prevalence vary between settings and across geographical location but the majority of studies have found that substance use disorders are more prevalent in people with psychosis than in the general population. The largest US study, the Epidemiologic Catchment Area Study [3], found that more than a quarter (27%) of those with schizophrenia had experienced a drug abuse disorder in comparison to 6.1% of the general population and one-third (33.7%) had experienced an alcohol disorder compared to 13.5% of the general population. Overall, 47% of people with schizophrenia had experienced substance abuse or dependence. The National Comorbidity Study [4] reported similar lifetime comorbidity rates for people with non-affective psychosis (45%).

The UK studies have generally reported lower rates of use than those in the USA. A recent review [5] recorded drug and alcohol misuse rates in psychosis of between 20 and 37% in mental health settings, 6–15% in addiction settings and 38–50% in inpatient, crisis team and forensic settings. The wide variations in prevalence rates and patterns of use reported in other European, Australian, Canadian and South American samples [6–11] suggests that substance use comorbidity may also depend on environmental and cultural differences including drug availability.

The types of substance used by people with psychosis vary widely. Alcohol and cannabis are the most commonly used substances in both US and UK samples [4, 12] but patterns of stimulant and opiate use vary across studies. Other substances abused by this client group include hallucinogens, hypnotics and prescription medications. Multiple drug and alcohol use is common, with a significant number of people using more than one substance [12, 13]. In general, people with psychotic disorders tend to use substances that are accessible and readily available in the community in which they live.

Consequences of Substance Use

Substance use by people with psychosis has a number of adverse consequences. As for people in the general population, substance use can lead to financial problems, with substance users spending money on drugs rather than other essentials, and to health problems, including liver, heart and lung damage. In addition to these direct health consequences, substance users with psychosis are also at an increased risk of indirect health consequences such as illness and injury [14] including the damage caused by risky behaviours such as unprotected sex and needle sharing, for example hepatitis and HIV [15].

People with psychosis and co-occurring substance use disorders are also more prone to violent victimisation. They are more likely to be exposed to people who may take advantage of them financially and sexually as a result of their substance use [16]. This is particularly true for women with combined problems, who are more likely to have experienced childhood sexual and physical abuse [17] and who are vulnerable to subsequent retraumatisation in adulthood. People with psychotic disorders are also vulnerable to a range of other adverse outcomes relating to substance use including increased rates of suicidal ideation [18, 19], increased aggression and violence [20, 21] and increased levels of criminal activity and incarceration. Interpersonal conflict and stress such as conflict with family members and service providers who disapprove of substance use and its effects are also increased for this client group [22–24] and as a result of these negative consequences of substance use, people with psychosis who use drugs or alcohol are more likely to experience social exclusion [25], homelessness and housing instability [26].

Clinically, there is evidence to suggest that people with psychosis who use drugs and alcohol have poorer long-term outcomes than their non-substance using counterparts [8, 27] and significantly, studies have shown that even relatively minor use can have an adverse impact [28–30]. Substance use has been associated with higher rates of treatment non-compliance [31–34] including medication adherence and appointment attendance; with more positive symptoms [35] and with more relapses and hospitalisations [36, 37]. The study by Menezes et al. [27] reported that inpatient admission rates among dually diagnosed patients were almost double those of patients with psychosis alone. People with combined problems also make greater use of emergency services [38] and these increased service utilisation rates are associated with greater economic costs.

Why Do People with Psychotic Disorders Use Drugs and Alcohol?

As we have already seen, people with psychosis are more likely to use substances than people in the general population and a number of negative outcomes result from this use. If treatments designed to help people with psychotic disorders are to be successful we need a better understanding of the factors that contribute to these increased rates of substance use disorders.

A number of demographic correlates of substance use have been documented for people with psychosis. Although there is some variation according to the type of substance used [39], there is some consistency in the main correlates identified. Like people in the general population of substance users, people with psychosis who use substances are more likely to be male. They tend to be younger (apart from alcohol users who are generally older), less well educated and are more likely to have a family history of substance use problems [27, 40–43].

Relatively few studies have investigated the relationship between substance use and psychiatric history, but there is evidence to suggest that substance use is associated with an earlier onset of schizophrenia [44] and with an earlier age at first hospitalisation [24]. Substance use has also been associated with better premorbid social functioning [45–47]. People with schizophrenia who are more socially active are assumed to have increased exposure to substances through their social networks: people with better social functioning have more opportunities to use substances and are therefore more likely to develop substance use disorders [24].

The only reliable clinical correlate of substance use in psychosis to be identified to date is antisocial personality disorder (ASPD) [42] and its childhood correlate, conduct disorder. Studies have shown that patients with schizophrenia and ASPD are more likely to have comorbid substance use disorder than patients without ASPD [48, 49]. For people with schizophrenia and substance use disorder, ASPD is also associated with a more severe course of substance use disorder including earlier age of onset and larger quantities of substance use [50]. A recent study compared people with psychosis with no history of conduct disorder (CD)/ASPD to those with CD only; those with adult ASPD and those with full ASPD and found evidence for a late-onset ASPD subtype which may develop in clients with severe mental illness secondary to substance abuse. This late onset group tended to have the most severe drug abuse severity, the most homelessness and the most criminal justice involvement [51].

Comorbidity Models

A number of theories have been put forward to explain why people with psychosis are more likely to experience substance use disorders. There are four broad explanations: (1) substance use causes psychosis, (2) substance use is a consequence of psychosis, (3) substance use and psychosis (particularly schizophrenia) share a common origin and (4) substance use and psychosis are bidirectional, interacting and maintaining each other.

Secondary Psychosis Models

These models of comorbidity posit that substance use precipitates or causes psychotic disorders. We know that many of the substances people with psychosis use, including alcohol, cannabis, hallucinogens and stimulants are known to have acute psychotic effects. Studies have shown that alcohol and amphetamines may worsen the symptoms of people with schizophrenia or precipitate relapse but there is little evidence to suggest that they cause chronic psychosis or schizophrenia. There is, however, evidence to suggest that cannabis, the most frequently used drug by people with psychosis, can have a causal effect.

A number of large-scale prospective longitudinal cohort studies have shown that cannabis users are more likely to develop psychotic disorders than non-cannabis users [52–58]. Zammit et al. [59] found that people who were "heavy cannabis users" by the age of 18 (at least 50 occasions of use) were 6.7 times more likely to later be diagnosed with schizophrenia. Another study [56] found that cannabis use at age 15 and 18 increased the risk of presenting with psychotic symptoms or schizophreniform disorder at age 26 (OR = 11.4 for those who had used cannabis before the age of 15). This relationship was independent of the use of other substances.

Research on non-clinical samples provides additional support for the cannabis–psychosis link. A number of studies have found a relationship between cannabis use and psychosis proneness or schizotypy (e.g. [60–63]). For example, Barkus et al. [60] found that cannabis use per se was not related to schizotypy in their sample of healthy volunteers but that high-scoring schizotypes were more likely to report psychosis-like experiences and unpleasant after-effects associated with cannabis.

However, despite the apparent causal link between cannabis use and psychosis we know that the majority of people who smoke cannabis do not go on to develop schizophrenia or another psychotic disorder. In countries where an increase in rates of cannabis use in the general population has been documented (e.g. Australia) there has not been a corresponding increase in rates of schizophrenia [64]. It is probable, therefore, that some individuals are more vulnerable to the effects of cannabis than others, perhaps because of a gene–environment interaction [65], with some individuals being genetically vulnerable to the effects of cannabis. Caspi et al. [66] tested this hypothesis in a longitudinal birth cohort study and found that a functional polymorphism of the catechol-O-methyltransferase (COMT) gene moderated the influence of adolescent cannabis use on adult psychosis: Carriers of the COMT valine[158] allele were more likely to experience psychotic symptoms after consuming cannabis than carriers of the COMT methionine allele. Experimental work also supports this link. Henquet et al. [67] exposed patients with a psychotic disorder and their relatives to delta-9-tetrahydrocannabinol (Δ-9-THC, the major psycho-active component of cannabis) in a double-blind placebo controlled study and found that carriers of the valine allele were most sensitive to Δ-9-THC induced psychotic experiences. This finding was conditional on preexisting psychosis liability. Other research has shown that Δ-9-THC transiently increases positive, negative and general schizophrenia symptoms in patients with schizophrenia and that furthermore, patients with schizophrenia are more vulnerable to the effects of Δ-9-THC than those without [68].

Secondary Substance Use Models

These models suggest that psychotic disorders lead to substance use. The most well known of these is the self-medication hypothesis [69, 70] which suggests that substance use is an attempt to self-medicate psychiatric symptoms such as hallucinations, anxiety and depression. The literature does show that some individuals report using substances to decrease symptoms or to cope with them better (e.g. [71–75]) and one study has shown that people who use substances to self-medicate psychotic symptoms and medication side effects are more likely to be substance use dependent [74].

"Weaker" variants of the self-medication model postulate that people with psychosis use substances to self-medicate the extrapyramidal symptoms caused by neuroleptic medication [76] or to alleviate dysphoria. Dixon et al. [46] suggest that dysphoria might be the common factor underpinning increased comorbidity. "Perhaps only those patients whose symptoms (positive, negative or extrapyramidal) lead to distress or depression are the ones who abuse drugs" (p. 75).

According to Mueser et al. [30], three types of evidence would provide support for the self-medication hypothesis (1) if epidemiological studies suggested that clients with particular psychiatric diagnoses were more prone to abusing specific types of substances, (2) if psychiatric clients with more severe symptoms were more likely than less symptomatic clients to abuse substances and (3) if clients with combined problems described beneficial effects of substance use on symptoms. Empirical data do not suggest a consistent relationship between substance use and specific diagnoses and the studies assessing the link between of symptoms and levels of substance use have also been contradictory. Some studies have found that substance use is associated with more positive symptoms [35] and fewer negative symptoms [24, 77] whilst others have found no such relationships [78, 79].

Evidence from the self-report studies in which patients with psychosis have been asked to identify their reasons for substance use and to describe the effects of that use have provided some support for the self-medication hypothesis, in particular, the "alleviation of dysphoria" formulation. Many clients with dual disorders are able to point to some symptoms or negative emotional states that they report using alcohol or drugs to modify even though for some patients their stated reasons for substance use and their outcome expectancies for the effects of that substance are incongruous with the actual achieved effect. Some patients report using drugs and alcohol to make them feel better yet report feeling worse afterwards [46].

Other secondary substance use models highlight social risk factors such as peer pressure and poor social competence [80] and again, the self-report literature reveals that for many people with psychosis a key motivator for substance use is the desire to fit in with others and to facilitate social interaction [46, 71–75, 81–84].

Gregg et al. [75] found evidence for three distinct groups of substance users: a group who predominantly used for social and enhancement reasons, a group who used to regulate negative affect and to alleviate positive symptoms and a group who used substances to improve positive affect and to intensify their experiences. It is possible that these different profiles are related to patient symptomatology and patterns of substance use.

An understanding of the temporal relationship between the onset of schizophrenia and substance use may help to elucidate whether one of the two disorders is the primary disorder (if substance use is generally found to occur prior to schizophrenia the self-medication hypothesis would be less plausible) but the evidence to date has been contradictory. Hambrecht and Hafner [85] found that one-third of the people in their sample had a drug problem for more than 1 year before the schizophrenia began, for another third the onset of schizophrenia occurred at a similar time to the onset of substance use and for the final third they began more than a year before the substance use. These findings were interpreted in terms of a vulnerability-stress-coping model: the first group might have their vulnerability threshold reduced or their coping resources diminished as a result of their substance use. The second group might contain people who are already vulnerable to schizophrenia for whom substance misuse is a stress factor precipitating the onset of psychosis whilst the third group uses substances for self-medicating against or "coping with" the symptoms of schizophrenia.

Common Origin Models

Three main common origin models of substance use and psychotic disorders have been proposed highlighting biological, individual and social factors. Although there is evidence to suggest that genetic factors independently contribute to schizophrenia [86] and to substance use disorder [87], the extent to which the two disorders share a common genetic vulnerability is not known. The results of family history studies are conflicting—although some studies have reported that people with combined problems are more likely to have family members with substance use disorders than patients with schizophrenia alone [88, 89]; other studies have not found this to be the case [90].

Some authors [91] have emphasised the possible role of reward circuitry dysfunction and dopamine opioid neurotransmission systems (see Chambers et al. [92] for a review). In brief, people with psychosis might be biologically vulnerable to the rewarding effects of substance abuse. It has been suggested that this relationship might imply a common underlying vulnerability for both disorders in which the pathology of the cannabinoid system in schizophrenia patients is associated with both increased rates of cannabis use and increased risk for schizophrenia [93]. Further research is needed to determine the relevant underlying neuropathological processes before firm conclusions can be drawn.

A number of social and environmental factors could also potentially underpin both disorders, for example, family dysfunction [94] and economic and social disadvantage. Another possible mechanism is traumatic early childhood experience. Members of the general population who report abuse in childhood are more likely to abuse substances in adulthood [95] and for some, childhood abuse can also contribute to psychosis [96]. The available evidence suggests that the relationship may be bidirectional: trauma precedes the onset of substance use in some people with schizophrenia but may also put people with schizophrenia at increased risk of subsequent retraumatisation.

Impairments in cognitive functioning have also been hypothesised to have an impact on both substance use and psychosis [97] as have poorer coping skills, lower educational attainment, lower socioeconomic status, poor interpersonal and social problem-solving skills. It is unlikely that any of these cognitive and social risk factors operate independently to increase rates of comorbidity but their cumulative effects might. Few multiple risk factor models have been proposed but the cross-sectional literature does seem to suggest that some of these factors may play a part.

Bidirectional Models

Bidirectional models propose that psychotic and substance use disorders trigger and maintain each other. For example, substance use may serve as a stressor precipitating onset of schizophrenia in vulnerable individuals and mental health problems are then subsequently maintained by continued substance use due to socially learned cognitive factors such as beliefs, expectancies and motives for substance use [30]. Thus, bidirectional models tend to involve multiple risk factors. Examples include the affect regulation model put forward by

Blanchard et al. [98] which emphasises the role of enduring personality traits, coping and stress in the development and maintenance of substance use disorders. Barrowclough et al. [99] also highlight the role of coping in their proposed multiple risk factor model which incorporates Marlatt and Gordon's social-cognitive model of addiction [100]. In brief: certain situations and cues trigger drug or alcohol-related thoughts which, in the absence of alternative coping strategies and in the context of low self-efficacy for resisting use and positive expectancies about the effects of that use, make the person with psychosis vulnerable and more likely to use substances. In this model, deficiencies in coping skills and positive expectancies about the effects of drug and alcohol operate independently and jointly to contribute to the use of substances as a coping model. There is a significant literature demonstrating that motivations and beliefs about the effects of substance influence substance use [74, 101] and research shows that people with schizophrenia experience difficulty coping with stresses and may experience a limited repertoire of coping strategies [102, 103] but there has not been an empirical test of this model.

Although the four types of model presented help clarify our understanding of the reasons for increased rates comorbidity, it is clear that no single model can adequately explain all comorbidity. The hypothesis that substance use causes schizophrenia is not supported sufficiently or consistently. Evidence from prospective cohort studies suggests that cannabis can have a causal role in the development of psychotic disorder but there is little evidence to suggest that other substances are a causative factor in chronic psychosis or schizophrenia. Little support is found in the literature for the self-medication hypothesis although the self-report studies of reasons for use do show that some people with schizophrenia report using substances in an attempt to alleviate specific psychopathological symptoms or medication side effects. Common origin models have implicated both genetics and neuropathology but no common gene has yet been identified and the neurobiological evidence is not consistent. Additional research is required. It is also possible that some other as yet unresearched variable or variables may account for the psychosis and substance use comorbidity. Bidirectional models which integrate aspects of the different causative models outlined above suggest that separate factors may be responsible for the initiation and maintenance of substance use by people with psychosis. It is possible, for example, that substance users whose drug use precipitated or caused the onset of psychotic symptoms (perhaps because of biological vulnerability) may continue using cannabis in order to alleviate or cope with the symptoms of schizophrenia better. To date, however, there have been no satisfactory empirical investigations of bidirectional models. Likewise, research has not yet tested the few multiple risk factors models that have been developed.

Treatment Approaches

Pharmacological Interventions

The overwhelming majority of people with psychotic disorders are prescribed antipsychotic medications. The two main classifications of medications, conventional "typical" antipsychotics (e.g. Haloperidol) and newer, "atypical" antipsychotics (e.g. aripiprazole, clozapine, olanzapine, quetiapine and risperidone) have both been shown to provide significant relief from psychotic symptoms and improve functioning. For people with comorbid substance use problems, however, typical antipsychotics have been found to be less effective [104]. They may even serve to worsen substance abuse in some people with psychosis [46, 105]. Better results have been reported for some of the newer atypical antipsychotics. There is preliminary evidence to suggest that clozapine, despite its many side effects, is effective at decreasing substance use in people with schizophrenia and schizoaffective disorder [106, 107] but no randomised controlled trials with this client group have been conducted to date. The evidence for the other atypicals whilst promising is either insubstantial or conflicting [108].

There are a number of pharmacological interventions for substance use disorders with two broad objectives: to manage withdrawal and to prevent relapse. Most medications work by targeting the neurotransmitters that are dysregulated in relation to a particular substance. Disulfiram, naltrexone and acamprosate have been shown to reduce the risk of relapse to specific substances (namely, alcohol and opioids) in the general population of substance users and methadone maintenance therapy (which seeks to stabilise chaotic lifestyles and reduce criminal activity and mortality) has been shown to be effective for opiate addiction. Tricyclic antidepressants (e.g. desipramine) have been found to reduce cravings for cocaine and dexamphetamine may be used to reduce amphetamine use. However, although all of these pharamacotherapies can be safely prescribed for people with psychotic disorders, research evidence is somewhat lacking for people with combined problems. Significantly, there are no pharmacological interventions for cannabis use, the main drug used by people with psychosis.

It is accepted that for people with psychosis, psychiatric medications must first be stabilised before adjunctive medications are added to the treatment regime [109]. It is also unlikely that pharmacological treatments can result in long-term abstinence without psychosocial intervention. However, we know that substance users with psychotic disorders are less likely to be compliant with medication and it is sometimes difficult to engage substance users with services. Barrowclough et al. [99] note that there is often a history of poor relationships with service providers; a reluctance to discuss substance use issues in anticipation of being criticised and lectured on the harmful consequences of substances and a bias towards suspiciousness or paranoid interpretation of relationships arising from psychotic symptoms and exacerbated by substance use. People with combined problems are also likely to have chaotic lifestyles making appointment scheduling and engaging in structured work difficult. Interventions must therefore seek to build alliance as a first step.

Psychosocial Interventions

Research into interventions for this client group can be broadly divided into two types: evaluations of service delivery models and individual client therapy approaches. The former originated in the US in the 1980s when mental health and substance abuse services began to be integrated at the clinical level with treatment for both the mental health problem and substance use problem being provided by the same team in a unified setting in order to avoid gaps in service delivery. Approaches within this framework often employ assertive community outreach and include both pharmacological and psychosocial treatments including intensive case management, residential treatment and contingency management. They may also make use of group and individual counselling, motivational interventions and family interventions. A number of reviews have reported modestly superior outcomes for integrated services [110–112] but it is probable that effects on substance use depend on the specific interventions chosen.

Common psychosocial interventions for people with both psychotic and substance use disorders include motivational interviewing, which aims to increase an individual's motivation for change; individual or group psychotherapy involving cognitive behavioural principles and group and individual social skills training [113]. These psychosocial treatments focus on engagement and building therapeutic alliance whilst recognising that motivation to change is often low and that relapse is common. Ongoing treatment works to increase motivation by enhancing desire to change, developing self-efficacy that change is possible, managing cognitive limitations and enhancing interpersonal skills [109].

Motivational Interviewing
Motivational interviewing (MI) seeks to help people understand the impact of substance use by helping them to recognise the relationship of the substance use to their personal life goals. MI takes a non-confrontational approach to treating substance misuse and is intended to enhance the individual's intrinsic motivation for change [114]. As Barrowclough et al. [99] note "rarely does the client come to therapy asking for help with reducing alcohol consumption or drug taking. Rather the therapist approaches the client and works towards getting substance use on a shared agenda for change".

Although a handful of studies have shown that motivational interviewing can be used successfully with people with psychosis and substance use disorders to reduce levels of substance use [115, 116], others have found no difference in substance use outcomes or any other outcomes [117, 118].

Cognitive Behavioural Therapy

Cognitive behavioural approaches emphasise functional analysis of drug use: understanding the reasons for use and consequences of that use and involve skills training for recognising the high-risk situations (including moods and symptoms) which lead to substance use and to develop alternative coping skills for handling those situations and avoiding substance use in future.

Although there is ample evidence to suggest that CBT can result in significant clinical benefit for people with psychosis, only two randomised controlled trials have compared CBT to treatment as usual in people with psychosis and comorbid substance use to date [119, 120]. Edwards et al. [119] evaluated a cannabis-focused CBT intervention for with a first episode of psychosis against an active control involving psychoeducation and treatment as usual and found no differences in substance use outcomes after 3 months of individual CBT. The study by Naeem et al. [120] combined CBT with psychoeducation and also found no difference between groups after 3 months.

Three studies have combined MI with CBT [121–123]. The first of these found superior outcomes for a longer-term intervention (9 months duration) which combined MI with CBT and a family intervention. Positive symptoms and relapse rates were decreased at 12 months and there was decreased abstinence from all substances; global functioning was also improved although not all of these benefits were maintained at 18 months. The second [122] compared 10 sessions of MI plus CBT with routine care plus self-help books. The intervention group had improved global function at 12 months and decreased depressive symptoms but there were no differences in substance use outcomes. The final study [123] compared group behavioural treatment (combing MI and CBT approaches with skills training and contingency management) with supportive group therapy and found increased substance use abstinence for the intervention group. Thus it appears that motivational interviewing combined with other interventions appears to offer some benefit for this client group. Further research is required to determine which combinations of intervention are most useful and cost-effective long term.

Social Skills Training

Social skills training usually takes place in a group setting. Structured sessions, using role play and corrective feedback aim to help people develop the necessary interpersonal skills for building and maintaining relationships with others; dealing with conflict and handling social situations involving substance misuse.

Two randomised controlled trials have evaluated social skills training for people with combined problems, with conflicting results. Hellerstein et al. [124] found no difference across groups whilst Jerrell and Ridgely [125] reported decreased drug and alcohol use, decreased psychiatric symptoms and improved functioning for skills training groups when compared to 12 step-based groups.

The recent Cochrane review of psychosocial interventions [113] reviewed 25 randomised controlled trials assessing the effectiveness of a number of psychosocial interventions (total $N = 2,478$) and found "no compelling evidence to support any one psychosocial treatment over another to reduce substance use (or improve mental state) by people with serious mental illnesses". A broader review, which included 45 psychosocial interventions [111] reported that no psychosocial interventions showed consistent results on either substance use or mental health outcomes. It should be noted, however, that it is difficult to pool results because of sampling and methodological differences. Furthermore, both reviews evaluated interventions for people with "severe mental illness" and included research involving people with bipolar disorder. The majority of participants in the studies reviewed will also have been taking antipsychotics and other medications but this was not accounted for in the analyses. To our knowledge there has not been a systematic review of psychosocial interventions for people with psychotic disorders and substance use only.

Summary and Conclusions

Large numbers of people with schizophrenia and other psychotic disorders use drugs and alcohol. This comorbidity has been associated with a range of adverse clinical and social outcomes including more positive symptoms, more relapses and hospitalisations, increased aggression and violence and higher rates of homelessness and housing instability. Although the correlates of substance use have been well documented, the causes are less well understood. A number of aetiological models have been proposed but no single model can explain all comorbidity. The dually diagnosed population is a heterogeneous group and it is probable that different models may account for comorbidity in different groups of people and multiple models may apply for some individuals.

A number of treatments for people with psychosis and combined substance use disorders are available. Typical antipsychotics are less effective for people with comorbid substance use problems but there is preliminary evidence to suggest that some newer atypical antipsychotics may decrease substance use, e.g. Clozapine. A number of psychosocial interventions have been developed for use with this client group, and there is promising evidence to suggest that motivational interviewing may be effective when combined with cognitive behavioural therapy although there is currently little evidence to support any one psychosocial intervention over another.

Substance use by people with psychosis is a significant concern and there is a clear need for good quality long-term research to further elucidate the causes of substance use and to identify the best treatment methods if we are to help people with psychosis reduce their substance use.

References

1. Perälä J, Suvisaari J, Saarni SI, Kuoppasalmi K, Isometsä E, Pirkola S, et al. Lifetime prevalence of psychotic and bipolar I disorders in a general population. Arch Gen Psychiatry. 2007;64:19–28.
2. American Psychiatric Association. Diagnostic and statistical manual of mental disorders. 4th ed. Washington, DC: APA; 1994.
3. Regier DA, Farmer MF, Rae DS, Locke BZ, Keith SJ, Judd LL, Goodwin FK. Comorbidity of mental disorders with alcohol and other drug abuse: results from the Epidemiologic Catchment Area (ECA) Study. JAMA. 1990;264:251–2518.
4. Kessler RC, Crum RM, Warner LA, Nelson CB, Schulenberg J, Anthony JC. Lifetime occurrence of DSM-III-R alcohol abuse and dependence with other psychiatric disorders in the National Comorbidity Survey. Arch Gen Psychiatry. 1997;54:313–21.
5. Carra G, Johnson S. Variations in rates of comorbid substance use in psychosis between mental health settings and geographical areas in the UK. A systematic review. Soc Psychiatry Psychiatr Epidemiol. 2008;44(6):429–47.
6. Jablensky A, McGrath J, Herrman H, Castle D, Gureje O, Evans M, et al. Psychotic disorders in urban areas: an overview of the Study on Low Prevalence Disorders. Aust NZ J Psychiatry. 2000;34:221–36.
7. Korkeila JA, Svirskis T, Heinimaa M, Ristkari T, Huttunen J, Ilonen T, et al. Substance abuse and related diagnoses in early psychosis. Compr Psychiatry. 2005;46:447–52.
8. Margolese HC, Malchy L, Negrete JC, Tempier R, Gill K. Drug and alcohol use among patients with schizophrenia and related psychoses: levels and consequences. Schizophr Res. 2004;67:157–66.
9. Mauri M, Volonteri L, De Gaspari I, Colasanti A, Brambilla M, Cerruti L. Substance abuse in first-episode schizophrenic patients: a retrospective study. Clin Pract Epidemiol Ment Health. 2006;23: 2–4.
10. Rossi Menezes P, Ratto LR. Prevalence of substance misuse among individuals with severe mental illness in Sao Paulo. Soc Psychiatry Psychiatr Epidemiol. 2004;39:212–7.
11. Soyka M, Albus M, Kathmann N, Finelli A, Hofstetter S, Holzbach R, et al. Prevalence of alcohol and drug abuse in schizophrenic inpatients. Eur Arch Psychiatry Clin Neurosci. 1993;242:362–72.
12. Weaver T, Madden P, Charles V, Stimson G, Renton A, Tyrer P, et al. Comorbidity of substance misuse and mental illness in community mental health and substance misuse services. Br J Psychiatry. 2003;183:304–13.
13. Baigent M, Holme G, Hafner RJ. Self reports of the interaction between substance abuse and schizophrenia. Aust NZ J Psychiatry. 1995;29:69–74.
14. Dickey B, Azeni H, Weiss R, Sederer L. Schizophrenia, substance use disorders and medical co-morbidity. J Ment Health Policy Econ. 2000;3:27–33.
15. Mahler JC. HIV, substance use and mental illness. In: Lehman AF, Dixon LB, editors. Double jeopardy, chronic mental illness and substance use disorders. London: Harwood Academic; 1995.
16. Goodman LA, Salyers MP, Mueser KT, Rosenberg SD, Swartz M, Essock SM, et al. Recent victimization in women and men with severe mental illness: prevalence and correlates. J Trauma Stress. 2001;14:615–32.
17. Alexander MJ. Women with co-occurring addictive and mental disorders: An emerging profile of vulnerability. Am J Orthopsychiatry. 1996;661:61–70.
18. Bartels SJ, Drake RE, McHugo GJ. Alcohol abuse, depression, and suicidal behavior in schizophrenia. Am J Psychiatry. 1992;149: 394–5.
19. Kamali M, Kelly L, Gervin M, Browne S, Larkin C, O'Callaghan E. The prevalence of comorbid substance misuse and its influence on suicidal ideation among in-patients with schizophrenia. Acta Psychiatr Scand. 2000;101:452–6.
20. Cuffel BJ, Shumway M, Choulgian TL, MacDonald T. A longitudinal study of substance use and community violence in schizophrenia. J Nerv Ment Dis. 1994;182:704–8.
21. Fulwiler C, Grossman H, Forbes C, Ruthazer R. Early onset substance use an d community violence by outpatients with chronic mental illness. Psychiatr Serv. 1997;48:1181–5.
22. Kashner TM, Rader LE, Rodell DE, Beck CM, et al. Family characteristics, substance abuse, and hospitalization patterns of patients with schizophrenia. Hosp Commun Psychiatry. 1991;42:195–7.
23. Barrowclough C, Ward J, Wearden A, Gregg L. Expressed emotion and attributions in relatives of schizophrenia patients with and without substance misuse. Soc Psychiatry Psychiatr Epidemiol. 2005;40:884–91.
24. Salyers MP, Mueser KT. Social functioning, psychopathology, and medication side effects in relation to substance use and abuse in schizophrenia. Schizophr Res. 2001;48:109–23.
25. Todd J, Green G, Harrison M, Ikuesan BA, Self C, Pevalin DJ, Baldacchino. Social exclusion in clients with comorbid mental health and substance use problems. Soc Psychiatry Psychiatr Epidemiol. 2004;39:581–7.
26. Drake RE, Osher FC, Wallach MA. Homelessness and dual diagnosis. Am Psychol. 1991;46:1149–58.
27. Menezes POR, Johnson S, Thornicroft G, Marshall J, Prosser D, Bebbington P, Kuipers E. Drug and alcohol problems among individuals with severe mental illnesses in South London. Br J Psychiatry. 1996;168:612–9.
28. Drake RE, Osher FC, Wallach MA. Alcohol use and abuse in schizophrenia: a prospective community study. J Nerv Ment Dis. 1989;177:408–14.
29. Gonzalez VM, Bradizza CM, Vincent PC, Stasiewicz PR, Paas ND. Do individuals with a severe mental illness experience greater alcohol and drug-related problems? A test of the supersensitivity hypothesis. Addict Behav. 2007;32:477–90.
30. Mueser KT, Drake RE, Wallach MA. Dual diagnosis: a review of etiological theories. Addict Behav. 1998;23:717–34.
31. Coldham EL, Addington J, Addington D. Medication adherence of individuals with a first episode of psychosis. Acta Psychiatr Scand. 2002;106:286–90.
32. Hipwell AE, Singh K, Clark A. Substance misuse among clients with severe and enduring mental illness: service utilisation and implications for clinical management. J Ment Health. 2000;9: 37–50.
33. Janssen B, Gaebel W, Haerter M, Komaharadi F, Lindel B, Weinmann S. Evaluation of factors influencing medication compliance in inpatient treatment of psychotic disorders. Psychopharmacology. 2006;187:229–36.
34. Owen RR, Fischer EP, Booth BM, Cuffel BJ. Medication noncompliance and substance use among patients with schizophrenia. Psychiatr Serv. 1996;47:853–8.

35. Pencer A, Addington J. Substance use and cognition in early psychosis. J Psychiatry Neurosci. 2003;28:48–54.
36. Linszen DH, Dingemans PM, Lenior ME. Cannabis use and the course of recent onset schizophrenic disorders. Arch Gen Psychiatry. 1994;51:273–9.
37. Swofford CD, Kasckow JW, Scheller-Gilkey G, Inderbitzin LB. Substance use: a powerful predictor of relapse in schizophrenia. Schizophr Res. 1996;20:145–51.
38. Bartels SJ, Teague GB, Drake RE, Clark RE, Bush PW, Noordsy DL. Substance abuse in schizophrenia: service utilization and cost. J Nerv Ment Disord. 1993;181:227–32.
39. Mueser KT, Yarnold PR, Bellack AS. Diagnostic and demographic correlates of substance abuse in schizophrenia and major affective disorder. Acta Psychiatr Scand. 1992;85:48–55.
40. Barnes TR, Mutsatsa SH, Hutton SB, Watt HC, Joyce EM. Comorbid substance use and age at onset of schizophrenia. Br J Psychiatry. 2006;188:237–42.
41. Cantwell R. Substance use and schizophrenia: effects on symptoms, social functioning and service use. Br J Psychiatry. 2003;182: 324–9.
42. Kavanagh DJ, Waghorn G, Jenner L, Chant DC, Carr V, Evans M, et al. Demographic and clinical correlates of comorbid substance use disorders in psychosis: multivariate analyses from an epidemiological sample. Schizophr Res. 2004;66:115–24.
43. Mueser KT, Bennet M, Kushner MG. Epidemiology of substance use disorders among persons with chronic mental illnesses. In: Lehman AF, Dixon LB, editors. Double-jeopardy: chronic mental illness and substance use disorders. London: Harwood; 1995.
44. Kovasznay B, Fleischer J, Tanenberg-Karant M. Substance use disorder and the early course of illness in schizophrenia and affective psychosis. Schizophr Bull. 1997;23:195–201.
45. Carey KB, Carey MP, Simons JS. Correlates of substance use disorder among psychiatric outpatients: focus on cognition, social role functioning, and psychiatric status. J Nerv Ment Dis. 2003;191:300–8.
46. Dixon L, Haas GH, Weiden PJ, Frances AJ. Drug abuse in schizophrenic patients: clinical correlates and reasons for use. Am J Psychiatry. 1991;148:224–30.
47. Sevy S, Robinson DG, Solloway S, Alvir JM, Woerner MG, Bilder R, Goldman R, Lieberman J, Kane J. Correlates of substance misuse in patients with first-episode schizophrenia and schizoaffective disorder. Acta Psychiatr Scand. 2001;104:367–74.
48. Caton CL, Shrout PE, Eagle PF, Opler LA, Felix A. Correlates of codisorders in homeless and never homeless indigent schizophrenic men. Psychol Med. 1994;24:681–8.
49. Mueser KT, Yarnold PR, Rosenberg SD, Swett C, Miles KM, Hill D. Substance use disorders in hospitalised severely mentally ill psychiatric patients: prevalence, correlates and subgroups. Schizophr Bull. 2000;26:179–92.
50. Mueser KT, Drake RE, Ackerson TH, Alterman AI, Miles KM, Noordsy DL. Antisocial personality disorder, conduct disorder, and substance abuse in schizophrenia. J Abnorm Psychol. 1997;106:473–7.
51. Mueser KT, Crocker AG, Frisman LB, Drake RE, Covell NH, Essock SM. Conduct disorder and antisocial personality disorder in persons with severe psychiatric and substance use disorders. Schizophr Bull. 2006;32:626–36.
52. Andreasson S, Allebeck P, Engstrom A, Rydberg U. Cannabis and schizophrenia: a longitudinal study of Swedish conscripts. Lancet. 1987;2:1483–6.
53. Ferdinand RF, Sondeijker F, van der Ende J, Selten JP, Huizink A, Verhulst FC. Cannabis use predicts future psychotic symptoms, and vice versa. Addiction. 2005;100:612–8.
54. van Os J, Bak M, Hanssen M, Bijl RV, de Graaf R, Verdoux H. Cannabis use and psychosis: a longitudinal population-based study. Am J Epidemiol. 2002;156:319–27.
55. Henquet C, Krabbendam L, Spauwen J, Kaplan C, Lieb R, Wittchen HU, van Os J. Prospective cohort study of cannabis use, predisposition for psychosis, and psychotic symptoms in young people. Br Med J. 2005;330(7481):11.
56. Arseneault L, Cannon M, Poulton R, Murray R, Caspi A, Moffitt TE. Cannabis use in adolescence and risk for adult psychosis: longitudinal prospective study. Br Med J. 2002;325:1212–3.
57. Fergusson DM, Horwood LJ, Ridder EM. Tests of causal linkages between cannabis use and psychotic symptoms. Addiction. 2005; 100:354–66.
58. Weiser M, Knobler HY, Noy S, Kaplan Z. Clinical characteristics of adolescents later hospitalized for schizophrenia. Am J Med Genet. 2002;114:949–55.
59. Zammit S, Allebeck P, Andreasson S, Lundberg I, Lewis G. Self reported cannabis use as a risk factor for schizophrenia in Swedish conscripts of 1969: historical cohort study. BMJ. 2002; 325:1199.
60. Barkus EJ, Stirling J, Hopkins RS, Lewis S. Cannabis-induced psychosis-like experiences are associated with high schizotypy. Psychopathology. 2006;39:175–8.
61. Dumas P, Saoud M, Bouafia S, Gutknecht C, Ecohard R, Dalery J, Rochet T, D'Amato T. Cannabis use correlates with schizotypal personality traits in health students. Psychiatry Res. 2002;109: 27–35.
62. Verdoux H, Gindre C, Sorbara F, Tournier M, Swendsen JD. Effects of cannabis and psychosis vulnerability in daily life: an experience sampling test study. Psychol Med. 2003;33:23–32.
63. Williams JH, Wellman JN, Rawlins JNP. Cannabis use correlates with schizotypy in healthy people. Addiction. 1996;91:869–77.
64. Degenhardt L, Hall W, Lynskey M. Testing hypotheses about the relationship between cannabis use and psychosis. Drug Alcohol Depend. 2003;71:37–48.
65. van Os J, Krabbendam L, Myin-Germeys I, Delespaul P. The schizophrenia envirome. Curr Opin Psychiatry. 2005;18:141–5.
66. Caspi A, Moffitt TE, Cannon M, McClay J, Murray R, Harrington H, et al. Moderation of the effect of adolescent-onset cannabis use on adult psychosis by a functional polymorphism in the catechol-O-methyltransferase gene: longitudinal evidence of a gene X environment interaction. Biol Psychiatry. 2005;57:1117–27.
67. Henquet C, Rosa A, Krabbendam L, Papiol S, Fananas L, Drukker M, Ramaekers JG, van Os J. An experimental study of catechol-o-methyltransferase Val158Met moderation of delta-9-tetrahydrocannabinol-induced effects on psychosis and cognition. Neuropsychopharmacology. 2006;31:2748–57.
68. D'Souza DC, Abi-Saab WM, Madonick S, Forselius-Bielen K, Doersch A, Braley G, Gueorguieva R, Cooper TB, Krystal JH. Delta-9-tetrahydrocannabinol effects in schizophrenia: implications for cognition, psychosis and addiction. Biol Psychiatry. 2005;57:594–608.
69. Khantzian EJ. The self-medication hypothesis of addictive disorders: focus on heroin and cocaine dependence. Am J Psychiatry. 1985;142:1259–64.
70. Khantzian EJ. The self-medication hypothesis of substance use disorders: a reconsideration and recent applications. Harv Rev Psychiatry. 1997;4:231–44.
71. Addington J, Duchak V. Reasons for substance use in schizophrenia. Acta Psychiatr Scand. 1997;96:329–33.
72. Gearon JS, Bellack AS, Rachbeisel J, Dixon L. Drug-use behavior and correlates in people with schizophrenia. Addict Behav. 2001;26:51–61.
73. Goswami S, Mattoo SK, Basu D, Singh G. Substance-abusing schizophrenics: do they self-medicate? Am J Addict. 2004;13: 139–50.
74. Spencer C, Castle D, Michie PT. Motivations that maintain substance use among individuals with psychotic disorders. Schizophr Bull. 2002;28:233–47.

75. Gregg L, Haddock G, Barrowclough C (2009) Self reported reasons for substance use in Schizophrenia: a Q methodological investigation. Ment Health Subst Use (Dual Diagnosis). 2(1):eScholar ID:1d18011.

76. Schneier FR, Siris SG. A review of psychoactive substance use and abuse in schizophrenia: patterns of drug choice. J Nerv Ment Dis. 1987;175:641–652.

77. Talamo A, Centorrino F, Tondo L, Dimitri A, Hennen J, Baldessarini RJ. Comorbid substance-use in schizophrenia: relation to positive and negative symptoms. Schizophr Res. 2006; 86:251–5.

78. Brunette MF, Mueser KT, Xie H, Drake R. Relationships between symptoms of schizophrenia and substance abuse. J Nerv Ment Dis. 1997;185:13–20.

79. Dervaux A, Baylé FJ, Laqueille X, Bourdel M, Le Borgne M, Olié J, Krebs M. Is substance abuse in schizophrenia related to impulsivity, sensation seeking, or anhedonia? Am J Psychiatry. 2001;158:492–4.

80. Bellack AS, Morrison RL, Wixted JT, Mueser KT. An analysis of social competence in schizophrenia. Br J Psychiatry. 1990;156: 809–18.

81. Baker A, Bucci S, Lewin TJ, Kay-Lambkin F, Constable PM, Carr VJ. Cognitive–behavioural therapy for substance use disorders in people with psychotic disorders: randomised controlled trial. Br J Psychiatry. 2006;188:439–48.

82. Fowler IL, Carr VJ, Carter NT, Lewin TJ. Patterns of current and lifetime substance use in schizophrenia. Schizophr Bull. 1998;24: 443–55.

83. Green B, Kavanagh DJ, Young RMCD. Reasons for cannabis use in men with and without psychosis. Drug Alcohol Rev. 2004;23: 445–53.

84. Schofield D, Tennant C, Nash L, Degenhardt L, Cornish A, Hobbs C, Brennan G. Reasons for cannabis use in psychosis. Aust NZ J Psychiatry. 2006;40:570–4.

85. Hambrecht M, Hafner H. Substance abuse and the onset of Schizophrenia. Biol Psychiatry. 1996;40:1155–63.

86. Gottesman II, Shields JA. A critical review of recent adoption, twin and family studies of schizophrenia: behavioural genetics perspectives. Schizophr Bull. 1976;2:360–401.

87. Tsuang MT, Bar JL, Harley RM, Lyons MJ. The Harvard Twin Study of Substance Abuse: what we have learned. Harv Rev Psychiatry. 2001;9:267–79.

88. Noordsy DL, Drake RE, Biesanz JD, McHugo GJ. Family history of alcoholism in schizophrenia. J Nerv Ment Dis. 1994;182:651–5.

89. Smith MJ, Barch DM, Wolf TJ, Mamah D, Csernansky JG. Elevated rates of substance use disorders in non-psychotic siblings of individuals with schizophrenia. Schizophr Res. 2008;106: 294–9.

90. Gershon ES, DeLisi LE, Hamovit J, Nurnberger JI, Maxwell ME, Schreiber J, Dauphinais D, Dingman CW, Guroff JJ. A controlled family study of chronic psychoses. Schizophrenia and schizoaffective disorder. Arch Gen Psychiatry. 1988;45:328–36.

91. Green AI, Drake RE, Brunette MF, Noordsy DL. Schizophrenia and substance use disorder. Am J Psychiatry. 2007;164:402–8.

92. Chambers RA, Krystal JH, Self DW. A neurobiological basis for substance abuse comorbidity in schizophrenia. Biol Psychiatry. 2001;50:71–83.

93. Weiser M, Noy S. Interpreting the association between cannabis use and increased risk for schizophrenia. Dialogues Clin Neurosci. 2005;7:81–5.

94. Fergusson DM, Horwood LJ, Lynskey MT. Parental separation, adolescent psychopathology, and problem behaviors. J Am Acad Child Adolesc Psychiatry. 1994;33:1122–31.

95. Kessler RC, Davis CG, Kendler KS. Childhood adversity and adult psychiatric disorder in the US national comorbidity survey. Psychol Med. 1997;27:1101–19.

96. Briere J, Woo R, McRae B, Foltz J, Sitzman R. Lifetime victimization history, demographics, and clinical status in female psychiatric emergency room patients. J Nerv Ment Dis. 1997;185:95–101.

97. Tracy JI, Josiassen RC, Bellack AS. Neuropsychology of dual diagnosis: understanding the combined effects of schizophrenia and substance use disorders. Clin Psychol Rev. 1995;15:67–97.

98. Blanchard JJ, Brown SA, Horan WP, Sherwood A. Substance use disorders in schizophrenia: review, integration and a proposed model. Clin Psychol Rev. 2000;20:207–34.

99. Barrowclough C, Haddock G, Lowens I, Allott R, Earnshaw P, Fitzsimmons M, Nothard S. Psychosis and drug and alcohol problems. In: Baker A, Velleman R, editors. Clinical handbook of co-existing mental health and drug and alcohol problems. London: Bruner Routledge; 2007.

100. Marlatt GA, Gordon JR. Relapse prevention: maintenance strategies in the treatment of addictive behaviours. New York: Guildford; 1985.

101. Hides L, Kavanagh DJ, Dawe S, Young RM. The influence of cannabis use expectancies on cannabis use and psychotic symptoms in psychosis. Drug Alcohol Rev. 2008;28(3):250–6.

102. Corrigan PW, Toomey R. Interpersonal problem solving and information processing in schizophrenia. Schizophr Bull. 1995;21:395–403.

103. Rollins AL, Bond GR, Lysaker PH. Characteristics of coping with the symptoms of schizophrenia. Schizophr Res. 1999;36:30.

104. Bowers MB, Mazure CM, Nelson JC, Jatlow PI. Psychotogenic drug use and neuroleptic response. Schizophr Bull. 1990;16: 81–5.

105. Brady KT, Anton R, Ballenger JC, Lydiard RB, Adinoff B, Selander J. Cocaine abuse among schizophrenic patients. Am J Psychiatry. 1990;147:1164–7.

106. Drake RE, Xie H, McHugo GJ, Green AI. The effects of clozapine on alcohol and drug use disorders among patients with schizophrenia. Schizophr Bull. 2000;26:441–9.

107. Zimmet SV, Strous RD, Burgess ES, Kohnstamm S, Green AI. Effects of clozapine on substance use in patients with schizophrenia and schizoaffective disorder: a retrospective survey. J Clin Psychopharmacol. 2000;20:94–8.

108. Green AI, Noordsy DL, Brunette MF, O'Keefe C. Substance abuse and schizophrenia: pharmacotherapeutic intervention. J Subst Abuse Treat. 2008;34:61–71.

109. Ziedonis DM, Smelson D, Rosenthal RN, Batki SL, Green AI, Henry RJ, Montoya I, Parks J, Weiss RD. Improving the care of individuals with schizophrenia and substance use disorders: consensus recommendations. J Psychiatr Pract. 2005;11:315–39.

110. Drake RE, Mueser KT, Brunette M, McHugo GJ. A review of treatments for people with severe mental illness and cooccurring substance use disorder. Psychiatr Rehabil J. 2004;27:360–74.

111. Drake RE, O'Neal EL, Wallach MA. A systematic review of psychosocial interventions for people with co-occurring substance use and severe mental disorders. J Subst Abuse Treat. 2008;34: 123–38.

112. Mueser KT, Drake RE, Sigmon SC, Brunette M. Psychosocial interventions for adults with severe mental illnesses and cooccurring substance use disorders: a review of specific interventions. J Dual Diagn. 2005;1:57–82.

113. Cleary M, Hunt GE, Matheson SL, Siegfried N, Walter G. Psychosocial interventions for people with both severe mental illness and substance misuse. Cochrane Database Syst Rev. 2008;Issue 1.

114. Tsuang J, Fong TW, Lesser I. Psychosocial treatment of patients with schizophrenia and substance abuse disorders. Addict Disord Their Treat. 2006;5:53–66.
115. Graeber DA, Moyers TB, Griffiths C, Guajardo E, Tonigan S. A pilot study comparing motivational interviewing and an educational intervention in patients with schizophrenia and alcohol use disorders. Commun Ment Health J. 2003;39:189–202.
116. Hulse GK, Tait RJ. Six-month outcomes associated with a brief alcohol intervention for adult in-patients with psychiatric disorders. Drug Alcohol Rev. 2002;21:105–12.
117. Kavanagh DJ, Young R, White A, Saunders JB, Wallis J, Shocklewy N, et al. A brief motivational intervention for substance misuse in recent-onset psychosis. Drug Alcohol Rev. 2004;23:151–5.
118. Swanson AJ, Pantalon MV, Cohen KR. Original interviewing and treatment adherence among psychiatric and dually diagnosed patients. J Nerv Ment Dis. 1999;187:630–5.
119. Edwards J, Elkins K, Hinton M, Harrigan SM, Donovan K, Athanasopoulos O, et al. Randomized controlled trial of a cannabis-focused intervention for young people with first-episode psychosis. Acta Psychiatr Scand. 2006;114:109–17.
120. Naeem F, Kingdon D, Turkington D. Cognitive behaviour therapy for schizophrenia in patients with mild to moderate substance misuse problems. Cogn Behav Ther. 2005;34:207–15.
121. Barrowclough C, Haddock G, Tarrier N, Lewis SW, Moring J, O'Brien R, Schofield N, McGovern J. Randomised controlled trial of cognitive behavioural therapy plus motivational intervention for schizophrenia and substance use. Am J Psychiatry. 2001;158:1706–13.
122. Baker A, Lewin T, Reichler H, Clancy R, Carr V, Garrett R, Sly K, Devir H, Terry M. Motivational interviewing among psychiatric in-patients with substance use disorders. Acta Psychiatr Scand. 2002;106:233–40.
123. Bellack AS, Bennett ME, Gearon JS, Brown CH, Yang Y. A randomized clinical trial of a new behavioral treatment for drug abuse in people with severe and persistent mental illness. Arch Gen Psychiatry. 2006;63:426–32.
124. Hellerstein DJ, Rosenthal RN, Miner CR. Integrated outpatient treatment for substance-abusing schizophrenics: a prospective study. Am J Addict. 1995;4:33–42.
125. Jerrell JM, Ridgely MS. Comparative effectiveness of three approaches to serving people with severe mental illness and substance abuse disorders. J Nerv Ment Dis. 1995;183:566–76.

Posttraumatic Stress Disorder and Psychological Trauma

Julian D. Ford

Abstract

Community and clinical epidemiologic studies indicate that adults and adolescents with substance use disorders (SUD; especially involving opiates or cocaine) are highly likely (as high as 90% prevalence in treatment-seeking samples) to have experienced psychological trauma at some time in their lives and as much as 11 times more likely than persons who do not have a SUD to meet diagnostic criteria for posttraumatic stress disorder (PTSD). Adults and adolescents with PTSD are as much as 14 times more likely to meet criteria for SUD (including alcohol or other drugs) than those without PTSD. SUD and PTSD may occur prior to the other, but research indicates that it is more likely that SUD develop or are worsened as a result of attempts to cope with PTSD than the reverse. PTSD and SUD also exacerbate and sustain each other over time. An evidence-based screening measure and promising treatments have been developed and preliminarily validated for PTSD in SUD treatment populations, including integrated approaches to simultaneous SUD/PTSD treatment rather than sequential or compartmentalized treatments. Implications for clinical identification and treatment of SUD/PTSD are presented.

Learning Objectives
- Posttraumatic stress disorder (PTSD) and substance use disorders (SUD) often co-occur
- As many as 90% of SUD treatment recipients report a history of psychological trauma
- PTSD and SUD exacerbate each other's severity when they co-occur
- PTSD is more likely to predate SUD than vice versa, although the timing is variable
- Screening for PTSD in SUD treatment samples can be accomplished with a brief tool
- Promising psychoeducational and psychotherapeutic treatments have been developed and preliminarily validated for the simultaneous treatment of PTSD and SUD
- Complex PTSD symptoms have a negative prognostic effect in SUD treatment

Issues that Need to Be Addressed by Future Research
- Studies are needed to determine the different sequences of onset of SUD and PTSD within high-risk samples such as adolescents, homeless persons, and military personnel
- Studies are needed to determine the prevalence of exposure to a variety of types of psychological trauma and of PTSD and complex PTSD across a range of populations
- Studies are needed to refine and definitively establish the evidence base for integrated treatments for comorbid SUD/PTSD, across a range of populations

J.D. Ford (✉)
Department of Psychiatry, Division of Child and Adolescent Psychiatry, University of Connecticut Health Center, Farmington, CT 06030-1410, USA
e-mail: jford@uchc.edu

J.C. Verster et al. (eds.), *Drug Abuse and Addiction in Medical Illness: Causes, Consequences and Treatment*,
DOI 10.1007/978-1-4614-3375-0_26, © Springer Science+Business Media, LLC 2012

In the National Comorbidity Study-Replication (NCS-R; [1, 2]), SUD were approximately twice as prevalent (15% lifetime; 4% past year) as posttraumatic stress disorder (PTSD; 7% lifetime, 1–2% current), and these disorders frequently occurred comorbidly. Epidemiologic studies indicate that adults with SUD (especially involving opiates or cocaine) are 2.6–10.8 times more likely to have PTSD than adults who do not have a SUD [3]. Comparable findings are reported in epidemiologic studies with adolescents, with alcohol, marijuana, and "hard drug" abuse or dependence associated with a 1.6–2.9 times increased risk of PTSD. When the focus is shifted to the risk of SUD conferred by PTSD, studies indicate that adults with PTSD are between 1.4 and 4.5 times more likely to have a SUD (including alcohol or other drugs) than adults without PTSD. Among adolescents, PTSD is associated with a 3–14 times greater risk of SUD [3].

In the present chapter, the scientific and clinical literatures on the relationship of SUD with exposure to psychological trauma and PTSD will be summarized, highlighting the bidirectional effects of SUD and PTSD on each other. Research on the impact of trauma exposure and PTSD on SUD treatment will be discussed, followed by implications for SUD treatment providers.

Psychological Trauma, Posttraumatic Stress Disorder, and Substance Use Disorders

Psychological trauma is defined in the American Psychiatric Association's [4] *Diagnostic and Statistical Manual, Fourth Edition Text Revision* (DSMIV-TR) as:

> "a traumatic event in which both of the following were present (1) the person experienced, witnessed, or was confronted with an event or events that involved actual or threatened death or serious injury or a threat to the physical integrity of self or others (2) the person's response involved intense fear, helplessness, or horror."

Psychological trauma thus is a special case of the larger class of life stressors which is defined by objective threat of death (directly or as a witness) or of physical integrity (i.e., sexual assault or abuse) and intense subjective distress at the time of or shortly after the event(s).

PTSD is further defined in the *DSMIV-TR* as present if, for more than 1 month, three types of symptoms occur and cause "clinically significant distress or impairment in social, occupational, or other important areas of functioning." The PTSD symptoms are as follows:

- *Intrusive re-experiencing*—unwanted disturbing memories of traumatic event(s), including but not limited to flashbacks (experiencing the event as if it was occurring at the present moment) and psychologically or physically distressing reminders of past traumatic events, while awake or asleep (e.g., nightmares)

- *Avoidance and emotional numbing*—efforts to avoid thoughts, feelings, discussion, people, places, or activities that are reminders of past traumatic events, amnesia for important portions of those events (which must be "psychogenic," that is, not due to physical injury or illness), generalized anhedonia, emotional numbing, detachment from relationships, and a sense that life will be cut short ("foreshortened future")

- *Hyperarousal*—sleep difficulties, anger or irritability, problems concentrating, extreme watchfulness ("hypervigilance"), and an exaggerated startle response

In order to qualify for a diagnosis of PTSD at least one intrusive re-experiencing symptom, three avoidance and emotional numbing symptoms, and two hyperarousal symptoms must occur.

As adults, survivors of early childhood victimization traumas are at risk for not only PTSD and SUD but also for other anxiety, affective, psychotic, and personality disorders and re-victimization. These adverse outcomes reflect disruptions of psychobiological self-regulation [5] that have been labeled "complex" PTSD [6]. Although complex PTSD was not included as a distinct diagnostic category in the *DSM-IV*, it is under consideration again as both an adult and childhood [7] diagnosis in the *DSM-5* (which will not be finalized until 2012). Complex PTSD involves emotional dysregulation, dissociation, somatization, risk-taking, and distrust/alienation, which are similar to criteria for some personality disorder diagnoses such as borderline personality disorder [6, 8, 9]. Complex PTSD may interfere with engagement in treatment, participation in and learning from structured treatment activities, and with the ability to inhibit substance cravings and impulsive substance-seeking behaviors while sustaining substance-free relationships, motivational commitments, and relapse prevention behaviors [10, 11].

Histories of exposure to traumatic violence (e.g., physical or sexual assault or abuse) are common and often lead to PTSD (i.e., 30–59% prevalence) among women with chronic SUD [12, 13]. Recent violence is prevalent among women with comorbid PTSD–SUD: more than 50% of women seeking treatment for comorbid PTSD–SUD reported involvement in physically assaultive behavior with a primary partner in the past year, and 45% reported being exposed to sexual coercion by a partner [14]. In community epidemiological studies of men and women, traumatic violence was with associated substantially greater risk of developing PTSD (e.g., 46–65%) than other forms of trauma (e.g., nonviolent traumas; 8–20% risk of PTSD) [3]. PTSD and SUD often co-occur after traumatic violence: women in a national survey of crime victims were three times more likely to have a SUD if they had PTSD than if they did not [15]. Adolescents with PTSD also are at four to eight times increased risk of SUD [16].

Across both genders and diverse ethnocultural backgrounds, as many as 90% of SUD treatment recipients report a history of sexual or physical assault, and as many as 59% have PTSD, including adults [3, 13, 15] and adolescents [17]. Moreover, women seeking SUD treatment who had comorbid PTSD–SUD had more extensive trauma histories and severe PTSD symptoms (particularly avoidance, emotional numbing, and sleep difficulties) than women with PTSD only [18]. Additionally, higher substance use levels or problems are associated with worse intrusive and avoidance PTSD [19] and dissociative [20] symptoms.

Several hypotheses have been advanced to explain why PTSD and SUD co-occur, with the strongest empirical support accrued for a "self-medication hypothesis" proposing that SUD are the result of attempts by people with PTSD to use substances to cope with PTSD symptoms such as intrusive memories, hypervigilance, sleep disturbance, irritability, and physical reactivity. Both epidemiological [3] and SUD treatment [21] studies indicate that PTSD more often (i.e., in 53–85% of cases) predates SUD than vice versa, with only one exception in which 18-year olds were slightly more likely (54%) to report that alcohol dependence preceded PTSD than vice versa (46%) [16]. A prospective study of primarily white middle-class adults in a health maintenance organization (age 21–35 years) found that PTSD led to a fourfold increased risk of developing SUD independent of the influence of prior conduct problems or depression, but SUD did not increase the risk of either exposure to trauma or developing PTSD [3]. The strongest relationship between PTSD and SUD was with abuse or dependence upon prescription drugs but not street drugs, consistent with the higher levels of use of prescription drugs versus street drugs by this particular subgroup of young adults. Similar findings of SUD leading to an increased risk of PTSD (but not of trauma exposure per se) have been reported with alcohol and street drugs in studies of women, military veterans, and disaster victims [21]. Both epidemiological and SUD treatment studies indicate that PTSD predates SUD more often (in 53–85% of cases) than vice versa, with only one exception in which 18-year olds were slightly more likely (54%) to report that alcohol dependence preceded PTSD than vice versa (46%). A longitudinal study of primarily white middle-class adults in a health maintenance organization (age 21–35 years) found that PTSD led to a fourfold increased risk of developing SUDs independent of the influence of prior conduct problems or depression, but SUDs did not increase the risk of either exposure to trauma or developing PTSD [3]. The strongest relationship between PTSD and SUDs was with abuse or dependence upon prescription drugs but not street drugs, consistent with the higher levels of use of prescription drugs versus street drugs by this particular subgroup of young adults. Similar findings of SUD leading to an increased risk of PTSD (but not increased risk of exposure to traumatic stressors) have been reported in studies of women, military veterans, and disaster victims [3].

Thus, SUD may predate PTSD, but it is more likely that SUD develop or are worsened as a result of attempts to cope with PTSD and SUD also may exacerbate and sustain each other over time. Men and women with alcohol- or cocaine-related SUD who had PTSD were more likely than those without PTSD to report a craving for substances if reminded of past trauma or substance use [22]. Accident survivors or women who have been raped were more likely to have persistent PTSD if they had prior alcohol disorders than those with no alcohol disorder [21].

Treatment for Comorbid SUD and PTSD

Despite these consistent findings of PTSD–SUD comorbidity, most adults receiving SUD treatment are neither evaluated for PTSD nor offered PTSD treatment, or PTSD services are provided only after lengthy periods of substance use abstinence [23]. Yet, adults with co-occurring PTSD and SUD often want to receive treatment for both PTSD and SUD and to do so in an integrated manner rather than addressing one disorder at a time [24]. Moreover, SUD treatment recruitment, retention [24], and outcomes [23, 25, 26] may be adversely affected if co-occurring PTSD is undetected and untreated.

PTSD appears to negatively influence the course and outcome of treatment for SUDs. Co-occurring PTSD and SUDs are associated with poorer SUD treatment recruitment and retention [24] and outcomes [23, 25, 26]. However, these findings were not replicated in two other studies. Chart-diagnosed PTSD was not associated with differential opiate substitution treatment outcomes with military veterans [27], nor with SUD residential treatment retention among adolescents [28]—although trauma exposed adolescents in the latter study were more likely to discontinue SUD residential treatment than adolescents with no history of psychological trauma.

Although persons with co-occurring PTSD and SUD often request integrated treatment for PTSD and SUD [24], most SUD treatment recipients are neither evaluated for PTSD nor offered PTSD treatment—or PTSD services are provided only after lengthy periods of substance use abstinence [23]. On the positive side, PTSD treatment has been shown to reduce not only immediate but also long-term risk of SUD relapse if provided during the transitional period beginning soon after discharge from inpatient SUD treatment and during the long-term recovery period [23]. When PTSD treatment was provided to military veterans immediately after discharge from inpatient SUD treatment, reduced immediate and long-term risk of SUD relapse was reported [23]. While they did not provide integrated PTSD–SUD treatment, Ouimette and colleagues' [23] findings suggest that SUD and PTSD recovery and treatment are not incompatible—indeed they may be essential to one another (see also Dansky et al., [15]). Consistent with the self-medication model of co-occurring PTSD/SUD, recent re-analyses of data from a large randomized controlled trial indicate that an integrated PTSD/SUD therapy was effective in reducing SUD with participants who had severe initial SUD problems only if PTSD symptoms also improved in treatment [29]. Improvement in substance use problems, however, did not appear to lead to reductions in PTSD. Although several models of PTSD treatment have been empirically validated in the past two decades, most PTSD therapies have not been adapted for co-occurring SUD [30]. Fortunately, integrated PTSD–SUD therapies have been developed (see Ford et al. [30]), with promising preliminary outcomes [31–35].

However, the Cohen and Hien [32] study found that, although cognitive behavior therapy for comorbid SUD and PTSD had positive results for PTSD and substance use outcomes, there were no differences between persons receiving cognitive behavior therapy and those who received no active treatment on measures of depression, dissociation, or social and sexual functioning. They note that sequelae of complex histories of interpersonal trauma (e.g., dissociation, affect dysregulation) may be particularly refractory to treatment [32]. Therefore, secondary analyses were conducted of data from a multisite study testing the efficacy of contingency management (CM) in community-based clinics to examine PTSD and complex PTSD symptom severity as separate prognostic indicators [36].

Over and above the strong effect of CM intervention, the severity of complex PTSD symptoms—but *not* history of trauma exposure, PTSD symptom severity, or overall psychiatric symptom severity—predicted poorer outcomes in terms of retention in treatment and objectively verified continuous abstinence from cocaine and heroin use during treatment. Brief measures of PTSD and complex PTSD symptoms were used which did not permit inferences about either PTSD or complex PTSD as diagnostic syndromes, and a more definitive test of the study hypotheses would require the use of a structured interview (for PTSD or complex PTSD) or questionnaire (for PTSD) with continuous scores based upon the full set of PTSD and complex PTSD symptoms. Nevertheless, complex PTSD symptoms emerged as an independent prognostic factor for cocaine- and heroin-use disorder treatment outcomes. Although there was not an interaction effect for complex PTSD symptoms and type of treatment (the comparison condition was supportive therapy, ST), closer inspection of the results for each treatment condition showed that complex PTSD symptoms were predictive of outcome only in the CM condition. Complex PTSD symptoms also appeared to impact, and to largely account for, a relationship between having witnessed an assault and poorer treatment retention. Thus, although CM has shown consistent positive outcomes in SUD treatment, strategies for successfully engaging and facilitating sustained abstinence with patients who have complex PTSD symptoms may be needed to enhance their CM outcomes. The absence of a predictive effect for complex PTSD symptoms in ST may be due to the lesser amount of change achieved by ST with most patients, effectively limiting the variance in change and thus reducing the likelihood of detecting prognostic relationships in the ST condition.

PTSD and complex PTSD symptoms were interrelated [36], but only complex PTSD symptoms predicted immediate treatment outcome, consistent with Ford and Kidd's [37] finding that complex PTSD rather than PTSD predicted chronic PTSD treatment outcome. Comorbid PTSD–SUD is particularly likely to occur following severe trauma exposure and may involve particularly severe PTSD symptoms [18, 38]. These studies have not, however, distinguished between PTSD and complex PTSD symptoms. Thus, the documented tendency of PTSD and SUDs to exacerbate and sustain each other over time (e.g., increased craving for substances when reminded of past traumatic stressors or substance use [22]) may be due in part to complex PTSD symptoms. Further, complex PTSD symptoms also have been found to be most strongly associated with severe intrusive re-experiencing symptoms (i.e., unwanted memories, flashbacks) than PTSD alone [5], which may elicit substance use as an attempt to self-medicate posttraumatic distress [21]. However, complex PTSD symptoms were unrelated to the number of CM-contracted activities completed; thus, interference with CM activity completion by complex PTSD symptoms does not appear to account the negative prognostic relationship.

Not only did PTSD symptom severity not predict immediate treatment outcomes, but a *high* level of baseline PTSD symptoms was the strongest predictor of achieving abstinence at 9-month follow-up assessments [36]. This finding is the opposite of prior studies' findings suggesting that higher levels of PTSD related to substance use problems and are negative predictors of SUD treatment outcomes [23, 24], but consistent with a recent study with adolescents in SUD treatment [39]. Upon closer inspection in bivariate analyses, this prognostic effect held only for patients receiving CM, a higher percent of whom achieved abstinence at 9-month follow-up (84%) than in the overall CM cohort or in ST. It is also possible that patients with severe PTSD symptoms receive more services than those with less severe PTSD [27]. Thus, trauma history and PTSD may not constitute a problem for successful SUD treatment, but instead may be addressed with integrated PTSD/SUD treatment [24]. Further research is needed to determine how SUD treatment retention and outcomes can be enhanced for patients with complex PTSD symptoms, for example by extending or adapting some of the recently developed manualized treatments for complex PTSD [30] and for severe comorbid PTSD and SUD [11, 25, 34].

Implications for the Treatment of Comorbid SUD and PTSD

Recovery from PTSD is complementary with recovery from SUD because recovery from PTSD involves learning how to deal with unfinished emotional business from trauma without denial and with personal responsibility (i.e., sobriety). Psychological trauma survivors with PTSD are not "fragile," but rather are highly resilient because they have had to develop ways of coping with extreme stressors, or else they would not be seeking sobriety [11]. Psychologcal trauma survivors with PTSD or complex PTSD have developed highly reactive bodily stress response systems that can precipitate or exacerbate SUD [40]. Awareness of and skills for managing PTSD symptoms, therefore, is an integral component of SUD relapse prevention [32].

Although there is a strong empirical evidence base for "prolonged exposure" and related therapies for PTSD which involve repeated re-telling of specific traumatic memories, treatment for PTSD—and particularly for complex PTSD [30]—involves substantial work on skills for managing traumatic stress symptoms that is an essential prerequisite to therapeutic "trauma memory work." Skills for managing traumatic stress symptoms—of both PTSD and complex PTSD—provide a foundation for psychological trauma survivors to make thoughtful choices about if, how, when, and with whom to re-examine trauma memories. Moreover, there is no way to eradicate memories of traumatic experiences nor necessarily any total permanent "cure" for PTSD or complex PTSD—but this is no different than for SUD. Most treatment recipients never completely eliminate traumatic stress symptoms, but they can reduce the distress caused by these symptoms by learning how to manage them rather than feeling powerless in the face of unwanted traumatic memories and the associated stress reactions.

Fundamental to integrated PTSD–SUD treatment is addressing how PTSD and SUD are understood by the clinician and client—their "meta-models" for conceptualizing PTSD and SUD [11]. From a "disease model" perspective, PTSD and SUD are the result of psychobiological vulnerability and reactions to environmental stressors that can become chronic disabilities. From a cognitive-behavioral standpoint, PTSD and SUD result from dysfunctional (i.e., threat-based or addiction-based) beliefs, cognitive biases, and reactive behavior patterns that lead to an escalating sense of anxiety, anger, and helplessness. From a stress and coping perspective, PTSD and SUD involve maladaptive coping in response to stressors that range in intensity from mild to traumatic [21]. From a resilience perspective, PTSD and SUD involve a loss or breakdown of the person's psychological and interpersonal resources (e.g., sense of safety, self-efficacy, motivation). From a developmental

viewpoint, PTSD and SUD involve disrupted learning and maturation, such that the person does not develop self-regulatory capacities and healthy attachments [5]. From a cultural perspective, PTSD and SUD involve larger sociocultural forces, barriers, and norms that influence the impact that traumatic events have upon entire communities or societies and people's core ways of life.

Treatments for co-occurring PTSD–SUD tend to address some but not all of these factors [11]. In order to retain streamlined interventions that are efficient and do not overload either the provider or the recipient with information and activities, two domains have been identified that cut across all metamodels of PTSD and SUD, memory and emotion regulation. PTSD and SUD involve a loss of control over one's own memory. In PTSD, this takes the form of unwanted, persistent, and fragmented memories of traumatic experiences. In SUD, memory tends to be fragmented, overwhelmingly painful and at times frustratingly elusive (e.g., when cues or cravings lead to impulsive substance seeking despite experiential knowledge of the adverse consequences). Therefore, integrated PTSD–SUD treatment must enable survivors to remember not only the traumatic stressors and addictive behaviors that they have experienced, but moreover to make fundamental developmental shift in personal identity from viewing self as a victim or failure to as a survivor whose life is enriched by sustained efforts toward recovery.

Although traumatic stressors and addictive behaviors are painful to remember, the major barrier to memory is not the events themselves but the extreme emotion dysregulation that traumatic memories or reminders evoke [5]. Chronic PTSD and SUD both involve mood shifts that encompass intense rage, grief, fear, despair, guilt, and shame, as well as profound emotional "cutoffs" such as dissociation, alexithymia, and numbing. Integrated PTSD–SUD treatment therefore focuses on enhancing emotional regulation, in order to increase clients' ability to recognize and manage both SUD and PTSD symptoms and their often complex interplay (e.g., intense denial, rage, and urges to use substances when experiencing painful unwanted memories or hypervigilance [11, 30]).

Based on the goal of memory recovery and emotional self-regulation, Ford and colleagues [11] have suggested several best practice guidelines for integrated PTSD/SUD services. For most SUD treatment recipients, the potential link between PTSD or complex PTSD symptoms and SUD symptoms typically has never been identified or discussed by a treatment provider, as if the two sets of symptoms were totally separate concerns. A brief (<5 min) screening questionnaire has been found to have strong sensitivity and specificity for the identification of SUD treatment recipients with undetected PTSD [41]. In addition to providing information about clients' current functioning and treatment needs, initial PTSD screening provides an opportunity to begin educating the recipient about how PTSD and SUD symptoms can be addressed in tandem. For example, during a screening interaction, the provider can briefly explain that unwanted traumatic memories are actually signs of biological and psychological self-protection that can be made more effective by viewing them as such rather than as signs of biological or psychological breakdown. For example, Ford and colleagues suggest the following explanation: "These unwanted memories and the feeling of being tense and in danger all the time actually are your body's alarm system trying to protect you, but the problem is that you're not in control of the alarm because you do not know how to turn it off when you really are safe. The treatment will help you learn some skills for controlling your body's alarm reactions without slipping up and using alcohol to try to turn off the alarm." Such empathic and practical approaches to PTSD/SUD psychoeducation can enhance engagement in and motivation for treatment by giving the recipient a new way to think of PTSD and SUD symptoms which has practical relevance and resonates with personal experiences and goals.

In addition, as a result of chronic SUD, persons with PTSD or complex PTSD often are not able to gauge the severity of these symptoms, and thus may unintentionally under- or over-report them [11]. Education about PTSD and SUD in the screening process can facilitate a more accurate identification and estimation of PTSD and complex PTSD symptoms. The provider can explain that trying not to avoid emotional and bodily "alarm reactions" such as anger or craving for substances is an understandable attempt to cope with these reactions that provides short-term relief ("helps you get through the day, or the night"), but that unfortunately makes the stress reactions and addictive cravings more frequent and disruptive in the long run. The provider can then offer the recipient an encouraging new perspective by explaining that the PTSD–SUD treatment is designed to teach new skills for giving the client more control over the body's stress system to enable the recipient to alter the vicious cycle of feeling distressed, avoiding or denying stress signals, and then feeling worse and seeking substances.

A thorough review of traumatic stressors and PTSD/complex PTSD symptoms can be upsetting or demoralizing. Therefore, screening does not automatically involve obtaining a detailed trauma history or survey of PTSD symptoms. The brief screen validated by Kimerling and colleagues [41] does not specifically ask about any traumatic stressors and inquires only about the four types of PTSD symptoms (subdividing avoidance and emotional numbing into two separate items, consistent with research on the factor structure of PTSD) in general. Many PTSD–SUD treatment recipients do not feel ready to disclose more than small amounts of information about traumatic experiences or PTSD symptoms until they have established a strong therapeutic alliance. In some cases, they may not be able to tolerate the intensity of their own reactions to disclosing the details of terrible personal memories. For others, this is merely a fairly rote recitation of a familiar list of problems that they believe will never change. Still others feel compelled to "tell all" either to justify their distress and their right to treatment, or because they do not know how to select manageable amounts of past memories and how to regulate the associated emotions. Screening therefore should not focus singularly on past traumatic events, but on how current stress reactions interfere with the current relationships and the attainment of life goals—and how treatment can help with this. Screening and follow-up assessment also should take into consideration diagnoses other than PTSD (e.g., depression, panic disorder) instead of assuming that stress-like symptoms always are due to PTSD or that the only sequela of exposure to traumatic stressors is PTSD [42].

Although it can be difficult logistically, Ford and colleagues [11] recommend that each PTSD–SUD treatment recipient has a primary counselor, clinician, or case manager to ensure that this is complementary with all other aspects of the treatment plan. Frequency of contact with a primary provider can be individualized and may differ depending on the stage of treatment (e.g., frequent regular individual visits or phone check-ins may be helpful early in treatment or when symptoms or lapses are severe). The goal of a primary provider is to provide recipients with enough therapeutic structure and support to enable them to focus on recovery and life management in an organized manner despite the interference caused by PTSD and SUD. The treatment may involve group or individual therapy or case management (or both). Ford and colleagues [11] recommend that PTSD–SUD groups should be gender specific, at least in the initial phases of treatment. Many trauma survivors have never (or only rarely or intermittently) had the opportunity to reflect on the impact that traumatic stress symptoms have had on their lives, as well as the chance to give and receive support with others of their gender. There are as many differences as similarities among same-sex trauma survivors, but a key similarity not shared with members of the opposite sex is the impact that traumatic stressors have upon each person's sense of self. Same-gender groups provide an opportunity for men or boys as well as for women or girls to experience counseling in ways that add depth and richness to recovery both from traumatic stress and addiction. Recipients may feel greater confidence in moving to mixed-gender groups after having had the opportunity to develop skills and a commitment to PTSD as well as SUD recovery first gender-specific PTSD–SUD groups. However, research is needed to validate these clinical observations, and to determine if, and for whom, same- or mixed-gender PTSD/SUD treatment groups are optimal.

Prior to, and possibly instead of, delving in great detail into specific traumatic memories or situations, PTSD–SUD clients benefit from learning skills that enhance their mastery of memory and emotion regulation in their current lives. These skills can be applied to incidents in which they are troubled by unwanted traumatic memories or PTSD symptoms. Focusing on helping treatment recipients to make, and successfully implement, self-enhancing choices when faced with PTSD or complex PTSD symptoms enables them to make connections between current stress reactions and substance use cues or cravings with past traumatic experiences while maintaining an adaptive here-and-now focus on current functioning, symptom management, sobriety, and personal goals.

Vicarious traumatization (VT), also referred to as secondary traumatization or compassion fatigue, refers to the emotional impact providers experience from the clients' intense traumatic stress reactions. Empathy, the ability to take another person's internal frame of reference seriously, involves personal and professional boundaries that do not prevent a clinician from feeling the impact of patients' suffering, but does help the clinician reflect on and work through that impact, rather than just absorbing it as inchoate distress. On the other hand, sympathy, while laudable and probably inevitable, involves excessively permeable emotional boundaries that can lead to overidentification or enmeshment with clients. Empathy may protect against extreme VT, but it is not an "antidote" for VT [11]. Intense sympathy (e.g., feeling a need to rescue a client), however, may intensify VT and is best addressed by regaining an empathic balance of involvement and separateness in relation to clients and clinical work.

VT also is most likely to occur and to be heightened when a clinician's personal issues are activated (affectively or symbolically) by patients' current suffering or traumatic memories. Working through personal issues is the responsibility of every helping professional, as well as deciding when it is necessary to place limits on the amount or type of therapeutic work being done for the sake of self-care and the well-being of clients. When providing SUD/PTSD treatment, it is particularly important to monitor and proactively prepare for VT.

Conclusion

In light of the extensive and growing empirical database demonstrating a bidirectional relationship between SUD and PTSD, and suggesting that not only PTSD but also complex PTSD symptoms may require systematic attention in SUD treatment, integrated SUD/PTSD represents a challenging but evidence-based paradigm shift [43]. Fortunately, a psychometrically and clinically promising brief screening measure is available for substance abuse (or primary care) providers to use in identifying patients for whom traumatic stress symptoms are particularly relevant in planning and

delivering SUD treatment [41]. Promising interventions for comorbid SUD/PTSD have a developing evidence base with these often highly impaired adults and adolescents [33, 35]. The clinician in practice can draw upon these resources to enhance healthcare outcomes for patients with comorbid SUD/PTSD, as researchers continue to refine and validate evidence-based tools for screening, assessment, and treatment of this challenging type of co-occurring disorder.

References

1. Kessler RC, Berglund P, Demler O, Jin R, Merikangas KR, Walters EE. Lifetime prevalence and age-of-onset distributions of DSM-IV disorders in the National Comorbidity Survey Replication. Arch Gen Psychiatry. 2005;62(6):593–602.
2. Kessler RC, Chiu WT, Demler O, Merikangas KR, Walters EE. Prevalence, severity, and comorbidity of 12-month DSM-IV disorders in the National Comorbidity Survey Replication. Arch Gen Psychiatry. 2005;62(6):617–27.
3. Chilcoat HD, Menard C. Epidemiological investigations: comorbidity of posttraumatic stress disorder and substance use disorder. In: Ouimette P, Brown PJ, editors. Trauma and substance abuse: causes, consequences, and treatment of comorbid disorders. Washington, DC: American Psychological Association; 2003. p. 9–28.
4. APA. Diagnostic and statistical manual of mental disorders: DSM-IV-TR. 4th ed. Washington, DC: American Psychiatric Association; 2000.
5. Ford JD. Treatment implications of altered affect regulation and information processing following child maltreatment. Psychiatr Ann. 2005;35(5):410–9.
6. van der Kolk BA, Roth S, Pelcovitz D, Sunday S, Spinazzola J. Disorders of extreme stress: the empirical foundation of a complex adaptation to trauma. J Trauma Stress. 2005;18(5):389–99.
7. van der Kolk BA. Developmental trauma disorder: toward a rational diagnosis for children with complex trauma histories. Psychiatr Ann. 2005;35(5):401–8.
8. Ford JD, Fisher P, Larson L. Object relations as a predictor of treatment outcome with chronic posttraumatic stress disorder. J Consult Clin Psychol. 1997;65(4):547–59.
9. Roth S, Newman E, Pelcovitz D, van der Kolk B, Mandel FS. Complex PTSD in victims exposed to sexual and physical abuse: results from the DSM-IV Field Trial for Posttraumatic Stress Disorder. J Trauma Stress. 1997;10(4):539–55.
10. Allen JG, Coyne L, Huntoon J. Complex posttraumatic stress disorder in women from a psychometric perspective. J Pers Assess. 1998;70(2):277–98.
11. Ford JD, Russo EM, Mallon SD. Integrating treatment of posttraumatic stress disorder and substance use disorder. J Counsel Dev. 2007;85(4):475–89.
12. Marcenko MO, Kemp SP, Larson NC. Childhood experiences of abuse, later substance use, and parenting outcomes among low-income mothers. Am J Orthopsychiatry. 2000;70(3):316–26.
13. Najavits LM, Weiss RD, Shaw SR. The link between substance abuse and posttraumatic stress disorder in women: a research review. Am J Addict. 1997;6(4):273–83.
14. Najavits LM, Sonn J, Walsh M, Weiss RD. Domestic violence in women with PTSD and substance abuse. Addict Behav. 2004;29(4):707–15.
15. Dansky BS, Brady KT, Saladin ME, Killeen T. Victimization and PTSD in individuals with substance use disorders: gender and racial differences. Am J Drug Alcohol Abuse. 1996;22(1):75–93.

16. Giaconia RM, Reinherz HZ, Hauf AC, Paradis AD, Wasserman MS, Langhammer DM. Comorbidity of substance use and post-traumatic stress disorders in a community sample of adolescents. Am J Orthopsychiatry. 2000;70(2):253–62.

17. Stevens SJ, Murphy BS, McKnight K. Traumatic stress and gender differences in relationship to substance abuse, mental health, physical health, and HIV risk behavior in a sample of adolescents enrolled in drug treatment. Child Maltreat. 2003;8(1):46–57.

18. Saladin ME, Brady KT, Dansky BS, Kilpatrick DG. Understanding comorbidity between PTSD and substance use disorder: two preliminary investigations. Addict Behav. 1995;20(5):643–55.

19. Read JP, Brown PJ, Kahler CW. Substance use and posttraumatic stress disorders: symptom interplay and effects on outcome. Addict Behav. 2004;29(8):1665–72.

20. Seedat S, Stein DJ, Carey PD. Post-traumatic stress disorder in women: epidemiological and treatment issues. CNS Drugs. 2005; 19(5):411–27.

21. Stewart SH, Conrod PJ. Psychosocial models of functional associations between posttraumatic stress disorder and substance use disorder. In: Ouimette P, Brown PJ, editors. Trauma and substance abuse: causes, consequences, and treatment of comorbid disorders. Washington, DC: American Psychological Association; 2003. p. 29–55.

22. Saladin ME, Drobes DJ, Coffey SF, Dansky BS, Brady KT, Kilpatrick DG. PTSD symptom severity as a predictor of cue-elicited drug craving in victims of violent crime. Addict Behav. 2003; 28(9):1611–29.

23. Ouimette P, Moos RH, Finney JW. PTSD treatment and 5-year remission among patients with substance use and posttraumatic stress disorders. J Consult Clin Psychol. 2003;71(2):410–4.

24. Brown PJ, Read JP, Kahler CW. Comorbid posttraumatic stress disorder and substance use disorders: treatment outcomes and the role of coping. In: Ouimette P, Brown PJ, editors. Trauma and substance abuse: causes, consequences, and treatment of comorbid disorders. Washington, DC: American Psychological Association; 2003. p. 171–88.

25. Najavits LM, Harned M, Gallop R, Butler S, Barber J, Thase ME. Six-month treatment outcomes of cocaine-dependent patients with and without PTSD in a multisite national trial. J Stud Alcohol. 2008;68:353–61.

26. Palacios WR, Urmann CF, Newel R, Hamilton N. Developing a sociological framework for dually diagnosed women. J Subst Abuse Treat. 1999;17(1–2):91–102.

27. Trafton JA, Minkel J, Humphreys K. Opioid substitution treatment reduces substance use equivalently in patients with and without posttraumatic stress disorder. J Stud Alcohol. 2006;67(2):228–35.

28. Jaycox LH, Ebener P, Damesek L, Becker K. Trauma exposure and retention in adolescent substance abuse treatment. J Trauma Stress. 2004;17(2):113–21.

29. Hien DA, Jiang H, Campbell AN, et al. Do treatment improvements in PTSD severity affect substance use outcomes? A secondary analysis from a randomized clinical trial in NIDA's Clinical Trials Network. Am J Psychiatry. 2010;167(1):95–101.

30. Ford JD, Courtois CA, Steele K, Hart O, Nijenhuis ER. Treatment of complex posttraumatic self-dysregulation. J Trauma Stress. 2005;18(5):437–47.

31. Coffey SF, Dansky BS, Brady KT. Exposure-based, trauma-focused therapy for comorbid posttraumatic stress disorder-substance use disorder. In: Ouimette P, Brown PJ, editors. Trauma and substance abuse: causes, consequences, and treatment of comorbid disorders. Washington, DC: American Psychological Association; 2003. p. 127–46.

32. Cohen LR, Hien DA. Treatment outcomes for women with substance abuse and PTSD who have experienced complex trauma. Psychiatr Serv. 2006;57(1):100–6.

33. Frisman L, Ford JD, Lin H, Mallon S, Chang R. Outcomes of trauma treatment using the TARGET model. J Groups Addict Recover. 2008;3(3/4):285–303.

34. Hien DA, Cohen LR, Miele GM, Litt LC, Capstick C. Promising treatments for women with comorbid PTSD and substance use disorders. Am J Psychiatry. 2004;161(8):1426–32.

35. Desai RA, Harpaz-Rotem I, Najavits LM, Rosenheck RA. Impact of the seeking safety program on clinical outcomes among homeless female veterans with psychiatric disorders. Psychiatr Serv. 2008;59(9):996–1003.

36. Ford JD, Hawke J, Alessi S, Ledgerwood D, Petry N. Psychological trauma and PTSD symptoms as predictors of substance dependence treatment outcomes. Behav Res Ther. 2007;45(10):2417–31.

37. Ford JD, Kidd P. Early childhood trauma and disorders of extreme stress as predictors of treatment outcome with chronic posttraumatic stress disorder. J Trauma Stress. 1998;11(4):743–61.

38. Riggs DS, Rukstalis M, Volpicelli JR, Kalmanson D, Foa EB. Demographic and social adjustment characteristics of patients with comorbid posttraumatic stress disorder and alcohol dependence: potential pitfalls to PTSD treatment. Addict Behav. 2003;28(9): 1717–30.

39. Williams JK, Smith DC, Gotman N, Sabri B, An H, Hall JA. Traumatized youth and substance abuse treatment outcomes: a longitudinal study. J Trauma Stress. 2008;21(1):100–8.

40. Jacobsen LK, Southwick SM, Kosten TR. Substance use disorders in patients with posttraumatic stress disorder: a review of the literature. Am J Psychiatry. 2001;158(8):1184–90.

41. Kimerling R, Trafton JA, Nguyen B. Validation of a brief screen for Post-Traumatic Stress Disorder with substance use disorder patients. Addict Behav. 2006;31(11):2074–9.

42. Read JP, Bollinger AR, Sharkansky E. Assessment of comorbid substance use disorder and posttraumatic stress disorder. In: Ouimette P, Brown PJ, editors. Trauma and substance abuse: causes, consequences, and treatment of comorbid disorders. Washington, DC: American Psychological Association; 2003. p. 111–25.

43. Simpson DD. A conceptual framework for transferring research to practice. J Subst Abuse Treat. 2002;22(4):171–82.

Seizures, Illicit Drugs, and Ethanol

John C.M. Brust

Abstract

Seizures can occur in recreational drug users by indirect mechanisms, including CNS infection, ischemic or hemorrhagic stroke, cerebral trauma, or metabolic derangements such as hypoglycemia, hyponatremia, or renal failure. With some drugs, seizures are a feature of acute toxicity. Cocaine-induced seizures often occur without other evidence of toxicity; seizures in users of other psychostimulants—such as methamphetamine or methylenedioxymethamphetamine (ecstasy)—are usually accompanied by additional signs of overdose. Sedative drugs and ethanol cause seizures as a withdrawal phenomenon, but ethanol-related seizures appear to be of more than one type, some lacking a close temporal relationship to withdrawal. Clinicians should consider substance abuse when dealing with unexplained seizures and should consider seizures when encountering unusual symptoms in recreational drug users.

Learning Objectives
- Seizures in recreational drug users can be associated with either withdrawal or toxicity, or they can have indirect mechanisms such as CNS infection, stroke, cerebral trauma, or metabolic derangement.
- With psychostimulant drugs, including cocaine and methamphetamine, seizures are most often the result of direct toxicity.
- With sedatives and ethanol, seizures are most often a withdrawal phenomenon.

Issues that Need to Be Addressed by Future Research
- Basic mechanisms for seizures that occur in association with drug toxicity or withdrawal need to be elucidated.

Most recreationally used drugs increase the risk of seizures. Mechanisms are both indirect and direct, the latter involving either toxicity or withdrawal. Especially in polysubstance abusers, different mechanisms are not mutually exclusive. For example, a drug user might be intoxicated with one agent while simultaneously withdrawing from another [1].

Indirect Mechanisms

Parenteral drug users are subject to systemic and central nervous system (CNS) infection. Immunocompromise associated with some agents (e.g., ethanol) confers additional risk. Of particular importance are endocarditis and AIDS. CNS

J.C.M. Brust, M.D. (✉)
Department of Neurology, Columbia University College
of Physicians & Surgeons, New York, NY, USA
e-mail: jcb2@columbia.edu

complications of endocarditis include cerebral infarction, septic (mycotic) aneurysm rupture, brain abscess, and meningoencephalitis, each of which may produce seizures. CNS complications of AIDS, especially toxoplasmosis, lymphoma, herpes simplex encephalitis, and tuberculous or fungal meningitis, also cause seizures, often as the presenting symptom.

Independent of endocarditis, recreational drug users are at risk for ischemic stroke. Mechanisms include embolization of foreign material, coagulopathy, and vasculitis. In cocaine users hemorrhagic stroke is most often the result of hypertensive surges, whereas most ischemic strokes are probably the result of direct cerebral vasoconstriction [2]. Low-to-moderate doses of ethanol appear to reduce the risk of ischemic stroke, whereas heavy doses increase the risk. Any dose increases the risk of hemorrhagic stroke [3]. Seizures are especially likely to occur when stroke occurs in the presence of drug intoxication or withdrawal.

Cerebral trauma in alcoholics is usually associated with intoxication and in illicit drug users with lawlessness and violence. Post-traumatic seizures can occur early (impact seizure) or late (post-traumatic epilepsy), and as with stroke, intoxication (e.g., with cocaine) or withdrawal (e.g., with ethanol) can further lower seizure threshold.

Metabolic derangements frequently encountered in drug users include hypoglycemia, hyponatremia, and liver or kidney failure. Hypoglycemia is often overlooked in alcoholics when seizures during a binge are attributed to ethanol withdrawal [4].

Direct Mechanisms: Individual Agents

Opiates

Opiate drugs include a large number of agonists, antagonists, and mixed agonist/antagonists acting variably at μ, δ, κ receptors. In animals opiates are proconvulsant or anticonvulsant depending on species, seizure model, dose, rate of administration, and particular agent [5, 6].

Heroin, the most commonly abused opiate, is injected, snorted, or smoked, often combined with cocaine or an amphetamine-like psychostimulant. Street preparations contain a variety of pharmacologically active and inactive ingredients, some of which are epileptogenic [7]. Heroin overdose, with coma, pinpoint pupils, and respiratory depression, is sometimes associated with seizures, but their occurrence in such a setting is so unusual that an alternative explanation such as concomitant ethanol withdrawal or CNS infection should be sought. In a case–control study heroin users were at increased risk for new-onset seizures, either unprovoked (OR = 2.57) or provoked (stroke, infection, trauma; OR = 3.65). OR was 6.61 for same day use, but seizures were

not associated with overdose, and the risk persisted after a year of abstinence [8].

Except in newborns, seizures are not associated with opiate withdrawal, which causes flu-like symptoms (fever, myalgia, rhinorrhea, lacrimation, sweating, piloerection, abdominal cramps, vomiting, and diarrhea) and is seldom dangerous. By contrast, withdrawal symptoms in neonates can be severe or even fatal [9]. Seizures and myoclonus are described but can be difficult to distinguish from jitteriness. Coexisting conditions that must be considered include hypoglycemia, hypocalcemia, intracerebral hemorrhage, meningitis, sepsis, and withdrawal from other drugs or ethanol.

Seizures and myoclonus, as well as tremor, agitation, and hallucinations, are well-recognized features of meperidine toxicity, attributable to its active metabolite normeperidine [10]. The combination of meperidine and a monoamine oxidase inhibitor exacerbates symptoms and can be lethal [11].

During the 1970s parenteral abuse of pentazocine (Talwin) and tripelennamine (Pyribenzamine)—"T's and blues"—became popular in the American midwest [12]. Seizures were often encountered, and the antihistamine probably contributed to lowered seizure threshold.

Seizures are anecdotally described in recreational users of propoxyphene [13]. Myoclonus is described during withdrawal from fentanyl [14].

Psychostimulants

Abusers of amphetamine, methamphetamine, and related psychostimulant drugs usually experience seizures in the setting of obvious overdose—agitation, psychosis, fever, hypertension, cardiac arrhythmia, delirium, or coma [15]. By contrast, seizures often occur in cocaine users in the absence of other symptoms [16–19]. The reason is unclear. The principal pharmacological action of amphetamine-like agents is a release of monoamine from synaptic terminals, and in animals methamphetamine-induced hyperthermia causes blood–brain barrier disruption and neuronal degeneration in the amygdala and hippocampus, probably contributing to seizures [20]. The principal action of cocaine is monoamine reuptake blockade; in addition, cocaine has local anesthetic properties, and other local anesthetics are also proconvulsant. In animals cocaine-induced seizures display "kindling"—that is, repeated subthreshold doses of the drug eventually trigger seizures [21, 22]. Cocaine users can experience seizures hours after use, perhaps attributable to pharmacologically active metabolites [16–18]. Seizures are usually generalized tonic–clonic; focality suggests an underlying structural lesion such as brain contusion or stroke. Cocaine-related seizures can follow parenteral or nasal use; new-onset seizures are especially likely in heavy "crack" smokers. Consistent with kindling, seizures can occur after repeated use of cocaine, but they can also affect first-time users. Cocaine can trigger seizures in known epileptics [19]. Status epilepticus in cocaine users is often difficult to control [17].

In different reports the prevalence of seizures among cocaine users ranged from 1% to 9.3% [17, 19, 23, 24]. The higher figure is from a phone survey. Higher prevalences among crack smokers probably reflect a dosage effect.

A case-report described bizarre behavior which was considered cocaine intoxication but turned out to be partial complex status epilepticus [25].

Seizures, as well as stroke, were well-recognized complications in users of phenylpropanolamine, which, until such products were banned by the Food and Drug Administration (FDA) in 2000, was available in over-the-counter diet pills and decongestants [26]. Seizures and stroke also occurred in users of "dietary supplements" containing ephedra alkaloids (ma huang) [27]. In 2003 the FDA banned these products.

Methylenedioxymethamphetamine (MDMA, "ecstasy") has pharmacological properties of both amphetamine-like psychostimulants and mescaline-like hallucinogens. The use of ecstasy at "rave" parties, in which frenetic dancing drives up body temperature, is especially dangerous. Seizures are described either in the setting of obvious intoxication (especially severe hyperthermia) or without any other symptoms [28, 29]. In animals MDMA-induced seizures display a kindling pattern [30].

Sedatives and Hypnotics

Acting indirectly as GABA agonists, barbiturates, benzodiazepines, and non-barbiturate non-benzodiazepine sedatives produce in chronic users withdrawal symptoms similar to those associated with ethanol. In a study with volunteers, withdrawal after several months of ingesting amobarbital or secobarbital 400 mg daily caused electroencephalographic paroxysmal changes in one-third of subjects but no seizures. 600 mg daily resulted in seizures in 10% of subjects. 900 mg daily resulted in seizures in three-fourths of subjects and delirium tremens in two-thirds [31].

Symptoms following abrupt discontinuation of benzodiazepine drugs—principally anxiety and tremor—can be difficult to tell from symptoms that led to benzodiazepine use in the first place, but seizures, hallucinations, and delirium tremens do occur [32]. Withdrawal symptoms usually appear between 3 and 10 days after stopping a long-acting agent and within 24 h after stopping a short-acting agent. As with barbiturates, seizures are dose-related and unlikely in patients taking recommended therapeutic doses [33].

Like barbiturates, glutethimide (often taken parenterally with codeine) can produce withdrawal seizures, but seizures or myoclonus can also occur with overdose, perhaps related to the drug's anticholinergic actions [34]. Seizures also occur

as a toxic effect of methaqualone (often taken with an antihistamine, and banned in the United States) [35].

Withdrawal seizures are described in users of zolpidem, the most widely prescribed sedative in the United States [36].

γ-hydroxybutyrate (GHB) and its precursors γ-butyrolactone and 1,4-butanediol are popular among participants at "rave" parties and as a "date-rape" drug [37, 38]. Physical dependence results in abstinence symptoms similar to those observed during withdrawal from ethanol, including seizures [39, 40]. GHB is often taken with ethanol, and the combination can produce a more severe and protracted withdrawal syndrome [41]. It is also often co-ingested with psychostimulants, including ecstasy and cocaine, making it difficult to interpret reports of seizures or myoclonus during GHB intoxication. GHB binds to specific GHB receptors and to GABA receptors, and its principal clinical effect is CNS depression. Although GHB-induced petit mal-like epileptiform EEG discharges are described in rodents and non-human primates, epileptogenicity has not been documented in humans [42].

Marijuana

In animals cannabinoid compounds (including the principal psychoactive ingredient, δ-9-tetrahydrocannabinol, THC) are variably proconvulsant or anticonvulsant depending on species and seizure model [43]. Although agonists at CNS endocannabinoid receptors inhibit synaptic release of both glutamate and GABA, their preponderant effect on experimental seizures is anticonvulsant [44]. The non-psychoactive compound, cannabidiol, is most consistently anticonvulsant [45, 46].

A case–control study found marijuana use to be protective against new-onset seizures in men (OR = 0.42). For women there was a trend toward risk reduction that did not reach statistical significance [8].

Anecdotal reports describe either improved or worsened seizure control temporally associated with marijuana use [47–49]. In a survey of 12 epileptic marijuana smokers, one subject reported increased seizure frequency and one decreased frequency [50]. A study of 16 refractory epileptics found that seven of eight subjects receiving cannabidiol became seizure-free compared to only one of eight receiving placebo [51].

Hallucinogens

The hallucinogenic drugs most popular in North America and Europe—peyote cactus containing mescaline, mushrooms containing psilocin and psilocybin, and the synthetic ergot alkaloid D-lysergic acid diethylamide (LSD)—produce similar perceptual, psychological, and somatic symptoms. Visual distortions and hallucinations are not considered epileptic in nature, and neither is their spontaneous recurrence days or weeks later (flashbacks) [52]. True seizures can follow very high doses, however, often accompanied by hypertension, fever, delirium, respiratory depression, or coma [53].

Inhalants

Volatile substance abuse involves a large number of commercial products and organic compounds, yet recreational inhalation of such substances produces similar effects that resemble ethanol intoxication. Inhalant abuse is addictive, yet a well-defined abstinence syndrome is not described in chronic users. Seizures and hallucinations can occur during severe intoxication, however [54, 55].

Phencyclidine and Ketamine

Phencyclidine (PCP, "angel dust") and the related compound ketamine block glutamatergic neurotransmission and therefore should have anticonvulsant properties. In overdose, however, they can cause myoclonus and seizures, including status epilepticus [56, 57]. Additional signs of intoxication—fever, tachycardia, hypertension, nystagmus, psychosis, delirium, dystonia, and stupor or coma with a blank stare—usually precede or accompany the seizures. The degree to which glutamatergic blockade contributes to the proconvulsant effects of PCP and ketamine, as opposed to actions at more specific "PCP receptors" and sigma receptors, is unclear. Tolerance and craving develop in PCP and ketamine users, but except in neonates an abstinence syndrome is not defined.

Anticholinergics

Plants containing atropine and scopolamine are used recreationally worldwide; in Europe and North America *Datura stramonium* is especially popular. Symptoms of intoxication—mydriasis, fever, dry mouth and skin, tachycardia, and restlessness—may progress to hallucinatory psychosis, delirium, and coma, with extensor posturing, myoclonus, or seizures [58]. The use of physostigmine in treating anticholinergic poisoning is reserved for those with severe symptoms, for physostigmine itself can cause seizures and cardiac arrhythmia [59].

Ethanol

The term "alcohol-related seizures" refers to seizures occurring in heavy drinkers in the absence of any other explanation such as cerebral trauma, stroke, CNS infection, metabolic derangement, pre-existing neurological disease, or a history of epilepsy. Alcohol-related seizures are considered a direct effect of ethanol, and they most often occur during withdrawal [60, 61].

In a study of over 200 alcoholics with seizures, either incident (new onset) or prevalent, 78% occurred 7–30 h after the last drink, and except for 2 whose seizures occurred after 2 or more weeks, 99% occurred within 72 h [62]. Some occurred while drinking. Seizures were single in 41% and more than 3 in 21%, usually occurring within a few hours. Status epilepticus was present in 3%. Seizures were generalized tonic–clonic in 95% and had a focal onset in 5%. They could occur alone or with other withdrawal signs such as tremor or hallucinosis. In a third of patients symptoms progressed to delirium tremens. (During delirium tremens, however, seizures are uncommon.) In this study the amount and duration of ethanol consumption were not determined. The authors concluded that seizures in alcoholics are a withdrawal phenomenon and that subjects with seizures occurring beyond the withdrawal period or with focal features probably have underlying structural pathology.

In a study of volunteers, six subjects drank ethanol around the clock (including a 3:00 AM dose) for at least 48 days [63]. Withdrawal symptoms included seizures in two and delirium tremens in two. One subject with seizures had had prior ethanol abuse. The pattern of drinking in these subjects was atypical; alcoholics do not awaken themselves in the middle of the night to have a drink. Moreover, the high percentage of subjects who experienced seizures was not encountered in other studies. In a report of over a thousand alcoholics detoxified without psychoactive drugs, only 1% had seizures [64]. In another study, abrupt withdrawal from ethanol produced abstinence symptoms including hallucinosis, but no subject had a seizure [65].

A case–control study of new-onset seizures found that the amount of absolute ethanol sufficient to raise the odds ratio for seizure risk above one was 50 g daily [66]. (12 ounces of beer, 5 ounces of wine, and 1.5 ounces of liquor each contain roughly 15–20 g absolute ethanol.) At 200 g daily the OR was 20, but the minimal duration of drinking that conferred increased risk of seizures could not be determined. In that study, many seizures occurred either during active drinking or more than a week after stopping, and statistical analysis failed to demonstrate a clear-cut temporal relationship between seizures and early abstinence. Moreover, those who had recently increased their ethanol consumption tended to have seizures sooner after the last drink than those who decreased their consumption.

Another case–control study of new-onset seizures similarly found an increased risk of seizures above 50 g daily absolute ethanol for men and 25 g daily for women [67]. That study did not address temporal relationships between seizures and active drinking.

Animal studies confirm that ethanol withdrawal can cause seizures [68, 69]. Such seizures tend to be dissimilar to what is observed in humans, however, for example occurring after very little ethanol consumption, having high fatality rates, or requiring that the animal be dropped onto a hard surface or subjected to a loud noise. As with humans, their variable time courses and semiology suggest more than a single mechanism. In both animals and humans, repeated bouts of ethanol withdrawal increase the likelihood of eventual ethanol-related seizures [70–72].

Both withdrawal seizures and non-withdrawal seizures in alcoholics might involve the excitatory neurotransmitter glutamate. Ethanol acutely inhibits glutamatergic neurotransmission and facilitates inhibitory GABAergic neurotransmission with consequent up-regulation of postsynaptic glutamate receptors and down-regulation of GABA receptors [73–75]. Abrupt cessation of ethanol intake would then produce a hyperactive glutamatergic state and a hypoactive GABAergic state, resulting in withdrawal symptoms, including seizures. Repeated bouts of withdrawal might, in turn, cause excitotoxic neuronal damage via N-methyl-D-asparte (NMDA) receptors and excessive calcium entry. Such damage could set the stage for the development of seizures independent of acute abstinence. (Glutamatergic neurotoxicity has been similarly offered as an explanation for alcoholic dementia.)

The diagnosis of alcohol-related seizures requires exclusion of additional brain pathology, and patients with new-onset seizures should undergo neuroimaging [76, 77]. Of 259 patients with seizures temporally related to ethanol consumption and with normal neurological examinations, 16 (6.2%) had intracranial lesions identified by CT scan: four subdural hematoma, four subdural hygroma, two vascular malformation, three cysticercosis, and one each aneurysm, neoplasm, skull fracture with subarachnoid hemorrhage, and cerebral infarction. In 10 patients management was affected by the CT findings [78]. More problematic are patients with prior alcohol-related seizures. Although imaging may not be necessary in every instance, the clinician must always consider the possibility of an underlying new treatable lesion in such patients.

Because alcohol-related seizures tend to occur singly or in a brief cluster, for many patients the need to treat has often passed by the time a patient is medically evaluated. On the other hand, in a controlled trial either intravenous lorazepam 2 mg or placebo was given to alcoholic patients after a single generalized seizure, and over the next 6 h 3% of those receiving lorazepam had a second seizure compared to 24% of those receiving placebo (OR = 10.4). Of those not admitted to the hospital, one patient receiving lorazepam and seven receiving placebo had a second seizure over the next 48 h [79]. As for primary prevention, a Cochrane review of 57 trials concluded that benzodiazepines are more effective than

placebo against ethanol withdrawal symptoms, especially seizures [80]. The use of a benzodiazepine in this setting follows the principle that prevention of withdrawal symptoms from any drug is best achieved using an agent from the same pharmacological class or with a degree of cross-tolerance [81]. Ethanol itself, being a direct neurotoxin, is an inappropriate agent for preventing ethanol withdrawal, even though it would be the alcoholic's drug of choice.

Although only a small percentage of alcohol-related seizures progress to status epilepticus, a large percentage of patients seen in emergency departments with status epilepticus have ethanol as the sole cause. In a series of 82 consecutive admissions for status epilepticus, 29 episodes (35.4%) occurred in alcoholics, and 16 had no other obvious precipitating factor [82]. Status epilepticus in such patients is treated by conventional means, with lorazepam the initial drug of choice.

Electroencephalography in patients with alcohol-related seizures is usually normal. A report that photomyoclonic or photoconvulsive responses were frequent during early withdrawal was not borne out by later studies [83].

Anticonvulsant prophylaxis is usually not indicated in patients with alcohol-related seizures and no additional pathology [76]. Subjects actively drinking are not likely to take their medications, and those not actively drinking do not usually need their medications. Animal and human studies, moreover, suggest that neither phenytoin, carbamazepine, nor valproate is effective in preventing alcohol-related seizures [76, 84–87]. When seizures in a heavy drinker are not temporally linked to active drinking or recent abstinence, when they occur in the presence of cerebral pathology such as brain contusion or epileptiform activity on EEG, or when seizures in an epileptic are mostly or entirely triggered by drinking, management considerations must be individualized. In such patients treatment may be indicated even though compliance is unlikely.

Relevant to the question of anticonvulsant prophylaxis are observations that some anticonvulsants, including carbamazepine, valproic acid, gabapentin, and especially topiramate, reduce craving and ethanol consumption [88–91].

Whether epileptics can safely drink ethanol is disputed. In one study, one or two drinks per day appeared to precipitate seizures in 5% of epileptic patients, and five or six drinks per day precipitated seizures in 85% [92]. In another study, epileptic patients drank 1–3 glasses of vodka over a 2 h period daily for 16 weeks, and there was no change in their seizure frequency or their EEG patterns [93]. Generalized epilepsies, especially juvenile myoclonic epilepsy in sleep-deprived individuals, appear to be especially sensitive to ethanol [94]. Guidelines from a European task force advise that most patients with partial epilepsy and controlled seizures and without a history of alcohol overuse can safely consume 1–3 standard drinks 1–3 times per week [76].

References

1. Brust JCM. Neurological aspects of substance abuse. 2nd ed. Butterworth-Heinemann: Boston; 2004.
2. Kaufman MJ, Levin JM, Ross MH, et al. Cocaine-induced cerebral vasoconstriction detected in humans with magnetic resonance angiography. JAMA. 1998;279:376–80.
3. Reynolds K, Lewis LB, Nolen JDL, et al. Alcohol consumption and risk of stroke. A meta-analysis. JAMA. 2003;289:579–88.
4. Malouf R, Brust JCM. Hypoglycemia: causes, neurological manifestations, and outcome. Ann Neurol. 1985;17:421–30.
5. Bohme GA, Stutzmann JM, Rouges BP, et al. Effects of selective mu- and delta-opioid peptides on kindled amygdaloid seizures in rats. Neurosci Lett. 1987;74:227–31.
6. Tortella FC. Endogenous opioid peptides and epilepsy: quieting the seizing brain? Trends Pharmacol Sci. 1988;9:366–72.
7. O'Neal CL, Poklis A, Lichtman AH. Acetylcodeine, an impurity of illicitly manufactured heroin, elicits convulsions, antinociception, and locomotor stimulation in mice. Drug Alcohol Depend. 2001;65:37–43.
8. Ng SKC, Brust JCM, Hauser WA, Susser M. Illicit drug use and the risk of new onset seizures. Am J Epidemiol. 1990;132:47–57.
9. Fulroth R, Phillips B, Durand DJ. Perinatal outcome of infants exposed to cocaine and/or heroin in utero. Am J Dis Child. 1989;143:905–10.
10. Kaiko RF, Foley K, Grabinski PY, et al. Central nervous system excitatory effects of meperidine in cancer patients. Ann Neurol. 1983;13:180–5.
11. Meyer D, Halfin V. Toxicity secondary to meperidine in patients on monoamine oxidase inhibitors: a case report and critical review. J Clin Psychopharmacol. 1981;1:319–21.
12. Caplan LR, Thomas C, Banks G. Central nervous system complications of addiction to "T's and Blues". Neurology. 1982;32:623–8.
13. Finkle BS. Self-poisoning with dextropropoxyphene and dextropropoxyphene compounds: the USA experience. Hum Toxicol. 1984;3(Suppl):115S.
14. Han PK, Arnold R, Bond G, et al. Myoclonus secondary to withdrawal from transdermal fentanyl: case report and literature review. J Pain Sympt Manage. 2002;23:66–72.
15. Alldredge BK, Lowenstein DH, Simon RP. Seizures associated with recreational drug abuse. Neurology. 1989;39:1037–9.
16. Harden CL, Montjo GE, Tuchman AJ, et al. Seizures provoked by cocaine use. Ann Neurol. 1990;28:263–4.
17. Lowenstein DH, Masse SM, Rowbotham MC, et al. Acute neurologic and psychiatric complications associated with cocaine. Am J Med. 1987;83:841–6.
18. Myers JA, Earnest MP. Generalized seizures and cocaine abuse. Neurology. 1984;35:675–6.
19. Pascual-Leone A, Dhuna A, Altafallah I, et al. Cocaine-induced seizures. Neurology. 1990;40:404–7.
20. Bowyer JF, Ali S. High doses of methamphetamine that cause disruption of the blood-brain barrier in limbic regions produce extensive neuronal degeneration in mouse hippocampus. Synapse. 2006;60:521–32.
21. Miller KA, Witkin JM, Ungard JT, et al. Pharmacological and behavioral characterization of cocaine-kindled seizures in mice. Psychopharmacology. 2000;148:74–82.
22. Dhuna A, Pascual-Leone A, Langendorf F. Chronic habitual cocaine abuse and kindling-induced epilepsy. A case report. Epilepsia. 1991;32:890–4.
23. Choy-Kwong M, Lipton RB. Seizures in hospitalized cocaine users. Neurology. 1989;39:425–7.
24. Schwartz RH, Luxenberg MG, Hoffman NG. Crack use by American middle-class adolescent polydrug abusers. J Pediatr. 1991;118:150–5.
25. Ogunyemi AO, Locke GE, Kramer LD, et al. Partial complex status epilepticus provoked by "crack" cocaine. Ann Neurol. 1989;26:785–6.
26. Mueller SM, Solow EB. Seizures associated with a new combination "pick-me-up" pill. Ann Neurol. 1982;11:322.
27. Haller CA, Benowitz N. Adverse cardiovascular and central nervous system events associated with dietary supplements containing ephedra alkaloids. N Engl J Med. 2000;343:1833–8.
28. Kalant H. The pharmacology and toxicology of "ecstasy" (MDMA) and related drugs. Can Med Assoc J. 2001;165:917–28.
29. Zagnoni PG, Albano C. Psychostimulants and epilepsy. Epilepsia. 2002;43 Suppl 2:28–31.
30. Giorgi FS, Pizzanelli C, Ferrucci M, et al. Previous exposure to (+/-)3,4-methylenedioxymethamphetamine produces long-lasting alterations in limbic brain excitability measured by electroencephalogram spectrum analysis, brain metabolism, and seizure susceptibility. Neuroscience. 2005;136:43–53.
31. Fraser HF, Wikler A, Essig EF, et al. Degree of physical dependence induced by secobarbital or pentobarbital. JAMA. 1958;166:126–9.
32. Fialip J, Aumaitre O, Eschalier A, et al. Benzodiazepine withdrawal seizures. Analysis of 48 case reports. Clin Neuropharmacol. 1987;10:538–44.
33. Busto U, Sellers EM, Naranjo CA, et al. Withdrawal reaction after long-term therapeutic use of benzodiazepines. N Engl J Med. 1986;315:854–9.
34. Myers RR, Stockard JJ. Neurologic and electroencephalographic correlates in glutethimide intoxication. Clin Pharmacol Ther. 1975;17:212–20.
35. Hoaken PCS. Adverse effects of methaqualone. Can Med Assoc J. 1975;112:685–6.
36. Madrak LN, Rosenberg M. Zolpidem abuse. Am J Psychiatry. 2001;158:1330–1.
37. McGinn CG. Close calls with club drugs. N Engl J Med. 2005;352:2671–2.
38. Snead OC, Gibson KM. Gamma-hydroxybutyric acid. N Engl J Med. 2005;352:2721–32.
39. McDonough M, Kennedy N, Glasper A, et al. Clinical features and management of gamma-hydroxybutyrate (GHB) withdrawal: a review. Drug Alcohol Depend. 2004;75:3–9.
40. Wojtowicz JM, Yarema MC, Wax PM. Withdrawal from gamma-hydroxybutyrate, 1,4-butanediol and gamma-butyrolactone: a case report and systematic review. Can J Emerg Med Care. 2008;10:69–74.
41. Thai D, Dyer JE, Benowitz NL, et al. Gamma-hydroxybutyrate and ethanol effects and interactions in humans. J Clin Psychopharmacol. 2006;26:524–9.
42. Mason PE, Kerns WP. Gamma-hydroxybutyric acid (GHB) intoxication. Acad Emerg Med. 2002;9:730–9.
43. Pertwee RG. The central neuropharmacology of psychotropic cannabinoids. Pharmacol Ther. 1988;36:189–261.
44. Wallace MJ, Blair RE, Falenski KW, et al. The endogenous cannabinoid system regulates seizure frequency and duration in a model of temporal lobe epilepsy. J Pharmacol Exp Ther. 2003;307:129–37.
45. Consroe P, Benedito MA, Leite R, et al. Effects of cannabidiol on behavioral seizures caused by convulsant drugs or current in mice. Eur J Pharmacol. 1982;83:293–8.
46. Perez-Reyes M, Winfield M. Cannabidiol and electroencephalographic epileptic activity. JAMA. 1974;230:1635.
47. Consroe PF, Wood GC, Buchsbaum A. Anticonvulsant nature of marijuana smoking. JAMA. 1975;234:306–7.
48. Ellison JM, Gelwan E, Ogletree J. Complex partial seizure symptoms affected by marijuana abuse. J Clin Psychiatry. 1990;51:439–40.
49. Gordon E, Devinsky O. Alcohol and marijuana: effects on epilepsy and use by patients with epilepsy. Epilepsia. 2001;42:1266–72.

50. Feeney DM. Marijuana use among epileptics. JAMA. 1976;235:1105.

51. Cunha JM, Carlini EA, Periera AE, et al. Chronic administration of cannabidiol to healthy volunteers and epileptic patients. Pharmacology. 1980;21:175–85.

52. Abraham HD, Duffy H. EEG coherence in post-LSD visual hallucinations. Psychiatry Res. 2001;107:151–2.

53. Fisher D, Underleider J. Grand mal seizures following ingestion of LSD. Calif Med. 1976;106:210–2.

54. Meredith TH, Ruprak M, Little A, Flanagan RJ. Diagnosis and treatment of acute poisoning with volatile substances. Hum Toxicol. 1989;8:277–86.

55. Skuse D, Burrell S. A review of solvent abusers and their management by a child psychiatric outpatient service. Hum Toxicol. 1982;1:321–9.

56. Kessler GF, Demers LM, Brennan RW. Phencyclidine and fatal status epilepticus. N Engl J Med. 1974;291:979.

57. McCarron MM, Schulze BW, Thompson GA, et al. Acute phencyclidine intoxication: clinical patterns, complications, and treatment. Ann Emerg Med. 1981;10:290–7.

58. Mickolich JR, Paulson GW, Cross CJ, Calhoun R. Neurologic and electro- encephalographic effects of jimson weed intoxication. Clin Electroencephalogr. 1976;7:49–57.

59. Oberndorfer S, Grisold W, Hinterholzer G, et al. Coma with focal neurological signs caused by Datura stramonium intoxication in a young man. J Neurol Neurosurg Psychiatry. 2002;73:458–9.

60. Brathen G, Brodtkorp E, Helde G, et al. The diversity of seizures related to alcohol use. A study of consecutive patients. Eur J Neurol. 1999;6:697–703.

61. Hillbom M, Pieninkeroinen I, Leone M. Seizures in alcohol-dependent patients. Epidemiology, pathophysiology and management. CNS Drugs. 2003;17:1013–30.

62. Victor M, Brausch CC. The role of abstinence in the genesis of alcoholic epilepsy. Epilepsia. 1967;8:1–20.

63. Isbell H, Fraser HF, Wikler A, et al. An experimental study of rum fits and delirium tremens. Q J Stud Alcohol. 1955;16:1–33.

64. Whitfield CL, Thompson G, Lamb A, et al. Detoxification of 1024 alcoholic patients without psychoactive drugs. JAMA. 1978;239:1409–10.

65. Mendelson JH, LaDou R. Experimentally induced chronic intoxication and withdrawal in alcoholics. Q J Stud Alcohol. 1964;2(Suppl):1–127.

66. Ng SKC, Hauser WA, Brust JCM, Susser M. Alcohol consumption and withdrawal in new-onset seizures. N Engl J Med. 1988;319:666–73.

67. Leone M, Bottacchi E, Beghi E, et al. Alcohol use is a risk factor for a first generalized tonic-clonic seizure. Neurology. 1997;48:614–20.

68. Goldstein DB. The alcohol withdrawal syndrome. A view from the laboratory. Rec Dev Alcohol 1986;4:231–40.

69. Crabbe JC, Phillips TJ. Selective breeding for alcohol withdrawal severity. Behav Genet. 1993;23:171–7.

70. Lechtenberg R, Warner TM. Seizure risk with recurrent alcohol detoxification. Arch Neurol. 1990;47:535–8.

71. Duka T, Gentry J, Malcolm R, et al. Consequences of multiple withdrawals from alcohol. Alcohol Clin Exp Res. 2004;28:233–46.

72. Mayo-Smith MF, Bernard D. Late onset seizures in alcohol withdrawal. Alcohol Clin Exp Res. 1995;19:656–9.

73. Dodd PR, Beckmann AM, Davidson MS, et al. Glutamate-mediated transmission, alcohol, and alcoholism. Neurochem Int. 2000;37:509–33.

74. Tsai G, Coyle JT. The role of glutamatergic neurotransmission in the pathophysiology of alcoholism. Annu Rev Med. 1998;49:173–84.

75. Roberto M, Schweitzer P, Madamba SG, et al. Acute and chronic ethanol alter glutamatergic transmission in rat central amygdala: an in vitro and in vivo analysis. J Neurosci. 2004;24:233–46.

76. Brathen G, Ben-Menachem E, Brodtkorp E, et al. The EFNS Task Force on Diagnosis and Treatment of Alcohol-Related Seizures. EFNS guidelines on the diagnosis and management of alcohol-related seizures; report of an EFNS task force. Eur J Neurol. 2006;12:575–81.

77. Schoenenberger RA, Heim SM. Indication for computed tomography of the brain in patients with first uncomplicated generalized seizure. BMJ. 1994;309:986–9.

78. Earnest MP, Feldman H, Marx JA, et al. Intracranial lesions shown by CT scans in 259 cases of first alcohol-related seizures. Neurology. 1988;38:1561–5.

79. D'Onofrio G, Rathlev NK, Ulrich AS, et al. Lorazepam for the prevention of recurrent alcohol withdrawal seizures. Ann Emerg Med. 1994;23:513–8.

80. Ntais C, Pakos E, Kyzas P, et al. Benzodiazepines for alcohol withdrawal. Cochrane Database Syst Rev. 2005;(3):CD005063.

81. Mayo-Smith MF. for the American Society of Addiction Medicine Working Group on Pharmacological Management of Alcohol Withdrawal. Pharmacological management of alcohol withdrawal. A meta-analysis and evidence-based practice guideline. JAMA. 1997;278:144–51.

82. Pilke A, Partinen M, Kovanen J. Status epilepticus and alcohol abuse: an analysis of 82 status epilepticus admissions. Acta Neurol Scand. 1984;70:443–50.

83. Fisch BJ, Hauser WA, Brust JCM, et al. The EEG response to diffuse and patterned photic stimulation during acute untreated alcohol withdrawal. Neurology. 1989;39:434–6.

84. Alldredge BK, Lowenstein DH, Simon RP. Placebo-controlled trial of intravenous diphenylhydantoin for short-term treatment of alcohol withdrawal seizures. Am J Med. 1989;87:645–8.

85. Hilbom M, Tokola R, Kuusela V, et al. Prevention of alcohol withdrawal seizures with carbamazepine and valproic acid. Alcohol. 1989;6:223–6.

86. Rathlev NK, D'Onofrio G, Fish SS, et al. The lack of efficacy of phenytoin in the prevention of recurrent alcohol-related seizures. Ann Emerg Med. 1994;23:513–8.

87. Pruett P. Prevention of alcohol withdrawal seizures with carbamazepine and valproic acid. Ann Emerg Med. 1989;18:11.

88. Mueller TI, Stout RL, Rudden S, et al. A double-blind placebo-controlled pilot study of carbamazepine for the treatment of alcohol dependence. Alcohol Clin Exp Res. 1997;21:86–92.

89. Brady KT, Myrick H, Henderson S, et al. Use of divalproex in alcohol relapse prevention: a pilot study. Drug Alcohol Depend. 2002;67:323–30.

90. Voris J, Smith NL, Rao SM, et al. Gabapentin for the treatment of ethanol withdrawal. Subst Abuse. 2003;24:129–32.

91. Johnson BA, Ait-Daoud N, Bowden CL, et al. Oral topiramate for treatment of alcohol dependence: a randomized controlled trial. Lancet. 2003;361:1677–85.

92. Mattson RH, Sturman JK, Gronowski ML, Gaico H. Effect of alcohol intake in nonalcoholic epileptics. Neurology. 1975;25:361–2.

93. Hoppener RJ, Kuyer A, van der Lugt PJM. Epilepsy and alcohol: the influence of social alcohol intake on seizures and treatment in epilepsy. Epilepsia. 1983;24:459–71.

94. Pedersen SB, Peterson KA. Juvenile myoclonic epilepsy: clinical and EEG features. Acta Neurol Scand. 1998;97:160–3.

Medication Overuse Headache: Causes, Consequences, and Treatment

28

Letizia M. Cupini, Paola Sarchielli, and Paolo Calabresi

Abstract

All primary headache subtypes (migraine, tension-type headache, cluster headache) may become complicated by medication overuse headache (MOH). MOH has developed into the third most common type of headache after tension-type headache and migraine. The prevalence reaches approximately 1% of the world's population and shows an increasing trend. MOH is a condition in which headaches become increasingly frequent as a patient begins to use more and more acute headache medications. The initial headache frequency is one of the factors that may play a role in the development of MOH. However, the reasons why some patients overuse acute treatments of headaches whereas others do not are not clearly understood. MOH might be prompted and sustained by some psychological states and behavioral disorders, including fear of headache, anticipatory anxiety of attacks, and psychological drug dependence. A range of behaviors presumed to be related to excessive medications are being increasingly recognized in MOH disease. These behaviors are linked by their reward-based and repetitive natures. Whether these behaviors are simply related to medications interacting with an underlying individual vulnerability or whether the primary pathological features of MOH play a role is not known. Neurobiological mechanisms underlying drug dependence and reward system (i.e. endocannabinoids, dopamine, orexins) might also be involved in MOH. The study of these neurobiological mechanisms and behaviors might allow not only a greater insight into the pathophysiology of MOH but also an improved clinical management of this disorder. Although many questions remain unanswered, it is encouraging that several clinical and experimental advances have shed new light on the neuropharmacology of nociception and have prompted new hope for more effective treatments of such diverse problems as chronic headache pain, migraine, and drug dependency.

Learning Objectives
- Primary headache subtypes may become complicated by MOH.
- The initial headache frequency is related to the development of MOH.
- MOH prevalence reaches approximately 1% of the world's population.

(continued)

L.M. Cupini (✉)
Centro Cefalee, Clinica Neurologica, Dipartimento Cranio Spinale,
U.O.C. Neurologia, Ospedale S. Eugenio, P.le dell'Umanesimo 10,
00144 Roma, Italy
e-mail: lecupini@tin.it

P. Sarchielli • P. Calabresi
Clinica Neurologica, Università degli Studi di Perugia, Perugia, Italy

J.C. Verster et al. (eds.), *Drug Abuse and Addiction in Medical Illness: Causes, Consequences and Treatment*,
DOI 10.1007/978-1-4614-3375-0_28, © Springer Science+Business Media, LLC 2012

(continued)

- Drugs inducing MOH: analgesics, ergotamine, triptans, combination analgesics with codeine or caffeine.
- Psychological and behavioral disorders have been reported in MOH.
- Neuroimaging studies have shown orbitofrontal hypofunction in MOH.
- Possible neurobiological mechanisms underlying drug dependence and reward system (i.e. endocannabinoids, dopamine, orexins) might also be involved in MOH.
- A detoxification program is needed in MOH.
- Relapse after MOH treatment may occur.
- Different pharmacological preventive strategies can be considered.
- Cognitive and behavioral therapeutic approaches might be helpful.

Issues that Need to Be Addressed by Future Research
- The reasons leading to different classes and amounts of medication overuse in headache patients must be further investigated.
- Neurobiological substrates underlying induction and maintenance of MOH, and in particular neurotransmitter systems, have to be explored.
- Genetic mechanisms leading to selective vulnerability to MOH should be further analyzed.
- Gender differences in MOH have been observed. The possible influence of estrogen in MOH needs to be explored.
- Future studies should assess whether patients with MOH need withdrawal of acute medication in order to respond to prophylactic medication.
- Future clinical studies dealing with the efficacy and tolerability of AEDs in MOH and possibly identification of further therapeutic and behavioral strategies are needed.

Introduction

In the 1988 International Headache Society (IHS) classification, drug-induced headache was defined as (1) headache appearing at least 15 days per month, (2) regular intake of analgesics or ergot alkaloids, and (3) headache disappearing after withdrawal of substance [1]. The term "drug-induced headache" has been replaced by the term "medication

Table 28.1 Revised criteria for medication overuse headache

Appendix 8.2 Medication overuse headache
Diagnostic criteria:
A. Headache present on ≥15 days per month
B. Regular overuse for >3 months of one or more acute/symptomatic treatment drugs as defined under subforms of 8.2
1. Ergotamine, triptans, opioids, or combination analgesic medications on ≥10 days per month on a regular basis for >3 months
2. Simple analgesics or any combination of ergotamine, triptans, analgesics, opioids on ≥15 days per month on a regular basis for >3 months, without overuse of any single class alone
C. Headache has developed or markedly worsened during medication overuse

overuse headache" (MOH) in the 2004 International Classification of Headache Disorders (ICHD-II) [2].

MOH is a condition in which headaches become increasingly frequent as a patient begins to use more and more acute headache medications. The revised criteria were more specific with regard to headache features and type of medication overuse and required that the headache worsened or increased in frequency during symptomatic medication overuse and resolved or reverted to its previous episodic pattern within 2 months after withdrawal of the overused medication [2]. However, the mandatory requirement of headache improvement following drug withdrawal has proven problematic in clinical practice. Using these criteria, the diagnosis of MOH could never be made during the initial evaluation as a withdrawal period was necessary to make the diagnosis. Furthermore, if patients improved after drug withdrawal, the diagnosis could be made only in retrospect, since the patient improved and the condition no longer existed. In addition, these criteria were difficult to apply in large epidemiologic studies [3]. Thus, a revised version of these diagnostic criteria has been published in the 2005 on behalf of the International Headache Society [4, 5]. According to the revised ICHD-IIR guidelines MOH should be diagnosed in patients who fulfill the criteria for a headache on ≥15 days per month, who overuse medications on a regular basis for >3 months, and for whom headache has developed or markedly worsened during medication overuse (Table 28.1) [6].

All primary headache subtypes (migraine, tension-type headache, cluster headache) may become complicated by MOH [6, 7]. MOH has developed into the third most common type of headache after tension-type headache and migraine. The initial headache frequency is one of the factors that may play a role in the development of MOH. However, other factors than initial headache frequency may play a role in the development of this complex neurobiological and behavioral disorder.

ICHD-II states primary episodic headaches as chronic when attacks appear for more than 15 days per month, for at least 3 months [2]. Not all patients with chronic daily headaches develop medication overuse. The reasons why some patients overuse acute treatments of headaches whereas others do not are not clearly understood.

Moreover, the reasons why patients with headaches using analgesics are more prone to developing chronic headache than patients with other pains remain unknown [8, 9]. It has been suggested that MOH might be prompted and sustained by some psychological states and behavioral disorders, including fear of headache, anticipatory anxiety of attacks, fear of disability with desire to relieve pain to continue function and psychological drug dependence. Psychiatric comorbidities (major depression, anxiety) and substance abuse disorders might also play a role in MOH [10, 11]. MOH is a complex neurobiological and behavioral disorder not completely understood [12]. MOH seemingly shares with other kinds of drug dependence some common neurobiological pathways, including those that modulate motivation, reward, novelty seeking, behavioral control, response to stress, and relapse [12–14]. The significantly increased familial risk for chronic headache, drug overuse, and substance abuse suggests that a genetic factor might be involved in the process of headache chronification [15]. The goal of treatment is to detoxify patients, to reduce headache frequency by preventive measures, and to prevent the relapse of MOH.

The implications of current pathophysiological hypothesis as well as available clinical data on MOH will be discussed.

Epidemiology

Epidemiological studies show that the prevalence of MOH reaches approximately 1% of the world's population and shows an increasing trend [3, 16–19]. Interestingly, MOH is not only prevalent in Europe and North America but it is a growing problem also in some Asian countries where the prevalence is the same as in Europe.

In a large cross-sectional population-based study conducted in Norway (The Head-HUNT study), the prevalence of chronic headache associated with analgesic overuse in relation to age and gender as well as the relation between analgesic overuse duration and chronic headache (both migraine and nonmigrainous headache) was examined [3]. This relationship was also examined for other common chronic pain conditions like neck and low-back pain.

The authors observed that the prevalence of chronic headache associated with analgesic use daily or almost daily for ≥1 month was 1% (1.3% for women and 0.7% for men) and for analgesic overuse duration of ≥3 months 0.9% (1.2% for women and 0.6% for men). Chronic headache was more than seven times more likely among those with analgesic overuse (≥1 month) than those without (odds ratio [OR]=7.5, 95%

CI: 6.6–8.5). Upon analysis of the different chronic pain subgroups separately, the association with analgesic overuse was strongest for chronic migraine (OR = 10.3, 95% CI: 8.1–13.0), intermediate for chronic nonmigrainous headache (OR=6.2, 95% CI: 5.3–7.2), and weakest for chronic neck (OR=2.6, 95% CI: 2.3–2.9) and chronic low-back (OR=3.0, 95% CI: 2.7–3.3) pain.

The association became stronger with increasing duration of analgesic use for all groups and was most evident among those with headache, especially those with migraine [3]. Thus, the overall prevalence of chronic headache associated with analgesic overuse was 1%, in accordance with previous population-based studies. The prevalence increased until middle age and declined after that, with a peak at 40–49 years of age in women and at 50–59 years of age in men. Interestingly, analgesic overuse and MOH can also become a problem in early adolescence and even in childhood [20, 21]. It has been shown that many adolescents consult neither their parents nor their physician when taking over-the-counter medication [22]. In a population of 5,471 adolescents, 13–18 years of age, who were interviewed about their headache complaints and completed a comprehensive questionnaire including use of analgesics, the prevalence of daily headache associated with analgesic use was estimated 0.5%, with a higher rate for girls (0.8%) than for boys (0.2%). There was a significant association for both genders between analgesic use and headache, although most pronounced for migraine and a significant linear relationship between analgesic use and headache frequency [20].

Classes of Overused Drugs and Dependence

The ICHD-2 suggests that MOH occurs as an interaction between a therapeutic agent used excessively and a susceptible patient. There is evidence that all drugs used for the treatment of headache can cause MOH in patients with primary headache disorders. In some patients, it is difficult to identify a single causal substance since many patients take more than one compound at a time and each component of antimigraine drugs might induce headache. The use of drugs that lead to MOH varies from country to country since their availabilities in the market differ and cultural-related factors influence people's attitudes.

In the past combination analgesics with codeine or caffeine, or ergots combined with codeine were the most common headache therapies in many countries. The introduction of triptans changed this picture. In a large retrospective study conducted in the United States, it was observed that medications associated with overuse changed substantially in the last 15 years [23]. There was a significant decrease in the frequency of ergotamine (from 18.6% to 0%) and combination analgesic overuse headache (from 42.2% to 13.6%), whereas the frequency of simple analgesic (from 8.8% to 31.8%), combination of acute medications (from 9.8% to 22.7%) and triptan (from 0% to 21.6%) overuse headache increased significantly. Interestingly, the frequency of opioid overuse headache did not change significantly over the time [23].

It seems that all available triptans can cause MOH [24]. Overuse of triptans has been shown to cause MOH faster and with lower dosages compared with ergots and analgesics, the interval between first intake and daily headache was 1.7 years for triptans, 2.7 years for ergots, and 4.8 years for analgesics [25]. Current recommendations suggest that drugs are taken as soon as possible in migraine. Although the degree of drug efficacy (triptans in particular) may improve with early use, this method increases the likelihood that the patient will take more drug than effectively necessary and thus develop MOH [24].

Headache patients have been reported to develop physical dependence on codeine and other opioids [26, 27]. Up to 10% of codeine is metabolized to morphine. Opioids are definitely behaviorally active substances, but ergotamine, triptans, as well as simple and combined analgesics are not included in DSM-IV criteria. Nevertheless, patients with MOH show symptoms of tolerance and withdrawal [28, 29]. Accordingly, ergotamine and dihydroergotamine may lead to physical dependency characterized by a self-sustaining, rhythmic headache/medication cycle, with daily or almost daily migraine headaches [28].

The reason for the physical dependency on ergotamine is unknown. One study found that the tyramine-induced mydriasis after ergotamine dose was increased during abuse but not after withdrawal of ergotamine, which would indicate a central inhibition of pupillary sympathetic activity during abuse [30]. Thus, a possible CNS effect of ergotamine might be observed after chronic use but not after a single dose of the drug.

Interesting is the role of caffeine in the development of CDH because of wide exposure to dietary and medicinal caffeine. Caffeine is a common ingredient in both over-the-counter and prescription headache medications since it may increase the analgesic action of aspirin and paracetamol [24]. As well known, caffeine increases vigilance, relieves fatigue, and improves performance and mood [31, 32]. Caffeine has been shown to cause withdrawal headache under placebo-controlled double-blind conditions [33].

The typical symptoms of caffeine withdrawal, such as irritability, nervousness, restlessness, and especially "caffeine withdrawal headache" [33] which may last for several days, encourage patients to continue their overuse. However, in a population-based study conducted in a sample of episodic and chronic headache sufferers, it has been shown that dietary and medicinal caffeine consumption appears to be a modest risk factor for CDH onset, regardless of headache type [34]. The results of this study are limited by the way in which pre-chronic daily headache caffeine consumption was measured

(patients' past caffeine consumption recall). Nevertheless, the study suggests that caffeine consumption is a risk factor for CDH as caffeine consumption was increased in the period prior to CDH onset. Conversely, this study is not consistent with the hypothesis that caffeine consumption increases as a consequence of increasing headache frequency.

Eventually, it has also be outlined the risk of having clinically significant pharmacokinetic drug–drug interactions in patients with medication overuse [35]. Overuse of indomethacin, prochlorperazine, and caffeine combination in chronic headache patients was found associated with increased plasma levels of indomethacin and caffeine, and with delayed elimination of indomethacin [36]. The authors suggested that high and sustained concentrations of these drugs may cause rebound headache, organ damages, and perpetuate MOH [36].

Possible Genetic Mechanisms

Both environmental and genetic factors may contribute to patient's vulnerability to intoxication, substance overuse, dependence, and withdrawal in MOH. Abnormalities of dopaminergic and serotoninergic innervation, possibly genetically determined, might play a role in dysfunction of the cerebral pain network in MOH patients [13].

Interestingly, the risk of substance overuse or dependence was found increased among MOH patients' relatives suggesting transmitted vulnerability to drug overuse [10, 15, 37]. In addition, a family history for chronic headache was found to represent a risk factor for the chronification of headaches [37]. On the other hand, it is worth of nothing that data on family history of psychopathological traits such as anxiety and depression in patients with MOH are not univocal [10, 15].

However, molecular genetic studies in the field of MOH are still scarce and preliminary.

A genetic association study of chronic headache with drug abuse versus the dopamine metabolism genes found that the allele 4 of the exon III VNTR polymorphism of the dopamine receptor 4 gene DRD4 was associated with CDH [38]. Moreover, the allele 9 of the dopamine transporter (DAT) gene SLC6A3 was more common in CDH associated with drug abuse than in episodic migraine [38]. Since the function of the DAT is the presynaptic reuptake of dopamine, reduced availability of DAT may translate into enhanced dopaminergic synaptic transmission. DAT knockout mice, indeed, display an increased dopaminergic tone and behavioral activation [39]. Thus, we can assume that genetic variability at the DAT gene modifies behavior and reactivity to medication overuse also in MOH.

An increased frequency of the short allele of the serotonin transporter gene and a different genotypic distribution was found in chronic tension-type headache patients with analgesic overuse in comparison with chronic tension-type headache patients without analgesic overuse and healthy controls. These data suggested that serotonergic activity might be involved in the development of analgesic overuse in chronic tension-type headache patients [40].

Moreover, wolframin polymorphism was analyzed in MOH patients [41]. Wolframin is a transmembrane protein mainly located in the endoplasmic reticulum, and involved in membrane trafficking, protein processing and the regulation of calcium homeostasis. Wolfram syndrome (WS) is a neurodegenerative disorder associated with diabetes mellitus, diabetes insipidus, hearing loss, progressive blindness, and a heterogeneous combination of psychiatric disorders [41]. Heterozygous WS carriers are more prone to psychiatric illness than the general population [41]. In particular, a number of studies suggested that common polymorphisms of WFS1 are associated with psychiatric illnesses, in the absence of other WS manifestations [41]. To test the influence of wolframin WFS1 polymorphisms on MOH, Di Lorenzo et al. analyzed MOH patients for the WFS1 polymorphism. The authors observed that wolframin polymorphism was the only significant predictor of drug consumption in a population of MOH and suggested that wolframin appears as facilitating factor in addictive behavior development [41].

Behavioral and Psychiatric Disorders Comorbidity

Compulsive drug seeking in MOH can be understood as involving both cognitive and behavioral mechanisms. Positive reinforcing effects of analgesic use during bouts of headaches may ultimately lead the patients to take the medication nearly ritualistically for fear that an attack might occur or worsen. The reinforcing psychotropic properties of opiates may accentuate this phenomenon. On the other hand, the negative reinforcing effects of withdrawal symptoms may contribute to the maintenance of dependence.

A limited number of studies addressed dependence on acute treatments of headaches according to DSM-IV criteria in patients with frequent headaches. Studying a group of MOH patients with preexisting primary migraine and a group of patients with episodic migraine, it was observed that MOH patients were at increased risk of developing overuse or dependence on psychoactive substances other than analgesics or acute treatments of headaches [10].

In a large Asian clinical-based study, a significant dependence on migraine-abortive drugs in 68% MOH patients vs. only 20% of CDH patients without medication overuse was observed [42]. Accordingly, in a French cross-sectional, multicenter study it was observed that two-thirds of the MOH patients were dependent on acute treatments of headaches according to the DSM-IV criteria [11].

Similarly, in an Italian study, using the Leeds Dependence Questionnaire, a markedly enhanced substance need in CDH patients with overuse of analgesics compared with patients with episodic headaches was reported [43]. The substance need was comparable in intensity to that noted in drug addicts despite some differences in dependence profiles (drug addicts had higher scores at items assessing compulsive use) [43].

Certain behaviors and psychological states seem particularly important in prompting and sustaining the overuse of medication [12]. These include fear of headache, anticipatory anxiety, obsessional drug-taking behaviors, and psychological drug dependence, among others. Additionally, persons with Axis II personality disorders exhibit certain behaviors that promote medication overuse [12].

Psychological comorbidities such as depression, anxiety, and failure of pain-coping abilities may contribute to headache chronification. Furthermore, there is some evidence that psychiatric comorbidity is higher in chronic migraine than in episodic migraine (particularly in the case of chronic substance abuse) [10, 44].

Psychiatric comorbidity (mood and anxiety disorders) in MOH with preexisting episodic tension-type headache as well as in those with preexisting migraine headache was observed [45]. In addition, borderline personality disorder associated with MOH has been observed [46, 47].

Higher symptomatic drug consumption and more severe depressive symptoms on the Beck Depression Inventory questionnaire in MOH were also observed [41].

Possible Neurobiological Mechanisms

Different neurotransmitters might be involved in MOH [13]. Glutamate is implicated in cortical spreading depression, trigeminovascular activation, central sensitization, and might be linked to migraine chronification. A significant increase in glutamate and nitrite levels in the cerebrospinal fluid, of CDH patients, without a significant difference between patients without and those with analgesic overuse headache was observed [48]. Accordingly, to test the hypothesis that glutamate might be related to triptan response and influence central sensitization, cerebrospinal fluid glutamate levels of patients diagnosed with chronic migraine overusing analgesics, those without overuse, and those overusing triptans were studied [49]. Cerebrospinal fluid glutamate levels were similar in patients overusing acute medications compared to those without overuse. In contrast, patients overusing triptans had cerebrospinal fluid glutamate levels significantly lower than that observed in nonoverusers, and significantly higher than controls. In triptan overusers, cerebrospinal fluid glutamate levels, although lower, were not significantly different from patients overusing other types of analgesics. This study showed lower glutamate levels in cerebrospinal fluid of chronic migraine patients overusing triptans. The authors suggest that glutamate may be implicated in triptan response mechanisms, triptans might also work in part by reducing extracellular glutamate levels in the brain [49]. Interestingly, a case report concerning a patient diagnosed with drug-resistant chronic migraine who unexpectedly reported full remission of headache after memantine, a commonly used NMDA receptor antagonist, administered for treating concomitant mild cognitive impairment, was recently reported [50].

In order to clarify the hypothesis that serotonin may be involved in MOH, the serotonin system in platelets of migraine patients with analgesic abuse headache compared to migraine patients and nonheadache controls was studied [51]. Significant decrease in platelet serotonin content in MOH patients compared to migraine patients and controls was observed. Based on this platelet model, the authors suggested that excessive use of analgesics alters the central serotonin system by depleting serotonin from its storage sites and results in the hyposerotonergic state. The authors hypothesized that this analgesic-induced serotonin alteration represents a possible mechanism of headache transformation observed in this condition [51]. The same group investigated, in an animal model, the effect of chronic analgesic exposure on the central serotonin system and the relationship between the serotonin system and the analgesic efficacy [52]. Chronic paracetamol administration resulted in a significant decrease in the maximum number of 5-HT2A binding sites and an increase in the maximum number of serotonin transporter binding sites in frontal cortical membrane [52]. Changes in the central serotonin system were associated with a rise in platelet serotonin levels. The degree of receptor down-regulation, as well as transporter up-regulation, became less evident after more prolonged drug administration. Plastic changes of serotonin receptors and transporters coincided with the decrease in the analgesic efficacy of paracetamol, as well as a fall in platelet serotonin levels. These findings provided further evidence in support of an involvement of the serotonin system in the antinociceptive activity of paracetamol [52]. The authors hypothesized that plasticity of this neurotransmitter system after chronic analgesic exposure may lead to the loss of analgesic efficacy and, in its more extreme form, may produce analgesic-related painful conditions, for example, analgesic abuse headache [52].

Moreover, the effect of chronic administration of different pain medications on the activity of the serotonin transporter (SERT) in patients with MOH was investigated [53]. The authors studied the kinetic of platelet serotonin uptake in patients with overuse of triptans or analgesics before and after drug withdrawal, as well as in headache-free healthy subjects and patients with episodic migraine. They observed a transient increase of SERT activity in patients with analgesic and triptan-induced MOH. However, these data do not allow to differentiate whether the increase of serotonin uptake is caused by either regular intake of analgesics and triptans or is a consequence of frequent headache attacks [53].

A dopaminergic hypothesis of migraine has been postulated [54] and a hypothalamic involvement with a possible hyperdopaminergic state was found indeed in patients with chronic migraine overusing analgesic drugs [55]. Endocannabinoid system plays a role in modulating pain including headache and this system is involved in the common neurobiological mechanism underlying drug addiction and reward system mainly interacting with dopamine [56–58]. In fact, cannabinoids regulate mesocortical as well as striatal DA systems [59]. Anandamide (AEA) and 2-arachidonoylglycerol (2-AG) are the most biologically active endocannabinoids, which bind to both central and peripheral cannabinoid receptors. The level of AEA in the extracellular space is controlled by cellular uptake via a purported AEA membrane transporter (AMT), followed by intracellular degradation by the enzyme fatty acid amide hydrolase (FAAH). AMT and FAAH have been also characterized in human platelets [60, 61].

Interestingly, reduced levels of AEA in the cerebrospinal fluid of chronic migraine and chronic migraine plus probable analgesic overuse in respect of control subjects have been found [62]. Moreover, to test the hypothesis of an impairment in the endocannabinoid system in patients with MOH and chronic migraine and to assess its relationship with any disruption of the serotonergic system, the levels of the two main endogenous cannabinoids, AEA and 2-AG, and the serotonin levels in platelets of chronic migraine patients, MOH patients and control subjects were investigated. 2-AG and AEA levels were significantly lower in MOH patients and chronic migraine patients than in the control subjects. Serotonin levels were also strongly reduced in the two patient groups and were correlated with 2-AG levels, with higher values for MOH patients. These data support the potential involvement of an imbalance of the endocannabinoid and serotonergic systems in the pathology of chronic migraine and MOH. These systems appear to be mutually related and able to contribute to headache chronification and MOH [63]. Accordingly, FAAH and AMT activities (the two main systems controlling AEA levels) are significantly reduced in chronic migraine and MOH in respect of either controls or episodic migraine group [64]. Thus, it can be hypothesized that a lowered AEA level in chronic migraine and MOH induces a reduction in FAAH and AMT as an adaptative response.

The orexins (hypocretins), hypothalamic neuropeptides, play a crucial role in arousal, feeding and reward [65]. Orexin-containing neurons from the lateral hypothalamus project densely to the ventral tegmental area, which is the origin of dopamine projections implicated in motivation and reward [65]. Orexin A is able to inhibit neurogenic dural vasodilation via activation of the OX1 receptor, resulting in inhibition of prejunctional release of CGRP from trigeminal neurons [66]. Moreover, orexins could be involved in the abnormalities of feeding, sleep, and neuroendocrine functions often observed in some chronic headaches.

Interestingly, significantly higher levels of orexin-A and corticotrophin-releasing factor were found in the cerebrospinal fluid of MOH and to a lesser extent in patients with chronic migraine compared with control subjects [67]. These findings support the involvement of the hypothalamus in both chronic migraine and MOH. Ventral tegmental area (VTA) is the origin of dopamine projections implicated in motivation and reward [68]. Orexins project densely to VTA where they exert long-term excitatory modulation on dopaminergic neurons of this area [65].

Interestingly, also endocannabinoids exert a strong modulatory control on VTA neurons [58]. In fact, the dopaminergic neurons of the VTA release endocannabinoids that, acting in a retrograde manner on presynaptic CB1 receptors, inhibit both inhibitory GABAergic and excitatory glutamatergic inputs to VTA neurons. Thus, we can speculate that both orexin and endocannabinoids selectively target VTA dopaminergic neurons to exert their control on the mechanisms of reward and dependence possibly implicated in the pathophysiology of MOH.

Neuroimaging Studies

A few neuroimaging studies have been conducted in MOH. Periaqueductal gray matter is considered the center of a powerful descending antinociceptive neuronal network. Interestingly, iron homeostasis in the periaqueductal gray was found selectively, persistently, and progressively impaired in episodic migraine and CDH with medication overuse [69]. The authors suggested that this finding was possibly caused by repeated migraine attacks [69].

Moreover, using MRI and voxel-based morphometry, a population of MOH, chronic tension-type headache patients and controls without headache history, was studied. Unexpectedly, morphometric alterations in MOH were not found [70].

On the other hand, glucose metabolism with 18-FDG PET has been measured in chronic migraineurs with analgesic overuse before and a few weeks after medication withdrawal. These data were compared with those obtained from a control population [14]. The authors observed that before withdrawal, the bilateral thalamus, orbitofrontal cortex (OFC), anterior cingulate gyrus, insula/ventral striatum and right inferior parietal lobule were hypometabolic, while the cere-

bellar vermis was hypermetabolic. All dysmetabolic areas recovered to almost normal glucose uptake after withdrawal of analgesics, except the OFC where a further metabolic decrease was found. A subanalysis showed that most of the orbitofrontal hypometabolism was due to eight patients overusing combination analgesics and/or an ergotamine-caffeine preparation. These data indicate that MOH is associated with reversible metabolic changes in pain processing structures like other chronic pain disorders, but also with persistent orbitofrontal hypofunction. The authors hypothesized that the hypoactivity of the OFC may be induced by the repeated drug intake, but it could also reflect an underlying, genetically determined, liability to medication overuse. Thus, the authors suggest that orbitofrontal hypofunction, known to occur in drug dependence, could predispose subgroups of migraineurs to recurrent analgesic overuse.

Neurophysiological Studies

The so-called "wind up" phenomenon, consisting of sensitization of central nociceptive neurons following prolonged stimulation of peripheral nociceptive pathways, has been implicated in the development of chronic pain including MOH [71].

The authors observed that a nociceptive stimulus was able to induce a second pain in chronic migraine with medication overuse. After discontinuation of the overused drug, an attenuation of the intensity of the second pain was observed [71]. In line with this study, pathophysiological mechanisms of impaired trigeminal pain processing in patients with MOH and migraine have been hypothesized [72]. Thus, trigeminal and somatic nociceptive systems in controls, episodic migraine, analgesics, and triptan-induced MOH before and after withdrawal were studied [72]. Trigeminal nociception was investigated by simultaneous registration of pain-related cortical potentials; nociceptive blink reflex was analyzed following nociceptive-specific electrical stimulation of the forehead; and somatic nociception was evaluated using pain-related cortical potentials of upper limbs. Facilitation of both trigeminal and somatic pain-related cortical potentials, but not of nociceptive blink reflex in MOH, which normalized after withdrawal were found. No differences were found comparing analgesics vs. triptan MOH. A transient facilitation was found of trigeminal and somatic nociceptive systems in MOH, which was more pronounced on a supraspinal level. Both trigeminal and somatic nociceptive systems that were found activated in patients with chronic migraine normalized again after withdrawal and consequent reduction of headache frequency. The authors did not find evidence that facilitation depends on the class of overused medication or the coexistence of depressive symptoms [72].

Detoxification

There is a general agreement that the patient should stop all medication and undergo a medication-free period of weeks to return to the initial headache frequency before medication overuse [73, 74]. Withdrawal may be necessary anyway because of serious health hazards associated with medication overuse. In fact, there are well-known potential secondary effects of chronic drug overuse on other organ system including analgesic nehropathy, nonsteroidal anti-inflammatory drug gastropathy, or ergotism. Moreover, the rare but potentially serious occurrence of the serotonin syndrome with triptan monotherapy has been recently pointed out [75].

However, when the patient tries to stop or reduce the drug intake, the preexisting headache usually worsens. The main symptom of withdrawal is headache, often associated with nausea, vomiting, arterial hypotension, tachycardia, sleep disturbances, restlessness, anxiety, and nervousness. The duration and severity of withdrawal headache and accompanying symptoms depends on the type of overused headache drug and appears to be shorter in patients overusing triptans than in those overusing ergots or analgesics [76]. Medication withdrawal strategies are not univocal [77–84].

It is generally believed that most patients can be treated on an outpatient basis [24]. Moreover, effective treatment of MOH involving ergots and triptan agents is more easily achieved than that which involves opioid or barbiturate-containing analgesics [12]. In order to improve the management of MOH, some authors have suggested dividing MOH into simple and complex subtypes to discriminate between cases with little behavioral influence from more complex ones [12, 47].

Definitely, MOH depends on primary headache type, the pattern and severity of medication overuse, the types of drug overused, the psychiatric comorbidities, patients' sociodemographic characteristics and patients' past therapeutic experiences. Thus, the effectiveness of strong advice to withdraw the overused medication versus the effectiveness of two pharmacological detoxification approaches (outpatients: advice + prednisone + preventive treatment; inpatients: advice + prednisone + preventive treatment + fluid replacement + antiemetics) in patients diagnosed with MOH and migraine has been investigated [85]. After 2 months, 85% of patients had reverted to an episodic pattern of migraine, and intake of acute medication was less than 10 days per month. No statistically significant difference was found between the groups [85]. These data suggest that advice and education about the risk of MOH and its consequences may be as effective as structured inpatient and outpatient detoxification programs in achieving withdrawal of the overused medication at least in patients with low medical need. Accordingly, it is important to outline that patients with previous detoxification treatments, coexistent medical

or psychiatric illnesses and overuse of agents containing opioids, benzodiazepines and barbiturates were excluded from this study [85].

However, there is a general agreement that inpatient detoxification is advisable for patients who use tranquillizers, opioids or barbiturates, especially in large daily doses [24, 86]. Due to a lack of treatment recommendations, therapeutical strategies to alleviate withdrawal symptoms vary among centers and countries. Among those agents suggested for withdrawal therapy are analgesics, tranquillizers, neuroleptics, antidepressant drugs, antiepileptic drugs, corticosteroids, intravenous dihydroergotamine, subcutaneous sumatriptan, oxygen, and behavioral treatment [24, 77–84, 87]. However, most of these treatments have not been investigated in a proper randomized, placebo-controlled trial. In a recent double-blind, placebo-controlled, randomized, single-center pilot study it was observed that 100 mg prednisone given daily for 5 days decreases the duration of withdrawal headache significantly compared with placebo-treated patients and is well tolerated [88]. However, a previous Norwegian placebo-controlled study has shown that 60 mg prednisone given for 2 days and tapering the dose the following 4 days had no effect on withdrawal headache in patients with CDH and medication overuse [89]. Additional studies to address the effectiveness of prednisone on withdrawal headache are needed.

Relapse in Medication Overuse Headache

After treatment of medication overuse and withdrawal of the overused medications, relapse occurs within months or years in a relatively high proportion of patients [90–96]. The relapse rate is lower for individuals overusing triptans rather than analgesics [92]. Predictors of relapse may include tension-type headache [92], overuse of combined analgesics [92], number of analgesic doses per day [91], duration of MO [91], overuse of butalbital and opioids [95], male sex [94] duration of migraine with more than eight headache days per month, a higher frequency of migraine after drug withdrawal, and a greater number of previous preventive treatments [96].

Pharmacological Treatments

Standardized, overall accepted, international and evidence-based guidelines for the treatment of MOH are not currently available. It partially depends on the absence of controlled clinical trials. It is generally believed that patients with MOH do not respond to prophylactic medications until the overused medications are withdrawn, and detoxification strategies are advocated prior to the initiation of preventive medications. The early introduction of prophylactic medication without a detoxification program in a randomized, open-label, 1-year follow-up study of patients with MOH was recently performed [97]. This program was found to be an effective way to reduce headache days and total headache burden during the first 3 months. The improvement was sustained during the whole follow-up period [97].

Accordingly, data from previous clinical trials of preventive migraine treatment in patients with chronic migraine, including those with medication overuse, provided similar suggestion [98–102]. Among treatment options the use of preventive medications such as sodium valproate (divalproex sodium) and topiramate, in order to reduce dependency on acute care medication in MOH, had previously provided to have beneficial effects in episodic migraine [87]. A general feature of the antiepileptic drugs (AEDs) effective in the prevention of migraine attacks is the ability to target multiple pre- and postsynaptic mechanisms [103]. In particular, the negative modulation of voltage-gated Na^+ and Ca^{2+} channels is a common feature of these drugs. Moreover, these AEDs share the ability to inhibit, although through different mechanisms, glutamate-mediated transmission in specific brain areas, to increase endogenous GABA tone and to modulate GABA receptors. Modulation of these multiple molecular targets can interfere with gene regulation and increase the threshold for the activation of pain sensitization, a pathophysiological mechanism presumably involved in MOH.

Future clinical studies dealing with the efficacy and tolerability of AEDs in MOH and possibly identification of further therapeutic strategies are needed.

Cognitive and Behavioral Therapeutic Approaches

Strategies for behavioral management of comorbid psychopathology in headache patients including MOH have been suggested [104]. An investigation to determine the role of behavioral therapy in the management of MOH has been conducted [105]. In a prospective study, patients with transformed migraine and analgesic overuse received either pharmacological therapy alone or pharmacological therapy supplemented with biofeedback-assisted relaxation. Both treatment groups achieved similar levels of improvement for up to 1 year following treatment. However, at the 3-year follow-up point, patients who had received biofeedback-assisted relaxation in addition to pharmacological therapy had greater sustained improvement on two out of three outcome measures (i.e. fewer headache days and reduced intake of analgesic medications) and fewer relapses [105].

Combined pharmacological and short-term psychodynamic psychotherapy for probable MOH has also been investigated [106]. Patients underwent a standard inpatient detoxification protocol, lasting a mean of 7 days. Preventive therapy was initiated during detoxification. The short-term psychodynamic psychotherapy protocol comprised the Brief Psychodynamic Investigation (BPI) and psychoanalysis-inspired psychotherapy. All patients (groups A and B) underwent the BPI and pharmacological therapy. Half of the patients (group B) also not randomly underwent psychoanalysis-inspired psychotherapy. At 12-month follow-up, a statistically greater decrease in headache frequency and medication intake was observed in group B than in group A. The relapse rate was much lower in group B patients at both 6 and 12 months than in group A. The risk of developing chronic migraine during follow-up was higher in group A than in group B at 6 and 12 months. The study suggests that short-term psychodynamic psychotherapy in conjunction with drug withdrawal and prophylactic pharmacotherapy relieves headache symptoms in MOH, reducing both long-term relapses and the burden of chronic migraine.

Conclusion

Apparently, MOH shares with other kinds of drug dependence some common neurobiological pathways, including those that modulate reward, novelty seeking, behavioral control, response to stress, and relapse. Dysfunction in the orbitofrontal cortex and the striato-thalamo-orbitofrontal circuits has been found in MOH patients possibly reflecting an underlying liability to medication overuse. A combination of environmental and genetic factors might play a role in MOH.

In all phases of drug abuse, females seem to be more sensitive to the rewarding effects of drugs than males, and estrogen is a major factor that underlies these sex differences [107]. MOH indeed was found to affect a higher rate of girls than boys as well as an higher rate of women than men [3, 20]. The possible influence of estrogen in MOH has not been properly explored so far.

For prevention of MOH, education of patients is the most important factor. Multidisciplinary approaches to support patients who are under withdrawal treatment are necessary.

Further research is needed in order to address the issue of medication overuse in headache patients. The reasons leading to different classes and amounts of medication overuse must be investigated.

References

1. Headache Classification Committee of the International Headache Society. Classification and diagnostic criteria for headache disorders, cranial neuralgias and facial pain. Cephalalgia. 1988;8 suppl 7:1–96.
2. The international classification of headache disorders, 2nd edn. Cephalalgia 2004;24 (suppl 1):1–160.

3. Zwart JA, Dyb G, Hagen K, Svebak S, Stovner LJ, Holmen J. Analgesic overuse among subjects with headache, neck, and low-back pain. Neurology. 2004;62:1540–4.

4. Silberstein SD, Olesen J, Bousser MG, Diener HC, Dodick D, First M, Goadsby PJ, Göbel H, Leinez MJA, Lance JW, Lipton RB, Nappi G, Sakai F, Schoenen J, Steiner TJ, On behalf of the International Headache Society. The international classification of headache disorders, 2nd Edition (ICHD-II)-revision of criteria for 8.2 Medication-overuse headache. Cephalalgia. 2005;25:460–5.

5. Headache Classification Committee of the International Headache Society. Classification and diagnostic criteria for headache disorders, cranial neuralgias and facial pain. 2nd ed. 1st Revision ICHD-IIR1. 2005. http://www.i-h-s.org.

6. Headache Classification Committee, Olesen J, Bousser MG, Diener HC, Dodick D, First M, Goadsby PJ, Gobel H, Lainez MJ, Lance JW, Lipton RB, Nappi G, Sakai F, Schoenen J, Silberstein SD, Steiner TJ. New appendix criteria open for a broader concept of chronic migraine. Cephalalgia. 2006;26:742–6.

7. Paemeleire K, Bahra A, Evers S, Matharu MS, Goadsby PJ. Medication-overuse headache in patients with cluster headache. Neurology. 2006;67:109–13.

8. Wilkinson SM, Becker WJ, Heine JA. Opiate use to control bowel motility may induce chronic daily headache in patients with migraine. Headache. 2001;41:303–9.

9. Bahra A, Walsh M, Menon S, Goadsby PJ. Does chronic daily headache arise de novo in association with regular use of analgesics? Headache. 2003;43:179–90.

10. Radat F, Creac'h C, Swendsen JD, et al. Psychiatric comorbidity in the evolution from migraine to medication overuse headache. Cephalalgia. 2005;25:519–22.

11. Radat F, Creac'h C, Guegan-Massardier E, Mick G, Guy N, Fabre N, Giraud P, Nachit-Ouinekh F, Lantéri-Minet M. Behavioral dependence in patients with medication overuse headache: a cross-sectional study in consulting patients using the DSM-IV criteria. Headache. 2008;48:1026–36.

12. Saper JR, Hamel RL, Lake III AE. Medication overuse headache (MOH) is a biobehavioural disorder. Cephalalgia. 2005; 25:545–6.

13. Calabresi P, Cupini LM. Medication-overuse headache: similarities with drug addiction. Trends Pharmacol Sci. 2005;26:62–8.

14. Fumal A, Laureys S, Di Clemente L, et al. Orbitofrontal cortex involvement in chronic analgesic-overuse headache evolving from episodic migraine. Brain. 2006;129:543–50.

15. Cevoli S, Sancisi E, Grimaldi D, Pierangeli G, Zanigni S, Nicodemo M, Cortelli P, Montagna P. Family history for chronic headache and drug overuse as a risk factor for headache chronification. Cevoli Headache. 2008. doi:10.1111/j.1526-4610.2008.01257.

16. Scher AI, Stewart WF, Liberman J, Lipton RB. Prevalence of frequent headache in a population sample. Headache. 1998;38: 497–506.

17. Castillo J, Munoz P, Guitera V, Pascual J. Epidemiology of chronic daily headache in the general population. Headache. 1999;39: 190–6.

18. Wang SJ, Fuh JL, Lu SR, et al. Chronic daily headache in Chinese elderly: prevalence, risk factors, and biannual follow-up. Neurology. 2000;54:314–19.

19. Lu SR, Fuh JL, Chen WT, Juang KD, Wang SJ. Chronic daily headache in Taipei, Taiwan: prevalence, follow-up and outcome predictors. Cephalalgia. 2001;21:980–6.

20. Dyb G, Holmen TL, Zwart JA. Analgesic overuse among adolescents with headache: the Head-HUNT-Youth Study. Neurology. 2006;24(66):198–201.

21. Wang S-J, Fuh J-L, Lu S-R, Juang K-D. Chronic daily headache in adolescents: prevalence, impact, and medication overuse. Neurology. 2006;66:193–7.

22. Stoelben S, Krappweis J, Rossler G, Kirch W. Adolescents' drug use and drug knowledge. Eur J Pediatr. 2000;159:608–14.

23. Meskunas CA, Tepper SJ, Rapoport AM, Sheftell FD, Bigal ME. Medications associated with probable medication overuse headache reported in a tertiary care headache center over a 15-year period. Headache. 2006;46:766–72.

24. Diener HC, Limmroth V. Medication-overuse headache: a worldwide problem. Lancet Neurol. 2004;3:475–83.

25. Limmroth V, Katsarava Z, Fritsche G, Przywara S, Diener HC. Features of medication overuse headache following overuse of different acute headache drugs. Neurology. 2002;59:1011–14.

26. Fisher MA, Glass S. Butorphanol (Stadol): a study in problems of current drug information and control. Neurology. 1997; 48:1156–60.

27. Ziegler DK. Opiate und opioid use in patients with refractory headache. Cephalalgia. 1994;14:5–10.

28. Saper JR, Jones JM. Ergotamine tartrate dependency: features and possible mechanisms. Clin Neuropharmacol. 1986;9:244–56.

29. Schnider P, Aull S, Baumgartner C, Marterer A, Wober C, Zeiler K, Wessely P. Long-term outcome of patients with headache and drug abuse after inpatient withdrawal: five-year follow-up. Cephalalgia. 1996;16:481–5.

30. Fanciullacci M, Alessandri M, Pietrini U, Briccolani-Bandini E, Beatrice S. Long-term ergotamine abuse: effect on adrenergically induced mydriasis. Clin Pharm Ther. 1992;51:302–07.

31. Griffiths RR, Woodson PP. Caffeine physical dependence: a review of human and laboratory animal studies. Psychopharmacology. 1988;94:437–51.

32. Griffiths RR, Woodson PP. Reinforcing properties of caffeine: studies in humans and laboratory animals. Pharmacol Biochem Behav. 1988;29:419–27.

33. Silverman K, Evans SM, Strain EC, Griffiths RR. Withdrawal syndrome after the double-blind cessation of caffeine consumption. N Engl J Med. 1992;327:1109–14.

34. Scher AI, Stewart WF, Lipton RB. Caffeine as a risk factor for chronic daily headache: a population-based study. Neurology. 2004;63:2022–7.

35. Sternieri E, Coccia CP, Pinetti D, Ferrari A. Pharmacokinetics and interactions of headache medications, part I: introduction, pharmacokinetics, metabolism and acute treatments. Expert Opin Drug Metab Toxicol. 2006;2:961–79.

36. Ferrari A, Savino G, Gallesi D, Pinetti D, Bertolini A, Sances G, Coccia CP, Pasciullo G, Leone S, Loi M, Sternieri E. Effect of overuse of the antimigraine combination of indomethacin, prochlorperazine and caffeine (IPC) on the disposition of its components in chronic headache patients. Pharmacol Res. 2006;54:142–9.

37. Ferrari A, Leone S, Vergoni AV, et al. Similarities and differences between chronic migraine and episodic migraine. Headache. 2007;47:65–72.

38. Cevoli S, Mochi M, Scapoli C, Marzocchi N, Pierangeli G, Pini LA, Cortelli P, Montagna P. A genetic association study of dopamine metabolism-related genes and chronic headache with drug abuse. Eur J Neurol. 2006;13:1009–13.

39. Giros B, Jaber M, Jones SR, Wightman RM, Caron MG. Hyperlocomotion and indifference to cocaine and amphetamine in mice lacking the dopamine transporter. Nature. 1996;379: 606–12.

40. Park JW, Kim JS, Kim YI, Lee KS. Serotonergic activity contributes to analgesic overuse in chronic tension-type headache. Headache. 2005;45:1229–35.

41. Di Lorenzo C, Sances G, Di Lorenzo G, Rengo C, Ghiotto N, Guaschino E, Perrotta A, Santorelli FM, Grieco GS, Troisi A, Siracusano A, Pierelli F, Nappi G, Casali C. The wolframin His611Arg polymorphism influences medication overuse headache. Neurosci Lett. 2007;424:179–84.

42. Fuh JL, Wang SJ, Lu SR, Juang KD. Does medication overuse headache represent a behavior of dependence? Pain. 2005;119: 49–55.

43. Ferrari A, Cicero AF, Bertolini A, Leone S, Pasciullo G, Sternieri E. Need for analgesics/drugs of abuse: a comparison between headache patients and addicts by the Leeds Dependence Questionnaire (LDQ). Cephalalgia. 2006;26:187–93.

44. Baskin SM, Lipchik GL, Smitherman TA. Mood and anxiety disorders in chronic headache. Headache. 2006;46 Suppl 3: S76–87.

45. Atasoy HT, Atasoy N, Unal AE, Emre U, Sumer M. Psychiatric comorbidity in medication overuse headache patients with pre-existing headache type of episodic tension-type headache. Eur J Pain. 2005;9:285–91.

46. Rothrock J, Lopez I, Zweifler R, Andress-Rothrock D, Drinkard R, Walters N. Borderline personality disorder and migraine. Headache. 2007;47:22–6.

47. Lake 3rd AE. Medication overuse headache: bio-behavioural issues and solutions. Headache. 2006;46 Suppl 3:S88–97.

48. Gallai V, Alberti A, Gallai B, Coppola F, Floridi A, Sarchielli P. Glutamate and nitric oxide pathway in chronic daily headache: evidence from cerebrospinal fluid. Cephalalgia. 2003;23:166–74.

49. Vieira DS, Naffah-Mazzacoratti Mda G, Zukerman E, Senne Soares CA, Cavalheiro EA, Peres MF. Glutamate levels in cere-brospinal fluid and triptans overuse in chronic migraine. Headache. 2007;47:842–7.

50. Spengos K, Theleritis C, Paparrigopoulos T. Memantine and NMDA antagonism for chronic migraine: a potentially novel ther-apeutic approach? Headache. 2008;48:284–28.

51. Srikiatkhachorn A, Maneesri S, Govitrapong P, Kasantikul V. Derangement of serotonin system in migrainous patients with analgesic abuse headache: clues from platelets. Headache. 1998;38:43–9.

52. Srikiatkhachorn A, Tarasub N, Govitrapong P. Effect of chronic analgesic exposure on the central serotonin system: a possible mech-anism of analgesic abuse headache. Headache. 2000;40:343–50.

53. Ayzenberg I, Obermann M, Leineweber K, Franke L, Yoon MS, Diener HC, Katsarava Z. Increased activity of serotonin uptake in platelets in medication overuse headache following regular intake of analgesics and triptans. J Headache Pain. 2008;9:109–12.

54. Akerman S, Goadsby PJ. Dopamine and migraine: biology and clinical implications. Cephalalgia. 2007;27:1308–14.

55. Peres MF, Sanchez del Rio M, Seabra ML, et al. Hypothalamic involvement in chronic migraine. J Neurol Neurosurg Psychiatry. 2001;71:747–51.

56. Pertwee RG. Cannabinoid receptors and pain. Prog Neurobiol. 2001;63:569–611.

57. Akerman S, Holland P, Goadsby PJ. Cannabinoid (CB1) receptor activation inhibits trigeminovascular neurons. J Pharmacol Exp Ther. 2007;320:64–71.

58. Maldonado R, Valverde O, Berrendero F. Involvement of the endocannabinoid system in drug addiction. Trends Neurosci. 2006;29:225–32.

59. Giuffrida A, Parsons LH, Kerr TM, Rodriguez de Fonseca F, Navarro M, Piomelli D. Dopamine activation of endogenous cannabinoid signaling in dorsal striatum. Nat Neurosci. 1999; 2:358–63.

60. Maccarone M, Bari M, Battista N, Finazzi-Agrò A. Estrogen stimulates arachidonoylethanolamide release from human endothe-lial cells and platelet activation. Blood. 2002;100:4040–8.

61. Cupini LM, Bari M, Battista N, Argirò G, Finazzi-Agrò A, Calabresi P, Maccarone M. Biochemical changes in endocan-nabinoid system are expressed in platelets of female but not male migraineurs. Cephalalgia. 2006;26:277–81.

62. Sarchielli P, Pini LA, Coppola F, Rossi C, Baldi A, Mancini ML, Calabresi P. Endocannabinoids in chronic migraine: CSF findings

63. Rossi C, Pini LA, Cupini ML, Calabresi P, Sarchielli P. Endocannabinoids in platelets of chronic migraine patients and medication-overuse headache patients: relation with serotonin levels. Eur J Clin Pharmacol. 2008;64:1–8.

64. Cupini LM, Costa C, Sarchielli P, Bari M, Battista N, Eusebi P, Calabresi P, Maccarone M. Degradation of endocannabinoids in chronic migraine and medication overuse headache. Neurobiol Dis. 2008;30:186–9.

65. Bonci A, Borgland S. Role of orexin/hypocretin and CRF in the formation of drug-dependent synaptic plasticity in the mesolimbic system. Neuropharmacology. 2009;56 Suppl 1:107–11.

66. Holland PR, Akerman S, Goadsby PJ. Orexin 1 receptor activa-tion attenuates neurogenic dural vasodilation in an animal model of trigeminovascular nociception. J Pharmacol Exp Ther. 2005;315:1380–5.

67. Sarchielli P, Rainero I, Coppola F, Rossi C, Mancini M, Pinessi L, Calabresi P. Involvement of corticotrophin-releasing factor and orexin-A in chronic migraine and medication-overuse headache: findings from cerebrospinal fluid. Cephalalgia. 2008;28:714–22.

68. Fields HL, Hjelmstad GO, Margolis EB, Nicola SM. Ventral teg-mental area neurons in learned appetitive behavior and positive reinforcement. Annu Rev Neurosci. 2007;30:289–316.

69. Welch KM, Nagesh V, Aurora SK, Gelman N. Periaqueductal gray matter dysfunction in migraine: cause or the burden of illness? Headache. 2001;41:629–37.

70. Schmidt-Wilcke T, Leinisch E, Straube A, Kämpfe N, Draganski B, Diener HC, Bogdahn U, May A. Gray matter decrease in patients with chronic tension type headache. Neurology. 2005;65(9):1483–6.

71. Fusco BM, Colantoni O, Giacovazzo M. Alteration of central excitation circuits in chronic headache and analgesic misuse. Headache. 1997;37:486–91.

72. Ayzenberg I, Obermann M, Nyhuis P, Gastpar M, Limmroth V, Diener HC, Kaube H, Katsarava Z. Central sensitization of the trigeminal and somatic nociceptive systems in medication overuse headache mainly involves cerebral supraspinal structures. Cephalalgia. 2006;26:1106–14.

73. Silberstein SD, Welch KM. Painkiller headache. Neurology. 2002;59:972–4.

74. Zeeberg P, Olesen J, Jensen R. Probable medication-overuse head-ache: the effect of a 2-month drug-free period. Neurology. 2006;66:1894–8.

75. Soldin OP, Tonning JM, Obstetric-Fetal Pharmacology Research Unit Network. Serotonin syndrome associated with triptan mono-therapy. N Engl J Med. 2008;358:2185–6.

76. Katsarava Z, Fritsche G, Muessig M, Diener HC, Limmroth V. Clinical features of withdrawal headache following overuse of triptans and other headache drugs. Neurology. 2001;57:1694–8.

77. Relja G, Granato A, Bratina A, Antonello RM, Zorzon M. Outcome of medication overuse headache after abrupt in-patient with-drawal. Cephalalgia. 2006;26:589–95.

78. Andrasik F. Behavioral treatment approaches to chronic headache. Neurol Sci. 2003;24 Suppl 2:S80–5.

79. Silberstein SD, Schulman EA, Hopkins MM. Repetitive intrave-nous DHE in the treatment of refractory headache. Headache. 1990;30:334–9.

80. Raskin NH. Repetitive intravenous dihydroergotamine as therapy for intractable migraine. Neurology. 1986;36:995–7.

81. Krymchantowski AV, Moreira PF. Out-patient detoxification in chronic migraine: comparison of strategies. Cephalalgia. 2003; 23:982–93.

82. Evans RW, Young WB. Droperidol and other neuroleptics/antiemet-ics for the management of migraine. Headache. 2003;43:811–3.

83. Mathew NT. Amelioration of ergotamine withdrawal symptoms with naproxen. Headache. 1987;27:130–3.

suggest a system failure. Neuropsychopharmacology. 2007;32: 1384–90.

84. Schwartz TH, Karpitskiy VV, Sohn RS. Intravenous valproate sodium in the treatment of daily headache. Headache. 2002;42:519–22.

85. Rossi P, Di Lorenzo C, Faroni J, Cesarino F, Nappi G. Advice alone vs. structured detoxification programmes for medication overuse headache: a prospective, randomized, open-label trial in transformed migraine patients with low medical needs. Cephalalgia. 2006;26:1097–105.

86. Katsarava Z, Jensen R. Medication-overuse headache: where are we now? Curr Opin Neurol. 2007;20:326–30.

87. Dodick DW, Silberstein SD. How clinicians can detect, prevent and treat medication overuse headache. Cephalalgia. 2008; 28:1207–17.

88. Pageler L, Katsarava Z, Diener HC, Limmroth V. Prednisone vs. placebo in withdrawal therapy following medication overuse headache. Cephalalgia. 2008;28:152–6.

89. Boe MG, Mygland A, Salvesen R. Prednisolone does not reduce withdrawal headache: a randomized, doubleblind study. Neurology. 2007;69:26–31.

90. Fritsche G, Eberl A, Katsarava Z, Limmroth V, Diener HC. Drug induced headache: long-term follow-up of withdrawal therapy and persistence of drug misuse. Eur Neurol. 2001;45:229–35.

91. Pini LA, Cicero AF, Sandrini M. Long-term follow-up of patients treated for chronic headache with analgesic overuse. Cephalalgia. 2001;21:878–83.

92. Katsarava Z, Muessig M, Dzagnidze A, Fritsche G, Diener HC, Limmroth V. Medication overuse headache: rates and predictors for relapse in a 4-year prospective study. Cephalalgia. 2005;25:12–5.

93. Tribl GG, Schnider P, Wober C, Aull S, Auterith A, Zeiler K, Wessely P. Are there predictive factors for long-term outcome after withdrawal in drug-induced chronic daily headache? Cephalalgia. 2001;21:691–6.

94. Suhr B, Evers S, Bauer B, Gralow I, Grotemeyer KH, Husstedt IW. Drug-induced headache: long-term results of stationary versus ambulatory withdrawal therapy. Cephalalgia. 1999;19:44–9.

95. Young WB. Medication overuse headache. Curr Treat Options Neurol. 2001;3:181–8.

96. Rossi P, Faroni JV, Nappi G. Medication overuse headache: predictors and rates of relapse in migraine patients with low medical needs. A 1-year prospective study. Cephalalgia. 2008; 28:1196–200.

97. Hagen K, Albretsen C, Vilming S, Salvesen R, Grønning M, Helde G, Gravdahl G, Zwart JA, Stovner L. Management of medication overuse headache: 1-year randomized multicentre open-label trial. Cephalalgia. 2009;29(2):221–32.

98. Silvestrini M, Bartolini M, Coccia M, Baruffaldi R, Taffi R, Provinciali L. Topiramate in the treatment of chronic migraine. Cephalalgia. 2003;23:820–4.

99. Mei D, Ferraro D, Zelano G, Capuano A, Vollono C, Gabriele C, Di Trapani G. Topiramate and triptans revert chronic migraine with medication overuse to episodic migraine. Clin Neuropharmacol. 2006;29:269–75.

100. Dodick DW, Bigal M, Silberstein SD, Mathew NT, Hulihan J, Ascher S, et al. Efficacy of topiramate treatment for chronic migraine in patients with medication overuse. Headache. 2007; 47:761.

101. Diener HC, Bussone G, Van Oene JC, Lahaye M, Schwalen S, Goadsby PJ, TOPMAT-MIG-201 (TOP-CHROME) Study Group. Topiramate reduces headache days in chronic migraine: a randomized, double-blind, placebo-controlled study. Cephalalgia. 2007; 27:814–23.

102. Landy SH, Baker JD. Divalproex ER prophylaxis in migraineurs with probable chronic migraine and probable medication-overuse headache: a case series. Pain Pract. 2004;4:292–4.

103. Calabresi P, Galletti F, Rossi C, Sarchielli P, Cupini LM. Antiepileptic drugs in migraine: from clinical aspects to cellular mechanisms. Trends Pharmacol Sci. 2007;28:188–95.

104. Smitherman TA, Maizels M, Penzien DB. Headache chronification: screening and behavioural management of comorbid depressive and anxiety disorders. Headache. 2008;48:45–50.

105. Grazzi L, Andrasik F, D'Amico D, Leone M, Usai S, Kass SJ, Bussone G. Behavioral and pharmacologic treatment of transformed migraine with analgesic overuse: outcome at 3 years. Headache. 2002;42:483–90.

106. Altieri M, Di Giambattista R, Di Clemente L, Fagiolo D, Tarolla E, Mercurio A, Vicenzini E, Tarsitani L, Lenzi GL, Biondi M, Di Piero V. Combined pharmacological and short-term psychodynamic psychotherapy for probable medication overuse headache: a pilot study. Cephalalgia. 2009;29(3):293–9. doi:10.1111/j.1468-2982.2008.01717.x.

107. Carroll ME, Lynch WJ, Roth ME, Morgan AD, Cosgrove KP. Sex and estrogen influence drug abuse. Trends Pharmacol Sci. 2004;25:273–9.

Addiction and Parkinson's Disease

29

Tatiana Witjas, Jean Philippe Azulay,
and Alexandre Eusebio

Abstract

Parkinson's disease (PD) is a neurodegenerative disease characterized by tremor, rigidity, and akinesia. PD patients are commonly treated by dopamine replacement therapy (DRT). The degeneration of the dopaminergic system and the longstanding exposure to DRT may cause, in a group of vulnerable patients, dysregulation of the brain reward system. These patients develop DRT-related compulsions, which include addiction to levodopa or dopamine dysregulation syndrome (DDS), punding, and impulse control disorders (ICDs). ICDs or behavioral addiction reported in PD include pathological gambling, hypersexuality, compulsive buying, and binge eating. Although the underlying pathophysiology is still poorly understood, these behaviors are linked by their reward-based and repetitive nature. Such behaviors may result in psychosocial impairment for the patients and are often hidden. The recognition of these behaviors is important and allows a better clinical management. Although the limited data do not permit particular therapeutic strategies, some approaches are worth considering: DRT reduction, trials of nondopaminergic medications and subthalamic chronic stimulation.

Abbreviations

DBS   Deep brain stimulation
DDS   Dopamine dysregulation syndrome
DRT   Dopamine replacement therapy
ICD   Impulse control disorder
OCD   Obsessive–compulsive disorder
PD   Parkinson's disease
STN   Subthalamic nucleus
VTA   Ventral tegmental area

Learning Objectives
- Addictive behaviors have been increasingly recognized in Parkinson's disease
- Recognition of the phenomenology, risk factors, and pathophysiology is important for an optimal management
- Clinicians should be aware of these symptoms in order to prevent potentially disabling psychosocial impact

Issues that Need to Be Addressed by Future Research
- The true prevalence of these DRT-related behaviors needs to be determined as well as the predisposing factors
- Screening tools for identifying PD patients at risk and rating scales to measure syndrome severity are needed for prevention and clinical assessment

T. Witjas (✉) • J.P. Azulay • A. Eusebio
Clinical Neurosciences Department, Movement Disorders Unit,
CHU Timone, 264 rue Saint Pierre, 13385 Marseille, France
e-mail: tatiana.witjas@ap-hm.fr

(continued)

J.C. Verster et al. (eds.), *Drug Abuse and Addiction in Medical Illness: Causes, Consequences and Treatment,*
DOI 10.1007/978-1-4614-3375-0_29, © Springer Science+Business Media, LLC 2012

(continued)

- Further research on the pathogenesis of these disruptive behaviors may allow a better understanding of primary addictive disorders in non-PD patients
- Outstanding questions are related to the management of these disabling behaviors: prospective studies and long-term follow-up should help to clarify the true association between dopaminergic treatment and the precipitation of such symptoms; the role of functional neurosurgery requires further investigations

Parkinson's disease (PD) is a progressive neurodegenerative disease characterized by the loss of pigmented neurons of the brainstem, mainly the dopaminergic cells of the substantia nigra. The prevalence rate has been estimated at 120–180 per 100,000, which places PD as the second most frequent neurodegenerative disorder after Alzheimer disease. James Parkinson in his monograph "an Essay on the Shaking Palsy" first described the disease in 1817 [1]. The cardinal motor features of PD are rest tremor, cogwheel rigidity, and brady/akinesia. However, a broad spectrum of nonmotor symptoms also complicates PD, encompassing autonomic, sensory, neuropsychiatric, and sleep disorders. The substitutive therapy by L-dopa or other dopaminergic agents dramatically improves the motor symptoms. However, with time the patient's condition inexorably deteriorates with the development of adverse events that include motor fluctuations, "on" and "off" state, dyskinesia, neuropsychiatric complications, and the progressive development of axial symptoms. These axial symptoms, which include falls, freezing of gait, speech disturbances are less responsive to dopamine-related therapy (DRT). In addition, a minority of PD patients develops compulsive behaviors that are triggered by dopaminergic drug therapy. In the past decade, these behaviors are being increasingly recognized and include pathological gambling, hypersexuality, compulsive shopping or eating, punding, and compulsive medication use. Such behaviors may result in devastating psychosocial consequences and are therapeutic challenges for physicians.

Historical Background

PD patients typically do not exhibit a predisposition to addictive and reward-seeking behaviors. The classical personality traits have been described as meticulous, anxious, anhedonic, more introverted, cautious, socially alert, and tense than controls [2, 3]. They have lower novelty-seeking than that of age-matched control subjects with a poor novelty-seeking character [4]. These characters may explain the lower incidence of tobacco and caffeine use among PD patients [5].

However, hyperlibidinous behaviors have been reported early after the discovery of levodopa therapy and later with the use of dopamine agonists or other antiparkinsonian drugs [6, 7]. Long-term dopamine replacement therapy (DRT) is associated with series of motor complications (dyskinesia and on–off phenomenon). It also induces psychomotor activation and behavioral disorders similar to those seen after excessive use of psychostimulants such as amphetamines and cocaine. Surprisingly, the addictive potential of DRT on PD patients was not investigated. In 1994, Friedman first identified a levodopa-related punding in PD patients [8]. Originally, punding describes stereotyped, senseless motor behaviors in amphetamine and cocaine addicts. Nevertheless, these hyperdopaminergic, disinhibitory behaviors were not widely recognized. In 2000, Giovannoni et al. reported a case series of young PD patients with behavioral disorders characterized by self-medication and addiction [9]. They named the syndrome "hedonistic homeostatic dysregulation." Since then, a succession of reports described different aspects of these repetitive and reward-based behaviors. Different names have been proposed: hedonistic homeostatic dysregulation, dopamine dysregulation syndrome, impulse control disorders syndrome in PD, dopamimetic drug addiction, compulsive dopaminergic drug use, dopamine replacement therapy dependence syndrome, repetitive and reward-seeking behaviors, medication-related impulse control and repetitive behaviors, dopamine-replacement-therapy-related compulsions. There is much disagreement surrounding the classification of these behaviors. However, although they encompass a broad spectrum of symptoms, these behaviors are linked by their repetitive and reward-based nature. Recently, Ferrara and Stacy proposed to divide these dopamine-related compulsions into three categories: impulse control disorder (ICD), punding behaviors, and dopamine dysregulation syndrome (DDS) [10].

Dopamine-Related Compulsions in Parkinson's Disease: Definitions, Prevalence, and Risk Factors

ICD, punding, and DDS may occur in combination in the same patient or independently. Some patient experienced one or two types of ICD (e.g. pathological gambling and hypersexuality) and do not use dopamine replacement therapy compulsively. Punding is often associated with DDS but can be isolated. Most patients with DDS develop punding and/or ICD. However, few of them may have only compulsive medication use.

Impulse Control Disorders

According to the *Diagnostic and Statistical Manual of Mental Disorders*, Fourth Edition-Text Revision, ICDs are characterized by a "failure to resist an impulse, drive or temptation to perform an act that is harmful to the person or to others" [11]. Only pathological gambling was formally defined in this category yet other types of excessive reward-seeking behaviors can be considered to be impulse-control disorders. The definition overlaps with substance use disorders thus such behaviors are commonly viewed as "behavioral addictions." There is a considerable variability in the clinical expression of each ICD. In Parkinson's disease, reported ICDs include pathological gambling, hypersexuality, compulsive buying, compulsive eating, kleptomania, impulsive-aggressive behaviors, and trichotillomania. The lifetime prevalence of ICDs (pathological gambling, hypersexuality, excessive shopping, or a combination) is estimated at 6.1% [12]. Weintraub et al. reported similar prevalence rates of 6.6% [13]. On a recent study using a directed questionnaire administered to the patient and spouse, which included also compulsive eating, the prevalence rate was 14% [14]. There is a strong association with dopamine receptor agonists and ICDs. The prevalence with levodopa alone is 0.7% whereas with dopamine agonists, it raised to 13.7% [12]. A recent study found that 25% of the patients taking dopamine agonists experienced a subjective increase in ICD but less than 20% of them estimated that the change was deleterious [15].

Pathological Gambling

Pathological gambling is one of the most frequently reported ICD, with hypersexuality in Parkinson's disease. Its prevalence is estimated between 3 and 8%, whereas the lifetime prevalence in the general population in North America is 1.7% [13, 16–18]. Pathological gambling occurs more frequently in young PD patients (at least younger age at PD onset). Gender plays also a role in prevalence as 75.6% of the gamblers were male in a literature review on pathological gambling in PD [19]. There is no specific characteristic with the profile of the Parkinson's disease but Voon et al. reported that right-sided Parkinson's disease onset was more frequently associated with pathological gambling [20]. Alcohol abuse and impulsivity are the associated comorbidities [13, 21]. The association of depression and pathological gambling is controversial [19, 20]. There is an association between novelty-seeking personality and pathological gambling in PD [20]. A personal or first-degree familial history of alcohol use disorder was found to be a predictive factor for pathological gambling [20]. The majority of the patients did not gamble before the diagnosis of PD [19]. The preferred gambling activities are slot machines (33%), casino attendance (unspecified activities) (21.3%), Internet gam-

bling (20%), lottery/scratch cards (16%), horse/greyhound racing (13.3%), bingo (5.3%), and stock market (1.3%). The increasing availability of Internet gambling has become an emerging problem [22]. Most reports indicate that pathological gambling is associated with the use of dopamine agonists as a monotherapy or as an adjuvant to levodopa [23]. Some studies have suggested a particular agonist whereas other studies found no difference between different agonists [13, 16, 17, 19, 24]. The mean latency of pathological gambling from dopamine agonist initiation was 23 months [19].

Hypersexuality

The abnormal behaviors of hypersexuality have a large variability in their expression. It may manifest as a sexual thoughts, excessive demands for sex from their partner, uncontrollable masturbation, compulsive use of pornography, exhibitionism, and paraphilias. Hypersexuality may occur in spite of impotence [6]. The prevalence is estimated between 2.4 and 7% but may be underestimated due to patient reluctance to discuss these symptoms [25]. Hypersexuality has been reported to be more common in men and in those with early-onset PD [12, 26]. Hypersexuality has been reported early with the initial levodopa therapy [27]. Later dopamine agonists and selegiline, monoamine oxidase B inhibitors, have also been implicated in these behaviors [6, 26, 28]. Like in pathological gambling, hypersexuality predominates in patients using dopamine receptor agonists [12, 13].

Compulsive Shopping

Compulsive shopping or excessive buying is less reported in PD. Its prevalence is estimated between 0.4% and 1.5% in PD whereas the estimated prevalence of compulsive buying in the general population in the United States is 5.8% [12, 13, 29].

Compulsive Eating

Compulsive or binge eating is less reported than pathological gambling or hypersexuality in PD and its prevalence is unknown. It affects mainly women. In a study in one clinic population, nine patients were identified with compulsive eating with undesired weight gain. They were all treated with dopamine agonists. Four had other comorbid compulsive behaviors; five patients were overweight at baseline [29].

Other Reported ICDs

There are two reports of kleptomania in PD, one of trichotillomania associated with other compulsive behaviors [30–32]. Recently, reckless driving has been reported in two PD patients as a result of excessive use of L-dopa. This behavior can be considered as a compulsive risk-seeking behavior [33].

Punding

Punding is a complex stereotyped behavior characterized by intense fascination with repetitive meaningless movements. Punding was first described in amphetamine and cocaine users [34]. The term itself comes from Swedish slang and literally translates into "block-head." It consists of repetitive aimless activities. Friedman described the first case of punding in Parkinson's disease with levodopa use [8]. Later, several similar cases of punding in PD patients under dopamine replacement therapy were reported [9, 35–37]. Punding consists in a constellation of purposeless ritualistic behaviors such as sorting and resorting objects, shuffling papers, grooming, hoarding, dismantling objects without being able to complete the tasks, doodling without producing artwork. Other unusual behaviors may be considered as punding, such as compulsive singing or humming [38, 39], inordinate writing or blogging [40], walkabouts or purposeless driving [9], and long meaningless monologue. Indeed, some authors consider punding as an excessive involvement with a hobby or activity as these behaviors are repetitive and difficult to disengage from. Activities usually remain selective for one or few types of behavior over time [8]. The phenomenology of punding is shaped by previous occupation or hobbies. Office workers stereotypically shuffle papers, carpenter collect tools and do senseless home repairs, women repetitively sort through their handbags or brush their hair [36, 41]. Punding is usually associated with feelings of relief or calmness but attempts to stop the activity by others results in irritability and frustration. However, Kurlan described PD patients who engaged in aimless, compulsive rituals but were agitated while carrying out the activity [42]. These behaviors are recognized as inadequate and socially disruptive. The punders recognized that time spent on their activities is inappropriate and excessive. They typically complained of difficulty in finishing their projects. However, some patients with punding lack awareness regarding the senseless nature of their behaviors [43]. These behaviors often resulted in isolation from or conflict with other people. It often caused disintegration of family relationships. PD patients with punding tend to pursue their activities overnight. Punding seems to occur mostly during "on" state. Punding is different from OCD as the punders do not report intrusive thoughts and anxiety [44]. Punding is distinct from mania as the patients withdraw into themselves instead of being enthusiastic with flight of ideas and engaging in multiple activities [36].

The prevalence of punding is difficult to assess due to difference in ascertainment. In one study on PD patients identified as taking high doses of dopaminergic medication (>800 mg levodopa equivalents per day), the prevalence was as high as 14% [36]. A second study conducted in a tertiary center in Canada found a prevalence of only 1.4% [43]. This disparity can be explained by the contrasting referral and assessment procedures used. The former study was based on a clinician interview of patients taking high dosages of DRT, the latter used a patient-rated questionnaire to an unselected population of PD patients. Furthermore, the variation in treatment practice may account for this discrepancy, as apomorphine is not available in Canada. Apomorphine is a potent rapid-onset dopamine agonist used as "rescue medication" or by continuous subcutaneous infusion. It is conceivable that greater dopaminergic stimulation may result in a higher punding incidence. Indeed, PD patients with punding require large dose of DRT, frequent rescue dose and use of rescue medication overnight [36]. Punding is associated with several neuropsychiatric comorbidities including previously treated psychosis, hypersexuality, pathological gambling, and compulsive overuse of DRT [8, 9, 35, 36]. Insomnia is a common comorbidity and query to determine a relative decrease in daily sleep-time may aid in making the diagnosis [23]. There is a correlation between punding and younger age of disease onset, but not with gender. Punding is associated with higher personality impulsivity (Barrat Impulsivity Scale score) and a poorer disease-related quality of life (PDQ-39 score) [45]. The severity of the punding correlated with Parkinson's disease's severity, especially with dyskinesia severity. The relationship between dyskinesia and punding severity suggest the two arise from analogous mechanisms. They may both relate to drug-induced sensitization of neural systems mediating motor and behavioral functions that seem to be favored by a pulsatile administration of DRT (e.g. apomorphine and L-dopa).

Unlike ICD, punding does not appear to be related to the type of DRT used (dopamine agonists or L-dopa). It has been reported exclusively in patients with high medication dosage using frequent rescue doses. Short-acting medications such as L-dopa and apomorphine, which induce pulsatile dopaminergic stimulation, may be important to the development of punding behaviors. However, punding may be underreported and the prevalence in PD patients on lower dosage of DRT is unknown.

Dopamine Dysregulation Syndrome

DDS relates to a pattern of compulsive medication use that results in psychosocial dysfunction and severe dyskinesia. Giovannoni and colleagues reported the first case series of 15 predominantly early-onset PD patients who take DRT in excess far beyond that required for motor control [9]. These patients were insistent on a rapid increase of medication dosage and resisted attempts to reduce the dose. Adverse effects were disabling dyskinesia and neuropsychiatric disturbances including mood disorders and social or legal difficulties. The term "hedonistic homeostatic dysregulation" was applied in reference to a model of substance dependence that interprets the motivation to take drugs in terms of escape from withdrawal [46]. With the observation that many of these behaviors improved with a reduction to DRT, the term dopaminergic dysregulation syndrome (DDS) was preferred [47, 48].

Levodopa addiction has been described in parkinsonian as well as in nonparkinsonian patients [49]. DDS occurs in a vulnerable group of PD patients who typically experience an excellent initial therapeutic motor response from levodopa. However, these patients report transient euphoria after each dose of DRT, which may result in the development of a pathological wanting for the drug. From an early stage of the disease, patients with DDS take extra medication complaining of tolerance or intolerable motor and affective symptoms. A pattern of compulsive drug-seeking through multiple sources develops leading to a rapid increase in DRT (>2 g per day levodopa equivalent) [50, 51]. Attempts at dose reduction are unsuccessful and may lead to a hoarding of medication and a search for alternative clandestine supplies [49]. Patients ignore medical advices and self-medicate using idiosyncratic cues. They perceived the "on" state only when disabling dyskinesia occurs. With higher DRT dosage, intense "off" period dysphoria or "on" period euphoria becomes evident. Patients often identify aversive "off" period as the reason for their compulsive medication use. In DDS, "off" period dysphoria (depression, anxiety, panic attacks) appears to be disproportionate in comparison to the "off" period motor disability [52]. Somatic complaints may be associated, which include abdominal pain, palpitations, painful limb, or profuse sweating [53, 54]. Euphoria, grandiose ideation, hyperactivity, or hypomania can appear during "on" period. Compulsive DRT use may lead to dopaminergic reversible psychosis. Delirium, paranoid ideation, and hallucinations are commonly associated with hypomania, severe dyskinesia, and sleep disturbances. This psychosis is very similar to psychostimulant (amphetamine or cocaine) psychosis. Punding is often associated with DDS [9, 36]. Hypersexuality, pathological gambling, compulsive shopping, and binge eating may also be features of hypomanic phases in DDS patients. Heightened aggression is common, and includes irritability, low tolerance of frustration, angry outbursts, use of insulting language or gesture, aggressive threats, and occasional violence. There is a lack of insight to the harm caused to themselves and to the people around them. These behavioral disorders may have devastating consequences to the patient with social isolation, marital breakdown, and legal or financial difficulties. Relapses are frequent after enforced medication reduction.

PD patients with DDS fulfill DSM IV clinical criteria for maladaptive substance dependence [55]. There are difficulties in applying the criteria for dependence to the use of medication in a chronic illness. PD patients require daily use of DRT and are unable to stop it. However, patients with DDS have a pathological use, as overdosing is a main characteristic.

There is a severe impairment in social functioning, which is also affected by the disease but usually less intensively and later. The tolerance is difficult to apply in PD as the dose requirements increase with time as motor disability progresses. Patients with DDS have a compulsive pattern of DRT-seeking leading to the intake of very large total daily doses of levodopa equivalents in the early course of the disease. Bearn and colleagues applied a semi-structured questionnaire designed to distinguish adaptive therapeutic dependence from maladaptive dependence on DRT [55]. The most common unifying feature was the withdrawal dysphoria in the group with DDS. PD patients with DRT misuse report anxiety and depression when unmedicated, which was the reason given for drug-seeking behavior. Panic attack and psychic off symptoms may represent withdrawal phenomena due to recurrent depletion of levodopa in the mesolimbic regions [56]. Some patients with DDS also report euphoriant effects as a reason for excess use.

The prevalence of DDS is estimated between 3.4 and 4% [9, 57]. However, in a prospective study on 85 PD patients (candidates) for subthalamic nucleus (STN) deep brain stimulation (DBS), 14 patients (16%) fulfilled the DDS criteria [58]. Candidates for surgery are at risk for DDS as they usually have young age of onset, high DRT dosage with disabling dyskinesia. Furthermore, the therapeutic management is uneasy in this population, as long-term DRT reduction is incompatible without sacrificing motor benefits. The prevalence of behavioral compulsions (hypersexuality, excessive shopping, or pathological gambling) and punding in DDS patients was found to be, respectively, 64% and 88% [45].

Compulsive DRT use is more prevalent in men with younger age of PD onset [9, 32]. Independent predictors for DDS are current alcohol intake, depressive symptoms, and novelty-seeking personality traits [59]. Other predisposing factors may be past history of drug abuse and family history of psychiatric problems [9, 57].

Short-acting medications such as subcutaneous apomorphine or fast-acting formulations of L-dopa (dispersible oral formulation) are more prone to compulsive use [9, 47, 54, 59]. Higher levodopa dosage with or without adjunctive dopamine agonist therapy in association with frequent need for "rescue" medication may be predictive for the development of DDS. DDS on dopamine agonist monotherapy is very rare [47, 60].

Physiopathology

Neuroanatomy and Sensitization Theory

There is a general consensus that dopamine is pivotal in the development and persistence of addiction [46, 61, 62]. It has been suggested that the use of dopamine in PD might abnormally

Fig. 29.1 Dopamine release
within the ventral striatal
reward circuit (from Evans
and Lees [48])

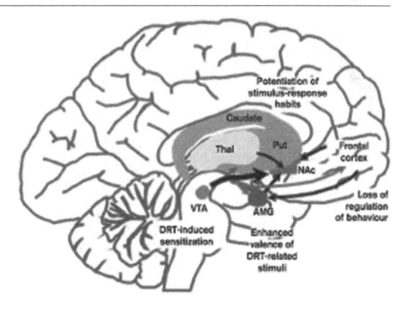

stimulate the mesolimbic pathways leading to behavioral disorders similar to that associated with psychostimulant addiction. The pathophysiologic processes underlying behavioral or substance addiction in PD are not clear. There is a debate whether behavioral and chemical addictions share the same substrates [3, 32, 63]. There may be a common pathophysiologic basis for the observed features as DDS, punding, and ICD are linked by their reward or incentive-based and repetitive nature.

Parkinson's disease is characterized primarily by loss of dopaminergic neurons in the substantia nigra pars compacta. In addition to the nigrostriatal motor pathway, dopaminergic neuronal circuitry also includes the mesolimbic and mesocortical systems, with fibers from the ventral tegmental area (VTA), which is relatively spared in PD, to the nucleus accumbens and frontal cortex. These neuronal circuits are involved in memory, reward and motivation and may be implicated in the pathogenesis of dopamine-related compulsions. Dopamine input to the nucleus accumbens is central to the sensitization to the motivational effects of drugs. It has been hypothesized that an overstimulation of the mesolimbic system may promote the development of these reward behaviors (Fig. 29.1). In PD, patients with compulsive medication use have enhanced dopamine release in the ventral striatum after taking levodopa in an 11C-raclopride PET study [3]. These results suggest that VTA neurons releasing dopamine in the ventral striatum might be sensitized to exogenous dopamine in DDS patients and support the neural sensitization theory [47, 64]. Similar observations have been made in the striatum of rodents after behavioral sensitization to psychostimulants [61]. Behavioral sensitization, which is an increase in behavioral drug effects with repeated exposure, reflects an increase in the incentive salience assigned to a drug. This leads to compulsive drug "wanting" dissociated from drug "liking." In line with this

finding, Evans and colleagues reported that the subjective "wanting" but not the "liking" of L-dopa was correlated with the ventral striatal dopamine release [3]. Furthermore, drug "wanting" predicted levels of drug use in DDS patients. This reflects an incentive salience for levodopa use rather than a rewarding hedonic impact. The effect of chronic pulsatile dopaminergic medication has been postulated to underlie dyskinesia. Levodopa-induced dyskinesia is generally thought to be also a sensitization phenomenon. The development of dyskinesia in animal models of PD requires the same drug schedule as that necessary to induce psychomotor sensitization by psychostimulants [65]. It has been hypothesized that pulsatile dopaminergic medications may induce dyskinesia by sensitization of the dorsal striatum and DRT-related compulsions by sensitization of the ventral striatum.

The Role of Dopamine Receptors and Dopaminergic Medications

The administration of dopaminergic medications may be associated with DRC-related compulsions by several mechanisms. ICDs are strongly associated with dopamine agonists as a class but not with any specific agonists [12, 13, 17]. Patients without PD taking dopamine agonists for restless leg syndrome, multiple system atrophy, or multiple sclerosis also develop ICD or punding [66–69]. The association between dopamine agonist therapy and ICDs has been attributed to an excessive stimulation off particular dopamine receptors, thus resulting in aberrant activity of specific regions. Dopamine D3 receptors are found predominantly in limbic regions, whereas D1 and D2 receptors are widely expressed in all dopaminergic areas. Dopamine agonists have a relative affinity for D3 receptors.

Phasic release of dopamine from the VTA to the nucleus accumbens occurs with unexpected reward with variation according to reward magnitude [70]. Conversely, phasic suppression occurs when an expected reward is not received. In contrast to phasic release, tonic dopamine release occurs with anticipation of the greatest reward uncertainty. High uncertainty such as slot machines or other gambling may itself be rewarding [70]. Thus, excessive levodopa doses in DDS, with its pulsatile (or phasic) stimulation or postsynaptic dopamine receptors tonic stimulation with dopamine agonists may result in loss of the physiological pattern of dopamine activity. This interference with the pattern of dopamine release may increase the expected value of stimuli by indicating reward in the absence of reward or by the absence of feedback indicating the lack of reward [20].

Underlying Vulnerability and Parkinson's Disease-Related Factors

Individual Risk Factors

The occurrence of DRT-related compulsions in a small subgroup of PD patients suggests an underlying susceptibility. It remains unclear what predispose some PD patients to develop ICDs, DDS, or punding while determination of risk factors may help to prevent the troubles. In PD, ICD and DDS are associated with a younger age of onset of the disease [9, 14, 19, 20]. The relations between age and punding are less striking and vary within the different studies [36, 45]. However, the greater use of dopamine agonists and higher dosage of levodopa equivalent medications in this group of patients may act as confounder. The link between disinhibitory behaviors and younger age could reflect an age-related susceptibility. Concerning personality traits, "novelty-seeking," impulsivity, and risk-taking are correlated with ICDs in PD and non-PD populations [20, 71] and with DDS in PD patients [59]. Higher impulsivity score is predictive for the occurrence of punding or ICDs [45, 72]. It has been hypothesized that although dopaminergic medications return dorsal striatum dopamine levels to more normal levels improving motor impairment, the relative preservation of ventral striatal dopamine may result in overdosing the ventral striatum and ventral prefrontal cortex [32, 73]. This may increase impulsivity in PD patients. Gender is also influencing the prevalence of ICDs and it seems that especially hypersexuality and gambling are more frequent in men than in women even if some sociologic bias may exist [12, 74]. Punding seems independent from sex while compulsive eating and weight gain may be more frequent in women [60].

Genetic factors are estimated to contribute to 50% of the vulnerability to substance addiction [75]. Genetic factors are associated with younger illness onset in PD. A history of previous addiction and/or alcohol abuse seems much more frequent in PDs patients and ICDs or DDS [12, 20, 47, 76]. A young age of onset and a personal or a family history of mood disorder have also been strongly associated with DDS and ICDs [12, 20, 57, 59].

Underlying potential predisposing personal, genetic, and disease subtype-related factors need to be assessed in order to prevent the emergence of these disabling behaviors in Parkinson's disease.

Dopaminergic Treatment as a Risk Factor

ICDs are strongly associated with dopamine agonists' intake often in the first months following initiation or after a dosage increase [13, 16, 19–21]. Initial reports incriminated mainly pramipexole, a dopamine receptor agonist with a high D3 receptor affinity, as a causing agent of ICDs but further reports have demonstrated that all the dopamine receptor agonists can induce the same disorders. ICDs are for most of the authors dose-dependent but in some patients dose reduction may not be sufficient and patients must stop the treatment intake. This fact may suggest an "all-or-none" phenomenon rather than a dosage-dependent mechanism as suggested by the occurrence in patients with restless leg syndrome of increased gambling (6%) and sexuality (4%) while they are treated with very low dosages of dopamine agonist associated or not with levodopa [24]. A few reports suggest that levodopa may induce ICDs in PD patients [26, 77].

DDS is related to short-acting dopaminergic medications such as levodopa or apomorphine subcutaneous injections [59]. Punding does not appear to be related to any type of dopaminergic treatment.

Management

There are limited data to support any particular therapeutic strategy for the management of DRT-related compulsions. Several approaches should be considered.

Prevention: Identifying Patients at Risk

The management of DRT-related compulsions consists of patients and caretaker education. The potential for behavioral addictions should be discussed with patients and caretaker in the context of potential side effects of the medication for Parkinson's disease before the initiation of treatment especially with dopamine agonists. Each case should be systematically evaluated for the presence of DRT misuse, ICD, or other signs consistent with punding or DDS.

Patients should be inquired about their pastimes and the quality of their sleep [32]. Most patients with DRT-related compulsions have sleep reduction secondary to nocturnal activities. Particular attention should be given to patients with dopamine agonists and higher dosage of L-dopa. The identification of patients at greater risk, which include younger age at PD onset, being male, depressed mood, increased novelty-seeking trait and personal or familial history of alcohol use, would allow for a closer follow-up [20, 57, 59, 78].

Pharmacological Approach

Several case reports and series indicate improvement of ICDs with decrease or discontinuation of dopamine agonist therapy or switching to a different agonist [13, 19, 24, 60, 79]. A recent study assessed the long-term outcome of ICDs in Parkinson's disease. At a mean follow-up period of 29 months, 83% of the patients no longer met the ICD criteria after cessation or reduction of dopamine agonist, without worsening in motor symptoms [80]. Punding behaviors may improve with reduction or cessation of dopamine agonist or levodopa [35, 43]. DDS requires enforced medication reduction with the cooperation among physicians (neurologist, psychiatrist, general practitioner) and family members or healthcare providers [10]. The lowest doses of DRT that control the motor symptoms should be used with cessation of rescue dose (subcutaneous apomorphine or liquid form of levodopa) [48]. Avoiding pulsatile dopaminergic stimulation by apomorphine subcutaneous infusion can be a successful compromise in some patients [9]. However, ICD and punding may sometimes be resistant to dopaminergic therapy reduction. The prognosis of DDS is generally poor with high rate of relapse [47, 59].

There are several case reports of various medications tried in order to control the DRT-related compulsions. However, data are limited and do not permit treatment guidelines. The atypical antipsychotics have been found to be of some benefit. Clozapine successfully treat hypersexuality and punding [35, 42]. In patients with DDS and/or punding, use of quetiapine was found to reduce or stop punding [36, 37]. However, quetiapine can also trigger punding [40]. Valproate, lithium, and selective serotonine reuptake inhibitors have been used successfully with PD patients with ICD and/or punding and/or DRT addiction [12, 26, 36]. Antiandrogen (cyproterone) may be considered for severe hypersexuality [33]. Topiramate was associated with the resolution of ICDs (pathological gambling, hypersexuality, excessive shopping, and binge eating) in seven PD patients [81]. Amantadine was found to be effective for severe punding in one patient [82]. However, amantadine has also been linked with ICDs [13] (Table 29.1).

Nonpharmacological Approach

Several reports note improved behaviors with multiple therapeutic approaches [23]. Counseling, including Gamblers Anonymous can be useful in some patients [13]. Restricting money or Internet access, requesting to be on the casino-banned list can have beneficial effects. Restriction in medications in patients with DDS and/or punding has been advocated [9, 36, 47]. Family involvement and psychotherapy may be beneficial.

Surgical Treatment

STN DBS, an effective therapy for treating disabled parkinsonian patients improves motor impairment and reduces dopaminergic treatment with a long-term efficacy [83]. However, data regarding its effects on addiction in PD remain controversial. Some authors emphasized the deleterious effects of STN DBS on behavioral disorder including DDS and ICDs. Houeto and colleagues reported two cases with worsening levodopa addictions after STN DBS [84]. Romito reported five cases with transient postoperative hypersexuality that occurred although DRT reduction [85]. PD patients may develop pathological gambling after STN DBS although these behaviors can be improved with change in parameters setting [86, 87]. However, STN DBS can be effective in controlling behavioral and DRT addiction in some patients. Pathological gambling, associated in some patients with DDS, has been reported to improve postoperatively [76, 80, 88, 89]. Two patients with severe DDS associated with hypersexuality had a dramatic improvement of their disruptive behaviors after STN DBS coupled with medication reduction [90]. In a recent prospective study, 11 out of 12 patients fulfilling DDS criteria had a complete resolution of their DRT addiction after STN DBS [91].

Some hypothesis may explain the efficacy of surgical therapy of these DRT-related compulsions [88]: (1) the massive reduction in DRT with dopamine agonist withdrawal, (2) the replacement of pulsatile stimulation with chronic stimulation which may decrease neural sensitization (as it does with dyskinesia), (3) the relative specificity of DBS for motor regions compared to medications which overflow all the brain and its dopamine receptors, (4) the improvement of nonmotor fluctuations with less mood swings, and (5) a possible direct effect of the STN on addiction. Concerning this last hypothesis, some recent data on animals showed that STN lesions reduced the rewarding efficacy of cocaine [92]. The mechanism by which such changes occurred remains to investigate.

Table 29.1   Diagnostic criteria for DRT-related compulsions (from Ferrara and Stacy [10])

Diagnostic criteria for pathological gambling [11]

A. Persistent and recurrent maladaptive gambling behavior as indicated by five or more of the following

   1. Is preoccupied with gambling (e.g. preoccupied with reliving past gambling experiences, handicapping or planning the next venture, or thinking of ways to get money with which to gamble)

   2. Needs to gamble with increasing amount of money in order to achieve the desired excitement

   3. Has repeated unsuccessful efforts to control, cut back or stop gambling

   4. Is restless or irritable when attempting to cut down or stop gambling

   5. Gables as a way of escaping from problems or of relieving a dysphoric mood (e.g. feelings of helplessness, guilt, anxiety, depression)

   6. After loosing money gambling, often returns another day to get even ("chasing" one's losses)

   7. Lies to family members, therapists, and others to conceal the extent of involvement with gambling

   8. Has committed illegal acts such as forgery, fraud, theft, or embezzlement to finance gambling

   9. Has jeopardized or lost a significant relationship, job, or educational or career opportunity because of gambling

   10. Relies on others to provide money to relieve a desperate financial situation caused by gambling

B. The gambling behavior is not better accounted for by a manic episode.

Proposed diagnostic criteria for pathological hypersexuality [12]

A. The sexual thoughts or behaviors are excessive or an atypical change from baseline marked by one or more of the following:

   1. Maladaptive preoccupation with sexual thoughts

   2. Inappropriately or excessively requesting sex from spouse or partner

   3. Habitual promiscuity

   4. Compulsive masturbation

   5. Telephone sex lines or pornography

   6. Paraphilias

B. The behavior must have persisted for at least 1 month

C. The behavior causes at least one of the following:

   1. Marked distress

   2. Attempts to control thoughts or behaviors are unsuccessful or result in marked anxiety or distress

   3. Are time-consuming

   4. Interfere significantly with social or occupational functioning

D. The behavior does not occur exclusively during period of hypomania or mania

E. If all criteria except C are fulfilled, the disorder is subsyndromal

Proposed diagnostic criteria for compulsive buying [12]

A. Maladaptive preoccupation with buying or shopping, or maladaptive buying or shopping impulses or behaviors, as indicated by at least one of the following:

   1. Frequent preoccupation with buying or impulses to buy that is/are experienced as irresistible, intrusive, and/or senseless

   2. Frequent buying of more that can be afforded, frequent buying of items that are not needed, or shaping for longer periods of time than intended

B. The buying preoccupations, impulses or behaviors cause marked distress, are time-consuming, significantly interfere with social or occupational functioning or results in financial problems (e.g. indebtedness or bankruptcy)

C. The excessive buying or shopping behavior does not occur exclusively during period of hypomania or mania

Proposed diagnostic criteria for dopamine dysregulation syndrome [9]

A. Parkinson's disease with documented levodopa responsiveness

B. Need for increasing doses o dopamine-related therapy (DRT) in excess of those normally required to relieve parkinsonian symptoms

C. Pattern of pathological use: expressed need for increased DRT in the presence of excessive and significant dyskinesia, despite being "on," drug-hoarding or drug-seeking behavior, unwillingness to reduce DRT, or absence of painful dystonia

D. Impairment in social and occupational functioning: fights, violent behavior, loss of friends, absence from work, loss of job, legal difficulties, arguments, or difficulties with family

E. Development of hypomanic, manic, or cyclothymic affective syndrome in relation with DRT

F. Development of a withdrawal state characterized by dysphoria, depression, irritability, and anxiety on reducing level of DRT

G. Duration of disturbance of at least 6 months

Conclusion

There is an extensive evidence to link addiction and dopamine and Parkinson's disease provides a unique condition with a chronic disturbance of dopamine regulation. There is an increasing recognition of behavioral and DRT addiction in a significant minority of PD patients. ICDs, punding, and DDS may result in devastating physical, social, and financial repercussions. The anatomic substrate for these behaviors is not fully elucidated but clearly involves changes in the dopaminergic pathways within the mesolimbic brain reward circuits.

Underlying potential predisposing personal, genetic and disease subtype-related factors need to be assessed. The optimal management of DRT-related compulsions in PD patients is not defined yet and awaits prospective data. Prevention is obviously most important. Clinicians treating PD patients should be aware of these behavioral disorders and systematically enquire about risk factors. While reduction of dopaminergic therapy is the main treatment strategy, other nondopaminergic agents, psychosocial interventions, and STN DBS are worth considering. However, these behaviors may be incompletely responsive and relapses are frequent. Active areas of research are done to determine the true prevalence, predisposing factors, and future treatment strategy for these addictive behaviors in Parkinson's disease.

References

1. Parkinson J. An essay on the shaking palsy. London: Sherwood Neely & Jones; 1817.
2. Menza M, Golbe L, Cody RA, Forman N. Dopamine-related personality traits in Parkinson's disease. Neurology. 1993;43:505–8.
3. Evans AH, Pavese N, Lawrence AD, et al. Compulsive drug use linked to sensitized ventral striatal dopamine transmission. Ann Neurol. 2006;5:852–8.
4. Jacobs H, Heberlein I, Vieregge A, Vieregge P. Personality traits in young patients with Parkinson's disease. Acta Neurol Scand. 2001;103:82–7.
5. Ishihara L, Brayne C. What is the evidence for a premorbid Parkinsonian personality: a systematic review. Mov Disord. 2006;21:1066–72.
6. Uitti RJ, Tanner C, Rajput AH, et al. Hypersexuality with antiparkinsonian therapy. Clin Neuropharmacol. 1989;12:375–83.
7. Vogel HP, Schiffter R. Hypersexualty—a complication of dopaminergic therapy in Parkinson's disease. Pharmacopsychiatria. 1983;16:107–10.
8. Friedman J. Punding on levodopa. Biol Psychiatry. 1994;36:350–1.
9. Giovannoni G, O'Sullivan JD, Turner K, Manson AJ, Lees AJ. Hedonistic homeostatic dysregulation in patients with Parkinson's disease on dopamine replacement therapies. J Neurol Neurosurg Psychiatry. 2000;68(4):423–8.
10. Ferrara JM, Stacy M. Impulse-control disorders in Parkinson's disease. CNS Spectr. 2008;13(8):690–8.
11. American Psychiatric Association. Diagnostic and statistical manual of mental disorders (DSM-IV-TR). 4th ed. Washington, DC: American Psychiatric Publishing; 2000.
12. Voon V, Hassan K, Zurowski M, de Souza M, Thomsen T, Fox S, Lang AE, Miyasaki J. Prevalence of repetitive and reward-seeking behaviors in Parkinson disease. Neurology. 2006;67:1254–7.
13. Weintraub D, Siderowf AD, Potenza MN, Goveas J, Morales KH, Duda JE, Moberg PJ, Stern MB. Association of dopamine agonist use with impulse control disorders in Parkinson disease. Arch Neurol. 2006;7:969–73.
14. Giladi N, Weitzman N, Schreiber S, Shabtai H, Peretz C. New onset heightened interest or drive for gambling, shopping, eating or sexual activity in patients with Parkinson's disease: the role of dopamine agonist treatment and age at motor symptoms onset. J Psychopharmacol. 2007;21(5):501–6.
15. Ondo WG, Lai D. Predictors of impulsivity and reward seeking behavior with dopamine agonists. Parkinsonism Relat Disord. 2008;14(1):28–32.
16. Voon V, Hassa K, Zurowski M, et al. Prospective prevalence of pathological gambling and medication association in Parkinson's disease. Neurology. 2006;66:1750–2.
17. Avanzi M, Baratti M, Cabrini S, Uber E, Brighetti G, Bonfà F. Prevalence of pathological gambling in patients with Parkinson's disease. Mov Disord. 2006;21(12):2068–72.
18. Shaffer HJ, Hall MN, Vander Bilt J. Estimating the prevalence of disordered gambling behavior in the United States and Canada: a research synthesis. Am J Public Health. 1999;89(9):1369–76.
19. Gallagher DA, O'Sullivan SS, Evans AH, Lees AJ, Schrag A. Pathological gambling in Parkinson's disease: risk factors and differences from dopamine dysregulation. An analysis of published case series. Mov Disord. 2007;22(12):1757–63.
20. Voon V, Fox S. Medication-related impulse control and repetitive behaviours in Parkinson disease. Arch Neurol. 2007;64(2):1089–96.
21. Pontone G, Williams JR, Bassett SS, Marsh L. Clinical features associated with impulse control disorders in Parkinson disease. Neurology. 2006;7:1258–61.
22. Larner AJ. Medical hazards of the Internet: gambling in Parkinson's disease. Mov Disord. 2006;21:1789.
23. GalpernWR WR, Stacy M. Management of impulse control disorders in Parkinson's disease. Curr Treat Options Neurol. 2007;9(3):189–97.
24. Driver-Dunckley E, Samanta J, Stacy M. Pathological gambling associated with dopamine agonist therapy in Parkinson's disease. Neurology. 2003;61(3):422–3.
25. Aarsland D, Alves G, Larsen JP. Disorders of motivation, sexual conduct, and sleep in Parkinson's disease. Adv Neurol. 2005;96:56–64.
26. Klos KJ, Bower JH, Josephs KA, Matsumoto JY, Ahlskog JE. Pathological hypersexuality predominantly linked to adjuvant dopamine agonist therapy in Parkinson's disease and multiple system atrophy. Parkinsonism Relat Disord. 2005;6:381–6.
27. Gisselmann A. Hypersexualité et L-dopa. Nouv Presse Med. 1973;2:1616.
28. Shapiro M, Chang Y, Munson SK, Okun MS, Fernandez HH. Hypersexuality and paraphilia induced by selegiline in Parkinson's disease: report of 2 cases. Parkinsonism Relat Disord. 2006;12(6):392–5.
29. Koran LM, Faber RJ, Aboujaoude E, Large MD, Serpe RT. Estimated prevalence of compulsive buying behavior in the United States. Am J Psychiatry. 2006;163(10):1806–12.
30. Sensi M, Eleopra R, Cavallo MA, et al. Explosive-aggressive behavior related to bilateral subthalamic stimulation. Parkinsonism Relat Disord. 2004;10(4):247–51.
31. Machado AG, Hiremath GK, Salazar F, Rezai AR. Fracture of subthalamic nucleus deep brain stimulation hardware as a result of compulsive manipulation: case report. Neurosurgery. 2005;57(6):E131.
32. Lim SY, Evans AH, Miyasaki JM. Impulse control and related disorders in Parkinson's disease: review. Ann NY Acad Sci. 2008;1142:85–107.
33. Avanzi M, Baratti M, Cabrini S, Uber E, Brighetti G, Bonfà F. The thrill of reckless driving in patients with Parkinson's disease: an additional behavioural phenomenon in dopamine dysregulation syndrome? Parkinsonism Relat Disord. 2008;14(3):257–8.
34. Rylander G. Psychoses and the punding and choreiform syndromes in addiction to central stimulant drugs. Psychiatr Neurol Neurochir. 1972;75(3):203–12.
35. Fernandez HH, Friedman JH. Punding on L-dopa. Mov Disord. 1999;14(5):836–8.
36. Evans AH, Katzenschlager R, Paviour D, O'Sullivan JD, Appel S, Lawrence AD, Lees AJ. Punding in Parkinson's disease: its relation to the dopamine dysregulation syndrome. Mov Disord. 2004;4:397–405.

37. Fasano A, Elia AE, Soleti F, Guidubaldi A, Bentivoglio AR. Punding and computer addiction in Parkinson's disease. Mov Disord. 2006;21(8):1217–8.

38. Micheli F, Fernandez Pardal M, Fahn S. What is it? Case 3, 1991: moaning in a man with Parkinsonian signs. Mov Disord. 1991;6(4): 376–8.

39. Bonvin C, Horvath J, Christe B, Landis T, Burkhard PR. Compulsive singing: another aspect of punding in Parkinson's disease. Ann Neurol. 2007;62(5):525–8.

40. Miwa H, Kondo T. Increased writing activity in Parkinson's disease: a punding-like behavior? Parkinsonism Relat Disord. 2005; 11(5):323–5.

41. O'Sullivan SS, Evans AH, Lees AJ. Punding in Parkinson's disease. Pract Neurol. 2007;7(6):397–9.

42. Kurlan R. Disabling repetitive behaviors in Parkinson's disease. Mov Disord. 2004;19(4):433–7.

43. Miyasaki JM, Al Hassan K, Lang AE, Voon V. Punding prevalence in Parkinson's disease. Mov Disord. 2007;22(8):1179–81.

44. Voon V. Repetition, repetition, and repetition: compulsive and punding behaviors in Parkinson's disease. Mov Disord. 2004; 19(4):367–70.

45. Lawrence AJ, Blackwell AD, Barker RA, Spagnolo F, Clark L, Aitken MR, Sahakian BJ. Predictors of punding in Parkinson's disease: results from a questionnaire survey. Mov Disord. 2007; 16:2339–45.

46. Koob GF, Le Moal M. Drug abuse: hedonic homeostatic dysegulation. Science. 1997;278:52–8.

47. Lawrence AD, Evans AH, Lees AJ. Compulsive use of dopamine replacement therapy in Parkinson's disease: reward systems gone awry? Lancet Neurol. 2003;2:595–604.

48. Evans AH, Lees AJ. Dopamine dysregulation syndrome in Parkinson's disease. Curr Opin Neurol. 2004;17(4):393–8.

49. Nausieda PA. Sinemet "abusers". Clin Neuropharmacol. 1985; 8(4):318–27.

50. Merims D, Galili-Mosberg R, Melamed E. Is there addiction to levodopa in patients with Parkinson's disease? Mov Disord. 2000;15(5):1014–6.

51. Borek LL, Friedman JH. Levodopa addiction in idiopathic Parkinson disease. Neurology. 2005;65(9):150.

52. Sanchez-Ramos J. The straight dope on addiction to dopamimetic drugs. Mov Disord. 2002;17(1):223–5.

53. Witjas T, Kaphan E, Azulay JP, Blin O, Ceccaldi M, Pouget J, Poncet M, Ali Chérif A. Nonmotor fluctuations in Parkinson's disease: frequent and disabling. Neurology. 2002;59(3):408–13.

54. Téllez C, Bustamante ML, Toro P, Venegas P. Addiction to apomorphine: a clinical case-centred discussion. Addiction. 2006;101(11): 1662–5.

55. Bearn J, Evans A, Kelleher M, Turner K, Lees A. Recognition of a dopamine replacement therapy dependence syndrome in Parkinson's disease: a pilot study. Drug Alcohol Depend. 2004;76(3):305–10.

56. Merims D, Giladi N. Dopamine dysregulation syndrome, addiction and behavioral changes in Parkinson's disease. Parkinsonism Relat Disord. 2008;14(4):273–80.

57. Pezzella FR, Colosimo C, Vanacore N, et al. Prevalence and clinical features of hedonistic dysregulation syndromein Parkinson's disease. Mov Disord. 2005;20:77–81.

58. Azulay JP, Witjas T, Cantiniaux S, Régis J, Péragut JC. Dopaminergic dysregulation syndrome in Parkinson's disease : a prospective study in patients treated with deep brain stimulation. Neurology. 2008;P04.024.

59. Evans AH, Lawrence AD, Potts J, Appel S, Lees AJ. Factors influencing susceptibility to compulsive dopaminergic drug use in Parkinson disease. Neurology. 2005;65:1570–4.

60. Nirenberg MJ, Waters C. Compulsive eating and weight gain related to dopamine agonist use. Mov Disord. 2006;21:524–9.

61. Robinson TE, Berridge KC. The psychology and neurobiology of addiction: an incentive-sensitization view. Addiction. 2000;95 Suppl 2:S91–117.

62. Franken IH, Booij J, van den Brink W. The role of dopamine in human addiction: from reward to motivated attention. Eur J Pharmacol. 2005;526(1–3):199–206.

63. Potenza MN. Should addictive disorders include non-substance-related conditions? Addiction. 2006;101 Suppl 1:142–51.

64. Bonci A, Singh V. Dopamine dysregulation syndrome in Parkinson's disease patients: from reward to penalty. Ann Neurol. 2006;59(5): 733–4.

65. Graybiel AM, Canales JJ, Capper-Loup C. Levodopa-induced dyskinesias and dopamine-dependent stereotypies: a new hypothesis. Trends Neurosci. 2000;23(10 Suppl):S71–7.

66. Tippmann-Peikert M, Park JG, Boeve BF, Shepard JW, Silber MH. Pathologic gambling in patients with restless legs syndrome treated with dopaminergic agonists. Neurology. 2007;68(4):301–3.

67. Driver-Dunckley ED, Noble BN, Hentz JG, Evidente VG, Caviness JN, Parish J, Krahn L, Adler CH. Gambling and increased sexual desire with dopaminergic medications in restlesslegs syndrome. Clin Neuropharmacol. 2007;5:249–55.

68. McKeon A, Josephs KA, Klos KJ, Hecksel K, Bower JH, Michael Bostwick J, Eric Ahlskog J. Unusual compulsive behaviors primarily related to dopamine agonist therapy in Parkinson's disease and multiple system atrophy. Parkinsonism Relat Disord. 2007;13(8): 516–9.

69. Evans AH, Butzkueven H. Dopamine agonist-induced pathological gambling in restless legs syndrome due to multiple sclerosis. Mov Disord. 2007;22(4):590–1.

70. Fiorillo CD, Tobler PN, Schultz W. Discrete coding of reward probability and uncertainty by dopamine neurons. Science. 2003; 299(5614):1898–902.

71. Brewer JA, Potenza MN. The neurobiology and genetics of impulse control disorders: relationships to drug addictions. Biochem Pharmacol. 2008;75:63–75.

72. Isaias IU, Siri C, Cilia R, De Gaspari D, Pezzoli G, Antonini A. The relationship between impulsivity and impulse control disorders in Parkinson's disease. Mov Disord. 2008;23(3):411–5.

73. Cools R. Dopaminergic modulation of cognitive function-implications for L-DOPA treatment in Parkinson's disease. Neurosci Biobehav Rev. 2006;30(1):1–23.

74. Singh A, Kandimala G, Dewey Jr RB, O'Suilleabhain P. Risk factors for pathologic gambling and other compulsions among Parkinson's disease patients taking dopamine agonists. J Clin Neurosci. 2007;12:1178–81.

75. Volkow N, Li TK. The neuroscience of addiction. Nat Neurosci. 2005;8(11):1429–30.

76. Molina JA, Sainz-Artiga MJ, Fraile A, et al. Pathological gambling in Parkinson's disease: a behavioural manifestation of pharmacologic treatment. Mov Disord. 2000;15:869–72.

77. Drapier D, Drapier S, Sauleau P, Derkinderen P, Damier P, Allain H, Vérin M, Millet B. Pathological gambling secondary to dopaminergic therapy in Parkinson's disease. Psychiatry Res. 2006; 144(2–3):241–4.

78. Silveira-Moriyama L, Evans AH, Katzenschlager R, Lees AJ. Punding and dyskinesias. Mov Disord. 2006;21:1214–7.

79. Dodd ML, Klos KJ, Bower JH, Geda YE, Josephs KA, Ahlskog JE. Pathological gambling caused by drugs used to treat Parkinson disease. Arch Neurol. 2005;62(9):1377–81.

80. Mamikonyan E, Siderowf AD, Duda JE, Potenza MN, Horn S, Stern MB, Weintraub D. Long-term follow-up of impulse control disorders in Parkinson's disease. Mov Disord. 2008;23(1):75–80.

81. Bermejo PE. Topiramate in managing impulse control disorders in Parkinson's disease. Parkinsonism Relat Disord. 2008;14(5): 448–9.

82. Kashihara K, Imamura T. Amantadine may reverse punding in Parkinson's disease–observation in a patient. Mov Disord. 2008; 23(1):129–30.

83. Krack P, Batir A, Van Blercom N, et al. Five-year follow-up of bilateral stimulation of the subthalamic nucleus in advanced Parkinson's disease. N Engl J Med. 2003;349(20):1925–34.

84. Houeto JL, Mesnage V, Mallet L, et al. Behavioural disorders, Parkinson's disease and sub-thalamic stimulation. J Neurol Neurosurg Psychiatry. 2002;72:701–7.

85. Romito LM, Raja M, Daniele A, et al. Transient mania with hypersexuality after surgery for high frequency stimulation of the subthalamic nucleus in Parkinson's disease. Mov Disord. 2002;17(6):1371–4.

86. Lu C, Bharmal A, Suchowersky O. Gambling and Parkinson disease. Arch Neurol. 2006;63(2):298.

87. Smeding HM, Goudriaan AE, Foncke EM, Schuurman PR, Speelman JD, Schmand B. Pathological gambling after bilateral subthalamic nucleus stimulation in Parkinson disease. J Neurol Neurosurg Psychiatry. 2007;78(5):517–9.

88. Ardouin C, Voon V, Worbe Y, et al. Pathological gambling in Parkinson's disease improves on chronic subthalamic nucleus stimulation. Mov Disord. 2006;21(11):1941–6.

89. Bandini F, Primavera A, Pizzorno M, Cocito L. Using STN DBS and medication reduction as a strategy to treat pathological gambling in Parkinson's disease. Parkinsonism Relat Disord. 2007; 13(6):369–71.

90. Witjas T, Baunez C, Henry JM, Delfini M, Regis J, Cherif AA, Peragut JC, Azulay JP. Addiction in Parkinson's disease: impact of subthalamic nucleus deep brain stimulation. Mov Disord. 2005;20(8):1052–5.

91. Azulay JP, Witjas T, Cantiniaux S, Régis J, Péragut JC. Dopaminergic dysregulation syndrome in Parkinson's disease: a prospective study in patients treated with deep brain stimulation. Neurology. 2008;P04.024.

92. Baunez C, Dias C, Cador M, Amalric M. The subthalamic nucleus exerts opposite control on cocaine and 'natural' rewards. Nat Neurosci. 2005;8(4):484–9.

Sleep and Sleep Disorders

30

Timothy Roehrs and Thomas Roth

Abstract

Nearly all drugs of abuse and alcohol have considerable effects on sleep efficiency, sleep continuity, sleep stages, and consequent next-day alertness. It has been hypothesized that such drug effects on sleep and wake function may act as contributing factors in maintaining compulsive and excessive drug use, as well as factors that increase the risk for relapse. Alcohol at high doses disrupts sleep continuity and suppresses REM sleep. In abstinent alcoholics, a REM sleep disturbance is predictive of relapse. Stimulants, which have daytime alerting effects, have been shown to increase alertness and wakefulness at night, and suppress REM sleep. Analgesics have been found to decrease REM sleep and total sleep time, as well as increase daytime sleepiness. Hallucinogens have varying effects on sleep. MDMA has been shown to reduce sleep time without having major effects on REM sleep, whereas marijuana has been found to decrease REM sleep while increasing slow wave sleep. Older sedative-hypnotics like the barbiturates are also REM suppressant. In fact, virtually all drugs of abuse have REM suppressant properties, at least acutely. In contrast, the newer sedative-hypnotics (i.e., the benzodiazepine receptor agonists) which have a low abuse liability have been shown to have little effect on REM sleep.

Learning Objectives
- Nearly all drugs of abuse and alcohol affect sleep efficiency, sleep continuity, sleep stages, and consequent next-day alertness
- These sleep and daytime alertness alterations, although not the primary reinforcing mechanism, function as contributing factors in initiating and maintaining drug abuse
- The clinician must determine whether chronic use of sleep or alertness altering drugs is therapy-seeking or drug-seeking behavior

T. Roehrs, Ph.D. (✉) • T. Roth
Sleep Disorders and Research Center, Henry Ford Health System, 2799 West Grand Blvd, CPF-3, Detroit, MI 48202, USA

Department of Psychiatry and Behavioral Neurosciences, School of Medicine, Wayne State University, Detroit, MI, USA
e-mail: TARoehrs@aol.com

Introduction

Alcohol and all drugs of abuse have effects on sleep efficiency and continuity, as well as sleep stages (e.g., most typically suppressing REM sleep) and consequent next-day alertness. It has been suggested that these sleep and daytime alertness alterations, although not the primary reinforcing mechanism, function as contributing factors in initiating and maintaining drug abuse and as factors that increase the risk for relapse. Except for alcohol little is known about the effects of other drugs of abuse on prevalent sleep disorders such

J.C. Verster et al. (eds.), *Drug Abuse and Addiction in Medical Illness: Causes, Consequences and Treatment*, DOI 10.1007/978-1-4614-3375-0_30, © Springer Science+Business Media, LLC 2012

as sleep-disordered breathing, restless legs/periodic leg movements (RLS/PLMS), and primary insomnia. After briefly reviewing the normal physiology of sleep and describing the more common primary sleep disorders relevant to drugs of abuse, this chapter will discuss the known effects of alcohol and drugs of abuse on sleep and alertness. The role these sleep and alertness alterations play in initiating and maintaining alcohol and drug abuse will be discussed.

Normal and Pathological Sleep

Normal NREM and REM Sleep

While sleep is a biologically motivated behavior, sleep research made its major advances after the discovery of the electrophysiological correlates of sleep, especially REM sleep. The simultaneous recording of the electroencephalogram (EEG), the electro-oculogram (EOG), and the electromyogram (EMG) are the accepted standard measures of sleep state and waking. In contrast to the low voltage (10–30 µV) and fast frequency (16–35 Hz) of activated wakefulness, the cortical EEG of relaxed, eyes-closed, wakefulness is characterized by increased voltage (20–40 µV) and an 8–12 Hz frequency (alpha). During the transition to sleep, sometimes called drowsy sleep or transitional sleep, the EEG frequency becomes mixed while the voltage remains at the level of relaxed wakefulness. In NREM sleep, EEG voltage is further increased and frequency is further slowed. When arousal threshold is highest, the EEG of NREM sleep has a predominance of 0.5–2 Hz frequency with voltages of 75 µV and higher which is termed slow wave sleep. The EMG, highest in wakefulness, is gradually reduced during NREM sleep, although limb and body movements occur aperiodically during NREM and there is voluntary control of musculature. The EOGs of wakefulness reveal rapid eye movements, which during the transition to NREM sleep become slow and rolling. Importantly, the rolling eye movements mark the onset of the functional blindness all humans experience during sleep. The EOG becomes quiescent during slow wave sleep. After 90–120 min of NREM sleep, the healthy normal enters REM sleep.

The EOG of REM sleep, for which this sleep state is named, is characterized by rapid conjugate eye movements. The cortical EEG of REM reverts to the low voltage, mixed frequency pattern of drowsy sleep. The second defining characteristic of REM sleep is its skeletal muscle atonia, which is reflected in the EMG showing a total absence of muscle tone. The muscle atonia of REM sleep occurs through a process of postsynaptic inhibition of motor neurons at the dorsal horn of the spinal cord. Another important feature of REM sleep is its tonic and phasic components. The tonic components of

REM sleep are the persistent muscle atonia and the desynchronized EEG. The phasic components include bursts of eye movements occurring against a background of EOG quiescence. Coupled with the eye movement bursts are muscle twitches, typically involving peripheral muscles. These twitches are superimposed on the tonic muscle atonia of REM and probably reflect sympathetic drive breaking through the postsynaptic inhibition. The autonomic nervous system also shows activity with increased and more variable respiration, heart rate and blood pressure. It is important to recognize that while REM/NREM are differentiated by EOG, EMG, and EEG activity, all systems are influenced including sexual function, control of respiration, thermoregulation, mentation, and a host of other parameters. These two distinct brain states, NREM and REM sleep, cycle every 90–120 min for 4–5 cycles each night.

Common Sleep Disorders

Insomnia

Insomnia complaints are reported by approximately 33% of the population, and about 10% meet DSM IV diagnostic criteria for an insomnia disorder and these are predominantly women. It is defined by both the Diagnostic and Statistical Manual, Fourth Edition Revised (DSM-IVR) and the International Classification of Sleep Disorders (ICSD) as difficulty initiating sleep, maintaining sleep, or nonrestorative sleep that is associated with daytime distress or impairment. The sleep problem must be present 2–4 weeks depending on diagnostic system. Exclusion of other primary sleep disorders, psychiatric disorders, and medical disorders is required in both classifications for the diagnosis of primary insomnia. Behavioral treatment and pharmacotherapy with hypnotics are the two well documented effective treatment modalities.

Restless Legs/Periodic Leg Movement Disorder

Restless legs/periodic leg movement disorder (RLS/PLMD) is estimated to occur in 3–15% of the population. RLS is a complaint of an irresistible urge to move the leg because of a dysthesia, uncomfortable, crawling sensations in the lower limbs that mostly occurs in the evening and when at rest. RLS is typically accompanied, during sleep, by periodic leg movements (PLMs), rhythmic (15–45 s), slow (0.5 s) dorso-flexions of the leg at the knee during sleep. PLMs usually cease during REM sleep due to the atonia of REM sleep. RLS delays sleep onset and a rapid return to sleep after nighttime awakenings and PLMs fragment sleep with brief arousals. The first line of treatment is dopaminergic agonists. Benzodiazepine, anticonvulsants, and opiates are also reported as being effective as second- and third-line treatments.

Sleep-Related Breathing Disorders

Sleep-related breathing disorders are found in approximately 4–10% of the population with sleep apnea syndrome being present in 3% of the population, typically obese men (a 2:1 ratio). It is characterized by frequent 10–30 s episodes of apnea (e.g., complete airflow cessation) or hypopnea (e.g., reduced airflow). The respiratory disturbance is due to obstruction of the airway associated with excessive tissue in the airway, the reduced muscle tonus of NREM sleep, the atonia of REM sleep, and an altered metabolic control of breathing during sleep. Hypoxemia and EKG changes occur during events and brief arousals from sleep occur to break the obstruction, restore upper airway tone, and open the airway and allow for resaturation. These frequent arousals fragment sleep, disrupt its restorative capacity, and produce excessive daytime sleepiness. Apnea is associated with hypertension, stroke, and an increased risk of accidents. The most common treatment is continuous positive airway pressure (CPAP) which serves as an airway splint blocking the airway collapse. Stimulants (i.e., modafinil) are used as adjuncts when the excessive sleepiness is not resolved with CPAP.

Narcolepsy

While not as common as the previous disorders, it is among the more disabling due to severity of the excessive daytime sleepiness, its principle symptom. In addition to sleepiness, the narcolepsy syndrome consists of cataplexy, sleep paralysis, and hypnagogic hallucinations. Cataplexy is a reversible short-lived loss of muscle tone occurring during the wake state and triggered by intense emotion. At transitions from wake to sleep, the person with narcolepsy experiences sleep paralysis, an inability to move or speak, and visual hallucinations. The clinical symptoms of cataplexy, sleep paralysis, and hypnagogic hallucination are all pathological manifestations of REM sleep. Today, it is recognized that the pathophysiology of narcolepsy involves the loss of orexin-producing cells in the hypothalamus. Orexin is a critical transmitter in the maintenance of wakefulness. Sleep onset REM periods are now considered the pathognomonic sign of narcolepsy. The principle treatments of narcolepsy are stimulants for the excessive daytime sleepiness and REM suppressing antidepressants for the cataplexy.

Alcohol and Alcoholism

Alcohol in Healthy Adults

Studies of alcohol effects on sleep typically administer alcohol 30–60 min before sleep resulting in peak concentrations at or just prior to bedtime. The doses used range from 0.16 to 1.0 g/kg, the rough equivalent of one to six standard drinks producing breath ethanol concentrations (BrEC) up to 0.105% at bedtime [1]. Sleep latency is reduced over this dose range. However, at a low 0.16 g/kg dose increased sleep time was reported, but not at the higher 0.32 and 0.64 g/kg doses. Improved sleep only at low doses is likely due to a second-half of the night sleep disruptive rebound wakefulness that occurs with higher doses. The typical BrEC at lights out for higher doses is between 0.05% and 0.09%, and given that ethanol is metabolized at a rate of 0.01–0.02% BrEC per hour, within the first 4–5 h of the sleep period ethanol has been completely metabolized. This leads to rebound wakefulness, as well as REM sleep, during the last hours of the sleep period [2]. Thus, for the whole night total sleep time at high doses is actually decreased and thus has profound clinical implications of alcohol used as a self-treatment for insomnia/sleep disturbance.

In addition to sleep induction and maintenance effects, ethanol alters the normal 90–120 min cycling of sleep stages [3]. A dose-dependent suppression of REM sleep, at the least in the first half of the night (i.e., with ethanol present in plasma), and in some studies increased slow wave sleep in the first half of the night is reported. After first-half of the night with REM sleep suppression, a second-half of the night REM sleep rebound is typically reported. As with the rebound wakefulness noted above, the second-half REM sleep rebound likely relates to the timing of complete ethanol elimination from the body. Repeated nightly administration of ethanol leads to tolerance development to both the sleep induction and sleep stage effects. Finally, discontinuation of short-term nightly ethanol is followed by a REM sleep rebound, although the appearance of a REM sleep rebound is likely related to dose, duration of use, basal level of REM sleep, and the extent of prior REM sleep suppression and tolerance development.

Some clinical implications of the studies on ethanol effects in healthy nonalcoholics can be mentioned. The association of regular heavy drinking and chronic insomnia complaints should be easily identifiable. But, occasional insomnia can be related to a patient's occasional heavy drinking. One- or two-week sleep diaries that query about social drug use, as well as, the sleep complaints can help identify for the clinician and patient the relation of their alcohol use and sleep problems. Inquiry as to the quantity and timing of the patient's alcohol consumption relative to the attempt to sleep may reveal the sleep-disruptive potential of the alcohol use.

Alcohol Effects in Primary Sleep Disorders

About 30% of individuals with insomnia in the general population report using alcohol to help them sleep and 67% of them report the alcohol was effective in inducing sleep [4]. The healthy normal studies showing sleep-disruptive ethanol effects used higher doses (about 5–6 drinks) than the doses (e.g., 1–2 drinks) reportedly used by insomniacs. In laboratory studies of primary insomniacs ethanol (BrEC 0.04% at bedtime) improved sleep without producing a second-half wakefulness rebound [5]. Compared to age-matched noninsomniac controls with a similar social drinking history, the insomniacs chose to self-administer alcohol before sleep more frequently. The risk associated with using alcohol as a sleep aid is that tolerance to its initial beneficial effect develops within 5 nights and insomniacs increase their self-administered dose to compensate [6], potentially leading to the use of doses which produce sleep-disruptive effects.

In the wake state alcohol is a mild respiratory depressant and during sleep it decreases upper airway tone leading to snoring, exacerbating obstructive sleep apnea syndrome (OSA), and possibly precipitating sleep-disordered breathing in at-risk persons (e.g., snorers, obese). Patients with moderate OSA, defined as an average respiratory disturbance index (RDI: number of apnea and hypopneas per hour of sleep) of 22, received 300 ml of bourbon 2 h before bedtime and their RDI was increased to 28 [7]. Patients with a range of sleep-related breathing disorders (baseline RDIs of 14–54) were given an unspecified dose and BrEC of ethanol which increased the RDIs of every patient [8]. In several patients with COPD ethanol worsened the degree of hypoxemia and in several patients with only a snoring history it induced apnea [8]. That an asymptomatic snorer with no apnea will develop apnea after ethanol was convincingly shown in a later study [9]. In another study, ethanol (BrEC=0.08%) in snoring men increased their RDIs to a pathological level (i.e., RDI >10) [10]. On the other hand, the findings in asymptomatic individuals without risk factors have been inconsistent.

The risk for PLMS is increased in association with self-reported alcohol consumption in a sample of sleep disorders clinic patients [11]. But, in abstinent alcoholics the rate of PLMs was not different than a general sleep disorders clinic sample rate of PLMS [12]. Alcoholism is associated with deficiencies in iron, ferritin, magnesium, and vitamin B_{12}, and polyneuropathy, all of which are also associated with PLMs and RLS. To the extent that the alcoholic has any of these deficiencies, RLS and PLMS may be precipitated and/or exacerbated.

Sleep of Alcoholics and Alcohol Effects in Alcoholics

Patients with alcoholism commonly complain of sleep problems, daytime sleepiness, and parasomnias. Alcoholics report polyphasic sleep patterns with short sleep periods followed by short wake periods that are distributed across the 24-h day during drinking binges. This type of sleep pattern is seen in organisms without a circadian pacemaker. It is possible that during these binges the sleep–wake cycles and light–

dark exposure of alcoholics are so chaotic that they are arrhythmic. Laboratory studies of patients with alcoholism show that sleep latency and total sleep time are disturbed on both drinking, as well as on nondrinking nights [13]. Prolonged sleep latency in alcoholics when drinking contrasts with the reduced sleep latency that alcohol produces in nonalcoholics and suggests tolerance development and possible neurobiological changes in sleep–wake mechanisms. In addition, as in healthy normals, drinking in alcoholics is associated with increased slow wave sleep and REM sleep suppression with rapid tolerance development to these effects [13].

The acute alcohol abstinence phase lasts 1–2 weeks, although some of the withdrawal symptoms such as mood instability, disturbed sleep, and craving remain beyond this period. During the acute abstinence phase slow wave sleep is reduced, sometimes to minimal levels, and REM sleep continuity is disrupted [3]. There are frequent and fragmented REM episodes and shortened NREM–REM cycles during the acute abstinence.

Recovery and Long-Term Abstinence in Alcoholics

Abnormal sleep patterns can persist for up to 3 years in some patients with alcoholism. Sleep remains shortened and REM sleep pressure elevated reflected in elevated REM percents, shortened latencies to REM sleep and higher REM densities [14]. While it is tempting to attribute these sleep abnormalities to the excessive alcohol drinking of the patients, the sleep problems could have preceded the development of the alcoholism or they could be secondary to the development of other medical and psychiatric disorders that develop during the alcoholic drinking of the patient.

Irrespective of the cause, both objective and subjective measures of sleep after acute abstinence predict the likelihood of relapse during long-term abstinence. Early laboratory studies suggested that low levels of slow wave sleep are predictive of alcoholism relapse [15]. Other more recent studies have identified REM sleep disturbances, either elevated REM sleep percent or shortened REM sleep latency as predictive of relapse [16]. Interestingly, sleep-predictive relapse risk was greater than that associated with other variables such as age, marital status, employment, duration and severity of alcoholism, hepatic enzymes, and depression ratings.

Stimulants

Caffeine

Many do not consider caffeine a drug of abuse; even within the medical community its potential for abuse is not fully appreciated. Laboratory data indicate there are conditions under which caffeine is persistently self-administered and it has abuse liability, albeit a relatively low liability compared to other recognized drugs of abuse [17]. Caffeine in doses of 150–400 mg administered immediately before sleep prolongs the onset of sleep and reduces total sleep time and sleep continuity in healthy normals [18–23]. The sleep-disruptive effects of caffeine were compared to that of the psychomotor stimulants. In that study 300 mg caffeine reduced sleep efficiency from 89 to 74%, while 40 mg pemoline reduced it to 80% and 20 mg methylphenidate to 61% [20]. As to sleep stage effects, some studies report reductions of stage 3–4 sleep [19, 20], but unlike the psychomotor stimulants, stage REM sleep is not affected. There are data indicating that heavy caffeine use is associated with RLS/PLMS.

Discontinuing the chronic use of caffeine is associated with mood and performance disturbances. A withdrawal syndrome was observed after a double-blind, placebo-controlled cessation of chronic, but moderate (235 mg daily on average), caffeine consumption [21]. Putting the dose in context, an 8 oz cup of coffee contains 100 mg caffeine, but some of the more recent "branded" coffees have as much as 500 mg. On the second day of caffeine cessation (20 h post-caffeine use), in addition to the ubiquitous headache, reduced vigor and increases in sleepiness, fatigue, and drowsiness were experienced. For moderate to heavy caffeine users, the morning cup of coffee immediately after arising probably restores caffeine levels and alertness. The 8-h sleep period is essentially a caffeine discontinuation and thus morning sleepiness is, in part, a caffeine discontinuation effect.

Nicotine

Study of nicotine's effects on sleep has been facilitated with the development of nicotine delivery systems (i.e., nicotine gum and patches) for use in clinical smoking cessation programs. Transdermal nicotine (7–14 mg) in normals produced a dose-dependent increase in wakefulness during the sleep period and a reduction in percent REM sleep relative to a placebo patch [24]. Another study of nonsmoking normals found that 17.5 mg transdermal nicotine increased wake time and decreased REM sleep percent [25]. In obese, non-smoking patients with sleep-disordered breathing 15 mg transdermal nicotine reduced both total sleep time and percent REM sleep. But, it did not improve the sleep-disordered breathing of these patients which was the study's primary purpose [26].

In nicotine-dependent individuals, its discontinuation is associated with a disturbance of sleep and alertness. Smokers were studied during the week prior to and following cessation of chronic smoking and the number of arousals, awakenings, and sleep stage changes were all increased during the cessation week [27]. In a double-blind study using a placebo vs. nicotine patch discontinuation of average daily use of 30

cigarettes, the number of arousals was increased relative to the smoking baseline in the placebo group, while in the nicotine (22 mg) patch group arousals were reduced and stage 3/4 sleep was increased relative to the smoking baseline [28]. Given the pharmacokinetics of nicotine, any smoking baseline is a partial discontinuation during the usual 8 h sleep period of nonsmoking. Since the nicotine patch was worn continuously, it is probable that sleep was improved relative to a partial discontinuation (i.e., a smoking baseline). These data are consistent with the several questionnaire studies that find smokers are more likely than nonsmokers to report problems falling asleep and staying asleep [29].

Psychomotor Stimulants

Cocaine

Very few laboratory studies have assessed the effects of cocaine and its discontinuation on sleep and daytime alertness. Clinical assessments describe continued and prolonged wakefulness during "cocaine runs." The cocaine runs are then followed by "crashes" characterized by excessive sleep and sleepiness [30]. Sleep laboratory studies of cocaine discontinuation in cocaine-dependent persons have shown elevated total sleep time and REM sleep rebound during the initial abstinence. The acute abstinence was followed by a persisting insomnia and REM sleep disturbance over the 3-week study duration [31]. A laboratory study of cocaine administration and discontinuation found that 600 mg per day intranasal cocaine (insufflated from 19:00 to 21:00 h) severely disrupted sleep, delaying its onset at the 23:00 h bedtime for up to 3–4 h and then suppressing REM sleep [32]. During the first two discontinuation days, average daily sleep latency on the multiple sleep latency test (MSLT) was less than 5 min (i.e., a pathological level of sleepiness), most probably due to the severely shortened sleep over the prior 5 days of cocaine use. The MSLT also showed multiple sleep onset REM periods (SOREMPs), probably due to a REM rebound secondary to the prior REM sleep suppression during the cocaine administration nights. After 14 days of abstinence, a nocturnal sleep and REM sleep disturbance remained, although the MSLTs were free of SOREMPs and the latencies returned to slightly elevated levels.

Amphetamine

While not the drug of choice, amphetamine is indicated for the treatment of narcolepsy and attention-deficit hyperactivity disorder (ADHD). Few sleep studies of amphetamine administration and discontinuation have been done. In an early study, 10 or 15 mg D-amphetamine administered at night doubled sleep latency and suppressed REM sleep in healthy young adults [33]. Another study of healthy adults and patients with narcolepsy reported that a 7–8 am administration of methamphetamine (10 mg) reduced sleep efficiency that night (11 pm bedtime) in control subjects and similarly at 40–60 mg doses in the narcoleptics [34]. With this morning administration, no REM sleep effects were observed in the normals. But, the patients who received higher doses showed prolonged REM latencies and reduced REM sleep times. Amphetamine-dependent subjects assessed during the drug's discontinuation showed a REM sleep rebound on the second night of discontinuation which lasted for 3–5 nights [35]. This amphetamine-related REM sleep rebound was delayed relative to that associated with cocaine discontinuation, which is probably due to the pharmacokinetic differences between the drugs (i.e., the longer half-life of amphetamine). The rebound also was longer lasting, which may be due to differences in the duration or amount of prior use, or the level and duration of REM sleep suppression. Total sleep time also was elevated over the same 3- to 5-day time period, probably recovery sleep due to the prior drug-induced sleep loss, but subsequently sleep time became shorter than normal, suggesting continuing insomnia. As in abstinence from cocaine dependence, the continued insomnia in amphetamine abstinence raises questions regarding a stimulant-induced persisting alteration of sleep–wake mechanisms.

No studies of the effects of amphetamine discontinuation on daytime levels of sleepiness–alertness have been done in amphetamine-dependent persons. One would predict amphetamine discontinuation is associated with increased daytime sleepiness and multiple sleep onset REM periods on the MSLT similar to that reported for the discontinuation of cocaine.

Methylphenidate

Methlyphenidate is indicated for ADHD and narcolepsy. It is the drug of choice for ADHD and a second choice drug for narcolepsy. While it is considered to have a lesser abuse liability than amphetamine, case studies of abuse have been reported and its neuropharmacology is similar to that of amphetamine. In healthy normals, 20 mg reduced total sleep time, increased the latency to REM sleep, and reduced the min of REM sleep, while 10 mg only increased REM sleep latency [36]. In an earlier study, 5 mg was reported to increase the latency to REM sleep and reduce the percent of REM sleep without affecting other sleep measures [37]. In children with ADHD, studies of the effects of methylphenidate taken during the day on subsequent sleep are inconclusive. Sleep time was shortened in one study [38] and increased in another [39] and in one study REM sleep was fragmented [39]. But, these studies can be questioned for a variety of methodological and control issues.

We are unaware of sleep studies that have documented the discontinuation effects of methylphenidate in dependent individuals. To the extent that sleep time and REM sleep was reduced during drug use, increased daytime sleepiness with multiple sleep onset REM periods would be predicted. The

role that the excessive sleepiness following discontinuation of any of these stimulant drugs may have in their continued use and abuse is illustrated by self-administration studies done in healthy normals. When given an opportunity to self-administer methylphenidate (20 mg), healthy normals, with no current or previous substance abuse history, choose active drug on only 20% of the opportunities after 8 h time-in-bed (TIB) the previous night, but on 80% of the opportunities (i.e., 20% placebo choice) when sleepiness was present due to a restriction of time in bed to 4 h [40].

Opioids

The opioids are disruptive of sleep continuity and sleep staging. Heroin (3, 6, and 12 mg/70 kg), administered IM in a double-blind placebo controlled design to abstinent opioid addicts, produced dose-related decreases in total sleep time, stage 3–4, and REM sleep [41]. Heroin is metabolized to morphine and morphine (7.5, 15, and 30 mg/70 kg) also produced a dose-related decrease in sleep time, stage 3–4 and REM sleep in the abstinent opioid addicts [42]. Similarly, methadone (7.5, 15, and 30 mg/70 kg) decreased total sleep time, stage 3–4 and REM sleep in abstinent opioid addicts [43]. All these opioids also produced increased brief arousals and frequent sleep stage changes, a disruption of sleep referred to as sleep fragmentation. Studies have indicated that tolerance to the sleep disruptive effects develops within weeks [44]. With tolerance development, the sleep fragmentation is lessened and the REM sleep suppressive effects tend to diminish.

The discontinuation of chronic opioid use is associated with sleep disturbance. Heroin addicts being maintained on methadone in an outpatient research treatment program were discontinued from their treatment and sleep was recorded in the laboratory [45]. Sleep latency and latency to REM sleep were prolonged and percent stage 3–4 sleep was reduced compared to normals. Interestingly, after a week of buprenorphine 4 mg, a partial mu opioid agonist, the sleep patterns normalized.

Opioids have important effects on sleep disorders. Although not the first line of treatment, opioids improve RLS and or often used in patients to do not respond to dopamine agonists, the first treatment choice. In contrast, given their negative effects of respiratory drive they are contraindicated in sleep-related breathing disorders.

Sedative-Hypnotics

The benzodiazepine receptor agonists (BzRAs) are indicated for the treatment of insomnia and studies clearly show they improve sleep with the newer non-BzRAs also not altering normal sleep staging. However, they are considered to have a relatively high abuse liability within the medical community. Epidemiological and laboratory studies indicate the abuse liability of modern sedative-hypnotics is relatively low. The distinction "modern" is critical in that, the early sedative-hypnotics, barbiturates and ethanol-based drugs (i.e., eth-chlorvynol, choral hydrate) clearly produce both physical and behavioral dependence. BzRAs are not as likely to do such.

Daytime self-administration studies were done in normals, persons with substance abuse histories, and patients with anxiety disorders. These studies showed a generally low behavioral dependence liability. The BzRAs were self-administered by substance abusers at low and declining rates over time [46] and were not differentially self-administered relative to placebo by the normals or patients with anxiety disorders [47, 48]. Recent research has found that some patients with anxiety disorders self-administered alprazolam relative to placebo [49]. Our own studies of presleep triazolam or placebo self-administration in patients with insomnia have found that triazolam and placebo are self-administered at similar rates (67–88%) in a single-choice paradigm (i.e., choice of taking the available capsule or not) [50–52]. When forced to choose on a given night between triazolam and placebo, triazolam is preferred 80% of the time [52]. But critical to assessing abuse liability, when given an opportunity, in a single-choice paradigm, to self-administer multiple capsules on the same night, a 0.27 mg average nightly triazolam dose was self-administered (i.e., 0.25 mg is the clinical dose), while the placebo dose was escalated to the three capsule maximum. Normal volunteers in these studies self-administered capsules at a 20–40% nightly rate, significantly lower than that of the insomniacs. This high hypnotic self-administration of insomniacs and active drug preference of some anxiety patients raise questions about distinguishing between therapy-seeking and drug-seeking behavior, an issue discussed below.

Hallucinogens

Tetrahydrocannabinol

Marijuana remains the most frequently abused illicit drug in the United States, although its popularity appears to cycle, trending up and down over decades. Tetrahydrocannabinol (THC) is one of the principle active ingredients in marijuana and THC is classified as a mild sedative at low doses and a hallucinogen at high doses.

Study of THC's effects on sleep and wakefulness occurred predominately during the 1970s. Low doses of THC, 4–20 mg, in either experienced marijuana users or nonusers had mildly REM sleep suppressive effects [53–55]. Some studies found total sleep time and stage 3–4 sleep were increased [52, 54], which then decreased after a week of repeated nightly use [55]. At high doses, 50–210 mg, in naive or experienced marijuana users THC suppressed REM sleep, but effects on total sleep time were not observed [56] and stage 3–4 sleep was reduced in one report [57]. Some of the studies report a REM sleep rebound on the THC discontinuation nights [53, 56] and some a reduction in sleep time or an increase in sleep latency [54, 56]. These studies all involved presleep laboratory administration of THC. Several studies in situ or semi-controlled laboratory situations with moderate and heavy marijuana users smoking their usual marijuana cigarettes during the day or early evening have also been done. Self-reported or rater-observed sleep time was increased in two such studies [58, 59]. But in one sleep laboratory study, little or no effects on sleep measures were observed [60]. These mild sedative effects have also been observed during daytime studies using performance assessments. In situ assessment of daily activity levels also show reduced activity during moderate or heavy marijuana use [59].

(±)3,4-Methylenedioxymethamphetamine

An amphetamine derivative that has become increasingly popular as a recreational and drug of abuse is (±)3,4-methylenedioxymethamphetamine (MDMA), or "Ecstasy." This drug has hallucinogenic properties and acts indirectly by stimulating the release of brain monoamines [61]. Exposure to MDMA decreases total sleep time with a decrease in NREM sleep, but no significant effects on REM sleep. Within the NREM sleep, individuals who use MDMA have less stage 2 sleep, but there are no apparent differences in stage 1 or slow wave sleep (stages 3 and 4) [62]. In a placebo-controlled study, acute MDMA shortened sleep primarily by increasing sleep initiation and it reduced stage 3–4 sleep and suppressed REM sleep [63]. The MDMA-reduced sleep time was not associated with increased daytime sleepiness the following day as seen in a 4-h sleep restriction condition. Average daily sleep latency on the MSLT the day after nighttime placebo was increased in MDMA users compared to age-matched controls and MDMA users had an elevated number of sleep onset REM periods compared to controls.

Sleep–Wake Disturbance in Alcoholism and Drug Abuse

As the review above indicates alcohol and all drugs of abuse alter sleep, its staging, and consequent daytime alertness. The role of sleep–wake disturbance in alcoholism and drug abuse is not well understood. It is known that insomnia is a risk factor for substance abuse. Yet, the extent to which insomnia or daytime sleepiness leads to new cases of alcoholism or drug abuse is not known. Furthermore, the degree to which treatment of insomnia or daytime sleepiness in abstinent alcoholics and drug abusers reduces risk of relapse is not known. To date the few alcoholism treatment trials have failed to clearly demonstrate that improved sleep reduces relapse and the only available drug abuse treatment trial, while encouraging, is not conclusive. There is the inherent assumption in this discussion that sleep disturbance is causally related to alcoholism or drug abuse, either as the precipitant or consequent. But, it may be co-morbid and independent or related to a third common factor.

In the above review of the sleep effects of alcohol and drugs of abuse, the reader may have noted that most all of the drugs of abuse suppress REM sleep, with tolerance to the REM suppression developing rapidly. The significance of these effects is not clear. Most antidepressants (tricyclics, MAOIs, and SSRIs) are much more potent REM suppressants, typically driving REM sleep to below 10% of the night and tolerance does not develop to the REM suppression even with chronic use. The degree of REM suppression in depressed patients is associated with improvement in mood [64]. Further, total sleep deprivation and REM sleep deprivation by awakening on entry to REM sleep has antidepression effects in patients with depression [64].

Studies have shown that acute REM deprivation by awakening enhances pain sensitivity [65]. Thus, whether the REM suppression of opiates is reducing their analgesic effect is a critical question. And, whether the reduced analgesic effect then leads to the need for higher opiate doses and to development of physical dependence is also a critical issue.

At the very least the REM effects may reflect the development of physical dependence and an altered CNS neurobiology. Chronic alcohol and drug use likely alters the neurobiology of sleep and the control of REM sleep, a predominately pontine cholinergeric phenomenon. In abstinent alcoholics, a REM sleep disturbance remaining after the acute discontinuation is predictive of relapse. We are unaware of studies regarding the presence of a REM disturbance following abstinence for other drugs of abuse and the predictive value of such a disturbance, if present, to relapse.

It also should be noted that some of the medications used to treat various sleep disorders (i.e., stimulants for narcolepsy, BzRAs for insomnia, opiates for RLS/PLMS) have known abuse liability. It is not fully known what the risk of abuse of these drugs is in sleep disorder patients. Earlier it was noted that there is risk for insomniacs who use alcohol as a sleep aid. Tolerance to ethanol's sleep inducing effects develops rapidly which then leads to dose escalation. Virtually all sleep disorders are chronic and hence require long-term therapy. The question then arises as to whether chronic use of these medications represents drug-seeking or therapy-seeking.

Drug-Seeking Versus Therapy-Seeking

It is often difficult to differentiate drug-seeking from therapy-seeking in clinical practice. In drug-seeking the drug and its effects, typically its "euphorogenic" effect, is the focus of the drug use, while in therapy-seeking the alleviation of disease-related symptoms is the focus of the drug use. However, in the clinic drug-seeking and therapy-seeking can become closely intertwined and what was once therapy-seeking can shift to drug-seeking. The clinical challenge for clinicians is to differentiate the two phenomena. Some of the potentially differentiating and defining characteristics of drug-seeking versus therapy-seeking are presented in Table 30.1. The defining characteristic of drug-seeking is evidence that the drug is taken in excessive amounts (supratherapeutic doses), in nontherapeutic contexts, and is preferred over other commodities (e.g., money) and various social and occupational activities. To the degree that the drug is chosen over other commodities or social activities is evidence for the extent of its risk for abuse. Supportive of its reinforcing capacity is evidence in the scientific literature that the drug is readily discriminated from placebo by behavioral and subjective assessment. These assessments typically rate the drug for it "euphorogenic" and drug-liking effects. That is, the drug's subjective effects are the focus of its use. Then, to the degree that the dose is escalated over time, one has evidence of the development of tolerance and possible physical dependence.

In contrast, therapy-seeking is evident if the drug has demonstrated efficacy for the disorder or condition being treated. As well, the patient has the signs and symptoms and the appropriate diagnosis for the indicated use of the drug. The pattern of drug taking, its dose and duration of use, is consistent with its therapeutic effects. Finally, the patient believes that the drug is effective and readily experiences its

Table 30.1 Drug-seeking vs. therapy-seeking behavior

Drug-seeking behavior
- Drug chosen over other commodities or activities
- Drug taken in excessive, nontherapeutic amounts
- Drug taken on chronic basis leading to tolerance and physical dependence
- Drug taken in nontherapeutic context

Therapy-seeking behavior
- Drug has demonstrated efficacy for the indicated condition
- Duration and dose of self-administration is limited to therapeutic effects
- Patient has signs and symptoms for which drug is indicated
- Drug is believed to be and is experienced as being efficacious

therapeutic effects. But, the drug-seeking versus therapy-seeking distinction becomes difficult in situations where therapy-seeking shifts to drug-seeking behavior. For example, one is concerned regarding the use of ethanol as a hypnotic by an insomniac. While presleep ethanol use may initially be effective in improving sleep, rapid tolerance development is likely which may lead to dose escalation. Further, other of ethanol's reinforcing effects (i.e., its "euphorogenic" effects) may be discovered by the person, especially as dose is escalated, and its use may then extend beyond the therapeutic context and dose (i.e., before sleep as a hypnotic). A similar shifting pattern can be described for stimulant or opiate use. On the other hand, drug-seeking may be maintained because the drug, in addition to its mood altering and "euphorogenic" effects, also has therapeutic effects (i.e., the stimulant effects of cocaine or amphetamine do reverse the excessive sleepiness that is experienced during drug discontinuation). Thus, the dependence is maintained by both its mood altering effects and its therapeutic effects, what others have termed "self-medication."

References

1. Stone BM. Sleep and low doses of alcohol. Electroencephalogr Clin Neurophysiol. 1980;48:706–9.
2. Roehrs T, Roth T. Sleep, sleepiness, sleep disorders and alcohol use and abuse. Sleep Med Rev. 2001;5:287–97.
3. Hyde M, Roehrs T, Roth T. Alcohol, alcoholism, and sleep. In: Lee-Chiong T, editor. Sleep: a comprehensive handbook. Philadelphia, PA: Wiley; 2006. p. 867–71.
4. Ancoli-Israel S, Roth T. Characteristics of insomnia in the United States: Results of the 1991 National Sleep Foundation Survey I. Sleep. 2000;22:S347–53.
5. Roehrs T, Papineau K, Rosenthal L, Roth T. Ethanol as a hypnotic in insomniacs: self administration and effects of sleep and mood. Neuropsychopharmacology. 1999;20:279–86.
6. Roehrs, Blaisdell B, Cruz N, Roth T. Tolerance to hypnotic effects of ethanol in insomnias. Sleep. 2004;27:352 (ab).
7. Guilleminault C. Sleep apnea syndromes: impact of sleep and sleep states. Sleep. 1980;3:227–34.
8. Issa FG, Sullivan CE. Alcohol, snoring and sleep apneas. J Neurol Neurosurg Psychiatry. 1982;45:353–9.
9. Mitler MM, Dawson A, Henriksen SJ, Sobers M, Bloom FE. Bedtime ethanol increases resistance of upper airways and produces sleep apneas in asymptomatic snorers. Alcohol Clin Exp Res. 1988;12:801–5.
10. Herzog M, Riemann R. Alcohol ingestion influences the nocturnal cardio-respiratory activity in snoring and non-snoring males. Eur Arch Otorhinolarygol. 2004;261:459–62.
11. Aldrich MS, Shipley JE. Alcohol use and periodic limb movements of sleep. Alcohol Clin Exp Res. 1993;17:192–6.
12. LeBon O, Verbanck P, Hoffmann G, et al. Sleep in detoxified alcoholics: impairment of most standard sleep parameters and increased risk for sleep apnea, but not for myclonias—a controlled study. J Stud Alcohol. 1997;58:30–6.
13. Brower KJ. Alcohol's effects on sleep in alcoholics. Alcohol Res Health. 2001;25:110–25.
14. Drummond SPA, Gillin JC, Smith TL, Demondena A. The sleep of abstinent pure primary alcoholic patients: natural course and relation to relapse. Alcohol Clin Exp Res. 1998;22:1796–802.
15. Allen RP, Wagman AM, Funderburk FR, Well DT. Slow wave sleep: a predictor of individuals differences in response to drinking? Biol Psychiatry. 1980;15:345–8.
16. Gillin JC, Smith TL, Irwin M, et al. Increased pressure for rapid eye movement sleep at time of hospital admission predicts relapse in nondepressed patients with primary alcoholism at 3-month follow-up. Arch Gen Psychiatry. 1994;51:189–97.
17. Arnedt JT, Conroy D, Rutt J, Aloia MS, Brower KJ, Armitage R. An open trial of cognitive-behavioral treatment for insomnia comorbid with alcohol dependence. Sleep Med. 2007;8:176–80.
18. Griffiths RR, Mumford GF. Caffeine—a drug of abuse? In: Bloom FE, Kupfer DJ, editors. Psychopharmacology: the fourth generation of progress. New York: Raven; 1995. p. 1699–713.
19. Brezinova V. Effect of caffeine on sleep: EEG study in late middle age people. Br J Clin Pharmacol. 1974;1:203–8.
20. Karacan I, Thornby JI, Anch M, Booth GH, Williams RL, Salis PJ. Dose-related sleep disturbances induced by coffee and caffeine. Clin Pharmacol Ther. 1977;20:682–9.
21. Nicholson AN, Stone BM. Heterocyclic amphetamine derivatives and caffeine on sleep. Br J Clin Pharmacol. 1980;9:195–203.
22. Okuma T, Matsuoka H, Matuse Y, Toyomura K. Model insomnia by methylphenidate and caffeine and use in the evaluation of temazepam. Psychopharmacology. 1982;76:201–13.
23. Bonnet MH, Arand DL. Caffeine use as a model of acute and chronic insomnia. Sleep. 1992;15:526–36.
24. Gillin LC, Lardon M, Ruiz C, Golshan S, Salin-Pascual RJ. Dose-dependent effects of transdermal nicotine on early morning awakening and rapid eye movement sleep time in non-smoking normal volunteers. J Clin Psychopharmacol. 1994;14:264–7.
25. Salin-Pascual RJ, de la Fuente JR, Galicia-Polo L, Drucker-Colin R. Effects of transdermal nicotine on mood and sleep in nonsmoking major depressed patients. Psychopharmacology. 1995;121:476–9.
26. Davila DG, Hurt RD, Offord KP, Harris CD, Shepard JW. Acute effects of transdermal nicotine on sleep architecture, snoring, and sleep-disordered breathing in nonsmokers. Am J Respir Crit Care Med. 1994;1560:469–74.
27. Prosise GI, Bonnet MH, Berry RB, Dickel ML. Effects of abstinence from smoking on sleep and daytime sleepiness. Chest. 1994;105:1136–41.
28. Wetter DW, Fiore MC, Baker TB, Young TB. Tobacco withdrawal and nicotine replacement influence objective measures of sleep. J Consult Clin Psychol. 1995;63:658–67.
29. Phillips BA, Danner FJ. Cigarette smoking and sleep disturbance. Arch Intern Med. 1995;155:734–7.
30. Gawin FH, Kleber HD. Abstinence symptomatology and psychiatric diagnosis in cocaine abusers. Gen Psychiatry. 1986;43:107–13.
31. Kowatch RA, Schnoll SS, Knisely JS, Green D, Elswick RK. Electroencephalograpic sleep and mood during cocaine withdrawal. J Addict Disorders. 1992;11:21–45.
32. Johanson CE, Roehrs T, Schuh K, Warbasse L. The effects of cocaine on mood and sleep in cocaine-dependent males. Exp Clin Psychopharm. 1999;4:338–46.
33. Rechtschaffen A, Maron L. The effect of amphetamine on the sleep cycle. Electroencephalogr Clin Neurophysiol. 1964;16:438–45.
34. Mitler MM, Hajdukovic R, Erman MK. Treatment of narcolepsy with methamphetamine. Sleep. 1993;16:306–17.
35. Watson R, Hartmann E, Schildkraut JJ. Amphetamine withdrawal: affective state, sleep patterns and MHPG excretion. Amer J Psychiat. 1972;129:262–9.
36. Nicholson AN, Stone BM. Stimulants and sleep in man. Agressologie. 1981;22:73–8.
37. Braekeland F. The effect of methylphenidate on the sleep cycle in man. Psychopharmacologia. 1966;10:179–83.
38. Tirosh E, Sadeh A, Munvez R, Lavie P. Effects of methylphenidate on sleep in children with attention-deficit hyperactivity disorder. Am J Dis Child. 1993;147:1313–5.

39. Greenhill L, Puig-Antich J, Goetz R, Hanlon C, Davies M. Sleep architecture and REM sleep measures in prepubertal children with attention deficit disorder with hyperactivity. Sleep. 1983;6:91–101.

40. Roehrs T, Papineau K, Rosenthal L, Roth T. Sleepiness and the reinforcing and subjective effects of methylphenidate. Exp Clin Psychopharm. 1999;7:145–50.

41. Kay DC, Pickworth WB, Neidert GL. Morphine-like insomnia from heroin in non-dependent human addicts. Br J Clin Pharmacol. 1981;11:159–69.

42. Kay DC, Eisenstein RB, Jasinski DR. Morphine effects on human REM state, waking state, and NREM sleep. Psychopharmacologia. 1969;14:404–16.

43. Pickworth WB, Neidert GL, Kay DC. Morphine-like arousal by methadone during sleep. Clin Pharmacol Ther. 1981;30:796–804.

44. Kay DC. Human sleep during chronic morphine intoxication. Psychopharmacologia. 1975;44:117–24.

45. Mello NK, Mendelson JH, Lukas SE, Gastfriend DR, Teoh SK, Homan L. Buprenorphine treatment of opiate and cocaine abuse: clinical and preclinical studies. Harv Rev Psychiatry. 1993;1:168–83.

46. Griffiths RR, Weerts EM. Benzodiazepine self-administration in humans and laboratory animals. Implications for problems of long-term use and abuse. Psychopharmacology. 1997;134:1 37.

47. deWit H, Pierri J, Johanson CE. Reinforcing and subjective effects of diazepam in nondrug-abusing volunteers. Pharm Biochem Behav. 1989;33:205–13.

48. deWit H, Uhlenhuth EH, Hedeker D, McCracken SG, Johanson CE. Lack of preference for diazepam in anxious volunteers. Arch Gen Psychiatry. 1986;43:533–41.

49. Oswald LM, Roache JD, Rhoades HM. Predictors of individual differences in alprazolam self-medication. Exp Clin Psychopharm. 1999;7:379–90.

50. Roehrs T, Merlotti L, Zorick F, Roth T. Rebound insomnia and hypnotic self administration. Psychopharmacology. 1992;107:480–4.

51. Roehrs T, Pedrosi B, Rosenthal L, Zorick F, Roth T. Hypnotic self administration and dose escalation. Psychopharmacology. 1996;127:150–4.

52. Roehrs T, Pedrosi B, Rosenthal L, Zorick F, Roth T. Hypnotic self administration: forced-choice versus single-choice. Psychopharmacology. 1997;133:121–6.

53. Pivick RT, Zarcone V, Dement WC, Hollister LE. Delta-9-tetrahydrocannabinol and synhexl: effects on human sleep patterns. Clin Pharmacol Ther. 1972;13:426–35.

54. Freemon FR. The effect of delta-9-tetrahydrocannabinol on sleep. Psychopharmacologia. 1974;35:39–44.

55. Barratt ES, Beaver W, White R. The effects of marijuana on human sleep patterns. Biol Psychiat. 1974;8:47–53.

56. Feinberg I, Jones R, Walker JM, Cavness C, March J. Effects of high dosage delta-9-tetrahydrocannabinol on sleep patterns in man. Clin Pharmacol Ther. 1976;17:458–66.

57. Tassinari CA, Ambrosetto G, Peraita-Adrados MR, Gastaut H. The neuropsychiatric syndrome of delta-9-tetrahydrocannabinol and cannabis intoxication in naive subjects: a clinical and polygraphic study during wakefulness and sleep. In: Braude MC, Szara S, editors. The pharmacology of marijuana. New York: Raven; 1976. p. 357–82.

58. Babor TF, Mendelson JH, Kuehnle J. Marijuana and human physical activity. Psychopharmacology. 1976;50:11–9.

59. Chait LD. Subjective and behavioral effects of marijuana the morning after smoking. Psychopharmacology. 1990;100:328–33.

60. Karacan I, Fernandez-Salas A, Coggins WJ, Carter WE, Willians RL, Thornby JI, Salis PJ, Okawa M, Villaume JP. Sleep electroencephalographic-electrooculographic characteristics of chronic marijuana users: Part I. Ann NY Acad Sci. 1977;103:348–74.

61. Schmidt CJ, Levin JA, Lovenberg W. In vitro and in vivo neurochemical effects of methylenedioxymethamphetamine on striatal monoamine systems in the rat brain. Biochem Pharmacol. 1987;36:747–55.

62. Allen RP, McCann UD, Ricaurte GA. Persistent effects of (±)3,4-Methylenedioxymethamphetamine (MDMA, "Ecstasy") on human sleep. Sleep. 1993;16(6):560–4.

63. Randall S, Johanson CE, Tancer M, Roehrs T. Effects of acute 3, 4-methylenedioxymethaphetamine on sleep and daytime sleepiness. Sleep. 2009;32(11):1513–9.

64. Benca RM. Mood disorders. In: Kryger MH, Roth T, Dement WC, editors. Principles and practice of sleep medicine. 4th ed. Philadelphia, PA: Elsevier Saunders; 2005. p. 1311–26.

65. Roehrs TA, Hyde M, Blaisdell B, Greenwalk M, Roth T. Sleep loss and REM sleep loss are hyperalgesic. Sleep. 2006;29:145–51.

Brian Johnson

Abstract

Craving is a concept with good face validity and poor construct validity. The difficulties measuring craving includes that it varies by time, by environment, by the amount of stress, by one's state of mood, that it may be partially unconscious and that there is no clearly established concept of what exactly is being measured. Neural mechanisms of drug craving are reviewed. The ventral tegmentum is central to craving. It is connected to limbic and cortical structures that help the organism learn to find alcohol and drugs via the establishment of drug cues that intensify craving. The "dream on" mechanism and the subcortical pathways of addiction are identical (Solms, Behav Brain Sci 23:843–850, 2000). Specimen drinking/drug dreams are provided. A possible neural mechanism of transition from heavy drinking of alcohol to physical addiction is described and tied to the onset of drinking dreams. Therefore, drinking dreams would represent a biological marker of the transition from psychological to physical addiction. With more empirical work, it is possible that drug dreams would be established as the psychological readout of the "switch mechanism" to physical addiction and persistent craving for alcohol or drugs. Drug dreams might then represent the "gold standard" for craving research because they are a direct readout of midbrain function, and become the basis of construction of scales to capture the phenomenon of craving. Drinking and drug dreams represent a biological manifestation of addiction that can be used in psychotherapy to help the patient to be conscious of their persistent urge to relapse and to understand that their brain has been permanently captured by the addictive drug; whether they use or not. Nightmares are a subset of dreams defined by the presence of alarm on awakening. Nightmares are common in the addicted population because of an increased incidence of childhood abuse and posttraumatic stress disorder. Despite the wishes of some patients to avoid using nightmares in their psychotherapy, addressing the issues raised by the nightmare is essential as part of helping the patient remain abstinent.

Learning Objectives
- Why craving for alcohol and drugs has high face validity and low construct validity
- The relationship between craving and subcortical mechanisms of addiction
- The relationship between subcortical mechanisms of addiction and dreaming about alcohol and drugs
- The nature of nightmares and why their use is essential in treating addicted patients

B. Johnson, M.D. (✉)
Department of Psychiatry, Suny Upstate Medical University,
Syracuse, NY 13210, USA
e-mail: johnsonb@upstate.edu

Issues to Be Addressed by Future Research

- When in the course of addictive illness do drug dreams and drinking dreams begin?
- How many exposures are required for each addictive drug?
- Is route of administration relevant?
- Are men or women more susceptible to developing this marker of craving?
- Is there a vulnerable age? Might later onset of use of drugs or alcohol make development of drug dreams less likely?
- In a population of heavy drinkers, for example persons convicted of drunk driving, might the presence of drinking dreams have a prognostic meaning such as persons who cannot resume drinking without further consequences?
- Might a verbally-administered craving scale be developed that was correlated with the presence or absence of drug dreams?
- Once one type of drug dream was established, indicating craving for that drug, how many exposures of a second addictive drug would be needed to provoke the new onset of dreams about the second drug?

Addiction specialists face a formidable problem in terms of measuring craving for alcohol and drugs. Craving has high face validity and poor construct validity [1]. By face validity is meant that there is plausibility to this measure. Anyone who has spoken to addicted persons knows that craving is central to perpetuation of addictive behaviors. Persons who are addicted to nicotine smoke cigarette after cigarette hour after hour for years because they are prompted by craving for another [2]. So according to face validity, we all know what craving is.

And yet, putting into words what craving might be is almost impossible. It seems to vary over time, and yet it is unusual to have a craving scale that can account for this. Craving varies according to environment; there are drug cues that accelerate it. For example, one person reported that he was comfortably and reliably sober 6 years after his last use of cocaine, but when he returned to his old neighborhood he was assailed by intense urges to buy cocaine and pick up prostitutes [3]. But cue-induced craving represents a specific subset of studies and these studies show that craving can be accelerated in a second [4–7]. No craving scale accounts for this [1]. Stress can increase craving; apparently via binding of corticotrophin releasing factor at ventral tegmental and nucleus accumbens shell sites [8, 9], and yet stressors are not incorporated into any craving scale. Craving is worsened by depression; the mechanism is not known [2, 10, 11], and yet

mood state is not part of any craving scale. Berridge and Robinson [12, 13] suggest that craving may be unconscious, which might put it beyond any measure. There is no reliable way to measure absolute craving, no "gold standard" of craving that could be used to validate a particular scale [1].

Construct validity refers to the explanatory power of a scientific concept. We could measure craving only if we had a theoretical framework to help us select measures that are conceptually relevant. If we do not know what causes craving, we are in a poor position to evaluate it. In fact, the problem of constructing a valid craving scale has yet to be accomplished [1].

The solution to the craving problem may lay in the use of dreams. What use are dreams? Isn't dream analysis some holdover from antiquated Freudian practitioners who used to think that listening to dreams had some relevance for understanding "the unconscious"—whatever that might be?

This chapter will take a neuropsychoanalytic approach. By this is meant that by having a brain science framework in listening to patients, one begins to understand more about the patient, and also more about the brain science. In order for a thought to achieve consciousness, it probably needs some cortical input [14, 15]. Freud's use of dreams to understand the unconscious thinking of his patients can be adapted in the twenty-first century to our use of dreams to help patients become aware of previously unconscious midbrain phenomena [16]. Psychoanalysis has been moving forward like any other field. It has a tradition of using brain science in its work since it was started by that neuroscience researcher Freud.

By combining the face validity of craving with the neuroscience of addiction and the phenomenon of drug dreams, we are in a position to receive readout from subcortical areas whose function has been distorted by exposure to alcohol and drugs. By adding brain science to dream observation, we will be able to suggest a solution to the problem of articulating and measuring craving. In turn, the improved appreciation of what craving for alcohol and drug represents should put practitioners into a better position to help their patients.

Subcortical Mechanisms of Physical Addiction

The addictive use of alcohol or drugs has two aspects. The first, the reason for initiation [17], and to some extent for persistent use, has to do with "psychological addiction," the use of the intoxicated state to supplant intolerable affect [3, 18–20]. Drinking or drug use becomes a typical response to difficulties from within or from outside the person—a character trait [20].

In addition to the wish to remove feelings by supplanting them with a state of intoxication is the demand of various neural systems that have been altered by repeated alcohol and/or drug exposure. Although it would be reductionistic to assume specific and concrete neural centers or pathways that result in the drive to compulsively perpetuate drinking or drug-taking, there is substantial evidence that the initial predisposition to accelerating alcohol and drug-taking has to do with aberrant salience created by sensitization of the ventral tegmental dopaminergic-SEEKING system [12, 21–26]. Over the course of the illness more frontal–cortical areas become important, such as the amygdala, hippocampus, anterior cingulate, and prefrontal cortex [27–30]. One way to summarize the neural process of addiction is that one falls ill unconsciously as the SEEKING system demands continuing alcohol and/or drug use. Secondarily, the frontal areas that control modulation of drive become overstimulated and compromised so that the addicted person automatically turns their attention to alcohol and drug cues, while eschewing natural rewards and becoming increasingly incapable of producing survival behaviors.

The diagram shows the pharmacological mechanism of three addictive drugs whose action on the ventral tegmental area (VTA) of the midbrain is best known.

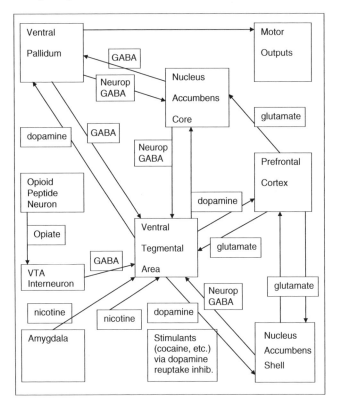

Craving/Dreaming Pathways: *Neurop* neuropeptides, *GABA* gamma amino butyric acid
- Nicotinic receptors for acetylcholine on the VTA and cholinergic inputs from the amygdala to VTA nicotinic receptors accelerate dopaminergic transmission to the nucleus accumbens shell.
- Cocaine and methamphetamine disrupt the dopamine reuptake transporter protein recycling of dopamine that

impinges on the nucleus accumbens shell. This provokes increased depolarization of nucleus accumbens shell neurons.
- Opiates inhibit a gamma amino butyric acid (GABA) inhibiting interneuron, which disinhibits the VTA, allowing increased dopaminergic stimulation of the nucleus accumbens shell [31].

In turn, the nucleus accumbens shell interacts with frontal areas: medial orbitofrontal cortex, frontal eye fields, etc., so that learning occurs. Desire for something with survival value is created by the experience of dopaminergic signals originating in the VTA. The system was created in animals so that they would be alert to the possible availability of food, water, or sex [12]. The mechanism of anticipation of a sought entity is instantiated by prefrontal areas detecting cues in the environment that suggest the availability of the desired drug. The perception is relayed to the VTA, which in turn increases dopaminergic tone to the nucleus accumbens shell, creating a sense of excitement. Learning is reinforced as glutamatergic inputs to frontal areas, and experience, guide and tone the prefrontal/VTA/nucleus accumbens shell system via long-term potentiation. The brain learns by asking, "Did the cue lead to gratification?"

The nucleus accumbens core is oriented to rote experiences. As experiences become well-worn by constant use of addictive drugs, neural circuits become well-connected via long-term potentiation. Eventually the core can take stimulation directly from the VTA alert system, and turn it into motor actions [30]. Nucleus accumbens core activation can dominate behaviors so that they become automatic. Obtaining drugs becomes routine, and deviating from established behaviors becomes more difficult [32].

It is only conscious inhibition of drug seeking that can oppose these subcortical mechanisms. Consciousness of the consequences of alcohol and drug use, and/or alliances with others who will help the individual maintain sobriety, is the only remedy for this constant unconscious stimulation from the midbrain that produces inchoate urge. Craving cannot have a standard word definition because of the subcortical brain system that provokes it. Addicted persons want alcohol or drugs for the same reasons that anyone wants sex or food; the desire just is. In Alcoholics Anonymous the aphorism that describes this midbrain mechanism is, "You drink because you are an alcoholic."

So the common mechanism of craving is dopaminergic tone in the SEEKING system provoked by exposure to addictive drugs, leading to a constant sense of drug hunger. Abstinence moderates the craving. But once established, it is unlikely that craving will disappear completely. As the neural system diagrammed above is sculpted by repeated drug exposure leading to long-term potentiation of connections that alert the vulnerable person to the availability of alcohol or drugs, there is a midbrain signal to obtain the substance provoked by drug cues. Craving varies according to environment—such as in the story at the beginning of the man who was 6 years sober and confident of remaining so until he entered his old neighborhood. Drug cues accelerate drug hunger by provoking glutamatergic stimulation from frontal areas to VTA. Stress can increase craving by virtue of corticotrophin releasing factor receptors on the VTA [8]. VTA/nucleus accumbens dopamine functioning is involved in depressive illness [33] and although the mechanism of increased craving during depressive illness is not yet described, there is a plausible interaction because of the shared substrate. Berridge and Robinson's [12] suggestion that craving may be unconscious would simply be a reflection of the craving pathway being subcortical, whereas it requires cortical activity to make a stimulus conscious [14, 15]. So we have now described a neural system that reflects all the problems that exist with the craving literature. Now, how might we solve the problem of measuring it?

Drug Dreams as a Marker of Exposure to Addictive Drugs

This is a dream from a sober patient who was addicted to alcohol and no other drugs (age 28).

> We were drinking a champagne toast. Then I begin to go around the room and drink leftover champagne from glasses. Then I am on my fourth glass of red wine and I forget to cover up my drinking. My mother says, "Have you been drinking? Tell the truth" [20].

This is a dream from a sober patient who came to treatment after heroin detoxification, and who had been addicted to nicotine, amphetamines, cocaine, benzodiazepines, barbiturates, and marijuana in addition to alcohol (age 50).

> My mother and I were in our summer house. There were three of us celebrating. My mother says, "We'll have to drink to that." She poured expensive champagne. I thought, "I already did Redi Whip. That will really be relapsing." Maybe I could hide it. I didn't think I could say no to her. I said fuck it and drank the champagne. I thought, "What does this mean? Should I take Percs?" I was thinking, "Why is she giving me booze?" The third person is a he, balancing my mother's morals, caring [16].[1]

Drug dreams have been observed recurrently, but there is no consensus in the addiction literature regarding their origin, utility, or persistence. According to Colace [34], "…drug dreams as biological-drive-related dreams may contribute to reducing the intensity of frustrated drives in the post-dream period. Patients who have drug dreams show a better ability

to deal with drug-craving stimulation than those who do not have drug dreams." However, there has been no systematic study of how common such dreams are in the addicted population, when in the course of addiction and/or treatment they are first reported, whether they persist over a lifetime, and how they are related to age, gender, cognitive functioning, or specific drug exposure.

> **Reports of Dreams About Alcohol and Drugs**
> *Alcohol* [16, 20, 35–38]
> *Nicotine* [16, 39, 40]
> *Cocaine* [16, 41–45]
> *Opiates* [16, 34, 46–48]
> *Benzodiazepines* [16, 49]
> *Marijuana* [50]
> *Benzodiazepines* [16, 49]
> *Multiple drugs appearing in multiple dreams* [16, 51]
> *Drug dreams reported to correlate with or be helpful for maintaining abstinence* [16, 36, 38–40, 43, 49, 51]

How might drug dreams be connected with drug craving? We know that drug dreams do not appear to be present while addicted persons are actively using their drug [34, 36, 39, 40, 48]. Rather, they appear as withdrawal and drug craving begin. Colace [34] showed that subjects who used heroin constantly did not have drug dreams, whereas subjects who became abstinent began to have frequent dreams of seeking or using heroin, apparently correlated with physical withdrawal. Araujo, Oliveira and Piccoloto [52] found that the 27% of their subjects who dreamed of alcohol had significantly higher scores on a craving scale. This increase of alcohol and drug dreams is greatest in the period immediately following cessation of use; Reid and Simeon [43] found that 89% of cocaine-dependent subjects had drug dreams within the first month of abstinence, while only 57% reported them at 6 months.

The Reid and Simeon study confirms the common clinical observation that abstinence facilitates the reduction of craving. But it appears likely that drug craving and drug dreams never go away. In my study of a single patient treated four times per week over 5 years of abstinence, drug dreams persisted at a constant rate [16]. What the dreams seemed to do was help the patient be conscious of her persistent urges to use alcohol and drugs. In a 6-month study, treatment outcomes were better for the 57% of subjects reporting drug dreams 6 months after intake [43].

As to why alcohol and drug dreams appear during abstinence rather than while using, one explanation is a variant of Freud's "dreams are the guardian of sleep"; that dreaming of alcohol and drugs allows the addicted individual to postpone

---

[1] "Redi Whip" is a pressurized whipped cream product. The patient had guilt over experimenting with inhaling a small amount of the gas vehicle the day before the analytic hour. "Percs" is the street name of a frequently abused compound of oxycodone and acetaminophen.

motor activity until they complete needed restorative sleep by giving an illusion of wish-fulfillment [16]. A second explanation might be that the user is now trying to develop new strategies and schemas for maintaining abstinence by rehearsing activities during the motor paralysis of sleep. This would lead to better outcomes.

In terms of clinical practice, listening to drug dreams is an effective way to help patients be conscious of their daily preoccupation with using drugs or drinking, and any connections, stressors or cues that may be provoking the urge. For example, in the sample dreams given above, the patients are acknowledging their continuing urge to drink. It may be helpful for the therapist to make an interpretation that this urge is apparent in the dreams, and ask if the patient were aware of these urges and any associated issues. In each dream, the patient is also expressing a wish to be helped with their alcohol craving. The therapist would inquire regarding the first dream about the patient's thoughts about her mother. In the second dream, the therapist would ask about the patient's thoughts about the therapist. In both cases, one interpretation might be that the dreams show that the patient has crossed over from alcohol abuse to physical addiction to alcohol. This means that having one drink would intensify craving to such an extent that many more drinks would be likely to follow.

Subcortical Mechanisms of Drug Dreams

Patients will often state that they have no more craving; even patients who subsequently relapse back to active addiction. Could it be that relapse after sustained sobriety is a manifestation of psychological addiction; that the addicted person was confronted by an issue that they felt helpless about, or they experienced intolerable isolation, and their use of the substance was purely an emotional response in the same neurotic direction that originally provoked their addiction? That may be the reason for relapse in some cases. But it would not explain the commonly observed phenomenon that a person has been abstinent from cigarettes for years, finds they have "just one," and then quickly resumes smoking at the frequency of previous years. Without denying the reality of relapse for emotional reasons, there must be a second cause of relapse; the kind that has no plausible emotional cause.

A link here is the persistence of drug dreams during sobriety. In my study of persistent drug dreams over 5 years of sobriety [16], despite the psychoanalysis of this patient 4 days per week, we rarely could find a plausible emotional cause. Solms [53] used a sophisticated analysis of patients with brain lesions in diverse areas to show that the dream-on mechanism and the drug craving mechanism share the identical medial forebrain pathways, originating in the VTA. Although there are many accounts of the meaning of dreams,

the one that fits here is that with the motor system paralyzed, the dreamer is able to make wide connections throughout the brain to consider possible strategies for survival and prosperity in the world [54]. But the initiation of the dreaming mechanism flows from the VTA and involves our basic quest for food, water, sex and relationships.

In other words, the origin of Freud's aphorism that every dream contains a wish is like the aphorism from Alcoholics Anonymous that "I drink because I'm an alcoholic." The brain system that exists to have us animals seek food, water, sex and relationships (the wish), and that is taken over by exposure to addictive drugs so that alcohol and drugs are sought, provokes dreams that allow the individual to experiment with potential actions while their motor system is paralyzed. Everyone since Freud has recognized that hunger [16, 55] and thirst [54] will provoke dreams of eating or drinking water. So of course when there is alcohol or drug hunger, the dreamer will seek alcohol and/or drugs. One characteristic of these dreams while patients are in treatment is that the treaters may also be part of the dream; notice that in the specimen dreams that there is a protective agent who comes in to help with the drive to drink.

The first specimen dream of the 28-year-old woman whose mother asked if she was drinking was produced by a woman who had left detox to drink in a motel. Her mother called me, asked if I would see her, and brought her from the motel to my office. In a memorable first visit I demonstrated the presence of alcoholic myopathy to the patient and her mother. In the dream, the urge to drink is modulated by the image of the mother.

The second specimen dream is from the 5-year study of this patient who had an absence of protective, nurturing figures both during childhood and in her adult life. As the analysis progressed, the dreams shifted from pure seeking to seeking with a protective male figure who reliably was described by the patient as the analyst [16].

The careful reader will notice that while the diagram shows the mechanisms of physical addiction to nicotine, cocaine (and methamphetamine) and opioids, there is not a diagram of how this might happen with alcohol. Alcohol can be drunk in large quantities, and daily, without the appearance of drinking dreams. For example, only one drinking dream was found during "The psychoanalysis of a man with active alcoholism" [56] despite daily heavy drinking before and during some of the treatment, and analytic observation over 1,580 treatment hours. The patient engaged in heavy daily drinking, with consequences, but did not ever show alcohol withdrawal. This is consistent with the critique of O'Brien, Volkow and Li [57] that dependency and withdrawal are not directly related to addiction.

But it seems that drinking dreams have an onset at about the same time as physical withdrawal begins. As seen in the craving/dreaming diagram, ventral tegmental dopamine activity is tonically inhibited by GABAergic input. The alcohol withdrawal syndrome is a product of the release of driving neurotransmitters from ordinary GABAergic modulation. While we are used to monitoring this phenomenon in the periphery by its manifestations as increased pulse, blood pressure, sweating, agitation, etc., decreased GABAergic tone is also present in the central nervous system. Due to the downregulation of GABAergic tone by blanketing of GABAergic neurons with alcohol, it may be that during withdrawal there is a corresponding increase in ventral tegmental dopamine now released from tonic GABA interneuron inhibition. Therefore, unlike other drugs, alcohol craving would begin to be seen some time after chronic heavy use had already been extent for a period of time. One can drink every day without provoking craving and drug dreams, as long as the amount is sufficiently small that GABAergic tone is unaffected because most of the day is spent in a homeostatic state unaffected by the alcohol.

This time course, that the transition from psychological to physical dependence on alcohol requires progression of drinking to the point where the alcohol will blanket GABAergic receptors takes away the explanation that alcohol dreams are simply a manifestation of emotionally-relevant experiences or daily experiences being represented in dreams. The dreams are therefore a marker of a brain change produced by the alcohol taken in large enough amounts over sufficient time to cause downregulation of GABAergic tone. The development of drinking dreams then would be a psychological manifestation of the "switch" mechanism from alcohol abuse to alcohol dependence and a direct readout of a permanent brain alteration of the dynamic balance of the SEEKING system against other competing and modulating systems.

All psychotherapies feature as a central component the need of the patient to be conscious of various factors that predispose to relapse into recurrent drinking and drug-taking. In this model, drinking and drug dreams are a measure of ability to be conscious of the activity of the ventral tegmental dopaminergic SEEKING system. The need to inhibit the drive to continue to use addictive drugs as the central feature of the process of recovery from active addiction is derived from the Berridge and Robinson [13] model of conscious and unconscious systems of motivation, learning, and memory. In their model, conscious cognitive incentives have an autobiographical (hippocampal) nature linked to ability to predict outcome and understand causation. Ventral tegmental dopaminergic seeking is connected to learning via Pavlovian-conditioned responses and instrumental-conditioned responses. In this model, not all wanting is conscious. Thus, addicted individuals may begin to seek alcohol and drugs for reasons of which they are not conscious. Berridge and Robinson [13] state, "For example, drug addicts in some circumstances will work for low doses of stimulants

or morphine, doses that produce no subjective effects and even no autonomic responses, without being aware that they are doing so." The process of recovery from this form of addiction requires that individuals be constantly conscious of their urge to relapse, constantly make conscious decisions regarding alcohol or drug use, and to be aware of the need to protect themselves from stress and loneliness.

Nightmares

A nightmare is simply a dream with unpleasant emotion. Hartmann [58] suggests that they are ubiquitous in childhood and that adult nightmares are not necessarily related to trauma. However, Hartmann has also followed the course of nightmares after trauma and suggests that their content becomes less frightening as the traumatic event is worked through.

The problem for therapists who treat addicted patients with nightmares is that the patients awaken terrified, the nature of addictive illness is that patients are intolerant of feeling, and the patients often demand that rather than use the dreams to help them understand what they have been through, the patients insist that the dreams be suppressed. Added to this is the problem that many addicted patients have been horribly brutalized as children, especially sexually, and frequently suffer from posttraumatic stress disorder [59, 60]. This situation can create a difficult countertransference in the therapist. Sometimes the material is so anxiety-provoking for the therapist as well as the patient that they also may want to escape from the experience of listening to the patients' memories. Some practitioners see nightmares as a symptom to be suppressed [61], for example with prazocin [62].

However, most psychotherapists would value nightmares and have their patients make associations that allow the issues that come up in the dreams to be discussed. Dreams allow past events to be remembered and compared with current circumstances [63]. No matter how horrible, memories of abuse or of life-threatening trauma need to be contextualized into the safer present. The danger of suppressing an urgent signal that a memory needs to be metabolized and the distress ameliorated via witnessing by the therapist and re-evaluation within discussions of the patient and therapist is that the patient will use alcohol or drugs persistently in an effort to distance themselves from experiences that are forever encoded in their brains. Late-stage patients can be irreversibly ill. They have gone decades since the original traumatic event, drinking or using drugs to try to get away from their memories, suffering cognitive decline from the cumulative effects of active addiction, and still having nightmares and other symptoms of posttraumatic stress disorder. They live as if the event had just happened.

Nightmares are a complex phenomenon involving many internal factors rather than simply being a manifestation of real external danger [64]. There would be no particular reason in a psychological treatment to work with a nightmare in any different way than any other dream. Any dream is a communication from the dreamer to the treater to be decoded via associations. By bringing a nightmare to treatment, the patient is asking for help from the therapist.

Summary and Conclusion

This chapter on dreams and nightmares is based on literature from craving studies, neurobiology, and drug dreams. Assembled together they provide a context for understanding each other so that it becomes clearer how to study and treat addicted patients. The model presented has the construct validity that has been missing from craving scales. By following dreams we have a direct readout of neural changes caused by exposure to alcohol and drugs. But it is evident from what has been presented that much more work needs to be done. It would follow from this material that drug dreams might form the "gold standard" for craving research; but that assertion could only be substantiated by more empirical studies of dreams and eventually correlation of dreams with scales constructed to capture the activity of the subcortical SEEKING pathway. This approach would require some innovative thinking.

In addition, if the hypothesis that drinking dreams represent a psychological manifestation of a biological change from psychological to physical addiction is supported by empirical data, the diagnostic criteria for alcohol dependence might be rewritten to include this biological marker rather than merely descriptions of behaviors related to drinking. If this hypothesis were confirmed, it would have significant implications for prevention, psychoeducation, and stigma-reduction. We would be able to show that the biological disease of alcoholism can be seen by a change in an everyday biologically-driven experience, dreams, and that this experience represents a permanent change in the brains of persons who use drink alcoholically. It would give addicted persons a way to know that they can never use again because they can observe this change in themselves.

Addicted persons can experience the urges to relapse by telling their dreams to people who care about them; psychotherapists, addiction counselors or fellow members of Alcoholics Anonymous. By discussing drug dreams, the reality that the patient has gone through an irreversible change, and will crave alcohol and/or drugs for the rest of their lives, becomes more integrated into the identity of the addicted person. Nightmares, even in the context of overwhelming physical trauma or sexual abuse, are an urgent signal that a memory is causing current stress; stress that could provoke a relapse to active addiction; unless the nightmare can be used to work through the trauma.

References

1. Sayette MA, Shiffman S, Tiffany ST, Niaura RS, Martin CS, Shadel WG. The measurement of drug craving. Addiction. 2000;95 Suppl 2:S189–210.
2. Xu J, Azizian A, Monterosso J, Domier CP, Brody AL, London ED, et al. Gender effects on mood and cigarette craving during early abstinence and resumption of smoking. Nicotine Tob Res. 2008;10(11):1653–61.
3. Johnson B. Three perspectives on addiction. J Am Psychoanal Assoc. 1999;47:791–815.
4. Wise RA. Ventral tegmental glutamate: a role in stress-, cue-, and cocaine-induced reinstatement of cocaine-seeking. Neuropharmacology. 2009;56:174–6.
5. Bordnick PS, Traylor A, Copp HL, Graap KM, Carter B, Ferrer M, et al. Assessing reactivity to virtual reality alcohol based cues. Addict Behav. 2008;33(6):743–56.
6. Volkow ND, Wang GJ, Telang F, Fowler JS, Logan J, Childres AR, et al. Dopamine increases in striatum do not elicit craving in cocaine abusers unless they are coupled with cocaine cues. Neuroimage. 2008;39(3):1266–73.
7. Schneider F, Habel U, Wagner M, Franke P, Salloum JB, Shah NJ, et al. Subcortical correlates of craving in recently abstinent alcoholic patients. Am J Psychiatry. 2001;158(7):1075–83.
8. Koob GF. A role for brain stress systems in addiction. Neuron. 2008;59(1):11–34.
9. Koob GF. Neurobiological substrates for the dark side of compulsivity in addiction. Neuropharmacology. 2009;56:18–31.
10. Elman I, Karlsgodt KH, Gastfriend DR, Chabris CF, Breiter HC. Cocaine-primed craving and its relationship to depressive symptomatology in individuals with cocaine dependence. J Psychopharmacol. 2002;16(2):163–7.
11. Nakama H, Chang L, Cloak C, Jiang C, Alicata D, Haning W. Association between psychiatric symptoms and craving in methamphetamine users. Am J Addict. 2008;17(5):441–6.
12. Robinson TE, Berridge KC. The neural basis of drug craving: an incentive-sensitization theory of addiction. Brain Res Rev. 1993;18:247–91.
13. Berridge KC, Robinson TE. Parsing reward. Trends Neurosci. 2003;26:507–13.
14. Freud S. Beyond the pleasure principle. Standard Edition 18. 1920.
15. Barbas H, Ghashghaei HT, Rempel-Clower NL, Xiao D. Anatomic basis of functional specialization in prefrontal cortices in primates. In: Segalowitz SJ, editor. Handbook of neuropsychology, vol. 7. 2nd ed. Amsterdam: Elsevier; 2002.
16. Johnson B. Drug dreams: a neuropsychoanalytic hypothesis. J Am Psychoanal Assoc. 2001;49:75–96.
17. Johnson B. A developmental model of addiction and its relationship to the Twelve Step Program of Alcoholics Anonymous. J Subst Abuse Treat. 1993;10:23–32.
18. Khantzian EJ. The self-medication hypothesis of substance use disorders: a reconsideration and recent applications. Harv Rev Psychiatry. 1997;4:231–44.
19. Dodes L. Compulsion and addiction. J Am Psychoanal Assoc. 1996;44:815–35.
20. Johnson B. Psychological addiction, physical addiction, addictive character, addictive personality disorder: a new nosology of addiction. Can J Psychoanal. 2003;11:135–60.
21. Panksepp J. Affective neuroscience. New York: Oxford University Press; 1998.
22. Ikemoto S, Panksepp J. The role of nucleus accumbens dopamine in motivated behavior: a unifying interpretation with special reference to reward-seeking. Brain Res Rev. 1999;31:6–41.

23. Nocjar C, Panksepp J. Chronic intermittent amphetamine pretreatment enhance future appetitive behavior for drug- and natural-reward: interaction with environmental variables. Behav Brain Res. 2002;128:189–203.

24. Berridge KC, Robinson TE. What is the role of dopamine in reward: hedonic impact, reward learning, or incentive salience? Brain Res Rev. 1998;28:309–69.

25. Robinson TE, Berridge KC. The psychology and neurobiology of addiction: an incentive-sensitization view. Addiction. 2000;95 Suppl 2:91–117.

26. Goldsmith RJ. What's the big deal about sensitization? J Addict Dis. 2001;20:1–5.

27. Volkow ND, Fowler JS, Wang G-J. The addicted human brain viewed in the light of imaging studies: brain circuits and treatment strategies. Neuropharmacology. 2004;47:3–13.

28. Kalivas PW, Volkow NP. The neural basis of addiction: a pathology of motivation and choice. Am J Psychiatry. 2005;162: 1403–13.

29. Kalivas PW, Volkow NP, Seamans J. Unmanageable motivation in addiction: a pathology in prefrontal-accumbens glutamate transmission. Neuron. 2005;45:647–50.

30. Everitt BJ, Robbins TW. Neural systems of reinforcement for drug addiction: from actions to habits to compulsion. Nat Neurosci. 2005;8:1481–9.

31. Nestler EJ. Is there a common molecular pathway for addiction? Nat Neurosci. 2005;8:1445–9.

32. Bechara A. Decision making, impulse control and loss of will power to resist drugs: a neurocognitive perspective. Nat Neurosci. 2005;8:1458–63.

33. Nestler EJ, Carlezon Jr WA. The mesolimbic dopamine reward circuit in depression. Biol Psychiatry. 2006;59(12):1151–9.

34. Colace C. Dreaming in addiction, a study on the motivational bases of dreaming process. NeuroPsychoanalysis. 2004;6:165–79.

35. Scott EM. Dreams of alcoholics. Percept Mot Skills. 1968;26: 1315–8.

36. Choi SY. Dreams as a prognostic factor in alcoholism. Am J Psychiatry. 1973;130:699–702.

37. Fiss H. Dream content and response to withdrawal from alcohol. Sleep Res. 1980;9:152.

38. Denizen NK. Alcoholic dreams. Alcohol Treat Q. 1988;5:133–9.

39. Hajek P, Belcher M. Dream of absent-minded transgression: an empirical study of a cognitive withdrawal symptom. J Abnorm Psychol. 1991;100:487–91.

40. Persico AM. Predictors of smoking cessation in a sample of Italian smokers. Int J Addict. 1992;27:683–95.

41. Jerry PA. Psychodynamic psychotherapy of the intravenous cocaine abuser. J Subst Abuse Treat. 1997;14:319–32.

42. Flowers LK, Zweben JE. The changing role of "using" dreams in addiction recovery. J Subst Abuse Treat. 1998;15:193–200.

43. Reid SD, Simeon DT. Progression of dream of crack cocaine as a predictor of treatment outcome: a preliminary report. J Nerv Ment Dis. 2001;189:854–7.

44. Yee T, Perantie DC, Dhanani N, Brown ES. Drug dreams in outpatients with bipolar disorder and cocaine dependence. J Nerv Ment Dis. 2004;192:238–42.

45. Colace C. Drug dreams in cocaine addiction. Drug Alcohol Rev. 2006;25:177.

46. Looney M. The dreams of heroin addicts. Social Work. 1972;17:23–8.

47. Colace C. Dreams in abstinent opiate drug addicts: a case reports study. Sleep. 1999;22 Suppl 1:175–6.

48. Colace C. Dreams in abstinent heroin addicts: four case reports. Sleep Hypn. 2000;2:160–3.

49. Johnson B. Commentary on "Freudian Dream Theory, Dream Bizarreness, and the Disguise-Censor Controversy". NeuroPsychoanalysis. 2006;8:33–40.

50. Jones DS, Krotick S, Johnson B, Morrison AP. Waiting for rescue: an attorney who will not advocate for himself. Harv Rev Psychiatry. 2005;13:244–56.

51. Christo G, Franey C. Addicts' drug-related dreams: their frequency and relationship to six-month outcomes. Subst Use Misuse. 1996;31:1–15.

52. Araujo RB, Oliveira M, Piccoloto LB. Dreams and craving in alcohol addicted patients in the detoxification stage. Rev Psychiatr Clin. 2004;31:63–9.

53. Solms M. Dreaming and REM sleep are controlled by different mechanisms. Behav Brain Sci. 2000;23:843–50.

54. Hartmann E. Dreams and nightmares: the new theory on the origin and meaning of dreams. New York: Plenum; 1998.

55. Freud S. The interpretation of dreams: Freud's seminal exploration of human nature. Standard Edition 18, 1900.

56. Johnson B. The psychoanalysis of a man with active alcoholism. J Subst Abuse Treat. 1992;9:111–23.

57. O'Brien CP, Volkow N, Li T-K. What's in a word? Addiction versus dependence in DSM-V. Am J Psychiatry. 2006;163:764–5.

58. Hartmann E. Nightmare after trauma as paradigm for all dreams: a new approach to the nature and functions of dreaming. Psychiatry. 1998;61(3):223–38.

59. Triffleman EG, Marmar CR, Delucchi KL, Ronfeldt H. Childhood trauma and posttraumatic stress disorder in substance abuse inpatients. J Nerv Ment Dis. 1995;183(3):172–6.

60. Plotzker RE, Metzger DS, Holmes WC. Childhood sexual and physical abuse histories, PTSD, depression, and HIV risk outcomes in women injection drug users: a potential mediating pathway. Am J Addict. 2007;16(6):431–8.

61. Mohamed S, Rosenheck RA. Pharmacotherapy of PTSD in the U.S. Department of Veterans Affairs: diagnostic- and symptom-guided drug selection. J Clin Psychiatry. 2008;69(6):959–65.

62. Miller LJ. Prazosin for the treatment of posttraumatic stress disorder sleep disturbances. Pharmacotherapy. 2008;28(5):656–66.

63. Palombo SR. Dreaming and memory: a new information processing model. New York: Basic Books; 1978.

64. Malcolm-Smith S, Solms M, Turnbull O, Tredoux C. Threat in dreams: an adaptation? Conscious Cogn. 2008;17(4):1281–91.

Drug Abuse in Cardiovascular Diseases

32

F. Furlanello, L. Vitali Serdoz, L. De Ambroggi, and R. Cappato

Abstract

A large amount of substances and their association can lead to worsening of latent or active cardiovascular diseases and, sometimes, to ex-novo cardiovascular diseases.

Negative cardiovascular effects are mainly due to pharmacokinetics of substances, in particular if drugs are administered in combination, or if intake, distribution, and elimination processes are altered; moreover, negative effects can be due to pharmacodynamics of drugs as in the presence of an interaction between an otherwise non-toxic substance and a morphofunctional altered cardiac substrate.

In the first part of this chapter, we systematically describe cardiovascular effects of illicit drugs, as listed by the World Anti-Doping Agency and including different classes of substances, namely, anabolic androgenic steroids, hormones and related substances, β2-agonists, diuretics, stimulants, narcotics, cannabinoids, glucocorticosteroids, alcohol, and β-blockers. The second part is dedicated to cardiovascular effects that can occur during the use and abuse of most common prescription drugs as antipsychotic, antibiotics, anti-viral, antihistaminic, and antineoplastic drugs.

Learning Objectives

1. The intake of illicit drugs could be particularly dangerous in athletes and in common people, especially in the presence of the following:
   - Pre-existing arrhythmic or structural primary disease also in an early or latent stage.
   - Latent form of some inherited arrhythmogenic molecular heart disease due to genetic defects related to cytoskeleton, sarcomere, cell junctions, ion channels, etc.
   - Cardiac disease presenting with ventricular tachycardia during physical effort.
   - Ex-novo cardiac diseases due to long-term intake of illicit drugs, especially at high doses and in multiple associations.
2. Caution should be always taken because some drugs, routinely prescribed in daily practice, can bring unexpected danger and cause severe cardiac arrhythmias (i.e. histamine receptor antagonists and antibiotics).

F. Furlanello (✉) • L. Vitali Serdoz • L. De Ambroggi • R. Cappato
Center of Clinical Arrhythmology and Electrophysiology,
Istituto Policlinico San Donato, IRCCS, University of Milan,
San Donato Milanese, Milan, Italy
e-mail: ffurlanello@villabiancatrento.it

J.C. Verster et al. (eds.), *Drug Abuse and Addiction in Medical Illness: Causes, Consequences and Treatment*,
DOI 10.1007/978-1-4614-3375-0_32, © Springer Science+Business Media, LLC 2012

Issues that Need to Be Addressed by Future Research
The main arrhythmologic, pathophysiologic, and epidemiologic aspects of cardiovascular adverse effects of illicit drugs and common prescription drugs are an excitant challenge for cardiologists activating serious prevention actions.

Background

A large amount of substances and their association can lead to worsening of latent or active cardiovascular diseases and, sometimes, to ex-novo cardiovascular diseases.

Negative cardiovascular effects are mainly due to both pharmacokinetics of substances, in particular if drugs are administered in combination or if intake, distribution, and elimination processes are functionally or anatomically altered, and their pharmacodynamics as in the presence of an interaction between an otherwise non-toxic substance and a morphofunctional altered cardiac substrate (e.g., Long QT syndrome).

This chapter is divided in two main sections:

1. Cardiovascular effects of illicit drugs are systematically described in this section. Illicit drugs are listed by World Anti-Doping Agency (WADA list 2011, yearly updated http://www.wada-ama.org) and comprise all the substances that can be assumed by common people and by athletes, both very young and master athletes, with ergogenic scope during all lifetime. Many of these drugs can induce cardiovascular effects during short-, mid-, and long-time use [1–6]. The description of those drugs offers the chance to understand and to acquire knowledge in the less-known but widespread field of modern sport cardiology [7–9]. We will describe cardiovascular changes that can potentially occur during treatment with these substances both in healthy subjects and in patients with preclinical or clinical manifestation of cardiovascular diseases. The different classes of WADA list also include substances that are taken without ergogenic effect but as recreational drugs that are often listed in abuse drugs registries.

2. The second section of this chapter is dedicated to cardiovascular effects that can occur during the use and abuse of the most common prescription drugs as antibiotics, antiviral, antihistaminic, antineoplastic, and anti-psychotic drugs. Many of these substances have been extensively treated in the other chapters of this book.

Cardiovascular Diseases in User of Illicit Drugs

The current medical survey of athletes is complicated by the large use of "illicit drugs" taken, at any age, by both professional and non-professional athletes [4, 6, 8, 9].

We prefer the term "illicit drugs," rather than "doping," because they comprise the following:

1. Drugs taken as true "doping," or "performance enhancing drugs (PEDs)," anabolic-androgenic steroids (AAS), stimulants, beta-2-agonist, erythropoietin (EPO), growth hormone (GH), insulin-like growth factor (IGF-1).

2. "Masking agents," i.e., drugs taken in order to cover the presence of other specific drugs in tests for doping control. (e.g., diuretic, plasma expanders, chemical and physical manipulations probenecid, alfa reductase inhibitor finasteride, etc.)

3. "Antagonists of side effects," to counteract the adverse effects of abuse of AAS (e.g., gonadotropins), agents with anti-estrogenic activity, and aromatase inhibitors (e.g., letrazole).

4. "Recreational drugs" (or drugs of abuse) including ecstasy (MDMA) and other amphetamines and other very new synthetically derived formulations, several classified as "designer drugs."

In fact, the spreading of the use of PEDs is often associated with an increased assumption of "recreational drugs" in athletic population [10, 11].

Several illicit drugs, banned by International Olympic Committee (IOC) and since 1999 yearly updated by the World Anti-Doping Agency, may cause cardiac collateral effects, through a direct or indirect cardiac action, and may provoke especially arrhythmogenic effect, during short, medium, or long term.

The cardiovascular (CV) effects comprise a wide spectrum of diseases: hypertrophic, dilated, ischemic cardiomyopathies, myocarditis, thromboembolic diseases, and also a wide range of supraventricular and/or ventricular cardiac arrhythmias, focal or re-entry type, that are often symptomatic and potentially lethal even in healthy subjects with no previous history of cardiac diseases. The risk of lethal arrhythmias and sudden death is very high in subjects with pre-existing cardiac diseases, particularly latent arrhythmogenic substrate or primary arrhythmic disorders, including some inherited cardiomyopathies at risk for sudden cardiac death (SCD) [12–14] or with structural disease caused by the long-lasting assumption of the illicit drugs, e.g., cocaine, stimulants, and AAS.

The 2011 IOC list of the "Prohibited classes of substances" (http://www.wada-ama.org—World Anti-Doping CODE—Valid 1 January 2011—International Standard) is reported in Table 32.1.

Table 32.1 The 2011 prohibited list world anti-doping code

I.   Substances and Methods Prohibited at All Times (in- and out-of-competition)

Prohibited Substances

S1. Anabolic agents

   1. Anabolic Androgenic Steroids (AAS)

      a. Exogenous AAS

      b. Endogenous AAS

   2. Other Anabolic Agents, including but not limited to clenbuterol, selective androgen receptor modulators (SARMs), tibolone, zeranol, zilpaterol

S2. Peptide hormones, growth factors, and related substances

   1. Erythropoiesis-Stimulating Agents [e.g., erythropoietin (EPO), darbepoetin (dEPO), hypoxia-inducible factor (HIF) stabilizers, methoxy polyethylene glycol-epoetin beta (CERA), peginesatide (Hematide)].

   2. Chorionic Gonadotrophin (CG) and Luteinizing Hormone (LH) in males.

   3. Insulins.

   4. Corticotrophins.

   5. Growth Hormone (GH), Insulin-like Growth Factor-1 (IGF-1), Fibroblast Growth Factors (FGFs), Hepatocyte Growth Factor (HGF), Mechano Growth Factors (MGFs), Platelet-Derived Growth Factor (PDGF), Vascular-Endothelial Growth Factor (VEGF), as well as any other growth factor affecting muscle, tendon, or ligament protein synthesis/degradation, vascularization, energy utilization, regenerative capacity or fiber type switching and other substances with similar chemical structure or similar biological effect(s)

S3. Beta-2-agonists

S4. Hormone antagonists and modulators

S5. Diuretics and other masking agents

Prohibited methods

M1. Enhancement of oxygen transfer

M2. Chemical and physical manipulation

M3. Gene doping

II. Substances and Methods Prohibited In-Competition

S6. Stimulants

S7. Narcotics

S8. Cannabinoids

S9. Glucocorticosteroids

III. Substances Prohibited in Particular Sports

P1. Alcohol

P2. Beta-blockers

http://www.wada-ama.org—World Anti-Doping CODE 2011

Table 32.2 Reported findings in users of AAS with severe C V events/SD

– Hypertrophic CMP with necrosis, fibrosis, inflammatory changes	
– Dilated CMP; Myocarditis	
– Myocardial infarction with or without thrombotic occlusion	
– Vasospasm in susceptible subjects	
– Systemic and cardiac thromboembolic events	
– Coronary atheroma, cardiac steatosis	
– Micropathology:	a. Focal myocardial necrosis
	b. Regional myocardial fibrosis
	c. Contractions band necrosis
	d. myocardial fibrosis
	e. myocardial coagulation necrosis

Arrhythmias occur often during physical activity

Anabolic-Androgenic Steroids

The IOC 2011 WADA list of AAS includes the more recent pharmaceutical products and contains also designer drugs in order to provide a complete spectrum for anti-doping controls (http://www.wada-ama-org) (Table 32.2).

The AAS are listed as "exogenous" (e.g., androstendiol, nandrolone, stanozolol, thetrahydrogestrinone) and "endogenous" defined as AAS when administered exogenously (e.g., prasterone and testosterone). Anabolic steroids are derived from modified testosterone to enhance anabolic rather than androgenic action and may be used in oral, 17alpha-alkylated, or intramuscular, 17beta-esterified, preparations. They represent the most used illicit drugs and the most frequently discovered drugs in anti-doping controls, often taken by very young athletes [3, 15, 16]. Their administration is often associated with other substances, to mask the identification in anti-doping controls or in pharmacological cocktails. They are taken in order to increase protein synthesis, muscle mass, level of aggressiveness, and to obtain a rapid recovery after effort. In sport activities based on prevalent use of muscular strength, such as bodybuilding and weight lifting, the dose of anabolic steroids taken by the athletes may be very high, up to 100-fold the therapeutic levels. Not infrequently, various anabolic steroids are used in combination, a practice known as "stacking" [17]. Moreover, pro-hormones and steroid hormones may be present in some dietary supplements for athletes, who, therefore, are exposed to the drug action [18–20].

Various cardiac adverse events have been reported with the use of these drugs: pathologic cardiac hypertrophy without a concomitant increase in microvascular circulation that is associated with fibrosis, necrosis, inflammatory infiltrates that are arrhythmogenic [2, 3, 21], myocardial infarction

Substances and Methods Prohibited at All Times (In- and Out-of-Competition)

Non-approved Substances

The 2011 WADA list points out the illicit role of any pharmacological substance which is not addressed by any section of the List and without current approval for human therapeutic use.

without coronary thrombus [6, 22], dilated cardiomyopathy [23, 24], and progressive myocardial hypertrophy not completely reversible [25, 26].

Moreover, their use is associated with intraventricular thrombi that can cause cerebral and peripheral thromboembolism [27], with myocardial infarction with and without coronary thrombus, with sudden death due to hypertrophic cardiomyopathy and myocarditis during sport activity [9, 25, 28–32]. Most of these fatal events were reported in power lifters and bodybuilders [29, 31].

Anabolic steroids produce several changes in lipid metabolism, with increase in LDL and decrease in HDL cholesterol levels [9, 21, 33, 34], as well as thromboembolic events due to an increase in platelet adhesion, to pro-thrombotic modification of endothelium, and to interferences with coagulation factors.

Many different arrhythmias may be induced by the anabolic steroids with different direct or indirect mechanisms. Among them are myocell injury and necrosis, inflammatory infiltrates, fibrosis, and hypertrophy [2, 3, 21].

AAS may present sympathetic effect during physical activity. Arrhythmias occur often during physical activity and may be due to myocellular alterations and increasing sympathomimetic activity.

Anabolic steroids are often administrated along with masking agents as diuretics, tamoxifene (to reduce gynecomastia), chorionic gonadotropin (which increases endogenous testosterone levels) [33], cocaine, and growth hormone (hGH) for its well-known anabolic effect [34].

The side effects of anabolic steroids intake are multiple: serious alterations of liver function with hepatocellular alterations, hepatitis, hepatic neoplasm, modification of connective tissue structure with decreased collagen, decrease in tension of tendons with susceptibility to ruptures [35], insulin resistance, sterility, gynecomastia, testicular hypotrophy, and acne; moreover immune depression, virilization in women, and aggressive behavior including sexual aberrations and crimes have been reported [2, 35, 36].

The arrhythmias frequently reported during assumption of anabolic steroids also in combination are atrial fibrillation [37], supraventricular and ventricular ectopic beats, sustained and not sustained ventricular tachycardia, and ventricular fibrillation [37, 38]. Arrhythmias occur often during physical activity. QT prolongation can also occur, particularly in genetically predisposed individuals [39]. Some reported findings in users of AAS with severe cardiovascular events and SD are listed in Table 32.2.

Erythropoietin

In clinical practice, erythropoietin (EPO) became available as a drug, recombinant human erythropoietin (rHuEPO), synthesized from ovary cells of hamster since 1988, thanks to genetic engineering techniques based on recombinant DNA. Its administration as medical therapy is mainly used in anemia, in chronic renal disease and heart failure (HF), and in some surgical and cardiosurgical fields. On the contrary, it is widely used as "blood doping" [40, 41] in place of former autologous or heterologous blood transfusion doping. Athletes often take EPO, to provide a sense of strength and stamina while engaged not only in physical activities as cycling, skiing, marathon running, and swimming, but also in competitive short duration performances. It is deemed that up to 3–7% of elite endurance athletes have used it [42].

The general aim of "blood doping" is the enhancement of oxygen tissue availability and thereby increasing its arterial blood concentration, by raising hemoglobin and red cell levels with EPO administration. In the bone marrow, it stimulates erythroid precursors and regulates apoptosis, according to physiologic inputs of oxygen requirements from interstitial renal tubular cells and from hepatic level.

The long-term use of HuEPO α β and darbopoietin, a synthetic derived of EPO, is characterized by many side effects. Increasing total number of red cells leads to a rise in blood viscosity, which in athletes could be further increased by natural perspiration during intense sport performances, especially in endurance sports. Besides, due to their actions on endothelium and platelets, thromboembolic risk could be raised in predisposed subjects, and cases of hypertension, myocardial infarction and stroke, and sudden death were reported in cyclists and other endurance athletes [1, 2, 10, 43].

More recently, a new drug for refractory anemia as the continuous erythropoiesis receptor activator (CERA) is used as a PED by the athletes. The administration of CERA induces a strong stimulation of red cells production and has the advantage of every 3 weeks intake (website 22-4-2004, F.Hoffmann-La Roche Ltd). Moreover, the 2011 list introduces a new erythropoiesis stimulator, namely hypoxia-inducible factor (HIF)-stabilizers.

Arrhythmias occurring in athletes with "blood doping" are usually "secondary" to circulatory effects induced by increased erythroid mass, increased blood viscosity, altered endothelial and platelet function with possible pulmonary and cerebral thromboembolic events, and hypertension during effort [44], as well as to frequent concomitant administration of PEDs such as stimulants, anabolic steroids, or masking agents like diuretics.

Growth Hormone and Insulin-Like Growth Factor I

Hypophysis produced growth factor (GH) acts on specific receptors present in almost all human tissue and especially in the heart, immune system, glucose metabolism, muscles, bone, and cartilaginous and fat tissue.

GH stimulates, in particular at the hepatic level, the production of IGF-I, that is, GH effectory factor, on many target organs which acts on specific IGF-I receptors. This is the reason why both GH and IGF-I are responsible for various tissue stimulating actions. The large physiological effects explain the polymorphism of collateral effects due to illicit intake of both GH and IGF-I as PED. Therapeutic clinical use of GH and IGF-I is quite limited, being indicated in some nutritional and endocrine disorders, congenital or acquired, with clear indications for GH established by law. Instead, exogenous rhGH and rhIGF-I are widely used by athletes as anabolic agents to decrease body fat and to increase muscle mass, cardiac performance, and stamina on the job [45–48]. The real effect on muscle strength is still subject to debate [49–51] and is under investigation.

Up to now, the side effects related to rhGH and rhIGF-I "ergogenic" abuse are not clarified in athletes, which usually present a wide individual and stress variability of GH plasmatic levels, but a significant increase in mortality was reported in clinical treatment for catabolic diseases [52].

In athletes taking these drugs for a long time and at high dosages, the following side effects are possible: myalgia, asthenia, headache, arthralgia, diabetes mellitus, metabolic–ionic alterations, disthyroidism, visceral acromegaly (liver, heart, bladder), osteoarthritis, pulmonary diseases, lipid metabolism disorders, and higher risk of rectal and breast cancer, hypertension, cardiomyopathy (hypertrophic or dilated), with interstitial fibrosis, linfo-monocytic infiltrates, and necrosis similar to the histological alterations observed in acromegaly [53]. Also, different types of supraventricular and ventricular arrhythmias, focal or re-entry, can occur, particularly when other arrhythmogenic conditions are present, as metabolic disorders, hypertension, or hypertrophic or dilated cardiomyopathy, especially in athletes with genetic susceptibility to arrhythmias or latent cardiomyopathy.

Some research models for hypertrophic cardiomyopathy suggest that genetic mutations of sarcomeric function can induce a reduction in velocity and strength of contraction that can be a trigger for GH release with secondary compensatory hypertrophy and fibroblastic growth [54]. The question about the negative role of GH abuse, for PDE effect, in athletes with latent HCM is still unclear. Adverse effects of IGF-I are similar to that of GH. IGF-I is thought to have analogous actions on muscle mass and function as the GH [44, 55].

Beta-2-Agonists

β_2-receptor agonists were both previously considered in the WADA lists, in the list of "anabolic agents," and in the list of "stimulants," and are used by athletes in order to increase muscle mass and physical strength. β_2-agonists are reported in the WADA list 2011 as S3 (http://www.wada-ama.org). Salbutamol and salmeterol inhalatory administration is allowed in accordance with the manufacturers' recommended therapeutic regime. The 2011 list abolished the requirement of β_2-agonists Declaration of Use. Another β_2-agonist clenbuterol included in the WADA list among other anabolic agents is banned "at all times" (Table 32.1).

β_2-Agonists might induce supraventricular and ventricular ectopic beats, as well as other focal and re-entry arrhythmias [56], particularly in subjects with underlying cardiomyopathies and in case of concomitant administration with other drugs.

The arrhythmogenic effect of these drugs is related both to their direct β_2-adrenergic action, particularly when inhaled, and, at long-term, to cardiac abnormality due to anabolic action, especially with systemic administration often in association with other anabolic agents.

β_2-Agonists' collateral effects are muscle mass increase with body fat loss, trembling, insomnia, headache, hypertension, nausea, excitement, and agitation.

Diuretics and Other Masking Agents

"Diuretics" are a class of heterogeneous substances prohibited by IOC that act both as masking agents and as diuretics, reported in the WADA list 2011 as S5 (http://www.wada-ama.org).

Diuretics are often taken to mask assumption of other drugs having renal excretion: the purpose is to attempt to dilute the cut-off urinary concentration of those drugs which is evaluated in tests for doping control (e.g., stimulants, narcotics, and anabolic steroids such as nandrolone, methandienone metabolites, methyltestosterone, and stanazolol). Probenecid is a typical drug used for this purpose.

Diuretics are also used to lose weight temporarily in many types of sports sorted by weight categories. Furosemide is often used by intravenous injection by bodybuilders before competitions, to get better shaped muscles by washing out all subcutaneous tissue water.

Administration of diuretics may cause supraventricular and ventricular arrhythmias due to hypokalemia, dehydration, severe hypotension, and electrolytic imbalances, which are further facilitated by concomitant intake of stimulants, steroids, and peptidic anabolic agents or β-agonists. Moreover, these arrhythmias might be particularly severe if underlying primary or "toxic" cardiac diseases are present. In the athletes with silent genetic mutations of sodium and potassium channels, induction of torsades des pointes, due to electrolytic imbalance and subsequent QT interval prolongation, may be particularly dangerous.

Substances and Methods Prohibited In Competition

Stimulants

The heterogeneous group of stimulants includes many classes of drugs, widely used in order to obtain performance enhancement, a raise of aggressiveness and competitiveness level, and reduction of fatigue perception, or for "recreational" purposes, systematically reported in the WADA list

(Table 32.3). Amphetamines are widely used among competitive athletes because of their well-known effects, which include performance enhancement, raise of aggressiveness, and reduction of fatigue perception [48, 57, 58]. Ephedrine and other similar alkaloids are also contained in the herbal product "ephedra," marketed as a dietary supplement [59, 60]. The 2011 List includes the stimulant "methylhexaneamine," another substance marketed as a nutritional supplement (commonly known as geranium oil). In addition, methylenedioxymethamphetamine and other synthetic analogues contained in the recreational drug "ecstasy" are commonly used by young people, including athletes [61, 62].

Stimulants are a frequent cause of atrial flutter/fibrillation, ventricular tachycardia [63], in athletes, particularly during physical activity. In subjects predisposed, the intake of stimulants can exacerbate the sympathetic effects due to physical exercise associated with the arrhythmogenic effect of illicit drugs administrated to athletes.

A meta-analysis [64] on the efficacy and safety of ephedra and ephedrine, taken for weight loss and improvement of physical performance, showed that there are not sufficient data to support the use of these compounds for enhancing athletic performance. By contrast, risks of psychiatric, autonomic, and gastrointestinal symptoms as well as heart palpitations were increased up to two- to threefold. QTc prolongation was observed in healthy young men who were taking ephedra and caffeine products [65]. Re-entry arrhythmias may be due to adrenergic activity on myocardial refractory periods [66, 67]. Some cases of myocardial infarction and ventricular tachycardia were reported in amphetamine-addicted individuals, even with normal coronary angiography [68]. Several cases of cardiac arrest and sudden death were reported in users associated with coronary artery disease, cardiomyopathy, and myocarditis and others with direct myocyte toxicity [61, 66].

In the long term, the abuse of stimulants may cause dilated cardiomyopathy and related arrhythmias [69, 70]. The consumption of stimulants might result as particularly hazardous in athletes with Wolf–Parkinson–White syndrome because of increasing atrial and ventricular excitability and shortening of accessory pathway refractoriness, with possible consequent fast atrial fibrillation and ventricular fibrillation [8].

Sympathomimetic amines are also used to treat the attention deficit hyperactivity disorder (ADHD), a typical disorder of school-age boys with increased activity, inability to concentrate, and poor school performance. Cases of myocardial infarction, stroke, and sudden death were reported in young people and adults treated for ADHD, particularly with methylphenidate [71], drug inserted in the WADA list 2009 as a specified stimulant. Caution in the long-term treatment of young subjects with ADHD [72] for pre-existing asymptomatic cardiovascular abnormality is strongly

Table 32.3 The 2011 prohibited list of stimulants (S6) WADA code

All stimulants (including both optical isomers where relevant) are prohibited, except imidazole derivatives for topical use and those stimulants included in the 2011 Monitoring Program.[a]

Stimulants include:

a: Nonspecified stimulants
Adrafinil; amfepramone; amiphenazole; amphetamine; amphetaminil; benfluorex; benzphetamine; benzylpiperazine; bromantan; clobenzorex; cocaine; cropropamide; crotetamide; dimethylamphetamine; etilamphetamine; famprofazone; fencamine; fenetylline; fenfluramine; fenproporex; furfenorex; mefenorex; mephentermine; mesocarb; methamphetamine(*d*-); p-methylamphetamine; methylenedioxyamphetamine; methylenedioxymethamphetamine; modafinil; norfenfluramine; phendimetrazine; phenmetrazine; phentermine; 4-phenylpiracetam (carphedon); prenylamine; prolintane.

   A stimulant not expressly listed in this section is a Specified Substance.

b: Specified stimulants (examples)
Adrenaline[b]; cathine[c]; ephedrine[d]; etamivan; etilefrine; fenbutrazate; fencamfamin; heptaminol; isometheptene; levmetamfetamine; meclofenoxate; methylephedrine[d]; methylhexaneamine (dimethylpentylamine); methylphenidate; nikethamide; norfenefrine; octopamine; oxilofrine; parahydroxyamphetamine; pemoline; pentetrazol; phenpromethamine; propylhexedrine; pseudoephedrine[e]; selegiline; sibutramine; strychnine; tuaminoheptane; and other substances with a similar chemical structure or similar biological effect(s).

[a]The following substances included in the 2011 Monitoring Program (bupropion, caffeine, phenylephrine, phenylpropanolamine, pipradol, synephrine) are not considered as *Prohibited Substances*
[b]*Adrenaline* associated with local anesthetic agents or by local administration (e.g., nasal, ophthalmologic) is not prohibited
[c]*Cathine* is prohibited when its concentration in urine is greater than 5 μg per mL
[d]Each of *ephedrine* and *methylephedrine* is prohibited when its concentration in urine is greater than 10 μg per mL
[e]*Pseudoephedrine* is prohibited when its concentration in urine is greater than 150 μg per mL
http://www.wada-ama.org — World Anti-Doping CODE 2011

recommended, and need of pre-treatment assessment and long-term monitoring is suggested.

Cocaine

The connection between cocaine use, sport, and arrhythmogenic effects is well established. This drug, included in the "illicit drug" list as "nonspecified stimulants S6" (Table 32.3), is usually taken for its euphoric effects rather than to improve physical performance. There are no scientific documentations about the efficacy of cocaine in improving physical activity, even though it is well known that it may alter fatigue perception by its euphoric effects. Furthermore, its use represents a serious social problem: millions of addicted in the world, including many athletes [6, 73]. For this reason, cocaine collateral effects have been extensively studied, both with experimental research and with clinical effects on humans, also in athletes, and those

Table 32.4 Arrhythmias and sudden death reported with cocaine use

- Any types of supra or ventricular arrhythmias, focal and re-entry, VT and VF.
- "Chaotic atrial arrhythmia," like in severe respiratory insufficiency or in acute myocarditis.
- 24-Fold increase in the risk of MI within the first hour after use.
- Typical toxic "wide complex VT" (high doses like in "body packers" with ruptured packet of cocaine in intestines) or "body stuffing" (ingestion of drugs for evasion of arrest).
- Wide QRS complex with large R′ wave in aVR (typical hallmark of Na channel blockade) in massive overdose.
- Torsade de pointes due to long QT syndrome frequently related to hERG IKr channel block in subjects with or without congenital silent susceptibility.
- Brugada-like ECG patterns (ST segment elevation "coved types" in leads V1, V2, and V3 due to selective block of Na channel).

studies represent an optimal model that can be extrapolated to the more complex phenomenon of illicit drugs including arrhythmias and sudden death (Table 32.4).

Cocaine, an alkaloid derived from Erythroxylon coca, has an important acute action, especially if inhaled or smoked, and also many important long-term effects has been demonstrated in both men and animals [74, 75]. Indeed, this alkaloid may cause different kinds of focal or re-entry supraventricular and ventricular arrhythmias, as ectopic beats, atrial fibrillation, AV node re-entry tachycardia, WPW arrhythmias, and non-sustained and sustained VT and VF. Arrhythmias are frequently associated with physical effort. The association of the sympathetic effects of physical exertion with cocaine addiction may play an important role in the genesis of these arrhythmias [73].

Clinical and experimental animal studies on cocaine effects showed prolongation of PR, QT, and QTc intervals; a wide QRS; supraventricular and ventricular ectopic activity; ventricular tachycardia; and ventricular fibrillation [74, 76–78].

Cocaine can lead to cardiac side effects, through multiple arrhythmogenic mechanisms:

(a) Local anesthetic effect with block of sodium and potassium channels

(b) Sympathomimetic effect with α- and β-receptors stimulation and consequent heart rate and atrial and ventricular excitability increase

(c) Intracellular calcium overload (after-depolarization arrhythmias)

(d) Arrhythmias due to ischemia/reperfusion

(e) Increase in heart rate due to vagolytic effect

(f) Inhibitor of generations and conduction of the action potential, with prolongation of QRS due to sodium channel-blocking effects [79]

Arrhythmias may also be "secondary" to systemic effects of the drug such as hyperthermia, acidosis, and stroke, which are favored by particular environmental conditions (high temperature, high humidity, and air pollution).

The ability of cocaine to cause myocardial infarction frequently with severe complications is well known [73, 75, 80, 81] with the risk in the first hour after use as much as 24-fold [82].

Myocardial infarction as well as various arrhythmias can occur even after the first administration of cocaine, regardless of dosage. Cases of young athletes involved in physical activity soon after cocaine inhalation are typical, and many types of arrhythmias have been observed either in the setting of ischemic/reperfusion events or not: supraventricular tachycardia, atrial fibrillation, ventricular tachycardia/fibrillation, torsades des pointes due to "secondary" long QT syndrome, asystole (sporadic reports of asystole treated with emergency cardiac pacing), and cardiac arrest. "Chaotic atrial arrhythmia," similar to that observed in severe respiratory insufficiency or acute myocarditis, is considered a typical toxic cocaine-related arrhythmia [8]. Also, cocaine-induced wide complex VT may be considered as typical toxic arrhythmia, frequently due to high doses of the drugs [75], and the treatment is based on administration of sodium bicarbonate [83].

Cocaine can induce electrocardiographic modifications as a V1–V3 ST elevation (coved type) typical for Brugada syndrome, due to a selective block of myocardial Na channels probably in subjects with latent arrhythmic disease [84]. Long QT syndrome with possible torsade des pointes/VT is a well-reported collateral complication of cocaine intake, especially in subjects with congenital silent susceptibility [78, 85] frequently related to hERG potassium channel blockade [77, 86].

Long-term abuse of cocaine could result in myocardial hypertrophy [87], myocarditis, dilated cardiomyopathy [75, 81, 87], rupture of aortic aneurysm, stroke, and in accelerating the course of atherosclerosis [88, 89]. Post-mortem examination of some patients has shown areas of myocardial necrosis with "contraction bands" due to strong adrenergic stimulation [75, 90]. Different arrhythmias due to the underlying diseases have been observed, with lethal events often during physical exertion.

Narcotics

In the WADA list 2011, the following narcotics are prohibited: *buprenorphine, dextromoramide, diamorphine (heroin), fentanyl and its derivatives, hydromorphone, methadone, morphine, oxycodone, oxymorphone, pentazocine, and pethidine.*

Narcotics are not PEDs but are usually used by athletes when unable to participate in trainings or competitions for traumatic reasons. Use of these substances may cause dangerous psychological reactions, a decrease in sensitivity to pain, and a disproportionate and false increase in the sense of courage, which may prove dangerous in certain situations.

Table 32.5 P1. Alcohol

Alcohol (ethanol) is prohibited *In-Competition* only, in the following sports. Detection will be conducted by analysis of breath and/or blood. The doping violation threshold (hematological values) is 0.10 g/L

- Aeronautic (FAI)
- Archery (FITA, IPC)
- Automobile (FIA)
- Karate (WKF)
- Motorcycling (FIM)
- Ninepin and Tenpin Bowling (FIQ)
- Powerboating (UIM)

http://www.wada-ama.org—World Anti-Doping CODE 2011

Table 32.6 P2. β-Blockers

Unless otherwise specified, beta-blockers are prohibited *in-Competition* only, in the following sports

- Aeronautic (FAI)
- Archery (FITA) (also prohibited *Out-of-Competition*)
- Automobile (FIA)
- Billiards and Snooker (WCBS)
- Bobsleigh and Skeleton (FIBT)
- Boules (CMSB)
- Bridge (FMB)
- Curling (WCF)
- Darts (WDF)
- Golf (IGF)
- Motorcycling (FIM)
- Modern Pentathlon (UIPM) for disciplines involving shooting
- Ninepin and Tenpin Bowling (FIQ)
- Powerboating (UIM)
- Sailing (ISAF) for match race helms only
- Shooting (ISSF, IPC) (also prohibited *Out-of-Competition*)
- Skiing/Snowboarding (FIS) in ski jumping, freestyle aerials/halfpipe, and snowboard halfpipe/big air
- Wrestling (FILA)

Beta-blockers include, but are not limited to, the following: Acebutolol, alprenolol, atenolol, betaxolol, bisoprolol, bunolol, carteolol, carvedilol, celiprolol, esmolol, labetalol, levobunolol, metipranolol, metoprolol, nadolol, oxprenolol, pindolol, propranolol, sotalol, timolol

http://www.wada-ama.org—World Anti-Doping CODE 2011

Some narcotics can have arrhythmogenic effects. In particular, methadone was found to have a pro-arrhythmic effect (torsade des pointes), most likely owing to a block of the IKr current with QT prolongation [91–93].

A list of side effects due to narcotics in athletes has been proposed, psychological (dizziness, mood changing), systemic (nausea, vomiting, depression, and sweating), and cutaneous (skin itching, skin redness, and skin irritations).

Among narcotics, oxycodone, a potent opioid analgesic drug, is increasingly used among high-school students and young athletes [94].

Cannabinoids

They include marijuana and hashish and can induce exercise-related sinus tachycardia, atrial fibrillation, paroxysmal supraventricular tachycardia, supra and/or ventricular ectopic beats, and severe ventricular arrhythmias [95, 96] mediated by catecholamines. An increase in cannabinoids addiction has been reported in every kind of sport, mostly because of a social recreational usage rather than for an ergogenic effect [97, 98]. Moreover, cannabinoids seem to cause drug dependence, psychomotor changes, antimotivational syndrome, and deficiencies of the immune system, which are often present in athletes after extreme physical efforts. A 4.8-fold increase in the risk of myocardial infarction in the first hour following marijuana use was described [99]. Some adverse CV events including vascular complications, cerebral ischemic events, and stroke were observed [100].

Substances Prohibited in Particular Sports

Alcohol

Alcohol is included in the classes of substances prohibited in particular sports and only in competition by some International Sports Federations (Table 32.5). Alcohol produces well-known depressive effects on central nervous systems, movement in-coordination, and difficulties in careful concentration. Moreover, alcohol intake may be a cause of

atrial flutter/fibrillation [101]. Chronic alcohol intake may provoke a late occurrence of alcoholic cardiomyopathy and atrial flutter/fibrillation, ventricular tachycardia, and heart failure.

Alcohol is often assumed in association with other illicit drugs. The combined use of ethanol and cocaine has been most frequently found in emergency departments and it can produce deleterious cardiovascular effects [102]. The risk of sudden death was found to be much higher in individuals who were taking both alcohol and cocaine than cocaine alone [103]. This additive effect was likely because of the production of a metabolite, coca-ethylene, which can block the dopamine reuptake, enhancing the toxic effect of the cocaine used alone.

Beta-Blockers

β-Blockers are a class of substances prohibited only in competition by IOC in specific sports that require high degree of concentration and steadiness and in which the intake of these drugs can minimize tremors, anxiety, and emotional tachycardia (Table 32.5, P2 WADA list 2011).

These drugs may induce bradyarrhythmias with atrioventricular blocks of various degrees, sinus bradycardia, junctional and ventricular escape rhythms, ventricular ectopic beats bradycardia-dependent, especially in patients with underlying structural and electrical disorders (Table 32.6).

Cardiovascular Effects During Use and Abuse of Common Prescription Drugs

Anxiety and Mood Disorders

Patients with anxiety or mood disorders are a patient population at risk for drug abuse and dependence. In this section, we will describe the cardiovascular adverse effect of the main drugs classes used to treat these disorders.

Anxiety disorders are the most common psychiatric illnesses, with a prevalence of up to 20% in medical patients. Anxiety can be a primary psychiatric disorder or it can be a concomitant illness or a reaction to a primary medical disease or a medication side effect.

Mood disorders are the second main family of mental disorders and comprise depressive disorders, bipolar disorders and depression associated to medical illness or alcohol and substance abuse. A depressive disorder can be diagnosed in 20–30% of patients suffering from cardiovascular diseases, especially after myocardial infarction or in patients with chronic heart failure.

Depressed patients seem to be predisposed to cardiac arrhythmias, one of the proposed mechanisms involve a reduced parasympathetic nervous system activity often present as a decreased heart rate variability [104].

Benzodiazepines

Benzodiazepines (BDZ) are useful and commonly used, often in combination with other drug classes, in different phases of the course of treatment planning.

BDZ differ in terms of kinetics, metabolic pathways, and active metabolites; BDZ should not be prescribed for more than 4–6 weeks because of tolerance development and risk of abuse and dependence.

Cardiovascular effects of chronic use of BDZ may be due to respiratory depression during night sleeping time that can affect negatively tissue oxygenation, a critical point in patients with heart failure or congenital heart diseases [105].

On the other side, discontinuation of BDZ assumption can cause a withdrawal syndrome with reactions that vary in severity and duration. Withdrawal syndrome is more common with triazolam and short-intermediate half-life BDZ, in particular if taken in repeated doses during daytime, while the syndrome is rare with long half-life BDZ and virtually absent with BDZ analogs as zolpidem and zopiclone. Time delay between last BDZ assumption and reactions onset is proportional to BDZ half-life (i.e., 24 h for lorazepam and 3–7 days for diazepam).

Cardiovascular reactions during withdrawal syndrome include rhythm disorders, as tachycardia and ectopic beats, and blood pressure imbalance (orthostatic hypotension and mild systolic hypertension); moreover, autonomic arousal

due to sympathetic hyperactivity conditions and different symptoms as diaphoresis, delirium, and tremors also occur. The administration of beta-blockers or clonidine can help in the management of reactions due to sympathetic hyperactivity [106].

Tricyclic Antidepressant Agents

Classic tricyclic antidepressant (TCA) agents, as imipramine, amitriptiline, and clomipramine, act as nonselective monoamino reuptake inhibitors. TCA present quinidine-like effects that are frequently encountered in older patients and children.

These effects are (a) dose-dependent reduction of myocardial electrical tissue conduction velocity often leading to intraventricular block and AV conduction block of different degrees with an increase in QRS width and PR interval on surface ECG; (b) negative inotropic effect with a reduction on left ventricular ejection fraction; (c) repolarization abnormalities with QT interval lengthening and negative T waves; and rarely also a QT interval reduction has been described, likely due to antimuscarinic effect and noradrenalin reuptake block at adrenergic cardiac terminations.

QT lengthening should be monitored for the risk of ventricular arrhythmias, in particular torsade des pointes (secondary long QT syndrome).

TCA can lead to other cardiovascular effects, especially in older patients: (a) sinus tachycardia (5% up to 20% of patients treated), with a mean increase of 15–20 bpm, probably due to peripheral anticholinergic activity; (b) peripheral vasospastic manifestations as Raynaud-like phenomena; and (c) orthostatic arterial hypotension in 5–25% of patients treated, in particular in patient treated with antihypertensive drugs [107–110].

Patients with cardiac diseases treated with class IC antiarrhythmic drugs (flecainide, propafenone) or quinidine should be highly monitored also because the interaction between these drugs can lead to an increase in TCA blood concentration. Moreover, in patients with hypertension treated with α_2-agonist (clonidine, metildopa), TCA act as antagonists of these drugs.

Selective Serotonin Reuptake Inhibitors

The second mainstay class of drugs used for mood disorders is selective serotonin reuptake inhibitors (SSRI), including drugs as fluoxetine, sertraline, paroxetine, and citalopram.

Among cardiovascular effect, hypertension and sinus tachycardia are the most frequently recorded, and rarely palpitations and heart failure symptoms due to a negative inotropic effect on myocardium. In older patients, SSRI can lead to sinus bradycardia and rarely to lipotimias. In case of drug overdose, rhythm disorders (brady-tachycardias) and hypotension are frequently present [111].

Regarding drugs interaction, it is important to remember that SSRI inhibit hepatic CYP3A4 and it is necessary to avoid or administer with reduced doses antiarrhythmic drugs as amiodarone, flecainide, propafenone, sildenafil, and lidocaine (i.v.). Moreover, during SSRI intake, caution should be taken for patients in therapy with warfarin and quinidine. SSRI present also an antiplatelet activity that can lead to hemorrhagic disorders in patients taking aspirin or other drugs with antiplatelet effect [111, 112].

Monoamine Oxidase Inhibitors

Monoamine oxidase inhibitors (MAOI), phenelzine, tranilcipromine, and isocarboxazide, are the third main group of drugs used in clinical practice. Monoamine oxidase is a complex enzyme system, widely distributed throughout the body. Drugs that inhibit monoamine oxidase in the laboratory are associated with a number of clinical effects.

MAOI therapy is not recommended in patients with cardiovascular disease, in particular in ischemic heart disease [112].

Common cardiovascular side effect is postural hypotension; on the other side, the most serious reaction to phenelzine and MAOI, in general, involves changes in blood pressure with occurrence of hypertensive crises, which have sometimes been fatal. These crises are characterized by some or all of the following symptoms: headache, palpitation, neck stiffness or soreness, nausea, vomiting, sweating, dilated pupils and photophobia, either tachycardia or bradycardia can be recorded sometimes associated with constrictive chest pain. Moreover, intracranial bleeding has been reported as a complication of blood pressure rise.

Therapy with MAOI should be discontinued in patients presenting with blood pressure levels increase, palpitations, or frequent headaches.

During MAOI therapy, some drugs should be avoided in order to prevent cardiovascular complications: sympathomimetics including amphetamines, ephedrine, and over-the-counter preparations for colds, fever, and weight reduction that contain vasoconstrictors (e.g., phenylephrine, phenylpropanolamine) as well as methyldopa, dopamine, levodopa, and tryptophan, as such combinations may precipitate hypertension, severe headache, hyperpyrexia, and rarely even cerebral (subarachnoid) hemorrhage.

Moreover during MAOI therapy, the ingestion of cheese or other foods with high tyramine content should be avoided: hypertensive crises have sometimes been reported after ingestion of foods with high tyramine content. Tyramine is normally metabolized by monoamine oxidase in the intestinal and hepatic cells. During monoamine oxidase inhibition, tyramine absorbed from the gastrointestinal tract passes freely into the blood circulation and releases norepinephrine from adrenergic neurons, causing exaggerated hypertensive reactions, tachycardia, and other adrenergic effects [113–115].

Antibiotics

Macrolides, as erythromycin, clarithromycin, and azithromycin, are a commonly used antibiotics class acting through protein synthesis inhibition with binding to ribosomal 50S subunit of sensitive microorganisms [116].

The most important cardiovascular adverse effect is QT prolongation on ECG, which brings a high risk of ventricular arrhythmias as torsade des pointes.

The risk of QT prolongation is higher as H1 antagonist (as terfenadine and astemizolo) are administered at the same time.

QT prolongation has been described with erythromycin, spiramycin, and rarely with clarithromycin, and caution should be taken during intravenous administration; torsade des pointes has been described more frequently during therapy with erythromycin and clarithromycin, while rarely during therapy with azithromycin. Moreover, palpitations have been reported in patients taking azithromycin.

In patients receiving both erythromycin and digoxin, an increase in digoxin concentration has been described due to killing of digoxin-metabolizing bacteria [117].

Rarely ventricular arrhythmias due to QT prolongation have been described during fluoroquinolones therapy.

Anti-viral Drugs

Antiherpetic agents, acting as nucleoside analogs (acyclovir, ganciclovir, and brivudin), do not present cardiovascular toxicity, while among antiretroviral agents, acting as nucleoside analog reverse transcriptase inhibitors, a direct cardiotoxicity leading to heart failure has been rarely described with zalcitabine and didanosine. The use of zalcitabine has been also correlated with atrial fibrillation, hypertension, and palpitations [118, 119].

Antineoplastic Agents

Among antineoplastic agents, anthracyclines present a well-known cardiotoxicity through both an acute effect, rarely described, and a chronic cardiomyopathy, more commonly diagnosed. The acute toxic syndrome is not correlated with anthracyclines dose (doxorubicin is commonly used) and includes arrhythmic disorders, as supraventricular and ventricular arrhythmias, atrioventricular conduction block, and acute heart failure with a severe depression of ventricular systolic function.

Chronic toxic cardiomyopathy is dose-dependent, heart failure is progressive and present a negative prognosis; risk factors for anthracyclines cardiomyopathy are hypertension, ischemic cardiopathy, and advanced age. Heart failure risk is about 1–4% for cumulative doses up to 550 mg/m^2; above that dose level, the risk of heart failure development becomes rapidly very high.

Among anthracyclines, epirubicine presents a smaller risk of cardiotoxicity [120–122].

Among antineoplastic acting as pirimidine analogs, 5-fluorouracil (FU) can present a severe cardiotoxicity in 0.5% of treated patients, displaying severe arrhythmic disorders and cardiac arrest due to myocardial ischemia. New onset of both angina pectoris and asymptomatic ischemia on ECG tracings is sometimes reported during 5 FU therapy [122, 123].

Histamine Receptor Antagonists

Antihistamine agents are contraindicated in clinical subsets at risk of development of cardiac arrhythmias, especially ventricular arrhythmias as torsade des pointes; 1st- and 2nd-generation agents act by inhibition of Ik$_i$ current channels, leading to a prolongation of QT interval on ECG up to arrhythmogenic threshold [124–126].

Caution should be taken in case of severe heart failure, severe left ventricular hypertrophy, electrolytic disturbances, complete bundle branch block, digitalis intoxication, and ischemic cardiopathy. If necessary, agents as cetirizine, desloratadine, fexofenadine, or levocetirizine should be administered with ECG monitoring.

1st-generation agents and terfenadine present a total cardiovascular toxicity (t.t.) in about 0.2 pt/million doses and severe toxicity (s.t.) in 0.16% of treated patients; astemizolo presents t.t. in about 0.12 pt/million doses and s.t. in 0.04% of treated patients; while 2nd-generation agents present t.t. in <0.1 pt/million doses and s.t. <0.02% of treated patients.

Long QT prolongation is dose dependent and it is more frequently observed during treatment with terfenadine, astemizolo, difenidramine, idrossizina, and dimenidrinate.

Other cardiovascular effects include the following:
(a) ECG abnormalities as U waves on ECG, and ST abnormalities
(b) Conduction blocks as atrioventricular block, fascicular or bundle branch blocks
(c) Sinus bradycardia or tachycardia, ectopic beats
(d) Orthostatic hypotension and sometimes syncope (in older patients or after i.v. administration)
(e) Hypertension

Thyroid Hormones

Eating disorders and the associated behavioral problems are frequently related to drug abuse. Levotiroxine or thyroid hormones extracts are frequently used as illicit components of anti-obesity pills in subjects with normal thyroid function.

Cardiovascular symptoms and signs during levotiroxine intake are usually tachycardia, palpitations, increase in differential pressure, and arrhythmias; moreover, exogenous thyroid hormones intake causes an increase in metabolic demand and myocardial oxygen consumption which can determine myocardial ischemia. Angina pectoris should be treated conventionally with large use of beta-blockers, if left ventricular dysfunction is not present. Caution should be taken in patients with previous history of hypertension, ischemic cardiopathy, and heart failure.

Conclusions

The intake of illicit drugs included in the WADA list may cause a wide spectrum of cardiac arrhythmias, even in healthy subjects with no previous history of cardiac diseases. The assumption of illicit drugs could be particularly dangerous in competitive athletes with previous arrhythmic manifestations, such as atrial fibrillation, flutter, and AV node re-entry tachycardia, or with an underlying arrhythmogenic substrate, such as accessory AV pathways and latent structural heart diseases (concealed hypertrophic or dilated cardiomyopathies, myocarditis, segmental arrhythmogenic ventricular cardiomyopathy, and coronary artery anomalies). It is possible that athletes with latent inherited arrhythmogenic cardiac diseases due to defects of genes encoding cytoskeleton, sarcomere, cell junction, and ion channels are most likely at risk of severe arrhythmic events. For instance, subjects with "silent" mutations of long QT syndrome genes may be particularly sensitive to illicit drugs such as anabolic steroids, beta-2-agonists, diuretics, cocaine, or drugs prescribed in clinical practice such as specific antibiotics and histamine receptor antagonists. These drugs could produce a critical prolongation of action potential duration that can precipitate, in combination with other trigger conditions, episodes of VT/VF. Also, subjects with latent Brugada syndrome are particularly sensitive to cocaine intake. Catecolaminergic polymorphic ventricular tachycardias (CPVT) due to cardiac ryanodine receptor gene (hRyR2) defects (CPVT type I) or to calsequestrin (CASQ2) gene defects (CPVT type II) or related to ARVD type II are genetic arrhythmogenic diseases with characteristic "polymorphic VT" during physical or emotional stress. In athletes carrying these gene mutations, illicit drugs like anabolic steroids, beta-2-agonists, stimulants, cocaine, cannabinoids, as well as various combinations of them could be particularly dangerous. Finally, the prolonged assumption of several illicit drugs such as androgenic anabolic agents, GH, IGF-I, and stimulants, including cocaine, may induce the development of "ex novo" forms of hypertrophic or dilated cardiomyopathy, coronary artery disease, and myocarditis.

Moreover, among common prescription drugs, caution should be always taken regarding many agents used in the treatment of anxiety and mood disorders, which can lead to cardiac toxicity and collateral effects.

References

1. Tokish JM, Kocher MS, Hawkins RJ. Ergogenic aids: a review of basic science, performance, side effects, and status in sports. Am J Sports Med. 2004;32:1543–53.

2. Dhar R, Stout W, Link SM, Homoud MK, Weinstock J, Estes III M. Cardiovascular toxicities of performance-enhancing substances in sports. Mayo Clin Proc. 2005;80:1307–15.

3. Kutscher EC, Lund BC, Perry PJ. Anabolic steroids: a review for the clinician. Sports Med. 2002;32:285–96.

4. Gauthier J. The heart and doping. Arch Mal Coeur Vaiss. 2006;99: 1126–9.

5. Estes III M, Link MS, Cannom D, Naccarelli GV, Prystowsky EN, Maron BJ, et al. Report of the NASPE policy conference on arrhythmias and the athlete. J Cardiovasc Electrophysiol. 2001;12:1208–19.

6. Kloner AR. Illicit drug use in the athlete as a contributor to cardiac events. In: Estes NA, Salem DN, Wang PJ, editors. Sudden cardiac death in the athlete. Armonk, NY: Futura; 1998. p. 441–51.

7. Furlanello F, Bentivegna S, Cappato R, De Ambroggi L. Arrhythmogenic effects of illicit drugs in athletes. Ital Heart J. 2003;4:829–37.

8. Furlanello F, Vitali Serdoz L, Cappato R, De Ambroggi L. Illicit drugs and cardiac arrhythmias in athletes. Eur J Cardiovasc Prev Rehabil. 2007;14:487–94.

9. Deligiannis A, Bjornstand H, Carre F, Heidbuchel H, Kouidi E, Panhuyzen-Goedkoop NM, et al. on behalf of the ESC Study Group of Sports Cardiology. ESC study group of sports cardiology position paper on adverse cardiovascular effects of doping in athletes. Eur J Cardiovasc Prev Rehabil. 2006;13:687–94.

10. Noakes TD. Tainted glory. Doping and athletic performance. N Engl J Med. 2004;351(9):847–9.

11. Waddingyon I, Malcolm D, et al. Drug use in English professional football. Br J Sports Med. 2005;39(4):18–22.

12. Priori SG, Napolitano C, Memmi M, Colombi B, Drago F, Gasparini M, et al. Clinical and molecular characterization of patients with catecholaminergic polymorphic ventricular tachycardia. Circulation. 2002;106:69–74.

13. Postma AV, Denjoy I, Hoorntje TM, Lupoglazoff JM, Da Costa A, Sebillon P, et al. Absence of calsequestrin 2 causes severe forms of catecholaminergic polymorphic ventricular tachycardia. Circ Res. 2002;91:21–6.

14. Tiso N, Stephan DA, Nava A, Bagattin A, Devaney JM, Stanchi F, et al. Identification of mutations in the cardiac ryanodine receptor gene in families affected with arrhythmogenic right ventricular cardiomyopathy type 2 (ARVD2). Hum Mol Genet. 2001;10: 189–94.

15. Yesalis CE, Bahrke MS. Doping among adolescent athletes. Baillieres Best Pract Res Clin Endocrinol Metab. 2000;14:25–35.

16. Nilsson S, Baigi A, Marklund B, Fridlund B. The prevalence of use of androgenic anabolic steroids by adolescents in a county of Sweden. Eur J Public Health. 2001;11:195–7.

17. Trenton AJ, Currier GW. Behavioural manifestations of anabolic steroid use. CNS Drugs. 2005;19:571–95.

18. Green GA, Catlin DH, Starcevic B. Analysis of over-the-counter dietary supplements. Clin J Sport Med. 2001;11:254–9.

19. Congeni J, Miller S. Supplements and drugs used to enhance athletic performance. Pediatr Clin North Am. 2002;49:435–61.

20. Pipe A, Ayotte C. Nutritional supplements and doping. Clin J Sport Med. 2002;12:245–9.

21. Sullivan ML, Martinez CM, Gennis P, Gallagher EJ. The cardiac toxicity of anabolic steroids. Prog Cardiovasc Dis. 1998;41: 1–15.

22. Fineschi V, Baroldi G, Monciotti F, Pagliacci Reattelli L, Turillazzi E. Anabolic steroid abuse and cardiac sudden death: a pathologic study. Arch Pathol Lab Med. 2001;125:253–5.

23. Schollert PV, Bendixen PM. Dilated cardiomyopathy in a user of anabolic steroids. Ugeskr Laeger. 1993;155:1217–8.

24. Ferrera PC, Putnam DL, Verdile VP. Anabolic steroid use as the possible precipitation of dilated cardiomyopathy. Cardiology. 1997;88:218–20.

25. Payne JR, Kotwinski PJ, Montgomery HE. Cardiac effects of anabolic steroids. Heart. 2004;90:473–5.

26. Urhausen A, Albers T, Kindermann W. Are the cardiac effects of anabolic steroid abuse in strength athletes reversible? Heart. 2004;90:496–501.

27. McCarthy K, Tang A, Dalrymple-Hay M. Ventricular thrombosis and systemic embolism in bodybuilders: etiology and management. Ann Thorac Surg. 2000;70:658–60.

28. Melchert RB, Welder AA. Cardiovascular effects of androgenic-anabolic steroids. Med Sci Sports Exerc. 1995;27:1252–62.

29. Parssinen M, Kujala U, Vartiainen E, Sarna S, Seppala T. Increased premature mortality of competitive powerlifters suspected to have used anabolic agents. Int J Sports Med. 2000;21:225–7.

30. Thiblin L, Lindquist O, Rajs J. Cause and manner of death among users of anabolic androgenic steroids. J Forensic Sci. 2000;45: 16–23.

31. Hartgens F, Kuipers H. Effects of androgenic-anabolic steroids in athletes. Sports Med. 2004;34:513–54.

32. Dickerman RD, McConathy WJ, Zachariah NY. Testosterone, sex hormonebinding globulin, lipoproteins, and vascular disease risk. J Cardiovasc Risk. 1997;4:363–6.

33. Karila T, Hovatta O, Seppala T. Concomitant abuse of anabolic androgenic steroids and human chorionic gonadotrophin impairs spermatogenesis in power athletes. Int J Sports Med. 2004;25: 257–63.

34. Karila TA, Karjalainen JE, Mantysaari MJ, Viitasalo MT, Seppala TA. Anabolic androgenic steroids produce dose-dependant increase in left ventricular mass in power athletes, and this effect is potentiated by concomitant use of growth hormone. Int J Sports Med. 2003;24:337–43.

35. Lenders JW, Demacker PN, Vos JA. Deleterious effects of anabolic steroids on serum lipoproteins, blood pressure, and liver function in amateur bodybuilders. J Sports Med. 1988;9:19–23.

36. Laseter JT, Russel JA. Anabolic steroids induced tendon pathology: a review of the literature. Med Sci Sports Exerc. 1991;23: 1–3.

37. Sullivan ML, Martinez CM, Gallagher EJ. Atrial Fibrillation and anabolic steroids. J Emerg Med. 1999;17:851–7.

38. Nieminen MS, Ramo MP, Viitasalo M, Heikkila P, Karjalainen J, Mantysaari M, et al. Serious cardiovascular side effects of large doses of anabolic steroids in weight lifters. Eur Heart J. 1996; 17:1576–83.

39. Stolt A, Karila T, Viitasalo M, Mantysaari M, Kujala UM, Karjalainen J. QT interval and QT dispersion in endurance athletes and in power athletes using large doses of anabolic steroids. Am J Cardiol. 1999;84:364–6, A9.

40. Jlekmann W. Use of recombinant human erythropoietin as an anti-anemic and performance enhancing drug. Curr Pharm Biotechnol. 2000;1:11–31.

41. Wilber RL. Detection of DNA-recombinant human epoetin-alfa as a pharmacological ergogenic aid. Sports Med. 2002;32:125–42.

42. Hainline B. Blood doping, erytropoietin and drug testing in athletes. In: Waller BF, Harvey WP, editors. Cardiovascular evaluation of

athletes: toward recognizing athletes at risk for sudden death. Newton, NJ: Laennec; 1993. p. 129–37.

43. Scheen AJ. Pharma-clinics: doping with erythropietin or the misuse of therapeutic advances. Rev Med Liege. 1998;43:499–502.

44. Shulman DI, Root AW, Diamond FB, Bercu BB, Martinez R, Boucek Jr RJ. Effects of one year of recombinant human growth hormone (GH) therapy on cardiac mass and function in children with classical GH deficiency. J Clin Endocrinol Metab. 2003;88:4095–9.

45. Pirnary F. Doping in sports. Rev Med Liege. 2001;56:265–8.

46. De Paolo EF, Gatti R, Lancerin F, Cappellin E, Spinella P. Correlations of growth hormone (GH) and insulin-like growth factor I (IGF-I): effects of exercise and abuse by athletes. Clin Chim Acta. 2001;305:1–17.

47. Saugy M, Robinson N, Saudan C, Baume N, Avois L, Mangin P. Human growth hormone doping in sport. Br J Sports Med. 2006;40 Suppl 1:i35–9.

48. Calfee R, Fadale P. Popular ergogenic drugs and supplements in young athletes. Pediatrics. 2006;117:577–89.

49. Ehrnborg C, Bengtsson BA, Rosen T. Growth hormone abuse. Pract Res Clin Endocrinol Metab. 2000;14:71–7.

50. Dean H. Does exogenous hormone improve athletic performance? Clin J Sport Med. 2002;12:250–3.

51. Rosen T. Supraphysiological doses of growth hormone: effects on muscles and collagen in healthy active young adults. Horm Res. 2006;66 Suppl 1:98–104.

52. Takala J, Ruokonen E, Webster NR, Nielsen MS, Zandstra DF, Vundelinckx G, Hinds CJ. Increased mortality associated with growth hormone treatment in critically ill adults. N Engl J Med. 1999;341:785–92.

53. Clayton RN. Cardiovascular function in acromegaly. Endocr Rev. 2003;24:272–7.

54. Hipp AA, Heitkamp HC, Rocker K, Dickhuth HH. Hypertrophic cardiomyopathy – sports – related aspects of diagnosis, therapy and sports eligibility. Int J Sports Med. 2004;25:20–6.

55. Meyers DE, Cuneo RC. Controversies regarding the effects of growth hormone on the heart. Mayo Clin Proc. 2003;78:1521–6.

56. Kallergis EM, Manios EG, Kanoupakis EM, Schiza SE, Mavrakis HE, Klapsinos NK, Vardas PE. Acute electrophysiologic effects of inhaled salbutamol in human. Chest. 2005;127:2057–63.

57. Bouchard R, Weber AR, Geiger JD. Informed decision-making on sympathomimetic use in sport and health. Clin J Sport Med. 2002;12:209–24.

58. Gray SD, Fatovich DM, McCoubrie DL, Daly FF. Amphetamine-related presentations to an inner-city tertiary emergency department: a prospective evaluation. MJA 2007;186:336–9.

59. Krome CN, Tucker AM. Cardiac arrhythmia in a professional football player. Was ephedrine to blame? Phys Sports Med. 2003; 31:1–12.

60. Gee P, Richardson S, Woltersdorf W, Moore G. Toxic effects of BZP-based herbal party pills in humans: a prospective study in Christchurch, New Zealand. NZ Med J. 2005;18:1227–37.

61. Hall AP, Henry JA. Acute toxic effects of "Ecstasy" (MDMA and related compounds): overview of pathophysiology and clinical management. Br J Anaesth. 2006;96:678–85.

62. Ricaurte GA, McCann UD. Recognition and management of complications of new recreational drug use. Lancet 2005;365: 2137–45.

63. Rakovec P, Kozak M, Sebestjen M. Ventricular tachycardia induced by abuse of ephedrine in a Young healthy woman. Wien Klin Wochenschr 2006;118(17–18):558–61.

64. Shekelle PG, Hardy ML, Morton SC, Maglione M, Mojica WA, Suttorp MJ, et al. Efficacy and safety of ephedra and ephedrine for weight loss and athletic peformance: a meta-analysis. JAMA. 2003;289:1537–45.

65. McBride BF, Karapanos AK, Krudysz A, Kluger J, Coleman CI, White CM. Electrocardiographic and hemodynamic effects of a multicomponent dietary supplement containing ephedra and caffeine: a randomized controlled trial. JAMA. 2004;291:216–21.

66. Haller CA, Benowitz NL. Adverse cardiovascular and central nervous system events associated with dietary supplements contraining ephedra alkaloids. N Engl J Med. 2000;343:1833–8.

67. Zahn KA, Li RL, Purssell RA. Cardiovascular toxicity after ingestion of 'herbal ecstacy'. J Emerg Med. 1999;17:289–91.

68. Carson P, Oldroyd K, Phadke K. Myocardial infarction due to amphetamine. Br Med J Clin Res Ed. 1987;294:1525–6.

69. Clark BM, Schonfield RS. Dilated cardiomyopathy and acute liver injury associated with combined use of ephedra, gamma-hydroxybutyrate, and anabolic steroids. Pharmacotherapy. 2005; 25:756–61.

70. Naik SD, Freudenberger RS. Ephedra-associated cardiomyopathy. Ann Pharmacother. 2004;38:400–3.

71. Nissen SE. ADHD Drugs and cardiovascular risk. N Engl J Med. 2006;354:1445–8.

72. Vitellio B. Understanding the risk of using medications for attention deficit hyperactivity disorder with respect to physical growth and cardiovascular function. Child Adolesc Psychiatric Clin N Am. 2008;17:459–74.

73. Kloner RA, Hale S, Alker K, Rezkalla S. The effects of acute and chronic cocaine use on the heart. Circulation. 1992;85:407–19.

74. Billman GE. Cocaine: a review of its toxic actions on cardiac function. Crit Rev Toxicol. 1995;25:113–32.

75. Karch SB. Cocaine cardiovascular toxicity. South Med J. 2005;98: 794–9.

76. Hale SL, Lehmann MH, Kloner RA. Electrocardiographic abnormalities after acute administration of cocaine in the rat. Am J Cardiol. 1989;63:1529–30.

77. Taylor D, Paroish D, Thompson K, Cavaliere M. Cocaine induced prolongation of the QT interval. Emerg Med J. 2004;21:252–3.

78. Magnano AR, Talathoti NB, Hallur R, Jurus DT, Dizon J, Holleran S, et al. Effect of acute cocaine administration on the QTc interval of habitual users. Am J Cardiol. 2006;97:1244–6.

79. Fuller TE, Milling TJ, Price B, Spangle K. Therapeutic hypothermia in cocaine-induced cardiac arrest. Ann Emerg Med. 2008; 51:135–7.

80. Hollander JE, Hoffman RS. Cocaine-induced myocardial infarction: an analysis and review of the literature. J Emerg Med. 1992; 10:169–77.

81. Turhan H, Aksoy Y, Ozgun Tekin G, Yetkin E. Cocaine-induced acute myocardial infarction in young individuals with otherwise normal coronary risk profile: Is coronary microvascular dysfunction one of the underlying mechanisms? Int J Cardiol. 2007;114:106–7.

82. Mittleman MA, Mintzer D, Maclure M, Togler GH, Sherwood JB, Muller JE. Triggering of myocardial infaction by cocaine. Circulation. 1999;99:2737–41.

83. Parker RB, Perry GY, Horan LG, Flowers NC. Comparative effects of sodium bicarbonate and sodium chloride on reversing cocaine-induced changes in the electrocardiogram. J Cardiovasc Pharmacol. 1999;34:864–9.

84. Littmann L, Monroe Mh, Svenson RH. Brugada-type electrocardiographic pattern induced by cocaine. Mayo Clin Proc. 2000;75: 845–9.

85. Perera R, Kraebber A, Schwartz MJ. Prolonged QT interval and cocaine use. J Electrocardiol. 1997;30:337–9.

86. Guo J, Gang H, Zhang S. Molecular determinants of cocaine block of human ether-a-go-go-related gene potassium channels. J Pharmacol Exp Ther. 2006;317:865–74.

87. Brickner ME, Willard JE, Eichhorn EJ, Black J, Grayburn PA. Left ventricular hypertrophy associated with chronic cocaine abuse. Circulation. 1991;84:1130–5.

88. Su J, Li J, Li W, Altura B, Altura B. Cocaine induces apoptosis in primari cultured rat aortic vascular smooth muscle cells: possible relationship to aortic dissection, atherosclerosis, and hypertension. Int J Toxicol. 2004;23:233–7.

89. He J, Xiao Y, Zhang L. Cocaine induces apoptosis in human coronary artery endothelial cells. J Cardiovasc Pharmacol. 2000;35: 572–80.

90. Fineschi V, Silver MD, Karch SB, Parolini M, Turillazzi E, Pomara C, Baroldi G. Myocardial disarray: an architectural disorganization linked with adrenergic stress? Int J Cardiol. 2005;99: 277–82.

91. Fanoe S, Jensen GB, Ege P. Proarrhythmic effect of methadone: an alternative explanation of sudden death in heroine addicts. PACE 2006;29 (Suppl 1):S30.

92. Fanoe S, Hvidt C, Ege P, Boje Jensen G. Syncope and QT prolongation among patients treated with methadone for heroin dependence in the city of Copenhagen. Heart. 2007;93:1051–5.

93. Krants MJ, Lewkowiez L, Hays H, Woodroffe MA, Robertson AD. Torsade de pointes associated with very-high-dose methadone. Ann Intern Med. 2002;137:501–4.

94. Friedman RA. The changing face of teenage drug abuse. The trend toward prescription drugs. N Engl J Med. 2006;354:1448–50.

95. Lindsay AC, Foale RA, Warren O, Henry JA. Cannabis as a precipitant of cardiovascular emergencies. Int J Cardiol. 2005;104: 230–2.

96. Fisher BA, Ghuran A, Vadamalai V, Antonios TF. Cardiovascular complications induced by cannabis smoking: a case report and review of the literature. Emerg Med J. 2005;22:679–80.

97. Campos DR, Yonamine M, de Moraes Moreau RL. Marijuana as doping in sports. Sports Med. 2003;33:395–9.

98. Lorente FO, Peretti-Watel P, Grelot L. Cannabis use to enhance sportive and non-sportive performances among French sport students. Addict Behav. 2005;30:1382–91.

99. Mittleman MA, Lewis RA, Maclure M, Sherwood JB, Muller JE. Triggering myocardial infarction by marijuana. Circulation. 2001;103(23):2805–9.

100. Arash A, Mark AW. Marijuana as a trigger of cardiovascular events: speculation or scientific certainty? Int J Cardiol. 2007; 118:141–4.

101. Whyte G, Stephens N, Sharma S, Shave R, Budgett R, McKenna WJ. Spontaneus atrial fibrillation in a freestyle skier. Br J Sports Med. 2004;38:230–2.

102. Pirwitz MJ, Willard JE, Landau C, Lange RA, Glamann DB, Kessler DJ, et al. Influence of cocaine, ethanol, or their combination on epicardial coronary arterial dimensions in humans. Arch Intern Med. 1995;155:1186–91.

103. Randall T. Cocaine, alcohol mix in body to form even longer lasting, more lethal drug. JAMA. 1992;267:1043–4.

104. Mann JJ. The medical management of depression. N Engl J Med. 2005;353(17):1819–34.

105. Biberdorf DJ, Steens R, Millar TW, Kryger MH. Benzodiazepines in congestive heart failure: effects of temazepam on arousability and Cheyne-Stokes respiration. Sleep. 1993;16(6):529–38.

106. Shader RI, Greenblatt DJ. Use of benzodiazepines in anxiety disorders. N Engl J Med. 1993;328(19):1398–405.

107. Miller J. Managing antidepression overdoses. Emerg Med Serv. 2004;33(10):113–9.

108. Witchel HJ, Hancox JC, Nutt DJ. Psychotropic drugs, cardiac arrhythmia, and sudden death. J Clin Psychopharmacol. 2003; 23(1):58–77.

109. Shader RI, Greenblatt DJ. More on potassium, the heart, and antipsychotic agents. J Clin Psychopharmacol. 1999;19(3): 201–2.

110. Tatsumi M, Groshan K, Blakely RD, Richelson E. Pharmacological profile of antidepressants and related compounds at human monoamine transporters. Eur J Pharmacol. 1997;340:249–58.

111. Shader RI, Greenblatt DJ. Selective serotonin reuptake inhibitor antidepressants: cardiovascular complications–sorting through findings. J Clin Psychopharmacol. 2001;21(5):467–8.

112. Warrington SJ, Padgham C, Lader M. The cardiovascular effects of antidepressants. Psychol Med Monogr Suppl. 1989;16:i–iii, 1–40.

113. Yamada M, Yasuhara H. Clinical pharmacology of MAO inhibitors: safety and future. Neurotoxicology. 2004;25(1–2):215–21. Review.

114. Goldman LS, Alexander RC, Luchins DJ. Monoamine oxidase inhibitors and tricyclic antidepressants: comparison of their cardiovascular effects. J Clin Psychiatry. 1986;47(5):225–9.

115. Murray JB. Cardiac disorders and antidepressant medications. J Psychol. 2000;134(2):162–8. Review.

116. Alvarez-Elcoro S, Enzler MJ. The macrolides: erythromycin, clarithromycin, and azithromycin. Mayo Clin Proc. 1999;74(6): 613–34.

117. Periti P, Mazzei T, Mini E, Novelli A. Adverse effects of macrolide antibacterials. Drug Saf. 1993;9(5):346–64.

118. Rolan P. Pharmacokinetics of new antiherpetic agents. Clin Pharmacokinet. 1995;29(5):333–40.

119. Flexner C. HIV-protease inhibitors. N Eng J Med. 1998;338(18): 1281–92.

120. Watts RG. Severe and fatal anthracycline cardiotoxicity at cumulative doses below 400 mg/m^2: evidence for enhanced toxicity with multiagent chemotherapy. Am J Hematol. 1991;36(3):217–8.

121. Frishman WH, Sung HM, Yee HC, Liu LL, Keefe D, Einzig AI, Dutcher J. Cardiovascular toxicity with cancer chemotherapy. Curr Probl Cancer. 1997; 21(6):301–60.

122. Broder H, Gottlieb RA, Lepor NE. Chemotherapy and cardiotoxicity. Rev Cardiovasc Med. 2008;9(2):75–83.

123. Freeman NJ, Costanza ME. 5-Fluorouracil-associated cardiotoxicity. Cancer. 1988;61(1):36–45.

124. Yap YG, Camm AJ. Potential cardiac toxicity of H1-antihistamines. Clin Allergy Immunol. 2002;17:389–419.

125. DuBuske LM. Second-generation antihistamines: the risk of ventricular arrhythmias. Clin Ther. 1999;21(2):281–95.

126. Barbey JT, Anderson M, Ciprandi G, Frew AJ, Morad M, Priori SG, Ongini E, Affrime MB. Cardiovascular safety of second-generation antihistamines. Am J Rhinol. 1999;13(3):235–43.

Liver Disease

33

Samir Zakhari, Bin Gao, and Jan B. Hoek

Abstract

The profiles of liver disease associated with chronic alcohol consumption show a great deal of individual variability in severity and progression of the condition for comparable levels of alcohol consumption. It has traditionally been assumed that this variability may reflect individual genetic factors, such as the expression and activity of individual isoforms of ADH and ALDH that determine the pharmacokinetics of ethanol metabolism, but is also influenced by variations in temporal intake patterns (binge vs. steady drinking) or by nutritional status, gender, exposure to other damaging factors, such as smoking or use of other drugs of abuse. In addition, the onset and severity of alcoholic liver disease (ALD) is strongly influenced by other comorbid conditions such as infection with hepatitis B or C viruses, and/or human immunodeficiency virus (HIV), diabetes, hemochromatosis, or obesity, suggesting that chronic alcohol consumption may affect the susceptibility to other challenges. The origin of this increase in susceptibility to ALD is not due solely to intrahepatic factors, but may also involve alcohol-induced changes in other tissues, ranging from adipose tissue to the CNS, the gut, and the immune system. Thus, although the factors contributing to alcohol-induced liver disease remain poorly understood, they are complex and systemic.

Although abstinence from drinking can reverse alcoholic fatty liver and is helpful in the management of alcoholic hepatitis and cirrhosis, current treatment of ALD includes palliative therapy and nutritional support. There are no specific antifibrotic compounds available for the reversal of alcohol-induced liver fibrosis and cirrhosis.

S. Zakhari (✉)
Division of Metabolism and Health Effects, National Institute on Alcohol Abuse and Alcoholism, National Institutes of Health, Bethesda, MD 20852, USA
e-mail: szakhari@mail.nih.gov

B. Gao
Division of Intramural Clinical and Biological Research, National Institute on Alcohol Abuse and Alcoholism, National Institutes of Health, Bethesda, MD 20852, USA
e-mail: bgao@mail.nih.gov

J.B. Hoek
Department of Pathology, Anatomy and Cell Biology, Thomas Jefferson University, Philadelphia, PA 19107, USA
e-mail: jan.hoek@jefferson.edu

Learning Objectives
- Chronic alcohol consumption results in alcoholic liver disease, which encompasses fatty liver, steatohepatitis, fibrosis, cirrhosis, hepatocellular carcinoma, and acute alcoholic hepatitis
- Alcohol metabolism by the liver produces acetaldehyde (a highly reactive chemical that forms adducts with DNA, RNA, and proteins) and acetate; increases the formation of reactive oxygen species (ROS) and produces oxidative stress; and changes the redox state of hepatocytes by increasing the ratio of reduced to oxidized NAD

(continued)

J.C. Verster et al. (eds.), *Drug Abuse and Addiction in Medical Illness: Causes, Consequences and Treatment*,
DOI 10.1007/978-1-4614-3375-0_33, © Springer Science+Business Media, LLC 2012

- Heavy alcohol consumption accelerates liver damage due to infection with hepatitis C and/or HIV viruses
- Although alcohol-induced fatty liver could be reversible, no treatment is currently available for cirrhosis

Issues that Need to Be Addressed by Future Research
- What are the exact mechanisms by which alcohol induces fatty liver, fibrosis and cirrhosis, as well as hepatocellular carcinoma?
- Is steatosis a prerequisite for fibrosis?
- Why do only about 15% of heavy drinkers have cirrhosis? And why does it often take over 20 years to develop? Is there a role for alcohol and ageing?
- What is the role of alcohol-induced disturbances of gut microflora on liver disease? Can we use prebiotics or probiotics to treat alcoholic liver disease?
- What is the role of the endocannabinoid system in energy balance, metabolism, inflammation, and alcoholic liver disease?
- How do alcohol effects on the circadian rhythm influence liver metabolism and disease?

Introduction

Liver disease can result from a variety of causes, including infectious agents, medications, herbs, excessive alcohol consumption, inherited metabolic disorders, cholestatic and immune disorders, hemochromatosis, schistosomiasis, and obesity. This chapter focuses on alcohol-induced liver disease. The consumption of large quantities of alcoholic beverages over long periods is associated with diseases of many organs, but the liver stands out as the tissue that is generally most severely affected by this exposure. Numerous mechanisms have been advocated for alcohol-induced liver disease, including alcohol metabolism which results in the formation of reactive oxygen species (ROS) and oxidative stress, formation of acetaldehyde, as well as the changes in the redox state of hepatocytes. In addition, activation of hepatic stellate cells (HSC) and expression of inflammatory cytokines are involved. Four topics will be addressed: (1) alcohol metabolism and role in alcoholic liver disease (ALD); (2) consequences of alcohol consumption and various aspects of ALD; (3) comorbid factors; and (4) treatment.

Alcohol (Ethanol) Metabolism in the Liver

Ingested ethanol is readily absorbed from the gastrointestinal tract. Only about 2–10% of the absorbed alcohol is eliminated via lungs and kidneys; the remaining 90% is metabolized mainly in the liver by oxidative pathways, and by nonoxidative pathways mainly in extrahepatic tissues. Oxidative metabolism in the liver results in extensive displacement of the liver's normal metabolic substrates and the production of acetate which is preferentially used as energy source by tissues such as the brain and the heart. Alcohol metabolism produces 7.1 kcal/g and as such is the preferred fuel in the body.

Oxidative Pathways

The liver is the main organ for metabolizing ethanol. The major pathway of oxidative metabolism of ethanol in the liver involves cytosolic *alcohol dehydrogenase* (ADH, of which multiple isoenzymes exist; see Table 33.1) to produce acetaldehyde, a highly reactive and toxic molecule accumulation of which contributes to tissue damage. ADH also acts on a wide range of other substrates, e.g., mediating ω-oxidation of fatty acids, but its preferred substrate is ethanol. This oxidation is accompanied by the reduction of NAD^+ to NADH, and ethanol oxidation thereby generates a highly reduced cytosolic environment in cells where ADH is active (predominantly hepatocytes). The cytochrome P450 isozymes, including CYP2E1, 1A2, and 3A4, which are present predominantly in the endoplasmic reticulum (ER), also contribute to ethanol oxidation to acetaldehyde in the liver, particularly after chronic ethanol intake. CYP2E1 is induced by chronic ethanol consumption and assumes an important role in metabolizing ethanol to acetaldehyde at elevated alcohol concentration. It also produces highly ROS, including hydroxyethyl, superoxide anion, and hydroxyl radicals. Another enzyme, *catalase*, located in the peroxisomes, is capable of oxidizing ethanol in vitro in the presence of a hydrogen peroxide (H_2O_2) generating system, such as *NADPH oxidase* or *xanthine oxidase*, or during peroxisomal oxidation of very long-chain fatty acids (Fig. 33.1). Quantitatively, however, this is considered a minor pathway of ethanol oxidation.

Acetaldehyde, produced by ethanol oxidation through any of these mechanisms, is rapidly metabolized, mainly by mitochondrial *aldehyde dehydrogenase* (ALDH2) to form acetate and NADH. Mitochondrial NADH is oxidized by the electron transport chain. Other metabolic pathways are discussed elsewhere [1].

Acetaldehyde also has the capacity to react with lysine residues on a wide range of proteins including enzymes, ER proteins, microtubules, and affect their function. It can also

Table 33.1 Human ADH isozymes

Class	Gene nomenclature		Protein	K_m (mM)	Turnover (min⁻¹)	Tissue
	New	Former				
I	*ADH1A*	*ADH1*	α	4.0	30	Liver
	*ADH1B*1*	*ADH2*1*	$β_1$	0.05	4	
	*ADH1B*2*	*ADH2*2*	$β_2$	0.9	350	Liver, lung
	*ADH1B*3*	*ADH2*3*	$β_3$	40.0	300	
	*ADH1C*1*	*ADH3*1*	$γ_1$	1.0	90	Liver, stomach
	*ADH1C*2*	*ADH3*2*	$γ_2$	0.6	40	
II	*ADH4*	*ADH4*	π	30.0	20	Liver, cornea
III	*ADH5*	*ADH5*	χ	>1,000	100	Most tissues
IV	*ADH7*	*ADH7*	σ(μ)	30.0	1,800	Stomach
V	*ADH6*	*ADH6*		ND	ND	Liver, stomach

The α, β, and γ subunits of ADH are encoded by three closely linked loci on chromosome 4: ADH1A, ADH1B, and ADH1C. In addition to metabolizing ethanol, ADH is involved in the metabolism of physiological substrates such as steroids, oxidation of intermediary alcohols in mevalonate metabolism, and ω oxidation of fatty acids (K_m and Turnover values from Hurley et al. [66]); ND = Not Determined

Oxidative Pathways of Alcohol Metabolism

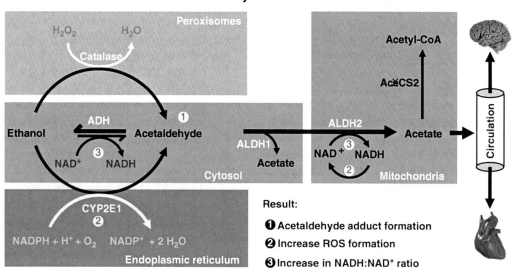

Fig. 33.1 *AceCS2* acetyl-CoA synthase 2; *ADH* alcohol dehydrogenase; *ALDH* aldehyde dehydrogenase; *NAD* nicotinamide adenine dinucleotide; *NADH* reduced NAD; *NADP* nicotinamide adenine dinucleotide phosphate; *H₂O₂* hydrogen peroxide; *ATP* adenosine 5′ triphosphate. Ethanol is metabolized mainly in hepatocytes cytosol by ADH, and the resultant acetaldehyde is mainly metabolized by the mitochondrial ALDH to form acetate. AceCS2, which metabolizes acetate to acetyl-CoA is not expressed in the liver, therefore acetate formed in the liver is released into the circulation to be metabolized by extrahepatic tissues to acetyl-CoA

react with biochemically active amines, e.g., in the CNS it can react with dopamine to form salsolinol, which has been suggested to play a role in the addictive effects of ethanol. Formation of protein adducts in hepatocytes may contribute to impaired protein secretion, resulting in hepatomegaly.

Consequences of Alcohol Metabolism by Oxidative Pathways

The following effects result from alcohol metabolism in the liver:

(a) *Acetaldehyde formation.* Oxidation of alcohol by ADH, CYP2E1, and *catalase* results in the formation of acetal-

dehyde, which is rapidly metabolized to acetate by ALDH mainly in the mitochondria. Acetaldehyde, if accumulates to high concentrations, can form adducts with DNA, RNA, and proteins resulting in enzyme inactivation and decreased DNA repair. There is evidence that more stable mixed adducts of acetaldehyde and malondialdehyde, a byproduct of oxidative stress, can form on reactive lysine residues on proteins which are immunogenic and can induce the production of specific antibodies that can contribute to immune-mediated tissue damage. The inactive form ALDH2*2 which is present in about 25–50% of Asians is ineffective in removing acetaldehyde resulting in facial flushing, tachycardia, headache, and nausea. This generally acts as a deterrent for developing alcohol dependence.

(b) *Acetate formation.* Most of the acetate resulting from ethanol metabolism escapes the liver to the blood and is eventually metabolized to CO_2 by way of the tricarboxylic acid (TCA) cycle in cells with mitochondria that contain enzymes to convert acetate to the metabolically active intermediate acetyl CoA. This occurs primarily in tissues such as heart, skeletal muscle, and brain. Acetate is not an inert product. Acetate has been suggested to activate a variety of metabolic processes in tissues where the formation of acetyl CoA is prominent [2], in part by serving as an energy substrate, in part through the formation of AMP. It should be noted that AMP formation may also activate intracellular signaling pathways through its effect on AMP-activated protein kinase (AMPK), which activates catabolic processes and inhibits synthetic processes, including protein synthesis and lipid synthesis. Acetate has also been reported to depress the central nervous system (CNS). It has been established that upon ethanol intake the brain starts using acetate as a substrate rather than glucose (analogous to the use of fatty acids in severe starvation when glucose levels from gluconeogenesis are low). However, the energy yield from acetate oxidation is relatively low compared to glucose.

(c) *Formation of reactive oxygen species (ROS) and oxidative stress.* ROS, including superoxide ($\cdot O_2^-$), hydrogen peroxide (H_2O_2), hypochlorite ion (OCl^-), and hydroxyl ($\cdot OH$) radicals, are generated by many reactions in multiple compartments in the cell, e.g., *NADPH oxidases* in the plasma membrane, cytochrome P450 isoforms in the ER, lipid metabolism within the peroxisomes; and various cytosolic *cyclooxygenases*. However, in most cells the vast majority of ROS results from electron transport by the mitochondria.

Ethanol-induced oxidative stress has been attributed to a decrease in the $NAD^+/NADH$ redox ratio, acetaldehyde formation, CYP2E1 induction, hypoxia, cytokine signaling, mitochondrial damage, LPS activation of Kupffer cells, reduction in antioxidants particularly mitochondrial and cytosolic glutathione, one electron oxidation of ethanol to 1-hydroxy ethyl radical, and the conversion of *xanthine dehydrogenase* to *xanthine oxidase*.

(d) *Change in Hepatocyte Redox State (Increase in NADH/ NAD+ Ratio).* Beginning in the late 1960s, Krebs and Veech have demonstrated that metabolic pathways in the liver are partly regulated by the ratio of the reduced and oxidized forms of nicotinamide adenine dinucleotide ($NADH:NAD^+$). A change in the levels of these metabolites, which results in a shift of the redox potential of hepatocytes, causes a marked alteration in various reversible metabolic pathways [3]. It has been demonstrated more than 50 years ago that both acute and chronic alcohol consumption shift the redox state of the liver to a more reduced level [4, 5], similar to, though much more pronounced than the shift observed in diabetes and during starvation. Rats fed alcohol for 4–6 weeks developed fatty livers, showed an increase in $NADH:NAD^+$ ratio from 1.2 to 8.6, and exhibited fourfold to fivefold increase in β-hydroxybutyrate, and double the level of α-glycerophosphate [6]. Alcohol metabolism produces a significant increase in the hepatic $NADH/NAD^+$ ratio in both the cytosol and the mitochondria, as evidenced by an increase in the lactate/ pyruvate and β-hydroxybutyrate/acetoacetate ratios, respectively [7]. The reducing equivalents of NADH in the cytosol are transported into the mitochondria primarily via the malate–aspartate shuttle. However, the activity of this process may be limited by the more reduced state of mitochondrial NAD due to the simultaneous oxidation of acetaldehyde. Formation of lactate functions in part as an overflow pathway to reoxidize cytosolic NADH in the liver. Thus, ethanol oxidation vastly increases the availability of oxidizable NADH to the electron transport chain in the mitochondria. The liver responds to ethanol exposure in part by increasing the rate of oxygen uptake, which may lead to periods of hypoxia, in particular in the downstream (pericentral) parts of the liver lobule. Interestingly, this is the region where tissue damage is often observed with chronic ethanol consumption. The change in NAD redox state may have many other consequences for metabolic regulation in the liver. NAD^+ influences many important cellular reactions, and the ratio of NADH to NAD^+ fluctuates in response to changes in metabolism. Redox changes that happen after binge drinking seem to be attenuated with chronic ethanol ingestion, although some changes, e.g., accumulation of fat in liver, continue with chronic consumption.

Consequences of Chronic Alcohol Consumption for Liver Function

Stages of Alcoholic Liver Disease

Alcoholic liver disease (ALD) incorporates a broad range of defects, with greatly variable degrees of severity. A common consequence of chronic alcohol consumption is the development of fatty liver, histologically evident by the occurrence of lipid droplets in hepatocytes (hepatocellular steatosis). Lipid droplets are vesicular structures formed at the endoplasmic reticulum by mechanisms that are still poorly understood and that function as intracellular lipid storage reservoirs. They consist of a lumen containing lipid esters, mostly triglycerides, surrounded by a single phospholipid monolayer and coated with proteins of the PAT family (perilipin, adipose differentiation-related protein (ADRP), and tail-interacting protein of 47 kDa (TIP47) are the founding members of this family), which control access to the lipid stores [8].

The condition of hepatocellular steatosis was long thought to be a relatively innocuous side effect of heavy drinking, because it is usually readily reversible upon cessation of alcohol consumption. However, fatty liver often develops in other clinical conditions characterized by significant metabolic defects, such as obesity, metabolic syndrome, and type 2 diabetes, and it is now generally recognized that fatty liver by itself reflects a condition of metabolic stress that is a risk factor for the development of more severe forms of liver disease. Some authors distinguish between macrovesicular (lipid droplets of several microns in diameter) and microvesicular (foamy) steatosis and suggest that the former is the more pernicious of these conditions, possibly associated with mitochondrial dysfunction and apoptotic cell death [9]. However, there is as yet no good understanding of the factors that differentiate these forms of steatosis or whether these are merely epiphenomena of different functional states of the tissue, e.g., related to conditions of more severe oxidative stress.

It is likely that steatosis predisposes the tissue to the development of hepatitis, an inflammatory condition characterized by moderate to severe tissue damage with a significant increase in serum levels of liver enzymes (ALT and AST) and histologically showing necrotic foci with neutrophil infiltration. Acute alcoholic hepatitis is a potentially fatal disease that develops in a significant fraction (30–40%) of chronic heavy drinkers, often after many years of alcohol consumption. However, subacute chronic hepatitis may be more widespread and often goes undetected.

A modest (10–15%) fraction of chronic heavy drinkers proceeds to develop fibrosis and cirrhosis. Fibrosis is a scarring response of the tissue that is characterized by the deposition of abnormal extracellular matrix. Excessive deposition of fibrotic material over many years leads to cross-linking and stabilization of the scar tissue that cannot be resolved by liver repair mechanisms and interferes with normal liver function.

Even though there is a clear relationship between lifetime alcohol consumption and the risk of developing liver cirrhosis, it is remarkable that only a small fraction of chronic heavy drinkers develop these more advanced stages of liver disease. The factors that facilitate the development of hepatitis and cirrhosis are not well characterized. It is often hypothesized that chronic alcohol consumption may be a predisposing factor that could sensitize the tissue to other injurious conditions (second-hit hypothesis). For instance, as discussed below, the existence of comorbid conditions, such as hepatitis B or hepatitis C infection, may contribute to the more severe forms of ALD. Fibrosis and cirrhosis also are

thought to be risk factors for hepatocellular carcinoma (HCC), which may occur in 10–15% of patients who develop liver cirrhosis. There is strong evidence from animal studies that chronic ethanol treatment causes both parenchymal and nonparenchymal cells to have different susceptibility to other damaging conditions. This may reflect a change in the cellular stress defense mechanisms, (e.g., oxidative stress defenses are reportedly impaired in hepatocytes from ethanol-fed animals) [10] or ethanol may affect the balance of autocrine or paracrine mediators that are critical in maintaining normal homeostatic conditions. In addition, chronic alcohol consumption interferes with liver regeneration, a highly effective repair mechanisms unique to the liver that avoids scar tissue formation. However, the second-hit hypothesis does not adequately account for the fact that the more advanced forms of ALD do not develop in a stochastic pattern and invariably take a minimum of 10–20 years to develop. This observation suggests that aging itself may constitute a conditioning factor that could enhance the risk of developing alcoholic liver fibrosis and cirrhosis. However, mechanisms to account for the age dependence of developing advanced forms of ALD remain to be explored.

Alcoholic Fatty Liver

Mechanisms That Promote Hepatocellular Steatosis
Metabolic factors: In the final instance, the development of fatty liver reflects a metabolic imbalance that involves deregulation of hepatic lipid metabolism. However, the metabolic pathways involved are complex and interact intricately with other metabolic demands in the liver (e.g., carbohydrate metabolism, energy supply and demand) and structural aspects of cell function (membrane function, vesicle trafficking). Also lipid metabolism in the liver is integrated with other tissues that regulate food intake, fat storage, and metabolism and that are controlled by hormones and other circulating mediators. Thus, it is not surprising that a wide variety of factors, nutritional, environmental, or metabolic, can result in a condition of hepatocellular steatosis. These include impairments in mitochondrial and peroxisomal fatty acid oxidation in the liver, enhanced release of fatty acids from storage sites in adipose tissue, increased uptake into the liver from the circulation, as well as increased hepatic de novo synthesis of fatty acids and triglycerides. In addition, sustained imbalances in nutritional supply of fat and the capacity to process it may lead to defects in lipoprotein metabolism and precipitate conditions that stretch the regulatory capacity of the body (largely dependent on the critical role of insulin) to its limits. Classically, this is reflected in a condition of insulin resistance, which commonly accompanies defects associated with the metabolic syndrome and type 2 diabetes mellitus.

Regulatory controls on lipid metabolism: Hepatic lipid metabolism is subject to short-term regulation at a large number of sites, mediated in large part by covalent modification (e.g., phosphorylation) of critical proteins that regulate the flux through distinct branches of the system. The cellular signals mediating these effects give the liver cell the capacity to respond to extracellular signals provided by hormones, cytokines, and adipokines that reflect the functional state of the organism. Major sites of regulation include the uptake of long-chain free fatty acids from the circulation into the liver cytosol where they can be bound to fatty acid binding proteins (FABP), which buffers their availability for interaction with other target proteins. Further metabolism largely requires activation of fatty acids to long-chain acyl-CoA esters and their binding to acyl-CoA binding protein (ACBP), which controls its delivery to major metabolic pathways, including mitochondrial or peroxisomal oxidation, triglyceride synthesis, or phospholipid synthesis and turnover. Additional sites of regulation involve the synthesis and processing of lipoprotein in the endoplasmic reticulum for export of triglycerides or their storage in lipid storage vesicles. Furthermore, de novo fatty acid synthesis responds to the availability of acetyl CoA produced from carbohydrate metabolism. A well-known example involves the regulation of the balance of mitochondrial fatty acid oxidation and de novo fatty acid synthesis from acetyl CoA at the level of acetyl CoA carboxylase (ACC). This enzyme mediates the formation of malonyl-CoA, the substrate for Fatty Acid Synthase. Malonyl-CoA simultaneously functions as an effective inhibitor of carnitine palmitoyl transferase-1 (CPT-1), the acylcarnitine transporter in the mitochondrial outer membrane that is required for mitochondrial β-oxidation of long-chain fatty acids. Thus, the level of malonyl-CoA is a major determinant of the balance of fatty acid synthesis and oxidation. Interestingly, ACC is subject to regulation by phosphorylation. The major protein kinase responsible for ACC regulation is AMPK, a system that is known to function as a sensor for metabolic demand. AMPK also regulates critical early steps in cholesterol biosynthesis and thereby is in a crucial position to affect lipid metabolism in the liver. Interestingly, recent studies on experimental animals have suggested that AMPK may be a target for ethanol [11]. A large number of additional regulatory controls on different steps of the lipid metabolic pathways have been described. However, there is as yet only a limited understanding as to how the multitude of control mechanisms integrates to generate a coherent response to the wide range of metabolic conditions encountered in the course of normal metabolism.

In large part, the adaptations to longer term deregulation of hepatic lipid metabolism involve two sets of transcription factors that exert predominant control over the expression of a diverse group of enzymes involved in hepatic lipid metabolism. PPAR-α is a transcriptional regulator that controls the expression of a broad range of critical enzymes required to enhance fatty acid oxidation through both peroxisomal and mitochondrial pathways. Upon activation, PPAR-α can be activated by heterodimerization with Retinoic acid X receptors (RXR) and migrate to the nucleus, where it can bind to promoter regions of its target genes. PPAR-α activity is regulated by a variety of drugs known as peroxisome proliferators, including clofibrate and its derivatives, but the predominant physiological regulators of PPAR-α are long-chain fatty acids. Transgenic animals that overexpress PPAR-α in the liver are resistant to steatosis and treatment with peroxisome proliferating drugs has a similar antisteatotic effect. The transcriptional response to PPAR-α activation is further enhanced by interaction with the coactivators protein PGC-1α. Interestingly, this protein has recently emerged as a major regulator of energy metabolism and its effects on cell metabolism closely interlink with the regulatory effects of AMPK [12].

Largely in opposition to PPAR-α, the enzymatic machinery of fatty acid synthesis and triglyceride formation is predominantly controlled by the SREBP-1c transcription factor. SREBP-1c is one of several isoforms encoded by two genes, *srebp1* and *serbp2*. SREBP-1 exists in two different splice forms, SREBP-1a and SREBP-1c, of which the latter isoform is the predominant form expressed in the liver. SREBP-2 also is active in the liver and controls the expression of enzymes of cholesterol metabolism. Precursor forms of SREBP-1c and SREBP-2 are intrinsic membrane proteins in the endoplasmic reticulum membrane. Upon activation SREBPs are proteolytically activated by SREBP-cleavage activating protein (SCAP), which enables the protein to migrate to the trans-Golgi apparatus, where it is further processed to the active form that can be translocated to the nucleus to control the expression of critical enzymes of fatty acid synthesis and triglyceride synthesis. Transcriptional activation of SREBP-1c is further stimulated by the coactivating protein p300/CBP. Among the significant target enzymes for SREBP-1c is Fatty Acid Synthase, which catalyzes de novo fatty acid synthesis, and stearoylCoA desaturase-1 (SCD-1), which functions as a desaturase to generate monounsaturated fatty acids from their saturated counterparts. Effective triglyceride formation requires a proper balance of saturated and unsaturated fatty acylCoA and a defect in SCD-1 expression impairs triglyceride synthesis with accumulation of free fatty acids. This condition is thought to contribute to cell injury even in the absence of triglyceride accumulation. These and other findings have been suggested to indicate that triglyceride synthesis and storage in the form of lipid droplets may be a protective mechanisms rather than a damaging factor itself [13].

SREBP-1c expression is responsive to insulin, possibly acting indirectly, through Liver X receptor (LXR), a nuclear receptor that also acts as a heterodimer with retinoic acid X receptor. The complementary role of RXR in the actions of SREBP-1c and PPAR-α may contribute to the corresponding complementarity in the regulation of fatty acid metabolizing enzyme systems. In addition, both SREBP-1 and SREBP-2 protein expression are subject to a positive feedback mechanism as a result of the mature protein activating its own transcription. Such mechanisms are typically subject to switch-like transitions that can result in very steep responses to critical levels of stimulatory input signals that persist even after the stimulus is removed. In addition, the strength of the stimulus that results in "throwing the switch" can be affected by secondary conditions that affect the system's sensitivity. Hence, conditions such as ethanol exposure may exert its effects indirectly by affecting the factors that determine the transition point for this switch.

A large number of additional regulatory controls on the multiple pathways of lipid metabolism are exerted at the level of covalent modification of these transcription factors and their coactivators and upstream regulatory proteins that affect their stability, localization, and activity. Considerable attention has been focused on the regulation of key regulatory factors by ε-acetylation on lysine residues. A broad range of proteins is regulated by reversible acetylation, and these include SREBP-1c, PGC-1α, and several other lipid metabolism regulatory proteins. Interestingly, the p300/CBP coactivator itself functions as an acetyltransferase that can acetylate SREBP-1c and activate its function. Conversely, among multiple classes of deacetylases, the NAD⁺-dependent protein deacetylase SIRT1 can act to remove the acetyl group from these (and multiple other) proteins. A direct involvement of SIRT1 in the regulation of hepatic lipid metabolism was recently corroborated by studies of mice with a hepatocyte-specific deletion of SIRT1 [14]. These mice are deficient in fatty acid β-oxidation and develop hepatocellular steatosis on a high-fat diet, predominantly through impaired PPAR-α function. Interestingly, these studies demonstrated that SIRT1 exerted these effects by direct binding to PPAR-α and deacetylating its coactivator PGC-1α. However, other studies have suggested that other proteins among the multitude of SIRT1 targets may contribute to the deregulation of lipid metabolism observed in SIRT1 knockout studies, or to the salutary effects of SIRT1 activators, such as the food additive resveratrol [15]. Importantly, SIRT1 and other deacetylases also contribute to the regulation of histone acetylation, one of the regulatory mechanisms that controls chromatin structure and its accessibility to transcription factors and other regulatory proteins. Thereby, factors that alter the activity of deacetylases, or the corresponding acetyl transferases that mediate the acetylation of protein lysine resides, may exert a multitude of indirect effects through epigenetic mechanisms. There is evidence that ethanol treatment affects the activity of both histone acetyl transferases and histone deacetylases [16], and ethanol treatment causes considerable alterations in the acetylation state of a multitude of cellular proteins [17]. The functional implications of these changes remain to be adequately analyzed.

Fatty liver and cellular stress: What is so disruptive about fatty liver that it causes damage to the liver? There is considerable evidence that the accumulation of free fatty acids themselves induces a stress condition in hepatocytes that is reflected in impaired function of intracellular organelles, notably the endoplasmic reticulum and mitochondrial damage, referred to as "lipotoxicity." However, the underlying mechanisms remain poorly characterized. Both free fatty acids and acyl CoA esters activate a variety of cell signaling pathways, including specific isoforms of protein kinase C, NF-κB, and JNK. It is likely that these signaling mechanisms also contribute to the endoplasmic reticulum and mitochondrial stress conditions, e.g., by their effect on pro- and anti-apoptotic Bcl2 family proteins that control the permeability of the mitochondrial outer membrane. These factors may contribute to the increased susceptibility to tissue damage that characterizes the fatty liver, irrespective of its origins. In fact, fatty liver is commonly associated with oxidative stress and triggers pro-inflammatory signals that invite infiltration with neutrophils and immune cells of different kinds.

What Is the Mechanism by Which Ethanol Treatment Promotes Steatosis?

The condition of hepatocellular steatosis that commonly develops with heavy alcohol consumption was classically attributed to a metabolic load imposed by the fact that the liver is the predominant site of ethanol metabolism. Possible mechanisms included the suppression of mitochondrial fatty acid β-oxidation resulting from the preferential oxidation of ethanol and acetaldehyde, which causes a highly reduced state of NAD in the cytosol and, to a more variable degree, in the mitochondria. This reductive effect of ethanol metabolism may be compounded by a limitation in the permeability of the outer mitochondrial membrane pore protein VDAC imposed by ethanol, which slows down the access of other substrates to the mitochondrial electron transport chain and facilitates preferential oxidation of acetaldehyde by mitochondrial low K_m ALDH [18]. In addition to the resulting impairments in mitochondrial and peroxisomal fatty acid oxidation, ethanol may enhance hepatic uptake of free fatty acids from the circulation, as well as increase de novo synthesis of fatty acids and triglycerides. Furthermore, there is evidence that ethanol treatment affects lipoprotein synthesis and secretion, contributing to the accumulation of lipids in the parenchymal cells of the liver.

More chronic exposure to ethanol induces a marked increase in alternative ethanol metabolic activities, most notably cytochrome P450 2E1 (CYP2E1), with a resultant increased demand for NADPH, an increased rate of formation of ROS, and a decrease in oxidative stress defense capacity. At the same time, an impairment of mitochondrial respiratory capacity becomes evident, caused by defects in the electron transport and ATP synthase complexes. Although the mechanisms responsible for the mitochondrial defects are not well characterized, this causes a further increase in ROS formation at the mitochondrial level [19]. Furthermore, the oxidative stress defense mechanisms are impaired with prolonged alcohol use, which may result in a decrease in glutathione levels, which appears to be more pronounced in mitochondria. The more oxidative environment can also promote a condition of endoplasmic reticulum stress. This condition is often associated with the activation of the Unfolded Protein Response, a cellular defense mechanism that results from an excess accumulation of defectively folded proteins [20]. It is possible that a more oxidized cellular environment impairs the proper folding of newly synthesized proteins. In addition, the ER stress is enhanced by defects in the methionine cycle, the cellular pathway that generates S-adenosylmethionine (SAMe). SAMe is the major methyl donor in the cell and its metabolism also provides precursors for the synthesis of glutathione. Defects in the methionine cycle therefore can also contribute to the decline in oxidative stress defenses. The resulting accumulation of stress conditions in the liver cell also brings with it an increased susceptibility to cell death signals.

However, the deregulation of the normal lipid metabolic balance in the liver can only partially be attributed to these direct consequences of ethanol metabolism. Accompanying the more chronic structural and functional changes in subcellular organelles, chronic ethanol treatment results in significant changes in the profile of transcription factors that regulate lipid homeostasis in the liver. Ethanol consumption elicits a decrease in PPAR-α activity, thereby suppressing the catabolic lipid metabolic pathways, including peroxisomal and mitochondrial fatty acid oxidation. At the same time, ethanol increases the activity of SREBP-1c and SREBP-2, which enhances lipid synthetic pathways.

Despite the observations from both animal experiments and cell line studies that chronic ethanol treatment affects the expression and activity state of the major transcriptional regulators involved in hepatic lipid homeostasis, the factors that are responsible for the changes in activity of these transcriptional regulatory systems remain poorly characterized. There has been some evidence from animal studies that the AMPK, one of the major metabolic stress sensors in the cells, itself is inhibited by ethanol. However, in these studies it is difficult to distinguish direct and indirect effects of ethanol. For instance, AMPK activity in the liver is regulated not only by the availability of AMP in the cell, but also responds to extracellular signals, including the adipose tissue-derived cytokine adiponectin. Chronic ethanol treatment has been found to decrease circulating adiponectin levels, at least in experimental animal models.

A related regulatory pathway affected by ethanol may involve the deacetylase SIRT-1. SIRT-1 belongs to the sirtuins, a family of deacetylases with homology to the yeast enzyme SIR-2, which have the characteristic of requiring activation by NAD+. Thus, the change in NAD redox state in the liver during ethanol oxidation may facilitate inhibition of SIRT-1. It has been reported that SIRT-1 activity in the liver of mice is decreased after ethanol treatment, although this may reflect a secondary adaptation to chronic exposure rather than being the result of a direct (and transient) effect of ethanol metabolism [21]. As mentioned earlier, among the targets of SITR-1 are several regulatory enzymes that affect lipid metabolism, including the transcriptional coregulators PGC-1a, deacetylation of which prevents its binding to PPAR-α and thereby suppresses its activity. Also, LKB1, the upstream protein kinase that controls AMPK activity requires acetylation and is a target for SIRT-1. Furthermore, SREBP-1c is a target for SIRT-1 and its acetylation state may affect its transcriptional activity. However, the broad range of proteins affected by SIRT-1 (and other deacetylases and acetyl transferases that may be affected by ethanol) and the potential for indirect effects through epigenetic mechanisms makes it difficult to gain a good perspective on the role of these proteins in ethanol-induced changes in the metabolic state of the liver based on the information currently available.

Extracellular Factors That Impact on the Liver to Promote Steatosis Under Conditions of Chronic Ethanol Treatment

Lipid metabolism in the liver is integrated with metabolic activities elsewhere in the body and a variety of signals from circulating hormonal, cytokines and other factors, combined with nutritional conditions impinge on the intrahepatic factors that cause steatosis. Not surprisingly, chronic ethanol consumption affects liver function in part through its impact on extracellular signaling mediators. Some of these factors are intrahepatic, e.g., cytokines released from Kupffer cells, endothelial cells, or stellate cells, others are dispatched by more remote tissues. Of particular relevance are factors that integrate the body's lipid metabolism. These include nutritional hormones (e.g., insulin) and the factors secreted from adipose tissue, notably adiponectin and leptin, as well as stress hormones and satiety factors that act through the hypothalamus or other brain structures affecting food intake. During the past decade, much evidence has accumulated that chronic ethanol consumption has a notable impact on the synthesis and secretion of several of these factors, in addition to affecting their capacity to impact lipid metabolic pathways in the liver.

In particular, the role of adiponectin has attracted considerable attention in recent years. Adiponectin is one of a diverse set of protein mediators that is secreted by adipose tissue to regulate the body's lipid homeostasis. Adiponectin acts on multiple tissues, including skeletal muscle, heart, and liver to sensitize the response to insulin and enhance fatty acid oxidation. Adiponectin acts through two types of cell surface receptor, AdipoR1 and AdipoR2, that are thought to activate AMPK and PPAR-α, respectively, both of which would enhance fatty acid oxidation and suppress lipid synthetic pathways. However, the intracellular signaling pathways by which the receptor activation is coupled to these pathways have not been clarified. Both receptors are expressed in liver. In animal experiments, there is evidence that adiponectin protects against the deleterious effects of steatosis and steatohepatitis and ethanol feeding tends to suppress adiponectin secretion from adipose tissue. However, the effects of ethanol on adiponectin levels may depend on the nutritional state of the animal, e.g., on the content of saturated and unsaturated fat [22]. This may have consequences for the susceptibility to liver damage. However, whether circulating adiponectin levels have similar correlations with liver damage in human alcoholics remains unclear [23].

The multiplicity of effects of adiponectin or other circulating factors on the susceptibility to alcohol-induced liver damage undoubtedly reflects the fact that these agents do not operate in isolation. For instance, adipokines such as leptin and adiponectin also act on, and interact with peptides released from the gut, the pancreas, or the hypothalamus that signal the nutritional state and other demands of the organism. The release of these peptides may themselves be affected by ethanol exposure.

Among the circulating factors that affect liver lipid metabolism, insulin is one of the dominant hormonal mediators that integrate fatty acid and carbohydrate metabolism in the liver with the energetic needs of other tissues. Nonalcoholic hepatocellular steatosis that occurs in the metabolic syndrome and type II diabetes are commonly associated with insulin resistance, i.e., a decreased capacity to respond to changes in circulating insulin, in multiple target tissues of insulin, not only the liver, but also in muscle, and adipose tissue. The factors that cause insulin resistance remain debated, but there is strong evidence that stress responses mediated by free fatty acid accumulation or ER stress result in activation of stress response protein kinases, including protein kinase C or JNK, which affect the intracellular signaling pathways through which insulin exerts its effects. Interestingly, although nonalcoholic fatty liver disease (NAFLD) is commonly characterized by insulin resistance, there is little evidence that insulin resistance is a common feature of the alcoholic fatty liver. Thus, despite many histological and functional similarities between the two conditions, the underlying profile of cellular changes that result in fatty liver is distinct.

In addition to these factors, there is ample evidence to suggest that hepatic steatosis is at least in part affected by the balance of pro- and anti-inflammatory cytokines that are released in the liver. Ethanol consumption affects both the release of these cytokines and the response of liver cells to these cytokines. These factors are also thought to contribute to the onset of alcoholic steatohepatitis.

Alcoholic Steatohepatitis

As described earlier, hepatocellular steatosis represents a common severe stress condition for the liver that is reflected in increased oxidative stress, endoplasmic reticular stress, and metabolic stress. Despite their different etiologies, alcoholic and NAFLD share many of these features. However, the mechanisms by which such stress conditions, at some point can lead to a more severe inflammatory condition remain only partly understood. In the case of alcoholic hepatocellular steatosis, several mechanisms have been identified by which alcohol consumption promotes inflammation. First among these is the increased intestinal wall permeability that can result from chronic alcohol consumption, allowing an increased circulating level of endotoxin and other bacteria-derived pro-inflammatory factors. Accumulation of high levels of acetaldehyde in the intestines caused by ethanol oxidation by the intestinal flora may contribute to this increased permeation. Endotoxin acts on toll-like receptor-4 (TLR4) in Kupffer cells and other resident cell types in the liver and activate these to promote activation of NADPH oxidase, resulting in the formation of superoxide and other reactive oxygen and nitrogen species and enhancing the oxidative stress environment in the liver. Activation of Kupffer cells also promotes the formation of the pro-inflammatory cytokine TNF-α. Furthermore, ethanol directly simulates the formation of TNF-α in activated Kupffer cells by enhancing its transcription and secretion. Early studies on animal models of alcoholic steatohepatitis demonstrated that TNF-α makes an important contribution to the pro-inflammatory environment in the liver through several mechanisms and alcohol-induced liver damage in experimental animal models could be suppressed by neutralizing TNF-α antibodies or TNF-receptor type 1 (TNFR1) knockout [24]. Additionally, ethanol consumption contributes to liver injury by suppressing survival signaling pathways and oxidative stress defense mechanisms in liver parenchymal cells that further exacerbate the damaging impact of elevated TNF-α levels and other cytokines. Increased cell death by necrosis or apoptosis sets in motion further pro-inflammatory responses in the tissue, resulting in the production of cytokines and chemokines that help mobilize neutrophils and other inflammatory cells that enhance tissue damage. Ethanol consumption further exacerbates the pro-inflammatory environment by suppressing the formation of protective cytokines, such as IL-10 and IL-4. Thus, the tissue response to control damage is impaired by a combination of extracellular mediators that promote inflammatory conditions and a suppression of intracellular survival signals that would normally contain their impact, resulting in progressive liver injury.

Fibrosis and Cirrhosis

Fibrosis is a common response of the liver to a chronic inflammatory condition. A critical (though not exclusive) role in fibrogenesis is played by HSC, which are in a quiescent state in the normal liver, but can be activated directly or indirectly in response to apoptotic or necrotic cell death. The program of cytokines released in the tissue as a result of injury further contributes to HSC activation resulting in the expression of a myofibroblast phenotype and stimulating the expression of extracellular matrix proteins, in particular collagen Type 1, which are not normally expressed in the liver. Under conditions of an acute tissue injury, the deposition of collagen fibers is a wound healing response that is transient and is followed by fibrinolysis mediated by metalloproteases that are activated as damaged tissue is replaced by newly generated liver cells resulting from the regenerative response. A continuing program of tissue damage and repair after chronic inflammation, accompanied by an imbalance in the normal liver repair mechanisms results in the excessive deposition of collagen fibers. In the absence of normal resolution of fibrosis, a gradual cross-linking and irreversible modification of collagen fibers occurs that can result in further impairment of normal liver function and lead to irreversible cirrhosis.

Chronic ethanol consumption can influence this program at multiple levels. First, ethanol consumption enhances the pro-inflammatory environment in the liver through several complementary mechanisms, including stimulating the release of pro-inflammatory cytokines by macrophages and decreasing the activity of protective cell types, including NK cells. Second, ethanol treatment enhances hepatocyte apoptosis and necrosis in response to other damaging conditions, both by the oxidative stress environment that commonly accompanies chronic ethanol exposure and by the shift in stress defense signaling pathways. Third, chronic ethanol treatment suppresses the regenerative response to tissue damage that is an essential component of the liver's repair mechanism and thereby facilitates the deposition of scar tissue that is the hallmark of fibrosis. This is probably accompanied by a suppression of metalloproteases, e.g., by the activation of inhibitor proteins, such as plasminogen activator inhibitor-1 (PAI-1), which normally would maintain the balance of ECM deposition and resolution to facilitate tissue repair. There is evidence that PAI-1 activation is associated with alcoholic liver injury, although its role is probably not restricted to the fibrotic stage [25]. In addition, there has been considerable evidence that ethanol directly affects the condition of HSC and promotes their activation and collagen formation. Although in the intact tissue it is difficult to distinguish direct effects of ethanol from the indirect contributions on the HSC response in a shifting cytokine balance, studies on isolated HSC have demonstrated that ethanol affects the response to TGF-β and IFN-γ, through effects on the intracellular signaling pathways or consequences of changes in the oxidative stress response, or through transcriptional effects of ethanol metabolites, such as acetaldehyde.

In the face of these multiple challenges brought about by chronic ethanol consumption to the normal repair response of the liver, it is all the more remarkable that the development of fibrosis and cirrhosis remains a relatively uncommon consequence of even long-term heavy drinking. In fact, much of the mechanistic insight into the actions of ethanol has resulted from studies on animal models, particularly rodents, who do not normally develop fibrosis or cirrhosis with ethanol consumption alone. Thus, it is common to consider that the onset of fibrosis and cirrhosis is often a reflection of comorbidity in which chronic ethanol consumption enhances disease patterns caused by other conditions.

Comorbid Factors

Chronic alcohol consumption accelerates progression of liver diseases in the presence of comorbid factors such as hepatitis C virus (HCV) or HBV and/or HIV infection, and NAFLD. A greater understanding of the interaction between alcohol and these comorbid factors on liver injury may help us design better therapies to treat chronic liver disease.

Alcohol and HCV Infection

Worldwide, about 170 million people are chronically infected with HCV, which is highly pronounced among alcoholic patients. In the United States, the reported prevalence of anti-HCV antibody in the general population is 1.8%, and for a subgroup of alcohol drinkers, the prevalence is much higher, ranging from 18.3 to 32.8% [26–28]. A significantly higher rate of HCV infection in alcoholics has also been reported in other countries, including Spain, Sweden, Germany, Israel, Japan, etc. [29–31]. While the principal cause of HCV infection in alcoholics is intravenous drug use, other causes are additionally responsible, as HCV infection remains particularly high even in those alcoholics without a history of intravenous drug use or blood transfusion.

The synergistic effects of HCV infection and alcohol consumption on the progression of liver diseases have been well documented by numerous studies conducted in many countries [29–31]. These studies have shown that the combination of alcohol abuse and HCV infection is associated with more severe liver fibrosis, greater risk of cirrhosis and HCC, hospitalizations at younger ages, and an increased risk of death compared with HCV infection or alcohol consumption separately [29–32]. Furthermore, standard antiviral therapy with IFN-α is reportedly less effective in alcoholics with HCV infection, thereby making treatment very difficult for these patients [33]. In clinical practice, HCV patients are asked to refrain from alcohol consumption while receiving treatment with IFN-α. However, it has been observed that despite a 6-month period of abstinence from alcohol, treatment efficacy with IFN-α was not improved in alcoholic patients [34].

The accumulating evidence suggests that multiple mechanisms may contribute to the synergistic effects of HCV and alcohol on the progression of liver diseases [29–32]. These include findings that show (1) ethanol inhibits innate immunity and viral acquired virus-specific immunity; (2) ethanol enhances HCV viral replication; (3) ethanol and HCV proteins synergistically induce production of ROS and nitrogen species; (4) ethanol potentiates HCV protein-activated inflammatory signals; [35] (5) ethanol inhibits the antifibrotic effects of natural killer cells/IFN-γ, thereby accelerating liver fibrosis in HCV patients [36].

Alcohol and HBV Infection

There are approximately more than 400 million HBV carriers worldwide. Most are found in Southeast Asia, China, the Pacific Islands, sub-Saharan Africa, and Alaska, affecting 10–20% of the general population for these geographical regions. Ranging between 3 and 5%, the level of HBV infection is intermediate within the Mediterranean basin, Eastern Europe, Central Asia, Japan, South America, and the Middle East [31]. The lowest prevalence of HBV infection at 0.1–2% is found in the United States, Canada, Western Europe, Australia, and New Zealand. Regardless of regional predominance, however, HBV infection is highly prevalent in alcoholics, affecting up to 55% of this subgroup of infected patients [31]. Although the heightened pervasiveness of HBV infection in alcoholic populations has been well documented, the reason for this has not been explored. One important factor contributing to the prevalent nature of HBV infection in alcoholic patients may be due to diminished innate and acquired immunity associated with long-term consumption of large amounts of ethanol.

The majority of HBV carriers (50–70%) do not show symptoms of viral infection or liver injury. However, several studies have shown that chronic asymptomatic HBV carriers are more susceptible to alcohol-induced liver injury, and that drinking alcohol may promote development of cirrhosis [31]. Nomura et al. [37] examined liver samples from 932 HBsAg carriers and 1,704 HBsAg-negative individuals in Japan.

The highest concentration of liver abnormalities was found in HBsAg-positive heavy drinkers (53.8%), followed by HBsAg-positive light drinkers and nondrinkers. Additionally, Ohnishi et al. [38] found that the average age at which cirrhosis developed in HBsAg-positive alcoholics was 38.8 years, which is 10.5 years earlier than HBsAg-positive nondrinkers, and 9.1 years younger than HBsAg-negative alcoholics.

Worldwide, HBV infection and alcohol consumption are two major risk factors resulting in the development of HCC. These two risk factors together have been shown to synergistically promote development of HCC [31]. Ohnishi et al. [38] observed that the average age at which HCC developed in nondrinkers infected with HBV was 57 years, but in HBV-infected alcoholic patients, HCC developed earlier at the average age of 48.9 years. Moreover, Yamanaka et al. [39] reported in alcoholic cirrhotic patients uninfected with HBV, the cumulative incidence of HCC at follow-up 5 and 10 years later was 7% and 15%, respectively. In comparison, 20% and 50% of the group of alcoholic cirrhotic patients with HBV or HCV infection showed evidence of HCC for each respective time point. The synergism produced by alcohol consumption and hepatitis infection on development of HCC may be attributed most simply to the active promotion of cirrhosis by these two factors, especially as cirrhosis is recognized as a major contributor to HCC development. However, other pathways, including alcohol-mediated immunosuppression may also promote development of HCC in HBV-infected patients [31].

Alcohol and HIV Infection/AIDS

An estimated 40 million people worldwide are infected with HIV; many of whom are alcoholics co-infected with HCV. Roughly 50% of HIV infected patients in the United States are alcoholics, and another 15–30% of these patients are infected with HCV [40, 41]. Alcohol consumption combined with HIV and HCV infection synergistically accelerate the progression of chronic liver disease, which has now become the second leading cause of death in AIDS patients [42, 43]. In addition, alcohol consumption reportedly reduces the efficacy of highly active antiretroviral therapy in HIV-infected patients and accelerates the hepatotoxicity of anti-HIV drugs [44]. This effect by alcohol is likely due to induction of cytochrome P450 expression, and subsequently, the acceleration of antiretroviral drug metabolism and generation of ROS.

Alcohol and Nonalcoholic Fatty Liver Disease/Obesity

In recent years, NAFLD has become another major cause of chronic liver disease due to an epidemic of obesity in Western countries. It is widely understood that moderate to heavy alcohol consumption potentiates liver injury and accelerates chronic liver disease progression in patients with NAFLD [45, 46]. Both Alatao et al. [45] and Ruhl et al. [46] recently reported that even moderate consumption of alcohol can significantly increase the risk of elevated serum levels of ALT liver enzymes in overweight and obese people. The observed synergistic effect on liver injury may be partially explained by the added effects of alcohol on obesity-induced mitochondrial dysfunction and oxidative stress. In contrast, one recent study showed that modest drinking of wine is associated with decreased prevalence of suspected NAFLD, implying that wine may exert beneficial effects in NAFLD [47]. The protective effects of modest wine drinking on NAFLD may be mediated by the polyphenol found in wine, resveratrol, which has been shown to reduce steatosis and improve insulin resistance and dyslipidemia [48].

Treatment

Abstinence and Nutritional Support

Abstinence and nutritional support are the first steps towards treating all forms of ALD. Abstinence can completely reverse alcoholic fatty liver, and it has been shown to yield beneficial effects in alcoholic hepatitis and cirrhosis [49]. Malnourishment is always associated with alcoholic patients, and therefore, nutritional support therapy is essential in the management of ALD.

Corticosteroids

Historically, corticosteroids were used to treat alcoholic hepatitis due to its broad anti-inflammatory effects. Corticosteroids have been shown to improve the short-term survival of selected patients with severe alcoholic hepatitis (as defined by Maddrey's discriminant function ≥32, and/or hepatic encephalopathy). Recent studies have attempted to uncover criteria that can be used to identify patients who may not benefit from corticosteroid treatment, also referred to as corticosteroid nonresponders. These include patients without early change in bilirubin levels (ECBL), who are patients that can be described as those with bilirubin levels scores lower on day 7 of treatment compared with day 1 [50], and with Lille scores ≥0.45 [51]. Treatment with corticosteroids is also not recommended for alcoholic hepatitis patients with active gastrointestinal bleeding, infection, and renal failure.

Anti-TNF-α Therapy

Studies using rodent models suggest that TNF-α plays an important role in alcohol-induced liver injury. These findings have led to human clinical investigations into the effects of several anti-TNF-α drugs for the treatment of alcoholic hepatitis. Drugs currently under study include pentoxifylline, infliximab, and etanercept. Pentoxifylline is a nonselective phosphodiesterase inhibitor that blocks synthesis of TNF-α. Treatment with pentoxifylline for 28 days has been shown to significantly improve survival in patients with severe alcoholic hepatitis (Maddrey's DF ≥32); however, the beneficial effects of pentoxifylline is likely attributed to a decreased risk in hepatorenal syndrome development and is unrelated to reductions in TNF-α [52]. Infliximab is a TNF-α antibody that binds soluble TNF in a stable complex. Two studies have reported that treatment with infliximab alone or infliximab plus prednisone significantly decreased Maddrey scores in patients with alcoholic hepatitis [53, 54], while a small French, multiple-dose, clinical trial has shown that treatment with high-dose infliximab plus prednisone caused more deaths and a higher incidence of infection [55]. Etanercept is a p-75-soluble TNF-α receptor that binds and neutralizes soluble TNF-α. Results from an early clinical trial have shown that etanercept treatment is associated with excellent short-term survival and decreased Maddrey scores in patients with moderate to severe alcoholic hepatitis [56]. However, a more recent trial showed that etanercept treatment is associated with a significantly higher 6-month mortality rate in patients with moderate to severe alcoholic hepatitis [57]. Thus, more studies are needed to clarify the therapeutic potential of anti-TNF-α therapy in alcoholic hepatitis.

Antioxidants

Accumulating evidence suggests that oxidative stress is a key mechanism contributing to alcoholic liver injury. Many antioxidants have been shown to effectively prevent and ameliorate alcoholic liver injury in rodent models. However, results from clinical trials using these antioxidants to treat patients with ALD have been mixed [58]. The antioxidants studied in clinical trials for ALD include SAMe, polyenylphosphatidyl-choline (PPC), silymarin, antioxidant vitamins, etc. The SAMe antioxidant functions by replenishing glutathione levels and serves as a methyl donor to maintain cell membrane fluidity. It was shown to reduce mortality and delay liver transplantation in patients with Child class A and B alcoholic cirrhosis [59]. Unfortunately, other trials failed to obtain findings that support the beneficial effect of SAMe treatment in ALD [60]. Unlike SAMe, PPC was not shown to exert any benefit in treating ALD [61]. Silymarin, an antioxidant component of the herb milk thistle, has been widely used by many patients with various types of liver disease. Results from clinical trials exploring silymarin as a therapy for alcoholic cirrhosis were inclusive. An early trial of silymarin on 91 patients with alcoholic cirrhosis revealed an increased 4-year survival in patients with Child class A cirrhosis [62], but a subsequent trial of 200 patients with alcoholic cirrhosis showed no survival benefit [63]. Several antioxidant vitamins such as vitamins A and E have been tested for the treatment of ALD, but results have been disappointing [64]. Treatment approaches for liver disease in alcoholics, patients with HCV or HIV infections are discussed in a recent article [65].

Liver Transplantation

Liver transplantation is currently the only curative treatment for patients with advanced alcoholic cirrhosis and is reserved for those patients that fail to recover after a period of alcohol abstinence. Patients that are candidates for surgery are required to abstain from alcohol for 6 months or longer before the surgery. The survival of patients with alcoholic cirrhosis after transplantation is comparable to patients with cirrhosis from other etiologies. Careful monitoring for relapse after transplantation is very important.

In summary, abstinence and nutritional support are essential in the management of all forms of ALD. Short-term treatment with corticosteroids may improve the survival of patients with severe acute alcoholic hepatitis, while long-term antioxidants may be useful in improving liver function and survival in patients with chronic ALD. Liver transplantation is an option of last resort to treat patients with end-stage alcoholic liver cirrhosis.

References

1. Zakhari S. Overview: how is alcohol metabolized by the body? Alcohol Research and Health. 2006;29:245–57.
2. Israel Y, Orrego H, Carmichael FJ. Acetate-mediated effects of ethanol. Alcohol Clin Exp Res. 1994;18:144–8.
3. Krebs HA, Veech RL. Regulation of the redox state of the pyridine nucleotides in rat liver. In: Sund H, editor. Pyridine nucleotide dependent dehydrogenase. New York: Springer; 1970. p. 439.
4. Smith ME, Newman HW. The rate of ethanol metabolism in fed and fasting animals. J Biol Chem. 1959;234:1544–9.
5. Rawat AK. Effects of ethanol infusion on the redox state and metabolite levels in rat liver in vivo. Eur J Biochem. 1968;6:585–92.
6. Gordon ER. The effect of chronic consumption of ethanol on the redox state of the rat liver. Can J Biochem. 1972;50:949–57.
7. Cunningham CC, Bailey SM. Ethanol consumption and liver mitochondria function. Biol Signals Recept. 2001;10:271–82.
8. Walther TC, Farese RV. The life of lipid droplets. Biochim Biophys Acta. 2009;1791:459–66.
9. Labbe G, Pessayre D, Fromenty B. Drug-induced liver injury through mitochondrial dysfunction: mechanisms and detection during preclinical safety studies. Fundam Clin Pharmacol. 2008;22:335–53.
10. Fernandez-Checa JC, Kaplowitz N. Hepatic mitochondrial glutathione: transport and role in disease and toxicity. Toxicol Appl Pharmacol. 2005;204:263–73.
11. You M, Matsumoto M, Pacold CM, Cho WK, Crabb DW. The role of AMPK-activated protein kinase in the action of ethanol on the liver. Gastroenterology. 2004;127:1798–808.
12. Canto C. Auwerx J PGC-1α, SIRT1 and AMPK: an energy-sensing network that controls energy expenditure. Curr Opin Lipidol. 2009;20:98–105.
13. Malhi H, Gores GJ. Molecular mechanisms of lipotoxicity in non-alcoholic fatty liver disease. Semin Liver Dis. 2008;28:360–9.
14. Purushotham A, Schug TT, Xu Q, Surapureddi S, Guo X, Li X. Hepatocyte-specific deletion of SIRT1 alters fatty acid metabolism and results in hepatic steatosis and inflammation. Cell Metab. 2009;9:327–38.
15. Ajmo JM, Liang X, Rogers CQ, Pennock B, You M. Resveratrol alleviates alcoholic fatty liver in mice. Am J Physiol Gastrointest Liver Physiol. 2008;295:G833–842.
16. Park PH, Lim RW, Shukla SD. Involvement of histone acetyltransferase (HAT) in ethanol-induced acetylation of histone H3 in hepatocytes: potential mechanisms for gene expression. Am J Physiol Gastrointest Liver Physiol. 2005;289:G1124–1136.
17. Shepard BD, Tuma PL. Alcohol-induced protein hyperacetylation: mechanisms and consequences. World J Gastroenterol. 2009;15:1219–30.
18. Holmuhamedov E, Lemasters JJ. Ethanol exposure decreases mitochondrial outer membrane permeability in cultured rat hepatocytes. Arch Biochem Biophys. 2009;481:226–33.
19. Hoek JB, Cahill A, Pastorino JG. Alcohol and mitochondria: a dysfunctional relationship. Gastroenterology. 2002;122:2049–63.
20. Kaplowitz N, Than TA, Shinohara M, Ji C. Endoplasmic reticulum stress and liver injury. Semin Liver Dis. 2007;27:367–77.
21. You M, Liang X, Ajmo JM, Ness GC. Involvement of mammalian sirtuin 1 in the action of ethanol in the liver. Am J Physiol Gastrointest Liver Physiol. 2008;294:G8920898.
22. You M, Considine RV, Leone TC, Kelly DP, Crabb DW. Role of adiponectin in the protective action of dietary saturated fat against alcoholic fatty liver in mice. Hepatology. 2005;42:568–77.
23. Adachi M, Ishii H. Hyperadiponectinemia in alcoholic liver disease: friend or foe? J Gastroenterol Hepatol. 2009;24:507–8.
24. Thurman RG. Alcoholic liver injury involves activation of Kupffer cells by endotoxin. Am J Physiol. 1998;275:G605–11.
25. Arteel GE. New role of plasminogen activators inhibitor-1 in alcohol-induced liver injury. J Gastroenterol Hepatol. 2008;23 Suppl 1:S54–9.
26. Mendenhall CL, Seeff L, Diehl AM, Ghosn SJ, French SW, Gartside PS, et al. Antibodies to hepatitis B virus and hepatitis C virus in alcoholic hepatitis and cirrhosis: their prevalence and clinical relevance. The VA Cooperative Study Group (No. 119). Hepatology. 1991;14:581–9.
27. Mendenhall CL, Moritz T, Rouster S, Roselle G, Polito A, Quan S, et al. Epidemiology of hepatitis C among veterans with alcoholic liver disease. The VA Cooperative Study Group 275. Am J Gastroenterol. 1993;88:1022–6.
28. Fong TL, Kanel GC, Conrad A, Valinluck B, Charboneau F, Adkins RH. Clinical significance of concomitant hepatitis C infection in patients with alcoholic liver disease. Hepatology. 1994;19:554–7.
29. Bhattacharya R, Shuhart MC. Hepatitis C and alcohol: interactions, outcomes, and implications. J Clin Gastroenterol. 2003;36:242–52.
30. Schiff ER. Hepatitis C and alcohol. Hepatology. 1997;26:39S–42S.
31. Gao B. Alcohol and hepatitis virus interactions in liver pathology, Comprehensive handbook of alcohol related pathology, vol. 2. 2005. p. 819–32.
32. Peters MG, Terrault NA. Alcohol use and hepatitis C. Hepatology. 2002;36:S220–225.
33. Ohnishi K, Matsuo S, Matsutani K, Itahashi M, Kakihara K, Suzuki K, et al. Interferon therapy for chronic hepatitis C in habitual drinkers: comparison with chronic hepatitis C in infrequent drinkers. Am J Gastroenterol. 1996;91:1374–9.
34. Tabone M, Sidoli L, Laudi C, Pellegrino S, Rocca G, Della Monica P, et al. Alcohol abstinence does not offset the strong negative effect

of lifetime alcohol consumption on the outcome of interferon therapy. J Viral Hepat. 2002;9:288–94.

35. Kim WH, Hong F, Jaruga B, Hu Z, Fan S, Liang TJ, et al. Additive activation of hepatic NF-kappaB by ethanol and hepatitis B protein X (HBX) or HCV core protein: involvement of TNF-alpha receptor 1-independent and -dependent mechanisms. FASEB J. 2001;15:2551–3.

36. Jeong WI, Park O, Gao B. Abrogation of the antifibrotic effects of natural killer cells/interferon-gamma contributes to alcohol acceleration of liver fibrosis. Gastroenterology. 2008;134:248–58.

37. Nomura H, Kashiwagi S, Hayashi J, Kajiyama W, Ikematsu H, Noguchi A, et al. An epidemiologic study of effects of alcohol in the liver in hepatitis B surface antigen carriers. Am J Epidemiol. 1988;128:277–84.

38. Ohnishi K, Iida S, Iwama S, Goto N, Nomura F, Takashi M, et al. The effect of chronic habitual alcohol intake on the development of liver cirrhosis and hepatocellular carcinoma: relation to hepatitis B surface antigen carriage. Cancer. 1982;49:672–7.

39. Yamanaka T, Shiraki K, Nakazaawa S, Okano H, Ito T, Deguchi M, et al. Impact of hepatitis B and C virus infection on the clinical prognosis of alcoholic liver cirrhosis. Anticancer Res. 2001;21:2937–40.

40. Galvan FH, Bing EG, Fleishman JA, London AS, Caetano R, Burnam MA, et al. The prevalence of alcohol consumption and heavy drinking among people with HIV in the United States: results from the HIV Cost and Services Utilization Study. J Stud Alcohol. 2002;63:179–86.

41. Cheng DM, Nunes D, Libman H, Vidaver J, Alperen JK, Saitz R, et al. Impact of hepatitis C on HIV progression in adults with alcohol problems. Alcohol Clin Exp Res. 2007;31:829–36.

42. Weber R, Sabin CA, Friis-Moller N, Reiss P, El-Sadr WM, Kirk O, et al. Liver-related deaths in persons infected with the human immunodeficiency virus: the D:A:D study. Arch Intern Med. 2006;166:1632–41.

43. Soto B, Sanchez-Quijano A, Rodrigo L, del Olmo JA, Garcia-Bengoechea M, Hernandez-Quero J, et al. Human immunodeficiency virus infection modifies the natural history of chronic parenterally-acquired hepatitis C with an unusually rapid progression to cirrhosis. J Hepatol. 1997;26:1–5.

44. Inductivo-Yu I, Bonacini M. Highly active antiretroviral therapy-induced liver injury. Curr Drug Saf. 2008;3:4–13.

45. Alatalo PI, Koivisto HM, Hietala JP, Puukka KS, Bloigu R, Niemela OJ. Effect of moderate alcohol consumption on liver enzymes increases with increasing body mass index. Am J Clin Nutr. 2008;88:1097–103.

46. Ruhl CE, Everhart JE. Joint effects of body weight and alcohol on elevated serum alanine aminotransferase in the United States population. Clin Gastroenterol Hepatol. 2005;3:1260–8.

47. Dunn W, Xu R, Schwimmer JB. Modest wine drinking and decreased prevalence of suspected nonalcoholic fatty liver disease. Hepatology. 2008;47:1947–54.

48. Baur JA, Pearson KJ, Price NL, Jamieson HA, Lerin C, Kalra A, et al. Resveratrol improves health and survival of mice on a high-calorie diet. Nature. 2006;444:337–42.

49. Pessione F, Ramond MJ, Peters L, Pham BN, Batel P, Rueff B, et al. Five-year survival predictive factors in patients with excessive alcohol intake and cirrhosis. Effect of alcoholic hepatitis, smoking and abstinence. Liver Int. 2003;23:45–53.

50. Mathurin P, Abdelnour M, Ramond MJ, Carbonell N, Fartoux L, Serfaty L, et al. Early change in bilirubin levels is an important prognostic factor in severe alcoholic hepatitis treated with prednisolone. Hepatology. 2003;38:1363–9.

51. Louvet A, Naveau S, Abdelnour M, Ramond MJ, Diaz E, Fartoux L, et al. The Lille model: a new tool for therapeutic strategy in patients with severe alcoholic hepatitis treated with steroids. Hepatology. 2007;45:1348–54.

52. Akriviadis E, Botla R, Briggs W, Han S, Reynolds T, Shakil O. Pentoxifylline improves short-term survival in severe acute alcoholic hepatitis: a double-blind, placebo-controlled trial. Gastroenterology. 2000;119:1637–48.

53. Tilg H, Jalan R, Kaser A, Davies NA, Offner FA, Hodges SJ, et al. Anti-tumor necrosis factor-alpha monoclonal antibody therapy in severe alcoholic hepatitis. J Hepatol. 2003;38:419–25.

54. Spahr L, Rubbia-Brandt L, Frossard JL, Giostra E, Rougemont AL, Pugin J, et al. Combination of steroids with infliximab or placebo in severe alcoholic hepatitis: a randomized controlled pilot study. J Hepatol. 2002;37:448–55.

55. Naveau S, Chollet-Martin S, Dharancy S, Mathurin P, Jouet P, Piquet MA, et al. A double-blind randomized controlled trial of infliximab associated with prednisolone in acute alcoholic hepatitis. Hepatology. 2004;39:1390–7.

56. Menon KV, Stadheim L, Kamath PS, Wiesner RH, Gores GJ, Peine CJ, et al. A pilot study of the safety and tolerability of etanercept in patients with alcoholic hepatitis. Am J Gastroenterol. 2004;99:255–60.

57. Boetticher NC, Peine CJ, Kwo P, Abrams GA, Patel T, Aqel B, Boardman L, Gores GJ, Harmsen WS, McClain CJ, Kamath PS, Shah VH. A randomized, double-blinded, placebo-controlled multicenter trial of etanercept in the treatment of alcoholic hepatitis. Gastroenterology. 2008;135(6):1953–60.

58. Lu SC. Antioxidants in the treatment of chronic liver diseases: why is the efficacy evidence so weak in humans? Hepatology. 2008;48:1359–61.

59. Mato JM, Camara J, Fernandez de Paz J, Caballeria L, Coll S, Caballero A, et al. S-adenosylmethionine in alcoholic liver cirrhosis: a randomized, placebo-controlled, double-blind, multicenter clinical trial. J Hepatol. 1999;30:1081–9.

60. Rambaldi A, Gluud C. S-adenosyl-L-methionine for alcoholic liver diseases. Cochrane Database Syst Rev 2006;CD002235

61. Lieber CS, Weiss DG, Groszmann R, Paronetto F, Schenker S. II. Veterans Affairs Cooperative Study of polyenylphosphatidylcholine in alcoholic liver disease. Alcohol Clin Exp Res. 2003;27:1765–72.

62. Ferenci P, Dragosics B, Dittrich H, Frank H, Benda L, Lochs H, et al. Randomized controlled trial of silymarin treatment in patients with cirrhosis of the liver. J Hepatol. 1989;9:105–13.

63. Pares A, Planas R, Torres M, Caballeria J, Viver JM, Acero D, et al. Effects of silymarin in alcoholic patients with cirrhosis of the liver: results of a controlled, double-blind, randomized and multicenter trial. J Hepatol. 1998;28:615–21.

64. Mezey E, Potter JJ, Rennie-Tankersley L, Caballeria J, Pares A. A randomized placebo controlled trial of vitamin E for alcoholic hepatitis. J Hepatol. 2004;40:40–6.

65. Zakhari S, LI T-K. Determinants of alcohol use and abuse: impact of quantity and frequency patterns on liver disease. Hepatology. 2007;46:2032–9.

66. Hurley TD, et al. Pharmacogenomics of alcoholism. In: Licinio J, Wong ML, editors. Pharmacogenomics—the search for individualized therapies. Weinheim: Wiley-VCH; 2002. p. 417–41.

Hyperkinetic Movement Disorders

34

Christopher Hess and Rachel Saunders-Pullman

Abstract

The relationship between movement disorders and substance abuse can be examined from two approaches: first, assessment of the movements which occur secondary to substance abuse, and second, review of the movement disorders that might increase the propensity for substance abuse. This chapter will first address the myriad of hyperkinetic movements that can be seen in drug abusers, followed by a discussion of alcohol and two movement disorders (myoclonus-dystonia and essential tremor) in which patients may be at increased risk of alcohol abuse and dependence due to self-treatment of the disorders with alcohol. Hyperkinetic movement disorders include tremor, myoclonus, dystonia, chorea, athetosis, tics, akathisia, and stereotypies. Amphetamines have been associated with dystonia, chorea, tics, and tremors, and may exacerbate underlying movement disorders. In addition to worsening pre-existing movements, cocaine may cause tics, dystonia, chorea, myoclonus, and tremor. Movements associated with opioid use usually occur in the setting of medically ill patients, and include myoclonus and chorea. Alcohol, in contrast, may dampen some hyperkinetic movement disorders, and people with essential tremor and myoclonus-dystonia may use alcohol to self-treat symptoms. In some situations this has led to abuse which has been more damaging to the lives of the affected individuals than the underlying movement disorders.

Learning Objectives
- Familiarization with the major categories of hyperkinetic movement disorders.
- Understanding that substances of abuse can produce transient disorders of movement during both use and withdrawal, and review of the types of movements they induce.

- Awareness that the disabling symptoms of some movement disorders, especially essential tremor and myoclonus-dystonia, may be reduced with alcohol ingestion, and this may increase the risk of alcohol misuse.

C. Hess, M.D. (✉)
Department of Neurology, Columbia University College
of Physicians and Surgeons, New York, NY 10032, USA
e-mail: ch2553@mail.cumc.columbia.edu

R. Saunders-Pullman, M.D., M.P.H.
Department of Neurology, Beth Israel Medical Center, New York,
NY 10003, USA

Department of Neurology, Albert Einstein College of Medicine,
Bronx, NY 10461, USA

Disorders of movement can be classified as those that are characterized by a paucity of movement (hypokinesias, which are primarily parkinsonian in nature) or a relative excess of movement (hyperkinesias) [1]. Movement disorders arise from perturbation of basal ganglia and cerebellar circuitry, and as such the dopaminergic, cholinergic, and glutamatergic systems may be affected. Hypokinetic and hyperkinetic movement disorders secondary to drugs of abuse are well described; however, our understanding of the clinical characteristics of these movements remains limited by the nature of drug abuse and the attributes and lifestyles of the abusers. Illegal substances of abuse often contain potentially neurotoxic impurities and can be contaminated by other drugs of abuse or toxic substances, which also may cause movement disorders (such as the "cutting" of cocaine with amphetamines). This is most vividly illustrated by the cases of parkinsonism induced by 1-methyl-4-phenyl-1,2,3,6-tetrahydropyridine (MPTP). This byproduct was created in the synthetic manufacture of the heroin analog 4'-methyl-alpha-pyrrolidinopropiophenone (MPPP) in a Northern California lab, and produced severe parkinsonism in a cluster of addicts using the substance. This led to the discovery of MPTP as one of the leading primate models of parkinsonism [2]. Abusers of street drugs may also not report side effects, may have difficulty giving accurate histories, often abuse multiple substances, and are frequently lost to follow-up. The descriptions of drug-induced movement disorders are thus based on case reports limited by these factors, and as such it is expected that the literature will continue to expand. This chapter will focus on the hyperkinetic movement disorders.

Types of Hyperkinesias

The major categories of hyperkinesias are reviewed below. While not all-encompassing, the major forms of hyperkinetic movement disorders are discussed [1].

Tremor

Tremor can be defined as an oscillatory rhythmic movement around a joint. Tremors can occur at rest or with movements. Parkinsonian tremor is typically 4–6 Hz and occurs in the arm or leg when one is seated and the limb is at rest or in the arm during walking. In contrast, essential tremor is a faster tremor, usually 6–10 Hz, and occurs with action such as eating or drinking. As the causes of tremor are varied, the pathophysiology of tremor is specific to etiology.

Myoclonus

Myoclonus is a sudden, brief jerk that can be due to active muscle contraction or sudden loss of postural tone (asterixis or negative myoclonus). It can be rhythmic or irregular and sometimes triggered by sensory stimuli. Unlike tics, it cannot be suppressed by conscious effort. Myoclonus can be cortical, subcortical, brainstem, or spinal in origin. As in tremor, the pathologic causes of myoclonic jerks are specific to etiology. It is seen in a number of primary neurologic

diseases, such as myoclonus-dystonia discussed later, as well as various metabolic derangements, including hepatic or uremic encephalopathy.

Dystonia

Dystonia is a syndrome of sustained muscle contractions involving both agonist and antagonist muscles, often producing torsional and repetitive movements that result in sustained abnormal twisting and postures. It may affect only one body region (e.g. the neck in cervical dystonia) or many body regions (e.g. both legs, trunk, and arms in early onset dystonia). It may be task specific, occurring with specific movements such as with walking or writing. When dystonia is the only neurologic feature other than tremor and there are no neuroimaging abnormalities or known toxic or metabolic etiologies, it is referred to as primary. The acute dystonic reactions sometimes associated with dopamine-blocking medications are examples of secondary dystonia. Impaired or abnormal neuronal firing of the globus pallidus giving rise to release of inhibition on the thalamus and subsequent changes involving thalamocortical neurotransmission is thought to play a role in the pathogenesis of dystonia.

Chorea and Athetosis

Choreiform movements or choreas are quick irregular movements that are brief in duration and can often be partially suppressed or hidden within voluntary movements. They flow from one body part to another, and are randomly distributed in time and body anatomy. The pathophysiology of choreas is not well understood, but in general is thought to involve disruptions in the direct and indirect pathways from the striatum to the basal ganglia output nuclei [1, 3]. Chorea is one of the characteristic movements seen in Huntington disease. Athetosis is a slow form of chorea that is torsional in quality like dystonia, but is not repetitive or sustained and is without consistent directionality. It can often be seen in patients with cerebral palsy. The coexistence of chorea and the slower athetosis is termed choreoathetosis.

Tics, Akathisia, and Stereotypies

Tics are brief, abrupt stereotyped behaviors that can manifest as movements or vocalizations, as seen in Tourette syndrome. Akathisia is an uncomfortable sensation of inner restlessness that compels the individual to carry out movements that reduce or relieve discomfort. Like dystonic reactions, they are a known complication of neuroleptic treatment. Stereotypies, which are behaviors that occur continually and identically, are often reported in animal models as repetitive sniffing or grooming behaviors, and are often considered part of the clinical spectrum of tics in humans. In contrast to tics, they are more continuous and are usually not associated with an irresistible urge [1]. While stereotypies may also be due to neuroleptic use, they are usually associated with other brain diseases, such as autism, Rett syndrome, mental retardation, or schizophrenia.

Movement Disorders Secondary to Substances of Abuse

Amphetamines

Amphetamine is a general term for a collection of compounds that act as peripheral sympathomimetics and central stimulants and increase the synaptic activity of dopamine (DA), norepinephrine (NE), and serotonin (5-HT). It is believed that the dopaminergic effects of amphetamines are responsible for the dyskinesias associated with their use [4]. Amphetamines act to increase DA in the synaptic cleft by a number of mechanisms, including competition with DA for uptake by the presynaptic DA transporter (DAT), induction of reverse transport of DA through the DAT into the synaptic cleft, and modulation of vesicular monoamine transporters [5, 6].

Since the 1970s, stereotyped complex repetitive movements known as punding have been associated with cocaine and amphetamine abuse. Punders find it soothing or fascinating to engage in basic activities such as repetitive grooming or handling of external objects or parts of the body, or more complex activities such as lining up small objects or taking apart mechanical devices. It is also commonly seen in patients with Parkinson disease who are treated with DA agonists or levodopa, underlying the role of DA dysregulation in its pathogenesis. However, these complex volitional behaviors (though possibly pathophysiologically related) are considered to be a form of compulsive disorder and do not represent abnormal hyperkinetic movements [1, 7, 8].

A number of cases of true dyskinesias have been reported. Acutely intoxicated patients often present hypertensive, tachycardic, and tachypneic [9]. Neck dystonia, and writhing choreoathetoid movements can sometimes be seen in the head, neck, and face [9, 10]. Abnormal movements often resolve spontaneously, but treatment with neuroleptics has been noted to resolve dyskinesias [9, 11]. Some long-term users have reported abnormal movements continuing after periods of abstinence. A 27-year-old man with almost daily amphetamine use for the better part of 6 years developed bruxism and choreiform movements of the face, mouth, and limbs, as well as athetoid movements of the limbs and trunk. Symptoms were reported to be worse with acute exposure

but still present during abstinence, and once abstinence was sustained abnormal movements of the limbs continued for at least a year in the limbs and longer in the face and mouth. Another long-term abuser reported continuation of choreiform movements during a year of abstinence [12]. Amphetamine use has also been considered as a risk factor for dystonia in patients treated with newer atypical antipsychotics [13]. Other hyperkinetic movements that have been described with amphetamines include tics and tremors [4]. In addition, the dyskinesias seen in Huntington disease, Tourette syndrome, Sydenham chorea, and lupus can all be worsened or precipitated by amphetamine abuse [14].

Cocaine

Cocaine is a local anesthetic and a central nervous system stimulant that produces feelings of euphoria and excitement [4]. It acts primarily through its inhibition of DA reuptake and the release of DA from granular storage vesicles, thereby increasing the neuromodulatory effects of DA on other neurons [15]. Recent studies have suggested that in addition to acutely blocking DAT leading to increased synaptic DA, cocaine increases DAT cell surface expression, which may cause a decrease in synaptic DA after cocaine has been metabolized [5].

Cocaine abusers can develop worsening of existing movement disorders, and develop de novo abnormal movements secondary to cocaine. As with amphetamine users, cocaine abusers often present to the emergency room hypertensive, tachycardic, and tachypneic.

Abnormal movements associated with cocaine include tics, dystonia, choreoathetosis, myoclonus, opsoclonus-myoclonus, and tremor. As with amphetamines, more complex movements such as bruxisms and stereotypies, as well as obsessive and/or compulsive behaviors can also be seen [4].

Patients with Tourette syndrome who abuse cocaine have reported a worsening of motor and vocal tics lasting hours before a return to baseline [16]. Another report described Tourette patients with cocaine-induced sustained worsening of tics and re-emergence of symptoms in remission even after cocaine abstinence, though the course of time was not specified [17]. Cocaine-induced tics have also been reported in patients without a prior history of motor or vocal tics [18, 19]. In one case the movements continued over a 2-year period with continued chronic use [18]. Paradoxically, one cocaine abuser with stuttering and facial motor tics who reported relief of symptoms with cocaine use has been reported in the literature as well [20].

Dystonia secondary to cocaine use has been described in multiple case reports [21–25]. Symptoms most often involved the facial and neck muscles [21–25], but limb involvement was reported as well [22, 24]. Most instances of dystonia seemed to occur in chronic users, with users of either intranasal or inhaled cocaine developing symptoms between 6 h and 3 days prior to the onset of symptoms. Most patients were initially treated successfully with intravenous diphenhydramine, and re-emergence of symptoms was common [21, 23, 24] and treated either with a repeat dose of diphenhydramine or benzodiazepines. Only one patient in the above case reports had a known history of prior (but not recent) neuroleptic exposure [21]. Other reports have indicated that cocaine should be considered as a risk factor for the development of dystonia in patients treated with both typical [26–28] and atypical [29, 30] antipsychotics.

Choreoathetoid movements secondary to cocaine use are well known to both abusers and physicians, and have been referred to as "crack attacks" or "crack dancing" [31]. First reported in 1991, Daras and colleagues described a woman who chronically abused cocaine who presented with "continuous slow abnormal involuntary movements of the head" with "purposeless writhing and uncoordinated movements of all four extremities" and rapid jerk-like movements as well, which resolved within 3 days without medical intervention. Another patient with choreoathetosis and orobuccal dyskinesias experienced resolution of symptoms after haloperidol treatment [32]. Subsequent reports of cocaine associated choreoathetoid movements have described similar symptoms [33, 34], and more mild dyskinesias have been reported as well [35].

Opioids

Opioids include a large group of naturally occurring and synthetic compounds that, like morphine, act centrally on the brain and spinal cord as agonists at endogenous opioid receptors to exert an analgesic effect [36]. Opioid receptors are also present in the basal ganglia and may modulate dopaminergic transmission, and are known to be altered in movement disorders such as Parkinson disease [1]. As different endogenous opioids are present in the different signaling pathways of the basal ganglia, it is thought that opioids might disrupt the balance between the inhibitory and excitatory output upon the thalamus [37]. Throughout the literature, most reports of movement disorders secondary to opiates have been in medically ill patients who are often on multiple medications or patients undergoing anesthesia that may also contribute to abnormal movements. Opiates have been associated with a number of hyperkinetic movement disorders, including myoclonus associated with fentanyl [38] and morphine [39, 40], and akathisia attributed to morphine has also been reported [41, 42]. Patients treated with intrathecal morphine have developed myoclonus and hyperalgesia that resolved with a reduction in morphine dose, and

the activity of opioids and related metabolites at the spinal cord level have also been hypothesized as a possible etiology for opioid-related myoclonus [43, 44]. Myoclonus has been reported in medically ill patients treated with meperidine, but this is thought to be secondary to its neurotoxic metabolite normeperidine [45]. Methadone-associated myoclonus in medically ill patients treated with methadone has been well described [46–48], and choreiform movements have also been attributed to methadone [49–51]. In patients who develop myoclonus secondary to opiates, gabapentin and dantrolene have been used to reduce symptoms [44, 47]. The relative lack of reports in otherwise healthy opiate abusers could be related to the decreased likelihood of abusers to present for such symptoms. However, patients presenting with acute heroin overdose can awaken with tremor, rigidity, myoclonus, dystonia, and ballistic movements in the setting of cerebral ischemia [14].

Ecstasy

3,4-Methylenedioxymethamphetamine (MDMA), also most commonly known as ecstasy, binds to a number of receptors in the CNS, but its main effects of euphoria and increased empathy and energy are thought to be secondary to the release of 5-HT (and inhibition of its reuptake) and the release of DA and norepinephrine [52, 53].

Rigidity, trismus, and bruxism have been described by ecstasy users [54–56], and two cases of acute dystonic reaction have also been reported [57, 58]. Heavy (more than 100 occasions) users of MDMA have self-reported experiencing tremors or twitches that they associated with MDMA use while abstinent [59], and one individual has described involuntary arm movements in between doses [60]. However, in addition to the general problems in studying drug users previously discussed, evaluation of MDMA is further complicated by the wide variety of compounds sold as ecstasy. Tablets contain varying amounts (0–100%) of MDMA, with related compounds such as 3,4 methylenedioxyethylamphetamine (MDE) and combinations of other drugs (such as amphetamine, ketamine, ephedrine, and caffeine) sometimes comprising a significant portion of pills sold as ecstasy [61, 62]. In addition to hyperkinetic movements, considerable controversy has been generated regarding a possible role of ecstasy as both a cause of parkinsonism and a possible treatment for dyskinesias in Parkinson disease (PD) [63–66].

Cannabinoids

The major psychoactive agents in marijuana, hashish, and other preparations derived from the cannabis plant are the tetrahydrocannabinols (THC) [4]. Though jitteriness is often experienced, neither typical nor large doses are associated with any true hyperkinetic movement disorders (though there is a single report of longstanding propriospinal myoclonus attributed to first time cannabis use) [67]. However, cannabinoids have been reported to be of benefit or have been evaluated for use in the treatment of a number of movement disorders, including Tourette syndrome, dystonia, PD-related dyskinesias, Huntington disease, and Wilson disease [68–73].

Other Substances of Abuse

Abnormal hyperkinetic movements can also be seen with a number of other drugs of abuse. Withdrawal from sedative and anxiolytic drugs such as benzodiazepines, barbiturates, and γ-aminobutyric acid agonists such as zolpidem can result in tremor and myoclonus [4, 14, 74]. A single report of transient choreoathetoid movements attributed to phenobarbital overdose in the setting of chronic diazepam use has also been reported [75]. The N-methyl-D-aspartate (NMDA) receptor antagonist phencyclidine (PCP) can cause rigidity, tremors, localized dystonias, and rarely athetosis [76], and is known to modulate a number of other neurotransmitters, including DA and 5-HT [4]. The significantly weaker NMDA antagonist ketamine has been shown to produce dystonia and bradykinesia in non-human primates [77]. Abuse of inhalants such as ethyl chloride can result in tremor [78] and lead-containing gasoline inhalation has resulted in myoclonus and chorea [4]. Toluene abuse has been associated with opsoclonus and cerebellar ataxia [4], and a single case of transient choreoathetoid movements after toluene sniffing has been described [79].

Alcohol and its Abuse in Patients with Hyperkinetic Movement Disorders

In addition to drug abuse leading to abnormal hyperkinetic movements, the relationship movement disorders and substance abuse can be more complex; substances of abuse that ameliorate the symptoms of movement disorders have the potential for abuse by patients self-medicating their disease. This is exemplified by the effects of alcohol on essential tremor (ET) and myoclonus-dystonia (M-D), two hyperkinetic movement disorders in which the symptoms of the disease are dramatically reduced with alcohol administration.

At doses comparable to those encountered clinically, ethyl alcohol or ethanol modulates multiple neurotransmitters, including glutamate, GABA, 5-HT, DA, acetylcholine, and opioids [4]. Tremor is the most common hyperkinetic movement disorder associated with alcohol abuse. A mild tremor can occur during the "hangover" period in sporadic drinkers [14]. In alcohol dependent subjects, tremor is characterized by large but variable amplitude and a frequency of 6–11 Hz,

as well its postural predominance and aggravation with movement [80]. It occurs most commonly in the early withdrawal period and affects the hands most noticeably. Its pathophysiology is likely multifactorial and may be related to enhanced physiologic tremor [14, 80]. Though rare, other movement disorders can sometimes be seen in alcoholics. Parkinsonism has been described during abuse or withdrawal in older patients (over 50 years of age) and is self-limited [81–84]. A follow-up to one of these reports [81] more than 9 years later showed no clinical evidence of parkinsonism to suggest nigrostriatal degeneration [85]. Transient dyskinesias involving the face, neck, and arms have also been described in younger patients during withdrawal or heavy use of alcohol, notably in the absence of liver disease [86]. Dyskinesias that followed parkinsonism during withdrawal [84] and akathisia and dystonia during acute intoxication have also been reported [80]. The mechanism of such disorders are not known, though ethanol-induced decreases in striatal dopamine may be related to transient parkinsonism and dyskinesias may be secondary to alterations in dopamine receptor sensitivity [4, 84, 87]. Usually pharmacologic treatment is not indicated in alcoholic tremor and treatment consists primarily of abstinence, but occasionally beta-blockers or benzodiazepines are used in severe cases or during acute withdrawal. Chronic abuse of alcohol is known to result in hepatic dysfunction and associated asterixis, a 3 Hz resting tremor secondary to alcoholic cerebellar degeneration can sometimes be seen in long-term abusers [1].

Alcohol and Essential Tremor

ET is one of the most common adult movement disorders and is a common neurologic disease in elderly patients [88]. It is characterized by a 4–12 Hz progressive kinetic tremor (usually an action and/or postural tremor) that decreases in frequency over time and is most often present in the arms but may also involve the neck and voice [89, 90]. The degree of resulting impairment and social embarrassment varies greatly between patients, and ranges from mild to significant, particularly in activities which require hand dexterity and coordination. Recently, possible psychiatric and cognitive features are being examined as well [90]. As indicated by its name, ET was traditionally considered a benign condition without neuropathologic correlate [91, 92]. However, recent research has raised the question as to whether ET is a pathologically heterogeneous and progressive neurodegenerative disorder [92]. Both environmental and genetic factors appear to play a role in its pathogenesis, and it can be inherited in an autosomal dominant pattern or in a more complex manner with variable penetrance [90, 93]. The pathophysiology underlying the disease is thought to involve abnormal oscillatory activity in the neural pathways between the olivary nuclei, cerebellum, and thalamus [94–98]. The first line treatments for essential tremor are propranolol and primidone, though anticonvulsants and benzodiazepines are sometimes used. In severe cases thalamotomy or thalamic deep brain stimulation may be undertaken [99].

Improvement of the symptoms of ET with alcohol was first described in 1949, and in patients who are responsive to alcohol, it is may be more efficacious than available pharmacologic treatments [100, 101]. Alcohol reduces the amplitude but not the frequency of tremor, though tremor may temporarily worsen when the effects of alcohol have subsided [89, 102, 103]. As many as 50–90% of patients will have improvement of symptoms with alcohol, and one study showed homogeneity of response within families with familial ET [102]. The mechanism of action by which alcohol decreases the amplitude of tremor in ET is not clear, though various mechanisms have been proposed. These include normalization of the abnormal olivocerebellar firing patterns, blocking the development of abnormal oscillations or modulating calcium currents in the olivary nucleus, or modulating GABA neurotransmission or NMDA-mediated glutamatergic neurotransmission in the cerebellum [89, 104–107].

Self-treatment with alcohol has been of concern since its effects on ET were first noted, particularly since the effect of alcohol are transient and repeated doses are required to maintain a reduction in tremor amplitude [100, 108]. This combined with the often increasing doses required to achieve the same ameliorative effect suggests that patients with ET might be at higher risk of abusing alcohol, and indeed alcoholism in ET patients has been reported [100, 108]. While the first systematic records-based study in a population of veterans indicated that males with ET abuse alcohol at higher rates than age-matched controls [109], two subsequent cross-sectional studies failed to find any significant increase in alcohol intake in ET patients compared to controls [110, 111]. Though there are no true prospective studies that address the possibility of an increased risk of alcoholism in ET patients and social alcohol intake is not discouraged for most patients with ET, it is prudent for the clinician to evaluate patients with ET for personal or family histories excessive alcohol intake that might increase their risk for self-medication leading to abuse [112].

Alcohol and Myoclonus-Dystonia

M-D is a hyperkinetic movement disorder that is genetically heterogeneous but most commonly associated with mutations in the epsilon sarcoglycan (SGCE) gene on chromosome 7q21. It is inherited in an autosomal dominant manner and is maternally imprinted (symptoms are present primarily when the abnormal gene is inherited paternally) [113, 114]. The function of SCGE proteins is not known, but it is suspected that disrupted neuronal architecture and/or synaptic structure, possibly interfering with monoaminergic transmission, are responsible for the symptoms of M-D [114–116]. The motor symptoms of M-D consist of early onset myoclonus, often with dystonia. Myoclonus is usually the more prominent feature, although dystonia can sometimes predominant or occur alone. The myoclonus of M-D most often affects the neck and arms, and similar to ET, may impair motor tasks of the upper limbs and cause considerable social embarrassment [113]. In addition, psychiatric symptoms including obsessive-compulsive disorder are also associated with the SGCE mutation [114, 117–123].

A marked decrease in the motor symptoms of M-D has long been known to occur with ingestion of alcohol [124, 125]. This response has been well reported in many families with SGCE mutations, though heterogeneity of response exists both between and within families and response to alcohol is not predictive of SGCE mutation or specific to the genetic etiology of the disease. Among family members from SGCE or chromosome 7 linked M-D families described in the literature between 1988 and 2004 (and for which alcohol responsiveness of family members was clearly stated), 81% of individuals experienced a reduction of motor symptoms with alcohol. Among families without linkage or mutation to the SGCE gene, 74% were alcohol-responsive [112].

A recent study of five M-D families demonstrated an increase in alcohol dependence but not abuse in symptomatic manifesting carriers of the SGCE mutation when compared to non-manifesting carriers and non-carriers of the mutation, which was attributed to the use of alcohol to self-treat motor symptoms [120]. However, a later study did not find an increase in substance abuse in manifesting carriers of the disease [118]. As current treatment options for M-D (anti-epileptics and anticholinergics) are of limited utility, the risk for self-treatment with alcohol in a population with co-morbid psychiatric disease is of great concern, and the consequences of alcohol dependence in such patients may be more disabling than the motor symptoms of the disease [112]. As with ET, it is important for the clinician to be cognizant of the possibility of self-treatment leading to misuse, and inquire about individual risk factors and counsel patients accordingly.

References

1. Fahn S, Jankovic J. Principles and practice of movement disorders. Philadelphia: Churchill Livingstone/Elsevier; 2007.
2. Ballard PA, Tetrud JW, Langston JW. Permanent human parkinsonism due to 1-methyl-4-phenyl-1,2,3,6-tetrahydropyridine (MPTP): seven cases. Neurology. 1985;35:949–56.
3. Bhidayasiri R, Truong DD. Chorea and related disorders. Postgrad Med J. 2004;80:527–34.
4. Brust JCM. Neurological aspects of substance abuse. 2nd ed. Philadelphia, PA: Elsevier; 2004.

5. Kahlig KM, Galli A. Regulation of dopamine transporter function and plasma membrane expression by dopamine, amphetamine, and cocaine. Eur J Pharmacol. 2003;479:153–8.

6. Fleckenstein AE, Volz TJ, Riddle EL, Gibb JW, Hanson GR. New insights into the mechanism of action of amphetamines. Annu Rev Pharmacol Toxicol. 2007;47:681–98.

7. Fasano A, Barra A, Nicosia P, et al. Cocaine addiction: from habits to stereotypical-repetitive behaviors and punding. Drug Alcohol Depend. 2008;96:178–82.

8. Rylander G. Psychoses and the punding and choreiform syndromes in addiction to central stimulant drugs. Psychiatr Neurol Neurochir. 1972;75:203–12.

9. Rhee KJ, Albertson TE, Douglas JC. Choreoathetoid disorder associated with amphetamine-like drugs. Am J Emerg Med. 1988;6:131–3.

10. Sperling LS, Horowitz JL. Methamphetamine-induced choreoathetosis and rhabdomyolysis. Ann Intern Med. 1994;121:986.

11. Downes MA, Whyte IM. Amphetamine-induced movement disorder. Emerg Med Australas. 2005;17:277–80.

12. Lundh H, Tunving K. An extrapyramidal choreiform syndrome caused by amphetamine addiction. J Neurol Neurosurg Psychiatry. 1981;44:728–30.

13. Shen YC. Amphetamine as a risk factor for aripiprazole-induced acute dystonia. Prog Neuropsychopharmacol Biol Psychiatry. 2008;32:1756–7.

14. Brust JCM. Substance abuse and movement disorders. Mov Disord. 2010;25(13):2010–20.

15. Nestler EJ. The neurobiology of cocaine addiction. Sci Pract Perspect. 2005;3:4–10.

16. Factor SA, Sanchez-Ramos JR, Weiner WJ. Cocaine and Tourette's syndrome. Ann Neurol. 1988;23:423–4.

17. Cardoso FE, Jankovic J. Cocaine-related movement disorders. Mov Disord. 1993;8:175–8.

18. Attig E, Amyot R, Botez T. Cocaine induced chronic tics. J Neurol Neurosurg Psychiatry. 1994;57:1143–4.

19. Pascual-Leone A, Dhuna A. Cocaine-associated multifocal tics. Neurology. 1990;40:999–1000.

20. Linazasoro G, Van Blercom N. Severe stuttering and motor tics responsive to cocaine. Parkinsonism Relat Disord. 2007;13:57–8.

21. Catalano G, Catalano MC, Rodriguez R. Dystonia associated with crack cocaine use. South Med J. 1997;90:1050–2.

22. Choy-Kwong M, Lipton RB. Dystonia related to cocaine withdrawal: a case report and pathogenic hypothesis. Neurology. 1989;39:996–7.

23. Farrell PE, Diehl AK. Acute dystonic reaction to crack cocaine. Ann Emerg Med. 1991;20:322.

24. Fines RE, Brady WJ, DeBehnke DJ. Cocaine-associated dystonic reaction. Am J Emerg Med. 1997;15:513–5.

25. Merab J. Acute dystonic reaction to cocaine. Am J Med. 1988;84:564.

26. Kumor K, Sherer M, Jaffe J. Haloperidol-induced dystonia in cocaine addicts. Lancet. 1986;2:1341–2.

27. Maat A, Fouwels A, de Haan L. Cocaine is a major risk factor for antipsychotic induced akathisia, parkinsonism and dyskinesia. Psychopharmacol Bull. 2008;41:5–10.

28. van Harten PN, van Trier JC, Horwitz EH, Matroos GE, Hoek HW. Cocaine as a risk factor for neuroleptic-induced acute dystonia. J Clin Psychiatry. 1998;59:128–30.

29. Duggal HS. Cocaine use as a risk factor for ziprasidone-induced acute dystonia. Gen Hosp Psychiatry. 2007;29:278–9.

30. Henderson JB, Labbate L, Worley M. A case of acute dystonia after single dose of aripiprazole in a man with cocaine dependence. Am J Addict. 2007;16:244.

31. Daras M, Koppel BS, Atos-Radzion E. Cocaine-induced choreoathetoid movements ('crack dancing'). Neurology. 1994;44:751–2.

32. Habal R, Sauter D, Olowe O, Daras M. Cocaine and chorea. Am J Emerg Med. 1991;9:618–20.

33. Kamath S, Bajaj N. Crack dancing in the United Kingdom: apropos a video case presentation. Mov Disord. 2007;22:1190–1.

34. Weiner WJ, Rabinstein A, Levin B, Weiner C, Shulman LM. Cocaine-induced persistent dyskinesias. Neurology. 2001;56:964–5.

35. Bartzokis G, Beckson M, Wirshing DA, Lu PH, Foster JA, Mintz J. Choreoathetoid movements in cocaine dependence. Biol Psychiatry. 1999;45:1630–5.

36. Pierce RC, Kumaresan V. The mesolimbic dopamine system: the final common pathway for the reinforcing effect of drugs of abuse? Neurosci Biobehav Rev. 2006;30:215–38.

37. Sethi KD. Drug-induced movement disorders. New York: Marcel Dekker; 2004.

38. Petzinger G, Mayer SA, Przedborski S. Fentanyl-induced dyskinesias. Mov Disord. 1995;10:679–80.

39. Ferris DJ. Controlling myoclonus after high-dosage morphine infusions. Am J Health Syst Pharm. 1999;56:1009–10.

40. Potter JM, Reid DB, Shaw RJ, Hackett P, Hickman PE. Myoclonus associated with treatment with high doses of morphine: the role of supplemental drugs. BMJ. 1989;299:150–3.

41. Gattera JA, Charles BG, Williams GM, Cavenagh JD, Smithurst BA, Luchjenbroers J. A retrospective study of risk factors of akathisia in terminally ill patients. J Pain Symptom Manage. 1994;9:454–61.

42. Mercadante S. Opioids and akathisia. J Pain Symptom Manage. 1995;10:415.

43. De Conno F, Caraceni A, Martini C, Spoldi E, Salvetti M, Ventafridda V. Hyperalgesia and myoclonus with intrathecal infusion of high-dose morphine. Pain. 1991;47:337–9.

44. Mercadante S. Pathophysiology and treatment of opioid-related myoclonus in cancer patients. Pain. 1998;74:5–9.

45. Latta KS, Ginsberg B, Barkin RL. Meperidine: a critical review. Am J Ther. 2002;9:53–68.

46. Ito S, Liao S. Myoclonus associated with high-dose parenteral methadone. J Palliat Med. 2008;11:838–41.

47. Mercadante S. Dantrolene treatment of opioid-induced myoclonus. Anesth Analg. 1995;81:1307–8.

48. Sarhill N, Davis MP, Walsh D, Nouneh C. Methadone-induced myoclonus in advanced cancer. Am J Hosp Palliat Care. 2001;18:51–3.

49. Bonnet U, Banger M, Wolstein J, Gastpar M. Choreoathetoid movements associated with rapid adjustment to methadone. Pharmacopsychiatry. 1998;31:143–5.

50. Clark JD, Elliott J. A case of a methadone-induced movement disorder. Clin J Pain. 2001;17:375–7.

51. Wasserman S, Yahr MD. Choreic movements induced by the use of methadone. Arch Neurol. 1980;37:727–8.

52. Hall AP, Henry JA. Acute toxic effects of 'Ecstasy' (MDMA) and related compounds: overview of pathophysiology and clinical management. Br J Anaesth. 2006;96:678–85.

53. Morton J. Ecstasy: pharmacology and neurotoxicity. Curr Opin Pharmacol. 2005;5:79–86.

54. Downing J. The psychological and physiological effects of MDMA on normal volunteers. J Psychoactive Drugs. 1986;18:335–40.

55. Peroutka SJ, Newman H, Harris H. Subjective effects of 3,4-methylenedioxymethamphetamine in recreational users. Neuropsychopharmacology. 1988;1:273–7.

56. Vollenweider FX, Gamma A, Liechti M, Huber T. Psychological and cardiovascular effects and short-term sequelae of MDMA ("ecstasy") in MDMA-naive healthy volunteers. Neuropsychopharmacology. 1998;19:241–51.

57. Cosentino C. Ecstasy and acute dystonia. Mov Disord. 2004;19:1386–7; author reply 1387.

58. Priori A, Bertolasi L, Berardelli A, Manfredi M. Acute dystonic reaction to ecstasy. Mov Disord. 1995;10:353.

59. Parrott AC, Buchanan T, Scholey AB, Heffernan T, Ling J, Rodgers J. Ecstasy/MDMA attributed problems reported by novice, moderate and heavy recreational users. Hum Psychopharmacol. 2002;17:309–12.

60. Parrott AC, Lasky J. Ecstasy (MDMA) effects upon mood and cognition: before, during and after a Saturday night dance. Psychopharmacology (Berl). 1998;139:261–8.

61. Cole JC, Sumnall HR. Altered states: the clinical effects of Ecstasy. Pharmacol Ther. 2003;98:35–58.

62. Kalant H. The pharmacology and toxicology of "ecstasy" (MDMA) and related drugs. CMAJ. 2001;165:917–28.

63. Iravani MM, Jackson MJ, Kuoppamaki M, Smith LA, Jenner P. 3,4-methylenedioxymethamphetamine (ecstasy) inhibits dyskinesia expression and normalizes motor activity in 1-methyl-4-phenyl-1,2,3,6-tetrahydropyridine-treated primates. J Neurosci. 2003;23:9107–15.

64. Mintzer S, Hickenbottom S, Gilman S. Parkinsonism after taking ecstasy. N Engl J Med. 1999;340:1443.

65. Ricaurte GA, Yuan J, Hatzidimitriou G, Cord BJ, McCann UD. Severe dopaminergic neurotoxicity in primates after a common recreational dose regimen of MDMA ("ecstasy"). Science. 2002; 297:2260–3.

66. Ricaurte GA, Yuan J, Hatzidimitriou G, Cord BJ, McCann UD. Retraction. Science. 2003;301:1479.

67. Lozsadi DA, Forster A, Fletcher NA. Cannabis-induced propriospinal myoclonus. Mov Disord. 2004;19:708–9.

68. Chatterjee A, Almahrezi A, Ware M, Fitzcharles MA. A dramatic response to inhaled cannabis in a woman with central thalamic pain and dystonia. J Pain Symptom Manage. 2002;24:4–6.

69. Consroe P, Laguna J, Allender J, et al. Controlled clinical trial of cannabidiol in Huntington's disease. Pharmacol Biochem Behav. 1991;40:701–8.

70. Fox SH, Kellett M, Moore AP, Crossman AR, Brotchie JM. Randomised, double-blind, placebo-controlled trial to assess the potential of cannabinoid receptor stimulation in the treatment of dystonia. Mov Disord. 2002;17:145–9.

71. Muller-Vahl KR. Cannabinoids reduce symptoms of Tourette's syndrome. Expert Opin Pharmacother. 2003;4:1717–25.

72. Muller-Vahl KR, Schneider U, Prevedel H, et al. Delta 9-tetrahydrocannabinol (THC) is effective in the treatment of tics in Tourette syndrome: a 6-week randomized trial. J Clin Psychiatry. 2003;64:459–65.

73. Uribe Roca MC, Micheli F, Viotti R. Cannabis sativa and dystonia secondary to Wilson's disease. Mov Disord. 2005;20:113–5.

74. Huang MC, Lin HY, Chen CH. Dependence on zolpidem. Psychiatry Clin Neurosci. 2007;61:207–8.

75. Lightman SL. Phenobarbital dyskinesia. Postgrad Med J. 1978;54: 114–5.

76. McCarron MM, Schulze BW, Thompson GA, Conder MC, Goetz WA. Acute phencyclidine intoxication: clinical patterns, complications, and treatment. Ann Emerg Med. 1981;10:290–7.

77. Shiigi Y, Casey DE. Behavioral effects of ketamine, an NMDA glutamatergic antagonist, in non-human primates. Psychopharmacology (Berl). 1999;146:67–72.

78. Finch CK, Lobo BL. Acute inhalant-induced neurotoxicity with delayed recovery. Ann Pharmacother. 2005;39:169–72.

79. Bartolucci G, Pellettier JR. Glue sniffing and movement disorder. J Neurol Neurosurg Psychiatry. 1984;47:1259.

80. Neiman J, Lang AE, Fornazzari L, Carlen PL. Movement disorders in alcoholism: a review. Neurology. 1990;40:741–6.

81. Carlen PL, Lee MA, Jacob M, Livshits O. Parkinsonism provoked by alcoholism. Ann Neurol. 1981;9:84–6.

82. Lang AE, Marsden CD, Obeso JA, Parkes JD. Alcohol and Parkinson disease. Ann Neurol. 1982;12:254–6.

83. Luijckx GJ, Nieuwhof C, Troost J, Weber WE. Parkinsonism in alcohol withdrawal: case report and review of the literature. Clin Neurol Neurosurg. 1995;97:336–9.

84. Neiman J, Borg S, Wahlund LO. Parkinsonism and dyskinesias during ethanol withdrawal. Br J Addict. 1988;83:437–9.

85. Shandling M, Carlen PL, Lang AE. Parkinsonism in alcohol withdrawal: a follow-up study. Mov Disord. 1990;5:36–9.

86. Mullin PJ, Kershaw PW, Bolt JM. Choreoathetotic movement disorder in alcoholism. Br Med J. 1970;4:278–81.

87. Balldin J, Alling C, Gottfries CG, Lindstedt G, Langstrom G. Changes in dopamine receptor sensitivity in humans after heavy alcohol intake. Psychopharmacology (Berl). 1985;86:142–6.

88. Louis ED, Barnes LF, Ford B, Pullman SL, Yu Q. Ethnic differences in essential tremor. Arch Neurol. 2000;57:723–7.

89. Klebe S, Stolze H, Grensing K, Volkmann J, Wenzelburger R, Deuschl G. Influence of alcohol on gait in patients with essential tremor. Neurology. 2005;65:96–101.

90. Louis ED. Environmental epidemiology of essential tremor. Neuroepidemiology. 2008;31:139–49.

91. Lambert D, Waters CH. Essential tremor. Curr Treat Options Neurol. 1999;1:6–13.

92. Louis ED, Vonsattel JP. The emerging neuropathology of essential tremor. Mov Disord. 2008;23:174–82.

93. Tan EK, Schapira AH. Hunting for genes in essential tremor. Eur J Neurol. 2008;15:889–90.

94. Deuschl G, Elble RJ. The pathophysiology of essential tremor. Neurology. 2000;54:S14–20.

95. Jenkins IH, Bain PG, Colebatch JG, et al. A positron emission tomography study of essential tremor: evidence for overactivity of cerebellar connections. Ann Neurol. 1993;34:82–90.

96. Louis ED, Shungu DC, Chan S, Mao X, Jurewicz EC, Watner D. Metabolic abnormality in the cerebellum in patients with essential tremor: a proton magnetic resonance spectroscopic imaging study. Neurosci Lett. 2002;333:17–20.

97. Pagan FL, Butman JA, Dambrosia JM, Hallett M. Evaluation of essential tremor with multi-voxel magnetic resonance spectroscopy. Neurology. 2003;60:1344–7.

98. Shin DH, Han BS, Kim HS, Lee PH. Diffusion tensor imaging in patients with essential tremor. Am J Neuroradiol. 2008;29:151–3.

99. Zesiewicz TA, Elble R, Louis ED, et al. Practice parameter: therapies for essential tremor: report of the Quality Standards Subcommittee of the American Academy of Neurology. Neurology. 2005;64:2008–20.

100. Critchley M. Observations on essential (heredofamial) tremor. Brain. 1949;72:113–39.

101. Koller WC. A new drug for treatment of essential tremor? Time will tell. Mayo Clin Proc. 1991;66:1085–7.

102. Bain PG, Findley LJ, Thompson PD, et al. A study of hereditary essential tremor. Brain. 1994;117(Pt 4):805–24.

103. Growdon JH, Shahani BT, Young RR. The effect of alcohol on essential tremor. Neurology. 1975;25:259–62.

104. Boecker H, Weindl A, Leenders K, et al. Secondary parkinsonism due to focal substantia nigra lesions: a PET study with [18F]FDG and [18F]fluorodopa. Acta Neurol Scand. 1996;93:387–92.

105. Kralic JE, Criswell HE, Osterman JL, et al. Genetic essential tremor in gamma-aminobutyric acidA receptor alpha1 subunit knockout mice. J Clin Invest. 2005;115:774–9.

106. Loewenstein Y. A possible role of olivary gap-junctions in the generation of physiological and pathological tremors. Mol Psychiatry. 2002;7:129–31.

107. Manto M, Laute MA. A possible mechanism for the beneficial effect of ethanol in essential tremor. Eur J Neurol. 2008;15:697–705.

108. Nasrallah HA, Schroeder D, Petty F. Alcoholism secondary to essential tremor. J Clin Psychiatry. 1982;43:163–4.

109. Schroeder D, Nasrallah HA. High alcoholism rate in patients with essential tremor. Am J Psychiatry. 1982;139:1471–3.

110. Koller WC. Alcoholism in essential tremor. Neurology. 1983;33:1074–6.

111. Rautakorpi I, Marttila RJ, Rinne UK. Alcohol consumption of patients with essential tremor. Acta Neurol Scand. 1983;68:177–9.

112. Hess CW, Saunders-Pullman R. Movement disorders and alcohol misuse. Addict Biol. 2006;11:117–25.

113. Saunders-Pullman R, Ozelius L, Bressman SB. Inherited myoclonus-dystonia. Adv Neurol. 2002;89:185–91.

114. Zimprich A, Grabowski M, Asmus F, et al. Mutations in the gene encoding epsilon-sarcoglycan cause myoclonus-dystonia syndrome. Nat Genet. 2001;29:66–9.

115. Chan P, Gonzalez-Maeso J, Ruf F, Bishop DF, Hof PR, Sealfon SC. Epsilon-sarcoglycan immunoreactivity and mRNA expression in mouse brain. J Comp Neurol. 2005;482:50–73.

116. Xiao J, LeDoux MS. Cloning, developmental regulation and neural localization of rat epsilon-sarcoglycan. Brain Res Mol Brain Res. 2003;119:132–43.

117. Asmus F, Zimprich A, Naumann M, et al. Inherited myoclonus-dystonia syndrome: narrowing the 7q21-q31 locus in German families. Ann Neurol. 2001;49:121–4.

118. Doheny DO, Brin MF, Morrison CE, et al. Phenotypic features of myoclonus-dystonia in three kindreds. Neurology. 2002;59:1187–96.

119. Hedrich K, Meyer EM, Schule B, et al. Myoclonus-dystonia: detection of novel, recurrent, and de novo SGCE mutations. Neurology. 2004;62:1229–31.

120. Hess CW, Raymond D, Aguiar Pde C, et al. Myoclonus-dystonia, obsessive-compulsive disorder, and alcohol dependence in SGCE mutation carriers. Neurology. 2007;68:522–4.

121. Kyllerman M, Forsgren L, Sanner G, Holmgren G, Wahlstrom J, Drugge U. Alcohol-responsive myoclonic dystonia in a large family: dominant inheritance and phenotypic variation. Mov Disord. 1990;5:270–9.

122. Marechal L, Raux G, Dumanchin C, et al. Severe myoclonus-dystonia syndrome associated with a novel epsilon-sarcoglycan gene truncating mutation. Am J Med Genet B Neuropsychiatr Genet. 2003;119B:114–7.

123. Nygaard TG, Raymond D, Chen C, et al. Localization of a gene for myoclonus-dystonia to chromosome 7q21-q31. Ann Neurol. 1999;46:794–8.

124. Mahloudji M, Pikielny RT. Hereditary essential myoclonus. Brain. 1967;90:669–74.

125. Quinn NP. Essential myoclonus and myoclonic dystonia. Mov Disord. 1996;11:119–24.

Alcohol and Cancer

35

Helmut K. Seitz and Sebastian Mueller

Abstract

Alcohol is a major risk factor for a variety of cancer sites including the upper gastrointestinal tract (oropharynx, oesophagus), the larynx, the colorectum, the liver, and the female breast. In animal experiments ethanol and acetaldehyde, the first metabolites of ethanol oxidation, are both carcinogenic. Acetaldehyde can bind to DNA forming various DNA adducts, some of them with high carcinogenic potential. Indeed, individuals with an increased accumulation of acetaldehyde due to changes in ethanol- or acetaldehyde metabolism have an increased cancer risk when they drink chronically. This includes individuals with a genetically determined increased acetaldehyde production due to alcohol dehydrogenase polymorphism and those with a decreased detoxification of acetaldehyde due to an acetaldehyde dehydrogenase mutation. In addition, oral bacterial overgrowth due to poor oral hygiene also increases salivary acetaldehyde, since bacteria and yeasts are capable to generate acetaldehyde from ethanol. Dietary deficiencies such as a lack of folate, riboflavine, and zinc may also contribute to the increased cancer risk in the alcoholic. It is of considerable importance that smoking and drinking act synergistically. Smoking increases the acetaldehyde burden following alcohol consumption since smoke itself contains acetaldehyde and drinking enhances the activation of various procarcinogens present in tobacco smoke due to increased metabolic activation by induction of the cytochrome P-4502E1 (CYP2E1)-dependent microsomal biotransformation system in the mucosa of the upper digestive tract and the liver. The induction of CYP2E1 by chronic ethanol consumption also results in the production of reactive oxygen species during ethanol metabolism via CYP2E1, and these oxygen species lead to lipid peroxidation. Lipid peroxidation products such as 4-hydroxynonenal can then bind to DNA, forming highly mutagenic and carcinogenic exocyclic etheno-DNA adducts. Subsequently, chronic ethanol ingestion results in severe alterations of the methyl transfer with hypomethylation of DNA and also in a decrease of retinoic acid concentrations associated with the activation of protooncogenes and hyperproliferation. All these mechanisms functioning in concert stimulate carcinogenesis and the intensity of the effect of various mechanisms may depend among others on tissue sensibility and susceptibility which is determined genetically and/or by the environment.

H.K. Seitz, M.D., Ph.D. (✉) • S. Mueller, M.D., Ph.D.
Department of Medicine and Center of Alcohol Research,
Liver Disease and Nutrition, Salem Medical Center,
University of Heidelberg, Zeppelinstraße 11-33,
69121, Heidelberg, Germany
e-mail: helmut_karl.seitz@urz.uni-heidelberg.de

J.C. Verster et al. (eds.), *Drug Abuse and Addiction in Medical Illness: Causes, Consequences and Treatment*,
DOI 10.1007/978-1-4614-3375-0_35, © Springer Science+Business Media, LLC 2012

Learning Objectives

1. Chronic alcohol consumption is a risk factor for the development of cancer of the oropharynx, larynx, oesophagus, liver, colorectum, and female breast.

2. Ethanol and acetaldehyde, the first metabolites of ethanol oxidation, are both carcinogenic in animals.

3. The cancer risk due to alcohol is modulated by a variety of individual factors and by the sensitivity of the target tissue. Thus, in healthy individuals, the daily alcohol intake should be limited to 2 drinks (approximately 20–25 g ethanol) in men and 1 drink in women.

4. Individuals with predisposing diseases for cancer such as chronic hepatitis B or C, hemochromatosis, cirrhosis of the liver, gastroesophageal reflux disease or chronic inflammatory bowel disease should avoid alcohol at all.

5. Other risk factors for alcohol mediated cancer development are smoking, poor oral hygiene with bacterial overgrowth, accumulation of acetaldehyde due to genetic changes in ethanol metabolism such as a decreased oxidation of acetaldehyde (low activity of acetaldehyde dehydrogenase) or an increased generation of acetaldehyde (high activity of alcohol dehydrogenase), folate deficiency, and additional vitamin A intake.

6. Ethanol mediated mechanisms of carcinogenesis may include the action of acetaldehyde, increased oxidative stress due to the induction of cytochrome P4502E1 resulting in reactive oxygen species with DNA damage (from the reaction with lipid peroxidation products), increased activation of various procarcinogens (e.g. in tobacco smoke) through induced CYP2E1, disturbed methyl transfer with DNA hypomethylation, and possibly reduced retinoic acid concentrations with hyperproliferation.

Issues that Need to Be Addressed by Future Research

1. Acetaldehyde may also occur from fermentation of carbohydrates via ethanol in the upper gastrointestinal tract, especially in the stomach in the presence of bacteria. What is the amount of acetaldehyde produced from carbohydrates in the atrophic stomach with bacterial overgrowth? Does this contribute to stomach cancer in atrophic gastritis, a risk factor for stomach cancer?

2. Acetaldehyde DNA adducts should be determined in human biopsies from the upper gastrointestinal tract and from the large intestine to finally demonstrate their role in ethanol mediated carcinogenesis.

3. The relative role of CYP2E1 in the generation of reactive oxygen species, in the degradation of retinoic acid and in the activation of procarcinogens should be characterized.

4. Non-toxic CYP2E1 inhibitors should be found for and they should be used to prevent tumour development in animal models of ethanol-mediated carcinogenesis.

5. The effect of ethanol on epigenetic factors needs to be focused on in more detail.

6. Since breast cancer is the most frequent cancer in women, the mechanisms of the effect of ethanol should be studied in detail, and especially women at risk should be identified.

Introduction

Alcohol misuse is in common in the U.S. and Western Europe and is increasing in Asia. In the U.S., 7% of the adult population meet the definition for alcohol misuse or dependence [1]. Similar data exist for some countries in Europe, including Germany, where 1.5 million individuals are alcohol-dependent and approximately three million people have alcohol-associated organ damage [2]. Chronic alcohol consumption has deleterious effects on almost every organ of the human body. One of the most severe consequences of alcohol misuse is cancer development.

The WHO's global burden of disease project estimates that more than 389,000 cases of cancer are attributable to alcohol drinking worldwide, representing 3.6% of all cancers (5.2% in men and 1.7% in women) [3]. In February 2007 the International Agency for Research on Cancer (IARC) has invited 26 scientists from 15 countries to evaluate the evidence of ethanol and ethanol containing beverages as cancer causing agents. These experts reviewed all epidemiological and experimental studies covering this topic and finally came to the following conclusion [4, 5]:

"Regular alcohol consumption is associated with an increased risk for cancer of the oral cavity, pharynx, larynx, oesophagus, liver, breast, and colorectum. There is substantial mechanistic evidence in humans deficient in aldehyde dehydrogenase that acetaldehyde derived from the metabolism of ethanol contributes to causing malignant oesophageal tumours". The studies demonstrate that ethanol and not the type of alcoholic beverage is responsible for the tumour risk.

In this chapter, epidemiology of alcohol and cancer with respect to cancer sites will be briefly discussed. Major emphasis, however, will be placed on general mechanisms by which ethanol affects carcinogenesis. Since it would be beyond the scope of this article to discuss all possible mechanisms, it will focus on acetaldehyde, the first and most toxic metabolite of ethanol oxidation and on oxidative stress generated during ethanol metabolism. For more detailed information, it is referred to recent review articles [6–8].

Epidemiology

Cancer of the Upper Aerodigestive Tract

Chronic alcohol consumption is also a major risk factor for cancer of the oropharynx and oesophagus [4]. It is estimated that 25–68% of upper aerodigestive tract (UADT) cancers can be attributed to alcohol and up to 80% of these tumours could be prevented by abstaining from alcohol and smoking [9–11]. In a metaanalysis including 235 studies, pooled relative risks for alcohol (25, 50 or 100 g per day) were 1.76, 2.87, and 6.10 for oral cavity and pharyngeal cancer and 1.51, 2.21, and 4.23 for oesophageal cancer respectively [12]. In a carefully designed French study, Tuyns was able to demonstrate that alcohol consumption of more than 80 g per day (approximately one bottle of wine) increases the RR of oesophageal cancer by a factor of 18, while smoking alone of more than 20 cigarettes leads to an increased RR of 5. Taken together, both factors act synergistically resulting in an increased RR of 44 [13]. An epidemiologic study by Maier et al. showed that 90% of all patients with head and neck cancer consumed alcohol regularly in quantities twice the amount of a control group with a significant dose–response relationship [14]. If the RR for an individual with a daily alcohol consumption of 25 g was assumed to be one, this figure rose to 32 if alcohol consumption exceeded 100 g. Bruguere and coworkers found RR values of 13.5 for oral cancer, 15.2 for oropharyngeal cancer, 28.6 for hypopharyngeal cancer when 100–159 g of alcohol were consumed daily [15]. It is noteworthy that even with these high daily alcohol dosages, the alcohol-associated cancer risk is not saturable. Alcohol consumption exceeding 1.5 bottles of wine daily results in a 100-fold increased RR for oesophageal cancer [16]. In an epidemiological study of the American Cancer Society (ACS) including more than 750,000 individuals, Bofetta and Garfinkel found an increased RR for oesophageal cancer already at a dose of 12 g alcohol daily (RR = 1.37) rising to an RR of 5.8 following 72 g of alcohol consumption daily [17]. A follow-up study of the ACS came to the same results [18]. Similar dose-dependent data have also been demonstrated in case control studies involving non-smokers.

It has been shown that the accumulation of acetaldehyde after alcohol consumption due to genetic polymorphisms of ethanol metabolizing enzymes was found to be associated with increased levels of acetaldehyde-derived DNA adducts as well as an increase in sister chromatide exchanges and micronuclei of peripheral lymphocytes [19–21], and that these individuals were at extreme by high risk when they consumed ethanol chronically [22].

Since acetaldehyde also occurs in tobacco smoke and since acetaldehyde can also be produced during bacterial ethanol metabolism in the oral cavity, smoking and poor oral hygiene are risk factors for ethanol-mediated carcinogenesis (see below). Other factors such as nutritional deficiencies of folate, retinoic acid, riboflavine, iron, and zinc may also contribute to the increased cancer risk in the alcoholic as well as gastroesophageal reflux disease (GERD), but these factors have not been studied in detail.

Hepatocellular Cancer

Case-control studies in countries with a high prevalence of alcohol use and a moderate prevalence of viral hepatitis, as well as studies from countries with a high prevalence of chronic viral hepatitis and a lower prevalence of alcohol use, report that chronic ethanol consumption is associated with an approximately twofold increased risk for hepatocellular cancer (HCC) [23]. The odds ratios increase further to five- to sevenfold when ethanol consumption exceeds 80 g per day for more than 10 years [24, 25]. In general, patients with alcoholic liver cirrhosis show an HCC incidence of 1–2% per year [8].

HCC in a non-cirrhotic liver is extremely rare. Chronic alcohol consumption also increases the HHC risk in patients with other liver diseases such as chronic hepatitis B and C, and possibly in hereditary hemochromatosis (HH) and non-alcoholic fatty liver disease (NAFLD).

A study in Taiwan showed a three- to fourfold increased odds ratio for HCC in patients with chronic hepatitis B when they consumed alcohol more than 3 times weekly for more than 15 years as compared to non-drinkers [26]. A longitudinal study in Japan in hepatitis B surface antigen-positive healthy blood donors found a fivefold increased risk for HCC when more than 27 g of alcohol were consumed by day [27]. In hepatitis B patients, ethanol in a dose of 40 g or more shortens the development of HCC by approximately 10 years [28, 29].

Patients with chronic hepatitis C have a threefold increased risk when they consume 80 g ethanol or more per day as compared to those patients who do not drink [23–25]. Chronic alcohol misuse also increases the risk of HCV infection. Whether this is due to an impaired function of the immune system following alcohol ingestion or whether it relates to the risky lifestyle of alcoholics is still unknown. In addition, alcohol may increase viral replication, possibly by immunosuppression. Finally, alcohol may stimulate inflammation and thus, oxidative stress.

Iron is an important factor in the generation of oxidative stress. Ethanol increases iron uptake from the gut and results in iron deposits in the liver with further negative effect on the prognosis in patients with HH [30].

With respect to NAFLD, it has become clear that type 2 diabetics are at any increased risk for HCC [31, 32]. The pathogenesis of NAFLD includes the accumulation of fat in the liver which may be predominantly induced by hyperinsulinemia due to peripheral insulin resistance. Free fatty acids induce cytochrome P4502E1 (CYP2E1) and lead to ROS. Alcohol also increases CYP2E1 and enhances this pathophysiological pathway. In addition, tumour necrosis factor-α (TNF-α) is elevated in NAFLD and alcoholic liver disease, resulting in a further aggravation of peripheral insulin resistance and in oxidative stress. It has been shown that the relative risk for HCC in type 2 diabetics is approximately 4, and it increases to almost 10 in those consuming more than 80 g alcohol per day [25].

It should be pointed out that 30–50% of individuals with HCC show a loss of heterozygosity of the long arm of chromosome 4 [33]. In French patients with HCC, a loss of 4q34-q35 in particular was reported [34]. However, a large proportion of these patients were infected with HCV. Various mechanisms may contribute to alcohol-associated carcinogenesis, including chronic inflammation resulting in increased oxidative stress, such as in alcoholic steatohepatitis, acetaldehyde and its detrimental effect on proteins and DNA [8, 35–38], induction of CYP2E1 leading to increased ROS production, lipid peroxidation and DNA damage [8, 35], a decrease in antioxidant defence and DNA repair [8, 35], a disturbed methyl transfer associated with DNA hypomethylation [39], decreased hepatic retinoic acid (RA) [40], iron overload [35], and a profound impairment of the immune system [41].

Breast Cancer

A clear-cut dose-dependent association between alcohol intake and breast cancer has been reported in more than 100 publications [42, 43]. The risk starts already at a dose of 18 g alcohol per day. According to a metaanalysis of 38 studies, 1–3 drinks per day increase breast cancer risk by 10, 20 and 40% [44]. Every additional 10 g of alcohol increase the breast cancer risk by 7% [43]. At a consumption of 50 g of alcohol daily, the cancer risk is enhanced by 50% [45]. In the US, it was calculated that 4% of all newly diagnosed breast cancer cases are due to alcohol, resulting in a total of approximately 8,000 cases per year [44]. Among others, the increase in estradiol mediated by ethanol may be one factor to explain the increased risk of breast cancer in alcohol-drinking women.

Colorectal Cancer

More than 50 prospective- and case-control studies found a positive association between colorectal cancer and alcohol

consumption [46]. Pooled data from eight cohort studies and data from a recent metaanalysis demonstrate a 1.4-fold increased cancer risk in patients with an alcohol intake of more than 50 g per day as compared to non-drinkers [47, 48]. Subsequently, a recent prospective follow-up study comprising more than 10,000 U.S. citizens concluded that the consumption of one or more alcoholic beverages per day at baseline is associated with an approximately 70% greater risk of colon cancer with a strongly positive dose–response relationship [49]. The most important factor for colorectal cancer appeared to be the consumption of alcohol.

Excessive alcohol consumption may also influence the adenoma–carcinoma sequence at different early steps as reported recently by Boutron et al. [50, 51]. It was also reported that a reduction in ethanol intake in individuals with genetic predisposition for colorectal cancer had a large beneficial effect on tumour incidence [52].

Five out of six studies also showed an increased risk for colorectal polyps following chronic alcohol consumption as compared to abstinence [46]. The same was observed regarding hyperplastic polyps. When more than 30 g alcohol per day were consumed, the relative risk for men was 1.8 and for woman 2.5 [53].

Epidemiological studies also underline the importance of the lack of dietary factors such as methionine and folate which modulate the ethanol-associated colorectal cancer risk [54]. More recently, it was reported that individuals who produce more acetaldehyde due to alcohol dehydrogenase (ADH) polymorphism are at higher risk for colorectal cancer when they consume more than 30 g of ethanol per day as compared to individuals who produce less acetaldehyde from ethanol [55].

All these data convinced the expert panel at the IARC that the colorectum should be included as a target site of ethanol-mediated carcinogenesis.

The mechanisms by which alcohol exerts its carcinogenic effect on the colorectal mucosa are not clear, but again acetaldehyde predominantly produced by faecal bacteria from ethanol may injure the mucosa leading to secondary hyper-regeneration, a precancerous condition [56–58]. Acetaldehyde may also interact with methyl transfer leading to DNA hypomethylation which is associated with increased cancer risk [59]. For more detail it is referred to most recent review articles [8, 41, 46].

Mechanisms of Alcohol Mediated Carcinogenesis

Acetaldehyde, a Carcinogen

Acetaldehyde is the first metabolite of ethanol oxidation. Acetaldehyde binds to proteins and DNA and is mutagenic and carcinogenic in animal experiments. It interferes with

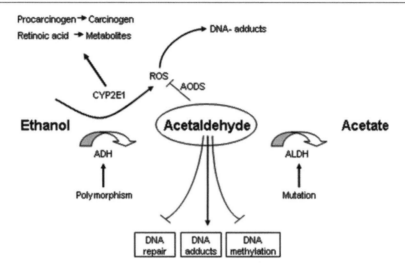

Fig. 35.1 Ethanol metabolism and its role in carcinogenesis: Ethanol is metabolized to acetaldehyde via alcohol dehydrogenase (ADH). Various ADH isozymes exist and two (ADH1B, ADH1C) reveal polymorphism associated with the generation of different amounts of acetaldehyde. Acetaldehyde is further metabolized via acetaldehyde dehydrogenase (ALDH) to acetate, which is non-toxic. The ALDH2 gene is mutated in approximately 50% of Asians resulting in low enzyme activity and the accumulation of acetaldehyde. When acetaldehyde accumulates, it exerts multiple toxic effects. With respect to carcinogenesis, it inhibits DNA repair and DNA methylation, and it leads to various carcinogenic DNA adducts. In a second pathway ethanol is metabolized to acetaldehyde via cytochrome P-4502E1 (CYP2E1). This pathway not only produces acetaldehyde, but also reactive oxygen species (ROS). These ROS lead to lipid peroxidation and lipid peroxidation products may bind to DNA resulting in carcinogenic exocyclic etheno-DNA adducts. Acetaldehyde also inhibits the antioxidative defence system (AODS) which further enhances the effect of ROS. Finally CYP2E1 also is involved in the activation of a variety of procarcinogens including those present in tobacco smoke and also leads to an enhanced degradation of retinoic acid to its metabolites resulting in low levels of hepatic retinoic acid associated with the activation of the AP1-gene and hyperproliferation

DNA synthesis and repair, injures the cellular antioxidative defence system, results in cellular hyperregeneration of the mucosa and finally, most importantly, binds to DNA forming stable adducts with mutagenic properties [19, 60, 61]. The generation of mutagenic adducts is especially enhanced in hyperregenerative tissues such as the upper and lower gastrointestinal mucosa (due to chronic ethanol consumption) due to the fact that biogenic amines present in hyperregenerative tissues favour the adduct formation [61].

Acetaldehyde is generated from ethanol oxidation and the enzyme responsible for this reaction is ADH (Fig. 35.1). Various ADH isozymes exist and two of them reveal polymorphism (ADH1B and ADH1C). While the ADH1B*2 allele encodes for an enzyme which is approximately 40 times more active than the enzyme encoded by the ADH1B*1 allele, ADH1C*1 transcription leads to an ADH isoenzyme 2.5 times more active than that from ADH1C*2 [62] (see below). Acetaldehyde accumulation is, however, also observed when its oxidation to acetate via acetaldehyde dehydrogenase (ALDH) is inadequate. Fifty percent of the Japanese population have a mutation of the ALDH 2 gene which codes for an ALDH enzyme with low activity. When these individuals drink alcohol, acetaldehyde accumulates in the blood, and they develop a flush syndrome with tachycardia, nausea, and vomiting. In addition, acetaldehyde also accumulates in the saliva, rinses the mucosa of

the UADT, and may enter the mucosal cells resulting in DNA adduct formation [63].

Ten percent of Japanese are homozygotes for ALDH2 2 (ALDH2 2/2) with zero ALDH activity. These individuals are incapable to consume alcohol, even at small doses, since they cannot oxidize acetaldehyde at all and develop severe side effects. Despite the unpleasant side effects of flushing, however, heterozygotes of the ALDH2 2/1 (40% of the Japanese population) with low ALDH activity may consume alcohol. These individuals have a significantly increased cancer risk for UADT cancer, in particular oesophageal cancer and for colorectal cancer [22, 64, 65]. Thus, their relative risk for oesophageal cancer is approximately 10 and for metachronic oesophageal cancer over 50 as compared to caucasians with the ALDH2 1/1 genotype [22].

ALDH2 gene mutation does not exist in Caucasians. However, Caucasians have a gene polymorphism for the ADH1B and ADH1C gene. Thus, heavy drinkers who are homozygous for the ADH1C*1 allele not only have an increased concentration of acetaldehyde in their saliva [66], but also seem to have an increased risk for UADT cancer [67, 68].

High levels of acetaldehyde occur in the saliva, and these levels are further increased in individuals with ADH1C*1 homozygosity [66] and ALDH2*1,2 heterozygosity [69], in smokers (smoke contains acetaldehyde) and in individuals with poor oral hygiene and bacterial overgrowth [70]. Saliva rinses the mucosa and acetaldehyde may enter the cell and result in DNA adduct formation. In addition, continuous contact of the mucosa with acetaldehyde derived from saliva leads to mucosal hyperproliferation, a precancerous condition [71, 72].

Acetaldehyde can also be generated by bacterial oxidation of ethanol. This can take place in the oral cavity and in the large intestine. In animal experiments it has been shown that acetaldehyde production in the colon was significantly reduced in germ free rats as compared to conventional animals following ethanol administration [56]. This was associated with mucosal injury and hyperregeneration [56, 57, 72]. Furthermore, salivary acetaldehyde concentrations are lower in humans after antiseptic mouthwash [63], emphasizing the role of oral bacteria in the production of acetaldehyde from ethanol.

Thus, in summary in vitro data, animal experiments and genetic linkage studies in humans strongly support the carcinogenic role of acetaldehyde in as a pathogenetic mechanism in gastrointestinal cancer development following chronic ethanol ingestion. As already pointed out, a working group of the IARC concluded that strong mechanistic evidence exists in humans that endogenous acetaldehyde derived from the consumption of ethanol in alcoholic beverages plays a causal role in the development of malignant oesophageal tumours in individuals who are deficient in aldehyde dehydrogenase [4].

Oxidative Stress

In the liver oxidative stress together with cirrhosis are important factors in ethanol-related carcinogenesis. The formation of ROS such as superoxide anion and hydrogen peroxide causes oxidative injury. Several enzyme systems are capable to produce ROS, including the cytochrome P-4502E1 (CYP2E1)-dependent microsomal mono-oxygenase system, the mitochondrial respiratory chain and the cytosolic enzymes xanthine oxidase, and aldehyde oxidase [73]. Ethanol-mediated ROS formation may be due to an increased electron leakage from the mitochondrial respiratory chain associated with the stimulation of reduced nicotinamide adenine dinucleotide (NADH) shuttling into mitochondria and to the interaction between N-acetylsphyngosine (from TNF-α) and mitochondria [74, 75]. The induction of sphingomyelinase by TNF-α increases the levels of ceramide, an inhibitor of the activity of the mitochondrial electron transport chain, leading to increased mitochondrial production of ROS. ROS can also be generated in alcoholic hepatitis with activated hepatic phagocytes [76]. Hepatic iron accumulation as observed in alcoholic liver disease increases ROS [37], and finally nitric oxide production due to ethanol-mediated

stimulation of inducible nitric oxide synthase results in the formation of peroxynitrite which is highly reactive [77].

Most important, however, is the production of ROS via CYP2E1 [37]. It has been shown that alcohol induces CYP2E1 in the liver. This induction is an adaptive process and is associated with an increased metabolism of ethanol to acetaldehyde and also to ROS [78]. The induction differs individually [79] and is most likely due to the fact that the degradation of CYP2E1 by the ubiquitin proteasome pathway is inadequate since alcohol has an effect on this pathway [80].

In animal experiments, the induction of CYP2E1 correlates with NAD phosphate (NADPH) oxidase activity, the generation of hydroxyethyl radicals, lipid peroxidation, and the severity of hepatic damage, all of which could be prevented by the CYP2E1 inhibitor chlormethiazole [81]. In addition, DNA lesions have been found to be lower in CYP2E1 knock-out mice as compared to wild type mice, and hepatic injury was significantly increased in transgenic mice that overexpressed CYP2E1 [82, 83].

ROS produced by CYP2E1 result in lipid peroxidation. Various lipid peroxidation products including 4-hydroxynonenal may bind to various purine and pyrimidine bases forming exocyclic DNA adducts. It has been shown that these adducts are highly mutagenic and carcinogenic. Such adducts have been described using immunohistochemistry, liver biopsies from patients with metal storage disorders such as Wilson's disease and haemotomachrosis, both of these diseases known to be associated with an increased risk for HCC [84]. We have investigated biopsies from patients with various degrees and severities of alcoholic liver disease and found that in these biopsies exocyclic DNA adducts are significantly increased. This already takes place at the stage of alcoholic fatty liver [84]. More recently we found a highly significant correlation between these adducts, CYP2E1 expression and 4 HNE in liver biopsies from patients with ALD [85].

By using CYP2E1 overexpressing cells, we also found that the generation of etheno-DNA adducts can be correlated with the degree of CYP2E1 expression and can be inhibited by the CYP2E1 inhibitor chlormethiazole [85]. In addition, etheno adduct formation also correlates with CYP2E1 as well as with lipid peroxidation products such as 4-hydroxynonenal in human liver biopsies [85] and in oesophageal biopsies from patients with oesophageal cancer [86]. However, another factor which may be of major importance is the presence of the antioxidative defence system. Most exocyclic etheno-DNA adducts have been observed in cells with a high expression of CYP2E1 and a low concentration of mitochondrial glutathione. Thus, both factors may play an important role in the production of this important mutagenic DNA adduct. In addition, this adduct can also be detected in the urine of patients. Using HPLC for determination of these adducts we found increased concentrations not only in patients with viral hepatitis such as hepatitis B and C, but also in patients with alcoholic liver disease [87]. Thus, measurement of exocylic etheno-DNA adducts in the urine of patients with alcoholic liver disease could be a predictive marker for risk assessment of HCC in the alcoholic.

Altered Methyl Transfer

In hepatocarcinogenesis, alcohol-related changes in hepatic methylation patterns appear to be a particular relevance. Alcohol interacts with absorption, storage, biological transformation, and excretion of compounds which are essential for methyl group transfer including folate, vitamin B6, and certain lipotropes [39]. In particular, the production of S-adenosyl-L-methionine (SAMe), the universal methyl group donor in methylation reaction, is impaired [88]. Alcohol interacts with SAMe synthesis through inhibition of crucial enzymes involved in SAMe generation [39, 86]. This can lead to a compromised formation of endogenous antioxidants such as glutathione and also lead to impaired cellular membrane stability due to impaired synthesis of phospholipids such as polyenylphosphatidylcholine [89]. In addition, alcohol may interact with the methylation of certain genes and thereby contribute to liver damage and tumour development. Accordingly, alcohol-induced depletion of lipotropes may cause hypomethylation of oncogenes, leading to their activation. The decrease in methylation capacity caused by chronic alcohol consumption may, therefore, contribute to epigenetic alterations of genes involved in carcinogenesis [8]. Whether and to what extend alcohol ingestion is sufficient to produce genetic hypomethylation and consequently tumour initiation has not been finally confirmed.

Reduced Retinoic Acid

Chronic ethanol consumption results in reduced hepatic vitamin A concentrations [90]. CYP2E1 enzyme induction by ethanol can lead to excessive catabolism of retinoic acid (RA) [91]. Chronic ethanol consumption results in a decrease of retinol and RA in the liver associated with an activation of the AP-1 gene leading to an increased expression of c-jun and c-fos and finally hepatocellular hyperproliferation which is associated with an increased cancer risk. It has been shown that the enhanced catabolism of retinol and retinoic acid in alcohol-fed rats can be inhibited by chlormethiazole both in vitro and in vivo [91, 92], indicating that CYP2E1 is the major enzyme responsible for the alcohol-enhanced catabolism of retinoids in hepatic tissue after exposure to alcohol. Since CYP2E1 enzyme induction in chronic intermittent drinking could continue to be a factor destroying retinol and

retinoic acid as well as mediating oxidative stress, even after withdrawal from alcohol, the inhibition of CYP2E1 induction by treatment with a CYP2E1 inhibitor could be a useful way to provide a protective effect against alcohol-related hepatic carcinogenesis.

In order to determine whether the restoration of the hepatic retinoid status in alcohol-fed rats by chlormethiazole protects against chemically induced, alcohol-promoted carcinogenesis of the liver, rats received a single injection of 20 mg diethylnitrosamine/kg body for tumour initiation and were then fed alcohol and control diets with or without chlormethiazole (Wang, personal communication). Hepatic amphophilic foci of cellular alteration, nodular regenerative hyperplasia, and hepatocellular adenoma were detected in the ethanol-fed rats after 10-months of treatment, but not control rats with the same dose of diethylnitrosamine treatment, including non-ethanol-fed rats and ethanol-fed rats with chlormethiazole treatment. In addition, chlormethiazole treatment prevented alcohol-induced CYP2E1 expression and activity, and restored alcohol-reduced retinoic acid to normal levels. These data demonstrate that chronic and excessive ethanol consumption alone promotes hepatic carcinogenesis by impairing hepatocyte regeneration in the rat liver. Furthermore, inhibition of CYP2E1 activation by a CYP2E1 inhibitor can counteract the tumour-promoting action of ethanol by restoring normal hepatic levels of retinoic acid. These data further support the notion that alcohol-promoted oncogenic transformation may be related to alcohol-impaired retinoic acid action. Although retinoid interventions which serve to restore normal retinoid signalling and functioning may offer protection at the cellular level and represent a means to modify cancer risk [93], high doses of vitamin A supplementation over a period of months are hepatotoxic, and chronic alcohol consumption enhances this intrinsic hepatotoxicity [94]. This is particularly true with respect to the potential detrimental effects of polar metabolites of retinoids generated during alcohol drinking [95]. Taking into account the efficacy and complex biological functions of retinoids in human cancer prevention, intervention using CYP2E1 inhibitors that target alcohol-induced CYP2E1 which is associated with the production of reactive oxygen species and carcinogenic acetaldehyde, the activation of procarcinogens as well as the enhanced catabolism of retinoid could provide complementary or synergistic protective effects against alcohol-related cancer risk.

Specific Mechanisms

In the liver, cirrhosis caused by chronic ethanol consumption is a prerequisite for the development of HCC due to mechanisms not clearly understood, but predominantly due to chronic inflammation with inflammation driven oxidative stress and proliferative changes during the development of cirrhosis. HCC in a non-cirrhotic alcoholic liver is extremely rare.

GERD is an additional factor which favours carcinogenesis in the oesophagus due to acid-mediated chronic inflammation of the oesophageal mucosa. GERD is favoured by alcohol since alcohol decreases the tonus of the lower oesophageal sphincter which facilitates GERD [8].

Increased oestrogen levels due to alcohol consumption, even at low doses, are most likely an important pathophysiological factor to explain the increased risk of breast cancer in regular drinkers [45]. The mechanism by which alcohol increases estradiol levels is not known.

Interaction Between Alcohol and Tobacco

Alcohol consumption and smoking have a synergistic effect on the risk of UADT cancer. This synergistic effect has been shown in countless studies. For example, a case control study of oral and pharyngeal cancer conducted in the U.S. regarding tobacco and alcohol use of 1,114 patients and 1,268 population-based controls demonstrated that the risk for these cancers among non-drinkers increased with the amount smoked, and conversely that the risks among non-smokers increased with the level of alcohol intake. In both groups, the risk of oropharyngeal cancer tended to be more in a multiplicative than additive fashion and was increased more than 35-fold among those who consumed two or more packs of cigarettes and more than four alcoholic drinks per day. Cessation of smoking was also associated with a sharply reduced risk of this cancer [96].

Various factors may contribute to this effect:

1. Local permeabilizing effects of alcohol on the penetration of tobacco-specific and other carcinogens across the oral mucosa [97].
2. Acetaldehyde is a known constituent of tobacco smoke. Smokers have been shown to have elevated breath acetaldehyde concentrations after acute cigarette smoking [98].
3. During ethanol ingestion smokers have about twice as high acetaldehyde levels in their saliva than non-smokers. This is due to a change in the capacity of oral bacteria to produce acetaldehyde from ethanol [96, 97]. Smokers have an increased incidence of yeast infections and occurrence of Gram-positive bacteria which are known to have a high capacity for ethanol oxidation [98, 99]. Thus, smoking increases the acetaldehyde load in the saliva following alcohol consumption.
4. Chronic alcohol consumption results in the induction of cytochrome P-4502E1 (CYP2E1) in various tissues including the mucosa of the UADT [78, 100] (see above). The CYP2E1-dependent ethanol oxidation not only produces acetaldehyde and ROS, but is also important in the activation of certain procarcinogens to ultimative carcinogens. Among these are some carcinogens present in

tobacco smoke such as polycyclic hydrocarbons and various nitrosamines. Due to the induction of CYP2E1 by ethanol, these procarcinogens are especially activated in the mucosal cells of the UADT and this may be another mechanism by which chronic ethanol exerts its carcinogenicity, particularly in smokers [101].

Conclusions

The aim of the present review was to summarize the current evidence for the important role of chronic alcohol consumption in the worldwide cancer development based on experimental and epidemiologic data, demonstrating a causal relationship between this lifestyle factor and various types of cancer. Considering the high frequencies of these cancers, especially in the Western World (colorectal cancer is the leading cancer in men and women in some countries), the link between drinking and these tumours has important consequences for prevention and early detection. Threshold levels for safe alcohol consumption are difficult to obtain and may vary interindividually since genetic and epigenetic risk factor have to be considered. The combination of smoking and alcohol drinking is an extremely strong risk factor for some types of cancer since smoking and alcohol consumption have a synergistic effect on cancer development in various tissues such as the mucosa of the UADT. Although difficult to implement, health authorities must introduce more effective measures in educating the public about the potential hazards of regular and excessive alcohol consumption, not only to avoid a variety of diseases associated with these behaviours, but also to prevent cancer development. While it is well-known even to the public that the liver is the major target organ for alcohol toxicity, it is less known that alcohol is a risk factor for certain cancers. Thus, chronic and heavy drinkers should not only be monitored for liver disease but also for the additional cancer sites discussed here. This means that extensive information about alcohol consumption and the risk for cancer development should be made accessible to various medical specialists as otorhinolaryngologists, gynaecologists and gastroenterologists.

Acknowledgement Original research was supported by grants of the Dietmar Hopp Foundation and the Manfred Lautenschläger Foundation to HKS.

References

1. Grant B, Harford T, Dawson D, Chou P, DuFour M, Pickering R. Prevalence of DSM-IV alcohol abuse and dependence: United States, 1992. Alcohol Res World. 1994;18:243–8.
2. Jahrbuch Sucht 08, Neuland Verlagsgesellschaft mbH, Geesthacht.2008

3. Rehm J, et al. In: Ezzati M, Murray C, Lopez AD, Rodgers A, editors. Comparative quantification of health risks: global and regional burden of disease attributable to selected major risk factors. Geneva: World Health Organization; 2004. p. 959–1108.

4. Baan R, et al. Carcinogenicity of alcoholic beverages. Lancet Oncol. 2007;8:292–3.

5. IARC. Alcohol consumption and ethyl carbamate (urethane). IARC monographs on the evaluation of carcinogenic risks to humans. International Agency for Research on Cancer, Vol. 96, IARC Library 2010

6. Boffeta P, Hashibe M. Alcohol and cancer. Lancet Oncol. 2006;7: 149–56.

7. Boffetta P, Hashibe M, La Vecchia C, Zatonski W, Rehm J. The burden of cancer attributable to alcohol drinking. Int J Cancer. 2006;119:884–7.

8. Seitz HK, Stickel F. Molecular mechanisms of alcohol mediated carcinogenesis. Nat Rev Cancer. 2007;7:599–612.

9. Tuyns AJ, Esteve J, Raymond L, Berrino F, Benhamou E, Blanchet F, Boffetta P, Crosignani P, Del Moral A, Lehmann W, Merletti F, Pequignot G, Riboli E, Sancho-Garnier H, Terracini B, Zubiri A, Zubiri L. Cancer of the larynx/hypopharynx, tobacco and alcohol: IARC international case-control study in Turin and Varese (Italy), Zaragoza and Navarra (Spain), Geneva (Switzerland) and Calvados (France). Int J Cancer. 1988;41:483–91.

10. Franceschi S, Talamini R, Barra S, Baron AE, Negri E, Bidoli E, Serraino D, La Vecchia C. Smoking and drinking in relation to cancers of the oral cavity, pharynx, larynx, and esophagus in northern Italy. Cancer Res. 1990;50:6502–7.

11. Blot WJ. Alcohol and cancer. Cancer Res. 1992;52(Suppl): 2119–23.

12. Bagnardi V, Blangiardo M, La Veccia C, Corrao G. A meta-analysis of alcohol drinking and cancer risk. Br J Cancer. 2001;85: 1700–5.

13. Tuyns A. Alcohol and cancer. Alcohol Health Res World. 1978;2: 20–31.

14. Maier H, Zöller J, Herrmann A, Kreiss M, Heller WD. Dental status and oral hygiene in patients with head and neck cancer. Otolaryngol Head Neck Surg. 1993;1088:655–61.

15. Brugere J, Guenel P, Leclerc A, Rodriguez J. Differential effects of tobacco and alcohol in cancer of the larynx, pharynx, and mouth. Cancer. 1986;57:391–5.

16. Tuyns A. Esophageal cancer in non-smoking drinkers and in non-drinking smokers. Int J Cancer. 1983;32:443–4.

17. Boffetta P, Garfinkel L. Alcohol drinking and mortality among men enrolled in an American Cancer Society prospective Study. Epidemiology. 1990;5:342–8.

18. Thun MJ, Peto R, Lopez A, Monaco JH, Henley SJ, Heath Jr CW, Doll R. Alcohol consumption and mortality among middle-aged and elderly U.S. adults. N Engl J Med. 1997;337:1705–14.

19. Fang JL, Vaca CE. Detection of DNA adducts of acetaldehyde in peripheral white blood cells of alcohol abusers. Carcinogenesis. 1997;18:627–32.

20. Morimoto K, Takeshita T. Low Km aldehyde dehydrogenase (ALDH2) polymorphism, alcohol drinking behaviour, and chromosome alterations in peripheral lymphocytes. Environ Health Perspect. 1996;104 Suppl 3:563–7.

21. Ishikawa H, Yamamoto H, Tian Y, Kawano M, Yamauchi T, Yokoyama K. Effect of ALDH2 gene polymorphism and alcohol drinking behaviour on micronuclei frequency in non-smokers. Mutat Res. 2003;541:71–80.

22. Yokoyama A, Muramatsu T, Ohmori T, Yokoyama T, Okoyama K, Takahashi H, Hasegawa Y, Higuchi S, Maruyama K, Shirakura K, Ishii H. Alcohol-related cancers and aldehyde dehydrogenase-2 in Japanese alcoholics. Carcinogenesis. 1998;19:1383–7.

23. Morgan TR, Mandayam S, Jamal MM. Alcohol and hepatocellular carcinoma. Gastroenterology. 2004;127:87–96.

24. Tagger A, Donato F, Ribero ML, Chiesa R, Portera G, Gelatti U, Alberini A, Fasola M, Moffetta P, Nardi G. Case control study on hepatitis C virus (HCV) as a risk factor for hepatocellular carcinoma: the role of HCV genotypes and the synergism with hepatitis B virus and alcohol Brescia HCC study. Int J Cancer. 1999;81: 695–9.

25. Hassan MM, Hwang LY, Hatten CJ, Swaim M, Li D, Abbruzzese JL, Beasley P, Patt YZ. Risk factors for hepatocellular carcinoma: synergism of alcohol with viral hepatitis and diabetes mellitus. Hepatology. 2002;36:1206–13.

26. Chen CJ, Liang KY, Chang AS, Cang YC, Lu SN, Liaw YF, Chang WY, Sheen MC, Lin TM. Effects of hepatitis B virus, alcohol drinking, cigarette smoking and familial tendency on hepatocellular carcinoma. Hepatology. 1991;13:398–406.

27. Oshima A, Tsukuma H, Hiyama T, Fujimoto I, Yamano H, Tanaka M. Follow up study of HbS-Ag-positive blood donors with special reference to effect of drinking and smoking on development of liver cancer. Int J Cancer. 1984;34:775–9.

28. Ohnishi K. Alcohol and hepatocellular cancer. In: Watson RR, editor. Alcohol and cancer. Boca Raton, FL: CRC; 1992. p. 179–202.

29. Pereira FE, Goncalves CS, Zago Mda P. The effect of ethanol intake on the development of hepatocellular carcinoma in HbS Ag carriers. Arq Gastroenterol. 1994;31:42–6.

30. Kowdley KV. Iron, hemochromatosis, and hepatocellular carcinoma. Gastroenterology. 2004;127:79–86.

31. El-Serag HB. Hepatocellular carcinoma: recent trends in the United States. Gastroenterology. 2004;127:27–34.

32. El-Serag HB, Tran T, Everhart JE. Diabetes increases the risk of chronic liver disease and hepatocellular carcinoma. Gastroenterology. 2004;126:460–8.

33. Laurent-Puig P, Legoix P, Bluteau O, Belghiti J, Franco D, Binot F, Monges G, Thomas G, Bioulac-Sage P, Zucman-Rossi J. Genetic alterations associated with hepatocellular carcinomas define distinct pathways of hepatocarcinogenesis. Gastroenterology. 2001;120:1763–73.

34. Bluteau O, Beaudoin JC, Pasturaus P, Belghiti J, Franco D, Bioulac-Sage P, Laurent-Puig P, Zacman-Rossi J. Specific association between alcohol intake, high grade of differentiation and 4q34-q35 deletions in hepatocellular carcinomas identified by high resolution allelotyping. Oncogene. 2002;21:1225–32.

35. Seitz HK, Stickel F. Risk factors and mechanisms of hepatocarcinogenesis with special emphasis on alcohol and oxidative stress. Biol Chem. 2006;387:349–60.

36. Seitz HK, Meier P. The role of acetaldehyde in upper digestive tract cancer in alcoholics. Transl Med. 2007;49:293–7.

37. Seitz HK. The role of acetaldehyde in alcohol-associated cancer of the gastrointestinal tract. In: Goode J, editor. Acetaldehyde-related pathology: bridging the transdisciplanary divide, Novartis Foundation Symposium No. 285. London: Wiley; 2007. p. 110–9.

38. Salaspuro M, Salaspuro V, Seitz HK. Alcohol and upper aerodigestive tract cancer. In: Cho CH, Purohit V, editors. Alcohol, tobacco and cancer. Basel: Karger; 2006. p. 48–62.

39. Stickel F, Herold C, Seitz HK, Schuppan D. Alcohol and transmethylation: implication for hepatocarcinogenesis. In: Ali S, Mann D, Friedman S, editors. Liver diseases: biochemical mechanisms and new therapeutic insights. New York: Plenum; 2006. p. 45–58.

40. Wang XD. Alcohol, vitamin A, and cancer. Alcohol. 2005;35: 251–8.

41. Pöschl G, Seitz HK. Alcohol and cancer (Review). Alcohol Alcohol. 2004;39:155–65.

42. Singletary KW, Gapstur SM. Alcohol and breast cancer: a review of epidemiologic and experimental evidence and potential mechanisms. JAMA. 2001;286:2143–51.

43. Hamajima N, et al. Alcohol, tobacco and breast cancer-collaborative reanalysis of individual data from 53 epidemiological studies, including 58 515 women with breast cancer and 95 067 women without the disease. Br J Cancer. 2002;87:1234–45.

44. Longnecker MP. Alcoholic beverage consumption in relation to risk of breast cancer: meta-analysis and review. Cancer Causes Control. 1994;5:73–82.

45. Seitz HK, Maurer B. The relationship between alcohol metabolism. Estrogen levels, and breast cancer risk. Alcohol Res Health. 2007;30:42–3.

46. Seitz HK, Pöschl G, Salaspuro MP. Alcohol and cancer of the large intestine. In: Cho CG, Purohit V, editors. Alcohol, tobacco and cancer. Basel: Karger; 2006. p. 63–77.

47. Cho E, Smith-Warner SA, Ritz J, van den Brandt PA, Colditz GA, Folsom AR, Freudenheim JL, Giovannucci E, Goldbohm RA, Graham S, Holmberg L, Kim DH, Malila N, Miller AB, Pietinen P, Rohan TE, Sellers TA, Speizer FE, Willett WC, Wolk A, Hunter DJ. Alcohol intake and colorectal cancer: a pooled analyses of 8 cohort studies. Ann Intern Med. 2004;140:603–13.

48. Corrao G, Bagnardi V, Zamborn A, Arico S. Exploring the dose response relationship between alcohol consumption and the risk of several alcohol-related conditions: a meta analysis. Addiction. 1999;94:551–73.

49. Su LJ, Arab L. Alcohol consumption and risk of colon cancer: evidence from the national health and nutrition examination survey I epidemiologic follow-up study. Nutr Cancer. 2004;50: 111–9.

50. Boutron MC, Faivre J, Dop MC, Quipourt V, Senesse P. Tobacco, alcohol, and colorectal tumors: a multistep process. Am J Epidemiol. 1995;141:1038–46.

51. Bardou M, Montembault S, Giraud V, Balian A, Borotto E, Houdayer C, Capron F, Chaput JC, Naveau S. Excessive alcohol consumption favours high risk polyp or colorectal cancer occurrence among patients with adenomas: a case control study. Gut. 2002;50:38–42.

52. Le Marchand L, Wilkens LR, Hankin JH, Kolonel LN, Lyu LC. Independent and joint effects of family history and lifestyle on colorectal cancer risk: implications for prevention. Cancer Epidemiol Biomarkers Prev. 1999;8:845–51.

53. Kearny J, Giovannucci E, Rimm EB, Stampfer MJ, Colditz GA, Ascherio A, Bleday R, Willett WC. Diet, alcohol, and smoking and the occurrence of hyperplastic polyps of the colon and rectum (United States). Cancer Causes Control. 1995;6:45–56.

54. Giovanucci E, Rimm EB, Ascherio A, Stampfer MJ, Colditz GA, Willett WC. Alcohol, low methionine-low folate diets, and risk of colon cancer in men. J Natl Cancer Inst. 1995;87:265–73.

55. Homann N, König I, Marks M, Benesova M, Stickel F, Millonig G, Mueller S, Seitz HK. Alcohol and colorectal cancer: role of alcohol dehydrogenase 1C polymorphism. Alcohol Clin Exp Res. 2009;33:551–6.

56. Seitz HK, Simanowski UA, Garzon FT, Rideout JM, Peters TJ, Koch A, Berger MR, Einecke H, Maiwald M. Possible role of acetaldehyde in ethanol-related rectal cocarcinogenesis in the rat. Gastroenterology. 1990;98:406–13.

57. Simanowski UA, Suter P, Russell RM, Heller M, Waldherr R, Ward R, Peters TJ, Smith D, Seitz HK. Enhancement of ethanol-induced rectal hyperregeneration with age in F344 rats. Gut. 1994;35:1102–6.

58. Simanowski UA, Homann N, Knühl M, Arce L, Waldherr R, Conradt C, Bosch FX, Seitz HK. Increased rectal cell proliferation following alcohol abuse. Gut. 2001;49:418–22.

59. Choi SW, Stickel F, Baik W, Kim YI, Seitz HK, Mason JC. Chronic alcohol consumption induces genomic, but not p53-specific DNA hypomethylation in the colon of the rat. J Nutr. 1999;129:1945–50.

60. Matsuda T, Terashima I, Matsumoto Y, Yabushita H, Matsui S, Shibutani S. Effective utilization of N2-ethyl-2'-deoxyguanosine triphospate during DNA synthesis catalyzed by mammalian replicative DNA polymerases. Biochemistry. 1999;38:929–35.

61. Theravathu JA, Jaruga P, Nath RG, Dizdaroglu M, Brooks PJ. Polyamines stimulate the formation of mutagenic 1, N2-propanodeoxyguanosine adducts from acetaldehyde. Nucleic Acids Res. 2005;33:3513–20.

62. Bosron WF, Li TK. Genetic polymorphism of human liver alcohol and aldehyde dehydrogenase and their relationship to alcohol metabolism and alcoholism. Hepatology. 1986;6:502–10.

63. Homann N, Jousimies-Somer H, Jokelainen K, Heine R, Salaspuro M. High acetaldehyde levels in saliva after ethanol consumption: methodological aspects and pathogenetic implications. Carcinogenesis. 1997;18:1739–43.

64. Yokoyama A, Watanabe H, Fukuda H, Haneda T, Kato H, Yokoyama T, Muramatsu T, Igaki H, Tachimori Y. Multiple cancers associated with esophageal and oropharyngolaryngeal squamous cell carcinoma and the aldehyde dehydrogenase-2 genotype in male Japanese drinkers. Cancer Epidemiol Biomarkers Prev. 2002;11:895–900.

65. Matsuo K, Hamajima N, Shinoda M, Hatooka S, Inoue M, Takezaki T, Tajima K. Gene-environment interaction between an aldehyde dehydrogenase-2 (ALDH2) polymorphism and alcohol consumption for the risk of esophageal cancer. Carcinogenesis. 2006;22:913–6.

66. Visapää J-P, Götte K, Benesova M, Li J, Homann N, Conradt C, Inoue H, Tisch M, Hörrmann K, Väkeväinen S, Salaspuro M, Seitz HK. Increased cancer risk in heavy drinkers with the alcohol dehydrogenase 1C*1 allele, possibly due to salivary acetaldehyde. Gut. 2004;53:871–6.

67. Harty LC, Caporaso NE, Hayes RB, Winn DM, Bravo-Otero E, Blott WJ, Kleinmen DV, Brown LM, Armenian HK, Fraumeni Jr JF, Shields PG. Alcohol dehydrogenase 3 genotype and risk of oral cavity and pharyngeal cancers. J Natl Cancer Inst. 1997;89:1689–705.

68. Homann N, Stickel F, König IR, Jacobs A, Junghanns K, Benesova M, Schuppan D, Himsel S, Zuberjerger I, Hellerbrand C, Ludwig D, Caselmann WH, Seitz HK. Alcohol dehydrogenase 1C*1 allele is a genetic marker for alcohol-associated cancer in heavy drinkers. Int J Cancer. 2005;118:1998–2002.

69. Väkeväinen S, Tillonen J, Agarwal DP, Svirastava N, Salaspuro M. High salivary acetaldehyde after a moderate dose of alcohol in ALDH2-deficient subjects: strong evidence for the local carcinogenic action of acetaldehyde. Alcohol Clin Exp Res. 2000;24:873–7.

70. Homann N, Tillonen J, Rintamäki H, Salaspuro M, Lindqvist C, Meurman JH. Poor dental status increases the acetaldehyde production from ethanol in saliva: a possible link to the higher risk of oral cancer among alcohol-consumers. Oral Oncol. 2001;37:153–8.

71. Homann N, Kärkkäinen P, Koivisto T, Nosova T, Jokelainen K, Salspuro M. Effects of acetaldehyde on cell regeneration and differentiation of the upper gastrointestinal tract mucosa. J Natl Cancer Inst. 1997;89:1692–7.

72. Simanowski UA, Suter P, Stickel F, Maier H, Waldherr R, Smith D, Russell RM, Seitz HK. Esophageal epithelial hyperproliferation following long term alcohol consumption in rats: effect of age and salivary function. J Natl Cancer Inst. 1993;85:2030–3.

73. Albano E. Alcohol, oxidative stress and free radical damage. Proc Nutr Soc. 2006;65:278–90.

74. Bailey SM, Cunningham CC. Contribution of mitochondria to oxidative stress associated with alcohol liver disease. Free Radic Biol Med. 2002;32:11–6.

75. Garcia-Ruiz C, Colell A, Paris R, Fernandez-Checa JC. Direct interaction of GD3 ganglioside with mitochondria generates

reactive oxygen species followed by mitochondrial permeability transition, cytochrome c release and caspase activation. FASEB J. 2000;14:847–50.

76. Bautista AP. Neutrophilic infiltration in alcoholic hepatitis. Alcohol. 2002;27:17–21.

77. Chamulitrat W, Spitzer JJ. Nitric oxide and liver injury in alcohol fed rats after lipopolysaccharide administration. Alcohol Clin Exp Res. 1996;20:1065–70.

78. Lieber CS. Alcohol and the liver. Update Gastroenterol. 1994;106:1085–105.

79. Oneta CM, Lieber CS, Li J, Rüttimann S, Schmid B, Lattmann J, Rosman AS, Seitz HK. Dynamics of cytochrome P-4502E1 activity in man: induction by ethanol and disappearance during with drawal phase. J Hepatol. 2002;36:47–52.

80. Bardag-Gorce F, Yuan QX, Li J, et al. The effect of ethanol-induced cytochrome P4502E1 on the inhibition of proteasome activity by alcohol. Biochem Biophys Res Commun. 2000;279: 23–9.

81. Gouillon Z, et al. Inhibition of ethanol-induced liver disease in the intragastric feeding rat model by chlormethiazole. Proc Soc Biol Med. 2000;224:302–8.

82. Bradford BU, et al. Cytochrome P-450 CYP2E1, but not nicotinamide adenine dinucleotide phosphate oxidase is required for ethanol-induced oxidative DNA damage in rodent liver. Hepatology. 2005;41:336–44.

83. Morgan K, Frensch SW, Morgan TR. Production of a cytochrome P-4502E1 transgenic mouse and initial evaluation of alcoholic liver damage. Hepatology. 2002;36:122–34.

84. Frank A, Seitz HK, Bartsch H, Frank N, Nair J. Immunohistochemical detection of 1, N6-ethenodeoxyadenosine in nuclei of human liver affected by diseases predisposing to hepatocarcinogenesis. Carcinogenesis. 2004;25:1027–31.

85. Wang Y, Millonig G, Nair J, Patsenkeer E, Stickel F, Mueller S, Bartsch H, Seitz HK. Ethanol induced cytochrome P-4502E12 causes carcinogenic etheno DNA lesions in alcoholic liver disease. Hepatology. 2009;50:453–61.

86. Millonig G, Wang Y, Homann N, Bernhardt F, Qin H, Mueller S, Bartsch H, Seitz HK. Ethanol induced carcinogenesis in the human esophagus implicates CYP2E1 induction and the generation of carcinogenic DNA lesions. Int J Cancer. 2010;128(3): 533–40.

87. Nair J, Srivatanakul P, Haas C, Jedpiyawongse A, Khuhaprema T, Seitz HK, Bartsch H. High urinary excretion of lipid peroxidation derived DNA damage in patients with cancer prone liver disease. Mutat Res. 2010;683:23–8.

88. Martinez-Chantar ML, et al. Importance of a deficiency in S-adenosyl-L-methionine synthesis in the pathogenesis of liver injury. Am J Clin Nutr. 2002;76:1177S–82S.

89. Schlemmer HPW, Sawatzki T, Dornacher I, Sammet S, Bachert P, Hellenschmitt M, van Kaick G, Seitz HK. Proton decoupled 31P MR-spectroscopy imaging of the liver: a new method for the assessment of altered hepatic phospholipid metabolism in patients with alcoholic liver disease. J Hepatol. 2005;42:752–59.

90. Leo MA, Lieber CS. Hepatic vitamin A depletion in alcoholic liver injury. N Engl J Med. 1982;304:597–600.

91. Liu C, Russell RM, Seitz HK, Wang XD. Ethanol enhances retinoic acid metabolism into polar metabolites in rat liver via induction of cytochrome P4502E1. Gastroenterology. 2001;120:179–89.

92. Liu C, et al. Chlormethiazole treatment prevents reduced hepatic vitamin A levels in ethanol-fed rats. Alcoholism Clin Exp Res. 2002;26:1703–9.

93. Chung IY, et al. Restoration of retinoic acid concentration suppresses ethanol induced c-jun overexpression and hepatocyte hyperproliferation in rat liver. Carcinogenesis. 2001;22:1231–19.

94. Albanes D, et al. α-Ttocopherol and β-carotene supplements and lung cancer incidents in the α-tocopherol, β-carotene cancer prevention study: effects of baseline characteristics and study compliance. J Natl Cancer Inst. 1996;88:1560–70.

95. Dan Z, et al. Alcohol-induced polar retinol metabolites trigger hepatocyte apoptosis via loss of mitochondrial membrane potential. FASEB J. 2005;19:1–4.

96. Blot WJ, McLaughlin JK, Winn DM, Austin DF, Greenberg RS, Preston-Martin S, Bernstein L, Schoenberg JB, Stemhagen A, Fraumeni JF. Smoking and drinking in relation to oral and pharyngeal cancer. Cancer Res. 1988;48:3282–7.

97. Du X, Squier CA, Kremer MJ, Wertz PW. Penetration of N-nitrosonornicotine (NNN) across oral mucosa in the presence of ethanol and nicotine. J Oral Pathol Med. 2000;29:80–5.

98. Salaspuro V, Salaspuro M. Synergistic effect of alcohol drinking and smoking on in vivo acetaldehyde concentration in saliva. Int J Cancer. 2004;111:480–3.

99. Salaspuro M. Acetaldehyde, microbes, and cancer of the digestive tract. Crit Rev Clin Lab Med. 2003;40:183–208.

100. Shimizu M, Lasker JM, Tsutsumi M, Lieber CS. Immunohistochemical localization of ethanol inducible cytochrome P4502E1 in the rat alimentary tract. Gastroenterology. 1990;93:1044–50.

101. Seitz HK, Osswald BR. Effect of ethanol on procarcinogen activation. In: Watson RR, editor. Alcohol and cancer. Boca Raton: CRC; 1992. p. 55–72.

Fetal Alcohol Spectrum Disorder

36

Andrea R. Kilgour and Albert E. Chudley

Abstract

One of the most tragic outcomes of a woman's addiction to or abuse of alcohol is the effects on the unborn child. Fetal Alcohol Spectrum Disorder (FASD) is common and preventable. Western estimates suggest that FASD affects 1% of the population, and in some communities, the frequency is much higher. FASD is caused by a mother's use of alcohol with or without other substances of abuse that can result in permanent physical and neurodevelopmental impairments to her unborn child. In addition to the primary effects of FASD, affected children are at risk of developing secondary disabilities, including drug and alcohol addictions. It is uncertain what factors, genetic and/or environmental, lead to this addiction. The individual, social, and financial costs are enormous. Multidisciplinary teams have been developed to improve ascertainment of, and standardized approaches to, FASD diagnosis. Strategies and mentorship programs have been developed to better recognize and support women at risk for having FASD children. We discuss issues specific to the treatment and management of FASD adolescents and adults who are struggling with addiction to alcohol and other substances.

Learning Objectives
- To understand and review the clinical presentation, diagnostic process, epidemiology, and prevention of FASD
- To become aware of the secondary disabilities, including addictions, suffered by FASD individuals
- To describe the treatment and management of addictions in FASD individuals

Issues that Need to be Addressed in Future Research
- To identify a means to separate genetic from prenatal and postnatal risk factors that lead to addictions in FASD individuals
- To compare the efficacy of various addiction treatment modules in FASD individuals.

A.R. Kilgour, Ph.D, C.Psych
Department Clinical Health Psychology, University of Manitoba, Winnipeg, MB R3E 3N4, Canada

A.E. Chudley, MD, FRCPC, FCCMG (✉)
Departments of Pediatrics and Child Health, Biochemistry and Medical Genetics, University of Manitoba, Winnipeg, MB R3A 1R9, Canada

WRHA Program in Genetics and Metabolism, Health Sciences Centre, FE 229 820 Sherbrook Street, Winnipeg, MB R3A 1R9, Canada
e-mail: achudley@hsc.mb.ca

Clinicians were first alerted to the risk of fetal harm from prenatal alcohol exposure in a French publication [1]. Since this paper was published in a French language journal with limited distribution, the significance of Lemoine's findings was largely hidden. In 1973, two key articles written by American investigators in the British Journal *The Lancet* alerted the world to this common and lifelong affliction [2]. The American authors were the first to use the term fetal alcohol syndrome (FAS). FAS children are recognized by prenatal and postnatal growth retardation, facial

Table 36.1 The IOM diagnostic categories and the corresponding DPN 4-Digit Code rankings

IOM nomenclature	Growth	Face	Brain[a]	Alcohol history
FAS (with confirmed exposure)	2,3, or 4	4	3 or 4	3 or 4
Partial FAS (with confirmed exposure)[a]	1, 2, 3, or 4	3 or 4	3 or 4	3 or 4
FAS (without confirmed exposure)	2, 3 or 4	4	3 or 4	2
ARND (with confirmed exposure)	1, 2, 3, or 4	1 or 2	3 or 4	3 or 4

[a]Occasionally a rank score of 2 for the brain for those less than age 6 years can be used in difficult cases or in whom no standardized scores are readily available; using clinical judgment, a rank of 3 or 4 implies at least three domains of neurological impairment. Modified from Chudley et al. [24]

anomalies characterized by short palpebral fissures, a smooth poorly formed philtrum, a thin vermillion border of the upper lip, and cognitive and behavioral difficulties. The clinician caring for the addicted woman now has to recognize that he has two patients at significant risk of harm, the mother and the fetus. What makes FAS different from other disorders is that this disorder is potentially preventable.

Since the original description of FAS, the spectrum of effects extended to include all subsets of affected individuals referred to as FASD. At one end of the spectrum is the subset of individuals with FAS. At the other end of the spectrum are those individuals with behavioral and cognitive deficits who exhibit minimal or no physical stigmata as a consequence of ethanol-induced prenatal brain injury, including those conditions using the terms described by the Institute of Medicine (IOM) review of FAS [3] (Table 36.1).

In FASD, addictions and substance abuse, and particularly the abuse of ethanol by the mother, not only lead to a child at high risk for learning difficulties, maladaptive behaviors, neuropsychological deficits, and birth defects, but the affected children themselves are at high risk for developing addiction and substance abuse themselves later in life [5–8]. Thus, FASD becomes a generational problem. A significant proportion of mothers of FASD children may be affected themselves. It is likely that the cycle may begin with genetic and social risk factors that predispose individuals to using and abusing a variety of substances including ethanol. In our society, the use of alcohol is widespread and promoted by commercial interests.

The term secondary disabilities was introduced by Streissguth et al. [9, 10] in a longitudinal study of children and adults with FAS and fetal alcohol effects (FAE). In contrast to the primary disabilities in FASD individuals (birth defects, cognitive impairments, etc.), secondary disabilities are disabilities the client was not born with and that could be ameliorated through earlier diagnosis, better understanding, and more appropriate interventions. Secondary disabilities are hypothesized to be the result of an interaction of behavioral and mental health problems associated with an adverse environment. Streissguth et al. defined six secondary disabilities for all ages: mental health problems, disrupted school experience, trouble with the law, confinement, inappropriate sexual behavior, and alcohol and drug problems.

Additionally, three secondary disabilities were defined as exclusive to adults: dependent living, problems with employment, and difficulties parenting. Other studies [11–13] have verified a common finding of these secondary disabilities in their study populations. Common manifestations in children include learning disability, immature or inappropriate social skills, hyperactivity, poor verbal abilities, conduct problems, and poor judgment. Adults may experience depression, anxiety, psychosis, sexual promiscuity, poor judgment, poor impulse control, restlessness, poor problem-solving skills, resistance to change, difficulty forming lasting and meaningful relationships, gullibility and victimization, inability to understand or conform to social norms, and unemployment.

Incidence and Prevalence

FAS is caused by excessive maternal alcohol use during pregnancy and is one of the leading causes of preventable congenital anomalies and developmental disabilities [3]. The incidence is highest among lower socioeconomic groups and in some minority populations, such as the Blacks in South Africa and Aboriginal peoples in North America and Australia. The full spectrum of prenatal alcohol effects is difficult to estimate, since there are no reliable biological markers that readily define those affected. The prevalence is related to the frequency of excessive alcohol use in pregnancy and thus will vary from population to population as demonstrated in the following table (Table 36.2).

In many countries, the frequency of the full spectrum is not known because of underreporting due to many factors including lack of awareness, lack of resources, and lack of trained and skilled professionals in diagnosis [22]. Ethnicity may also lead to variability in alcohol effects. An international research consortium in FAS assessed affected children from several different countries [23]. They showed measurements that reflected reduced size of the orbit to be a consistent feature discriminating between FAS and controls across each study population. Each population had a unique, though often overlapping, set of variables that discriminated the two groups, suggesting important ethnic differences in the presentation of the syndrome.

Table 36.2 Incidence and prevalence of FAS and FASD in various worldwide populations

Country	Population	Incidence (I) or prevalence (P)	Comments	References
European and other countries	FAS	$I = 1–3/10,000$	May be an underestimate; thought to be more related to poverty than ethnicity	[14]
USA	FAS	$P = 0.3–1.5/1,000$	Live births	[15, 16]
Seattle, USA	FAS & ARND	$P = 9.1/1,000$	1975–1981	[17]
Western Cape Community, South Africa	FAS	$P = 40.5–46.4/1,000$	Children aged 5–9 years	[18]
South Africa	FAS	$P = 65.2–74.2/1,000$	First grade children	[19]
Remote NE Manitoba, CAN	FAS	$I = 7.2/1,000$	All live births in one hospital, 1 year period	[20]
First Nations community, Manitoba, CAN	FASD	$P = 55–101/1,000$	Cross-sectional survey of 178 school-aged children from one community school	[74]
Lazio region of Italy	FAS FASD	$P = 3.7–7.4/1,000$ $P = 20.3–40.5/1,000$	First grade children randomly selected from pimary schools in two health districts	[21]

Diagnostic Process and Criteria

Given that these patients have a complex pattern of disabilities, we have advocated for a multidisciplinary approach to diagnosis. The assessments need to be comprehensive and encompass the evaluation of several factors that no one health discipline alone can provide, and therefore, the diagnostic team best involves the collaboration of a number of health professionals to make an accurate diagnosis and provide multidimensional recommendations for management [24]. The assessment process begins with the recognition of the need for diagnosis and ends with the implementation of appropriate recommendations. The multidisciplinary diagnostic team can be geographical/regional, virtual, or can accept referrals from distant communities and be evaluated using video conferencing or telehealth. The members of the team may vary according to the context of the diagnosis. The team could include knowledgeable physicians, psychologists, speech and language pathologists, social workers, and a coordinator. Clinical geneticists are key members of multidisciplinary diagnostic teams, who have unique training and skills in syndrome recognition, and sometimes the diagnosis may require excluding other genetic syndromes that may mimic FAS [24]. Multidisciplinary teams ideally work with community partners and resources to develop and implement management plans to maximize intervention for the affected individual.

The diagnosis of FAS depends on the presence of the cardinal findings of dysmorphic facial features, evidence of brain dysfunction, and prenatal and postnatal growth deficiency in the presence of prenatal alcohol exposure [4]. In the absence of characteristic growth impairment and facial dysmorphology, the diagnosis of partial FAS (pFAS) or

alcohol-related neurodevelopmental disorder (ARND) might be considered assuming cognitive impairments. However, only FAS can be reliably diagnosed without information on prenatal alcohol exposure. In individuals with cognitive and behavioral difficulties without facial dysmorphology and the absence of maternal history of prenatal alcohol exposure, an FASD-related diagnosis cannot be made with our current understanding and assessments.

Evaluating the Face and Other Physical Findings

Astley and Clarren, using data from the Washington State FAS Diagnostic and Prevention Network (DPN) of clinics, developed the 4-Digit Diagnostic Code [25–27]. The four digits in the code reflect the magnitude of expression of the four key diagnostic features of FAS in the following order: [1] growth deficiency; [2] the FAS facial phenotype, using the palpebral fissure length (pfl) percentiles (Fig. 36.1), and the shape of the philtrum and upper lip (Fig. 36.2); [3] central nervous system damage/dysfunction; and [5] gestational alcohol exposure. The third edition of the DPN 4-Digit Diagnostic Code Manual [29] is available and is being used for diagnosis, screening, and surveillance efforts in all Washington State FAS DPN clinics. Modifications of the 4-Digit Code using IOM diagnostic categories are being used in many clinics throughout North America for use in the diagnosis of children and adults [28, 30].

The sentinel facial features consist of short pfl, a poorly formed philtrum, and a thin vermillion border of the upper lip. Ideally and traditionally, a short pfl is considered to be less than 1.5–2 standard deviations (or approximately tenth

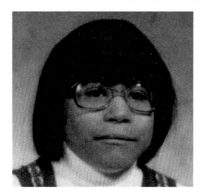

Fig. 36.1 A dysmorphic child with features consistent with FAS. Note the short palpebral fissures, the smooth and poorly formed philtrum, and thin upper lip

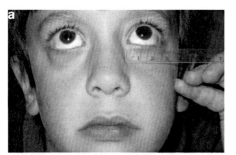

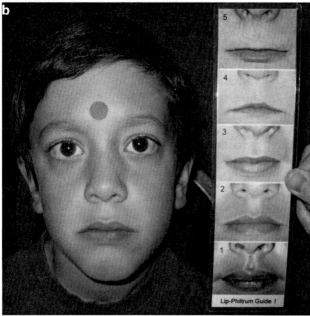

Fig. 36.2 Clinical assessment of a child for facial features that might indicate alcohol effects. (**a**) Using a clear flexible plastic ruler to assess palpebral fissure lengths. (**b**) Using the lip philtrum guide (Astley [28]) to assess the philtrum and upper lip form

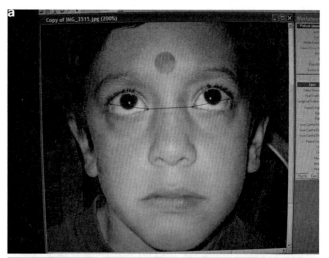

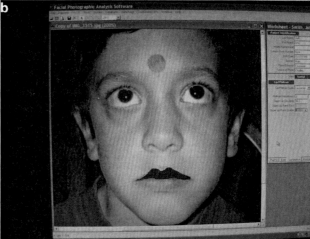

Fig. 36.3 The use of digital photographic analysis of the face (Astley [28]). (**a**) Note the size marker and landmarks used to measure the palpebral fissure lengths. (**b**) Note the assessment of the upper lip that will objectively determine the circularity of the upper lip (Astley [28])

%ile and second %ile); for an adult, this is typically pfl of less than 27 mm. We based this measurement on extensive experience with adults, as well as a study using three methods to evaluate the pfl: a clear plastic ruler, a slide precision

caliper, and the photographic analysis using the software program available through the University of Washington DPN [25]. The landmarks for pfl measurements are key in the evaluation (Fig. 36.3), and require training and practice. Standardized graphs by age are available and are based on data from Farcus who used calipers for the pfl measurements and were derived from Caucasian adolescents and adults from Southern Ontario, Canada [31, 32]. A recent publication from Canada provided reliable pfl measurements for school age children from ages 6 to 17 years [33]. Therefore, using the published graph standards when measurements involve the use of the ruler or the calculation from photographic computer program analysis gives a result that is about one standard deviation more than from our study and our clinical experience. To correct for this, one needs to add one standard deviation to the standard deviation calculated on the photographic computer program analysis or plotted on Hall et al. published graph [31]. The lesson here is that if one uses the published norms, the method or tool used to acquire the measurement needs to be the same as the method that generated the normative data! Clinically, we recommend the use of either the plastic clear ruler or the photographic tool, and correct for the one standard deviation difference in the published norms. Pfl do not change after 16 years of age. Reliable data for pfl in non-Caucasian individuals are not currently available.

Evaluating the Brain

There are several ways in which the brain in FASD needs a detailed evaluation, which is as critical as a proper evaluation searching for evidence of dysmorphic features. The Canadian and American guidelines for FASD assessment have recommended the evaluation of several brain domains [3, 24, 29, 34]. These domains include the documentation of structural, neurologic, and functional abnormalities.

The brain is vulnerable to the adverse effects of prenatal alcohol exposure through all three trimesters of pregnancy, although different effects may be observed depending on the amount of alcohol consumed, the blood alcohol level achieved, the duration of exposure, and the stage of gestation during which alcohol is consumed. No specific anatomical region of the brain appears to be targeted, although malformations seen include migration abnormalities including gray matter heterotopias or variable degrees of lissencephaly; abnormalities in the size, shape, and position of the corpus callosum; cerebellar vermis hypoplasia; hypoplasia of the basal ganglia and hippocampus, and microcephaly [35, 36]. Most individuals with FAS show no gross anatomical abnormalities on brain imaging. However, many may have neurologic damage, exhibit seizures, and show soft neurological signs such as poor coordination and balance, and visual motor difficulties. Thus a careful neurological examination is warranted [24, 34].

Neuropsychological Assessments

The Canadian guidelines [24] recommend assessment of hard and soft neurological signs (including sensory-motor) and brain structure (presence of microcephaly, abnormalities on MRI scans, etc.). In addition, neuropsychological assessment provides information regarding general intellectual ability (IQ), attention, visuospatial perception, receptive and expressive language skills, academic achievement, memory, executive functioning, and adaptive and social behavior. The assessment should include and compare basic and complex tasks in each domain, as appropriate. Although the domains are assessed as though independent entities, where there is overlap, experienced clinical judgment is required to decide

how many domains are affected. A domain is considered "impaired" when, on a standardized measure, scores are two standard deviations or more below the mean, or when there is a discrepancy of at least one standard deviation between subdomains (for example, there is a one standard deviation difference between verbal and perceptual indices on standard IQ tests). For areas where standardized measurements are not available, a clinical judgment of "severely abnormal" is made, taking into consideration that important variables, including age, mental health factors, social-economic factors, and disrupted family/home environment (e.g., multiple foster placements, history of abuse and neglect) that may affect development but do not indicate brain damage [24].

On neuropsychological assessments, FASD individuals typically show deficits on tasks related to the function of the prefrontal cortex and hippocampus, characterized by deficiencies in executive functions, working memory, information processing, complex attention, and place learning [35, 37, 38]. FAS adults who have an IQ in the normal range exhibit clear deficits in measures sensitive to complex attention, verbal learning, and executive function [39]. Research assessing functional memory in both adults and children with FAS and ARND shows impairments in spatial working memory on functional MRI analysis compared to that in controls [40]. Whether these findings are specific to FASD individuals and a potential tool in diagnosis is yet to be determined. Fagerlund et al. studied the brains of adolescents and adults with FASD using magnetic resonance spectroscopy, and suggested that prenatal alcohol exposure appears to alter brain metabolism in a long-standing or permanent manner in multiple brain areas [41]. These findings agreed with previous findings from structural and functional studies. Most of the metabolic alterations involved changes in glial cells rather than in the neurons.

From the neuropsychological perspective, the most difficult diagnoses are those in which severe deficits are not found across all diagnostic criteria. It is becoming more recognized that full-blown FAS will manifest with significant impairment across at least three domains of cognitive functioning [24], including reduced general intellectual ability (IQ), as well as at least two other areas mentioned below. Those individuals whose Full Scale IQ scores are below 70 and show impaired adaptive functioning may be diagnosed with mental retardation. However, many FASD-affected individuals do not meet these severe criteria. The Committee on Substance Abuse and Committee on Children with Disabilities recognized that cognitive, behavioral, and psychosocial manifestations of FASD may vary with age and life circumstances and that each individual may display a somewhat different constellation of deficits [42]. There is no neurocognitive profile specific to FASD, although some research is emerging that shows fairly consistent patterns [43].

Evidence of significant impairment in at least three cognitive domains is necessary for diagnosis and, in terms of diagnostic code for the brain, would be equated to a score of 3 or 4 in the 4-digit code depending on the severity. A score of 2 is reserved for the individuals with mild cognitive impairment that may or may not reflect brain dysfunction from prenatal alcohol exposure and would not normally lead to a diagnosis in any category of FASD. This approach is conservative and the threshold that has been established may exclude some individuals who may be mildly impaired from prenatal alcohol exposure. Until there are tests that can better differentiate alcohol brain injury from other etiologies, establishing a cut-off is justifiable. Furthermore, individuals who score 3 or 4 on the brain assessment may have other reasons for their impairment, and these could include genetic factors, brain injury from other pre- and postnatal environmental exposures, traumatic brain injury, and alcohol and drug abuse.

Addictions in FASD Individuals

Research on children of alcoholics is focused on studies of FAS, the transmission of alcoholism, psychobiologic markers of vulnerability, and psychosocial characteristics. Most studies suggest that prenatal exposed children, when compared with children of non-alcoholics, exhibit maladaptive behaviors later in life, such as academic failure or alcoholism, to a greater extent [44]. Famy et al. showed that adults with FAS or FAE were more likely to suffer mental illness, with the most common diagnosis being alcohol or drug dependence [12].

Streissguth reported a study on 61 adults with FAS. Mental health problems, alcoholism and drug abuse, antisocial behaviors, and repeated pregnancies (for the woman) were common problems [45]. A study on 197 adoptees was designed to determine the effects of fetal alcohol exposure and a diagnosis of substance abuse disorders including alcohol, nicotine, and other drug dependence. Comparing those adoptees who were exposed to prenatal alcohol to those who were not prenatally exposed showed a higher incidence of drug and alcohol dependence in the exposed adoptees [46]. The authors suggested that the possible effects of fetal alcohol exposure on development of adult substance use patterns need attention in genetic studies of substance abuse.

Alati et al. reported the results of a population-based birth cohort study conducted in Australia commencing in 1981 [5, 47]. Maternal alcohol consumption was assessed prepregnancy, in early and late pregnancy, and then at 5-year, 14-year, and 21-year follow-up intervals. Their work determined that in utero exposure to alcohol of three or more glasses was associated with later alcohol disorders in the exposed children.

Baer et al., in their population-based longitudinal studies, further suggested that prenatal alcohol exposure was more predictive of adolescent alcohol use than was family history of alcohol problems [6, 7]. That is, it was the prenatal exposure rather than exposure to alcohol use and abuse among family members as a young child that resulted in higher alcohol disorders in adolescents. Furthermore, prenatal alcohol exposure was significantly associated with alcohol disorders into young adulthood (cohort aged 21 years), but nicotine use in the mother during pregnancy was not associated with later alcohol problems by the offspring.

As such, there is emerging evidence that suggests a more biological origin of alcohol use, particularly in adolescents. Further studies, however, are needed to better extricate the nature of the association and the role of other more environmental factors.

Costs of FAS

The cost of FAS to affected individuals, their families, and society is staggering. In the USA, it is estimated that in 1992 the cost of treating affected infants, children, and adults was over $1.9 billion [48]. The lifetime cost per child affected with FAS is estimated to be $1.4 million. Recent data from Canada suggest that the lifetime cost of FASD was estimated at $1 million per case. With an estimated 4,000 new cases yearly, this translates to $4 billion annually [49, 50]. Using standard measures, children and youth with FASD were shown to have a significantly lower health-related quality of life when compared to the general Canadian population [51].

Mortality

There are no national statistics on mortality in adults affected by FASD. In children, the mortality rate has been suggested to be 6%, and the all-cause mortality in siblings of children diagnosed with FAS is increased by 530% compared to that in controls [52–54]. It is assumed that the mortality rate is high in FASD adults in light of the social chaos, their propensity to alcohol and drug dependency, and the high incidence of mental health problems these individuals face. Effective prevention strategies must include a variety of approaches involving the general population and targeting high-risk populations. Many mothers of individuals with FASD are also affected themselves by prenatal alcohol exposure, and this may have been present through several generations in some families. There appears to be a high rate of involvement of adolescents and adults affected with FAS in the criminal justice system [55–57]. Many end up in jail, having become perpetrators of crime, which is often violent.

Prevention

Public education, warning labels, family support groups, advocacy groups, early childhood intervention programs, specialized educational and career training, addiction counseling and treatment for women, and paraprofessional mentoring programs have been helpful in reducing the birth prevalence of affected individuals, thereby reducing the morbidity from this disorder. An early diagnosis is associated with a lower occurrence of secondary disabilities, thus more effort has to be made to diagnose the children as soon as possible.

There are several reliable and validated screening questionnaires that identify pregnant women with high-risk drinking patterns. The questionnaires are simple and are best administered by physicians, midwives, or nurse practitioners to all women prior to or early in their pregnancy. These include the TWEAK, T-ACE, CAGE, BMAST, SMAST, and AUDIT screening questionnaires [58–60]. Women who score high in these questionnaires can be offered counseling to help reduce drinking in pregnancy. Primary health care providers can identify and intervene on behalf of mothers at risk before they become pregnant, and thus prevent future affected children [60]. Primary prevention is achievable using a mentoring program and identifying mothers at risk after the birth of an affected child, thereby reducing the chance of birth of another affected child [61, 62].

Prevention of FASD is a tall order, but there is hope. The development of community support, drug and alcohol treatment centers, early childhood intervention programs, public education, and targeted intervention efforts all play a role in raising awareness and offering help. Warning labels on alcohol beverages do increase awareness about the risks of taking alcohol in pregnancy, but this must be tied to other strategies in order to be effective [63, 64]. A comprehensive approach to FASD prevention efforts in Washington State has resulted in a decrease in the prevalence of maternal use of alcohol during pregnancy and a reduction in the prevalence of FAS among foster children [65].

Treatment

Intervention strategies for those with FASD have been emerging as an understanding of FASD progresses and increasingly appropriate diagnosis is made. However, it is not within the scope of this paper to review the overall management of FASD individuals in terms of potential medical and mental health risks outside of the issue of addictions. The reader can consult other sources for these topics [66, 67]. When FASD is diagnosed in childhood, these intervention strategies can be introduced at an early age, and therefore, the likelihood of later addictions is reduced. However, if the diagnosis is not made until adulthood, then treatment and intervention must not only include targeting the primary, but also the secondary disabilities, including alcohol and drug abuse and addiction. In this latter case, the primary, cognitive deficits will interfere with successful treatment of the addiction, unless these deficits are recognized and accommodations in intervention strategies are made. Plainly speaking, standard addiction treatment programs that are designed for relatively cognitively intact individuals will not work for those with FASD.

Interventions for FASD in childhood have focused on recognition of and remediation of the cognitive deficits. For example, it is widely accepted that one of the cognitive skills that most affects an individual's ability to function adaptively within the environment is executive function. As Kalberg & Buckley point out, executive function can be broadly thought of as two sets of skills: cognition-based executive functioning and emotion-related cognitive functioning [68]. Cognition-based executive functioning limitations may manifest in the inability to (a) understand and remember the specific sequences required for numerous activities of daily living; (b) carry out the appropriate steps of social exchange; (c) learn sequences; (d) maintain attention to complete a goal; (e) planning a task; and (f) solving problems. An affected individual may need an environmental tool to help him or her stay on track during daily routines. Through role modeling and daily interactions, most children learn the steps of appropriate social communication without explicit instruction. However, for FASD-affected children, these steps are neither obvious nor easily understood. Therefore, the steps of social engagement must be taught. In many settings, difficulty in planning, problem solving, and sustaining attention can result in the inability to follow directions and generalize information from one situation to another. Emotion-related executive dysfunction may manifest as impulsivity and disinhibition, resulting in the individual being seen as speaking or acting inappropriately. The individual with FASD may also have difficulty regulating emotions and may act out toward others.

Other cognitive deficits commonly seen in FASD that negatively impact ability to engage in standard intervention programs are verbal and visuospatial learning and memory [69–71]. These individuals have difficulty taking in new verbal information through auditory channels and holding that information in memory for use at a later time. As such, intervention programs solely based on verbal sharing of information would not be ideally effective for the person with FASD.

Although the neuropsychological deficits have been well documented and many researchers in the field recognize the need to design interventions specifically to compensate for the cognitive deficits, those programs that have been developed have not been adequately evaluated [72]. In a step to resolve this problem, Grant et al. described a 1-year community pilot intervention program with FASD-affected women [73]. Their program included a community intervention model of targeted education and collaboration with key service providers, and used trained case managers as facilitators. Some of the skills taught to service providers were to talk in concrete terms and avoid using words with double meanings, to give simple step-by-step instructions, and then have the FASD patient demonstrate understanding of the directions by showing a skill, rather than relying on a verbal affirmation. It was also recommended that simple (fifth grade level) written instructions be given if necessary, and with illustrations if possible. Advocates and professional providers alike found it critical to re-teach and repeat important points at each visit, and to remember that instructions were unlikely to generalize to a different, albeit similar situation. In their work with service providers, advocates emphasized the importance of consistency both in the environment and in the people providing care. Finally, advocates emphasized that the aim of treatment should be to stabilize presenting problems rather than to pursue a cure for permanent disabilities in reasoning, judgment, and memory. One of the improved outcomes of this pilot project included decreased alcohol and drug use.

In another targeted community intervention program, May et al. evaluated the efficacy of providing case management enhanced with strategies derived from motivational interviewing to women at risk in four American Indian communities in Northern Plains states [74]. The project staff actively engaged each of the project participants in case management for an average of 17.2 months (SD = 16.6), and 31% of their participants also entered some type of formal alcohol or drug treatment. The investigators found that consumption of alcohol, as measured by both quantity and frequency measures, was reduced at 6 months.

Overall, there is a paucity of evaluated, efficacious general intervention programs for individuals with FASD, and specific alcohol and drug treatment programs have not been reviewed in the literature. It appears that the best course of action is to provide the FASD-affected individual with a case manager/advocate who can assist in educating staff of standard addictions treatment programs as to the particular requirements of their client. Accommodations for the specific cognitive deficits are required in order for the FASD-affected individual to benefit maximally from any program.

Conclusions

FASD are common, with Western estimates suggesting that at least 1% of the population is affected, with specific subpopulations showing higher prevalence. These disorders are preventable through minimizing, or ideally eliminating, maternal use of alcohol, which is the cause of this set of disorders. FASD can result in permanent physical and neurodevelopmental impairments to the unborn child, which requires the work of multidisciplinary teams for diagnosis and management. As well, the affected individuals are at risk of developing secondary disabilities, including drug and alcohol addictions. It is likely that both genetic and environmental factors lead to addictions within the affected individuals. In women with FASD and alcohol dependency, prevention of generational FASD is difficult to achieve. Although strategies and mentorship programs have been developed to better recognize and support women at risk for having FASD children, few addictions programs that have been modified to accommodate for the typical cognitive deficits observed have been evaluated.

References

1. Lemoine P, Harousseau H, Borteyru JP, Menuet JC. Les enfants de parents alcooliques: Anomalies observees. A propos de 127 cas. Ouest Med. 1968;21:476–82.
2. Jones KL, Smith DW. Recognition of the fetal alcohol syndrome in early infancy. Lancet. 1973;2(836):999–1001.
3. Stratton K, Howe C, Battaglia FC. Fetal alcohol syndrome: diagnosis, epidemiology, prevention, and treatment. Washington DC: Institute of Medicine; National Academy Press; 1996. http://www.nap.edu/books/0309052920/html/index.html.
4. Clarren SK, Smith DW. The fetal alcohol syndrome. Lamp. 1978; 35:47.
5. Alati R, Al Mamun A, Williams GM, O'Callaghan M, Najman JM, Bor W. In utero alcohol exposure and prediction of alcohol disorders in early adulthood: a birth cohort study. Arch Gen Psychiatr. 2006;63:1009–16.
6. Baer JS, Barr HM, Bookstein FL, Sampson PD, Streissguth AP. Prenatal alcohol exposure and family history of alcoholism in the etiology of adolescent alcohol problems. J Stud Alcohol. 1998;59: 533–43.
7. Baer JS, Sampson PD, Barr HM, Connor PD, Streissguth AP. A 21-year long longitudinal analysis of the effects of prenatal alcohol exposure on young adult drinking. Arch Gen Psychiatr. 2003; 60:377–85.
8. Williams S. Alcohol's possible covert role: brain dysfunction, paraphilias, and sexually aggressive behaviors. Sex Abuse. 1999;11: 147–58.
9. Streissguth A, Barr H, Kogan J, Bookstein F (1996) Understanding the occurrence of secondary disabilities in clients with fetal alcohol syndrome (FAS) and fetal alcohol effects (FAE). Final Report to CDC Grant No. R04/CCR008515. Seattle: University of Washington School of Medicine
10. Streissguth AP. Fetal Alcohol Syndrome: a guide for families and communities. Baltimore (MD): Paul H. Brookes Publishing Company; 1997.
11. Lemoine P. The history of alcoholic fetopathies. J FAS Int. 2003;3(1):e2.
12. Famy C, Streissguth AP, Unis AS. Mental illness in people with fetal alcohol syndrome or fetal alcohol effects. Am J Psych. 1998;155:552–4.
13. Clark E, Lutke J, Minness P, Ouellette-Kuntz H. Secondary disabilities among adults with fetal alcohol spectrum disorder in British Columbia. J FAS Int. 2004;2:e13.
14. Abel EL. An update on incidence of fetal alcohol syndrome: Fetal alcohol syndrome is not an equal opportunity birth defect. Neurotoxicol Teratol. 1995;17:427–43.

15. Abel EL. Fetal alcohol syndrome and fetal alcohol effects. New York: Plenum; 1984.

16. Centers for Disease Control and Prevention (CDC). Fetal Alcohol syndrome—Alaska, Arizona, Colorado, and New York, 1995–1997. MMWR. 2002;51:433–5.

17. Sampson PD, Streissguth AP, Bookstein FL, Little RE, Clarren SK, Dehaene P, Hanson JW, Graham Jr JM. Incidence of fetal alcohol syndrome and prevalence of alcohol-related neurodevelopmental disorder. Teratology. 1997;56(5):317–26.

18. Centers for Disease Control and Prevention (CDC). Fetal alcohol syndrome-South Africa, 2001. MMWR. 2003;52:660–2.

19. Viljoen DL, Gossage JP, Brooke L, Adnams CM, Jones KL, Robinson LK, Hoyme HE, Snell C, Khaole NC, Kodituwakku P, Asante KO, Findlay R, Quinton B, Marais AS, Kalberg WO, May PA. Fetal alcohol syndrome epidemiology in a South African community: a second study of a very high prevalence area. J Stud Alcohol. 2005;5:593–604.

20. Williams RJ, Odaibo FS, McGee JM. Incidence of fetal alcohol syndrome in northeastern Manitoba. Can J Public Health. 1999;90(3):192–4.

21. May PA, Fiorentino D, Gossage JP, Kalberg WO, Hoyme HE, Robinson LK, Coriale G, Jones Kl, Del Campo M, Tarani L, Romeo M, Kodituwakku PW, Deiana L, Buckley D, Ceccanti M. The epidemiology of FASD in a province in Italy: prevalence and characteristics of children in a random sample of schools. Alcohol Clin Exp Res. 2006;30:1562–75.

22. Chudley AE. Fetal alcohol spectrum disorder: counting the invisible—mission impossible? Arch Dis Child. 2008;93:721–2.

23. Moore ES, Ward RE, Wetherill LF, Rogers JL, Autti-Rämö I, Fagerlund A, Jacobson SW, Robinson LK, Hoyme HE, Mattson SN, Foroud T, CIFASD. Unique facial features distinguish fetal alcohol syndrome patients and controls in diverse ethnic populations. Alcohol Clin Exp Res. 2007;31(10):1707–13.

24. Chudley AE, Conry J, Cook JL, Loock C, Rosales T, LeBlanc N. Public Health Agency of Canada's National Advisory Committee on fetal alcohol spectrum disorder. Fetal alcohol spectrum disorder: Canadian guidelines for diagnosis. Can Med Assoc J. 2005;172(5 Suppl):S1–S21.

25. Astley SJ, Clarren SK. A case definition and photographic screening tool for the facial phenotype of fetal alcohol syndrome. J Pediatr. 1996;129:33–41.

26. Astley SJ, Clarren SK. Diagnostic guide for fetal alcohol syndrome and related conditions: the 4-digit diagnostic code. Seattle, WA: University of Washington Publication Services; 1997.

27. Astley SJ, Clarren SK. Diagnosing the full spectrum of fetal alcohol-exposed individuals: introducing the 4-digit diagnostic code. Alcohol. 2000;35(4):400–10.

28. Hoyme HE, May PA, Kalberg WO, Kodituwakku P, Gossage JP, Trujillo PM, Buckley DG, Miller JH, Aragon AS, Khaole N, Viljoen DL, Jones KL, Robinson LK. A practical clinical approach to diagnosis of fetal alcohol spectrum disorders: clarification of the 1996 institute of medicine criteria. Pediatrics. 2005;115:39–47.

29. Astley SJ. Diagnostic guide for fetal alcohol syndrome and related conditions. The 4-digit diagnostic code. 3rd ed. Seattle, WA: University of Washington Press; 2004.

30. Chudley AE, Kilgour A, Cranston M, Edwards M. Challenges of diagnosis in fetal alcohol syndrome and fetal alcohol spectrum disorder in the adult. Am J Med Genet C Semin Med Genet. 2007;145C(3):261–72.

31. Hall JG, Froster-Iskenius UG, Allanson JE. Handbook of normal physical measurements. Toronto: Oxford University Press; 1989. p. 149–50.

32. Farkas LG. Anthropometry of the head and face. 2nd ed. New York: Raven; 1994.

33. Clarren SK, Chudley AE, Wong L, Friesen J.Brant R. Normal distribution of palpebral fissure lengths in Canadian school-age children. Can J Clin Pharmacol (FAS Research) 2010;17:e67–e78.

34. Centres for Disease Control and Prevention (CDC). Guidelines for identifying and referring persons with fetal alcohol syndrome. MMWR. 2005;54(No. RR-11):1–15.

35. Mattson SN, Schoenfeld AM, Riley EP. Teratogenic effects of alcohol on brain and behavior. Alcohol Res Health. 2001;25:185–91.

36. Streissguth AP, Aase JM, Clarren SK, Randels SP, LaDue RA, Smith DF. Fetal alcohol syndrome in adolescents and adults. J Am Med Assoc. 1991;265:1961–7.

37. Mattson SN, Riley EP, Gramling L, Delis DC, Jones KL. Neuropsychological comparison of alcohol-exposed children with or without physical features of fetal alcohol syndrome. Neuropsychology. 1998;12:146–53.

38. Hamilton DA, Kodituwakku P, Sutherland RJ, Savage DD. Children with fetal alcohol syndrome are impaired at place learning but not cued-navigation in a virtual Morris water task. Behav Brain Res. 2003;143(1):85–94.

39. Kerns KA, Don A, Mateer CA, Streissguth AP. Cognitive deficits in non-retarded adults with fetal alcohol syndrome. J Learn Disabil. 1997;30:685–93.

40. Malisza KL, Allman AA, Shiloff D, Jakobson L, Longstaffe S, Chudley AE. Evaluation of spatial working memory function in children and adults with fetal alcohol spectrum disorders: a functional magnetic resonance imaging study. Pediatr Res. 2005;58:1150–7.

41. Fagerlund A, Heikkinen S, Autti-Rämö I, Korkman M, Timonen M, Kuusi T, Riley EP, Lundbom N. Brain metabolic alterations in adolescents and young adults with fetal alcohol spectrum disorders. Alcohol Clin Exp Res. 2006;30(12):2097–104.

42. Committee on Substance Abuse and Committee on Children with Disabilities. Fetal alcohol syndrome and alcohol-related neurodevelopmental disorders. Pediatrics. 2000;106:358–61.

43. Greenbaum R, Nulman I, Rovet J, Koren G. The Toronto experience in diagnosing alcohol-related neurodevelopmental disorder: A unique profile of deficits and assets. Can J Clin Pharmacol. 2002;9:215–25.

44. Johnson JL, Leff M. Children of substance abusers: overview of research findings. Pediatrics. 1999;103:1085–99.

45. Streissguth AP. Fetal alcohol syndrome in older patients. Alcohol. 1993;2:209–12.

46. Yates WR, Cadoret RJ, Troughton EP, Stewart M, Giunta TS. Effect of fetal alcohol exposure on adult symptoms of nicotine, alcohol, and drug dependence. Alcohol Clin Exp Res. 1998;22:914–20.

47. Alati R, Clavarino A, Najman JM, O'Callaghan M, Bor W, Mamun AA. Williams GM The developmental origin of adolescent alcohol use: findings from the Mater University Study of Pregnancy and its outcomes. Drug Alcohol Depend. 2008;98(1–2):136–43.

48. Harwood HJ, Fountain D, Livermore G. Economic costs of alcohol abuse and alcoholism. Recent Dev Alcohol. 1998;14:307–30.

49. Centers for Disease Control and Prevention (CDC). Identification of children with fetal alcohol syndrome and opportunity for referral of their mothers for primary prevention-Washington, 1993–1997. MMWR Morb Mortal Wkly Rep. 1998;47(40):861–4.

50. Stade B, Ungar WJ, Stevens B, Beyen J, Koren G. Cost of fetal alcohol spectrum disorder in Canada. Can Fam Physician. 2007;53:1303–4.

51. Stade BC, Stevens B, Ungar WJ, Beyene J, Koren G. Health-related quality of life of Canadian children and youth prenatally exposed to alcohol. Health Qual Life Outcomes. 2006;13(4):81.

52. Habbick BF, Nanson JL, Snyder RE, Casey RE. Mortality in fetal alcohol syndrome. Can J Public Health. 1997;88:181–3.

53. Burd L, Klug M, Martsolf J. Increased sibling mortality in children with fetal alcohol syndrome. Addict Biol. 2004;9:179–86. discussion 187–8.

54. Burd L, Wilson H. Fetal, infant, and child mortality in a context of alcohol use. Am J Med Genet C Semin Med Genet. 2004;27:51–8.

55. Fast DK, Conry J, Loock CA. Identifying fetal alcohol syndrome among youth in the criminal justice system. J Dev Behav Pediatr. 1999;20(5):370–2.

56. Conry J, Fast DK. Fetal alcohol syndrome and the criminal justice system. Vancouver: Fetal Alcohol Syndrome Resource Society; 2000.

57. Boland FJ, Chudley AE, Grant BA. The challenge of fetal alcohol syndrome in adult offender populations. Forum Corrections Res. 2003;14:61–4.

58. Russell M, Martier SS, Sokol RJ, Mudar P, Bottoms S, Jacobson S, Jacobson J. Screening for pregnancy-risk drinking. Alcohol Clin Exp Res. 1994;18(5):1156–61.

59. Bradley KA, Bush KR, McDonell MB, Malone T, Fihn SD, The Ambulatory Care Quality Improvement Project (ACQUIP). Screening for problem drinking: Comparison of CAGE and AUDIT. J Gen Intern Med. 1998;13(6):379–88.

60. Loock C, Conry J, Cook JL, Chudley AE, Rosales T. Identifying fetal alcohol spectrum disorder in primary care. Can Med Assoc J. 2005;172:628–30.

61. Astley SJ, Bailey D, Talbot C, Clarren SK. Fetal alcohol syndrome (FAS) primary prevention through FAS diagnosis: I Identification of high-risk birth mothers through the diagnosis of their children. Alcohol. 2000;35(5):499–508.

62. Astley SJ, Bailey D, Talbot C, Clarren SK. Fetal alcohol syndrome (FAS) primary prevention through fas diagnosis: II. A comprehensive profile of 80 birth mothers of children with FAS. Alcohol. 2000;35(5):509–19.

63. Kaskutas L, Greenfield TK. First effects of warning labels on alcoholic beverage containers. Drug Alcohol Depend. 1992;31(1):1–14.

64. Abel EL. Prevention of alcohol abuse-related birth effects—I Public education efforts. Alcohol. 1998;33(4):411–6.

65. Astley SJ. Fetal alcohol syndrome prevention in Washington State: evidence of success. Paediatr Perinat Epidemiol. 2004;18:344–51.

66. Chudley AE, Longstaffe S. Fetal alcohol syndrome and fetal alcohol spectrum disorder. In: Cassidy S, Alanson J, editors. Management of genetic syndromes. Thirdth ed. New York: Wiley; 2010. p. 363–80.

67. Chandrasena AN, Mukherjee RAS, Turk J. Fetal Alcohol Spectrum Disorders: An Overview of Interventions for Affected Individuals. Child and Adolescent Mental Health 2008 (early view) doi:10.1111/j.1475-3588.2008.00504.x

68. Kalberg WO. Buckley D FASD: What types of intervention and rehabilitation are useful? Neurosci Biobeh Rev. 2007;31(2):278–85.

69. Willford J, Richardson GA, Leech SL, Day NL. Verbal and visuospatial learning and memory function in children with moderate prenatal alcohol exposure. Alcohol Clin Exp Res. 2004;28(3):497–507.

70. Mattson SN, Roebuck TM. Acquisition and retention of verbal and nonverbal information in children with heavy prenatal alcohol exposure. Alcohol Clin Exp Res. 2002;26:875–82.

71. Streissguth A, Bookstein FL, Sampson PD, Barr HM. Neurobehavioral effects of prenatal alcohol: part III PLS analyses of neuropsychological tests. Neurotoxicol Teratol. 1989;11:493–507.

72. Coles CD, Lynch M. Adolescents with disabilities: Insights for individuals with FAS/E. In: Kleinfeld J, editor. Fantastic Antone grows up: adolescents and adults with fetal alcohol syndrome. Anchorage: University of Alaska Press; 2000. p. 247–58.

73. Grant T, Huggins J, Connor P, Pedersen JY, Whitney N, Streissguth A. A pilot community intervention for young women with fetal alcohol spectrum disorders. Commun Mental Health J. 2004;40(6):499–511.

74. May PA, Miller JH, Goodhart KA, Maestas OR, Buckley D, Trujillo PM, Gossage JP. Enhanced case management to prevent fetal alcohol spectrum disorders in Northern Plains communities. Matern Child Health J. 2008;12(6):747–59.

75. Square D. Fetal alcohol syndrome epidemic on Manitoba reserve. Can Med Assoc J. 1997;157(1):59–60.

Part IV

Current Issues in Drug Abuse and Addiction

Linda Simoni-Wastila and Hui-Wen Keri Yang

Abstract

Misuse and abuse of legal and illegal drugs constitute a current and growing problem among older adults. This chapter reviews the prevalence, risks and protective factors, screening and diagnosis, and treatment of drug abuse in older adults. Despite a wealth of information on the epidemiology and treatment of alcohol abuse in older adults, few data are available on drug abuse in this population. Limited evidence suggests that although illegal drug use among older adults is relatively rare compared to younger adults and adolescents, there is a growing problem of prescription drug misuse and abuse, with nonmedical use of prescription drugs among all adults aged ≥50 years estimated to increase to 2.7 million by 2020. Factors associated with drug misuse and abuse in older adults include female sex, social isolation, history of a substance use or mental health disorder, and medical exposure to prescription drugs with abuse potential. The paucity of validated screening and assessment instruments impedes the identification and diagnoses of substance use disorders in the older population. Thus, special approaches may be necessary when treating substance use disorders in older adults with multiple comorbidities and/or functional impairment, with the least intensive approaches considered first. In conclusion, psychoactive medications with abuse potential are used by at least one in four older adults. The treatment of substance use disorders in older adults may involve family and caretakers, and should take into account the unique physical, emotional, and cognitive factors associated with aging. Further research should focus on epidemiologic, health services, and screening and treatment aspects of drug abuse in older adults.

Learning Objectives
- Understand the prevalence of substance use disorders in older adults
- Describe the risk and protective factors uniquely associated with substance use disorders in older adults
- Identify symptoms and signs of substance use in older adults, and how to screen and assess their severity
- Understand the fundamentals of treating substance use disorders in geriatric patients

Issues that Need to be Addressed by Future Research
- Development and validation of screening, assessment, and diagnostic tools and instruments
- Epidemiological work to better estimate national and international prevalence of substance use in older populations
- Identification of risk and protective factors for substance use disorders in order to better develop effective prevention and intervention strategies
- Development of treatment approaches for substance-impaired older adults

L. Simoni-Wastila, B.S.Pharm., Ph.D. (✉) • H.-W.K. Yang, Ph.D.
Peter Lamy Center on Drug Therapy and Aging, School of Pharmacy,
University of Maryland Baltimore, Baltimore, MD, USA
e-mail: lsimoniw@rx.umaryland.edu

J.C. Verster et al. (eds.), *Drug Abuse and Addiction in Medical Illness: Causes, Consequences and Treatment*,
DOI 10.1007/978-1-4614-3375-0_37, © Springer Science+Business Media, LLC 2012

Introduction

The potential for misuse, abuse, and dependence on psycho-active drugs among older adults is a growing problem and there is considerable concern that the use of abusable drugs will grow as the baby-boom generation ages [1]. Unlike the illegal drugs of abuse among adolescents and younger adults (e.g., marijuana, cocaine, heroin), the substances abused by older adults are usually alcohol, nicotine, and prescription drugs. Also unlike use by younger individuals, the problem use of psychoactive substances by older adults is often unintentional rather than purposive.

In this chapter, we review the evidence for the abuse of prescription and illegal psychoactive drugs among older adults. The focus was on drugs with the potential for abuse, dependency, and/or addiction; we do not examine problem use of tobacco, alcohol, or medications available over-the-counter, although each of these substances (especially tobacco and alcohol) are sizable problems with significant clinical and economic ramifications. In this chapter, we cover: the current and projected prevalence of drug abuse in the older population; screening for, evaluating, and diagnosing drug abuse; treatment concerns specific to older adults; the health care and economic consequences of drug abuse; and recommendations to practitioners and researchers.

Definitions

For the purposes of this chapter, older adults include individuals aged 50 and older. In this review, we refer to "abuse" as problematic use of psychoactive drugs that could lead to adverse consequences such as diagnostically defined abuse or dependency, cognitive and/or physical impairment, limitations in social and daily living, and use that in any way impairs the normal functioning of older adults. Whenever possible, and as the literature allows, we identify those studies which use diagnostic definitions of abuse and dependency (such as those defined using DSM-IV criteria) [2]. In the older adult population, this standard definition may be overly broad; however, the reviewed literature of substance use lacks a standard definition of what constitutes psychoactive drug abuse in older adults. Indeed, many studies fail to provide a definition of abuse, dependency, or sufficient detail of how substance use is categorized. Finally, it is important to note that abuse does not necessarily connote "inappropriate use" as seen in a medical context and as defined by criteria such as those established by Beers [3, 4] and others [5, 6].

Drugs of Abuse and Dependence

Like their younger counterparts, younger adults are susceptible to abuse of both legal and illegal drugs. Illegal drugs include marijuana, hashish, heroin, cocaine and crack cocaine, methamphetamine, inhalants, hallucinogens such as LSD, Ecstasy, MDMA, and others. In general, the use of illegal drugs by older adults is limited to a small group of aging criminals and long-term heroin addicts, and new onset use disorders rarely develop in older age [7].

Legal drugs consist of medications obtainable by prescription or over-the-counter. As evidenced by research documenting the appropriateness of prescribed medicines in elders, much inappropriate use concerns psychoactive medications, many of which have addiction potential [3, 4, 8]. Inappropriate use of prescription drugs with addiction potential by elders encompasses a variety of behaviors ranging from sharing medications to using higher doses or for longer duration than prescribed to recreational use to persistent abuse and dependency. The therapeutic classes involved in prescription drug abuse include opioid analgesics, anxiolytics, sedative-hypnotics, and central nervous system stimulants. Table 37.1 summarizes the illegal and legal substances subject to abuse by older adults.

The two major classes of prescription drugs used by older adults include the opioid analgesics and benzodiazepine minor tranquilizers; less frequently, older adults misuse central nervous stimulants and non-benzodiazepine sedatives and hypnotics. When used appropriately, opioid analgesics provide pain relief and anesthesia; however, when used nonmedically, they can produce a sense of euphoria and well-being. As a result, opioid analgesics have the potential to produce physical and psychological dependency, sedation, and impair cognitive and physical functioning, especially when used in the long term [2, 9–11]. There is a common perception that abuse of illegal or prescription opioids is rare in the geriatric population except among those who have a history of abuse or when used with alcohol [12, 13].

In addition to the rapid development of tolerance and physiological dependence on the opioid analgesics, older patients using these medications are at increased risk of increased sedation, impairment of motor coordination (particularly with the weaker opioid analgesics such as codeine and propoxyphene), and substantial impairment of vision, attention, and motor coordination with stronger opioids such as oxycodone and intramuscular meperidine [11] (although no relation between increasing age and sedation has been noted in patients treated with morphine and pentazocine) [14, 15]. Although opioid analgesic withdrawal is uncomfortable (characterized by restlessness, nausea and/or vomiting, dysphoria, aching muscles, diarrhea, and insomnia), it is not potentially life threatening.

Table 37.1 Illegal and legal drugs subject to abuse and dependence in older adults

Illegal drugs	Marijuana and hashish	
	Heroin	
	Cocaine and crack cocaine	
	Hallucinogens	Lysergic acid diethylamide (LSD), Ecstasy (3,4-methylenedioxymethamphetamine
Prescription drugs	Benzodiazepines	Long-acting: flurazepam, diazepam
		Short-acting: alprazolam, lorazepam, triazolam, temazepam
	Barbiturate and nonbarbiturate sedative-hypnotics	Pentobarbital, secobarbital, aprobarbital/ and secobarbital, chloral hydrate, ethchlorvynol, glutethimide
	Opioid analgesics	Morphine, levorphanol, methadone, codeine, hydrocodone, oxycodone, propoxyphene, fentanyl, tramadol
	Central nervous system stimulants	Methylphenidate, methamphetamine, dextroamphetamine, amphetamine–dextroamphetamine

Primarily used to treat anxiety and sleep disorders, benzodiazepines have largely replaced barbiturate and nonbarbiturate sedatives and hypnotics due to their improved safety profile over these older products [7, 16]. Nevertheless, when use involves long-acting products, prolonged duration of use exceeding 4 months, and/or use exceeding ten diazepam-milligram equivalents per day, benzodiazepines can induce dependence [7, 17–19]. In older adults, this dependence may manifest itself in the absence of apparent abuse [20]. It is important to recognize that all benzodiazepines demonstrate physiological dependence even at therapeutic doses and for as short a duration as 2 months [21]. Because of this potential, longer half-life benzodiazepines such as flurazepam should be avoided in older adults due to their sedative effects and their association to adverse outcomes including falls, motor vehicle accidents, and worsened memory [7, 12, 22–24]. Benzodiazepines and other sedative-hypnotics should be used judiciously in older adults when prescribed for sleep disorders. No research has documented the long-term effectiveness of these drugs for insomnia beyond 30 days; thus, their use should be limited to 7–10 days in the lowest possible dose, with frequent monitoring and evaluation, and with no more than a 30-day supply [7]. The most commonly prescribed hypnotic benzodiazepine hypnotics in older adults are oxazepam, temazepam, triazolam, and lorazepam [25].

Benzodiazepine withdrawal should be carefully monitored. Symptoms of withdrawal include increased pulse, hand tremor, insomnia, nausea and/or vomiting, and rebound anxiety. Grand mal seizures occur in 20–30% of all dependent persons whose withdrawal symptoms are untreated [11, 17]. Another relatively common adverse effect of untreated benzodiazepine withdrawal is hallucinations, such as those associated with alcoholic delirium tremens (DTs) [11, 17]. Both seizures and DTs can be life threatening in individuals undergoing either involuntary or medical benzodiazepine withdrawal.

Prevalence

Little is known about the epidemiology of psychoactive drug use disorders in older adults. This is due to under-sampling of older adults in surveys that collect information on drug use, lack of standard definitions of abuse and dependency in this population, and prevalence estimates for narrowly defined populations and settings ranging from community to long-term care residences to emergency department and inpatient substance abuse treatment programs.

Illegal Drugs

Illegal drug use is rare among older adults, although illicit substance use is projected to rise as the baby-boom population enters retirement. In one of the few national studies of prevalence available, the Epidemiologic Catchment Area Study found that the lifetime prevalence rates of drug abuse and dependence is 0.12% for older men and 0.06% for women; the lifetime history of illegal drug use among older men and women was 2.88% and 0.66%, respectively [26].

There is a limited but growing literature that suggests illegal substance abuse is becoming more common in older adults seeking treatment. Indeed, the percentage of adults aged 55 and older receiving treatment for substance abuse nearly tripled between 1995 and 2002 (from 50,200 admissions to 66,500) [27]. Among patients aged 55 and older with diagnoses of both psychiatric and substance use disorders receiving services through Veteran's Administration, 26% reported a drug use disorder whereas the remaining 74% had an alcohol disorder [28]. Older methadone maintenance patients are relatively rare, most likely due to initial regulations (now removed) that capped maintenance at age 40, as well as the theory that heroin addicts "mature out" of addiction problems by age 40 [12]. Older methadone maintenance patients have higher rates of comorbid mental health disorders and worse physical health functioning than general population norms for their non-using peers [29]. Mortality rates among heroin users are high; in one 24-year follow-up study of heroin addicts, more than 27% of the study subjects had died [30]. In other words, older addicts may simply represent younger addicts who have survived their drug use disorder [31].

Cocaine use in older populations is not well documented in the literature. One study presented evidence of cocaine use in adults aged 60 and older presenting to a large urban emergency department over a 6-month period [32]. Among 911 visits, the urine samples of 18 older patients, or 2.0%, tested positive for cocaine. Rates of treatment for older adults entering treatment for cocaine abuse are estimated at 0.2% for patients aged 61–65 years, and 0.1% for those aged 65 and older [33]. In a second study of geriatric patients receiving a substance abuse consultation, 10.2% reported cocaine use [34]. Another study of 684 individuals aged 50 and older with a lifetime history of intravenous cocaine and/or heroin use found 13.0% were daily cocaine users [35]. One study of 565 geriatric inpatients in the Veterans Administration system found that 1.0% had an illegal drug use disorder [36], while another found 38% of older veterans in treatment reported recent illegal substance use [37].

Prescription Drugs

Although Americans aged 65 and older represent 13.0% of the total US population, they account for 36.0% of total outpatient prescription medication spending [38]. Furthermore, growth in prescription drug use and spending among older adults is increasing—at least one study estimates that drug spending among insured elders has increased by more than 18% annually between 1997 and 2000 [39]. In 2000, the average older citizen received more than 20 prescriptions per year, representing an average of 4.7 different therapeutic classes [39].

Older adults who abuse or become dependent upon prescription psychoactive drugs may be markedly different than older adults who purposively abuse marijuana, cocaine, heroin, and other illegal substances. Unlike use patterns demonstrated by younger adults, problematic prescription drug use by older adults is usually unintentional and is best described as a continuum that ranges from appropriate use for medical or psychiatric conditions through non-medical use, or misuse, to persistent abuse and dependence, as characterized by the Diagnostic and Statistical Manual of Mental Disorders, Fourth Edition (DSM-IV) [2]. Non-medical use encompasses a wide range of behaviors including a single incidence of medical misuse or medically inappropriate use (e.g., "borrowing" a product from a friend or relative who is legally prescribed the drug), periodic recreational use, and physiologic addiction [2, 7]. Other behaviors characteristic of misuse include using higher doses than prescribed, using for purposes other than indicated, hoarding drugs, and using with other substances and/or alcohol. These patterns of use can lead to addiction, which is marked by signs of tolerance, withdrawal, reduction in normal activities, and declines in home or work performance [2]. It is important to note that misuse behaviors can be promulgated by the patient, the provider, or both. In the geriatric population, medical exposure to abusable prescription medications is itself a risk factor for potentially problematic use.

Older adults can become physiologically dependent upon prescription medications without meeting dependence criteria. Tolerance and physical dependence can develop when prescription medications such as benzodiazepines and opioid analgesics are taken at appropriate doses for even short periods of time. Thus, withdrawal symptoms or an abstinence syndrome can occur if the drug is abruptly discontinued. In older adults, iatrogenically induced physiological dependence is usually not accompanied by purposive attempts of the patient to increase dosage during or after withdrawal, to experience craving after discontinuation, or to continue use or addictive behaviors [7, 21].

A growing body of literature has begun to document the prevalence of inappropriate prescription drug use in older adults [3, 4, 8, 40–44]. The most recently available research suggests that 7.2 million older adults, or 21.7% of older adults residing in the community, used at least one controlled prescription drug with abuse potential in 1999 [45]. This study found that 14.9% of the nation's older adults received at least one controlled opioid analgesic and 10.4% received at least one anxiolytic or sedative-hypnotic [45]. Other studies have confirmed the prevalent exposure of community-dwelling older adults to psychoactive prescription medications with abuse potential, with estimates ranging from 5% to 33%. [8, 13, 16, 46–48], depending upon the population sampled, the drugs defined as psychoactive, and the year the estimate was made. Although several studies note older adults are more likely to use psychoactive medications than their younger counterparts [21, 23], it should be noted that many of these studies do not differentiate between psychoactive drugs with dependency potential (e.g., benzodiazepines and opioid analgesics) and those without dependency potential (e.g., antidepressants and antipsychotics).

A population often overlooked in considering substance use disorders and risk of their development are older adults residing in nursing homes and other institutions, including hospitals. Exposure to abusable prescription medications is quite high in this particularly frail population; one study found that among nursing home residents in 878 facilities, 11% received an anxiolytic and 3% received a sedative-hypnotic medication [49].

There is considerably less information on the prevalence of prescription drug abuse and dependence among older adults. One report estimates that 300,000 older adults aged 55 and older reported past-month non-medical use of at least one prescription drug [50]. In a recent report, it is estimated 2.8 million (11.0%) of US women aged 60 and older misuse psychoactive prescription medications [51]. Among older adults seeking treatment for any substance use (excluding alcohol), it is estimated that one in ten clients reported used of at least one prescription drug in the 30 days prior to admission [52]; of these, 17.7% reported prescription drugs as their drugs of choice. In a recent report of treatment episodes, 50,700 persons aged 55 or older were admitted to publicly funded substance abuse treatment facilities [50]. Among this group, alcohol was the primary substance of abuse for 76%; legal and illegal opioid analgesics were the primary drug for 12.6%, and prescription sedatives, tranquilizers, and stimulants accounted for 1.3% of use.

Older adults will comprise a growing segment of the future treatment population. One study estimated the number of adults aged 50 and older requiring treatment for a substance use disorder will grow to 4.4 million in 2020, up from 1.7 million in 2001 [53]. Of these 2.3% of older adults at baseline who required treatment for substance use disorders in 2001, 10.2% were dependent upon or abusing drugs only, 4.0% were dependent upon or abusing both drugs and alcohol, and the remaining 85.8% were dependent upon or abusing alcohol. Among the 244,000 older adults dependent upon or abusing drugs, the most common drugs were marijuana (42%), cocaine (36%), pain relievers (25%), stimulants (18%), and sedatives (17%). A recently published analysis estimates the non-medical use of psychoactive prescription drugs by adults aged 50 and older will increase from 911,000 in 2001 to nearly 2.7 million in 2020 [54]. These projected estimates are due to: (1) the increase in the sheer number of older adults and (2) the increase in the rate of treatment need by this population [53, 54]. Estimates are also fuelled by the premise that the baby boom cohort is larger than earlier cohorts (although following cohorts are as large or larger than the baby-boom group) and the fact that this particular cohort is composed of heavy illegal and legal psychoactive drug users.

Factors Associated with Drug Abuse

Although mature adults are less likely than younger counterparts to abuse psychoactive drugs, once they use they may be particularly vulnerable to developing substance use dependence [55, 56]. This increased risk is due to several factors unique to older adults, including increased frailty, changes in body composition and drug metabolism, increased morbidity, and high utilization of prescription medications

Table 37.2 Risk factors for prescription drug abuse in older adults

Female sex
Social isolation (living alone or with nonspousal others)
Poor health status
Significant drug burden/polypharmacy
Chronic physical illness/polymorbidity
Previous and/or concurrent substance use disorder
Previous and/or concurrent psychiatric illness

(including their use of psychoactive medications with addiction potential). Collectively, these factors place older adults at increased risk for iatrogenic complications, including dependency and abuse.

There is a paucity of literature describing correlates associated with illegal drug use by older adults. In a small study of older cocaine users presenting to an urban emergency department, cocaine users were more likely to be younger (66.4 years vs. 76.0 years), males (88.9% vs. 46.6%), and more likely to be diagnosed with drug or alcohol abuse compared with the older adults negative for cocaine use [32]. Because late-life development of new psychoactive drug abuse is rare in older adults, it is likely, though unproven, that the most important correlate of use is prior abuse.

While little is understood about the risk and protective factors unique to prescription drug abuse in older adults, several variables emerge as predictors in the general population and may be generalizable to older adults as well. Table 37.2 lists the main risk factors associated with prescription drug abuse in older adults. These factors include female gender, younger and older ages, white race, poor health status, living in rural areas, and social isolation [11, 45, 57–70]. In a recent study that examined correlates of abusable prescription drug use in Medicare beneficiaries aged 65 and older, female sex, white race, those aged 65–79, those with one or more limitation in activities of daily living, increasing number of comorbid conditions, large drug burden, and those living with non-spousal others were significantly more likely to use one or more abusable prescription drugs in the past year [45].

Female gender is perhaps among the most studied risk factor for prescription drug problem use. Older women are prescribed more and consume more psychoactive medications than men, particularly benzodiazepines, and are more likely to be long-term users of these substances [7]. Among older women, use of psychoactive drugs is associated with recent divorce and widowhood, lower education, lower income, poorer health status, and depression and anxiety disorders [71–74]. Szwabo [75] suggests prescription drug misuse is a growing problem among older impoverished and minority women. Indeed, one study suggests that with increasing age, women are more likely to report 12-month dependency and meet dependence criteria than their older male peers [76]. Among older women, use of psychoactive drugs is associated with recent divorce and widowhood, lower education, lower income, and depression and anxiety disorders [72–74].

Several studies have examined gender differences in substance use and dependence, including prescription drugs with addiction potential. In a study based on the 1990–1992 National Comorbidity Survey (NCS), Anthony and colleagues found the prevalence of lifetime dependence on anxiolytics and sedative-hypnotics in women aged 15–54 was 12.3%, more than two times greater than the lifetime prevalence in men [71]. This finding stands in sharp contrast to men's generally higher risk for developing lifetime dependence on alcohol and marijuana. To the extent earlier psychoactive drug use in earlier years translates into later life use, this information may be useful in predicting treatment need resource differences for older men and women in the future. Reasons for drug-specific sex differences in dependence include men's preference for alcohol [77] and the possibility that among psychotherapeutic users, women use more heavily than men.

Other risk factors for developing prescription drug abuse include prior and concurrent substance use and psychiatric illness [58, 64, 78–81]. One study estimated that nearly 80% of the persons with a psychoactive drug disorder also had an alcohol or mental comorbidity [74]. Both historical and concurrent substance use are associated with non-medical prescription drug use [58, 59, 61, 70, 80–83]. Anxiety and affective disorders have been shown, along with alcohol-related disorders, to be highly correlated with lifetime drug dependency [78]. In one study, rates of mental health conditions among 100 older adults hospitalized for prescription drug dependence included mood disorders (32%), organic mental problems (28%), personality disorders (27%), somatoform disorders (16%), and anxiety (12%) [84]. Although research on older adults with substance dependence disorders is rare, one study indicates that older addicts are more likely than younger addicts to have a dual diagnosis, with 85% of older drug-dependent patients had a dual diagnosis compared with 36% of younger drug-dependent patients [15].

Benzodiazepine abuse liability, while generally rare [19, 78], may exist in individuals who are light-to-moderate alcohol drinkers, have a history of sedative abuse or poly-drug abuse, who were methadone-maintained, and who have developed physiologic dependence on benzodiazepines after long-term use and who experience acute withdrawal effects following abrupt discontinuation [18, 19, 78]. Also of importance are provider and economic variables. In particular, physician specialty influences drug prescribing, with primary care physicians prescribing more psychotropics of any type, including opioid analgesics and minor tranquilizers, than specialists [63].

Several studies also suggest a link between medical opioid analgesic exposure and eventual abuse and dependency

[2, 9, 11, 75, 85], with individuals suffering from chronic non-cancer pain more likely to develop opioid drug use disorders than individuals suffering acute or chronic cancer pain [85, 86]. Finally, there is limited evidence that problematic prescription opioid use may be differentiated from medically appropriate use based on drug, dose, formulation, and dosage form [87–89].

Screening and Assessment

The great majority of older adults (87%) see physicians regularly; however, 40% of those older adults at risk for developing substance use disorders do not self-identify or seek services for these problems on their own [13]. These patients are unlikely to be recognized by their physicians as having a substance use disorder, despite the frequency of provider contact. In one study of primary care physicians presented patient scenarios of older women indicative of potential substance abuse problems, only 1% accurately recognized these symptoms; the remainder diagnosed the patient with depression, anxiety, and/or stress problems [51]. Misdiagnoses of this sort can be medically dangerous, as the treatment for anxiety and other related disorders often is a benzodiazepine or other potentially abusable prescription medication, which only potentiates the drug abuse problem.

Similarly, comorbid conditions may complicate the diagnosis of substance abuse in older adults (Table 37.3). Many of these conditions may be antecedent or consequent to abuse, serving as warning signs to health care providers in detecting

Table 37.3 Comorbid conditions that may complicate the diagnosis of prescription drug abuse in older adults

Neuropsychological	Psychiatric conditions (depression, anxiety, mood disorders, schizophrenia, or psychotic disorders)
	Cognitive impairment (e.g., Alzheimer's disease, dementia)
	Delirium
	Personality changes
	Mood changes or swings (depression, agitation)
	Seizures
	Tremor
	Sleep complaints (insomnia or hypersomnia)
Medical	Chronic pain
	Gastrointestinal disorders
	Hepatic and/or renal disorders
Functional	Falls, fractures, or other trauma
	Functional decline
	Hygiene deterioration
	Motor vehicle accidents

abuse or masking its symptoms. For example, cognitive impairment, including dementia, is an important condition which makes screening for prescription drug abuse difficult. Some of the symptoms of dementia, such as agitation, delirium, combativeness, and mood shifts, are the same symptoms associated with substance abuse. Early signs of depressant misuse and abuse, for example, include such symptoms as decreased energy, weight loss, irritability, heart burn and other gastrointestinal distress, and insomnia [7, 20, 51].

A nonconfrontational approach with the collateral participation from family members or friends is suggested in this type of situation where an accurate response is unlikely to be obtained from the older adult [11].

Although there are a myriad of instruments available for screening and assessing alcohol and other substance use disorders, few instruments are pertinent to older adults and fewer still screen for problems relate to prescription drugs. The CAGE and the Michigan Alcoholism Screening Test_ Geriatric Version (MAST-G) are two well-known alcohol screening instruments whose use has been validated in older adults [11, 90]. Unfortunately, no similar screening instruments have been validated for use of illegal or prescription psychoactive drugs in general or specifically for use in older adults. Thus, screening for illegal and prescription drug abuse in older adults requires providers to ask questions about the drugs they are taking, the side effects the patient may experience, where the prescriptions are filled, the use of over-the-counter, and supplemental or alternative medications (including medical marijuana use and other herbal substances). Additional warning signs that may emerge in patient-provider conversations include: excessive worry about whether psychoactive medications are really working, display of detailed knowledge and attachment to a particular psychoactive medication, excessive worry about supply and timing of medications, continued use or refill request when the medical condition for which the medication was originally prescribed should have resolved, complaints about physicians who refuse to write prescriptions for preferred drugs, who reduce or taper dosages, or do not take symptoms seriously, excessive sleeping (especially during the day), changes in personal grooming and hygiene, withdrawal from family, friends and normal and life-long social activities, among others [11].

Once an older adult has screened positive for a potential drug problem, an assessment is needed to confirm the problem, to characterize the dimensions of the problem, and to develop an individualized treatment plan [11]. This is often accomplished using criteria established in the Diagnostic and Statistical Manual of Mental Disorders, Fourth Edition (DSM-IV) [2]. These criteria include: (1) failure to fulfill major role obligations at home, work or school; (2) physically hazardous situations; (3) substance-related legal problems; or (4) recurrent social or interpersonal problems.

It is significant, however, that these criteria often do not pertain to older adults—most older adults do not work or attend school, many no longer drive or operate dangerous equipment, which in turn may reduce legal consequences such as driving while impaired, and finally, many older adults live alone and/or have limited mobility, making substance-related interpersonal problems less apparent [20].

The current older geriatric patient often is loathe to discuss possible problems with substance use. Such reluctance is due to lack of knowledge or insight as prescription medication use might be within prescribed limits, as well as because they may not recognize symptoms, such as insomnia, as associated with drug misuse [16]. Among older adults who suspect drug use is associated with health and psychological complaints, few may admit it due to shame, guilt, and stigma associated with drug use in their age cohort [91, 92].

Treatment

Little information exists on the comparative efficacy of various approaches for the treatment of drug use disorders in older adults. A primary reason for the lack of clinical studies of treatment effectiveness in mature adults is the rarity of impaired older individuals presenting with possible drug use problems, resulting in difficulties in enrolling sufficient numbers of older adults [31]. This is unfortunate as a growing body of research suggests older adults admitted for treatment generally have a favorable prognosis [93, 94].

Older adults may require specialized treatment modalities due to their older age, the probability of more severe addiction, and the increased likelihood of comorbid conditions that makes detoxification riskier [12]. For example, opioid detoxification in older adults often requires a medical setting, and although the choice of medication may not differ from that of their younger counterparts, the dosage may differ due to differences in metabolism [12]. As well, clinicians need to pay close attention to potential drug–drug interactions and drug–disease interactions in the older adult receiving treatment [12].

Treatment of benzodiazepine dependence is accomplished by very gradual tapering to avoid withdrawal symptoms [15, 18, 19]. Benzodiazepine withdrawal symptoms in older adults are usually different from those seen in younger people; in older adults, withdrawal symptoms include confusion and disorientation rather than anxiety, insomnia, and perceptual changes and that withdrawal symptoms also are usually less severe in older adults who are gradually tapered [95].

Whatever the substance, when examining treatment options for impaired older adults, the least intensive treatment options should be the first explored [11]. These initial approaches can function as either pretreatment or treatment strategies, and include brief interventions, interventions,

Table 37.4 Strategies to improve the treatment of prescription drug abuse in older adults

Treatment Strategies	Summary
Brief interventions	One or more counseling sessions involving direct feedback on screening questions; patient education; approaches to motivational and behavioral change; use of written manuals and materials to reinforce message
Interventions	Counseling sessions with patient in the presence of family or friends to confront drug-use problems
Motivational counseling	Intensive meetings with counselor to understand patient's perspective on the situation, assess readiness to change behaviors, help patient shift perspective and consider alternative solutions
Specialized treatment	Inpatient/outpatient detoxification, inpatient/outpatient rehabilitation, outpatient services
Maintenance treatment	Psychotherapy, individual and/or group counseling, self-help and 12-step programs

motivational counseling, and specialized treatment approaches [11]. Table 37.4 summarizes strategies to improve treatment for older adults with prescription drug abuse problems. Brief interventions range from somewhat unstructured counseling to motivational and behavioral self-control psychological approaches. Interventions generally involve the presence of family members and friends who, under the guidance of a counselor, confront the impaired older adult with their experiences and perceptions of their drug use. Motivational counseling builds on an individual's recognition of the problem and his/her readiness to change behaviors to treat the problem [11]. In addition, an educational approach involving communication skills to help patients identify problem prescription drug use and motivate them to obtain treatment is especially important in prescription drug abuse. Strategies include identifying causes of noncompliance, educating and assisting patients to manage medications and use correct dosing instructions, and describing the consequences of prescription drug abuse on the patient's health and functional status.

If these modalities are not sufficient treatment strategies, more specialized treatment services including admission to medical or psychiatric inpatient facilities should be considered. Such intensive services include inpatient or outpatient detoxification, inpatient rehabilitation, outpatient rehabilitation, and specialized outpatient services. Detoxification is riskier for older adults; thus, it is advisable to provide them 24-h primary medical, psychiatric, and nursing [11]. Once stabilized and returned to the community, older adults, like their younger counterparts, may benefit from 12-step and other self-help groups, as well as individual and/or group counseling and psychotherapy.

Consequences of Use

There are medical and economic consequences associated with substance abuse by older adults. Clinical and functioning problems associated with the misuse and abuse of illegal and prescription drugs are numerous and include drowsiness, sedation, confusion, memory loss and other cognitive impairments, falls, and other accidents [7, 20]. These impairments, in turn, can lead to hospitalization and institutionalization [96].

Adverse consequences associated with many substances drugs are heightened when used with alcohol, which also is a depressant [97]. Indeed, although older adults generally have lower rates of heavy drinking than do their younger counterparts [98, 99], many older adults use alcohol in patterns that run counter to current guidelines [99]. Metabolic and physiologic changes that occur in older age can make even an occasional drink problematic [13]. Nearly all drugs with abuse potential, especially prescription drugs, tend to be cross-tolerant with alcohol; thus, the central nervous system depressant effects of benzodiazepines, other sedative-hypnotics, and the opioid analgesics tend to be markedly enhanced by the addition of even relatively small amounts of alcohol and can even be lethal [2, 11]. A recent study of older, low-to-moderate income adults enrolled in the Pennsylvania Pharmaceutical Assistance Contract for the Elderly (PACE) examined the potential for alcohol interactions with prescription drugs, many of which have abuse liability [100]. This study found that 77% of all drug users were exposed to prescription medications that interact with alcohol and of these, 19% reported concomitant alcohol use. Among narcotic analgesic users, 16.7% reported concomitant alcohol use and among users of anxiolytics and sedative-hypnotics, 16.8% reported concomitant alcohol use. Related to this is the potential for interactions with other drugs. This is particularly problematic in older adults, as they tend to consume more prescription and over-the-counter medications, on average, than do younger individuals.

Substance use adds considerably to the nation's health care expenditures. Although no research to date has attempted to quantify the economic costs explicitly associated with the drug use disorders among older adults, the annual total costs associated with all substance use disorders is estimated at $276 billion [101]. Almost 20% of all Medicaid hospital costs, and nearly $1 of every $4 of Medicare hospital costs, are associated with substance use [102]. Several studies have found that individuals with substance use disorders use more health care resources and incur higher health care costs than those without substance use problems [53]. Hospitals and emergency departments also are used more frequently by substance abusers, who may utilize these services in hopes of seeking prescription drugs or because they are suffering from adverse effects, such as overdose, associated with prescription drugs.

Illegal drug users make nearly 530,000 visits to expensive emergency departments each year for drug-related problems [103]. Emergency department episodes associated with involving prescriptions for opioid analgesics have increased markedly from 1994 to 2001, with visits involving oxycodone increasing 352%, methadone increasing by 230%, and morphine by 210% [53]. Further, individuals coming to emergency departments often use more than one drug; multiple drugs were mentioned in 72% of all emergency department visits involving opioid analgesics [53].

Conclusions

Although older adults are vulnerable to psychoactive drug abuse, especially prescribed medications, there is a paucity of evidence on factors associated with abuse, screening, assessment and diagnosis, and treatment. Current national and international prevalence estimates are lacking, due largely to the inability of adequate available data. More research on patient, provider, socioeconomic, environmental, and clinical factors associated with psychoactive drug abuse and dependence in older adults is necessary to understand how use progresses from medical exposure to problematic use, as well as to document factors that may contribute to—or protect from—the development of psychoactive drug abuse. Knowledge of such factors is necessary in order to develop and implement prevention and education resources for patients and providers. Considerably more study is required to develop and validate adequate screening and assessment instruments tailored to older individuals and the drugs that they abuse. Finally, resources need to be allocated to identify and test treatment modalities in older adults with psychoactive drug use disorders.

Practitioners need to be educated on potential psychoactive drug use problems in older adults. For physicians and other health care providers, this means being aware of and eliciting through conversation and medical workup the signs and symptoms of possible drug use disorders, including marked changes in demeanor and mood, increased use or seeking of psychoactive medications, changes in regular social activities, changes in functioning and activities of daily living, and evidence of growing cognitive and physical impairment. As well, evidence of falls, motor vehicle accidents, and other injury and trauma also should be reviewed for possible involvement of psychoactive medication use. Family members and other formal and informal caregivers should be attuned to the same issues as providers.

Acknowledgments The author would like to thank David Maccharia, PharmD and Nikki Mehdizadegan, B, both pharmacy students at the University of Maryland Baltimore School of Pharmacy, for their assistance in identifying, retrieving, and organizing relevant manuscripts.

References

1. Culberson J, Ziska M. Prescription drug misuse/abuse in the elderly. Geriatrics. 2008;63(9):22–31.
2. American Psychiatric Association. Diagnostic and statistical manual of mental disorders. 4th ed. Washington, DC: APA; 1994.
3. Beers MH. Explicit criteria for determining potentially inappropriate medication use by the elderly. An update. Arch Intern Med. 1997;157(14):1531–6.
4. Beers MH, Ouslander JG, Rollingher I, Reuben DB, Brooks J, Beck JC. Explicit criteria for determining inappropriate medication use in nursing home residents UCLA Division of Geriatric Medicine. Arch Intern Med. 1991;151(9):1825–32.
5. Briesacher B, Limcangco R, Simoni-Wastila L, Doshi J, Gurwitz J. Evaluation of nationally-mandated drug use reviews to improve patient safety in nursing homes: a natural experiment. J Am Geriatr Soc. 2005;53(6):991–8.
6. Charlson ME, Pompei P, Ales KL, MacKenzie CR. A new method of classifying prognostic comorbidity in longitudinal studies: development and validation. J Chronic Dis. 1987;40(5): 373–83.
7. SAMHSA. Substance abuse among older adults. Rockville, MD: Substance Abuse and Mental Health Services Administration. Center for Substance Abuse Treatment; 1998. DHHS Publication Number SMA 98–3179.
8. Zhan C, Sangl J, Bierman AS, et al. Potentially inappropriate medication use in the community-dwelling elderly: findings from the 1996 Medical Expenditure Panel Survey. J Am Med Assoc. 2001;286(22):2823–9.
9. Cowan C. Coverage, sample design, and weighting in three federal surveys. J Drug Issues. 2001;31:599–614.
10. Joranson DE, Ryan KM, Gilson AM, Dahl JL. Trends in medical use and abuse of opioid analgesics. J Am Med Assoc. 2000; 283(13):1710–4.
11. Blow FC. Substance abuse among older adults treatment protocol (TIP). Rockville, MD: USDHSS/PHS/SAMHSA Center for Substance Abuse Treatment; 2001.
12. Menninger JA. Assessment and treatment of alcoholism and substance-related disorders in the elderly. Bull Menninger Clin. 2002;66(2):166–83.
13. Jinks MJ, Raschko RR. A profile of alcohol and prescription drug abuse in a high-risk community-based elderly population. DICP. 1990;24(10):971–5.
14. Ray WA, Thapa PB, Shorr RI. Medications and the older driver. Clin Geriatr Med. 1993;9(2):413–38.
15. Solomon K, Manapelli J, Ireland G, Mahon G. Alcoholism and prescription drug abuse in the elderly: St Louis grand rounds. J Am Geriatr Soc. 1993;41(1):57–69.
16. Finlayson R. Misuse of prescription drugs. Int J Addict. 1995;301(13 and 14):1871–901.
17. Salzman C. Benzodiazepine dependence, toxicity, and abuse: a task force report of the American Psychiatric Association. Washington, DC: American Psychiatric Association; 1990.
18. Salzman C. Benzodiazepine treatment of panic and agoraphobic symptoms: use, dependence, toxicity, abuse. J Psychiatr Res. 1993;27:97–110.
19. Salzman C. Issues and controversies regarding benzodiazepine use. Washington, DC: NIDA; 1993. NIDA Research Monograph Series no. 131; NIH Pub. No. 93–3507.
20. Fingeld-Connett DL. Treatment of substance misuse in older women: using a brief intervention model. J Gerontol Nursing. 2004;30(8):30–7.
21. Woods J, Winger G. Current benzodiazepine issues. Psychopharmacology. 1995;118(2):107–15.

22. Hanlon JT, Horner RD, Schmader KE, et al. Benzodiazepine use and cognitive function among community-dwelling elderly. Clin Pharmacol Ther. 1998;64(6):684–92.

23. Sheahan SL, Coons SJ, Robbins CA, Martin SS, Hendricks J, Latimer M. Psychoactive medication, alcohol use, and falls among older adults. J Behav Med. 1995;18(2):127–40.

24. Leipzig RM, Cumming RG, Tinetti ME. Drugs and falls in older people: a systematic review and meta-analysis: I Psychotropic drugs. J Am Geriatr Soc. 1999;47(1):30–9.

25. Fouts M, Rachow J. Choice of hypnotics in the elderly. P and T News. 1994;14(8):1–4.

26. Anthony J, Helzer J. Syndromes of drug abuse and dependence. In: Robins L, Regier D, editors. Psychiatric disorders in America: the epidemiologic catchment area study. New York: The Free Press; 1991. p. 116–54.

27. SAMHSA. The DASIS Report: Older Adults in Substance Abuse Treatment. The DASIS Report; 2005.

28. Prigerson HG, Desai RA, Rosenheck RA. Older adult patients with both psychiatric and substance abuse disorders: prevalence and health service use. Psychiatr Quart. 2001;72(1):1–18.

29. Rosen D, Smith M, Reynolds C. The prevalence of mental and physical health disorders among older methadone patients. Am J Geriatr Psychiatr. 2008;16(6):488–97.

30. Hser Y, Anglin D, Powers K. A 24-year follow-up of California narcotics addicts. Arch Gen Psychiatr. 1993;50:577–84.

31. Oslin DW. Evidence-based treatment of geriatric substance abuse. Psychiatr Clin North Am. 2005;28(4):897–911.

32. Rivers E, Shirazi E, Aurora T, et al. Cocaine use in elder patients presenting to an inner-city emergency department. Acad Emerg Med. 2004;11(8):874–7.

33. SAMHSA. Treatment Episode Data Set (TEDS): 1994–1999 National Admissions to Substance Abuse Treatment Services. Rockville, MD: Office of Applied Studies, Substance Abuse and Mental Health Services Administration, Department of Health and Human Services; 2000.

34. Weintraub E, Weintraub D, Dixon L, et al. Geriatric patients on a substance abuse consultation service. Am J Geriatr Psychiatr. 2002;10(3):337–42.

35. McBride DC, Inciardi JA, Chitwood DD, McCoy CB. Crack use and correlates of use in a national population of street heroin users, The National AIDS Research Consortium. J Psychoactive Drugs. 1992;24(4):411–6.

36. Edgell R, Kunik M, Molinari V. Nonalcohol-related use disorders in geropsychiatric patients. J Geratr Psychiatr Neurol. 2000;13(1):33–7.

37. Schonfeld L, Dupree LW, Dickson-Euhrmann E, et al. Cognitive-behavioral treatment of older veterans with substance abuse problems. J Geriatr Psychiatr Neurol. 2000;13(3):124–9.

38. Cook AE. Strategies for containing drug costs: implications for a Medicare benefit. Health Care Financ Rev Spring. 1999;20(3):29–37.

39. Thomas CP, Ritter G, Wallack SS. Growth in prescription drug spending among insured elders. Health Aff (Millwood). 2001;20(5):265–77.

40. Stuart B, Kamal-Bahl S, Briesacher B, et al. Trends in the prescription of inappropriate drugs for the elderly between 1995 and 1999. Am J Geriatr Pharmacother. 2003;1(2):61–74.

41. Willcox SM, Himmelstein DU, Woolhandler S. Inappropriate drug prescribing for the community-dwelling elderly. J Am Med Assoc. 1994;272(4):292–6.

42. Zuckerman I. Inappropriate medication use and transition to nursing home among community-dwelling elders [Dissertation]. Baltimore: School of Medicine, University of Maryland Baltimore; 2005.

43. Zuckerman I, Byrns P, Baumgarten M, Orwig D, Langenberg P, Magaziner J. Inappropriate medication use and transition to nursing home. Paper presented at: Annual meeting of the Gerontological Society of America; 2005; Orlando, FL.

44. Kamal-Bahl S, Doshi J, Stuart B, Briesacher B. Propoxyphene use by community dwelling and institutionalized elderly Medicare beneficiaries. J Am Geriatr Soc. 2003;51:1099–104.

45. Simoni-Wastila L, Singhal PK, Hsu VD, Gardner JS, Briesacher B, Zuckerman I. Potentially problematic drug use in community-dwelling elders. Silver Spring, MD: Submitted to Johnson, Bassin, and Shaw, Inc. as part of project funded by the SAMHSA; June 24, 2003.

46. Simoni-Wastila L, Zuckerman I, Singhal PK, Briesacher B, Hsu VD. National estimates of exposure to prescription drugs with addiction potential in the Medicare population. Subs Abuse. 2005;26(1).

47. Moxey ED, O'Connor JP, Novielli KD, Teutsch S, Nash DB. Prescription drug use in the elderly: a descriptive analysis. Health Care Financ Rev. 2003;24(4):127–41.

48. Gleason PP, Schulz R, Smith NL, et al. Correlates and prevalence of benzodiazepine use in community-dwelling elderly. J Gen Intern Med. 1998;13(4):243–50.

49. Blazer D, Hybels C, Simonsick E, Hanlon JT. Sedative, hypnotic, and antianxiety medication use in an aging cohort over ten years: a racial comparison. J Am Geriatr Soc. 2000;48(9):1073–9.

50. Tobias D, Pulliam C. General and psychotherapeutic medication use in 878 nursing facilities. A 1997 national survey. Consultant Pharmacist. 1997;12(12):1401–1408

51. SAMHSA. Older adults in substance abuse treatment. The DASIS report. Drug and alcohol services information system. Rockville, MD: Office of Applied Statistics, Substance Abuse and Mental Health Service Administration, U.S. Department of Health and Human Services; 2001.

52. CASA. Under the rug: substance abuse and the mature woman. New York: CASA, Columbia University; 1998.

53. Batten H, Prottas J, Horgan C, et al. Drug services research survey. Phase II final report: NIDA; 1992.

54. Gfroerer J, Penne M, Pemberton M, Folsom R. Substance abuse treatment need among older adults in 2020: the impact of the aging baby-boom cohort. Drug Alcohol Depend. 2003;69(2):127–35.

55. Colliver J, Gfroerer J, Condon T. Projecting drug use among aging baby boomers in 2020. Ann Epidemiol. 2006;16(4):257–65.

56. Patterson TL, Jeste DV. The potential impact of the baby-boom generation on substance abuse among elderly persons. Psychiatr Serv. 1999;50(9):1184–8.

57. Sheahan SL, Hendricks L, Coons SJ. Drug misuse among the elderly: a covert problem. Health Values. 1989;13(3):22–9.

58. Simoni-Wastila L, Strickler G. Risk factors for problem use of prescription drugs. Am J Public Health. 2004;94(2):266–8.

59. Simoni-Wastila L, Strickler G, Ritter G. Gender and other factors associated with the non-medical use of abusable prescription drugs. Substance Use Misuse. 2004;39(1):1–14.

60. Simoni-Wastila L. Gender and psychotropic drug use. Med Care. 1998;36(1):88–94.

61. Simoni-Wastila L. The use of abusable prescription drugs: the role of gender. J Womens Health Gend Based Med. 2000;9(3):289–97.

62. Olfson M, Pincus HA. Use of benzodiazepines in the community. Arch Intern Med. 1994;154(11):1235–40.

63. Hohmann AA, Larson DB, Thompson JW, Beardsley RS. Psychotropic medication prescription in U.S. ambulatory medical care. DICP. 1991;25(1):85–9.

64. Takala J, Ryynanen OP, Lehtovirta E, Turakka H. The relationship between mental health and drug use. Acta Psychiatr Scand. 1993; 88(4):256–8.

65. Swartz M, Landerman R, George LK, Melville ML, Blazer D, Smith K. Benzodiazepine anti-anxiety agents: prevalence and correlates of use in a southern community. Am J Public Health. 1991;81(5):592–6.

66. NIDA. *Prescription drugs abuse and addiction*: DHHS/NIH/NIDA; 2001.

67. SAMHSA. *Summary of findings from the 1999 national household survey on drug abuse*. Rockville, MD: Office of Applied Studies, Substance Abuse and Mental Health Service Administration, U.S. Department of Health and Human Services; 2000.

68. Johnston L, O'Malley P, Bachman J. Monitoring the future: national survey results on drug use, 1975–1999: DHHS/NIH/NIDA; 2000.

69. SAMHSA. Substance use among women in the United States. Rockville, MD: Office of Applied Studies, SAMHSA, U.S. Department of Health and Human Services; 1997. DHHS Publication No. SMA 97–3162.

70. Zickler P. NIDA scientific panel reports on prescription drug misuse and abuse. NIDA Notes. 2001:16.

71. Anthony JC, Warner LA, Kessler RC. Comparative epidemiology of dependence on tobacco, alcohol, controlled substances, and inhalants: basic findings from the National Comorbidity Survey. Exp Clin Psychopharmacol. 1994;2:244–68.

72. Gomberg ESL. Older women and alcohol use and abuse. Recent developments in alcoholism. alcohol and women, vol. 12. New York: Plenum; 1995. p. 61–79.

73. Closser MH, Blow FC. Recent advances in addictive disorders. Special populations. Women, ethnic minorities, and the elderly. Psychiatr Clin North Am. 1993;16(1):199–209.

74. Regier DA, Farmer ME, Rae DS, et al. Comorbidity of mental disorders with alcohol and other drug abuse. Results from the Epidemiologic Catchment Area (ECA) Study. J Am Med Assoc. 1990;264(19):2511–8.

75. Szwabo P. Substance abuse in older women. Clin Geriatr Med. 1993;9:197–208.

76. Warner LA, Kessler RC, Hughes M, Anthony JC, Nelson CB. Prevalence and correlates of drug use and dependence in the United States. Results from the National Comorbidity Survey. Arch Gen Psychiatr. 1995;52(3):219–29.

77. Hilton ME. The demographic distribution of drinking patterns in 1984. In: Clark WB, Hilton ME, editors. Alcohol: drinking practices and problems. Albany, NY: State University of New York Press; 1991. p. 73–86.

78. Barnas C, Rossmann M, Roessler H, Riemer Y, Fleischhacker WW. Benzodiazepines and other psychotropic drugs abused by patients in a methadone maintenance program: familiarity and preference. J Clin Psychopharmacol. 1992;12(6):397–402.

79. Golub A, Johnson BD. Variation in youthful risks of progression from alcohol and tobacco to marijuana and to hard drugs across generations. Am J Public Health. 2001;91(2):225–32.

80. Kessler RC, Crum RM, Warner LA, Nelson CB, Schulenberg J, Anthony JC. Lifetime co-occurrence of DSM-III-R alcohol abuse and dependence with other psychiatric disorders in the National Comorbidity Survey. Arch Gen Psychiatr. 1997;54(4):313–21.

81. Kessler RC, Nelson CB, McGonagle KA, Edlund MJ, Frank RG, Leaf PJ. The epidemiology of co-occurring addictive and mental disorders: implications for prevention and service utilization. Am J Orthopsychiatr. 1996;66(1):17–31.

82. Dickey B, Normand SL, Weiss RD, Drake RE, Azeni H. Medical morbidity, mental illness, and substance use disorders. Psychiatr Serv. 2002;53(7):861–7.

83. Iguchi MY, Handelsman L, Bickel WK, Griffiths RR. Benzodiazepine and sedative use/abuse by methadone maintenance clients. Drug Alcohol Depend. 1993;32(3):257–66.

84. Finlayson RE, Davis Jr LJ. Prescription drug dependence in the elderly population: demographic and clinical features of 100 patients. Mayo Clin Proc. 1994;69(12):1137–45.

85. Fishbain D, Rosomoff H, Rosomoff R. Drug abuse, dependence, and addiction in chronic pain patients. Clin J Pain. 1992;8:77–85.

86. Harstell C, Ospina M. How prevalent is chronic pain? Pain Clin Update. 2003;11(2):1–4.

87. Zacny J, Bigelow G, Compton P, Foley K, Iguchi M, Sannerud C. College on problems of drug dependence taskforce on prescription opioid non-medcial use and abuse: position statement. Drug Alcohol Depend. 2003;69:215–32.

88. Zacny J. Characterizing the subjective, psychomotor, and physiological effects of a hydrocodone combination product (Hycodan) in non-drug-abusing volunteers. Psychopharmacology (Berl). 2003;165(2):146–56.

89. Zacny J, Gutuerrez S. Characterizing the subjective, psychomotor, and physiological effects of oral oxycodone in non-drug-abusing volunteers. Psychopharmacol Bull. 2003;170(3): 242–54.

90. Blow F, Brower K, Schulenberg J, Demo-Dananberg L, Young J, Beresford T. The Michigan alcoholism screening test - Geriatric Version (MAST-G): a new elderly-specific screening instrument. Alcoholism: Clin Exp Res. 1992;16:372.

91. Kail B, DeLaRosa M. Challenges to treating the elderly Latino substance abuser: A not so hidden research agenda. J Gerontol Soc Work. 1998;30:123–41.

92. Reid M, Anderson P. Geriatric substance use disorders. Med Clin North Am. 1997;81:999–1016.

93. Sarte D, Mertens J, Arean P, Weisner C. Five-year alcohol and drug treatment outcomes of older adults versus middle-aged and younger adults in a managed care program. Addiction. 2004;99: 1286–97.

94. Sarte D, Mertens J, Arean P, Weisner C. Contrasting outcomes of older versus middle-aged and younger adult chemical dependency patients in a managed care program. J Studies Alcohol. 2003;64: 520–30.

95. Kruse W. Problems and pitfalls in the use of benzodiazepines in the elderly. Drug Safety. 2000;5(5):328–44.

96. Roy W, Griffin M. Prescribed medicines and the risk of falling. Top Geriatr Rehabil. 1990;5(20):12–20.

97. Fink A, Elliott M, Tsai M, Beck J. An evaluation of an intervention to assist primary care physicians in screening and educating older adults who use alcohol. J Am Med Assoc. 2005;53(11): 1937–43.

98. Adams W, Cox N. Epidemiology of problem drinking among elderly people. Int J Addict. 1995;30:1693–716.

99. Liberto J, Oslin D, Ruskin P. Alcoholism in older persons. A review of the literature. Hosp Commun Psychiatr. 1992;43: 975–84.

100. Pringle K, Ahern F, Heller D, Gold C, Brown T. Potential for alcohol and prescription drug interactions in older people. J Am Geriatr Soc. 2005;53(11):1930–6.

101. Harwood H. Unpublished data. Falls Church, VA: The Lewin Group, Inc; 1995.

102. Harwood H, Fountain D, Livermore G. The economic costs of alcohol and drug abuse in the United States. Fairfax, VA: Prepared for the National Institute on Drug Abuse and the National Institute on Alcohol Abuse and Alcoholism; 1998.

103. SAMHSA. Year-end 1998 emergency department data from the drug abuse warning network. Rockville, MD: Office of Applied Studies, SAMHSA; 1999.

Drug Use and Abuse and Human Aggressive Behavior

38

Peter N.S. Hoaken, Vanessa L. Hamill, Erin H. Ross,
Megan Hancock, Megan J. Lau, and Jennifer L. Tapscott

Learning Objectives

- Drugs and violence co-occur, but there are a number of different reasons they co-occur and to assume direct pharmacological mechanisms is to oversimplify.
- The drug most consistently found to elicit aggression is alcohol; however, research also demonstrates that alcohol is more likely to provoke aggression in individuals who are already predisposed to behave in an aggressive manner.
- Recent research indicates that benzodiazepine use and aggression indeed co-occur; again, however, research suggests that those with a preexisting risk of aggression are at greater risk for the aggression-eliciting effects of these drugs.
- The link between anabolic/androgenic steroid use and aggressive behavior is complex, confounded, and putatively indirect.
- The effects of cannabis on aggression may be dose dependent, with low doses of cannabis contributing towards greater aggression than high doses; that being said, cannabis-dependent individuals may be at greatest risk of behaving aggressively during cannabis withdrawal.
- The correlation between stimulant (cocaine, amphetamine) use and aggression may be largely due to several indirect factors.
- The most proximal reason opiate users manifest aggression is as a means of accessing more drugs or accessing resources with which to attain drugs.

Issues that Need to be Addressed by Future Research

- Future research of individual factors will help researchers to determine who is more likely to behave in an aggressive manner when under the influence of alcohol, and thus delineate a "risk profile" which would be of tremendous benefit from both an academic and applied perspective
- Future research should systematically investigate the role of each of these confounding variables so that we may arrive at a clearer picture of the BZD–aggression link.
- Future research on the consequences of steroid use should utilize controlled designs rather than survey methods.
- Additional controlled studies, specifically examining the temporal relationship between drug use and aggression, are required before any definitive conclusions can be made regarding the aggression-eliciting properties of stimulants.

Introduction

That there is a relationship between drug use and/or abuse and human interpersonal violence cannot be denied. The relationship is profound, costly, and culturally non-specific. Epidemiological studies show substance abuse disorders rate among the most prevalent psychiatric disorders, for 1 month, yearly, or lifetime diagnoses [1]. Given that majority of drug abusers do not receive adequate treatment, become enmeshed in the legal system, seek alternative approaches, or never seek and/or receive treatment, the problem of drug-related aggression is likely to continue to prove problematic to clinicians and lawmakers alike. As has been previously illustrated [2, 3], there are at least four differential mechanisms through

P.N.S. Hoaken (✉) • V.L. Hamill • E.H. Ross • M. Hancock
• M.J. Lau • J.L. Tapscott
Department of Psychology, University of Western Ontario,
London, ON N6A 3K7, Canada
e-mail: phoaken@uwo.ca

J.C. Verster et al. (eds.), *Drug Abuse and Addiction in Medical Illness: Causes, Consequences and Treatment*,
DOI 10.1007/978-1-4614-3375-0_38, © Springer Science+Business Media, LLC 2012

which the relationship between drugs and aggression may come to be. These are: (1) Violent crimes can be committed to gain access to drugs or resources to purchase drugs; (2) violence is often a necessary means of resolving disputes in an illegal, and thus inherently lawless and unregulated business; (3) violent behavior and drug use can be the result of the same factors (e.g., high sensation seeking; antisociality) and exist coincidentally; and (4) certain drugs can increase the likelihood of violence because of their direct effects on the individual (i.e., that drug consumption has a causal relationship with aggressivity). These four mechanisms should in no way be considered mutually exclusive; however, in this paper when we talk about the relationship between aggression and drugs, the predominant focus is on the last. This mechanism we will specify in three categories: Direct pharmacological effects (intoxication), neurotoxic effects (damage caused by prolonged use), or withdrawal effects (abstinence immediately following prolonged use).

What follows is a discussion of the prominent drugs of use and abuse, and the evidence that each is related to heightened human aggressive behavior. In instances where the evidence for a relationship between the drug in question and aggression is strong, putative explanatory mechanisms will be discussed in the context of the four mechanisms described above. We will focus on the effects of proximal drug administration (notably intoxication), but when relevant studies are available, we will also discuss the drug–aggression relationship in terms of the effects of chronic-use (i.e., neurotoxic effects), and/or with some withdrawal syndrome. For each of the drug classes, we will begin with a reiteration of what conclusions were reached in our last review of this literature [3], and will then follow with an integration of what studies have emerged since that time, or were not included in that review, and then a statement about what new conclusions, if any, may be reached. We begin this review with alcohol, for three reasons: (1) it is the drug with the greatest prevalence of both use and abuse; (2) it is a pharmacologically complex drug, with several properties which might be seen as having the potential to increase aggressivity; and (3) it is, by far, the drug with the greatest amount of empirical evidence to support its direct aggression-inducing properties.

Legal/Prescriptive

Alcohol

There is little doubt that alcohol induces aggressive behavior; Hoaken and Stewart [3] referred to the alcohol–aggression relationship as "incontrovertible" and no evidence has since emerged to contradict this perspective. Research continues to demonstrate that alcohol consumption is associated with a wide range of types of violence, including sexual

aggression [4], family and marital violence [5], child abuse [6], and suicide [7, 8]. Since 2003, the focus of the alcohol–aggression literature has shifted from first determining the presence of such a relation, to later proposing explanatory theories. For example, psychopharmacological theories and alcohol expectancy theories have been predominately utilized to describe the alcohol–aggression relationship.

Recent research literature related to the psychopharmacological properties of alcohol focus primarily on the impact of intoxication on cognitive processing. Evidence suggests that, at moderate to high doses, alcohol impairs abilities which have been thought to be mediated by the prefrontal cortex (such as inhibition, working memory, and developing and monitoring strategy) while leaving capacities not traditionally associated with this area (such logical memory, vocabulary scores, spatial learning, and logical reasoning) relatively unaffected [9–11]. As such, much attention has been given to the construct of "executive functioning" as an explanatory factor for the alcohol–aggression relationship. Executive functioning is a higher order construct traditionally associated with the prefrontal cortex that is involved in the planning, initiation, and regulation of goal-directed behavior, and includes cognitive abilities such as attentional control, previewing, strategic goal planning, abstract reasoning, cognitive flexibility, and inhibition [9, 12]. Executive function has been shown to be related to, and even predictive of, aggressive and violent behavior (see [13] for a review). Recently it has been proposed that executive function is both a mediator and moderator of the alcohol–aggression relationship. Specifically, executive function has a mediating effect on the relationship in that acute alcohol consumption reduces executive capacity, which then increases the likelihood of aggressive behavior. Conversely, moderating effects are present in that acute alcohol consumption is less likely to facilitate aggressive behavior for individuals with above-average executive function [12, 14, 15]. In further support, a study by Giancola et al. [16] found that below-average executive function predicted increased aggression following alcohol consumption. Thus, earlier cognitive models may still be applicable, but better explained through the higher order construct of executive function.

In contrast to psychopharmacological theories, alcohol expectancy explanations have focused on beliefs regarding the effects of alcohol on behavior. Supporters of this theory suggest that aggressive behavior following alcohol consumption is partially a result of learned beliefs about the effects of alcohol. Alcohol expectancies can be thought of as cognitive templates for drinking behaviors, or representations of an "if–then" relationship, for example, "If I drink, then I will be more aggressive" [17]. Current theory suggests alcohol–aggression expectancies can be represented as complex associative networks in memory, where an association between alcohol and aggression is likely to form in an individual who frequently experiences or observes the co-occurrence of drinking and violence [17, 18]. Given that these alcohol–aggression expectancies are associated with increased rates of drinking [19, 20], we would expect to see a corresponding association with increased rates of aggression. However, the relationship between alcohol–aggression expectancies and aggressive behavior is ambiguous. Although several meta-analytic reviews found no support for the hypotheses that alcohol–aggression expectancies directly elicit aggression [21–23], it is important to note that the empirical studies did not actually examine the effects of alcohol or placebo on participants with different alcohol expectancies, instead assuming that placebos automatically triggered alcohol expectancy beliefs [24]. Conversely, other studies have found evidence to support the conclusion that there is a stronger association between alcohol and aggression for those with strong alcohol–aggression expectancies, but only in the presence of increased alcohol consumption [17, 25]. Such developments have led researchers to theorize that alcohol–aggression expectancies may interact with alcohol consumption to produce aggressive behavior [26–28].

The above paragraphs attempt to explain the mechanisms through which alcohol consumption can lead to aggression; however, it remains a fact that alcohol consumption does not lead to aggression in all persons. To explain this, theorists have speculated that alcohol is more likely to provoke aggression in individuals who are already predisposed to behave in an aggressive manner [29]. Several studies have attempted to determine what profile of personality characteristics is most likely to manifest an aggressive response while under the influence of alcohol. Various individual differences have been proposed as moderating the alcohol–aggression relationship. Alcohol consumption has been shown to increase aggression particularly for individuals with difficult temperaments [30], who have high levels of irritability [31], who are prone to anger [29, 32], and who have aggressive dispositions [26, 33]. It has been tentatively hypothesized that these dispositional traits may act as markers of heightened susceptibility to alcohol's effects on executive functioning, meaning individuals with these traits may be more likely to respond aggressively when intoxicated [32]. It is hoped that further study of such individual factors will help researchers to determine who is more likely to behave in an aggressive manner when under the influence of alcohol, and thus delineate a "risk profile" which would be of tremendous benefit from both an academic and applied perspective.

Benzodiazepines

Hoaken and Stewart [3] characterized the literature on the relationship between benzodiazepines (BZDs) and aggression as confusing and idiosyncratic; though some studies suggested that BZDs decrease aggression, others suggested BZDs increase aggression. This mixed review suggested that a number of factors may serve as moderators of the BZD–aggression relationship. For example, individuals appear to be at greater risk of the aggression-eliciting effects of BZDs if they have preexisting brain damage, concurrently use alcohol, intake relatively low doses of BZDs, or have a preexisting risk for aggression (i.e., a history of impulsivity or hostility). While acknowledging that many studies have demonstrated significant increases in aggression after BZD consumption, Hoaken and Stewart questioned the clinical significance of these findings.

Recent research indicates that BZD use and aggression indeed co-occur. For example, in a meta-analysis examining drug abuse and aggression between intimate partners, the weighted effect size for studies testing the relationship between physical abuse and BZD use was significantly greater than zero [34]. In addition, greater frequency of BZD use has been reported to be associated with a greater likelihood of assault outside of intimate relationships, even after controlling for 51 common risk factors [35]. Though such correlational research does little to suggest a possible mechanism that can account for the BZD–aggression link, these authors do provide data suggesting that the co-occurrence of BZD use and aggression is not a result of individuals' involvement in the drug trade. Specifically, BZD use was not related to frequency of drug sales and it was negatively related to gang and drug-war fighting [35]. To better understand the BZD–aggression link, Friedman and colleagues subsequently divided this sample into delinquent and nondelinquent groups; violent offenses were positively related to BZD use in the delinquent group only [36]. These results are consistent with Hoaken and Stewart's [3] conclusion that those with a preexisting risk of aggression are at greater risk for the aggression-eliciting effects of BZDs.

The dose-dependent effects of BZDs are also poorly understood. In one study, BZD of varying doses was administered to adult male parolees [37]. Aggression was low when doses were sufficiently high as to produce sedative effects; relatively low doses of BZDs had no effect on aggression. Conversely, in another study [38], while violent offenders were no more likely to engage in violence within 24 h of regular BZD use as compared to after periods of no BZD use, they were more likely to engage in violence in the 24 h following unusually high doses of BZDs. Discrepant results may be understood by noting that these studies did not all involve the same BZD and that different BZDs carry different risks for paradoxical aggressive reactions [39]. Another point to be made regarding the dose-dependent effects of BZDs is that deviations from an individual's typical dosage may have a greater impact on aggression than the absolute dosage itself.

A possible mechanism for the paradoxical aggressive reactions seen with some BZDs is an impaired ability to recognize human facial expressions. It has been demonstrated that acute doses of diazepam impair individuals' recognition of the threat-related facial expressions of anger [40] and fear [41]. This is important to understand, given that the ability to process threatening facial expressions may serve to prevent aggression [42]. Also interesting to note is that lorazepam, known to produce relatively fewer aggressive reactions than diazepam [39], does not produce impairment in emotion recognition [43]. Future studies might test whether impaired recognition of facial affect statistically mediates the BZD–aggression relationship.

The conclusion for this section of our review remains much the same as that reached by Hoaken and Stewart [3]; the relationship between BZD use and aggression remains poorly understood, largely because of uncontrolled individual differences, varying dosages, and the variety of BZDs available for study. Future research should systematically investigate the role of each of these confounding variables so that we may arrive at a clearer picture of the BZD–aggression link.

Anabolic/Androgenic Steroids

Anabolic–androgenic steroids are not typically considered drugs of abuse, but are certainly relevant to the discussion at hand, because: (a) they are often used for off-label (i.e., recreational) purposes, most often by young athletes for their performance-enhancing properties; (b) following the original demonstration by Lindstrom and colleagues [44], a number of retrospective reports have seemed to demonstrate a link between violence and the use of these drugs [45, 46]; and (c) the literature does contain case reports of extreme violence, including murder, in individuals who have been users of steroids [47]. However, in our 2003 review [3], we concluded that this literature was "largely confounded." That conclusion still seem reasonable, and is predicated on four considerations: first of these is the fact that the majority of anabolic and androgenic steroid users—and the vast majority of *abusers* of these drugs—are young, hypercompetitive men, a population that may well be prone to violence in the first place. Second, research demonstrates that these young men are also prone to high levels or alcohol consumption [48]. Third, continuing with the theme of the problem of differentiating drug effects, some have suggested that anabolic–androgenic steroids may act as so-called "gateway" drugs to wide ranges of illegal substances of use and abuse, which, like alcohol, may themselves have demonstrable aggression-eliciting properties [49, 50]. Lastly, there is a consistent belief among users of these drugs that a so-called "roids rage" phenomenon exists [51], bringing into question the possibility of expectancy effects.

All of that being said, the current manuscript will reject the phrase "largely confounded" and adopt instead "complex, confounded, and putatively indirect." In this section we will articulate some findings that have motivated this minor revision. In 2003 we called for more "controlled" investigations of this relationship; such a literature may hopefully now be in its infancy. One such study, which our previous review failed to mention, was conducted by Harrison Pope and his colleagues. In this study [52], the researchers ventured from retrospective non-controlled studies, and conducted a randomized, placebo-controlled, crossover study of the effects of testosterone cypionate on a variety of variables, including self-reported personality factors, anger, hostility, and verbal and physical aggression. They also utilized a laboratory measure of aggression, the Point-Subtraction Aggression Paradigm [53]. In this study, even with participants agreeing to consume no illicit drugs, and with minimal alcohol consumption, and with major psychopathology an exclusion criterion (which it clearly is not in vivo), participants receiving testosterone cypionate appeared more aggressive on the Point-Subtraction Paradigm ($P=0.03$). While this is clearly the most controlled study to date, there are some caveats: first, several have questioned the external validity of lab measures of aggression in general, and the Point-Subtraction Paradigm specifically (see [54, 55], for example). Additionally, there were no differences between the groups (placebo vs. drug) on the total score of the self-rated Buss-Perry Aggression Questionnaire (BPAQ), which is an idiosyncratic result given the retrospective self-report literature. Instead of anger or hostility (as measured by the BPAQ) perhaps one better explanation for the significant relationship between steroid use and the lab-based aggression paradigm might have been the most prominent effect shown in this study: that men currently taking the steroids had much higher scores on the Young Mania Rating Scale ($P=0.002$).

Another study [56], which consisted of post-mortem investigations of 34 fatalities of anabolic and/or androgenic steroid users, death was attributed to suicide in 11 cases, to homicide in 9 cases, to automobile accidents secondary to risky driving in two deaths, and to complications arising due to polysubstance use in 11 cases. These causes of death are evocative, and suggest poorly regulated, disinhibited lives; one might consider them evidence of more of a mania-eliciting property than a direct aggression-eliciting property of these drugs, per se.

Drawing conclusions based on the extant literature poses a challenging problem. The best conclusion about the anabolic and androgenic steroids is that they are dangerous. However, regarding the relationship between steroids and aggression, the best conclusion we can draw is that it is complex, that it is confounded, and that it is putatively indirect, and that more studies, particularly controlled studies, need to be conducted.

Illegal/Recreational

Cannabis

Hoaken and Stewart's [3] review of the literature on the relationship between aggression and cannabis led to the following conclusions: (1) the effects of cannabis on aggression may be dose dependent, with low doses of cannabis contributing towards greater aggression than high doses; and (2) cannabis-dependent individuals may be at greatest risk of behaving aggressively, not during cannabis intoxication, but during cannabis withdrawal.

Currently there is no shortage of studies demonstrating a cannabis–aggression relationship. To illustrate this point, a recent meta-analysis weighted 32 effect sizes from 14 studies on the relationship between marijuana use and physical abuse within the context of an intimate relationship and found a significant mean effect size of 0.21 [34]. However, much of the cannabis–aggression literature in humans suggests that the relationship may be spurious; as an illustration, two recent studies demonstrated that aggression–marijuana use correlations disappear when common risk factors such as deviance are controlled for [57, 58]. Thus, although marijuana use and violence tend to co-occur, there is no evidence of either behavior preceding the other [59].

Although much of the research to date suggests that the relationship between cannabis and aggression is either indirect or absent, there have been two studies that have found the relationship to persist after common risk factors were controlled for. In the first study, lifetime frequency of marijuana use was found to be positively associated with likelihood of weapon offenses and attempted homicides, despite controlling for 51 variables thought to predispose a person to act violently [35]. The second study, also controlling for possible confounds, found frequency of marijuana use to predict the variety and frequency of violent crimes of incarcerated, drug-abusing offenders [60]. However, both studies interpreted their findings by considering participants' involvement in drug trafficking. These interpretations are consistent with the mechanism discussed in the introduction of this chapter whereby the drug–violence relationship occurs as a result of violence being a necessary way to resolve disputes in the drug business.

Moreover, it must be noted that studies conducted to date that have tested the temporal relationship between cannabis use and aggression do not support a causal explanation. In one study, participants with mental illness who were identified as being at high risk for violence were followed for an average of 6 months [61]. Although serious violence was more likely to occur on days after marijuana had been consumed, results may not be generalizable to shorter lag periods. This limitation is of importance given that if violence is an acute

pharmacological effect of marijuana use, then episodes of violence would be expected to occur not on the day after use, but in the period of time immediately following use when the user is intoxicated or experiencing withdrawal. Fals-Stewart et al. [62] conducted a 15-month study using daily logs that examined the odds of male-to-female physical aggression occurring on days on which the male partner used cannabis. When controlling for male partners' antisocial personality and couples' average relationship satisfaction, cannabis use was not associated with increased likelihood of later same-day male-to-female aggression. Lastly, using a case-crossover design in which each participant could serve as his own control, Haggård-Grann et al. [38] found that the risk of participants (who were violent offenders) engaging in violence within 24 h of cannabis use was not significantly different than the risk of violence after periods of no cannabis consumption.

Though there is little evidence to suggest that cannabis intoxication leads to aggression, the same cannot be said of cannabis withdrawal. Current literature strongly supports the existence, reliability, and clinical significance of a cannabis withdrawal syndrome [63–65], and many researchers have argued for the inclusion of this syndrome in the next edition of the Diagnostic and Statistical Manual for Mental Disorders [65–67]. Although, Budney et al. [66] is the only study to have identified a specific time course for aggression as a result of cannabis withdrawal, other studies have found an increase in heavy cannabis users' self-reported aggression during periods of abstinence [63, 64, 68].

A final explanation for the cannabis–aggression link is the self-medication hypothesis which posits that individuals experiencing difficulties controlling their aggressive behavior use cannabis to reduce their aggression [63, 64, 69]. In a recent study by Arendt et al. [63, 64], although violent individuals reported using cannabis for many of the same reasons as did non-violent individuals (e.g., to decrease aggression, to relieve depression, to "get high"), the former group differed from the latter by being more likely to report using cannabis to decrease aggression. These results support the hypothesis that individuals with violent tendencies may use cannabis as self-medication for their behavioral problems. Though Moore and Stuart [70] suggest that these expectancy effects may cause marijuana use to decrease the likelihood of violence, the opposite appears to be true: the violent participants in the Arendt et al. study who reported using cannabis to decrease aggression were more likely to react with aggression after cannabis use than were the non-violent subjects who did not report using cannabis to decrease aggression. These paradoxical results do, however, support Moore and Stuart's contention that personality variables (e.g., individuals' antisociality) may moderate the marijuana–violence relationship.

To summarize our review of the cannabis–aggression literature, no existing literature suggests that cannabis intoxication causes aggression. Nonetheless, cannabis use appears to be associated with aggression as a result of common risk factors such as involvement in the drug trade and as a result of aggression being a common symptom of cannabis withdrawal. Controlled laboratory studies and prospective longitudinal studies remain necessary to better our understanding of the cannabis–aggression link.

Psychostimulants

Cocaine

Cocaine is a potent psychostimulant that has been reported to induce euphoria, enhance arousal and vigilance, reverse fatigue-induced deficits in performance, and increase blood pressure and heart rate [71]. In their review of the cocaine literature in 2003, Hoaken and Stewart reported that the relationship between cocaine and aggression was idiosyncratic, and that there had not been substantial evidence to support that the pharmacological effects of cocaine lead to aggression. While there was evidence of a correlation between cocaine use and aggression, the authors posited that this relationship may be due to several indirect factors.

Since the publication of this review, a number of new investigations have been carried out. Developmental studies have demonstrated that prenatal exposure to cocaine can be a predictor of childhood aggressive behavior [72–74]. Bendersky et al. found that prenatal exposure to cocaine was a predictor of childhood aggression at age 5, and they hypothesized that this aggression may be the result of cocaine's potential effects on the developing brain and the functions most likely affected, especially inhibitory control and emotional regulation. Furthermore, it is possible that cocaine exerts a similar effect on the brain functions of adolescent and adult users. Kemmis et al. [75] found that recreational users of cocaine exhibited impaired fear recognition accuracy compared to occasional users and non-users. Recreational users also correctly identified anger, fear, happiness, and surprise more slowly than the other participants. This impairment may have been the result of the direct neurotoxic effects of cocaine use on the brain; however, the performance of the recreational users resembled that of psychopathic individuals who have been reported to exhibit impaired recognition of fear and sadness [76, 77]. As Hoaken and Stuart [121] posited, an alternative explanation for these findings is that fear recognition is impaired due to psychopathic tendencies, as there is a high comorbidity between psychopathy and cocaine use.

Acutely, cocaine binds to the serotonin transporter and strongly inhibits serotonin (5-HT) reuptake [78]. Chronic administration of cocaine seems to downregulate several subtypes of postsynapic 5-HT receptors, possibly as a compensatory mechanism to increased synaptic 5-HT [79].

Aggression is a key component of a number of psychiatric disorders, and there is substantial evidence to suggest that 5-HT is a key component in this aggression [80–81]. As such, studies have begun to investigate the role of 5-HT as a potential mechanism underlying cocaine-induced aggression. In an examination of 35 cocaine abusers, Patkar et al. [84] found that central 5-HT function, as measured by prolactin (PRL) response to meta-chlorophenylpiperazine (m-CPP) a mixed 5-HT agonist/antagonist differed significantly between cocaine-dependent subjects and controls. A blunted response was pronounced in the subgroup of cocaine users with high disinhibition and aggression, while the response was not blunted in controls. Additional studies are necessary to clarify the extent to which the 5-HT disturbances signal a vulnerability to impulsive aggressive behavior or whether they are a consequence of cocaine dependence.

While the experimental literature on the causal nature of the relationship between cocaine use and aggression toward strangers is still somewhat equivocal, many studies on cocaine use and intimate partner violence (IPV) present a somewhat more explicit argument. Moore et al.'s [34] meta-analytic review of the literature on the relationship between drug use and IPV perpetration and victimization by both men and women demonstrated the overall effect size for cocaine ($d = 0.38$; 0.45 after outlier removal) was consistent across all types of aggression (physical, psychological, and sexual), and significantly larger than any of the other classes of drugs. Despite these impressive findings, an overall effect size in itself does not necessarily indicate that the significant effects for cocaine and aggression are due to the direct psychopharmacological effects of the substance [34]. The specific methodologies of these studies need to be examined in order to infer the exact mechanisms linking cocaine use to aggression. Fals-Stewart et al. [62] assessed the temporal relationship between cocaine use and partner aggression among men in substance abuse treatment. Results showed that after controlling for antisocial personality disorder and relationship discord there was greater chance (almost three times) of any male-to-female physical aggression on the days of cocaine use compared to days of no use. The majority of the physical aggression episodes occurred during or shortly after cessation of use, which may indicate that the aggression was directly related to pharmacological effects. Additional studies examining the temporal relationship are required before any definitive conclusions can be made.

Clearly additional research is needed before any definitive conclusions can be made about the relationship between cocaine and aggression. The manipulations required to evaluate whether cocaine has direct pharmacological effects on aggression in humans is difficult and many times unethical. Neuroimaging studies offer the most promise, however, they are expensive and technically elaborate and usually involve a small number of subjects.

Amphetamines

In 2003, Hoaken and Stewart's conclusion regarding the association between amphetamine use and aggression was that while there appeared to be a correlation, the controlled literature was "equivocal" about direct pharmacological action, instead suggesting a complex interplay of variables. Since then, amphetamines (and in particular methamphetamines) have become more commonly abused drugs [85], and the number of abusers seems to be steadily increasing worldwide [86, 87].

The notion that amphetamine use results in violence continues to be supported by a large body of literature, associating amphetamine use with aggression [88–90], domestic violence [34, 91], and violent criminal behaviors [85, 92, 93]. Evidence for an amphetamine–aggression association has continued to accumulate. Research employing self-report indicates that 33%–66% of methamphetamine users cite violent behavior as an outcome of their usage [94, 95]. Additionally, in a study surveying both in-treatment and non-treatment amphetamine users, 62% of the participants reported either violent, hostile behaviors, or involvement in violent crime, resulting from their drug use [96]. Moreover, evidence of amphetamine intoxication, assessed by urine toxicology screens, has also been linked to increased hospital admissions due to self-injury or physical altercations [97]. However, reliance on retrospective reports of use and behaviors, or indirect measures of behaviors, still cannot provide sufficient evidence of a causal relationship [86]. Furthermore, few studies fail to differentiate aggression as a consequence of intoxication versus withdrawal of methamphetamine (e.g., [98]), and few also determine whether the aggression was reactive or instrumental.

Since our last review, one randomized controlled amphetamine challenge, focused on aggression, has been conducted. White et al. [99] administered amphetamine or placebo to 70 non-drug abusing participants, who where blind to the administration. They discovered heightened levels of aggression reported by those who ingested amphetamine; however, not all amphetamine participants reported increases in aggression. This result is congruent with both controlled laboratory and field studies, where only select amphetamine users report or depict violent acts, suggesting that the relationship between amphetamines and violence is not due exclusively to pharmacological action, but is likely complex and multifactorial, and due to individual, situational, and cultural factors [96, 100]. Decreased ability to inhibit impulsive behavior, and deficits in other higher order cognitive functions, as a consequence of withdrawal or neurotoxicity of prolonged usage, have also been suggested as likely causes of increased aggression in amphetamine abusers [101–103].

A distinct discussion of a form of amphetamine, MDMA (3,4-methylenedioxymeth-amphetamine; "ecstasy") was absent from our 2003 review, but will be briefly discussed here. Usage of this drug has become extremely widespread [104], in large part to its reputation as a "safe drug" [105].

This reputation is the result of its perceived positive effects such as increased emotionality, empathy, extroversion, and euphoria [106, 107]. Nonetheless, aggression and hostility have been reported repeatedly in MDMA users [108, 109], even those who have abstained from use for an extended period of time [110]. A recent study indicated that in a sample of 260 MDMA users, those with a higher prevalence of lifetime ecstasy use exhibit higher levels of aggressive and violent behavior. Attempting to contribute to our understanding of cause, these authors also demonstrated that the effect of lifetime ecstasy use differs by levels of low self-control as a measure of propensity for aggression; those who exhibited low self-control were more affected by ecstasy use than those who did not, in terms of aggression [111].

Clearly, a relationship exists between amphetamine (and MDMA) and aggression; however, the conclusion that there is a direct causal link is perhaps too simplistic. Although heightened aggression may occur during intoxication, withdrawal, or subsequent to neurotoxicity, it is likely that other individual and social factors (such as family violence, poor parental supervision, early exposure to violence or to substance use, individual histories of aggressive behavior [93, 102, 112]) significantly affect which users will engage in aggressive acts.

Opiates

In 2003, Hoaken and Stewart argued that individuals who are abusers of opiates are likely to manifest aggressive behaviors, but may be more likely to be aggressive because of the reasons they abuse the drug, or because they are enmeshed in the drug trade, not because of the drug itself. Controlled laboratory studies on the effects of opiates on aggression in humans have found a positive relationship between opiate use and aggressive behavior; for example, in a study using the Taylor aggression paradigm, Berman et al. [113] found that individuals who were using morphine had a higher propensity to initiate attacks, and displayed more aggression at all levels of provocation than controls. Furthermore, Gerra et al. [114] found that heroin-dependent patients on methadone treatment reported higher levels of aggressiveness and hostility, in comparison to controls. However, Gerra et al. concluded that the level of aggressiveness demonstrated by the methadone patients seemed to be related more to the personality traits than to drug effects. The conclusion in Hoaken and Stewart [3] was also predicated on several studies demonstrating that opioid abusers demonstrate premorbid feelings of rage [115], and score high on self-report [116] and observer-report [117] measures of hostility.

Since 2003, there is little accumulated evidence from which to draw a different conclusion. In one study [118], abstinent heroin-dependant participants and controls competed on the Point-Subtraction Paradigm (discussed previously). Aggressive responses were significantly higher in the heroin-dependant participants; given that they were abstinent at the time, this again seems to be suggestive of a non-pharmacological cause for the heroin–aggression relationship. In another study of several hundred Spanish arrestees, those who were found to be currently heroin dependant were found to be less aggressive, and less resistant to arrest than the arrestees for whom no psychiatric diagnosis could be found. The authors argue against a cause–effect relationship for the opiate–crime relationship, and suggest instead that criminal activity perpetrated by heroin-dependant individuals is based on financial need.

Conclusion

Interpersonal violence and drug use are strongly linked, and constitute a significant public health challenge. That being said, the illegality of some types of drugs, relative to the widespread availability of others seems predicated on some abstruse and arcane rationalization. Clearly, any effort to invoke "safety" is absurd, considering that the drug we know to be most likely to induce aggressive behavior (alcohol) is legally available and typically a significant source of state profit, and also considering that the greatest amount of drug-related violence is likely due to indirect causes (i.e., dependant users committing violent crime to gain access to drugs or resources to buy drugs; and/or regulation by force of an illegal and highly profitable industry; [119, 120]). In no way do the authors advocate for any move towards global de-regulation, or legalization of drug classes that are currently proscribed. What we do advocate for is increases in funding for both research and treatment. If we were to better understand what drugs make individuals more aggressive, at what doses, and in what contexts, and were we better able to treat addiction, monitoring withdrawal and associated symptoms, then we may well be able to reduce the enormous costs of drug-related violence.

Is there a relationship between drugs and aggression? Clearly, the answer is a resounding yes. However, just as clearly, the nature of the relationship is interactional and multi-factorial, and, moreover, different for different classes of drug. Additionally, some drugs, at different doses, have paradoxical effects. There is only one thing that can be said unequivocally about the drug–aggression relationship: We do not know enough about it.

References

1. Eaton WW, Kramer M, Anthony JC, Drymon A, Locke BZ. the incidence of specific DIS/DSM-III mental disorders: Data from the NIMH Epidemiologic Catchment Area Program. Acta Psychiatr Scand. 1989;79:163–78.
2. Pihl RO, Hoaken PNS. Clinical correlates and predictors of violence in patients with substance use disorders. Psychiatr Annals. 1997;27:735–40.
3. Hoaken PNS, Stewart SH. Drugs of abuse and the elicitation of human aggressive behavior. Addict Behav Special Issue: Interpersonal Violence Substance Use. 2003;28:1533–54.
4. Testa M. The impact of men's alcohol consumption on perpetration of sexual aggression. Clin Psychol Rev. 2002;22:1239–63.
5. Caetano R, Schafer J, Fals-Stewart WO, O'Farrell TJ, Miller B. Intimate partner violence: New research on methodological issues, stability and change, and treatment. Alcohol Clin Exp Res. 2003; 27:292–300.
6. Dube SR, Anda RF, Felitti VJ, Croft JB, Edwards VJ, Giles WH. Growing up with parental alcohol abuse: exposure to childhood abuse, neglect, and household dysfunction. Child Abuse Negl. 2001;25:1627–40.
7. Giner L, Carballo JJ, Guija JA, Sperling D, Oquendo MA, Garcia-Parajua P, Sher L, Giner J. Psychological autopsy studies: The role of alcohol use in adolescent and young adult suicides. Int J Adolesc Med Health. 2007;19:99–113.
8. Modesto-Lowe V, Brooks D, Ghani M. Alcohol dependence and suicidal behaviour: from research to clinical challenges. Harv Rev Psychiatr. 2006;14:241–8.
9. Giancola PR. Executive functioning and alcohol-related aggression. J Abnorm Psychol. 2004;113:541–55.
10. Seguin JR, Nagin D, Assaad JM, Tremblay RE. Cognitive-neuropsychological function in chronic physical aggression and hyperactivity. J Abnorm Psychol. 2004;113:603–13.
11. Giancola PR, Corman MD. Alcohol and aggression: A test of the attentional-allocation model. Psychol Sci. 2007;18:649–55.
12. Pihl RO, Assaad JM, Hoaken PNS. The alcohol-aggression relationship and differential sensitivity to alcohol. Aggress Behav. 2003;29:302–15.
13. Fishbein D. Neuropsychological function, drug abuse, and violence: A conceptual framework. Criminal Justice Behav. 2000;27:139–59.
14. Hoaken PNS, Assaad J, Pihl RO. Cognitive functioning and the inhibition of alcohol-induced aggression. J Stud Alcohol. 1998;59: 599–607.
15. Giancola PR. Executive functioning: A conceptual framework for alcohol- related aggression. Exp Clin Psychopharmacol. 2000;8: 576–97.
16. Giancola PR, Parrott DJ, Roth RM. The influence of difficult temperament on alcohol-related aggression: Better accounted for by executive functioning? Addict Behav. 2006;31:2169–87.
17. McMurran M. The relationship between alcohol-aggression proneness, general alcohol expectancies, hazardous drinking, and alcohol-related violence in adult male prisoners. Psychol Crime Law. 2007;13:275–84.
18. Bartholow BD, Heinz A. Alcohol and aggression without consumption: Alcohol cues, aggressive thoughts, and hostile perception bias. Psychol Sci. 2006;17:30–7.
19. Goldman MS. Expectancy and risk for alcoholism: The unfortunate exploitation of a fundamental characteristic of neurobehavioral adaptation. Alcohol Clin Exp Res. 2002;26:737–46.
20. Jones BT, Corbin W, Fromme K. A review of expectancy theory and alcohol consumption. Addition. 2001;96:57–72.
21. Bushman BJ. Effects of alcohol on human aggression: Validity of proposed explanations. In: Galanter M, editor. Recent developments in alcoholism: Alcohol and violence, vol. 13. New York: Plenum; 1997. p. 227–43.
22. Bushman BJ, Cooper HM. Effects of alcohol on human aggression: An integrative research review. Psychol Bull. 1990;107:341–54.
23. Hull J, Bond C. Social and behavioral consequences of alcohol consumption and expectancy: A meta-analysis. Psychol Bull. 1986;99:347–60.
24. Quigley BM, Leonard KE. Alcohol expectancies and intoxicated aggression. Aggression Violent Behav. 2006;11:484–96.
25. Leonard KE, Senchak M. Alcohol and premarital aggression among newlywood couples. J Stud Alcohol. 1993;11:96–108.

26. Smucker Barnwell S, Borders A, Earleywine M. Aggression expectancies and dispositional aggression moderate the relationship between alcohol consumption and alcohol-related violence. Aggress Behav. 2006;32:517–25.

27. Leonard KE, Collins RL, Quigley BM. Alcohol consumption and the occurrence and severity of aggression: An event-based analysis of male to male barroom violence. Aggress Behav. 2003;29: 346–65.

28. Zhang L, Welte JW, Wieczorek WW. The role of aggression-related alcohol expectancies in explaining the link between alcohol and violent behavior. Subst Use Misuse. 2002;37:457–71.

29. Giancola PR, Saucier DA, Gussler-Burkhardt NL. The effects of affective, behavioural, and cognitive components of trait anger on the alcohol- aggression relation. Alcohol Clin Exp Res. 2003;27: 1944–54.

30. Giancola PR. Difficult temperament, acute alcohol intoxication, and aggressive behaviour. Drug Alcohol Depend. 2004;74: 135–45.

31. Giancola PR. Irritability, acute alcohol consumption and aggressive behavior in men and women. Drug Alcohol Depend. 2002;68: 263–74.

32. Parrott DJ, Giancola PR. A further examination of the relation between trait anger and alcohol-related aggression: The role of anger control. Alcohol Clin Exp Res. 2004;28:855–64.

33. Giancola PR. Alcohol-related aggression in men and women: The influence of dispositional aggressivity. J Stud Alcohol. 2002;63: 696–708.

34. Moore TM, Stuart GL, Meehan JC, Rhatigan D, Hellmuth JC, Keen SM. Drug abuse and aggression between intimate partners: A meta-analytic review. Clin Psychol Rev. 2008;28:247–74.

35. Friedman AS, Glassman K, Terras A. Violent behavior as related to use of marijuana and other drugs. J Addict Dis. 2001;20: 49–72.

36. Friedman AS, Terras A, Glassman K. The differential disinhibition effect of marijuana use on violent behavior: A comparison of this effect on a conventional, non-delinquent group versus a delinquent or deviant group. J Addict Dis. 2003;22:63–78.

37. Pietras CJ, Lieving LM, Cherek DR, Lane SD, Tcheremissine OV, Nouvion S. Acute effects of lorazepam on laboratory measures of aggressive and escape responses of adult male parolees. Behav Pharmacol. 2005;16:243–51.

38. Haggård-Grann U, Hallqvist J, Långström N, Möller J. The role of alcohol and drugs in triggering criminal violence: A case-cross-over study. Addiction. 2006;101:100–8.

39. Gutierrez MA, Roper JM, Hahn P. Paradoxical reactions to benzodiazepines. Am J Nurs. 2001;101:34–9.

40. Blair RJ, Curran HV. Selective impairment in the recognition of anger induced by diazepam. Psychopharmacology. 1999;147: 335–8.

41. Zangara A, Blair RJR, Curran HV. A comparison of the effects of a B-adrenergic blocker and a benzodiazepine upon the recognition of human facial expressions. Psychopharmacology. 2002;163: 36–41.

42. Blair RJ, Morris JS, Frith CD, Perrett DI, Dolan R. Dissociable neural responses to facial expressions of sadness and anger. Brain. 1999;122:883–93.

43. Kamboj SK, Curran HV. Scopolamine induces impairments in the recognition of human facial expressions of anger and disgust. Psychopharmacology. 2006;185:529–35.

44. Lindstrom M, Nilsson AL, Katzman PL, Janzon L, Dymlingt F. Use of anabolic-androgenic steroids among body builders-frequency and attitudes. J Int Med. 1990;227:407–411.

45. Pope HG, Katz DL. Psychiatric and medical effects of anabolic-androgenic steroid use: A controlled study of 160 athletes. Arch Gen Psychiatr. 1994;51:375–82.

46. Yates WR, Perry P, Murray S. Aggression and hostility in anabolic steroid users. Biol Psychiatr. 1992;31:1232–4.

47. Pope HG, Katz DL. Homicide and near-homicide by anabolic steroid users. J Clin Psychiatr. 1990;51:260.

48. DuRant RH, Richert VI, Ashworth CS, Newman C, et al. Use of multiple drugs among adolescents who use anabolic steroids. N Engl J Med. 1993;328:922–6.

49. Kanayama G, Cohane GH, Weiss RD, Pope Jr HG. Past anabolic-androgenic steroid use among men admitted for substance abuse treatment: An underrecognized problem? J Clin Psychiatr. 2003;64:156–60.

50. Hall R, Hall R, Chapman M. Psychiatric complications of anabolic steroid use. Psychosomatics. 2005;46:285–90.

51. Porcerelli JH, Sandler BA. Anabolic-androgenic steroid abuse and psychopathology. Psychiatr Clin North Am. 1998;21:829–33.

52. Pope HG, Kouri EM, Hudson JI. Effects of supraphysiologic doses of testosterone on mood and aggression in normal men: A randomized controlled trial. Arch Gen Psychiatr. 2000;57: 133–40.

53. Cherek DR, Schnapp W, Moeller FG, Dougherty M. Laboratory measures of aggressive responding in male parolees with violent and nonviolent histories. Aggress Behav. 1996;22:27–36.

54. Tedeschi J, Quigley B. Limitations of laboratory paradigms for studying aggression. Aggression Violent Behav. 1996;1:163–77.

55. Tedeschi JT, Quigley BM. A further comment on the construct validity of laboratory aggression paradigms: A response to Giancola and Chermack. Aggression Violent Behav. 2000;5: 127–36.

56. Thiblin I, Lindquist O, Rajs J. Cause and manner of death among users of anabolic androgenic steroids. J Forensic Sci. 2000;45: 16–23.

57. Macdonald S, Erickson P, Wells S, Hathaway A, Pakula B. Predicting violence among cocaine, cannabis, and alcohol treatment clients. Addict Behav. 2008;33:201–5.

58. Wei EH, Loeber R, White HR. Teasing apart the developmental associations between alcohol and marijuana use and violence. J Contemporary Crim Justice. 2004;20:166–83.

59. Wade TJ, Pevalin DJ. Adolescent delinquency and health. Can J Criminol Crim Justice. 2005;47:619–54.

60. Kinlock TW, O'Grady KE, Hanlon TE. Prediction of the criminal activity of incarcerated drug-abusing offenders. J Drug Issues. 2003;33:897–920.

61. Mulvey EP, Odgers C, Skeem J, Gardner W, Schubert C, Lidz C. Substance use and community violence: A test of the relation at the daily level. J Consult Clin Psychol. 2006;74:743–54.

62. Fals-Stewart W, Golden J, Schumacher JA. Intimate partner violence and substance use: A longitudinal day-to-day examination. Addict Behav Special Issue: Interpersonal Violence Substance Use. 2003;28(9):1555–74.

63. Arendt M, Rosenberg R, Fjordback L, Brandholdt J, Foldager L, Sher L, Munk-Jorgensen P. Testing the self-medication hypothesis of depression and aggression in cannabis-dependent subjects. Psychol Med. 2007;37:935–45.

64. Arendt M, Rosenberg R, Foldager L, Sher L, Munk-Jogensen P. Withdrawal symptoms do not predict relapse among subjects treated for cannabis dependence. Am J Addict. 2007;16:461–7.

65. Vandrey RG, Budney AJ, Hughes JR, Liguori A. A within-subject comparison of withdrawal symptoms during abstinence from cannabis, tobacco, and both substances. Drug Alcohol Depend. 2008;92:48–54.

66. Budney AJ, Moore BA, Vandrey RG, Hughes JR. The time course and significance of cannabis withdrawal. J Abnorm Psychol. 2003;112:393–402.

67. Crowley TJ. Adolescents and substance-related disorders: research agenda to guide decisions on Diagnostic and Statistical Manual of

Mental Disorders, fifth edition (DSM-V). Addiction. 2006;101 (Supplement 1):115.

68. Budney AJ, Vandrey RG, Hughes JR, Moore BA, Bahrenburg B. Oral delta-9-tetrahydrocannabinol suppresses cannabis withdrawal symptoms. Drug Alcohol Depend. 2007;86:22–9.

69. Khantzian EJ. The self-medication hypothesis of addictive disorders: Focus on heroin and cocaine dependence. Am J Psychiatr. 1985;142:1259–64.

70. Moore TM, Stuart GL. A review of the literature on marijuana and interpersonal violence. Aggression Violent Behav. 2005;10: 171–92.

71. Grilly DM. Drugs and human behavior. Boston: Allyn and Bacon; 2002.

72. Yolton KA, Bolig R. Psychosocial, behavioral, and developmental characteristics of toddlers prenatally exposed to cocaine. Child Study J. 1994;24:49–68.

73. Delaney-Black V, Covington C, Templin T, Ager J, Nordstrom-Klee B, Martier S. Teacher-assessed behavior of children prenatally exposed to cocaine. Pediatrics. 2000;106:782–91.

74. Bendersky M, Bennett D, Lewis M. Aggression at age 5 as a function of prenatal exposure to cocaine, gender, and environmental risk. J Pediatr Psychol Special Issue: Prenatal Substance Exposure: Impact on Children's Health, Dev School Perform Risk Behav. 2006;31:71–84.

75. Kemmis L, Hall JK, Kingston R, Morgan MJ. Impaired fear recognition in regular recreational cocaine users. Psychopharmacology. 2007;194:151–9.

76. Blair RJT. Neuro-cognitive models of aggression, the antisocial personality disorders and psychopathy. J Neurol Neurosurg Psychiatr. 2001;71:727–31.

77. Blair RJT. Facial expressions, their communicatory functions and neuro-cognitive substrates. Philos Transac R Soc B: Biol Sci. 2003;358:561–72.

78. Castanon N, Scearce-Levie K, Lucas JJ, Rocha B, Hen R. Modulation of the effects of cocaine by 5-HT1B receptors: a comparison of knockouts and antagonists. Pharmacol Biochem Behav. 2000;67:559–66.

79. King GR, Pinto G, Konen J, Castro G, Tran S, Hilburn C. The effects of continuous 5-HT(3) receptor antagonist administration on the subsequent behavioral response to cocaine. Eur J Pharmacol. 2002;449:253–9.

80. Coccaro EF, Kavoussi RJ, Hauger RL. Physiological responses to d-fenfluramine and ipsapirone challenge correlate with indices of aggression in males with personality disorders. Int Clin Psychopharmacol. 1995;10:177–9.

81. Goveas JS, Csernansky JG, Coccaro EF. Platelet serotonin content correlates inversely with life history of aggression in personality-disordered subjects. Psychiatr Res. 2004;126:23–32.

82. Stanley B, Molcho A, Stanley M, Winchel R, Gameroff MJ, Parsons B. Association of aggressive behavior with altered serotonergic function in patients who are not suicidal. Am J Psychiatr. 2000;157:609–14.

83. Twitchell GR, Hanna GL, Cook EH, Stoltenberg SF, Fitzgerald HE, Zucker RA. Serotonin transporter promoter polymorphism genotype is associated with behavioral disinhibition and negative affect in children of alcoholics. Alcohol Clin Exp Res. 2001;25: 953–9.

84. Patkar AA, Mannelli P, Peindl K, Hill KP, Gopalakrishnan R, Berrettini WH. Relationship of disinhibition and aggression to blunted prolactin response to meta-chlorophenylpiperazine in cocaine-dependent patients. Psychopharmacology. 2006;185(1): 123–32.

85. Iritani BJ, Hallfors DD, Bauer DJ. Crystal methamphetamine use among young adults in the USA. Addition. 2007;102(7): 1102–13.

86. Black E, Degenhardt L. Drug-related aggression among injecting drug users. NSW Public Health Bull. 2006;17:12–6.

87. Farrell M, Marsden J, Ali R, Ling W. Methamphetamine: Drug use and psychoses becomes a major public health issue in the Asia Pacific region. Addiction. 2002;97:771–2.

88. Brecht ML, O'Brien A, von Mayrhauser C, Anglin MD. Methamphetamine use behaviors and gender differences. Addict Behav. 2004;29(1):89–106.

89. Degenhardt L, Topp L. 'Crystal meth' use among polydrug users in Sydney's dance party subculture: Characteristics, use patterns and associated harms. Int J Drug Policy. 2003;14:17–24.

90. Gorman EM, Nelson KR, Applegate T, Scrol A. Club drug and poly-substance abuse and HIV among gay/bisexual men: Lessons gleaned from a community study. J Gay Lesbian Social Services: Issues Practice Policy Res. 2004;16(2):1–17.

91. Sommers I, Baskin DR. Methamphetamine use and violence. J Drug Issues. 2006;36(1):77–97.

92. Cartier J, Farabee D, Prendergast ML. Methamphetamine use, self-reported violent crime, and recidivism among offenders in California who abuse substances. J Interpers Violence. 2006;21: 435–45.

93. Zweben JE, Cohen JB, Christian D, Galloway GP, Salinardi M, Parent D, Iguchi MY. Psychiatric symptoms in methamphetamine users. Am J Addict. 2004;13(2):181–90.

94. Pennell S, Ellett J, Rienick C, Grimes J. Meth matters: report on methamphetamine users in five western cities. Washington, DC: U.S. Department of Justice; 1999.

95. von Mayrhauser C, Brecht M, Anglin MD. Use ecology and drug use motivation of methamphetamine users admitted to substance abuse treatment facilities in Los Angeles: An emerging profile. J Addict Dis. 2002;21(1):45–60.

96. Wright S, Klee H. Violent crime, aggression, and amphetamine: What are the implications for drug treatment services? Drugs Educ Prevention Policy. 2001;8:73–90.

97. Tominaga GT, Garcia G, Dzierba A, Wong J. Toll of methamphetamine on the trauma system. Arch Surg. 2004;139:844–7.

98. Nordahl TE, Salo R, Leamon M. Neuropsychological effects of chronic methamphetamine use on neurotransmitters and cognition: A review. J Neuropsychiatr Clin Neurosci. 2003;15:317–25.

99. White TL, Grover VK, de Wit H. Cortisol effects of D-amphetamine relate to traits of fearlessness and aggression but not anxiety in healthy humans. Pharmacol Biochem Behav. 2006;85:123–31.

100. Boles SM, Miotto K. Substance and violence: a review of the literature. Aggression Violent Behav. 2003;8:155–74.

101. Kim SJ, Lyoo IK, Hwang J, Sung YH, Lee HY, Lee DS, et al. Frontal glucose hypometabolism in abstinent methamphetamine users. Neuropsychopharmacology. 2005;30:1383–91.

102. Semple SJ, Zians J, Grant I, Patterson TL. Impulsivity and methamphetamine use. J Subst Abuse Treat. 2005;29:85–93.

103. Simonsa JS, Olivera MNI, Gahera RM, Ebelb G, Brummels P. Methamphetamine and alcohol abuse and dependence symptoms: Associations with affect lability and impulsivity in a rural treatment population. Addict Behav. 2005;30:1370–81.

104. Carapcioglu A, Ogel K. Factors associated with ecstasy use in Turkish students. Addiction. 2004;99:67–76.

105. Schwartz RH, Miller NS. MDMA (ecstasy) and the rave: A review. Pediatrics. 1997;100:705–8.

106. Pape H, Rossow I. Ordinary people with ordinary lives? A longitudinal study of ecstasy and other drug use among Norwegian youth. J Drug Issues. 2004;22:389–418.

107. Sloan JJ. It's all the rave: Flower power meets technoculture. Am Crim Justice Soc Today. 2000;19:3–6.

108. Parrot AC, Sisk E, Turner JD. Psychobiological problems in heavy "ecstasy" (MDMA) polydrug users. Drug Alcohol Depend. 2000;60:105–10.

109. Verheyden SL, Hadfield J, Calin T, Curran HV. Sub-acute effects of MDMA (3,4-methylenedioxymeth-amphetamine) on mood: Evidence of gender differences. Psychopharmacology. 2002;161: 23–31.

110. Gerra G, Zaimovic A, Moi G, Giusti F, Gardini S, Delsignore R, et al. Effects of 3,4-methylene-dioxymethamphetamine (ecstasy) on dopamine system function in humans. Behav Brain Res. 2002;134:403–10.

111. Reid L, Elifson K, Sterk C. Hug drug or thug drug? Ecstasy use and aggressive behavior. Violence Vict. 2007;22:104–19.

112. Cohen JB, Dickow A, Horner K, Zweben JE, Balabis J, Vandersloot D, et al. Abuse and violence history of men and women in treatment for methamphetamine dependence. Am J Addict. 2003;12:377–85.

113. Berman M, Taylor S, Marged B. Morphine and human aggression. Addict Behav. 1993;18:263–8.

114. Gerra G, Zaimovic A, Raggi M, Guish F, Delsignore R, Bertacca S, Brambilla F. Aggressive responding of male heroine addicts under methodone treatment: Psychometric and neuroendocrine correlates. Drugs Alcohol Depend. 2001;65:85–95.

115. Miczek KA, Weerts EM, DeBold JF. Alcohol, benzodiazepine-GABAA receptor complex and aggression: Ethological analysis of individual differences in rodents and primates. J Stud Alcohol. 1993(Suppl 11):170–179.

116. Lindquist CU, Lindsay JS, White GD. Assessment of assertiveness in drug abusers. J Clin Psychol. 1979;35:676–9.

117. Babor TF, Meyer RE, Mirin SM, Davies M, Valentine N, Rawlins M. Interpersonal behavior in a small group setting during the heroin addiction cycle. Int J Addict. 1976;11:513–23.

118. Gerra G, Zaimovic A, Raggi M, Moi G, Branchi B, Moroni M, Brambilla F. Experimentally induced aggressiveness in heroin-dependent patients treatment with buprenorphine: Comparison of patients receiving methadone and healthy subjects. Psychiatr Res. 2007;149:201–13.

119. Fagan J, Chin KL. Violence as regulation and social control in the distribution of crack. NIDA Res Monogr. 1990;103:8–43.

120. Moss HB, Tarter RE. Substance abuse, aggression, and violence: What are the connections? Am J Addict. 1993;2:149–60.

121. Hoaken PNS, Stewart SH. Drugs of abuse and the elicitation of human aggressive behaviour. Addict Behav. 2003;28:1533–1554.

Suicidal Behavior in Alcohol and Drug Abuse

39

Leo Sher

Abstract

Suicidal behavior is common among individuals with substance use disorders. The large population of individuals with alcohol and drug abuse and dependence, the relative frequency of suicides and suicide-related behaviors in this population, and the devastating effects of attempted and completed suicides on individuals, families, and society make this an important area for clinical and research work. Multiple lines of evidence suggest that lower serotonin activity is tied to increased aggression/impulsivity which in turn is presumed to enhance the probability of suicidal behavior. Dopaminergic dysfunction may play a role in the pathophysiology of suicidal behavior in alcoholism. Alcohol and drugs can damage the brain in many ways. The brain is vulnerable to the toxic effects of alcohol and drugs and can be affected by substance-related damage to other organs, including the liver, pancreas, and heart. Brain damage and neurobehavioral deficits are associated with suicidal behavior. It is possible that cognitive abnormalities contribute to increased suicidality in individuals with alcohol use disorders. Low selenium status is associated with depressed mood, anxiety, and cognitive decline. These symptoms are commonly observed in persons with alcohol use disorders. Selenium deficiency may play a role in the pathophysiology of depression and suicidal behavior in individuals with alcohol abuse. Cocaine use is associated with suicidal behavior. The management of the suicidal patient with substance abuse/dependence involves three components: first, the diagnosis and treatment of existing substance abuse and other psychiatric disorders; second, the assessment of suicide risk and limiting access to the most lethal methods for suicide; and third, specific treatment to reduce the diathesis or propensity to attempt suicide. Treatments designed to enhance social supports and foster abstinence from alcohol and drugs, together with those directed at the resolution of major depression, often reduce the risk of suicide.

L. Sher, M.D. (✉)
James J. Peters Veterans' Administration Medical Center
and Mount Sinai School of Medicine,
130 West Kingsbridge Road, Bronx,
New York 10468, USA
e-mail: Leo.Sher@mssm.edu

J.C. Verster et al. (eds.), *Drug Abuse and Addiction in Medical Illness: Causes, Consequences and Treatment*,
DOI 10.1007/978-1-4614-3375-0_39, © Springer Science+Business Media, LLC 2012

Learning Objectives
- Risk factors for suicide can be organized according to whether their effect is on the threshold for suicidal acts, or whether they serve mainly as triggers or precipitants of suicidal acts. A predisposition to suicidal behavior is a key element that differentiates patients who are at high risk versus those at lower risk.
- Alcohol and drug use disorders are associated with suicidal ideation, suicide attempts, and suicides.
- Careful assessment of suicide risk and appropriate treatment of comorbid psychiatric and medical disorders may reduce suicidal behavior in patients with substance abuse.

Issues that Need to Be Addressed by Future Research
- The investigation of genetic and rearing effects on the development of substance use disorders and suicidal behavior
- Development of pharmacological and psychological treatments to reduce substance abuse/dependence
- Testing pharmacological treatments to ameliorate aggressive/impulsive behavior that might reduce the probability of suicidal behavior

Suicidal Behavior as a Medical and Social Problem

Suicide is a major public health problem in many countries. The World Health Organization reported that self-inflicted injuries including suicide accounted for more than 800,000 deaths in 2001 [1]. If every suicide affects at least six family members or friends, then every year in the world there would be about five million new survivors. There are approximately 30,000 deaths per year by suicide in the United States every year [2].

Suicidal behavior refers to the occurrence of suicide attempts, which can be defined as self-directed injurious acts with at least some intent to end one's own life [3–5]. Suicidal behavior ranges from fatal acts (completed suicide), to highly lethal and failed suicide attempts (where high intention and planning are evident, and survival is fortuitous), and to low-lethality attempts (usually impulsive attempts that are triggered by a social crisis seem to be ambivalent and contain a strong element of an appeal for help).

Identifying individuals at imminent risk for suicidal behavior is a major challenge for clinicians [3–5]. However, prediction of suicidal behavior is difficult due to the relative rarity of the event as well as the multidetermined cause of such behavior. Cross-sectional and retrospective studies have identified numerous clinical risk factors for suicidal behavior including mood disorder, alcohol and substance use disorders, cluster B category personality disorders, aggressive and impulsive traits, pessimism, and cigarette smoking.

Suicide is generally a complication of a psychiatric disorder such as alcoholism or depression, but it requires additional risk factors, because most psychiatric patients never attempt suicide [3, 4]. The objective severity of psychiatric disorders does not assist in identifying patients at high risk

for suicide attempt. The stress-diathesis model of suicidal behavior suggests that risk factors for suicide can be organized according to whether their effect is on the threshold for suicidal acts, or whether they serve mainly as triggers or precipitants of suicidal acts [3–5]. A predisposition to suicidal behavior is a key element that differentiates patients who are at high risk versus those at lower risk. Risk factors affecting the diathesis for suicidal behavior include alcohol and/or substance abuse, marital isolation, not living with a child under age 18, family history of suicide, parental loss before age 11, childhood history of physical and/or sexual abuse, tobacco smoking, cluster B personality disorders, hopelessness, impulsiveness, aggression, low self-esteem, low cerebrospinal fluid (CSF) 5-hydroxyindolacetic acid (5-HIAA) levels, low blood cholesterol levels, and physical illnesses [3–5]. Most common precipitants of suicidal acts include the onset or acute worsening of a psychiatric disorder, interpersonal losses or conflicts, financial troubles, and job problems.

Alcohol Use Disorders and Suicide

Prevalence and the Model

Alcohol misuse is an important risk factor for suicidal behavior [6–10]. The large population of individuals with alcohol abuse and dependence, the relative frequency of suicides and suicide-related behaviors in this population, and the devastating effects of attempted and completed suicides on individuals, families, and society make this an important area for research. Some reports have found that lifetime mortality due to suicide in alcohol dependence is as high as 18% [7]. Murphy and Wetzel [8] reviewed the epidemiological literature and found that the lifetime risk of suicide among individuals with alcohol dependence treated in outpatient and inpatient settings was 2.2% and 3.4%, respectively. Nonetheless, individuals with alcohol dependence have a 60–120 times greater suicide risk than the nonpsychiatrically ill population.

High rates of suicide attempts among individuals with alcohol use disorders have also been reported [9, 10]. For example, in an urban community in the US, 24% of subjects with alcohol dependence attempted suicide, as compared with 5% with other psychiatric diagnoses [9]. Forty percent of a sample of depressed subjects with alcohol dependence who were hospitalized had attempted suicide in the prior week and 70% had attempted suicide at some point in their lives [10]. Depressed subjects with a history of alcohol dependence have higher current suicide ideation scale scores compared with depressed subjects without a history of alcohol dependence [6]. These data indicate that a lifetime diagnosis of alcohol dependence is a major risk factor for attempted or completed suicide.

A model of suicidal behavior among subjects with alcoholism has recently been proposed [11]. Predisposing factors that are presumed to increase (moderate) the risk for suicide among individuals with alcoholism are aggression/impulsivity and alcoholism severity, which represent predominantly externalizing constructs, and negative affect and hopelessness, which represent predominantly internalizing constructs. Major depressive episodes and stressful life events—particularly interpersonal difficulties—are conceptualized as precipitating factors. This model is consistent with the stress-diathesis model of suicidal behavior.

Serotonin

Multiple lines of evidence suggest that lower serotonin activity is tied to increased aggression/impulsivity which in turn is presumed to enhance the probability of suicidal behavior [12, 13]. Low CSF 5-hydroxyindolacetic acid 5-HIAA has been reported in suicide attempters with major depression, schizophrenia, and personality disorders as compared with people who do not attempt suicide but have the same psychiatric diagnosis [12–14]. The levels of 5-HIAA in CSF taken from abstinent individuals with a history of alcohol dependence of both sexes were shown to be lower than in controls [15]. Moreover, impulsive offenders with alcohol dependence had lower CSF 5-HIAA levels than nonimpulsive offenders with alcohol dependence [16]. High-lethality depressed suicide attempters with comorbid alcoholism have lower CSF 5-HIAA levels compared with low-lethality depressed suicide attempters with comorbid alcoholism [17]. In subjects with comorbid depression and alcoholism greater serotonergic impairment may be associated with higher risk of completed suicide.

Dopamine

Chen et al. [18] suggest that pathological aggression may be related to genetically determined abnormalities in the dopaminergic system. Suicidal behavior may be regarded as self-directed pathological aggression. Several lines of evidence suggest that the dopamine system is involved in the pathophysiology of suicidal behavior. Lower levels of CSF homovanillic acid (HVA) have been found in depressed patients with a history of either violent or nonviolent suicide attempts than in controls [19]. In our recent study, we compared CSF HVA levels in depressed suicide attempters without comorbid Axis II disorders, depressed nonattempters without comorbid Axis II disorders, and normal controls [20]. Depressed suicide attempters had lower CSF HVA levels compared to depressed nonattempters and to controls. There was no difference in CSF HVA levels between depressed nonattempters and controls. Several studies that did not involve CSF HVA measures also suggested that the dopaminergic system may be involved in the neurobiology of suicidal behavior. For example, Pitchot et al. [21] studied the growth hormone (GH) response to apomorphine, a selective dopaminergic agonist, in depressed patients with and without a history of suicide attempts and found that patients with a history of suicidal behavior exhibited a significantly lower GH response to apomorphine than patients who never attempted suicide. More recent reports from the same group confirmed their earlier finding. It has also been observed that dopamine abnormalities are associated with impulsivity, emotional dysregulation, and alcohol use disorders [22]. For example, a recent neuroimaging study suggests that alcoholism is associated with blunted dopamine transmission in the ventral striatum [23]. Alcoholism is also associated with high aggression, impulsivity, and suicidal behavior [24]. Therefore, it is reasonable to suggest that genetically determined dopaminergic dysfunction may play an important role in the pathophysiology of suicidal behavior in alcoholism.

Brain Damage

Alcohol can damage the brain in many ways [25, 26]. The brain is vulnerable to the toxic effects of alcohol itself and can be affected by alcohol-related damage to other organs, including the liver, pancreas, and heart. The risk of alcohol-induced brain damage and related neurobehavioral deficits varies from person to person and is influenced by factors such as age, gender, drinking history, and nutrition. In the US, up to two million individuals with alcoholism have permanent and debilitating conditions that require lifetime custodial care. Examples of such conditions include alcohol-induced persisting amnesic disorder (also called Wernicke–Korsakoff syndrome) and dementia, which seriously affect many mental functions in addition to memory (e.g., language, reasoning, and problem-solving abilities). Brain damage and neurobehavioral deficits are associated with suicidal behavior [27, 28].

Cognitive Impairment

Alcohol and Cognitive Dysfunction

Etiological models for alcohol use disorders have traditionally proposed trait and cognitive explanations for initiation, maintenance, and dependence [29]. Within this framework, temperament and personality models have often focused on trait disinhibition [30], including behavioral undercontrol [31], impulsivity, and sensation seeking [32], suggesting that deficits in interrupting ongoing behavior may be central to hazardous drinking. Numerous studies have shown that heavy drinkers and subjects suffering from alcohol dependence have reduced performance on neurocognitive tests such as Wisconsin Card Sorting Test, the Stroop Test, Trails A and B test/Trail Making, Tower of Hanoi/London, and the Go No-Go Test compared with controls [33–62]. These effects have been shown to persist after detoxification [36, 38, 44–47, 55, 56, 58, 59, 63], and may be based on hereditary predispositions [64, 65]. The effects appear to be correlated with years of alcohol use [35, 47], although some studies have not found such an effect [43]. Subjects suffering from alcohol dependence have been found to perform like subjects with frontal brain lesions in some investigations [34, 39]. It is not clear whether the results are general for substance abuse populations as two investigations have found similar effects when comparing subjects dependent on alcohol with subjects dependent on other substances [33, 34]. However, one study has found worse executive functioning among alcohol-dependent subjects [40]. A number of investigations have found worse performance among subjects suffering from alcohol dependence, former alcoholics, and heavy social drinkers compared with controls on the standard Stroop Test [34, 40, 41, 46, 49, 58] and the Stroop tests containing alcohol-related words [43, 51–53, 56]. Two studies have found that this difference may be specific for the alcohol-related version of the Stroop Test, while alcohol-dependent subjects had normal scores on the standard Stroop Test [28, 29]. Another study has found that Stroop performance may predict results of detoxification treatment [66]. A recent study found differences in tests' scores on the Go No-Go Test between detoxified polysubstance users with alcohol dependence and control subjects [46]. Another study found that subjects with alcohol dependence differ electrophysiologically from control individuals using the Go No-Go Test [36]. In summary, neuropsychological studies of alcohol use disorders overall suggest that individuals with alcohol abuse and dependence are cognitively impaired.

Suicide and Cognitive Impairment

Data suggest that neuropsychological dysfunction may play a role in determining risk for suicidal acts. Suicide attempters have been characterized as "cognitively rigid" on the basis of self-ratings and performance on mental flexibility tasks [67–69]. From case studies [70], Rourke et al. [71] suggested that a specific nonverbal learning disability may predispose individuals to suicidal behavior. Bartfai et al. [72], using standard neuropsychological measures, found poorer performance on measures of fluency (verbal as well as nonverbal) and reasoning in a small sample of recent suicide attempters compared to patients with chronic pain and nonpatients. Subjects with a history of high-lethality suicide attempts exhibited deficits in executive functioning that were independent of deficits associated with depression alone [27].

Alcohol use disorders are associated with both cognitive impairment and suicidal behavior. It is possible that cognitive abnormalities contribute to increased suicidality in individuals with alcohol use disorders. Future studies of the role of cognitive abnormalities in the pathophysiology of suicidal behavior are merited.

Selenium Deficiency

Selenium and Alcohol

Selenium is an essential trace element for humans and animals [73–77]. The four natural oxidation states of selenium are elemental selenium (0), selenide (−2), selenite (+4), and selenate (+6). Inorganic selenate and selenite predominate in water whereas organic selenium compounds (selenomethionine, selenocysteine) are the major selenium species in cereal and in vegetables. For the general population, the primary pathway of exposure to selenium is food, followed by water and air. Both selenite and selenate possess substantial bioavailability. Selenium is an essential component of glutathione peroxidase, which is an important enzyme for processes that protect lipids in polyunsaturated membranes from oxidative degradation.

The selenium content in human blood varies between different areas of the world due to the soil content of selenium with consequent variations in dietary intake. Blood selenium level appears to be an index of long-term selenium status and does not change from day-to-day. There is a consensus in the literature concerning the lower concentration of plasma selenium in patients with alcoholism, even in the absence of severe liver pathology as well as in some cases of modest alcohol consumption [78–84]. Serum, erythrocyte, and whole blood levels of selenium are also decreased in patients with alcoholism [82–89]. For example, Korpela et al. [85] measured serum selenium values in patients with alcoholism having various degrees of liver damage. As a percentage of healthy control level, the average serum selenium level of alcoholics with histologically normal liver was 60%, with fatty liver was 63%, with alcoholic hepatitis was 52%, and with cirrhosis was 46%. Decrease in selenium levels in patients with alcoholism may be related to insufficient dietary intake, reduced intestinal absorption, changes in plasma proteins (much of the circulating selenium is bound to glutathione peroxidase and other proteins), and increased requirements [80–82, 84, 90].

Selenium, Mood, and Behavior

Selenium is thought to play an important role in brain function, because its metabolism in the brain is vastly different than in other organs [91–93]. Specifically, during times of deficiency, the brain retains selenium at the expense of tissues, such as muscle, kidney, and liver. Indeed, selenium is an important modulator of mood. Effects of dietary selenium on mood in healthy men were assessed by the Profile of Mood States-Bipolar Form [94]. Eleven healthy men were confined in a metabolic research unit for 120 days. The diet of conventional foods provided 80 µg per day of selenium for the first 21 days, then either 13 or 356 µg per day for the remaining 99 days. There were no significant changes in any of the mood scales due to dietary selenium. However, in the low-selenium group, the changes in the agreeable-hostile and the elated-depressed subscales were correlated with initial erythrocyte selenium concentration; that is, the lower the initial selenium status, the more the mood scores decreased. Finley and Penland [95] investigated the effects of dietary selenium on healthy men who were fed either a low or a high selenium diet for 15 weeks. Subjects on the low selenium diet had significantly decreased clearheaded/confused and elated/depressed subscores, whereas those on the high selenium diet significantly improved in the clearheaded/confused, confident/unsure, and composed/anxious subscores.

The possibility that a subclinical deficiency of the trace element selenium might exist in a sample of the British population was examined by Benton and Cook [96]. A selenium supplement was given for 5 weeks. Using a double-blind cross-over design, 50 subjects received either a placebo or 100 µg of selenium on a daily basis. On three occasions they filled in the Profile of Moods States. Selenium intake was associated with a general elevation of mood and in particular, a decrease in anxiety. The change in mood when taking the active tablet was correlated with the level of selenium in the diet, which was estimated from a food frequency questionnaire. The lower the level of selenium in the diet the more the reports of anxiety, depression, and tiredness, decreased following 5 weeks of selenium therapy. Thus, selenium depletion may affect mood and behavior. Selenium influences compounds with hormonal activity and neurotransmitters in the brain, and this is postulated to be the reason why selenium affects mood in humans and behavior in animals [73, 91, 97].

In a randomized trial of HIV-infected patients, researchers found that supplementation with 200 µg per day selenium caused a 20-fold reduction of depressed–dejected mood state and a trend toward improvement in quality of life scores [98].

Selenium is required for appropriate thyroid hormone synthesis, activation, and metabolism [99]. Selenium status influences thyroid function. It has been suggested that the effects of selenium status on mood, behavior, and cognition may be partly mediated by changes induced by selenium deficiency or selenium supplementation in thyroid function.

Low selenium status is associated with depressed mood, anxiety, and cognitive decline. These symptoms are commonly observed in persons with alcohol use disorders. Selenium deficiency may play a role in the pathophysiology of depression and suicidal behavior in individuals with alcohol abuse. Healthy nutrition and possibly mineral supplementations should be a part of the treatment plan of patients with alcohol use disorders especially when alcohol misuse is comorbid with depression. Adequate nutrition is needed for many aspects of brain functioning. In general, greater attention to nutritional factors in psychiatry is warranted.

Suicidal Behavior in Individuals with Drug Abuse or Dependence Other than Alcohol

The prevalence of suicide-related deaths among drug users may be underestimated [100]. These suicides may be by opioid overdose as well as by other means. Currently, such deaths are not necessarily registered as "drug user's suicide."

Among substance abusers aged 15–19 years, the prevalence of suicidal ideations is 31% among men and 75% among women, whereas among college students of the same age who do not use drugs the prevalence is 11% and 8%, respectively [101, 102]. Multisubstance abusers report suicidal thoughts or suicide attempts in the last year twice as often as monosubstance abusers [103, 104]. Studies of suicide cases using the psychological autopsy method show that the proportion of suicide victims having a substance abuse problem varies between one-quarter and two-thirds [105, 106].

A study comparing drug users currently in the methadone maintenance treatment, abstinent drug users who completed the methadone maintenance treatment, and a community control group showed that the prevalence of suicide attempts was 18 and 16 times higher in the two drug user groups, respectively, compared to the control group [107]. Men and women who smoked marijuana before age 17 are 3.5 times as likely to attempt suicide as those who started later [108]. Individuals who are dependent on marijuana have a higher risk than nondependent individuals of experiencing major depressive disorder and suicidal thoughts and behaviors.

Cocaine use is associated with suicidal behavior [109, 110]. Risk factors across the life cycle are associated with suicidal behavior in cocaine-dependent patients [109]. Distal risk factors include a family history of suicide, childhood trauma, neuroticism, hostility, and introversion. More proximal risk factors include the comorbidities of other substance dependence, major depression, and physical disorders. These results suggest a stress-diathesis model of suicidal behavior in cocaine-dependent patients with distal threshold-affecting factors, including family, childhood, and personality variables. It has been shown that cocaine use is associated with an increased prevalence of suicidal behavior and suicidal ideation in depressed individuals with alcoholism [111]. There is no evidence that the use of sedative-hypnotics and amphetamines is associated with suicidal behavior [110].

Preventing Suicidal Behavior in Individuals with Substance Use Disorders

Substance abusers who commit suicide often see a physician or are psychiatrically hospitalized in the months prior to their deaths [3–5, 24, 110]. Those who talk of suicide may be ambivalent about their wish to die. They may thus be amenable to clinical interventions such as detoxification, substance-abuse rehabilitation, or psychiatric hospitalization. Conversely, those who take special precautions against discovery during a prior suicide attempt are much more likely to die in a subsequent suicide attempt. Beyond psychiatric diagnoses, the strongest indicator of suicide risk in substance abusers is such an interpersonal loss. Beyond these actual losses, anticipated losses, such as impending legal, financial, or physical demise, may also increase the risk of suicide among substance abusers. Availability of guns at home may contribute to suicide risk, especially in adolescents and young adults [110, 112, 113].

The management of the suicidal patient involves three components [5]: first, the diagnosis and treatment of existing substance abuse and other psychiatric disorders; second, the assessment of suicide risk and limiting access to the most lethal methods for suicide; and third, a specific treatment to reduce the diathesis or propensity to attempt suicide.

If there is any indication of suicidality, a clinician trained in assessing suicide risk should meet with the patient. If suicide risk is high, patients should be referred immediately for further evaluation. If patients are not an imminent threat for suicide, therapists should proceed with treatment as usual, but evaluate suicide risk at each patient contact. This evaluation should include standard clinical questions used to assess suicide risk. If possible, clinicians should obtain written agreements from patients to engage in "safe" behavior, which includes agreeing to call the therapist or designated agency

(e.g., crisis clinic) if feeling suicidal. Any time clinicians feel uncomfortable about a patient's level of risk, the patient should be referred to an appropriate service.

Prediction of those who will complete suicide remains poor in individual cases, even among high-risk groups such as substance abusers [2, 110]. Despite their high prevalence, alcoholism and drug abuse often go unrecognized by physicians and other health care professionals. People with psychiatric disorders, suicidal behavior, and/or substance abuse are frequently stigmatized. Even physicians and other health care professionals frequently have such negative attitudes. This detrimental approach compromises dual diagnosis patient evaluations, treatment, and prognosis. Clinicians should be educated about a risk of suicidal behavior among individuals with substance abuse. Clinicians' recognition of alcohol and drug use disorders and of risk factors such as major depression that increase the risk of suicide may assist them in making preventive interventions. The substance abuser with active suicide plans or a recent suicide attempt may need hospitalization, detoxification, and/or rehabilitation designed to foster abstinence from alcohol and drugs of abuse. Firearms should be removed from the homes of substance abusers with active suicide ideation, especially adolescents and young adults. Treatments designed to enhance social supports and foster abstinence from alcohol and drugs, together with those directed at the resolution of major depression, often reduce the risk of suicide. Careful assessment of suicide risk and appropriate treatment of comorbid psychiatric and medical disorders may reduce suicidal behavior in patients with substance abuse.

References

1. World Health Organization. Burden of mental and behavioral disorders. In: The World Health Report 2001. Mental health: new understanding, new hope. Geneva: World Health Organization; 2001. p. 19–45.
2. Sher L. Preventing suicide. QJM. 2004;97:677–80.
3. Sher L, Oquendo MA, Mann JJ. Risk of suicide in mood disorders. Clin Neurosci Res. 2001;1:337–44.
4. Sher L. Risk and protective factors for suicide in patients with alcoholism. ScientificWorldJournal. 2006;6:1405–11.
5. Mann JJ. Neurobiology of suicidal behaviour. Nat Rev Neurosci. 2003;4:819–28.
6. Sher L, Oquendo MA, Conason AH, Brent DA, Grunebaum MF, Zalsman G, Burke AK, Mann JJ. Clinical features of depressed patients with or without a family history of alcoholism. Acta Psychiatr Scand. 2005;112(4):266–71.
7. Roy A, Linnoila M. Alcoholism and suicide. Suicide Life Threat Behav. 1986;16(2):244–73.
8. Murphy GE, Wetzel RD. The lifetime risk of suicide in alcoholism. Arch Gen Psychiatry. 1990;47(4):383–92.
9. Weissman MM, Myers JK. Clinical depression in alcoholism. Am J Psychiatry. 1980;137(3):372–3.
10. Cornelius JR, Salloum IM, Day NL, Thase ME, Mann JJ. Patterns of suicidality and alcohol use in alcoholics with major depression. Alcohol Clin Exp Res. 1996;20(8):1451–5.

11. Conner KR, Duberstein PR. Predisposing and precipitating factors for suicide among alcoholics: empirical review and conceptual integration. Alcohol Clin Exp Res. 2004;28(5 Suppl):6S–17S.
12. Sher L, Mann JJ. Neurobiology of suicide. In: Soares JC, Gershon S, editors. Textbook of medical psychiatry. New York: Marcel Dekker; 2003. p. 701–11.
13. Placidi GP, Oquendo MA, Malone KM, Huang YY, Ellis SP, Mann JJ. Aggressivity, suicide attempts, and depression: relationship to cerebrospinal fluid monoamine metabolite levels. Biol Psychiatry. 2001;50:783–91.
14. Roy A, De Jong J, Linnoila M. Cerebrospinal fluid monoamine metabolites and suicidal behavior in depressed patients. A 5-year follow-up study. Arch Gen Psychiatry. 1989;46:609–12.
15. Ratsma JE, Van Der Stelt O, Gunning WB. Neurochemical markers of alcoholism vulnerability in humans. Alcohol Alcohol. 2002;37:522–33.
16. Virkkunen M, Rawlings R, Tokola R, et al. CSF biochemistries, glucose metabolism, and diurnal activity rhythms in alcoholic, violent offenders, fire setters, and healthy volunteers. Arch Gen Psychiatry. 1994;51:20–7.
17. Sher L, Oquendo MA, Grunebaum MF, Burke AK, Huang Y, Mann JJ. CSF monoamine metabolites and lethality of suicide attempts in depressed patients with alcohol dependence. Eur Neuropsychopharmacol. 2007;17(1):12–5.
18. Chen TJ, Blum K, Mathews D, et al. Are dopaminergic genes involved in a predisposition to pathological aggression? Hypothesizing the importance of "super normal controls" in psychiatric genetic research of complex behavioral disorders. Med Hypotheses. 2005;65:703–7.
19. Engstrom G, Alling C, Blennow K, Regnell G, Traskman-Bendz L. Reduced cerebrospinal HVA concentrations and HVA/5-HIAA ratios in suicide attempters. Monoamine metabolites in 120 suicide attempters and 47 controls. Eur Neuropsychopharmacol. 1999;9:399–405.
20. Sher L, Mann JJ, Traskman-Bendz L, Huang Y, Fertuck EA, Stanley BH. Lower cerebrospinal fluid homovanillic acid levels in depressed suicide attempters. J Affect Disord. 2006;90:83–90.
21. Pitchot W, Hansenne M, Moreno AG, Ansseau M. Suicidal behavior and growth hormone response to apomorphine test. Biol Psychiatry. 1992;31:1213–9.
22. Tupala E, Tiihonen J. Dopamine and alcoholism neurobiological basis of ethanol abuse. Prog Neuropsychopharmacol Biol Psychiatry. 2004;28:1221–47.
23. Martinez D, Gil R, Slifstein M, et al. Alcohol dependence is associated with blunted dopamine transmission in the ventral striatum. Biol Psychiatry. 2005;58:779–86.
24. Sher L. Alcoholism and suicidal behavior: a clinical overview. Acta Psychiatr Scand. 2006;113:13–22.
25. Rourke SB, Loeberg T. The neurobehavioral correlates of alcoholism. In: Nixon SJ, editor. Neuropsychological assessment of neuropsychiatric disorders. 2dth ed. New York: Oxford University Press; 1996. p. 423–85.
26. Oscar-Berman M, Marinkovic K. Alcoholism and the brain: an overview. Alcohol Res Health. 2003;27(2):125–33.
27. Keilp JG, Sackeim HA, Brodsky BS, Oquendo MA, Malone KM, Mann JJ. Neuropsychological dysfunction in depressed suicide attempters. Am J Psychiatry. 2001;158(5):735–41.
28. Oquendo MA, Friedman JH, Grunebaum MF, Burke A, Silver JM, Mann JJ. Suicidal behavior and mild traumatic brain injury in major depression. J Nerv Ment Dis. 2004;192(6):430–4.
29. Anderson KG, Schweinsburg A, Paulus MP, Brown SA, Tapert S. Examining personality and alcohol expectancies using functional magnetic resonance imaging (fMRI) with adolescents. J Stud Alcohol. 2005;66(3):323–31.
30. McGue M, Iacono WG, Legrand LN, Malone S, Elkins I. Origins and consequences of age at first drink. I. Associations with substance-use disorders, disinhibitory behavior and psychopathology, and P3 amplitude. Alcohol Clin Exp Res. 2001;25(8):1156–65.
31. Sher KJ, Walitzer KS, Wood PK, Brent EE. Characteristics of children of alcoholics: putative risk factors, substance use and abuse, and psychopathology. J Abnorm Psychol. 1991;100(4):427–48.
32. Grau E, Ordet G. Personality traits and alcohol consumption in a sample of non-alcoholic women. Pers Indiv Diff. 1999;27:1057–66.
33. Beatty WW, Katzung VM, Moreland VJ, Nixon SJ. Neuropsychological performance of recently abstinent alcoholics and cocaine abusers. Drug Alcohol Depend. 1995;37(3):247–53.
34. Bechara A, Dolan S, Denburg N, Hindes A, Anderson SW, Nathan PE. Decision-making deficits, linked to a dysfunctional ventromedial prefrontal cortex, revealed in alcohol and stimulant abusers. Neuropsychologia. 2001;39(4):376–89.
35. Brokate B, Hildebrandt H, Eling P, Fichtner H, Runge K, Timm C. Frontal lobe dysfunctions in Korsakoff's syndrome and chronic alcoholism: continuity or discontinuity? Neuropsychology. 2003;17(3):420–8.
36. Cohen HL, Porjesz B, Begleiter H, Wang W. Neurophysiological correlates of response production and inhibition in alcoholics. Alcohol Clin Exp Res. 1997;21(8):1398–406.
37. Demir B, Ucar G, Ulug B, Ulusoy S, Sevinc I, Batur S. Platelet monoamine oxidase activity in alcoholism subtypes: relationship to personality traits and executive functions. Alcohol Alcohol. 2002;37(6):597–602.
38. Fama R, Pfefferbaum A, Sullivan EV. Perceptual learning in detoxified alcoholic men: contributions from explicit memory, executive function, and age. Alcohol Clin Exp Res. 2004;28(11):1657–65.
39. George MR, Potts G, Kothman D, Martin L, Mukundan CR. Frontal deficits in alcoholism: an ERP study. Brain Cogn. 2004;54(3):245–7.
40. Goldstein RZ, Leskovjan AC, Hoff AL, Hitzemann R, Bashan F, Khalsa SS, Wang GJ, Fowler JS, Volkow ND. Severity of neuropsychological impairment in cocaine and alcohol addiction: association with metabolism in the prefrontal cortex. Neuropsychologia. 2004;42(11):1447–58.
41. Ihara H, Berrios GE, London M. Group and case study of the dysexecutive syndrome in alcoholism without amnesia. J Neurol Neurosurg Psychiatry. 2000;68(6):731–7.
42. Joyce EM, Robbins TW. Frontal lobe function in Korsakoff and non-Korsakoff alcoholics: planning and spatial working memory. Neuropsychologia. 1991;29(8):709–23.
43. Lusher J, Chandler C, Ball D. Alcohol dependence and the alcohol Stroop paradigm: evidence and issues. Drug Alcohol Depend. 2004;75(3):225–31.
44. Moriyama Y, Mimura M, Kato M, Yoshino A, Hara T, Kashima H, Kato A, Watanabe A. Executive dysfunction and clinical outcome in chronic alcoholics. Alcohol Clin Exp Res. 2002;26(8):1239–44.
45. Munro CA, Saxton J, Butters MA. The neuropsychological consequences of abstinence among older alcoholics: a cross-sectional study. Alcohol Clin Exp Res. 2000;24(10):1510–6.
46. Noel X, Van der Linden M, Schmidt N, Sferrazza R, Hanak C, Le Bon O, De Mol J, Kornreich C, Pelc I, Verbanck P. Supervisory attentional system in nonamnesic alcoholic men. Arch Gen Psychiatry. 2001;58(12):1152–8.
47. Oscar-Berman M, Kirkley SM, Gansler DA, Couture A. Comparisons of Korsakoff and non-Korsakoff alcoholics on neuropsychological tests of prefrontal brain functioning. Alcohol Clin Exp Res. 2004;28(4):667–75.
48. Ratti MT, Bo P, Giardini A, Soragna D. Chronic alcoholism and the frontal lobe: which executive functions are imparied? Acta Neurol Scand. 2002;105(4):276–81.

49. Rothlind JC, Greenfield TM, Bruce AV, Meyerhoff DJ, Flenniken DL, Lindgren JA, Weiner MW. Heavy alcohol consumption in individuals with HIV infection: effects on neuropsychological performance. J Int Neuropsychol Soc. 2005;11(1):70–83.

50. Schmidt KS, Gallo JL, Ferri C, Giovannetti T, Sestito N, Libon DJ, Schmidt PS. The neuropsychological profile of alcohol-related dementia suggests cortical and subcortical pathology. Dement Geriatr Cogn Disord. 2005;20(5):286–91.

51. Sharma D, Albery IP, Cook C. Selective attentional bias to alcohol related stimuli in problem drinkers and non-problem drinkers. Addiction. 2001;96(2):285–95.

52. Stetter F, Ackermann K, Bizer A, Straube ER, Mann K. Effects of disease-related cues in alcoholic inpatients: results of a controlled "Alcohol Stroop" study. Alcohol Clin Exp Res. 1995;19(3): 593–9.

53. Stormark KM, Laberg JC, Nordby H, Hugdahl K. Alcoholics' selective attention to alcohol stimuli: automated processing? J Stud Alcohol. 2000;61(1):18–23.

54. Sullivan EV, Mathalon DH, Zipursky RB, Kersteen-Tucker Z, Knight RT, Pfefferbaum A. Factors of the Wisconsin Card Sorting Test as measures of frontal-lobe function in schizophrenia and in chronic alcoholism. Psychiatry Res. 1993;46(2):175–99.

55. Sullivan EV, Rosenbloom MJ, Pfefferbaum A. Pattern of motor and cognitive deficits in detoxified alcoholic men. Alcohol Clin Exp Res. 2000;24(5):611–21.

56. Sullivan EV, Fama R, Rosenbloom MJ, Pfefferbaum A. A profile of neuropsychological deficits in alcoholic women. Neuropsychology. 2002;16(1):74–83.

57. Tapert SF, Brown SA. Substance dependence, family history of alcohol dependence and neuropsychological functioning in adolescence. Addiction. 2000;95(7):1043–53.

58. Tedstone D, Coyle K. Cognitive impairments in sober alcoholics: performance on selective and divided attention tasks. Drug Alcohol Depend. 2004;75(3):277–86.

59. Uekermann J, Daum I, Schlebusch P, Wiebel B, Trenckmann U. Depression and cognitive functioning in alcoholism. Addiction. 2003;98(11):1521–9.

60. Uekermann J, Daum I, Schlebusch P, Trenckmann U. Processing of affective stimuli in alcoholism. Cortex. 2005;41(2):189–94.

61. van Gorp WG, Altshuler L, Theberge DC, Wilkins J, Dixon W. Cognitive impairment in euthymic bipolar patients with and without prior alcohol dependence. A preliminary study. Arch Gen Psychiatry. 1998;55(1):41–6.

62. Zinn S, Stein R, Swartzwelder HS. Executive functioning early in abstinence from alcohol. Alcohol Clin Exp Res. 2004;28(9): 1338–46.

63. Smith ME, Oscar-Berman M. Resource-limited information processing in alcoholism. J Stud Alcohol. 1992;53(5):514–8.

64. Corral M, Holguin SR, Cadaveira F. Neuropsychological characteristics of young children from high-density alcoholism families: a three-year follow-up. J Stud Alcohol. 2003;64(2):195–9.

65. Nigg JT, Glass JM, Wong MM, Poon E, Jester JM, Fitzgerald HE, Puttler LI, Adams KM, Zucker RA. Neuropsychological executive functioning in children at elevated risk for alcoholism: findings in early adolescence. J Abnorm Psychol. 2004;113(2):302–14.

66. Cox WM, Hogan LM, Kristian MR, Race JH. Alcohol attentional bias as a predictor of alcohol abusers' treatment outcome. Drug Alcohol Depend. 2002;68(3):237–43.

67. Levenson M, Neuringer C. Problem-solving behavior in suicidal adolescents. J Consult Clin Psychol. 1971;37:433–6.

68. Neuringer C. Rigid thinking in suicidal individuals. J Consult Psychol. 1964;28:54–8.

69. Patsiokas AT, Clum GA, Luscomb RL. Cognitive characteristics of suicide attempters. J Consult Clin Psychol. 1979;47:478–84.

70. Bigler E. On the neuropsychology of suicide. J Learn Disabil. 1989;22:181–5.

71. Rourke BP, Young GC, Leenaars AA. A childhood learning disability that predisposes those afflicted to adolescent and adult depression and suicide risk. J Learn Disabil. 1989;22:169–75.

72. Bartfai A, Winborg I, Nordstrom P, Asberg M. Suicidal behavior and cognitive flexibility: design and verbal fluency after attempted suicide. Suicide Life Threat Behav. 1990;20:254–65.

73. Sher L. Role of selenium depletion in the etiopathogenesis of depression in patients with alcoholism. Med Hypotheses. 2002;59:330–3.

74. Rayman MP. The importance of selenium to human health. Lancet. 2000;356:233–41.

75. Barceloux DG. Selenium. J Toxicol Clin Toxicol. 1999;37(2): 145–72.

76. Flohe L, Andreesen JR, Brigelius-Flohe R, Maiorino M, Ursini F. Selenium, the element of the moon, in life on earth. Life. 2000;49:411–20.

77. Alertsen AR, Aukrust A, Skaug OE. Selenium concentrations in blood and serum from patients with mental diseases. Acta Psychiatr Scand. 1986;74:217–9.

78. Lecomte E, Herbert B, Pirollet P, Chancerelle Y, Arnaud J, Musse N, Paille F, Siest G, Artur Y. Effect of alcohol consumption on blood antioxydant nutrients and oxidative stress indicators. Am J Clin Nutr. 1994;60:255–61.

79. Ward RJ, Julta J, Peters TJ. Antioxidant status in alcoholic liver disease. Adv Biosci. 1989;76:343–51.

80. Tanner AR, Bantock I, Hinks L, Lloyd B, Turner NR, Wright R. Depressed selenium and vitamin E levels in a alcoholic population. Dig Dis Sci. 1986;31:1307–12.

81. Johansson U, Johnsson F, Joelsson B, Berglund M, Akesson B. Selenium status in patients with liver cirrhosis and alcoholism. Br J Nutr. 1986;55:227–33.

82. Girre C, Hispard E, Therond P, Guedj S, Bourdon R, Dally S. Effect of abstinence from alcohol on the depression of glutathione peroxidase activity and selenium and vitamins E levels in chronic alcoholic patients. Alcohol Clin Exp Res. 1990;14:909–12.

83. Dworkin BM, Rosenthal WS, Gordon GG, Jankowski RH. Diminished blood selenium levels in alcoholics. Alcohol Clin Exp Res. 1984;8:535–8.

84. Ringstad J, Knutsen SF, Nilssen OR, Thomassen Y. A comparative study of serum selenium and vitamin E levels in a population of male risk drinkers and abstainers. Biol Trace Elem Res. 1993;36:65–71.

85. Korpela H, Kumpulainen J, Luoma PV, Arranto AJ, Sotaniemi EA. Decreased serum selenium in alcoholics as related to liver structure and function. Am J Clin Nutr. 1985;42:147–51.

86. Watson RR, Mohs ME, Eskelson C, Sampliner RE, Hartmann B. Identification of alcohol abuse and alcoholism with biological parameters. Alcohol Clin Exp Res. 1986;10:364–85.

87. Välimäki MJ, Harju KJ, Ylikahri RH. Decreased serum selenium in alcoholics—a consequence of liver dysfunction. Clin Chim Acta. 1983;130:291–6.

88. Corrigan FM, Besson JAO, Ward NI. Red cell caesium, lithium and selenium in abstinent alcoholics. Alcohol Alcohol. 1991;26:309–14.

89. Bjorneboe GE, Johnsen J, Bjorneboe A, Bache-Wiig JE, Morland J, Drevon CA. Diminished serum concentration of vitamin E in alcoholics. Ann Nutr Metab. 1988;32:56–61.

90. Lieber CS. Alcohol and the liver. In: Arias IM, Frenkel MS, Wilson JHP, editors. Liver annual-VI. Amsterdam: Excerpta Medica; 1987. p. 163–240.

91. Dutta SK, Miller PA, Greenberg LB, Levander OA. Selenium and acute alcoholism. Am J Nutr. 1983;38:21–9.

92. Whanger PD. Selenium and the brain: a review. Nutr Neurosci. 2001;4:81–97.

93. Bodnar LM, Wisner KL. Nutrition and depression: implications for improving mental health among childbearing-aged women. Biol Psychiatry. 2005;58(9):679–85.

94. Hawkes WC, Hornbostel L. Effects of dietary selenium on mood in healthy men living in a metabolic research unit. Biol Psychiatry. 1996;39:121–8.

95. Finley JW, Penland JG. Adequacy or deprivation of dietary selenium in healthy men: clinical and psychological findings. J Trace Elem Exp Med. 1998;11:11–27.

96. Benton D, Cook R. Selenium supplementation improves mood in a double-blind crossover trial. Biol Psychiatry 1991;29: 1092–8.

97. Brtkova A, Brtko J. Selenium: metabolism and endocrines (minireview). Endocr Regul. 1996;30:117–28.

98. Shor-Posner G, Lecusay R, Miguez MJ, Moreno-Black G, Zhang G, Rodriguez N, Burbano X, Baum M, Wilkie F. Psychological burden in the era of HAART: impact of selenium therapy. Int J Psychiatry Med. 2003;33(1):55–69.

99. Sher L. Role of thyroid hormones in the effects of selenium on mood, behavior, and cognitive function. Med Hypotheses. 2001;57:480–3.

100. Mino A, Bousquet A, Broers B. Substance abuse and drug-related death, suicidal ideation, and suicide: a review. Crisis. 1999;20(1): 28–35.

101. Deykin EY, Buka SL. Suicidal ideation and attempts among chemically dependent adolescents. Am J Publ Health. 1994;4:634–9.

102. Felts WM, Chenier T, Barnes R. Drug use and suicide ideation and behavior among North Carolina public school students. Am J Publ Health. 1992;6:870–2.

103. Murphy SL, Rounsaville B, Eyre S, et al. Suicide attempts in treated opiate addicts. Compr Psychiatry. 1983;24:79–89.

104. Allison M, Hubbard RL, Ginzburg HM. Indicators of suicide and depression among drug abusers. NIDA Treatment Research Monograph. Rockville: National Institute on Drug Abuse; 1985.

105. Brent DA. Risk factors for adolescent suicide and suicidal behavior: mental and substance abuse disorders, family environmental factors, and life stress. Suicide Life Threat Behav. 1995; 25(suppl):52–63.

106. Graham C, Burvill PW. A study of coroner's records of suicide in young people, 1986–88 in Western Australia. Aust NZ J Psychiatry. 1992;26:30–9.

107. Frederick CJ, Resnik HLP, Wittlin BJ. Self-destructive aspects of hard core addiction. Arch Gen Psychiatry. 1973;28:579–85.

108. Lynskey MT, Glowinski AL, Todorov AA, Bucholz KK, Madden PA, Nelson EC, Statham DJ, Martin NG, Heath AC. Major depressive disorder, suicidal ideation, and suicide attempt in twins discordant for cannabis dependence and early-onset cannabis use. Arch Gen Psychiatry. 2004;61(10):1026–32.

109. Roy A. Characteristics of cocaine-dependent patients who attempt suicide. Am J Psychiatry. 2001;158(8):1215–9.

110. Bohn M, Sher L. Suicide and substance abuse. In: Kranzler HR, Korsmeyer P, editors. Encyclopedia of drugs, alcohol and addictive behavior. 3rd ed. New York: MacMillan Reference USA; 2008.

111. Cornelius JR, Thase ME, Salloum IM, Cornelius MD, Black A, Mann JJ. Cocaine use associated with increased suicidal behavior in depressed alcoholics. Addict Behav. 1998;23(1):119–21.

112. Sher L, Zalsman G. Alcohol and adolescent suicide. Int J Adolesc Med Health. 2005;17(3):197–203.

113. Heninger M, Hanzlick R. Nonnatural deaths of adolescents and teenagers: Fulton County, Georgia, 1985-2004. Am J Forensic Med Pathol. 2008;29(3):208–13.

Gambling and Drug Abuse

40

Nancy M. Petry and Robey Champine

Abstract

Pathological gambling shares many similarities to substance use disorders, including some diagnostic criteria and high rates of comorbidity. This chapter reviews epidemiological and treatment studies exploring the relationship between disordered gambling and substance use. It also delineates the increased problems experienced by individuals with both disorders. Further, this chapter describes treatment interventions for individuals with gambling problems. Existing research demonstrates the efficacy of cognitive-behavioral therapy for pathological gambling as well as motivational enhancement therapy for gambling behavior problems. Based on consideration of these findings, we suggest an integrated treatment approach to assist dually diagnosed clients in overcoming concurrent gambling and substance use problems. However, further empirical research is needed to evaluate the efficacy of treatments specifically for this dually diagnosis population.

Learning Objectives
- To define the diagnostic criteria for pathological gambling
- To understand the comorbidity between pathological gambling and substance use disorders
- To identify problems in individuals with substance use and gambling problems
- To describe efficacious treatment interventions for problem and pathological gamblers

Issues that Need to Be Addressed by Future Research
- Empirical data are needed to examine the longitudinal relationships between substance use and gambling disorders
- Additional research is needed to inform the development of treatment interventions that focus on individuals with substance use and gambling problems

Pathological gambling is characterized as "persistent and recurrent maladaptive gambling behavior that disrupts personal, family, or vocational pursuits" [1]. This disorder has many similarities to substance use disorders, and it also shares high rates of comorbidity with drug and alcohol abuse. This chapter describes the symptoms and criteria for pathological gambling. It also reviews the literature on comorbidity between gambling and substance use disorders. Finally,

N.M. Petry (✉) • R. Champine
Calhoun Cardiology Center, University of Connecticut Health Center,
263 Farmington Avenue, Farmington, CT 06030-3944, USA
e-mail: npetry@uchc.edu

J.C. Verster et al. (eds.), *Drug Abuse and Addiction in Medical Illness: Causes, Consequences and Treatment*,
DOI 10.1007/978-1-4614-3375-0_40, © Springer Science+Business Media, LLC 2012

the chapter describes efficacious treatment interventions for gambling and provides suggestions for treatment for individuals with combined gambling and substance use disorders.

Classification and Diagnosis

The Diagnostic and Statistical Manual of Mental Disorders, Revision III [2], was the first to introduce pathological gambling as a psychiatric disorder. It included this disorder as a Disorder of Impulse Control, Not Elsewhere Classified. Today in the DSM-IV [1], pathological gambling remains in the impulse control section, although discussions are ongoing about integrating it with substance use disorders [3].

In the DSM-IV, there are ten diagnostic criteria for pathological gambling, and an individual must meet at least five for a diagnosis [1]. Half of the ten pathological gambling criteria parallel diagnostic criteria for substance use disorders. They include: being preoccupied with gambling or ways to get money to gamble, increasing amounts of money or frequencies of gambling over time (i.e., tolerance), feeling irritable or restless when unable to gamble (i.e., withdrawal), having repeated unsuccessful attempts of stopping or reducing gambling, and giving up other activities or relationships because of gambling. The other five criteria for pathological gambling are: chasing lost money (or betting more money to re-coup losses), gambling to escape or relieve problems or adverse moods, lying to others to hide gambling, committing illegal acts to support gambling, and relying on others to relieve gambling-related financial difficulties.

The DSM-IV classification system does not include a subthreshold condition as exists for substance abuse versus dependence. However, many individuals have some gambling-related problems, but do not meet the full five criteria necessary for a diagnosis. Throughout this chapter, this subthreshold condition will be termed "problem gambling." Problem gambling refers to those who endorse fewer than five pathological gambling symptoms, and typically three to four symptoms. The term "disordered gambling" will be used to refer to the combined group of problem and pathological gamblers.

Prevalence Rates of Disordered Gambling in General Populations

A number of national and international epidemiological studies have evaluated the prevalence of disordered gambling. Initially, we describe studies from the United States (U.S.) and then include data from studies conducted around the world.

Five nationally based studies examining prevalence rates of problem and pathological gambling have been conducted in the USA. The first of these studies took place prior to the inclusion of the disorder in the DSM-III, and therefore it evaluated gambling behaviors and attitudes rather than

diagnoses. Kallick, Suits, Dielman, and Hybels [4] conducted a telephone survey of 1,749 randomly selected US residents. They reported that 0.8% of respondents had a lifetime gambling problem, and 2.3% had moderate gambling problems. The next nationally based survey occurred about 20 years later. As part of the National Gambling Impact Study Commission (NGISC), Gerstein, Hoffman, Larison, Engleman, Murphy, Palmer et al. [5] interviewed 2,417 randomly selected US residents by telephone. The lifetime prevalence rate of pathological gambling was estimated to be 0.8%, and the lifetime prevalence rate of problem gambling was estimated to be 1.3%. Past-year rates were 0.1% for pathological gambling and 0.4% for problem gambling. In an another independent telephone survey of 2,638 participants conducted around the same time, Welte, Barnes, Wieczorek, Tidwell, and Parker [6] reported lifetime prevalence rates of pathological and problem gambling to be slightly higher—2.0% and 2.8%, respectively. Rates of past-year pathological and problem gambling were 1.3% and 2.2%, respectively.

More recently, the National Comorbidity Survey Replication (NCS-R) evaluated 9,282 household respondents and found the rate of lifetime pathological gambling to be 0.6%, and the rate of problem gambling to be 2.3% [7]. The past-year prevalence rate of pathological gambling was 0.3% in this survey. The National Epidemiologic Survey on Alcohol and Related Conditions (NESARC) is the largest nationally based survey. Petry, Stinson, and Grant [8] reported results from this in-person survey of over 43,000 randomly selected adults. The lifetime prevalence rate of pathological gambling was 0.4%.

Thus, the lifetime prevalence rate of pathological gambling in the US varies from 0.4 to 2.0%, and past-year rates are substantially lower at 0.1 to 1.3%. Prevalence rates for lifetime problem gambling range from 1.3 to 2.8%, and past-year prevalence rates for problem gambling are about 0.4 to 2.2%.

The rates reported in US studies parallel prevalence rates from studies conducted in countries around the world. Stucki and Rihs-Middel [9] examined prevalence surveys from ten countries including Australia, Canada, China, Italy, New Zealand, Norway, Singapore, Sweden, Switzerland, and the USA. The weighted means across the studies for problem gambling ranged from 1.2 to 2.4%, and for pathological gambling it was 0.8 to 1.8%.

Comorbidities in General Population Surveys

Several of the studies outlined above not only assessed gambling disorders, but also substance use disorders. All of them found statistically significant increases in substance use disorders among individuals identified with problem or pathological gambling compared to those without gambling problems.

Gerstein et al. [5] found that 9.9% of individuals identified with pathological gambling and 12.4% identified with problem gambling met criteria for a lifetime substance use disorder, compared with 1.1% of nongamblers and 1.3% of recreational (nonproblem) gamblers. Kessler et al. [7] noted that 76.3% of pathological gamblers identified in the NCS-R study had a lifetime substance use disorder. These results are consistent with studies from other countries as well. For example, from a survey of 14,934 respondents in Canada, El-Guebaly, Pattern, Currie, Williams, Beck, Maxwell et al. [10] found that nearly 50% of those identified as "moderate-risk" or problem gamblers had substance dependence or reported harmful use of alcohol versus 7.6% of nonproblem gamblers.

In terms of alcohol use disorders specifically, Gerstein et al. [5] reported that 9.9% of the disordered gamblers identified in their survey met lifetime alcohol dependence criteria versus 1.1% of the nongamblers. Welte et al. [6] found that 25% of current pathological gamblers were also alcohol-dependent compared with 1.4% of nonpathological gamblers. The odds ratio of current alcohol dependence with current pathological gambling was extraordinarily high—23.1, suggesting a 23-fold risk of pathological gambling among those with alcohol dependence. In the NESARC study, Petry et al. [8] noted that 25.4% of those identified with lifetime pathological gambling also met criteria for lifetime alcohol abuse and 47.8% for lifetime alcohol dependence. The odds ratio was 6.0, indicating that those with an alcohol use disorder had a sixfold increased risk of pathological gambling compared to those without an alcohol use disorder.

Some studies, albeit fewer, have also examined comorbidity of gambling and drug use disorders. In the Gerstein et al. [5] study, formal drug use diagnoses were not made, but 8.1% of lifetime pathological gamblers and 16.8% of lifetime problem gamblers reported illicit drug use in the past year versus 4.2% of social gamblers and 2.0% of nongamblers. Petry et al. [8] noted that 26.9% of the pathological gamblers met criteria for lifetime illicit drug abuse and 11.2% for dependence, with odds ratios of 3.5.

Comorbidity of Disordered Gambling in Treatment-Seeking Substance Abusers

Consistent with the aforementioned epidemiological data, many individuals seeking treatment for substance use disorders also have disordered gambling. Below, we review rates of disordered gambling in patients seeking treatment for substance use disorders in general outpatient clinics and then in specific populations of substance abusers, including alcohol-, cocaine-, marijuana-, and opioid-dependent patients.

General Substance Abuse Patients

Several studies have evaluated rates of pathological gambling in general substance abuse treatment patients who were not differentiated by substance use diagnoses. These studies found rates of pathological gambling ranging from 5 to 33% [11–20]. In terms of problem gambling, the rates range from 5 to 22% [12, 13, 16, 18–20]. These rates are clearly much higher than the rates for problem and pathological gambling noted in the general population surveys reported earlier.

Specific Substance Use Disorders

Few studies exist that examine rates of disordered gambling in specific substance-abusing populations. Studies assessing patients seeking alcohol treatment generally find rates of pathological gambling between 4 and 13% [16, 17, 20–24]. Rates of pathological gambling among patients seeking treatment for cocaine abuse range from 8 to 15% [16, 20, 25, 26]. In methadone-maintained patients with opioid dependence, rates of pathological gambling vary from 5 to 18% [16, 20, 27–29]. Only one known study [20] examined patients seeking treatment for cannabis dependence for gambling problems, and 24% were identified as pathological gamblers and 14% as problem gamblers.

Onset and Severity of Problems in Dually Diagnosed Patients

The data reviewed above suggest that pathological gambling is a relatively common comorbid condition that should be routinely evaluated in substance abuse treatment settings. Most studies of treatment-seeking samples find that individuals with both substance abuse and disordered gambling have more severe problems than individuals with just substance abuse or gambling alone. Difficulties encountered by dually diagnosed patients include more severe substance use problems, along with psychosocial, legal, and psychiatric difficulties.

The severity and number of substance use problems appear to be greater in substance abusers with gambling problems compared to substance abusers without gambling problems. In comparison to cocaine abusers without pathological gambling, cocaine abusers with pathological gambling had increased prevalence of alcohol dependence and more drug abuse treatment attempts [26]. McCormick [17] found that substance abusers with gambling problems abused a greater number of substances than their counterparts without gambling problems, and Daghestani, Elenz, and Crayton [14] found that substance abusers with disordered gambling began using substances at an earlier age and reported more frequent alcohol use than those without disordered gambling. Langenbucher, Bavly, Labouvie, Sanjuan, and Martin [15] noted more frequent use of alcohol and more alcohol and drug dependence symptoms among substance abusers identified with gambling problems in comparison to those without gambling problems.

Disordered gambling substance abusers also tend to have more severe legal, employment, and family difficulties. Steinberg, Kosten, and Rounsaville [26] reported that cocaine abusers with pathological gambling had more arrests, convictions, and time in prisons than those without gambling problems. Hall, Carriero, Takushi, Montoya, Preston, and Gorelick [25] further reported that cocaine-dependent patients identified with pathological gambling were more often unemployed, were more likely to engage in illegal activities for profit, and had served more time in prison than cocaine-dependent patients without pathological gambling. Langenbucher et al. [15] found that substance abusers identified with pathological gambling scored higher on indices of social impairment than their counterparts who were not pathological gamblers. Petry [30] found that severity of gambling problems in substance abusers was predictive of high-risk sexual activities who spread HIV and other infectious diseases.

Finally, psychiatric symptoms are more severe and comorbid psychiatric disorders are more prevalent in substance abusers with gambling problems compared to those without gambling problems. Steinberg et al. [26] found increased rates of attention-deficit disorder among cocaine abusers with gambling problems. McCormick [17] reported that substance abusers with gambling problems scored higher on measures of hostility, negative effect, and impulsivity. Petry [31] found that those with both disorders had increased somatization, obsessive-compulsive, interpersonal sensitivity, hostility, and paranoia symptoms than those with substance use disorders alone. Hall et al. [25] and Langenbucher et al. [15] noted increased rates of attention deficit disorder, conduct disorder, and antisocial personality disorder among substance abusers with gambling problems compared to those without gambling problems.

While gambling and substance abuse are associated with increased problems, little research has addressed issues related to the onset and patterning of these problems. Spunt, Lesieur, Hunt, and Cahill [29] found that substances are often used in conjunction with gambling in methadone-maintained patients. These patients reported combining gambling and drug use to make money to buy drugs, increase their high from drugs, and celebrate after winning at gambling. Cunningham-Williams, Cottler, Compton, Spitznagel, and Ben-Abdallah [13] found that most of the pathological gamblers in their study began smoking cigarettes, drinking alcohol, and smoking marijuana prior to developing

gambling problems, but pathological gambling often preceded dependence on other drugs, especially stimulants. Similarly, Hall et al. [25] noted that gambling preceded onset of cocaine dependence in 72% of their cocaine-dependent sample from the Baltimore, MD, area, while in Korea, Cho, Hahm, Suh, Suh, Cho, and Lee [21] found that alcohol problems most often preceded gambling problems.

Only a couple of studies have examined the association of disordered gambling with substance abuse treatment outcomes. Hall et al. [25] did not find that pathological gambling status was associated with increased cocaine or opioid use or treatment retention in samples of cocaine-dependent outpatients. However, in another study of methadone-maintained patients, Ledgerwood and Downey [28] found that those identified as pathological gamblers were more likely to use cocaine during treatment and drop out of treatment prematurely than those without pathological gambling. Thus, limited data are available about how gambling impacts drug abuse treatment outcomes, but rarely are the two disorders concurrently addressed in substance abuse treatment programs.

Comorbidity of Substance Use Disorders in Treatment-Seeking Pathological Gamblers

Not only do treatment-seeking substance abusers evidence high rates of disordered gambling, but the converse relationship also holds. Treatment-seeking pathological gamblers have high rates of substance use disorders, as outlined below.

Prevalence Rates of Substance Use Diagnoses

Substance use disorders occur in about one-quarter or two-thirds of treatment-seeking gamblers. For example, in one of the earliest studies, Ramirez, McCormick, Russo, and Taber [32] assessed substance use disorders in 51 successive admissions to a Veterans Administration Gambling Treatment Program, and found that 39% had a past-year diagnosis of a drug or alcohol use disorder, and 47% had a lifetime substance use disorder. In small studies of Gamblers Anonymous (GA) members, Linden, Pope, and Jones [33] found 48% had alcohol dependence, and Lesieur and Blume [34] noted 26% had alcohol abuse. McCormick, Russo, Ramirez, and Taber [35] studied inpatient pathological gamblers, and 32% had alcohol use disorders and 4% had drug use disorders. Specker, Carlson, Edmonson, Johnson, and Marcotte [36] reported that 60% of 40 outpatient gamblers surveyed met lifetime criteria for a substance use disorder, with 50% meeting criteria for alcohol abuse or dependence, 23% for cannabis, 8% for stimulants, and 5% each for cocaine and sedatives.

Similar results are reported in other countries. For example, Ibanez, Blanco, Donahue, Lesieur, Castro, Fernandez-Piqueras et al. [37] found that 23% of 69 treatment-seeking pathological gamblers in Madrid, Spain, were currently abusing or dependent upon alcohol, and 35% had lifetime diagnoses of an alcohol use disorder. Maccallum and Blaszczynski [38] interviewed 75 poker-machine players who were receiving gambling treatment in Australia and noted that 16% met criteria for alcohol abuse, 8% for alcohol dependence, 37% for nicotine dependence, 5% for cannabis abuse, 5% for cannabis dependence, and 1% each for amphetamine and inhalant abuse. From a sample of 150 treatment-seeking pathological gamblers in Singapore, Teo, Mythily, Anantha, and Winslow [39] found that 4.7% were abusing or dependent on alcohol and 7.3% were abusing other substances.

From a large sample of 944 admissions at gambling outpatient treatment programs in Minnesota, Stinchfield and Winters [40] reported that 33% had previously received treatment for a substance use disorder. Similarly, we noted that about a third of outpatient gamblers in Connecticut had one or more substance abuse treatment episodes [41]. Of the pathological gamblers who had received substance abuse treatment, it was most often for alcohol, followed by cocaine and then others drugs, primarily marijuana. Thus, both treatment and epidemiological data concur that substance use disorders and pathological gambling are related.

Psychosocial Problems in Dually Diagnosed Pathological Gamblers

The studies outlined above all indicate that individuals seeking treatment for pathological gambling have high rates of substance use disorders. However, most substance use diagnoses were past, not current, with only about 10% of treatment-seeking gamblers reporting current use of illicit drugs or regular, heavy use of alcohol [40, 41].

Ladd and Petry [41] found that treatment-seeking gamblers with a history of substance use disorders (31%) tended to have more severe gambling problems, psychiatric symptoms, and other psychosocial difficulties than pathological gamblers with no prior substance abuse problems. Specifically, pathological gamblers with a history of substance abuse had more years of gambling problems, more frequent gambling activity, and more gambling problems in the month prior to initiating gambling treatment than pathological gamblers without prior substance abuse problems. Compared to those without substance abuse problems, gamblers with substance abuse treatment histories were also more likely to be receiving treatment for mental health problems.

These studies call for further investigation of the role of substance abuse in the development and course of pathological gambling and whether substance abuse problems affect the course of treatment or outcomes among gamblers. To date, few studies have systematically investigated the effects of substance use disorders on treatment outcomes in gamblers. Two reports suggest that pathological gamblers with a past or current substance use disorder were less likely to experience a gambling relapse than those without other addictive disorders [42, 43]. In contrast, other studies found no relationship between past or current substance use and gambling treatment outcomes [44–46]. These inconsistent findings highlight the need for more research examining the impact of substance use on gambling treatment outcomes.

Treatment of Disordered Gambling

Few randomized controlled trials of treatments for pathological gambling have been conducted, and no known randomized studies have examined interventions specifically for substance-abusing pathological gamblers. This lack of data makes treatment recommendations speculative, especially among dually diagnosed patients. Below, we briefly review the most common interventions for individuals seeking treatment for gambling, and we provide suggestions for treating substance-abusing gamblers.

Gamblers Anonymous

Gamblers Anonymous (GA) is a self-help fellowship modeled after Alcoholics Anonymous (AA), which is based on the premise that alcoholism (or gambling) is a disease that cannot be cured but managed only by complete abstinence. Twelve principles or steps are followed that include acceptance and powerlessness over drinking (or gambling) as well as surrendering to a Higher Power. Many substance abuse treatment programs in the US will refer substance-abusing gamblers to GA as they do AA, because the philosophies are similar. However, Petry [47] found that pathological gamblers with a substance use disorder were less likely to become involved in GA than gamblers without substance use problems.

By definition, individuals seeking treatment for drug use problems would be likely to have less severe gambling problems than substance abuse problems. They may be reluctant to endorse a complete abstinence goal for gambling and therefore less likely to relate to GA. Thus, referral to GA may be a useful option only among a relatively small number of treatment-seeking substance abusers with severe gambling problems. Further, even among severe pathological gamblers, Stewart and Brown [48] found that less than 10% of 232 attendees at GA became actively engaged and were abstinent a year later.

The effectiveness of GA may be enhanced when professionally delivered counseling is provided concurrently. Russo, Taber, McCormick, and Ramirez [49], Taber, McCormick, Russo, Adkins, and Ramirez [50], Lesieur and Blume [34], and Petry [47] followed treatment-seeking gamblers who received combined GA and professional therapy. Gambling abstinence rates at 6–14 months following treatment ranged from 25 to 50% across studies, and attendance at GA was positively associated with outcomes. However, in the above studies, the professional treatment was not standardized or well-described, and random assignment procedures were not used so efficacy of GA has not been established.

Cognitive-Behavioral Therapy

Cognitive-behavioral therapy (CBT) has been evaluated for the treatment of pathological gambling. In a number of studies [51–55], CBT was more efficacious in reducing gambling than a wait-list condition, no further treatment, or referral to GA alone. Several types of CBT for pathological gambling have been described, varying in emphasis on behavioral or cognitive aspects. Some approaches are relapse-prevention oriented and based on traditional models of CBT for substance use disorders [54], while others focus much more on altering irrational cognitions associated with gambling [52, 53].

Our CBT approach [56] attempts to restructure the environment to increase reinforcement from nongambling sources. Patients are taught to identify triggers of gambling, which in some cases may include substances. They are taught to conduct functional analyses of gambling behaviors, which consists of breaking gambling episodes into precipitants (or triggers), and evaluating the positive and negative consequences of wagering. In one session, gamblers are provided with a "leisure checklist," containing activities and hobbies, and patients check those they once liked to do or would like to try. Gamblers are then encouraged to engage in these activities during high-risk gambling times. In other sessions, gamblers brainstorm about methods for handling internal (or mood) triggers as well as external gambling triggers, such as viewing gambling advertisements. Interpersonal conflicts commonly trigger gambling urges, so skills training and role-playing for handling interpersonal conflict are included. One session addresses cognitive biases associated with gambling, such as overestimating the odds of winning and engaging in superstitious behaviors. Each session concludes with a weekly homework exercise to monitor and practice skills learned within the session. Many of the exercises can incorporate issues relevant to both substance use and gambling. For example, if drinking is a trigger for gambling, then scheduling alternative activities that do not involve either drinking or gambling would be important [57].

Motivational Enhancement Therapy and Brief Interventions

Motivational enhancement therapy (MET) is another approach used for treating both substance abuse and gambling behaviors [58–60]. MET is based on the conceptualization that behavior change occurs through stages: precontemplation, contemplation, action, and maintenance. The therapist elicits the patient's understanding of the consequences of substance use or gambling and strengthens his or her commitment to change. Motivational enhancement techniques are efficacious in reducing alcohol use in heavy alcohol users [58].

Hodgins, Currie, and El-Guebaly [61] evaluated the efficacy of MET in treating gamblers. In this study, 105 individuals with problem or pathological gambling were randomly assigned to one of three conditions: a 1-month wait-list, a cognitive-behavioral skills training workbook, or the same workbook plus a one-session telephone intervention with a therapist using motivational enhancement techniques. The workbook plus motivational intervention resulted in a significantly greater reduction of gambling than the wait-list control condition. In the follow-up periods, the patients assigned to the motivational intervention tended to maintain their gains better than those who received only the workbook [62].

Petry, Weinstock, Ledgerwood, and Morasco [45] screened patients from substance abuse treatment and other settings to identify problem and pathological gamblers who were not actively seeking gambling treatment. Those who were classified as problem or pathological gamblers ($n=180$) were randomized to one of four conditions: assessment only, ten minutes of Brief Advice, one session of MET, or one session of MET plus three sessions of CBT. In the Brief Advice condition, therapists informed patients of their level of gambling in relation to the general population and pointed out four specific strategies to ensure gambling did not progress to more problematic levels. In all conditions, gambling was assessed at baseline, 6 weeks later, and a 9-month follow-up. Relative to the assessment only, Brief Advice was the only condition that significantly decreased gambling between baseline and week 6, and it was also associated with clinically significant reductions in gambling at month 9. Between week 6 and month 9, the combination of MET and CBT demonstrated significantly reduced gambling on one index compared to the control condition. These results suggest the efficacy of a very brief intervention for reducing gambling among problem and pathological gamblers not actively seeking gambling treatment. Current substance use problems were not associated with gambling outcomes, suggesting the wide-spread potential benefits of this intervention.

These results demonstrate the possible efficacy of Brief Advice and MET in treating gamblers. Due to their brief durations and nonconfrontational approach, these interventions appear suitable for substance abusers who are identified as having a gambling problem during the course of substance abuse treatment. However, more research on these interventions is needed.

Summary

In summary, disordered gambling and substance use are common comorbid conditions, in both general epidemiological samples and in treatment-seeking populations. Individuals with both gambling and substance use problems tend to have more severe problems along a number of dimensions than individuals with either disorder alone. These high rates of comorbidities and compounded difficulties underscore the need to develop and test treatments for patients with both substance use and gambling problems. While little systematic research has evaluated treatments specifically for these dually diagnosed patients, Brief Advice appears to be a useful intervention for reducing gambling among substance abusers who are not actively seeking treatment for their gambling problems. In addition, an integrated treatment approach, focusing on both the substance use and gambling problems, may also assist in reducing problems associated with one or both disorders, but such interventions have yet to be well developed or empirically tested.

References

1. American Psychiatric Association. Diagnostic and statistical manual of mental disorders. 4th ed. Washington, DC: American Psychiatric Association Press; 1994.
2. American Psychiatric Association. Diagnostic and statistical manual of mental disorders. 3rd ed. Washington, DC: American Psychiatric Association Press; 1980.
3. Petry NM. Should the scope of addictive behaviors be broadened to include pathological gambling? Addiction. 2006;101 Suppl 1:152–60.
4. Kallick M, Suits D, Dielman T, Hybels J. A survey of American gambling attitudes and behavior. 1st ed. Washington, DC: U.S. Government Printing Office; 1976.
5. Gerstein D, Hoffman J, Larison C, Engleman L, Murphy S, Palmer A, et al. Gambling impact and behavior study report to the National Gambling Impact Study Commission. Chicago, IL: University of Chicago, National Opinion Research Center; 1999.
6. Welte J, Barnes G, Wieczorek W, Tidwell MC, Parker J. Alcohol and gambling pathology among U.S. adults: prevalence, demographic patterns and comorbidity. J Stud Alcohol. 2001;62:706–12.
7. Kessler RC, Hwang I, LaBrie R, Petukhova M, Sampson NA, Winters KC, et al. DSM-IV pathological gambling in the National Comorbidity Survey Replication. Psychol Med. 2008;38:1351–60.
8. Petry NM, Stinson FS, Grant BF. Comorbidity of DSM-IV pathological gambling and other psychiatric disorders: results from the National Epidemiologic Survey on Alcohol and Related Conditions. J Clin Psychiatry. 2005;66:564–74.
9. Stucki S, Rihs-Middel M. Prevalence of adult problem and pathological gambling between 2000 and 2005: an update. J Gambl Stud. 2007;23:245–57.
10. El-Guebaly N, Pattern SB, Currie S, Williams JV, Beck CA, Maxwell CJ, Wang JL. Epidemiological associations between gambling behavior, substance use, and mood and anxiety disorders. J Gambl Stud. 2006;22:275–87.
11. Castellani B, Wootton E, Rugle L, Wedgeworth R, Prabucki K, Olson R. Homelessness, negative affect, and coping among veterans with gambling problems who misused substances. Psychiatr Serv. 1996;47:298–99.
12. Ciarrocchi JW. Rates of pathological gambling in publicly funded outpatient substance abuse treatment. J Gambl Stud. 1993;9:289–93.
13. Cunningham-Williams RM, Cottler LB, Compton WM, Spitznagel EL, Ben-Abdallah A. Problem gambling and comorbid psychiatric and substance use disorders among drug users recruited from drug treatment and community settings. J Gambl Stud. 2000;16:347–76.
14. Daghestani AN, Elenz E, Crayton JW. Pathological gambling in hospitalized substance abusing veterans. J Clin Psychiat. 1996;57:360–63.
15. Langenbucher J, Bavly L, Labouvie E, Sanjuan PM, Martin CS. Clinical features of pathological gambling in an addictions treatment cohort. Psychol Addict Behav. 2001;15:77–9.
16. Lesieur HR, Blume SB, Zoppa RM. Alcoholism, drug abuse and gambling. Alcohol Clin Exp Res. 1986;10:33–8.
17. McCormick RA. Disinhibition and negative affectivity in substance abusers with and without a gambling problem. Addict Behav. 1993;18:331–36.
18. Rupcich N, Frisch GR, Govoni R. Comorbidity of pathological gambling in addiction treatment facilities. J Subst Abuse Treat. 1997;6:573–74.
19. Shaffer HJ, Freed CR, Healea D. Gambling disorders among homeless persons with substance use disorders seeking treatment at a community center. Psychiat Serv. 2002;53:1112–7.
20. Toneatto T, Brennan J. Pathological gambling in treatment-seeking substance abusers. Addict Behav. 2002;27:465–69.
21. Cho M, Hahm BJ, Suh T, Suh GH, Cho SJ, Lee CK. Comorbid mental disorders among patients with alcohol abuse and dependence in Korea. J Korean Med Sci. 2002;17:236–41.
22. Elia C, Jacobs D. The incidence of pathological gambling among Native Americans treated for alcohol dependence. Int J Addict. 1993;28:659–66.
23. Lejoyeux M, Feuché N, Loi S, Solomon J, Adès J. Study of impulse-control disorders among alcohol-dependent patients. J Clin Psychiatry. 1999;60:302–05.
24. Sellman JD, Adamson S, Robertson P, Sullivan S, Coverdale J. Gambling in mild-moderate alcohol-dependent outpatients. Subst Use Misuse. 2002;37:199–213.
25. Hall GW, Carriero NJ, Takushi RY, Montoya ID, Preston KL, Gorelick DA. Pathological gambling among cocaine-dependent outpatients. Am J Psychiatry. 2000;157:1127–33.
26. Steinberg MA, Kosten TA, Rounsaville BJ. Cocaine abuse and pathological gambling. Am J Addict. 1992;1:121–32.
27. Feigelman W, Kleinman PH, Lesieur HR, Millman RB, Lesser ML. Pathological gambling among methadone patients. Drug Alcohol Depend. 1995;39:75–81.
28. Ledgerwood DM, Downey KK. Relationship between problem gambling and substance use in a methadone maintenance population. Addict Behav. 2002;27:483–91.
29. Spunt B, Lesieur H, Hunt D, Cahill L. Gambling among methadone patients. Int J Addict. 1995;30:929–62.
30. Petry NM. Gambling problems in substance abusers are associated with increased sexual risk behaviors. Addiction. 2000;95:1089–100.

31. Petry NM. Psychiatric symptoms in problem gambling and non-problem gambling substance abusers. Am J Addict. 2000;9: 163–71.

32. Ramirez LF, McCormick RA, Russo AM, Taber JI. Patterns of substance abuse in pathological gamblers undergoing treatment. Addict Behav. 1983;8:425–28.

33. Linden RD, Pope HG, Jones JM. Pathological gambling and major affective disorder: preliminary findings. J Clin Psychiatry. 1986;47: 201–03.

34. Lesieur HR, Blume SB. Evaluation of patients treated for pathological gambling in a combined alcohol, substance abuse and pathological gambling treatment unit using the Addiction Severity Index. Br J Addict. 1991;86:1017–28.

35. McCormick RA, Russo AM, Ramirez LF, Taber J. Affective disorders among pathological gamblers seeking treatment. Am J Psychiatry. 1984;141:215–18.

36. Specker SM, Carlson GA, Edmonson KM, Johnson PE, Marcotte M. Psychopathology in pathological gamblers seeking treatment. J Gambl Stud. 1996;12:67–81.

37. Ibanez A, Blanco C, Donahue E, Lesieur H, Castro I, Fernandez-Piqueras J, et al. Psychiatric comorbidity in pathological gamblers seeking treatment. Am J Psychiatry. 2001;158:1733–35.

38. Maccallum F, Blaszczynski A. Pathological gambling and comorbid substance abuse. Aust NZ J Psychiatry. 2002;36:411–15.

39. Teo P, Mythily S, Anantha S, Winslow M. Demographic and clinical features of 150 pathological gamblers referred to a community addictions programme. Ann Acad Med Singapore. 2007;36: 165–8.

40. Stinchfield R, Winters K. Effectiveness of six state-supported compulsive gambling treatment programs in Minnesota. 3rd ed. Minneapolis, MN: Minnesota Department of Human Services; 1996.

41. Ladd GT, Petry NM. A comparison of pathological gamblers with and without substance abuse treatment histories. Exp Clin Psychopharmacol. 2003;11:202–09.

42. Hodgins DC, Peden N, Cassidy E. The association between comorbidity and outcome in pathological gambling: a prospective follow-up of recent quitters. J Gambl Stud. 2005;21:255–71.

43. Zion MM, Tracy E, Abell N. Examining the relationship between spousal involvement in Gam-Anon and relapse behaviors in pathological gamblers. J Gambl Stud. 1991;7:117–31.

44. Leblond J, Ladouceur R, Blaszczynski A. Which pathological gamblers will complete treatment? Br J Psychol. 2003;42(Pt2):205–9.

45. Petry NM, Weinstock J, Ledgerwood DM, Morasco B. A randomized trial of brief interventions for problem and pathological gamblers. J Consult Clin Psychol. 2008;76:318–28.

46. Stinchfield R, Kushner MG, Winters KC. Alcohol use and prior substance abuse treatment in relation to gambling problem severity and gambling treatment outcome. J Gambl Stud. 2005;21: 273–97.

47. Petry NM. Patterns and correlates of Gamblers Anonymous attendance in pathological gamblers seeking professional treatment. Addict Behav. 2003;28:1049–62.

48. Stewart RM, Brown RIF. An outcome study of Gamblers Anonymous. Br J Psychiatry. 1988;152:284–88.

49. Russo AM, Taber JI, McCormick RA, Ramirez LF. An outcome study of an inpatient treatment program for pathological gamblers. Hosp Community Psychiatry. 1984;35:823–27.

50. Taber J, McCormick R, Russo A, Adkins B, Ramirez L. Follow-up of pathological gamblers after treatment. Am J Psychiatry. 1987;144:757–61.

51. Echeburúa E, Fernández-Montalvo J, Báez C. Relapse prevention in the treatment of slot-machine pathological gambling: long-term outcome. Behav Ther. 2000;31:351–64.

52. Ladouceur R, Sylvian C, Boutin C, Lachance S, Doucet C, Leblond J, et al. Cognitive treatment of pathological gambling. J Nerv Ment Dis. 2001;11:774–80.

53. Ladouceur R, Sylvain C, Boutin C, Lachance S, Doucet C, Leblond J. Group therapy for pathological gamblers: a cognitive approach. Behav Res Ther. 2003;41:587–96.

54. Petry NM, Ammerman Y, Bohl J, Doersch A, Gay H, Kadden R, et al. Cognitive-behavioral therapy for pathological gamblers. J Consult Clin Psychol. 2006;74:555–67.

55. Sylvian C, Ladouceur R, Boisvert JM. Cognitive and behavioral treatment of pathological gambling: a controlled study. J Consult Clin Psychol. 1997;65:727–32.

56. Petry NM. Pathological gambling: etiology, comorbidity and treatments. Washington, D.C.: American Psychological Association Press; 2005.

57. Morasco BJ, Pietrzak RH, Blanco C, Grant BF, Hasin D, Petry NM. Health problems and medical utilization associated with gambling disorders: results from the National Epidemiologic Survey on Alcohol and Related Conditions. Psychosom Med. 2007;68:976–84.

58. Miller WR, Brown JM, Simpson TL, Handmaker NS, Bien TH, Luckie LF, editors. What works? A methodological analysis of the alcohol treatment outcome literature. Handbook of alcoholism treatment approaches: effective alternatives. 2nd ed. Boston, MA: Allyn and Bacon; 1995.

59. Prochaska JO, DiClemente CC. The transtheoretical approach: crossing traditional boundaries of therapy. Homewood, IL: Dow Jones/Irwin; 1984.

60. Prochaska JO, DiClemente CC. Toward a comprehensive model of change. Addictive behaviors: processes of change. New York: Plenum Press; 1986.

61. Hodgins DC, Currie SR, El-Guebaly N. Motivational enhancement and self-help treatments for problem gambling. J Consult Clin Psychol. 2001;69:50–7.

62. Hodgins DC, Currie S, El-Guebaly N, Peden N. Brief motivational treatment for problem gambling: a 24-month follow-up. Psychol Addict Behav. 2004;18:293–6.

The Role of Parents in Adolescents' Alcohol Use

Haske van der Vorst

Abstract

This chapter provides an overview of the existing literature on the role of parents in the development of adolescents' alcohol use. Numerous studies showed that adolescents model the drinking of their parents, particularly the drinking of the fathers. Other parental influences involve the way parents raise their children in general or specifically concerning alcohol use (alcohol-specific socialization). Parents being supportive toward their adolescent children and monitoring their daily lives have children who drink fewer amounts of alcohol. Also, parents who prohibit alcohol use at home and in other settings have strict attitudes about youth drinking, and supervising the drinking of adolescents lower the risk for their children to start using alcohol at an early age and to drink heavy later on in adolescence. However, parents are not rigid in their (alcohol-specific) parenting and adolescents are not passive recipients of the parenting. It seems that parents become more tolerant toward youth drinking over time which results in heavier drinking of the adolescents. The drinking of adolescents, on the other hand, affects their parents in the sense that parents withdraw in their parental efforts of controlling youth alcohol use. This in turn predicts an increase in adolescents' alcohol use. Implications for future research are discussed.

Learning Objectives

- Adolescents model the drinking behaviors of their parents, particularly the drinking of the father.
- General parenting practices, such as parental support and control, are protective factors in the development of adolescents' alcohol use.
- Alcohol-specific socialization referring to parenting practices specifically targeted to prevent, reduce, or control adolescents' alcohol use plays an important role in delaying the age of alcohol use onset and lowering the amount of drinking during adolescence.
- Setting rules about alcohol, having strict attitudes about youth drinking, supervising the alcohol use of adolescents, and prohibiting alcohol use in all settings predict less alcohol use of adolescents.
- Parents withdraw from their adolescent children when confronted with their drinking.

H. van der Vorst (✉)
Behavioural Science Institute, Radboud University Nijmegen,
P.O. Box 9104, 6500, Nijmegen, The Netherlands
e-mail: H.vandervorst@pwo.ru.nl

J.C. Verster et al. (eds.), *Drug Abuse and Addiction in Medical Illness: Causes, Consequences and Treatment*,
DOI 10.1007/978-1-4614-3375-0_41, © Springer Science+Business Media, LLC 2012

Issues that Need to be Addressed by Future Research

- Parental sanctions after an adolescent broke the house rule about alcohol use should be a topic of future research.
- The influence of the quality and frequency of parental alcohol-specific communication should be measured with longitudinal data.
- Bi-directional associations between parents and adolescents need to be included in future research on alcohol use.
- Future research should include both parents and peers to gain insight into how parents affect the influence of peers in youth drinking.
- Person–environment interactions should be tested in parenting and adolescents' alcohol use.
- In addition to longitudinal survey research, systematic observational research is needed on parenting and adolescents' alcohol use.

Introduction

In general, people start drinking alcohol in adolescence and their use sharply increases in the following years [1, 2]. On the individual level, however, there are substantial differences in drinking patterns [3–5]: Some adolescents merely experiment with alcohol, whereas others become heavy drinkers in a short period of time [6]. Nevertheless, it seems that adolescents who drink alcohol rarely will decrease their levels of use [4]. The short-term risks of heavy drinking, such as being involved in aggressive behaviors and unsafe sex [7–9], as well as the long-term risks (alcohol misuse) [10] stress the necessity to determine the factors that delay the age of onset and reduce alcohol use later on. In the last years, a considerable body of evidence has accumulated on the role of parents in adolescents' alcohol use: by the way parents raise their children [11–13] and their own use [8, 14, 15]. The current chapter provides an overview of the results of studies focusing on the influence of parents in adolescents' alcohol use (initiation and continuation). The following topics will be addressed: parental alcohol use, general parenting practices, alcohol-specific socialization, and bi-directionality.

Parental Alcohol Use

Intergenerational transmission of alcohol use and alcoholism has been well established [8, 14–17], and is the strongest between a parent and an adolescent who share gender [18, 19]. Parental drinking has been associated with the onset of

drinking [20], the amount of alcohol use [8], heavy drinking, and alcohol misuse in late adolescence and young adulthood [14, 15, 21]. Furthermore, parental alcoholism increases the risk for adolescents to develop heavy and binge drinking patterns later on [1]. It should be noted that only a few studies tested the influence of parental drinking separately for fathers and mothers. Those studies showed that the drinking of fathers is stronger related to adolescents' drinking than the drinking of mothers [19, 22].

Intergenerational transmission of alcohol use has been explained by social cognitive learning [23]. The social (cognitive) learning theory states that engagement in a behavior is more likely if one is exposed to significant (role) models of that behavior. Parents serve as role models for youth alcohol use [19, 24]. Observing parents drinking alcohol, for instance to relax or to celebrate, shapes adolescents' beliefs about when alcohol use is appropriate or what the consequences of drinking are [25]. Thus, through their own alcohol use, parents propagate their norms and attitudes toward alcohol use. This (positive) attitude might, in turn, motivate adolescents to use alcohol, also because adolescents might think that their parents will approve of their drinking. Moreover, adolescents will model the use when they find themselves in a similar situation as when they observed their parents drinking.

Apart from observing their parents, adolescents might also drink together with their parents [26]. This issue has received little attention in research on alcohol use. The few studies that examined whether drinking with parents is related to youth drinking showed that adolescents consume less and are less involved in binge drinking with their parents than with their friends [26, 27], perhaps because of parental supervision, or because adolescents do not feel comfortable being drunk in the presence of their parents [28, 29]. On the other hand, drinking with parents is shown to be positively correlated with youth drinking at home and drinking in settings outside the home, such as a pub or at a friend's house [30]. However, all these findings are based on cross-sectional data, and thus do not gain insight into the predictive effect of drinking with parents on youth alcohol use. Nevertheless, parental alcohol use seems to be a robust factor in the development of adolescents' alcohol use. In addition to parents' own alcohol use, parents influence adolescents' alcohol involvement in the way that they raise their children.

Parenting

General Parenting Practices

Parenting has been thought of as socialization, or a process whereby parents raise their children in a way that the children can conform to societies' demands, and meanwhile maintain a sense of autonomy [31, 32]. Thus, adolescents' alcohol use would be a result of their parents' efforts to shape and raise them. Socialization should take place in a safe, stimulating, and good family climate [31, 33]. Such a family climate is founded on two general parenting practices, parental support and parental control, which emerge from the literature as key constructs of parental socialization and the alcohol use of adolescents [11, 34–36]. Parental support refers to general parenting practices such as praising, nurturing, providing a warm relationship, encouraging, and giving physical and emotional affection. Parental control is a parenting practice that directs the adolescents' behavior in a manner that is acceptable for parents and society.

Parental Support and Adolescents' Alcohol Use

Parental support has been considered to be a protective factor in adolescents' alcohol use [37]. Adolescents are less likely to get involved in (heavy) alcohol use if their parents are supportive and warm and show physical and emotional affection [38–41]. Although the beneficial effects of parental support in the development of adolescents' drinking are well documented, less is known about possible underlying mechanism(s) [42, 43]. Based on previously proposed underlying mechanisms, it seems that at least some other factors mediate the association between parental support and adolescents' alcohol use, such as coping abilities, deviant peer affiliations, or deviance-prone attitudes. For instance, emotionally supported adolescents are better at coping with their problems and regulating their emotions, which in turn leads to controlling their own alcohol use [43]. Furthermore, parents who provide a supportive family climate have adolescent children who are more likely to be receptive to parental control efforts, which in turn prevents the adolescents from heavier alcohol use [11].

Parental Control and Adolescents' Alcohol Use

Ample studies have shown that parental control is effective in preventing adolescents' alcohol use [39]. Parental monitoring seems to be particularly important in reducing the amount and frequency of adolescents' alcohol use. Parents (actively) finding out what their adolescent children are doing, where and with whom, have children who are less likely to drink heavily [11, 13, 38, 44–47]. However, Stattin and Kerr [48] argued that the previously studied parental monitoring efforts do not really capture the meaning of monitoring, because the monitoring scales commonly used do not tap those parenting practices to track adolescents' whereabouts. These measurements rather refer to parents' awareness of what their children are doing, with whom and where. Thus, according to Stattin and Kerr (2002), parental *knowledge* would have been a better label than parental monitoring. Despite this meaningful critique, many studies on parental control and adolescents' drinking have used the term parental monitoring instead of parental knowledge.

In addition to parental monitoring or knowledge, parental discipline has been linked to adolescents' alcohol use. That is, inconsistent parental discipline promotes adolescents' alcohol use [49], and consistent discipline plays a preventive role in adolescents' drunkenness [17]. Coercive control, on the other hand, seems to predict heavy drinking in adolescence [38], while psychological control has not been associated with youth drinking [46].

To summarize, general parenting practices, such as parental control and parental support, are protective factors in adolescents' alcohol use. However, parental support and control do not provide insight into how parents exactly raise their children concerning alcohol use. For example, parents might monitor their adolescents' behavior in general, but they may be ignorant about their children's alcohol use at a friend's house. Therefore, it is important to take a step further when studying the role of parenting in adolescents' drinking, namely, to examine the role of the so-called alcohol-specific socialization.

Alcohol-Specific Socialization

Jackson and her colleagues [12] were one of the first introducing the term alcohol-specific socialization in alcohol research. They emphasized the importance of examining more precisely the way parents deal with the drinking behaviors of adolescents. Alcohol-specific socialization refers to parenting practices specifically targeted to prevent, reduce, or control adolescents' alcohol use [22]. In an attempt to uncover alcohol-specific socialization, researchers made a distinction between several alcohol-specific parenting practices, for instance, setting rules about adolescents' alcohol use, parent–child communication about alcohol use, expressing norms or attitudes toward youth drinking, or prohibiting adolescents' alcohol use at home [12, 22]. It seems that parents and adolescents have a different perception of the extent to which parents impose these alcohol-specific socialization practices [22, 50]. For example, parents reported to talk more often about alcohol with their children, punish their child more when he/she comes home drunk, and set stricter rules than what their children actually reported to experience. Despite these differences in perception on alcohol-specific socialization, alcohol-specific socialization has a strong influence in the development of youth drinking.

Setting Alcohol-Specific Rules

One of the most effective alcohol-specific parenting practices seems to be setting strict rules about adolescents' alcohol use. Prohibiting adolescents to drink alcohol delays the age of onset of alcohol use and prevents heavy drinking later on in adolescence [22, 50]. If parents set strict rules about alcohol, including at home, then those boys and girls start to drink later in adolescence, drink less, and less often than children of parents who are permissive toward youth alcohol use [12, 51–53]. Prohibiting alcohol will postpone the onset of drinking, which in turn decreases the risk for getting involved in alcohol abuse or alcohol-related problems later on [14]. However, it seems that the effect of setting strict alcohol-specific rules is the strongest for adolescents who have not yet started to drink alcohol or for those who are light drinkers (only one or two glasses a week) [4]. Research has shown that the more parents prohibit concerning alcohol at the start, the less likely it will be that adolescents will develop a heavy drinking pattern. Nevertheless, parents seem to keep their influence after the initiation phase of use, but the influence is not as strong as in the period when their adolescent children were not drinking regularly yet. Individual characteristics of the adolescents do not change the preventive effect of setting alcohol-specific rules. Extravert children, children who follow special education due to behavioral problems, or boys and girls are equally sensitive to the alcohol rules of their parents as their peers [50, 54].

Not all parents find it as important to set rules about their children's alcohol use. More specifically, parents who are (heavy) drinkers themselves have fewer rules and are less opposed to youth drinking. Moreover, parents who are generally tolerant toward youth alcohol use, or who monitor their children to a lesser extent in the first place, are less strict toward the drinking of their own children [54, 55]. However, also in these families, alcohol-specific rule setting is effective in lowering adolescents' drinking levels.

In general, it is difficult for all parents to maintain their strictness toward alcohol; most parents become significantly more tolerant over time [50]. Parents are also less strict toward younger children in the family than toward the oldest when he/she was the age of the youngest. This indicates that birth order plays a role in alcohol-specific rules setting. Perhaps that firstborns have already introduced youth alcohol use in the family, creating a more permissive family climate toward youth alcohol use in general. The next sibling in order may experience then less strict rules, which might put him/her at risk for drinking higher amounts of alcohol later on [4]. Another issue in alcohol-specific rules setting that is not clear yet is how parents react when their children are not obeying the rules. Research indicates that parents should continue prohibiting alcohol, but we lack the knowledge how parents should react at the moment they are confronted with the drinking of their children. Thus, it remains unclear how parents should sanction their child after he/she broke the house rules about alcohol. Not perceiving consequences after disobeying the rules might give adolescents the idea that their parents give them permission for drinking, which might, in turn, affect future alcohol use [50].

Parent–Child Communication About Alcohol

Verbal communication is considered to be the most direct way for parents to express to their adolescent children their rules, disapproval or attitudes toward adolescent drinking [56, 57], and thus a central feature in dealing with adolescents' alcohol use. This is, for instance, shown by European and North American prevention projects focusing on improvements of the communication about alcohol between parents and their children [58–60]. Surprisingly enough, empirical evidence supporting the relevance of parent–child communication in adolescents' drinking is lacking. The few, mainly cross-sectional, studies that examined alcohol-specific communication did not find a significant relation with adolescents' alcohol use [12, 56, 61], or found a positive association [22, 51, 52]. This positive association between parent–child communication about alcohol and adolescents' alcohol use seems to indicate that frequent conversations about alcohol lead to heavier drinking, meaning that parents talk in an unconstructive way with their children [12, 22], or as the authors also suggested, that it reflects a *forbidden fruit effect*. A forbidden fruit effect refers to that talking about alcohol (the forbidden fruit) triggers adolescents' curiosity about alcohol and consequently stimulates adolescents to try alcohol themselves [22]. Furthermore, some studies examined parent–child communication in general in the development of youth drinking [61, 62]. Again, the findings of the different studies did not correspond: Ackard and colleagues [62] showed that a low level of parent–child communication in general is associated with heavier substance use including alcohol, while Komro and colleagues [61] did not find an association at all. Taken all together, it seems that the results that are currently available about the role of parent–child communication (about alcohol) in adolescents' alcohol use are inconsistent. So it is clear that more longitudinal research is needed to determine how parents can talk effectively with adolescent children about alcohol in order to reduce youth drinking.

On the other hand, several studies have shown that most parents do not talk so often with their children about alcohol-related situations [22]. The topic of alcohol use tends to be a part of the ongoing discourse of family life [63]. In addition, parents talk less often with their children about alcohol issues when one of the parents drinks than when neither parent drinks alcohol [56]. In the case mothers do communicate with their children about drinking alcohol, they have a stronger tendency to ask the adolescent questions about alcohol than to lecture or to discuss negative consequences [64], although according to Miller-Day [65], parents usually encourage youth not to drink.

Parental Attitudes Toward Adolescents' Alcohol Use

Parents who show their disapproval of youth drinking, or their strict attitudes or norms about youth drinking, or who discourage adolescents not to drink has been related to less adolescent involvement in alcohol use [28, 29, 47, 66, 67], although some others have not found evidence [53, 68, 69]. Overall though, there is substantial support that parental attitudes about adolescents' alcohol use is negatively related to adolescents' alcohol use, indicating that strict parental attitudes prevent adolescents' from heavier drinking later on. However, one should be cautious with this conclusion since the results are based on mainly cross-sectional study designs. In addition, parental attitudes about adolescents' alcohol use have been indirectly related to youth drinking. Parental attitudes have an influence on, e.g., adolescents' own attitudes about alcohol [67, 70], perceived prototypes [71], or alcohol preferences [72], which in turn predict alcohol use in adolescents. Moreover, it seems that the attitudes of parents are linked to their own drinking behaviors: Parents who are heavy drinkers themselves tend to be more tolerant toward youth alcohol use [53, 55].

At Home

Most adolescents neither drink heavily nor become drunk, intoxicated, or get involved in alcohol-related problems at home, but in a setting outside the home without adult supervision [26, 27, 73–75]. This has led to a discussion whether parents should be advised to allow their adolescent children to drink alcohol at home (and not in other settings). However, there is empirical evidence that drinking at home results in negative outcomes as well. That is, most adolescents have their first alcohol experiences at home [76, 77], usually during a family gathering [78], and drinking at home is one of the most common drinking locations for early adolescents [27, 73]. Adolescents who drink at home or who are allowed to drink at home tend to drink more frequently [26], and are more likely to be drunk and involved in heavy episodic drinking later on [12, 61]. Moreover, a recent study of Van Der Vorst and colleagues [30] showed that at-home drinking predicted higher amounts of alcohol use at home and in settings outside home. At-home drinking also increased the risk for being involved in problematic alcohol use. Thus, drinking at home may have some benefits, such as the lower risk for intoxication or drunkenness, but the negative consequences seem to more pronounced: more frequent drinking, higher amounts of use, and a risk for problem drinking. Again, the results indicate that it is important to delay the age of onset of adolescents' alcohol use, whether the onset is at home or at a place outside the home.

Adolescents Influencing Their Parents

Most studies in alcohol research targeting parents seem to treat the adolescents as rather passive recipients of their parents' influences. However, a family is a dynamic system in which the members interact and influence each other. Concerning adolescents' alcohol use, there will come a time when parents are confronted with the drinking behavior of their children, e.g., an adolescent comes home drunk or tells the parent that he/she had been drinking with friends. It is likely that in such a case, adolescents also affect their parents. In general, cross-sectional parent–child associations have been interpreted as parents influencing their children,

although it is as logic to assume that parents are responding to the drinking behaviors of their children. Not taking this so-called bi-directionality [35, 79] into account may lead to overemphasizing the relevance of parents' contribution in youth drinking [80]. The few studies that took bi-directional effects into account support the idea of bi-directionality. That is, if adolescents drink alcohol, their parents are lenient in their attitudes for drinking at a young age [81]. Furthermore, parents lower their monitoring efforts of the daily lives of their adolescent children [49, 50]. It has been suggested that parents realize by their adolescents' drinking that their children are growing up and provide them, therefore, more autonomy [49]. It is also possible that parents are not accepting their children's alcohol use and consequently distance themselves from them. There is empirical support for this last explanation: Alcohol use of adolescents can lead to an emotional distance between parents and their children [50]. In addition, although it is a small effect, the alcohol use of mid-adolescents predicted increases in later alcohol use of both mothers and fathers [82]. This finding indicates that alcohol norms within the family change as soon as children start to experiment with alcohol. Studies like the aforementioned underline that bi-directionality should be included in future research.

Discussion and Implications for Future Research

It is clear that parents can play a significant role in the development of adolescents' alcohol use. On the one hand, parents should drink as less as possible in the presence of their children, also during family gatherings, or should avoid drinking alcohol with them in order to reduce youth drinking. That parents generally offer their children sips of alcohol or a first glass does not seem to be an effective strategy [76, 77], although it seems to be a common behavior in many families [83]. On the other hand, parents can delay the age of onset and subsequent drinking after initiation with their parenting efforts. That is, by monitoring and supporting their adolescents, they lower the increase of alcohol use during adolescence. Moreover, it has recently been shown that alcohol-specific socialization is important. Prohibiting alcohol use at home or in places outside the home, expressing strict attitudes about alcohol, and showing disapproval of youth alcohol use prevent heavy drinking in adolescents. Although all these outcomes are promising, and perhaps result in valuable tools for alcohol prevention programs, several issues remain unsolved.

Nowadays, it is clear that both parents and peers have an impact on youth drinking [4, 84], but parents and peers might also interact [51]. Parents might have an influence on the behaviors of the best friend (including their drinking) and other friends of their adolescent children [85, 86], for instance, by their own alcohol use, the rules about alcohol they set, or their monitoring efforts. When friends visit adolescents at home, they come in contact with the parents and subsequently with their parenting or alcohol use. Observing these family dynamics might affect peers' drinking attitudes, expectancies, or actual use. In addition, parents probably affect the selection of their offspring's potential friends by showing approval of certain peers (non-drinking peers) and disapproval of others (drinking peers). Parents also affect the selection of friends by the neighborhood or area they choose to live in [87]. Research on other youth problem behaviors has shown that high parental monitoring prevents adolescents from affiliating with deviant peers, and parents' negative reactions to friendships affect the continuation of those friendships. Thus, future longitudinal research on (alcohol-specific) socialization should take a broader network of social influential factors into account. Not only will this provide further insight into the complexity of the development of adolescents' alcohol use, but it may also provide a better understanding on the relative roles of peers and parents in youth drinking.

Although it is generally accepted that individual characteristics interact with the environment, alcohol research targeting at parents generally neglected to test person–environment interactions. It seems reasonable to assume that adolescents react differently to parental socialization efforts or parental alcohol use, simply because they differ in characteristics, such as their temperament, experiences of life events, genetic disposition for alcohol use, drinking history, and personality features. By unraveling person–environment interactions, alcohol prevention will get the knowledge to develop programs for specific groups of adolescents and parents, and consequently might be more effective in the future.

Furthermore, a shortcoming of longitudinal research is that it has a rather long interval between measurement points in which many things happen in the lives of the adolescents, but of which researchers lack insight. All these hidden factors (e.g., experiences, emotions, and social interactions) might affect the development of adolescents' alcohol use. As has been clearly shown, behaviors and attitudes of individuals change over time, including adolescents' drinking as well as parental behaviors. However, knowledge about the underlying processes that change these behaviors is limited with longitudinal panel designs based on surveys. Although certain parenting practice such as alcohol-specific rule setting seems to be very effective in reducing adolescents' drinking, clear insights into how mutual influence processes in families are operating and whether these are content dependent are still lacking. It seems therefore that survey research should be combined with observational studies. Using observational data, information can be gathered on about how processes are developing in the short term and in situations that reflect real life situations more accurately.

References

1. Chassin L, Pitts SC, Prost J. Binge drinking trajectories from adolescence to emerging adulthood in a high risk sample: Predictors and substance abuse outcomes. J Consult Clin Psychol. 2002;70: 67–78.
2. Duncan SC, Duncan TE, Strycker LA. Alcohol use from ages 9 to 16: A cohort-sequential latent growth model. Drug Alcohol Depend. 2006;81:71–81.
3. Jackson KM, Sher KJ, Schulenberg JE. Conjoint developmental trajectories of young adult alcohol use tobacco use. J Abnorm Psychol. 2005;114:612–26.
4. Van Der Vorst H, Vermulst AA, Meeus WH, Deković M, Engels RC. Identification and prediction of drinking trajectories in early and mid-adolescence. J Clin Child Adolesc Psychol. 2009; 38(3):329–41.
5. Zucker RA, Fitzgerald HE, Moses HD. Emergence of alcohol problems and the several alcoholisms: A developmental perspective on etiologic theory and life course trajectory. In: Cicchetti D, Cohen DJ, editors. Risk, disorder, and adaptation. New York: Wiley; 1995.
6. Colder CR, Campbell RT, Ruel E, Richardson JL, Flay BR. A finite mixture model of growth trajectories of adolescent alcohol use: Predictors and consequences. J Consult Clin Psychol. 2002;70: 976–85.
7. Cooper ML. Alcohol use and risky sexual behaviour among college students and youth: Evaluating the evidence. J Stud Alcohol. 2002;63:101–17.
8. Duncan SC, Alpert A, Duncan TE, Hops H. Adolescent alcohol use development and young adult outcomes. Drug Alcohol Depend. 1997;49:39–48.
9. Verdurmen J, Monshouwer K, Van Dorsselaer S, Ter Bogt T, Vollebergh W. Alcohol use and mental health in adolescence: Interactions with age and gender—Findings from the Dutch 2001 health behaviour in school-aged children survey. J Stud Alcohol. 2005;66:605–9.
10. Hawkins JD, Graham JW, Maguin E, Abbott R, Hill KG, Catalano RF. Exploring the effects of age of alcohol use initiation and psychosocial risk factors on subsequent alcohol misuse. J Stud Alcohol. 1997;58:280–90.
11. Barnes GM, Reifman AS, Farell MP, Dintcheff BA. The effects of parenting on the development of adolescent alcohol misuse: a six wave latent growth model. J Marriage Family. 2000;62:175–86.
12. Jackson C, Henriksen L, Dickinson D. Alcohol-specific socialization, parenting behaviors and alcohol use by children. J Stud Alcohol. 1999;60:362–7.
13. Simons-Morton B, Chen R. Latent growth analyses of parent influences on drinking progression among early adolescents. J Stud Alcohol. 2005;66:5–13.
14. Ellickson PL, Tucker JS, Klein DJ, McGuigan KA. Prospective risk factors for alcohol misuse in late adolescence. J Stud Alcohol. 2001;62:773–82.
15. Raskin-White H, Johnson V, Buyske S. Parental modeling and parenting behavior effects on offspring alcohol and cigarette use. A growth curve analysis. J Subst Abuse. 2000;12:287–310.
16. Chassin L, Curran PJ, Hussong AM, Colder CR. The relation of parent alcoholism to adolescent substance use A longitudinal follow-up study. J Abnorm Psychol. 1997;105:70–80.
17. Engels RMCE, Van Der Vorst H. The roles of parents in adolescent and peer alcohol consumption. The Netherlands' J Soc Sci. 2003;39:53–68.
18. Yu J, Perrine MW. The transmission of parent/adult-child drinking patterns: Testing a gender-specific structural model. Am J Drug Abuse. 1997;23:143–65.
19. Zhang L, Welte JW, Wieczorek WF. The influence of parental drinking and closeness on adolescent drinking. J Stud Alcohol. 1999;60:245–51.

20. Pedersen W, Skondal A. Alcohol consumption debut: Predictors and consequences. J Stud Alcohol. 1998;59:32–42.
21. Casswell S, Pledger M, Pratap S. Trajectories of drinking from 18 to 26 years: Identification and prediction. Addiction. 2002;97:1427–37.
22. Van Der Vorst H, Engels RCME, Meeus W, Dekovic M, Leeuwe J. The role of alcohol-specific socialization in adolescents' drinking behavior. Addiction. 2005;100:1464–76.
23. Bandura A. Social learning theory. Englewood Cliffs: Prentice-Hall; 1977.
24. Webb JA, Bear PE. Influence of family disharmony and parental alcohol use on adolescent social skills, self-efficacy, and alcohol use. Addict Behav. 1995;20:127–35.
25. Petraitis J, Flay B, Miller TQ. Reviewing theories of adolescent use: Organizing pieces in the puzzle. Psychol Bull. 1995;117:67–86.
26. Long Foley K, Altman D, Durant R, Wolfson M. Adults' approval and adolescents' alcohol use. J Adolesc Health. 2004;35:345–54.
27. Mayer RR, Forster JL, Murray DM, Wagenaar AC. Social settings and situations of underage drinking. J Stud Alcohol. 1998; 59:207–15.
28. Bahr SJ, Hoffman JP, Yang X. Parental and peer influences on the risk of adolescent drug use. J Primary Prevent. 2005;26:529–51.
29. Callas PW, Flynn BS, Worden JK. Potentially modifiable psychosocial factors associated with alcohol use during early adolescence. Addict Behav. 2004;29:1503–15.
30. van der Vorst H, Engels RC, Burk WJ. Do parents and best friends influence the normative increase in adolescents' alcohol use at home and outside the home? J Stud Alcohol Drugs. 2010;71(1): 105–14.
31. Baumrind D. Effects of authoritative control on child behavior. Child Dev. 1966;37:887–907.
32. Darling N, Steinberg L. Parenting style as context: An integrative model. Psychol Bull. 1993;113:487–96.
33. Baumrind D. New directions in socialization research. Am Psychol. 1980;35:639–52.
34. Foxcroft DR, Lowe G. Adolescent drinking behaviour and family socialization factors: A meta-analysis. J Adolesc. 1991;14:255–73.
35. Rollins BC, Thomas DL. Parental support, power, and control techniques in the socialization of children. In: Burr WR, Hill R, Nye FI, Reiss IL, editors. Contemporary theories about the family, vol. 1. New York: Free; 1979. p. 317–64.
36. Shucksmith J, Glendinning A, Hendry L. Adolescent drinking behaviour and the role of family life: A Scottish perspective. J Adolesc. 1997;20:85–101.
37. Howard Caldwell C, Sellers R, Hilkenen Berant D, Zimmerman MA. Racial identity, parental support, and alcohol use in a sample of academically at-risk African American high school students. Am J Commun Psychol. 2004;34:71–82.
38. Barnes GM, Farrell MP. Parental support and control as predictors of adolescent drinking, delinquency, and related problem behaviors. J Marriage Family. 1992;54:763–76.
39. Stice E, Barrera M, Chassin L. Relation of parental support and control to adolescent's externalizing symptomatology and substance use: A longitudinal examination of curvilinear effects. J Abnorm Child Psychol. 1993;21:609–29.
40. Stice E, Barrera M, Chassin L. Prospective differential prediction of adolescent use and problem use: Examining the mechanism of effect. J Abnorm Psychol. 1998;107:616–28.
41. Urberg K, Goldstein MS, Toro PA. Supportive relationships as a moderator of the effects of parent and peer drinking on adolescent drinking. J Res Adolesc. 2005;15:1–19.
42. Mason WA, Windle M. Family, religious, school and peer influences on adolescent alcohol use: A longitudinal study. J Stud Alcohol. 2001;62:44–53.
43. Wills TA, Cleary SD. How are social support effects mediated? A test with parental support and adolescent substance use. J Personal Soc Psychol. 1996;71:937–52.
44. Borawski EA, Ievers-Landis CE, Lovegreen LD, Trapl ES. Parental monitoring negotiated unsupervised time, and parental trust: The role of perceived parenting practices in adolescent health risk behaviors. J Adolesc Health. 2003;33:60–70.
45. Duncan SC, Duncan TE, Biglan A, Ary D. Contributions of the social context to the development of adolescent substance use: A multivariate latent growth modeling approach. Drug Alcohol Depend. 1998;50:57–71.
46. Van Der Vorst H, Engels RCME, Meeus W, Dekovic M, Vermulst A. Parental attachment, parental control and early development of alcohol use: a longitudinal study. Psychol Addict Behav. 2006;20:107–16.
47. Wood MD, Read JP, Mitchell RE, Brand NH. Do parents still matter? Parent and peer influences on alcohol involvement among recent high school graduates. Psychol Addict Behav. 2004; 18:19–30.
48. Stattin H, Kerr M. Parental monitoring: A reinterpretation. Child Dev. 2000;71:1072–95.
49. Stice E, Barrera M. A longitudinal examination of the reciprocal relations between perceived parenting and adolescents' substance use and externalizing behaviors. Dev Psychol. 1995;31:322–34.
50. Van Der Vorst H, Engels RCME, Deković M, Meeus W, Vermulst AA. Alcohol-specific rules, personality and adolescents' alcohol use: A longitudinal person-environment study. Addiction. 2007; 102:1064–75.
51. Engels RCME, De Leeuw R, Poelen E, Van Der Vorst H, Van Der Zwaluw C, Van Leeuwe J. The impact of parents on adolescent drinking and friendship selection processes. In: Järvinen M, Room R, editors. Youth drinking cultures. European experiences. Hampshire: Ashgate Publishing Limited; 2007.
52. Spijkerman R, Van Den Eijnden RJJM, Huib Ore A. Social economical differences in alcohol-specific parenting practices and adolescents' drinking patterns. Eur Addict Res. 2008;14:26–37.
53. Yu J. The association between parental alcohol-related behaviors and children's drinking. Drug Alcohol Depend. 2003;69:253–62.
54. Van Zundert R, Van Der Vorst H, Vermulst AA, Engels RMCE. Pathways to alcohol use among Dutch students in regular education and education for adolescents with behavioral problems: The role of parental alcohol use, general parenting practices, and alcohol-specific parenting practices. J Fam Psychol. 2006;20:456–67.
55. Van Der Vorst H, Engels RCME, Meeus W, Dekovic M. The impact of alcohol-specific rules, parental norms about early drinking and parental alcohol use on adolescents' drinking behavior. J Child Psychol Psychiatr. 2006;47:1299–306.
56. Ennett ST, Bauman KE, Foshee VA, Pemberton M, Hicks KA. Parent–child ommunication about adolescent tobacco and alcohol use: what do parents say and does it affect youth behavior. J Marriage Fam. 2001;63:48–62.
57. Jackson S, Bijstra J, Oostra L, Bosma H. Adolescents' perceptions of communication with parents relative to specific aspects of relationships with parents and personal development. J Adolesc. 1998;21:305–22.
58. Komro KA, Perry CL, Veblen-Mortenson S, Farbakhsh K, Toomey TL, Stigler MH, et al. Outcomes from a randomized controlled trial of a multi-component alcohol use preventive intervention for urban youth: Project Northland Chicago. Addiction. 2008;103:606–18.
59. Robertson EB, David SL, Rao SA. Preventing drug use among children and adolescents. A research based guide for parents, educators and community leaders. 2nd ed. Maryland: National Institute on Drug Abuse (NIDA); 2003.
60. Rueter MA, Conger RD, Ramisetty-Mikler S. Assessing the benefits of a parenting skills training program: A theoretical approach to predicting direct and moderating effects. Fam Relat. 1999; 48:67–77.
61. Komro KA, Maldonado-Molina MM, Tobler AL, Bonds JR, Muller KE. Effects of home access and availability of alcohol on young adolescents' alcohol use. Addiction. 2008;102:1597–680.

62. Ackard DM, Neumak-Sztainer D, Story M, Perry C. Parent–child connectedness and behavioral and emotional health among adolescents. Am J Prevent Med. 2006;30:59–66.

63. Miller-Day MA. Parent-adolescent communication about alcohol, tobacco, and other drug use. J Adolesc Health. 2002;17:604–16.

64. Boone TL, Lefkowitz ES. Mother-adolescent health communication: Are all conversations created equally? J Youth Adolesc. 2007;36:1038–47.

65. Miller-Day MA. Talking to youth about drugs: What do late adolescents say about parental strategies? Fam Relat. 2008;57:1–12.

66. Aas H, Klepp KI. Adolescents' alcohol use related to perceived norms. Scand J Psychol. 1992;33:315–25.

67. Webster RA, Hunter M, Keats JA. Peer and parental influences on adolescents' substance use: A path analysis. Int J Addict. 1994;29:647–57.

68. Ennett ST, Bauman KE. Mediators in the relationship between parental and peer characteristics and beer drinking by early adolescents. J Appl Soc Psychol. 1991;21:1699–711.

69. Wilks J, Callan VJ, Austin DA. Parent, peer and personal determinants of adolescents drinking. Br J Addict. 1989;84:619–30.

70. Brody GH, Flor DL, Hollett-Wright N, McCoy JK, Donovan J. Parent–child relationships, child temperament profiles and children's alcohol use norms. J Stud Alcohol. 1999;60:45–51.

71. Spijkerman R, Van Den Eijnden RJJM, Overbeek GJ, Engels RCME. The impact of peer and parental norms and behaviour on adolescent drinking: The mediating role of drinker prototypes. Psychol Health. 2007;22:7–29.

72. Biddle BJ, Bank BJ, Marlin MM. Social determinants of adolescent drinking. What they think, what they do and what I think and do. J Stud Alcohol. 1980;41:215–38.

73. Beck K, Treiman KA. The relationship of social context of drinking, perceived social norms, and parental influence to various drinking patterns of adolescents. Addict Behav. 1996;21:633–44.

74. Forsyth A, Barnard M. Preferred drinking locations of Scottish adolescents. Health Place. 2000;6:105–15.

75. Wells S, Graham K, Speechley M, Koval JJ. Drinking patterns, drinking context and alcohol related aggression among late adolescent and young adult drinkers. Addiction. 2005;100:933–44.

76. Engels R. M. C. E. Forbidden fruits. Social dynamics in smoking and drinking behavior of adolescents. Dissertation. Maastricht: Universitaire Pers Maastricht 1998.

77. Jackson C. Initial and experimental stages of tobacco and alcohol use during late childhood: Relation to peer, parent and personal risk factors. Addict Behav. 1997;22:685–98.

78. Warner LA, White HR. Longitudinal effects of age of onset and first drinking situations on problem drinking. Substance Use Misuse. 2003;38:1983–2016.

79. Bell RQA. reinterpretation of the direction of effects in studies of socialization. Psychol Rev. 1968;75:81–95.

80. O'Connor TG. Annotation: The effects of parenting reconsidered: Findings, challenges and applications. J Child Psychol Psychiatr. 2002;43:555–72.

81. Derkman MM, Engels RC, Kuntsche E, van der Vorst H, Scholte RH. Bidirectional associations between sibling relationships and parental support during adolescence. J Youth Adolesc. 2011 Apr; 40(4):490-501.

82. Otten R, Van der Zwaluw C, Van der Vorst H, Engels RCME. Partner effects and bi-directional parent–child effects in family alcohol use. Eur Addict Res. 2008;14:106–12.

83. Donovan JE, Molina BSG. Children's introduction to alcohol use: sips and tastes. Alcoholism: Clin Exp Res. 2008;32:108–19.

84. Poelen EAP, Scholte RHJ, Engels RCME, Boomsma DI, Willemsen G. Prevalence and trends of alcohol use and misuse among adolescents and young adults in the Netherlands from 1993 to 2000. Drug Alcohol Depend. 2005;79:413–21.

85. Brown BB, Mounts NS, Lamborn SD, Steinberg LD. Parenting practices and peer group affiliation in adolescence. Child Dev. 1993;64:467–82.

86. Mounts NS. Adolescents' perceptions of parental management of peer relationships in an ethnically divers sample. J Adolesc Res. 2004;19:446–67.

87. Engels RCME, Bot SM. Social influences on adolescent substance use: Insights into how parents and peers affect adolescent's smoking and drinking behavior. In: De Ridder DTD, De Wit JBF, editors. Self-regulation in health behavior. West Sussex: Wiley; 2006.

Legal Aspects of Drug Addiction

Malcolm Lader

Abstract

Human societies are regulated by social rules which can be formalised as laws. The principles and philosophy upon which laws are based often differ fundamentally from country to country. The law is so closely involved in the regulation of drug addiction because, firstly, the disorder follows the epidemiological model of a communicable, 'infectious disease', and needs containment. Secondly, drug addiction imposes enormous personal, social and economic burdens. The law may also govern the conduct of research into the problems of addiction, both animal and human studies. The debate concerning prohibition or liberalisation of drug legislation has been conducted fiercely for many years and has raised many issues.

The legal situation has unfortunately tended to become polarised with experts and lay people backing up their arguments with purblind opinions rather than firm factual evidence-based reasoning. For example, those enforcing the law may regard any use of illicit drugs as problematic or fundamentally undesirable; those seeking to legalise some forms of drug misuse consider that most such drug use does not raise problems: rather, the problems arise from the illegal designation of much widespread recreational drug use. A major difference between the two sides relates to the effectiveness or otherwise of drug enforcement measures. This is a contentious subject and opinions diverge radically. Whatever the differences, both sides agree that drug use is dangerous. They differ in how to lessen harm. One side advocates legislation, the other a medical approach. Research should be directed towards monitoring outcomes of legal measures to see if their effects in practice attain pre-specified goals, say lessening of overall usage or of a particular type of harm.

Learning Objectives
- Legal systems vary greatly from country to country.
- Scientists and physicians should be familiar with the law as it applies to their research and therapy.
- Debate continues as to whether to relax or tighten current drug laws.
- Workers in this area should be familiar with the complex arguments.

Issues that Need to be Addressed by Future Research
- What is the true impact of a change in the law as it relates to drug misuse?
- How can we reduce harm effectively—legal or medical measures?

M. Lader (✉)
Institute of Psychiatry, Kings College,
London, UK
e-mail: malcolm.lader@kcl.ac.uk

J.C. Verster et al. (eds.), *Drug Abuse and Addiction in Medical Illness: Causes, Consequences and Treatment*,
DOI 10.1007/978-1-4614-3375-0_42, © Springer Science+Business Media, LLC 2012

Introduction

Social rules govern and regulate human societies, even the most 'primitive'. In a wider context, they restrict our basic biological instincts. Among clinical medical disciplines, drug misuse, abuse or addiction—whatever the terminology—is one that is intimately influenced by legal measures. Indeed, clinical practice is often dictated by the law, and preclinical research may encounter difficulty gaining access to research drugs, if they are deemed to be Controlled Substances.

Legal precepts may be normative and lay down what ought or ought not to happen. The law lays down rules of behaviour to which we are expected to obey, and reserves sanctions, often severe or even swingeing, for miscreants who flout those laws. Most legal systems pay little heed to the psychological aspects of addiction, in particular the compulsive nature of the behaviour.

In this chapter, I will outline some of the principles by which the law addresses drug addiction, illustrating those principles where possible with examples drawn from a particular jurisdiction. I will not cover alcohol problems in any detail. I will conclude by setting out the arguments for and against relaxing some of the restrictive legislation. For a fuller account, please refer to Glaser and Warren [1].

Systems of Law

The different systems of law administered by each jurisdiction make it impossible for any review to be comprehensive. Not only do individual laws vary from country to country, but also the principles and philosophy upon which those laws are based may differ fundamentally. Most European countries base their legal system on Roman law as codified by Napoleon. By contrast, the USA and England (but not Scotland) rely on case-law, essentially judge-given interpretations of available legislation. If no legislation is extant, judges make up their own common law principles. Religious principles may operate in parallel or form the basis of the legal system, as in Sharia law. This is part of the wider issue of morality: does the law reflect public morals or seek to influence them? Does it designate certain behaviours as inherently undesirable morally and ethically, or provide instructions to discourage behaviour that society finds it has been educated to find unacceptable. Nowhere is the dual nature of the epistemology that governs our management of the problem more confusing than in the field of drug addiction and the law.

Determinism and Free Will

One legal concept which is fairly widespread is *mens rea* [2]. This is the intent of the person committing the crime. For example, typically a person committing an act of homicide, the *actus reus*, is assumed to have intent, mens rea, to kill or cause grievous bodily harm. This makes the crime one of murder. If intent cannot be proven, the crime may be 'reduced' to 'manslaughter'. But with respect to drug addiction, society is often split in its attitudes. Politicians, egged on by the media, particularly tabloid newspapers, take a punitive stance while paying lip service to treatment and rehabilitation. People engaged in the medical prevention and treatment of drug problems tend to be much more supportive. Politicians and drug enforcement agencies use a *volitional* approach— addicts know that they are breaking societal rules, but do so voluntarily, i.e. with appropriate mens rea, and must be punished. Drug addiction personnel take a more *biological* approach, regarding drug addiction as a disorder and use the classical nature-nurture model. Drug addiction is seen as the interaction of some degree of biological predisposition with environmental influences, particularly social ones. Thus, both factors must be operating to some extent.

The whole question of the compulsive nature of drug addiction governs public attitudes. The 'pull-yourself-together brigade' would regard the misuser of drugs of addiction as lacking moral fibre. The 'there-but-for-the-grace-of-God-go-I' liberals will regard the unacceptable behaviour as largely outside the addicts' control. Otherwise, why do addicts persist with their habits at the expense of their personal medical, occupational and social well-being?

Why Does the Law Intervene?

One reason is that addicts harm themselves. The most serious drug addiction in terms of both mortality and morbidity is smoking tobacco. Society has tried to educate smokers about the dangers of smoking, and finance departments in governments have tried to price cigarettes off the market, but suspicion grows that there is an irreducible minimum of smokers. The medical consequences are brushed aside by nicotine addicts. So are the medical consequences of alcohol ingestion, despite licensing laws of varying stringency. The users of addictive drugs often minimise or ignore the risks of transmission of viral and other infections, particularly when they are injecting.

But the main reasons that the law is so intimately involved in the regulation of drug addiction are at least twofold. Firstly, the disorder follows the epidemiological model of a communicable, 'infectious disease'. Peer pressures to abuse drugs are often intolerable for the neophyte. Hence the sections of the drug addiction laws and regulations dealing with 'supply' incorporate penalties which are much more stringent than those relating to 'possession' for personal use. Secondly, drug addiction exacts an enormous social and economic toll. Estimates generally place drug addiction as the second largest economic enterprise, after the oil industry. The cost to the USA is estimated at around $200 billion. Countless arguments have been put forward to justify drug laws in economic and social terms, and lie outside the scope of this chapter. Suffice it to say that attempts to suppress the trade in addictive substances are generally ineffectual because the profits are so substantial that the risks are generally worth taking by the criminally inclined. In turn, the price of feeding a habit, amphetamine, heroin or whatever, is beyond the legitimate earning capacity of most addicts, so they resort to crime. The proportion of crimes such as robbery, with or without violence, is variously estimated at 40–80% of total crimes. This has led to the suggestion that legalising a drug of 'addiction', for example cannabis, would actually benefit society. There might be some basis for this in social terms, but we cannot estimate the medical cost until more is known of the roots of addiction, for example how many people are at risk because of some genetic predisposition. Cannabis is a case in point where a minority of people have an allele gene that might predispose them to psychosis if they overuse cannabis [3]; but also see [4].

Research

Some legal points are apposite to the conduct of research into the problems of addiction. Legal systems, under pressure from animal rights activists, have mostly introduced measures to regulate research on animals. Regulations vary from country to country, reflecting the attitudes of the most vociferous activists. Many countries have a set of rules rather than guidelines. In some, registration of laboratories, projects and individual experimenters is required. Particular stringency is often applied to studies on primates. Research on Great Apes may be prohibited altogether, as may that on species deemed at risk of extinction, even if they are not primates.

In clinical matters, a series of declarations followed the abhorrent practices of the Nazis. The Declaration of Helsinki [5] states that 'It is the duty of the physician in medical research to protect the life, health, privacy and dignity of the human subject'. Ethical committees were set up, first in the USA, and then in other countries, to regulate human research, first voluntarily, but increasingly under statute. Based on a detailed protocol, a properly constituted ethical committee containing both professional and lay members should consider the proposal, modify it if necessary, and ensure that it is closely followed. Such committees have a special (fiduciary) duty to act properly and responsibly. Any researcher failing to submit an appropriate protocol would, depending on the jurisdiction, find himself subject to the criminal code for inflicting bodily harm, or to redress under the civil code for causing a personal injury ('tort'), or expulsion from the relevant professional body. With psychotropic drugs, psychological harm could be the basis for a court action.

Informed consent is typically a *sine qua non* for recruitment of experimental subjects. This requires that each potential participant be adequately informed of the purpose of the study, its methods, sources of funding, any possible conflicts of interest, institutional affiliations of the researcher, the expected risks and potential benefits of the study and the anticipated discomfort. The presence of a neutral witness during the recruitment process is a useful safeguard. The volunteer should be informed of the right to withdraw from the study at any time without explanation. The investigator must be sure that the potential subject has understood the information and has been encouraged to ask questions. Consent should be in writing, wherever possible. Special rules generally apply to subjects who suffer from a severe psychiatric disorder, or lack mental capacity to give informed consent, and to children. Recently, the question of genetic privacy has been raising concern.

Two European Directives, Clinical Trials Directive [6] and Good Clinical Practice [7], initiated change in medical research procedures across Europe to varying extents [2]. (A Directive sets out the broad goals of the legislation but allows each EU country to determine the form and precise content of that legislation.)

Therapeutics

It is a truism that every administration of a therapeutic substance is essentially an experiment. If that usage in that patient is grossly negligent, criminal proceedings may follow. If it falls short of that, then the injured party generally has to show that the drug administration was below acceptable clinical standards, and that it caused an injury that can be quantified, at least in financial terms. Standard rates are applied to gross physical injuries such as an amputation, but psychological or psychiatric damages are difficult to quantify. Often the functional impairments such as occupational handicap are evaluated, as well as symptomatic complaints.

In most jurisdictions, the development of an adverse effect, *ipso facto*, does not constitute grounds for action, as long as the drug was administered in accord with accepted clinical standards. These can change over time, and regulatory bodies may suggest different practices. Prescribers must be aware of the latest developments and even trends.

Service Issues

The duty of confidentiality is an important issue and pertains to substance misusers as to others under treatment. Professional training and codes of ethics, legal measures and regulations and social mores all emphasise the need for confidentiality in dealings with patients and clients. Confidentiality is a fundamental patient's right often enshrined in various codes of practice.

But in practice, maintaining confidentiality is not always straightforward [2]. The underlying problem is that the patient is undertaking illegal activities, such as possession and perhaps supply. This provides the opportunity and sometimes necessity for the law to intervene and to override medical considerations. In most countries, medical practitioners do not have an absolute right of doctor/patient confidentiality. They may be forced to break their oath of confidentiality, either voluntarily or by order of a legal authority.

Confidentiality issues extend to patients' records, written and videotaped, as well as to the personal confidences from the patient to the doctor. This has obvious counterproductive consequences. Addicts are aware of the illicit nature of their activities. They will accordingly be reluctant to confide in health-care professionals and may lie to protect themselves and their associates. Even examination of the patient technically constitutes an assault under many jurisdictions. A misuser presenting to a clinician can legitimately refuse a physical examination, for example for needle tracks. He can refuse to give a sample of blood for estimation of illicit substances, or detection of blood-borne disease antibodies. However, some jurisdiction may insist that appropriate tests are carried out. Perhaps the most widely applied example concerns measurement of breath alcohol levels where, in some countries, failure to provide a sample may in itself constitute a criminal offence.

These legal issues vary greatly from country to country. Each practitioner should be aware not only of the general principles but also of the legal technicalities. Special laws may apply to the workplace, for example driving while under the influence of alcohol or a drug. Compulsory screening of applicants for particularly sensitive jobs is also in place in some situations.

In some jurisdictions, courts may 'dispose' of a drug offender, not by imprisonment, but by compulsory participation in a treatment facility. Again, the health-care professional must be cognisant of her or his legal responsibilities under such a regimen.

In addiction, the health-care professional may have a duty of care under the civil code of law. If a drug misuser seeks help, what are the therapist's responsibilities concerning the response? Can he or she refuse to take on the care of the patient, or does the request automatically put the therapist in a position where the duty of care must be acknowledged?

The therapist may have a wider duty of care. For example what does she or he do to control a promiscuous addict who is HIV positive, or actively recruiting youngsters to experiment with increasingly dangerous drugs? Does the therapist have a duty of care to warn others, for example parents of a young girl who is consorting with older irresponsible addicts? In general, medical defence protection agencies can help with these legal conundrums.

Prohibition Versus Legalisation

This debate has been raging for many years and has raised many issues. The legal situation has tended to become polarised with experts and lay people backing up their arguments with opinions rather than firm factual evidence-based reasoning. The following is a resume of the main arguments, but space precludes a detailed analysis of the evidence, such as it is, that supports either side. This account is heavily based on the publication 'Tools for the Debate', recently published by the Transform Drug Policy Foundation [8]. Numerous issues will be enumerated:

1. The prohibitionists want illicit illegal drug use to be completely eliminated; reformers accept that people have used drugs for millennia, and always will.
2. Any use of illicit drugs is regarded as problematic by the law enforcers; the legalisers consider that most illicit drug use does not raise problems, rather the problems encountered stem from the illegal designation of much recreational drug use. The problems of drug use reflect underlying personal, social or occupational problems. Reformers admit that illicit drug use can worsen those underlying problems.
3. Problematic drug use and related harm have not lessened under draconian prohibitory measures. In many instances, it has risen dramatically, but this is an association and not necessarily proven case and effect.
4. Supporters of present legislation are concerned that decriminalisation or legalisation with regulation raises unknown consequences. Reformers riposte that governments have years of experience in legally regulating numerous drugs. Indeed, some major drugs of abuse have valuable therapeutic actions in the clinical context, diamorphine being the prime example. Drugs make people lose control, say the prohibitionists. The reformers agree, but this is a general problem regarding behaviour, particularly group behaviour.
5. Prohibition sends an important message, the 'no-tolerance' message about avoiding drugs and the harm they cause. The reformers believe the criminal justice system to be an inappropriate vehicle to put across public health messages. Attempts to legalise drugs, say the enforcers, with subsequent regulation make a mockery of the law. The reformers regard such legislation as ineffective and

counterproductive, and this is more likely to bring the law into disrepute.

6. A major difference between the two sides relates to the effectiveness or otherwise of drug enforcement measures. In some countries, especially the USA, major resources are devoted to preventing the supply of illicit substances. This has resulted in powerful vested interests supporting these policies, leaving few governmental agencies espousing the alternative approach of concentrating on the health aspects of the users. Enforcers reply that cutting off the supply of drugs must inevitably lead to harm reduction. But evidence that drug enforcement measures are effective is sadly exiguous. Some of the more vocal opposers of relaxing current legislation believe harm reduction itself to be counterproductive as it lulls the misusers into a false sense of security that his or her health will not be jeopardised, when in fact harm reduction itself is largely ineffective. It thus encourages drug use. Reformers regard such attitudes as immoral, unethical and unhelpful.

7. The moral position of those opposed to relaxing preventative measures is that drugs are unacceptable in modern society. Reformers believe in a Benthamite moral position of maximising well-being, both of the users and of the society in general. Prohibitionists are generally not concerned with the human rights of users; reformers are adamant that everyone has human rights, including users. The human rights of the users must be set into the context of the human rights of the wider community, including innocent bystanders.

8. Both sides agree that drug use is dangerous. Enforcers assert that they must be prohibited. Reformers point in despair at the continuing, perhaps rising, incidence of drug misuse (sometimes on scanty evidence). They assert that reform measures may indeed increase availability, but they will reduce harm. Most importantly, they should largely obviate the enormous criminal industry of illicit supply, with its vast profits. These, in turn, lead to extraordinary levels not only of organised crime down the supply chain but also of persistent minor criminal activity on the part of the end users. Those supporting the status quo regard the financial, social and even health costs of maintaining prohibition as a necessary societal cost that is well worth paying. Reformers regard such expenditure as excessive and unjustified, especially as they believe it to be ineffective and often counterproductive.

9. On a wider scale, prohibitionists are wary that legalisation and regulation would fall within health legislation, and thus would inevitably involve multinational corporations such as the pharmaceutical industry. The drug companies would want to maximise their profits by aggressively marketing their products, namely drugs of addiction. This would merely exchange one set of 'pushers' for another. Reformers consider that governmental control could minimise such adverse consequences, or governments could themselves market the drugs or set up disinterested agencies to do so. At least the gangsters would be marginalised. Internationally, producer countries are accused by the enforcers of deliberately ignoring illicit drug cultivation, manufacture and supply. In particular, corrupt politicians are heavily involved. Reformers counter that the profits from illicit drugs are so great that producers engage in such activities because there are few alternatives. Remaining economic incentives pale by comparison.

Prohibition Versus Harm Reduction

Further arguments revolve around the legal and moral issues concerning ways of facilitating harm reduction, both for the individual users and society. Prohibition results in the stigmatising and demonising of problem drug users. They are often already the neediest, most marginalised and mentally disturbed members of society. Prohibition hampers measures to help such unfortunates. The availability of treatment measures may be curtailed, for example needle exchange schemes may be frowned upon. As a first measure, funds could be diverted from enforcement to improved and proven educational measures.

The most cogent argument, say the reformers, is that seriously addicted individuals would not have to face the risks of impure 'street' preparations. Many blood-borne diseases such as HIV and hepatitis would be reduced if drugs of pharmaceutical purity were available, and safe injection procedures introduced, at the least as an initial step. Contact with users would be established and reinforced, and encouragement towards reduction and eventual abstinence initiated. Criminal activity should be greatly reduced as in heroin prescribing projects [9]. Illegal activities such as 'mugging', prostitution and street dealing should reduce dramatically. In the UK, it was estimated that the social and economic impact of class A drugs in 2000 was 10–17 million pounds sterling (16–25 million US dollars), 88% of which related to drug-related crime [10]. A huge burden would be lifted from the police, Customs and Excise, courts, prisons and probation services—in short, the entire Criminal Justice system of most countries. The prison population would plummet. Internationally, funding for criminal activity including terrorist activities in countries like Afghanistan would disappear.

There are numerous other health rather than legal issues that lie outside the scope of this chapter.

Future Research

Legal issues demand a different type of research from scientific and medical areas of drug addiction. Essentially, legislation can be enacted on legal, political or even economic grounds, hopefully compatible with evidence-based medicine and science. The effects of that legislation can be monitored to see if its effects in practice attain its goals, say lessening of overall usage or of a particular type of harm. The unit is not, however, a subject, client or patient. Instead it is a jurisdiction, not necessarily a whole country but often a police or judicial authority or even a locality or an area health service. Increasingly, such measures, administrative or health provisions or treatment, are being trialed in a systematic way. This enables the results to be analysed, conclusions drawn, and the decision taken by responsible authorities to jettison the innovation as a failure or to extend it to other area or nationwide.

The main problems arise not so much in designing useful studies, which can simulate as far as possible the gold standard in medical research, the randomized clinical trial (RCT), but in the development and utilization of valid, reliable and relevant outcome measures; those monitoring harm are relatively straightforward such as enumerating cases of hepatitis or general indicators of health. Those reflecting availability or usage of illicit drugs or their economic burden are more elusive. Indirect indicators such as seizures or the cost of an illicit drug 'on the street' may be the only feasible measures.

Nevertheless, whenever a legal intervention is applied, either in tightening or relaxing legislation or its application, monitoring or even quantification of its effects, after having established a reliable baseline, is essential in order to accumulate information if it is of use to the community, locally and nationally.

References

1. Glaser FB, Warren DG. Legal and ethical issues. pp 399–411 in TBC.
2. Brazier M, Cave E. Medicine, patients and the law. 4th ed. London: Penguin; 2007.
3. Caspi A, Moffitt T, Cannon M, McClay J, Murray R, Harrington H, Taylor A, Aresnault L, Williams B, Braithwaite A, Poulton R, Craig IW. Moderation of the effect of adolescent-onset cannabis use on adult psychosis by a functional polymorphism in the catechol-o-methyltransferase gene: longitudinal evidence of a gene X environment interaction. Biol Psychiatr. 2005;57:117–27.
4. Zammit S, Spurlock G, Williams H, Norton N, Williams N, O'Donovan M, Owen M. Genotype effects of CHRNA7, CNRI and COMT in schizophrenia; interactions with tobacco and cannabis use. Br J Psychiatr. 2007;191:402–7.
5. Frewer A, Schmidt U, editors. History and theory of human experimentation: the Declaration of Helsinki and modern medical ethics. Stuttgart: Franz Steiner Verlag; 2007.
6. European Union, Clinical Trials Directive 2001.
7. European Union, Good Clinical Practice 2005.
8. Transform Drug Policy Foundation. Tools for the Debate, Bristol, 2007.
9. Joseph Rowntree Foundation. Prescribing heroin: what is the evidence. 2003. http://www.jrf.org.uk
10. Godfrey, C et al. 2002. The economic and social costs of Class A drug use in England and Wales, 2000. http://www.homeoffice.gov.uk/rds/pdfs2/hors24.9.pdf.

Occupational Impact of Drug Abuse and Addiction

Valerie J. Slaymaker

Abstract

It may be surprising to learn that the majority of alcohol and drug-using individuals are gainfully employed full- or part-time. This equates to millions in the workforce whose substance use may create work-related problems and consequences. Studies have demonstrated the negative impact of substance use on worker productivity, safety, and functioning that result in substantial economic and societal costs. Strategies to address substance use among employees include workplace education and awareness campaigns, drug testing, Employee Assistance Programs, and other intervention efforts. Despite the popularity of such services, there is a relative lack of experimental study of their impact. Nonetheless, recent studies have begun to document the benefit of workplace programs on worker productivity and safety. Future study is needed to experimentally test workplace interventions, document cost–benefit ratios, and replicate findings across work sites. Additional work is necessary to address barriers faced by human resource professionals when identifying and addressing substance use problems among the workforce.

Learning Objectives
- Understand the prevalence of drug and alcohol use among the workforce.
- Identify the consequences of drug and alcohol use in the work place.
- Name a variety of workplace interventions available to address drug and alcohol use among employees.
- Summarize research findings related to work-place interventions for drug and alcohol use.

Issues that Need to Be Addressed by Future Research
- Additional randomized, experimental research studies are needed to assess the direct impact of workplace prevention and intervention programs on employee substance use and job functioning. Testing needs to be replicated across populations and work sites.
- Economic impact studies are also necessary to document cost–benefit ratios associated with workplace programs.
- Research is needed to elucidate the potential deterrent effect of drug-testing programs. The extent to which individuals who use alcohol and drugs avoid application to companies where drug testing is conducted is unclear. In a similar fashion, it is unknown to what extent alcohol- and drug-using employees may stop using substances when faced with drug testing.

V.J. Slaymaker (✉)
Butler Center for Research, Hazelden,
Center City, MN 55012-0011, USA
e-mail: vslaymaker@hazelden.org

J.C. Verster et al. (eds.), *Drug Abuse and Addiction in Medical Illness: Causes, Consequences and Treatment*,
DOI 10.1007/978-1-4614-3375-0_43, © Springer Science+Business Media, LLC 2012

- Controlled, experimental tests of EAP interventions are needed to address methodological concerns noted with earlier evaluations.
- Development and testing of educational and training programs for human resource professionals, specifically, are warranted given identified barriers in addressing substance use in the workplace.

Occupational Impact of Drug Abuse and Addiction

Contrary to pejorative, stereotyped images of drug users, the majority of people with substance problems are gainfully employed. According to the latest US government estimates [1], for example, 62% of adults with substance use problems, whether alcohol or drugs, are employed full-time. Among the estimated 17.4 million adults who use illicit drugs, approximately 75% are employed, and among heavy drinkers, specifically, 79% are employed full- or part-time [1].

This equates to millions of people in the workforce who may struggle with problematic drug and alcohol use. These substance use problems, in turn, negatively impact the workplace. Prevention, screening, intervention, and treatment can go a long way toward improving lives, productivity, and health.

Prevalence of Drug Use in the Workplace

Each year, a substantial national household survey is conducted by the Substance Abuse and Mental Health Services Administration (SAMHSA) to estimate rates of substance use among the US population. The National Survey on Drug Use and Health (NSDUH) utilizes independent, multistage area probability sampling to interview over 67,000 respondents who form a representative sample of the overall population in each state and the District of Columbia [1].

According to the 2007 NSDUH [1] estimates, 17.4 million people aged 18 years and older are current illicit drug users, with the highest prevalence rates found among those 18–20 years of age. While *rates* of drug use are highest among unemployed individuals (18.3%; see Fig. 43.1), the majority of drug users themselves are employed full- or part-time, numbering 13.2 million and comprising 75.3% of drug users, overall (see Fig. 43.2).

With regard to heavy alcohol use, specifically, similar findings emerge. For the purpose of the NSDUH, binge

Fig. 43.1 Percentage of persons ages 18 years and older using illicit drugs by employment status, 2007. Source: Substance Abuse and Mental Health Services Administration, Office of Applied Studies (2008). Results from the 2007 National Survey on Drug Use and Health: National Findings (NSDUH Series H-34, DHHS Publication No. SMA 08-4343). Rockville, MD

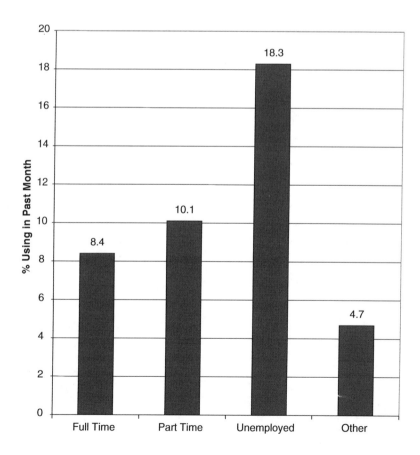

Fig. 43.2 Number of illicit drug users (in millions) by employment status, 2007. Source: Substance Abuse and Mental Health Services Administration, Office of Applied Studies (2008). Results from the 2007 National Survey on Drug Use and Health: National Findings (NSDUH Series H-34, DHHS Publication No. SMA 08-4343). Rockville, MD

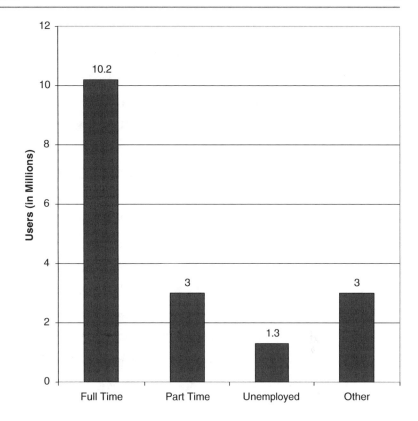

drinking was defined as five or more standard drinks on the same occasion on at least 1 day in the prior month. Heavy use was defined as binge drinking occurring on 5 or more days in the past month. According to the estimates, 55.3 million adults were classified as binge drinkers and 16.4 million were classified as heavy drinkers. Over 79% of binge or heavy drinkers were employed full- or part-time [1].

Rates of illicit drug use among the workforce vary by occupational category [2, 3]. Larson and colleagues [3] utilized NSDUH data obtained in 2002, 2003, and 2004 and calculated rates of illicit drug use in the past month among full-time workers representing 21 broad occupational areas. As shown in Fig. 43.3, the highest prevalences of illicit drug use were found among those in food service, construction, arts, design, entertainment, sports, and media occupations. The lowest rates were found among those in education, library, and social and protective services occupations. Similar patterns were found among those workers with heavy alcohol use in the past month (see Fig. 43.4).

As part of the National Survey of Workplace Health and Safety, Frone [2] analyzed data obtained from 2,829 respondents and found a similar pattern. Rates of illicit drug use were higher among arts, entertainment, sports, and media and food service occupations. Rates were also high among construction/extraction and buildings and grounds maintenance workers. Similar to NSDUH data, illicit drug use was higher among males compared to females. However, when analyses were controlled for demographic characteristics, construction/extraction and building and grounds maintenance occupations no longer exhibited elevated risk for illicit drug use.

Substance use among employees is problematic, no matter where the use occurs. However, some employees use substances shortly before reporting to work or at the work site itself. From a national survey of over 2,800 respondents, Frone [2] estimated that over 3.4 million workers used an illicit drug within 2 h of reporting to work at least once in the period spanning the prior year. Likewise, over 2.2 million were estimated to use illicit drugs during lunch breaks, 1.5 million were estimated to use illicit drugs during other breaks, and 2.1 million were estimated to use illicit substances during work itself. Alcohol use during work is also problematic, with over 7% of American workers reporting alcohol use during the workday and 9% reporting having worked during a hangover [4].

Impact on Employment Functioning

Not surprisingly, alcohol and drug use has a negative impact on employment productivity, which in turn results in economic costs to society. For 2002, the latest year for which data are available, the Office of National Drug Control Policy [5] estimated the economic impact of illicit drug use at

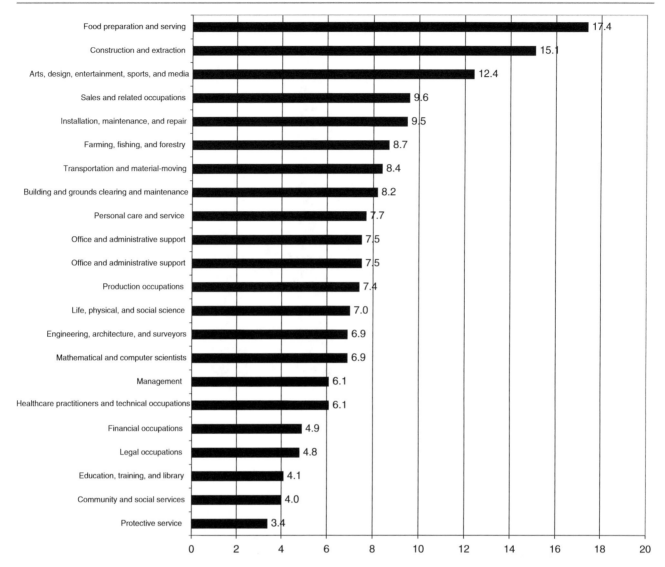

Fig. 43.3 Percentage of adult full-time workers with illicit drug use in the past month by occupational category. Source: Larson, S. L., Eyerman, J., Foster, M. S., & Gfroerer, J. C. (2007). *Worker Substance Use and Workplace Policies and Programs* (DHHS Publication No. SMA 07-4273, Analytic Services A-29). Rockville, MD: Substance Abuse and Mental Health Services Administration, Office of Applied Studies

$128.6 billion dollars in lost productivity alone in the USA. Latest estimates for alcohol-related lost productivity and earnings, updated for 1998, top $134 billion [6].

Specific analysis of workplace impact is difficult, given the numbers of industries and employers across the globe and the difficulty in assessing the complete impact of drug and alcohol use. However, the NSDUH includes workplace variables in a national survey of a representative sample of the US population. As shown in Fig. 43.5, workers with past month illicit drug use reported higher job turnover and absenteeism than those with no past month use of illicit substances [1]. Similar patterns are found among workers reporting heavy alcohol use (see Fig. 43.6).

Foster and Vaughan [7] combined two data sets obtained from the 2000 National Household Survey on Drug Abuse, collected by SAMHSA, and the 2000 National Occupational Employment Statistical Survey conducted by the US Bureau of Labor Statistics. Absenteeism due to substance use was calculated as the difference in absenteeism rates between employees with substance abuse or dependence and employees without substance use problems. The analysis of over 110,000 employees resulted in an estimate of $178 billion per year in wages lost to all absences, with over $8 billion in excess wages lost to substance-use related absences, specifically. Because this represents 4.54% of all absentee wages, and only 0.2% of total wages, the authors question whether the absenteeism-related expenses associated with substance use are sufficient to justify the expense of screening and prevention programs in the workplace. The authors recognize, however, that their analysis did not include

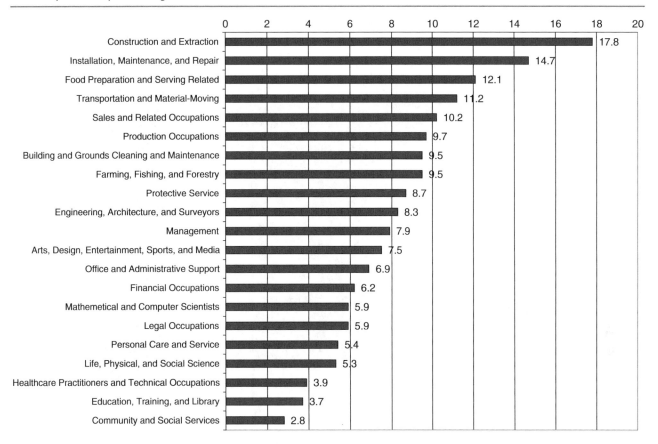

Fig. 43.4 Percentage of adult full-time workers with heavy alcohol use in the past month by occupational category, 2002–2004. Source: Larson, S. L., Eyerman, J., Foster, M. S., & Gfroerer, J. C. (2007). *Worker Substance Use and Workplace Policies and Programs* (DHHS Publication No. SMA 07-4273, Analytic Services A-29). Rockville, MD: Substance Abuse and Mental Health Services Administration, Office of Applied Studies

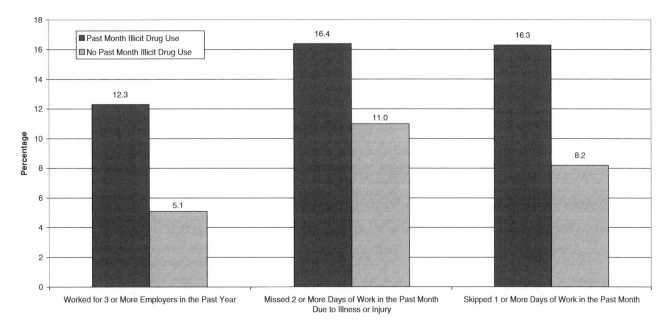

Fig. 43.5 Employment Indicators by Past Month Illicit Drug Use Status, 2002–2004. Source: Larson, S. L., Eyerman, J., Foster, M. S., & Gfroerer, J. C. (2007). *Worker Substance Use and Workplace Policies and Programs* (DHHS Publication No. SMA 07-4273, Analytic Services A-29). Rockville, MD: Substance Abuse and Mental Health Services Administration, Office of Applied Studies

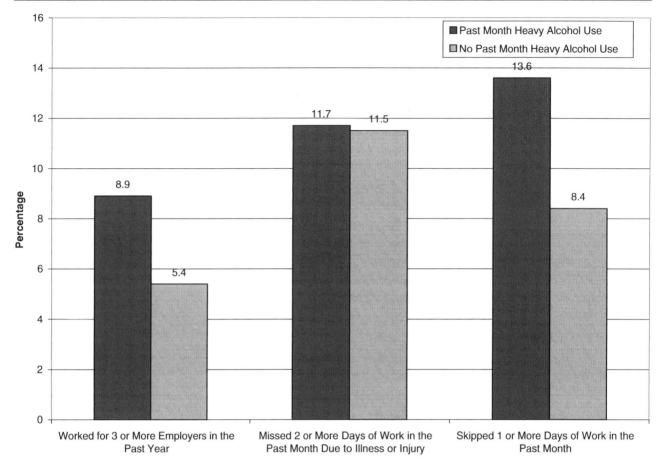

Fig. 43.6 Employment Indicators by Past Month Heavy Alcohol Use Status: 2002–2004. Source: Larson, S. L., Eyerman, J., Foster, M. S., & Gfroerer, J. C. (2007). *Worker Substance Use and Workplace Policies and Programs* (DHHS Publication No. SMA 07-4273, Analytic Services A-29). Rockville, MD: Substance Abuse and Mental Health Services Administration, Office of Applied Studies

costs related to decreased productivity, tardiness, or other disruptions to businesses related to substance use.

Employee substance use is also related to workplace injuries. In a matched case-controlled study of over 26,000 workers, Spicer, Miller, and Smith [8] found that the odds of injury among employees with alcohol or drug-related problems were 1.35 times greater than that among those without alcohol or drug involvement indicators, even when the results were controlled for job type, demographic characteristics, and exposure. Substance use is also involved in fatal work-related injuries. An analysis of toxicology reports found that approximately 5% were positive for alcohol and/or other drugs among fatal occupational injuries in the USA [9].

Creating Drug-Free Workplaces

Given the negative consequences of drug and alcohol use on occupational functioning, attention has turned toward reducing its impact. The focus to create drug-free workplaces was catalyzed by the 1986 presidential order in the USA that all

Federal agencies be drug free. Not long afterward, the US Congress passed the Drug-Free Workplace Act in 1988 requiring all federal grantees and contractors to implement written policies, employee education, and disclosures of drug-related offenses, among other activities. An additional act in 1991, known as the Omnibus Transportation Employee Testing Act, requires alcohol and drug testing among employees in transportation (e.g., aviation, trucking, and railroad) and pipeline industries.

Materials are readily available to business managers wanting to foster a drug-free work environment. Educational posters, policy development, and employee awareness campaign materials are available online. The SAMHSA [10] offers a free Drug-free Workplace Kit to provide employers with helpful tools and resources. Those organizations required to abide with the Drug Free Workplace Act of 1988 can access additional materials through the US Department of Labor's [11] website. Ensuring Solutions to Alcohol Problems [12], a public policy and awareness project of the George Washington University Medical Center, publishes a monograph titled "Workplace screening & brief intervention: What employers can and should do about excessive alcohol use" (2008) on their website, as well. The document provides guidance to employers who wish to implement screening and brief interventions to address alcohol problems, specifically.

Additional programs and curricula are readily available. SAMHSA's National Registry of Evidence-based Programs and Practices (NREPP) lists several workplace programs that have undergone the registry's rigorous review process [13]. Each program's methods, outcomes, and contact information are provided.

Workplace Prevention and Intervention

Workplace prevention and intervention programs vary greatly from job site to job site. Common components include employee education and awareness campaigns, pre-hire drug testing, random drug testing, and EAP to address problematic drug and alcohol use. Recent surveys show wide-spread implementation of these methods. Among full-time workers in the USA, for example, 79% report aware-ness of alcohol and drug use policies in their workplace and 44% report access to additional educational information [3]. With regard to drug testing, 43% work for employers who conduct "pre-hire" drug testing, while 30% work in random drug-testing environments. Overall, 58% had access to an EAP [3].

Despite their popularity, formal evaluations of workplace prevention or intervention programs are relatively sparse. Nonetheless, a growing number of studies have found posi-tive outcomes when testing efficacy via pre–post, quasi-experimental, and experimental methodologies.

Bennett and colleagues [14] surveyed the existing litera-ture and conducted a meta-analytic review of controlled studies published during the 1990s and early 2000s. Only 12 of 22 studies met the criteria for inclusion. The authors found a small but significant effect for workplace prevention pro-grams in reducing alcohol and other drug use, changing knowledge and beliefs associated with use, and overall func-tioning. Specifically, the mean effect size across studies was .299, suggesting that, while weak, the programs were effec-tive compared to the control conditions.

Using sophisticated univariate and bivariate statistical techniques, French and colleagues [15] estimated the relative benefit of drug testing among the workforce. The researchers utilized data obtained from the National Household Survey on Drug Abuse conducted by SAMHSA. Data were collected from over 50,000 households during 1997 and 1998. According to the estimates, workplaces with drug-testing programs experienced a 24% reduction in drug usage compared to workplaces without drug testing. In addition, employees at drug-testing workplaces were 38.5% less likely to be chronic drug users. As such, the authors suggest that

drug-testing programs may provide a deterrent effect whereby chronic drug users may be discouraged from seeking employ-ment at companies where drug testing takes place.

Given the potential positive effect of drug testing, it is unclear how much drug testing is necessary to achieve the desired impact. Ozminkowski and colleagues [16] examined the impact of urinalysis testing on the reduction of medical expenses and injuries at a large manufacturing firm with over 1,700 employees across 15 sites. Drug-testing rates did not significantly impact injury rates, which were very low at the outset. However, a significant impact was found for drug-testing rates and reductions in medical expenses. In order to minimize medical expenses among the workforce, statistical simulations estimated that a random testing rate of 42% of the workforce each quarter was needed. That rate translated to testing each employee an average of 1.68 times per year.

Web-based interventions can also be helpful in preventing or limiting problematic alcohol use among employees. Doumas and Hannah [17] examined the efficacy of a brief, web-delivered personal feedback system on the quantity and frequency of drinking among young adults in the workforce. Employees in the 18–24-year-old age group ($N = 196$) were randomly assigned to the web intervention, the web interven-tion plus a 15-min motivational counseling session, or a con-trol condition. Consistent with hypotheses, those assigned to the two web-based conditions reported significant decreases in weekend drinking, drinking to intoxication, and consump-tion levels at the 1-month follow-up compared to the control condition. Furthermore, those who were drinking at risky levels at baseline reported the greatest reductions over time compared to the control group. Among low-risk drinkers, the web and control conditions did not differ. The addition of the 15-min motivational counseling session did not provide any additive benefit.

Using time-series analyses, Miller and colleagues [18] examined the impact of a peer-based prevention program called PeerCare and random drug testing on work-related injury rates for a large, national transportation company employing 26,000 people. In this particular program, trained employees intervene when concerned about a peer's alcohol or drug usage. In addition, non-punitive approaches are taken to support those with substance use problems. According to analyses, the program reduced injury rates by approximately one-third, equating to an estimated $48 million in savings. Furthermore, the cost–benefit ratio of the program was 26:1, resulting in substantial savings related to program costs.

As mentioned earlier, the SAMHSA NREPP lists several workplace programs that have applied to the Registry and undergone their rigorous review criteria. The Healthy Workplace [19] program, for example, is comprised of five sections delivered via a small group format. The program has been demonstrated to reduce alcohol use and improve healthy lifestyle behaviors among participants compared to controls [19–21].

Team Awareness, developed by Bennett and colleagues [22], is also listed on the NREPP. An interactive group training program, Team Awareness is delivered via two 4-h sessions with an additional session for supervisors. Materials are also available specifically for small businesses. In one randomized study, over 200 municipal workers received either the 8-h training program or a 4-h informational session covering policies [23]. Those in the training session demonstrated positive change in help-seeking, support for others, and attitudes toward substance users, whereas little change was observed among control group participants. Another investigation of the program's impact on supervisors found an increase in responsiveness to substance use problems in the workforce among supervisors in the training group compared to those in the control condition [24]. The program has also worked to decrease alcohol use and alcohol-related absenteeism relative to controls.

As shown, a variety of prevention programs and techniques are demonstrating a positive impact on decreasing employee drug and alcohol use among staff. But what does an employer do once an employee is identified as an individual with substance use problems? Whether identified via drug testing, self-disclosure, or other means, a variety of intervention programs are available to address problematic drug or alcohol usage among the workforce.

One common intervention involves referral to an EAP. Provided as a benefit, these programs typically offer assessment and brief counseling to employees facing work- or life-related difficulties. Referral for more intensive mental health and/or substance use problem interventions is made when necessary. Research data on the impact of EAP referral on substance use and employment outcomes, specifically, are scarce. As noted by Merrick and colleagues in their review [25], few EAP evaluations have focused specifically on substance use and employment outcomes, and the majority of studies have been limited by methodological problems. As a result, Merrick and colleagues call for a new research agenda to address these issues. Specifically, they illustrate the need for large-scale studies utilizing experimental and quasi-experimental methodologies to examine substance use outcomes, changes in employment functioning, cost–benefits of programming, identification of barriers to EAP utilization, and development of EAP performance measures.

A study by Elliot and Shelley [26] examined the impact of EAP referral on workplace accident rates among employees who either tested positive for drugs or self-disclosed drug use. Drug test-positive employees were fired and considered for re-employment only after attending an EAP and being recommended for re-hire by treatment professionals. Those who self-disclosed drug-use problems were retained as employees and referred to the EAP. The records of 507 employees (334 drug-test positive workers who were re-hired and 173 self-referred who received treatment) were examined. Workplace accident rates decreased from pre- to posttreatment among both groups. However, drug test-positive employees had significantly higher workplace accident rates compared to those who were self-referred.

Among employees with alcohol and/or drug dependence, treatment is effective in reducing absenteeism and improving employment functioning. A study conducted by Slaymaker and Owen [27], for example, examined the impact of residential treatment for substance dependence among a sample of 212 full-time employed people. Significant improvement in alcohol, drug, legal, psychiatric, and family/social severity was observed from baseline to 6 and 12 months posttreatment. The proportion of the sample reporting unplanned absences from work decreased significantly from 78% at baseline to 30% at the 12-month follow-up. The number of employment problem days also dropped significantly from 5.20 to 0.14 days, on average, at the baseline and 12-month follow-up, respectively. Job disciplinary actions also reduced substantially from pre- to posttreatment.

Worner and colleagues [28] found economic benefits related to treatment among 123 employees. Specifically, union workers who entered treatment for substance use and received no other services for the 2-year follow-up period exhibited a 48% reduction in health-care costs from the pre- to posttest period. Those employees who entered treatment and continued to receive treatment during the follow-up period, however, had a 93% increase in health costs, and those who refused treatment services exhibited a 116% increase in costs. The pattern of findings persisted at the 5-year follow-up. Unfortunately, nearly one-fourth of the sample required ongoing care and the analyses were not adjusted for substance use disorder severity.

In a later study, Jordan and colleagues [29] analyzed data obtained from 498 outpatients in a large treatment system in southern California. As shown in Fig. 43.7, substantial reductions in the proportion reporting absenteeism, productivity problems, and workplace conflict following 1–2 months of care occurred from baseline to the follow-up periods. Furthermore, economic cost–benefit analyses found a net benefit to employers who offered treatment benefits. Specifically, returns on investment were conservatively estimated to range from 23% among employees with an income of $45K per year to 64% among those earning $60K per year.

The Perspective of Human Resource Professionals

Given the review above, it is no surprise to find that human resource professionals are concerned about substance use among the workforce. A nationwide telephone survey of over 300 senior human resources (HR) professionals found

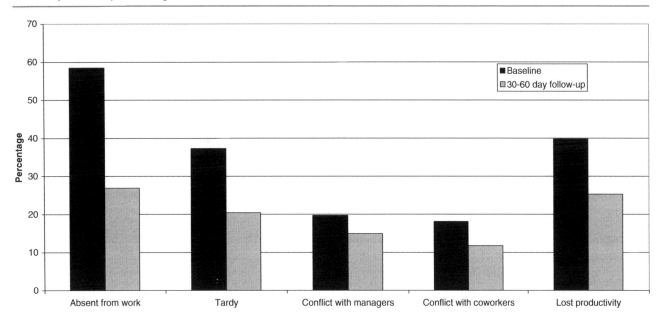

Fig. 43.7   Changes in job functioning from baseline to posttreatment follow-up among 468 employees. Data source: Jordan et al., 2008

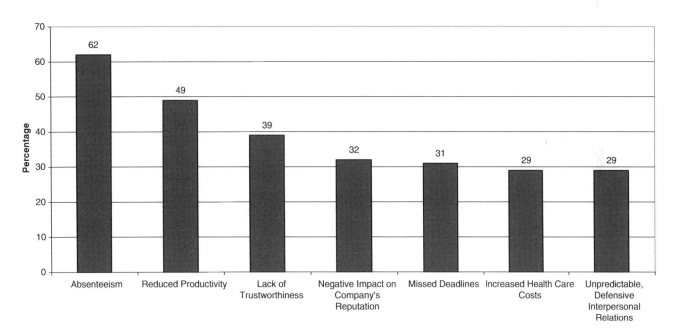

Fig. 43.8   Substance use-related problems in the workplace as identified by human resources professionals. Source: Hazelden Foundation, 2007

that 67% believe substance use is one of the most serious issues they face in their company [30]. As shown in Fig. 43.8, the most common problems related to substance use among employees included absenteeism, reduced productivity, and a negative impact on the company's reputation, among others.

Despite the widespread availability of workplace interventions, few HR professionals (22%) believed their companies proactively addressed addiction problems among employees. The most common hurdles faced by HR professionals in addressing addiction among employees included limited experience recognizing or identifying substance-related problems, discomfort addressing problems with employees, and a lack of knowledge of treatment resources. Despite these challenges, HR professionals readily acknowledged the positive impact of effective treatment, with 92% believing that effective treatment increases employee productivity. Two-thirds (67%) agreed that treatment resulted in reduced health-care costs to the employers.

Summary and Directions for Future Research

The occupational impact of employee substance use is profound, resulting in substantial economic and societal costs to individuals, families, and employers. As a result, a variety of workplace programs have been implemented to prevent, identify, and intervene ranging from drug-testing, educational campaigns, and EAP services. Despite the popularity of these services, relatively little experimental study of their impact has been conducted. Recent data, however, have begun to demonstrate the positive impact of workplace programming on reducing substance use, lowering costs, reducing injuries, and increasing employee productivity. Initial cost–benefit data suggest the programs can be economically feasible and effective. Nonetheless, future study is necessary to experimentally test workplace interventions, document cost–benefit ratios, and replicate findings across work sites. Additional work is needed to address barriers faced by human resource professionals when identifying and addressing substance use problems among the workforce. In the meantime, the data reviewed here demonstrate the important impact workplace programs can have on enhancing employee performance. Given the benefits to both the employer and the employee, it is in an employer's best interests to identify and address substance use problems among the workforce.

References

1. Substance Abuse and Mental Health Services Administration, Office of Applied Studies. Results from the 2007 National Survey on Drug Use and Health: national findings (NSDUH Series H-34, DHHS Publication No. SMA 08-4343). Rockville, MD: Substance Abuse and Mental Health Services Administration, Office of Applied Studies; 2008.
2. Frone MR. Prevalence and distribution of illicit drug use in the workforce and in the workplace: findings and implications from a U.S. national survey. J Appl Psychol. 2006;91(4):856–69.
3. Larson SL, Eyerman J, Foster MS, Gfroerer JC. Worker substance use and workplace policies and programs (DHHS Publication No. SMA 07-4273, Analytic Series A-29). Rockville, MD: Substance Abuse and Mental Health Services Administration, Office of Applied Studies. 2007. Available online http://www.oas.samhsa.gov/work2k7/work.pdf.
4. Frone MR. Prevalence and distribution of alcohol use and impairment in the workplace: a U.S. national survey. J Stud Alcohol. 2006;67:147–56.
5. Office of National Drug Control Policy. The economic costs of drug abuse in the United States, 1992–2002. Washington, DC: Executive Office of the President (Publication No. 207303). 2004. Available online http://www.whitehousedrugpolicy.gov/publications/economic_costs/.
6. Harwood H. Updating estimates of the economic costs of alcohol abuse in the United States: estimates, update methods, and data. Report prepared for the National Institute on Alcohol Abuse and Alcoholism, National Institutes of Health, Department of Health and Human Services. Rockville, MD: National Institutes of Health. 2000. Available online http://pubs.niaaa.nih.gov/publications/economic-2000/alcoholcost.PDF.
7. Foster WH, Vaughan RD. Absenteeism and business costs: does substance abuse matter? J Subst Abuse Treat. 2005;28:27–33.
8. Spicer RS, Miller TR, Smith GS. Worker substance use, workplace problems and the risk of occupational injury: a matched case-control study. J Stud Alcohol. 2003;64:570–8.
9. Greenberg M, Hamilton R, Toscano G. Analysis of toxicology reports from the 1993-94 census of fatal occupational injuries. Compensation and Working Conditions, pp. 26–28. 1999. Available online: http://www.bls.gov/iif/oshwc/cfar0032.pdf.
10. U.S. Department of Health and Human Services, SAMHSA, Center for Substance Abuse Prevention, Division of Workplace Programs. [Retrieved November, 2008] Making your workplace drug-free: a kit for employers. Available online http://www.workplace.samhsa.gov/WPWorkit/index.html.
11. U.S. Department of Labor. Working partners for an alcohol and drug-free workplace. 2008. Available online http://www.dol.gov/workingpartners/welcome.html.
12. Ensuring Solutions to Alcohol Problems. Workplace screening & brief intervention: what employers can and should do about excessive alcohol use. Washington, DC: Ensuring Solutions to Alcohol Problems. 2008. Available online http://www.ensuringsolutions.org/usr_doc/Workplace_SBI_Report_Final.pdf.
13. Substance Abuse and Mental Health Services Administration. NREPP: SAMHSA's national registry of evidence-based programs and practices. 2008. Retrieved November 25, 2008. Available online http://www.nrepp.samhsa.gov/index.asp.
14. Bennett JB, Reynolds S, Lehman WEK. Understanding employee alcohol and other drug use: toward a multilevel approach. In: Bennett JB, Lehman WEK, editors. Preventing workplace substance abuse: beyond drug testing to wellness. Washington: American Psychological Association; 2003. p. 29–56.
15. French MT, Roebuck MC, Alexandre PK. To test or no to test: do workplace drug testing programs discourage employee drug use? Soc Sci Res. 2004;33(45–63).
16. Ozminkowski RJ, Mark TL, Goetzel RZ, Blank D, Walsh JM, Cangianelli L. Relationships between urinalysis testing for substance use, medical expenditures, and the occurrence of injuries at a large manufacturing firm. Am J Drug Alcohol Abuse. 2003;29(1):151–67.
17. Doumas DM, Hannah E. Preventing high-risk drinking in youth in the workplace: a web-based normative feedback program. J Subst Abuse Treat. 2008;34:263–71.
18. Miller TR, Zaloshnja E, Spicer RS. Effectiveness and benefit-cost of peer-based workplace substance abuse prevention coupled with random testing. Accid Anal Prev. 2007;39:565–73.
19. Cook RF, Hersch RK, Back AS, McPherson TL. The prevention of substance abuse among construction workers: a field test of a social cognitive program. J Prim Prev. 2004;25(3):337–58.

20. Cook RF, Back AS, Trudeau J. Preventing alcohol use problems among blue-collar workers: a field test of the Working People program. Subst Abuse Misuse. 1996;31(3):255–75.

21. Cook RF, Back AS, Trudeau J. Substance abuse prevention in the workplace: recent findings and an expanded conceptual model. J Prim Prev. 1996;16(3):319–39.

22. Bennett JB, Patterson CR, Reynolds GS, Witala WL, Lehman WEK. Team awareness, problem drinking and drinking climate: workplace social health promotion in a policy context. Am J Health Promot. 2004;19(2):103–13.

23. Bennett JB, Lehman WEK. Workplace substance abuse prevention and help seeking: comparing team-oriented and informational training. J Occup Health Psychol. 2001;6(3):243–54.

24. Bennett JB, Lehman WEK. Supervisor tolerance-responsiveness to substance abuse and workplace prevention training: use of a cognitive mapping tool. Health Educ Res. 2002;17(1):27–42.

25. Merrick ESL, Volpe-Vartanian J, Horgan CM, McCann B. Revisiting employee assistance programs and substance use problems in the workplace: key issues and a research agenda. Psychiatr Serv. 2007;58(10):1262–4.

26. Elliott K, Shelley K. Effects of drugs and alcohol on behavior, job performance, and workplace safety. J Employment Couns. 2006;43:130–4.

27. Slaymaker VJ, Owen PL. Employed men and women substance abusers: job troubles and treatment outcomes. J Subst Abuse Treat. 2006;31:347–54.

28. Worner TM, Chen P, Ma H, Xu S, McCarthy EG. An analysis of substance abuse patterns, medical expenses and effectiveness of treatment in the workplace: long-term follow-up. Empl Benefits J. 1993;18(4):15–9.

29. Jordan N, Grissom G, Alonzo G, Dietzen L, Sangsland S. Economic benefit of chemical dependency treatment to employers. J Subst Abuse Treat. 2008;34:311–9.

30. Hazelden Foundation. Substance abuse and addiction among most serious workplace issues. 2007. Available http://www.hazelden.org/web/public/2007workplacesurvey.page.

Drugs of Abuse and Traffic Safety

44

Renske Penning, Janet Veldstra, Anne P. Daamen, Berend Olivier, and Joris C. Verster

Introduction

In most Western countries, alcohol prevalence in traffic crashes and fatalities has been declining since the early 1980s. This is probably due to successful public health campaigns and vigorous enforcement. In contrast, the number of drug-impaired drivers seems to increase and so is the prevalence of combined alcohol and drug driving. Roadside studies estimate the prevalence of drug-impaired drivers between 1 and 15% [1]. A report by the European Monitoring Centre for Drugs and Drugs Addiction (EMCDDA), [1] based on different driving studies in Europe, Australia, the USA, and Canada, estimates the prevalence of a combination of drugs and alcohol in the general driving population between 0.3% and 1.3%. These increasing numbers are of concern, since drugged drivers are, like alcohol-impaired drivers, significantly more likely to be culpable for a fatal accident [2, 3].

Drug Effects and Driving

The effects of drugs on driving can be determined using several methodologies, including driving tests in normal traffic or closed roads, driving simulators, and epidemiological studies.

The on-the-road driving test is currently considered as the gold standard to determine the effects of drugs on driving. This standardized test has a high ecological validity, since it is performed on a public highway in normal traffic. The test

was developed in the 1980s by O'Hanlon and colleagues [4]. Participants are instructed to drive for 100 km on a public highway, with a constant speed (usually 95 km/h) and a steady lateral position. The participant is allowed to take over slower vehicles and is accompanied by a driving instructor with dual controls. The lateral position of the vehicle relative to the left lane boundary is measured with a camera mounted on the roof of the car (see Fig. 44.1).

From these measurements, the standard deviation of the lateral position (SDLP) (e.g., weaving of the car) is calculated. The SDLP is the primary parameter of the test reflecting overall vehicle control. The on-the-road driving test is used in more than 60 clinical trials, and its primary parameter SDLP is able to differentiate dose-dependent impairment for various substances, including alcohol, hypnotics, anxiolytics, antidepressants, and antihistamines [5, 6].

Another test performed in normal traffic is the car-following test. In this test, two vehicles are driving in front of each other. The first vehicle is driven by an investigator and the second by the participant. The participant is instructed to maintain a steady distance of 50 m between the two cars, while the lead car now and then varies its speed. The primary outcome is the amount of time the participant needs to respond to these speed changes by adapting his own speed to maintain the 50-m distance between the cars. Decreased attention and impaired perception can be measured by this test, since these are involved in the drivers' ability to react properly on other vehicles [7].

Both the on-the-road driving test and the car-following test have their limitations in determining all aspects related to driving. For example, studies in which the acute effects of 3,4-methylenedioxymethamphetamine (MDMA) on driving performance were investigated show that MDMA improves driving performance in the on-the-road driving test, but risk taking was significantly increased [8–10]. This illustrates that it is important to test driving behavior at multiple levels, thus not only vehicle control, but also driving behavior itself (for example, risk taking). Driving simulators are a safe way to test these driving behaviors.

R. Penning (✉) • A.P. Daamen • B. Olivier • J.C. Verster
Division of Pharmacology, Utrecht Institute
for Pharmaceutical Sciences, Utrecht University,
Universiteitsweg 99, 3584 CG Utrecht, The Netherlands
e-mail: r.penning@uu.nl

J. Veldstra
Faculty of Behavioural and Social Sciences,
Section Experimental Psychology, University of Groningen,
Traffic and Environmental psychology,
Groningen, The Netherlands

J.C. Verster et al. (eds.), *Drug Abuse and Addiction in Medical Illness: Causes, Consequences and Treatment*,
DOI 10.1007/978-1-4614-3375-0_44, © Springer Science+Business Media, LLC 2012

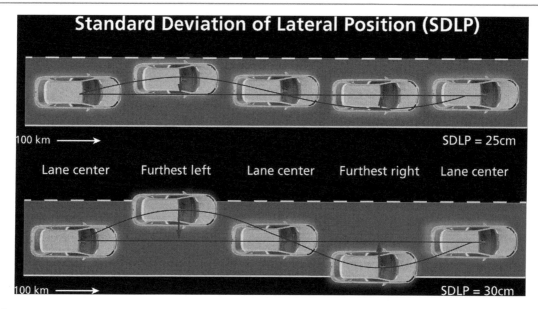

Fig. 44.1 Standard deviation of the lateral position (SDLP)

Other sources of information on drugs and traffic safety include epidemiological studies, roadside studies, and testing driving-related skills in a laboratory setting. The first two methodologies provide information on the incidence of drugged driving and risks of having accidents.

Laboratory tests provide information on driving-related skills. An advantage of these measurements is that they can be performed in a controlled setting. It is, however, difficult to predict actual driving performance of the laboratory test results. This is understandable from the fact that these tests examine driving-related skills in isolation, whereas during driving these skills are applied simultaneously [11]. In conclusion, different aspects of driving performance are covered by the available methodologies. Preferably, to draw conclusions on the effects of a specific drug on driving ability, the drug should therefore be tested applying more than one of these techniques. This chapter summarizes data from clinical trials examining the effects of drugs of abuse on driving ability and the risk of becoming involved in traffic accidents.

Alcohol

Alcohol is the most commonly detected substance in drivers. This is not surprising since alcohol is not prohibited in most countries and its use can be tested easily by police officers by applying a breath alcohol test.

Most epidemiological studies on alcohol investigated the prevalence of alcohol in (fatally) injured drivers. About 50 years ago, Borkenstein et al. [12] conducted a classic roadside study. His team stopped several thousand drivers and measured their blood alcohol concentration (BAC). After the drivers continued their way, they investigated the number of

the tested drivers who were involved in a traffic accident afterward. A dose–response relationship was found between BAC and the risk of involvement in traffic accidents. In this study, the risk of alcohol impairment was shown to begin at a BAC level of 0.5 g/l; therefore, many countries have this BAC level as their legal limit. Many studies confirmed these findings and form foundation of current traffic regulations and legal limits for driving after using alcohol. The most common legal limits are 0.5 g/l (experienced drivers) and 0.2 g/l (novice drivers). Some countries have lowered their BAC limits to 0.2 g/l. This is a consequence of findings in experimental studies showing that critical driving skills, such as divided attention, vigilance, psychomotor skills, and information processing, are impaired by a BAC as low as 0.2 g/l. Studies which have investigated the effects of the lower legal BAC limits all show a decrease in car accidents after lowering the limit [13, 14].

Alcohol involvement is reported in 20–38% of the traffic-related deaths [15, 16]. In Sweden, Ahlm et al. [15] recently found a comparable number of intoxicated drivers. They revealed that 38% of the fatally injured and 21% of the non-fatally injured drivers tested positive for alcohol. A Dutch study reported an adjusted 5.5 odds ratio for traffic accident injury after alcohol consumption [17]. A study in New Zealand tested 571 car-crash victims of which 36% tested positive for alcohol. In the control population (randomly stopped drivers), only 2% was under the influence of alcohol [18]. US studies show a decrease in the number of drivers with a BAC above the legal limit, from 36% in 1973 to 17% in 1996 [19]. This number is relatively high compared to that of Europe, especially when the legal BAC limits in some US states (0.8 g/l) is compared with the European limit (0.5 g/l) [20, 21].

Many experimental studies examined the effects of alcohol on driving performance. For example, Louwerens et al. [22] conducted an on-the-road driving study with different BAC levels. Examination of the effects of the three most common legal BAC limits shows an SDLP increment of +2.4 cm (0.5 g/l), +4.1 cm (0.8 g/l), and +5.3 cm for a BAC level of 1.0 g/l. Their study also found a dose-dependent impairment of alcohol on weaving and is frequently used as a reference study when assessing the effects of other drugs on driving.

Drivers with low BAC levels may show successful compensation for awareness of mild alcohol-induced impairment. Calhoun et al. [23] conducted a simulated driving study and found that at a low BAC (0.04%), performance slightly improved and drivers reduced their average speed. However, in the high BAC condition (0.08%), this compensation was absent: performance deteriorated and speed increased.

In conclusion, there is substantial evidence that alcohol negatively affects driving performance. Therefore, alcohol use before driving should be avoided.

Nicotine

Laboratory studies show that nicotine decreases reaction speed, but increases attention [24]. Taking this into account, it can be hypothesized that nicotine enhances driving performance. However, smoking can also be regarded as a secondary task while driving, which potentially distracts from the primary driving task.

There have been no studies on the prevalence of driving under the influence of nicotine or on nicotine's involvement in traffic accidents. In the few driving studies that have been performed, there was a focus on the impact of nicotine abstinence on driving performance. Two driving simulator studies show that smokers and nonsmokers perform equally in a testing situation [25, 26]. However, when smokers had to refrain from smoking, a significant decrease in driving performance was observed. After smoking a cigarette, driving performance restored to normal [25, 26].

Cannabis

Cannabis or Δ^9-tetrahydrocannabinol (THC) is, after alcohol, the most commonly found drug in drivers. A recent study in Scotland showed that in approximately half of the drug or alcohol driving offenders, cannabinoids were found [27]. A Norwegian roadside study randomly stopping drivers revealed that 0.6% of the 10.835 drivers tested positive for the use of THC [21]. A recent roadside study in Queensland, Australia, showed that of the 1,587 stopped drivers, 1.26% of the drivers tested positive for THC [28]. Several epidemiological studies, but not all [17], reveal that THC usage significantly elevates the chance to be involved in car accidents [17, 29–34]. However, when looking at culpability rates, various studies did not show a significant effect for THC alone on these rates [3, 5].

Klonoff [35] was the first who tested THC effects in real traffic. After taking THC or placebo, subjects drove under supervision of a professional driving instructor, who evaluated their performance. Subjects smoked a standardized cigarette containing 4.9 mg THC or 8.4 mg THC. Only in the highest dosage group the driving skills were affected. Sutton [36] conducted an on-the-road test on a closed course, investigating the effects of cannabis and alcohol (combined and alone). He used the same THC dosages as Klonoff [35]. The alcohol intake was sufficient to establish a BAC of 0.06%. Sutton [36] used official driver examination statutes, which makes his results more reliable than Klonoff's subjective assessments of driving performance. The results only showed a significant driving impairment when alcohol and THC were combined and no impairment when each substance was used alone. The relatively short circuit that was used for the driving tests may account for the absence of THC effects when administered alone [36]. In an early review on THC and on-road and driving simulator studies, Smiley [37] also concluded that THC impaired driving performance. Robbe [38] tested the effects of THC alone and in combination with alcohol on driving performance. Robbe [38] performed the on-the-road driving test, a car-following test, and a city driving test. Only the on-the-road driving test showed a significant dose-related decrease in driving performance. Results of the other two tests were not significant [38]. When alcohol was co-administered with THC, a dramatic decrease in driving performance was found. This effect was greater than when alcohol or THC was administered alone [39, 40]. Taking the results of these on-the-road studies into account, it can be said that THC alone impairs driving performance to some extent, whereas the combination of THC with alcohol has a clear negative effect on driving performance.

People seem aware of the impairing effects of THC and often compensate this impairment by a more conservative driving style (e.g., reducing speed) [37, 41]. This compensation might fail when cannabis is used in combination with alcohol. In conclusion, driving after cannabis use is unsafe, especially when combined with alcohol.

Cocaine

Studies show that the prevalence of cocaine-impaired drivers varies from less than 1 to 13%** [21, 42–45]. This wide range is probably caused by the fact that cocaine use is more popular among different subgroups, for example, partygoers, than in the general population. The percentage of cocaine-using drivers depends therefore on the time and place of the roadside survey.

Cocaine users often report that they feel the drug does not impair their driving. Only one-third of 300 injecting drug users in Australia indicated that they found driving after cocaine use dangerous [46]. Thus most subjects did not indicate cocaine-drugged driving as dangerous, probably because cocaine improves vigilance performance and reduces reaction speed [47]. Cocaine users also reported being more alert and euphoric when using cocaine [47]. This may explain the overconfidence in their driving skills, and may result in unsafe driving such as speeding and dangerous take-over maneuvers. Police records confirm that these dangerous driving behaviors are commonly seen in cocaine-impaired drivers [45, 47]. Experimental studies also show that cocaine impairs complex decision making and increases risk taking on tests such as the Iowa Gambling Task [48, 49]. This increased risk taking is also seen when participating in traffic. Misjudgment of driving ability and increased risk taking make driving after using cocaine unsafe.

Ecstasy or/and MDMA

Ecstasy or ±3,4-,methylenedioxymethamphetamine (MDMA) is a popular recreational drug that is frequently used at parties and festivals. It can be expected that after such events, a substantial number of ecstasy users will drive home under the influence of MDMA [50, 51]. Ecstasy is often used in combination with other drugs and alcohol. Interviews performed in Scotland and Australia revealed that 8–33% of the MDMA users would either drive themselves home under the influence of drugs, or would be driven by someone who had used drugs [52–55]. Interviews held with regular ecstasy users in Australia even revealed that 53% of the 573 users admitted to have driven under the influence of this drug within the last 6 months [56]. Roadside studies show that only a small percentage (1–2%) of the general population drives under the influence of ecstasy [57, 58]. Studies on car accident in Australia, Hong Kong, and France reveal that less than 5% of injured drivers tested positive for the use of MDMA [59, 60]. Thus, the use of ecstasy in traffic remains limited to a subgroup of partygoers.

Various studies have been conducted to examine the effects of MDMA on driving performance. Ramaekers and colleagues performed on-the-road driving tests in normal traffic to examine the effects of MDMA (with and without alcohol) [9, 10]. These studies showed a significant decrease in weaving of the car, indicating that MDMA improves performance in the on-the-road driving test. Performance on the car-following test yielded mixed results [9, 10]. MDMA partly counteracted the impairing effects of alcohol in the

on-the-road driving rest, an effect that was not seen in the car-following test.

Brookhuis et al. [8] investigated simulated driving performance of MDMA users before and after visiting a rave party. The results of this study indicate that driving performance decreases during the night after MDMA use. It was also shown that when MDMA was combined with other drugs, driving performance was further impaired. The results of this study can be influenced by the effects of sleep deprivation as the tested subjects did not sleep during the night. Almost all subjects indicated that they found themselves a better driver after MDMA intake. A recent study confirmed that more than half of regular ecstasy users indicate that ecstasy does not impair their driving ability, or actually improves it [56].

Although some researchers show that basic driving skills (lane keeping and reaction speed) improve after MDMA intake [9, 10], which can explain the experienced driving improvement, other researchers found increased risk-taking behavior, impaired decision making, and impulsivity (e.g., speeding and ignoring stop signs) [61, 62]. MDMA can thus result in overconfidence and corresponding unsafe driving behavior.

LSD

The prevalence of lysergic acid diethylamide (LSD) use is low in the general driving population [63]. However, as for cocaine and ecstasy, LSD use is high in specific populations. For example, Riley et al. interviewed 122 partygoers of whom 30.3% admitted using LSD in the past year. Of these partygoers, 36% confirmed they had driven after LSD intake on one or more occasions [53]. Neal [55] questioned 61 Scottish nightclub attendees about their drug usage and driving experiences. Eight percent of the questioned attendees admitted to have driven after the intake of LSD. Noteworthy, all interviewed drivers experienced driving after LSD usage as very dangerous. They reported distracting hallucinations and visual impairments as the most dangerous effects of LSD on driving performance.

No real driving or simulator tests have been performed with LSD and there is little experimental evidence on its effects on psychomotor functioning; besides that LSD significantly decreases reaction time [64].

Ketamine

Researchers suggest that driving after using ketamine is common among partygoers [65]. In Scotland, 15% of 122 partygoers admitted the use of ketamine; of them, 36% confirmed driving after ketamine use [53]. A study on the victims of fatal car-crashes in Hong Kong revealed that in

9% of the investigated cases, ketamine was found in the victim [65].

Several studies investigated the effects of ketamine on psychomotor and cognitive function, but driving itself has not been studied. Krystal et al. [66] reported an impairing effect of ketamine on executive cognitive function. Other studies reported impaired response inhibition, decreased attention, and impaired memory function after ketamine infusion in healthy volunteers [67, 68], and prolonged reaction time in choice reaction time tests [69]. Subjects are often aware of these effects and indicated that they feel more tired and clumsy [70]. In addition, ketamine can also cause "out of body" experiences, illusions, sometimes hallucinations, and misinterpretation of visual and auditory stimuli [71, 72]. These last effects are the main reason why people use ketamine as a recreational drug. However, these effects make driving after ketamine use unsafe.

Amphetamines

The incidence of methamphetamine use in the general driver population is about 2% [73]. The prevalence of methamphetamine in victims of traffic accidents ranges from 2 to 5% [59, 60, 74, 75]. Recent studies in Switzerland and Scotland revealed that approximately 7% of apprehended suspects of driving under the influence of drugs tested positive for amphetamine [27].

Truck drivers and other long-distance drivers are known to use methamphetamines and other stimulant drugs to stay awake during their long driving hours. Crouch et al. [76] investigated the use of drugs in fatally injured truck drivers. They found that 7% of them had used methamphetamines or amphetamine. A more recent study among 1,000 truck drivers in France revealed that 0.3% of the drivers tested positive for amphetamine [77]. Although percentages of users are relatively low, (meth)amphetamine use by professional drivers is of particular concern.

There are no on-the-road driving studies performed with amphetamine. A driving simulator study revealed that dexamphetamine, a drug with similar effects as methamphetamine, significantly improved driving performance during day-time testing. During night-time testing, no significant difference from placebo was found [78]. Miller et al. [79] investigated narcoleptic patients and healthy controls, who had to perform a simple computer-based driving simulator test. After the use of methamphetamine, the performance of the narcoleptic patients improved in a dose-dependent manner.

Gustavsen et al. [80] reviewed literature on amphetamine and methamphetamine use and the effects on psychomotor performance. They concluded that low dosages of amphetamine restore the performance of fatigue persons to baseline and significantly improve performance in normal subjects.

However, after reviewing data of the impaired driver registry of the Norwegian Institute of Public Health, they also concluded that there was a positive relationship between amphetamine concentration and driving impairment [80].

Logan [81] reviewed 28 cases where drivers were arrested or killed after methamphetamine use. This review examined the effects of low and high dosages of methamphetamine on driving performance. The results indicate that a low dose of methamphetamine increases alertness and reduces sleepiness and reaction time. Higher dosages (commonly used by drivers) can lead to euphoria, rapid flow of ideas, feelings of great mental capacity and physical strength, and sometimes hallucinations and delusions. When blood methamphetamine concentrations are declining, agitation replaces feelings of euphoria, the subject becomes very fatigue, and concentration problems may occur. Therefore, he concluded that methamphetamine at every concentration can cause impairment in driving performance. In another review, Logan [82] stated that most studies that examined the behavioral effects of stimulant drugs suggested an increase in risk-taking behavior and impaired decision making.

Taken together, driving after high dosages of methamphetamine is dangerous, especially in the withdrawal phase.

Inhalants

Only few studies have reported the use of inhalants in drivers, which is not surprising since inhalants are not a popular drug of abuse. Of 1,500 Spanish drivers, only 0.1% admitted to have driven after the non-medical use of an inhalant in the past week [83]. Five percent of 300 interviewed injecting drug users in Australia declared that they had at least once driven after non-medical inhalant use [46]. Bennet et al. [84] reported that among US students, 5.2% had abused inhalants before their eighteenth birthday; of them, 61.7% admitted to have driven after the use of drugs or alcohol. At present no simulator studies or actual driving test has been conducted to examine the effects of inhalants on driving performance.

Some studies have examined the psychomotor effects of inhalants. Korman et al. [85] compared inhalant abusers with other-drug-abusing controls on 67 neuropsychological measures. These tests show significantly more impairment in inhalant abusers on various tests, including impaired visual-perceptual skills and decreased psychomotor skills. More recent, Beckman et al. [86] investigated the direct effects of three inhalants (N_2O, isoflurane, and sevoflurane) on psychomotor functioning. Memory function, auditory reaction time, eye–hand coordination, and time estimation were significantly impaired after the use of these three inhalants. Subjects were also more tired after using isoflurane and sevoflurane.

Adverse effects of inhalant abuse can be hallucinations, delusions, and distortions in perception of size, color, and time [87]. Kurtzman et al. [88] confirmed these findings and added tremors, slurred speech, euphoria, and decreased reflexes as common side effects of inhalant abuse. More research is needed to establish the effects of inhalants on actual driving performance.

Anabolic Steroids

Anabolic steroids are used by athletes to enhance their sport performance. However, there are also cases in which anabolic steroids were used as a recreational drug [89].

Due to the small number of studies which are performed examining anabolic steroids, little is known about the effects of these drugs on driving performance. Ellingrod et al. [90] performed the only driving simulator study with a small number of subject. They compared driving performance and level of aggression of six subjects after administrating testosterone cypionate and placebo. The drugs were administrated daily for a period of 3 weeks to establish steady-state concentrations. They found no significant effects of the steroid on driving performance and aggressive behavior.

A review of Thiblin et al. [91] investigated the pharmacoepidemiology of anabolic steroid use. They report an increase in confidence, self-esteem, motivation, and energy as short-term consequences of steroid use. They also noticed that prolonged anabolic steroid use could cause deviant behavior such as aggressive behavior and reckless driving. Hall et al. [92] also reported an increase in aggression and symptoms as rage, depression, delirium, mania, and psychosis for anabolic steroid users. More recently, Mc Gabe et al. [93] confirmed these results. They also found a positive association between anabolic steroids intake and risk-taking behavior, such as combining drinking and driving. A study in Massachusetts (USA) revealed that students showed significantly more risk-taking behavior after using anabolic steroids. They drove more frequently after drinking and did not use seatbelts or helmets [94].

Since there is little known about the actual effects of anabolic steroids on driving and psychomotor performance, more research is needed to draw absolute conclusions on steroids and driving.

Conclusion

Many drugs of abuse have a negative effect on driving performance. The effects can be characterized as sedation or increasing risk-taking behavior.

The effects of alcohol, THC, and ecstasy are extensively investigated. In contrast, other common drugs of abuse such as cocaine and amphetamines received much less scientific attention. Future research should focus on these drugs, because they are commonly used in subgroups of drivers

(e.g., partygoers) who sometimes even claim that these drugs improve their driving. Another line of research that deserves further studying regards the effects of polydrug use on driving. Little is known about the effects of co-use of two or more drugs, or the effects of concurrent alcohol use. This research is important, because in real life the use of drugs is generally combined with alcohol, and not very often limited to a single drug [51].

References

1. Raes E, Van den Neste T, Verstraete AG. Drug use, impaired driving and traffic accidents. Luxembourg: EMCDDA Insights; 2008.
2. Drummer OH, Gerostamoulos J, Batziris H, Chu M, Caplehorn J, Robertson MD, et al. The involvement of drugs drivers of motor vehicles killed in Australian road traffic crashes. Accid Anal Prev. 2004;36:239–48.
3. Longo MC, Hunter CE, Lokan RJ, White JM, White MA. The prevalence of alcohol, cannabinoids, benzodiazepines and stimulants amongst injured drivers and their role in driver culpability: part ii: the relationship between drug prevalence and drug concentration, and driver culpability. Accid Anal Prev. 2000;32:623–32.
4. O'Hanlon JF, Haak TW, Blaauw GJ, Riemersma BJ. Diazepam impairs lateral position control in highway driving. Science. 1982;217:79–81.
5. Verster JC, Pandi-Perumal SR, Ramaekers JHG, De Gier JJ, editors. Drugs, driving and traffic safety. Basel: Birkhauser; 2009.
6. Verster JC, Roth T. Standard operation procedures for conducting the on-the-road driving test, and measurement of the Standard Deviation of Lateral Position (SDLP). Int J Gen Med. 2011;4:359–71.
7. Ramaekers JG, Robbe HWJ, O'Hanlon JF. Marijuana, alcohol and actual driving performance. Hum Psychopharmacol Clin Exp. 2000;15:551–8.
8. Brookhuis KA, de Waard D, Samyn N. Effects of MDMA(ecstasy), and multiple drugs use on (simulated) driving performance and traffic safety. Psychopharmacology. 2004;173:440–5.
9. Kuypers KPC, Samyn N, Ramaekers JG. MDMA and alcohol effects, combined and alone, on objective and subjective measures of actual driving performance and psychomotor function. Psychopharmacology. 2006;187:467–75.
10. Ramaekers JG, Kuypers KPC, Samyn N. Stimulant effects of 3,4-methylenedioxymethamphetamine (MDMA) 75 mg and methylphenidate 20 mg on actual driving during intoxication and withdrawal. Addiction. 2006;101:1614–21.
11. Verster JC, Roth T. Predicting psychopharmacological drug effects on actual driving (SDLP) from psychometric tests measuring driving-related skills. Psychopharmacology. 2012;220(2):293–301.
12. Borkenstein RF, Crowther RP, Shumate RP, Ziel HB, Zylman R. The role of the drinking driver in traffic accidents. Bloomington, IN: Department of police Administration, Indiana University; 1964.
13. Fell JC, Voas RB. The effectiveness of reducing illegal blood alcohol concentration (BAC) limits for driving: evidence for lowering the limit to.05 BAC. J Safety Res. 2006;37:233–43.
14. Mann RE, Macdonald S, Stoduto G, Bondy S, Jonah B, Shaikh A. The effects of introducing or lowering legal per se blood alcohol limits for driving: an international review. Accid Anal Prev. 2001;33:569–83.
15. Ahlm K, Björnstig U, Öström M. Alcohol and drugs in fatally and non-fatally injured motor vehicle drivers in northern Sweden. Accid Anal Prev. 2009;41:129–36.

16. Mercer GW, Jeffery WK. Alcohol, drugs, and impairment in fatal traffic accidents in British Columbia. Accid Anal Prev. 1995;27:335–43.

17. Movig KLL, Mathijssen MPM, Nagel PHA, van Egmond T, de Gier JJ, Leufkens HGM, et al. Psychoactive substance use and the risk of motor vehicle accidents. Accid Anal Prev. 2004;36:631–6.

18. Connor J, Norton R, Ameratunga S, Jackson R. The contribution of alcohol to serious car crash injuries. Epidemiology. 2004; 15:337–44.

19. Williams AF. Alcohol-impaired driving and its consequences in the United States: the past 25 years. J Safety Res. 2006;37:123–38.

20. Vanlaar W. Drink driving in Belgium: results from a third improved roadside survey. Accid Anal Prev. 2005;37:391–7.

21. Gjerde H, Norman PT, Pettersen BS, Assum T, Aldrin M, Johansen U, et al. Prevalence of alcohol and drugs among Norwegian motor vehicle drivers: a roadside survey. Accid Anal Prev. 2008; 40:1765–72.

22. Louwerens JW, Gloerich ABM, De Vries G, Brookhuis KA, O'Hanlon JF. The relationship between drivers' blood alcohol concentration (BAC) and actual driving performance during high travel speed. In: Noordzij PC, Roszbach R, editors. Alcohol, drugs and traffic safety. Amsterdam: Excerpta Medica; 1987. p. 183–92.

23. Calhoun VD, Pekar JJ, Pearlson GD. Alcohol intoxication effects on simulated driving: exploring alcohol-dose effects on brain activation using functional MRI. Neuropsychopharmacolgy. 2004; 29:2097–107.

24. Rycroft N, Rusted JM, Hutton SM. Acute effects of nicotine on visual search tasks in young adult smokers. Psychopharmacology. 2005;181:160–9.

25. Heimstra NW, Bancroft NR, DeKock AR. Effects of smoking upon sustained performance in a simulated driving task. Ann NY Acad Sci. 1967;142:295–307.

26. Sherwood N. Effects of cigarette smoking on performance in a simulated driving task. Neuropsychobiology. 1995;32:161–5.

27. Officer J. Trends in drug use of Scottish drivers arrested under Section 4 of the Road Traffic Act—a 10 year review. Sci Justice. 2009;49:237–41.

28. Davey J, Freeman J. Screening for drugs in oral fluid: drug driving and illicit drug use in a sample of Queensland motorists. Traffic Inj Prev. 2009;10:231–6.

29. Mura P, Kintz P, Ludes B, Gaulier JM, Marquet P, Martin-Dupont S. Comparison of the prevalence of alcohol, cannabis and other drugs between 900 injured drivers and 900 control subjects: results of a French collaborative study. Forensic Sci Int. 2003;133:79–85.

30. Hingson R, Heeren T, Mangione T, Morelock S, Mucatel M. Teenage driving after using marijuana or drinking and traffic accident involvement. J Safety Res. 1982;13:33–8.

31. Ferguson DM, Horwood LJ. Cannabis use and traffic accidents in a birth cohort of young adults. Accid Anal Prev. 2001;33:703–11.

32. Gerberich-Goodwin S, Sidney S, Braun BL, Tekawa T, Tolan KK, Quesenberry CP. Marijuana use and injury events resulting in hospitalisation. Ann Epidemiol. 2003;13:230–7.

33. Laumon B, Gadegbeku B, Martin JL, Biecheler MB, the SAM group. Cannabis intoxication and fatal road crashes in France: population base case–control study. BMJ. 2005;331:1371–7.

34. Blows S, Ivers RI, Connor J, Ameantunga S, Woodward M, Norton R. Marijuana use and crash injury. Addiction. 2005;100:577–8.

35. Klonoff H. Marijuana and driving in real-life situations. Science. 1974;186:137–54.

36. Sutton LR. The effects of alcohol, marihuana and their combination on driving ability. J Stud Alcohol. 1983;44:438–45.

37. Smiley A. Marijuana: on road and driving simulator studies. Alcohol Drugs Driving. 1986;2:121–34.

38. Robbe HWJ. Influence of Marijuana on driving. Maastricht, The Netherlands: University of Limburg; 1994.

39. Ramaekers JG, Berghaus G, van Laar M, Drummer OH. Dose related risk of motor vehicle crashes after cannabis use. Drug Alcohol Depend. 2004;73:109–19.

40. Lamers CTJ, Ramaekers JG. Visual search and urban city driving under the influence of Marijuana and Alcohol. Hum Psychopharmacol Clin Exp. 2001;16:393–401.

41. Liguori A, Gatto C, Robinson JH. Effects of marijuana on equilibrium, psychomotor performance, and simulated driving. Behav Pharmacol. 1998;9:599–609.

42. Fitzpatrick P, Daly L, Leavy CP, Cusack DA. Drinking, drugs and driving in Ireland: more evidence for action. Inj Prev. 2006;12:404–8.

43. Schmink BE, Ruiter B, Lusthof KJ, de Gier JJ, Uges DRA, Egberts ACG. Drug use and severity of a traffic accident. Accid Anal Prev. 2005;37:427–43.

44. Papadodima SA, Athanaselis SA, Stefanidou ME, Dona AA, Papoutsis I, Maravelias CP, et al. Driving under influence in Greece; A 7-year survey (1998–2004). Forensic Sci Int. 2008;174:157–60.

45. Jones AW, Holmgren A, Kugelberg FC. Concentrations of cocaine and it's major metabolite benzoylecgonine in blood samples from apprehended drivers in Sweden. Forensic Sci Int. 2008;17:133–9.

46. Darke S, Kelly E, Ross J. Drug driving among injecting drug users in Sydney, Australia: prevalence, risk factors and risk perceptions. Addiction. 2003;99:175–85.

47. Isenschmid DS. Cocaine—effects on human performance and behaviour. Forensic Sci Rev. 2002;14:61–100.

48. van der Plas EA, Crone EA, van den Wildenberg WP, Tranel D, Bechara A. Executive control deficits in substance-dependent individuals: a comparison of alcohol, cocaine, and methamphetamine and of men and women. J Clin Exp Neuropsychol. 2009;31:706–19.

49. Verdejo-Garcia A, Benbrook A, Funderburk F, David P, Cadet JL, Bolla KI. The differential relationship between cocaine use and marijuana use on decision-making performance over repeat testing with the Iowa Gambling Task. Drug Alcohol Depend. 2007; 90:2–11.

50. Kuypers KPC, Bosker W, Ramaekers J. Ecstasy, driving and traffic safety. In: Verster JC, Pandi-Perumal SR, Ramaekers JHG, De Gier JJ, editors. Drugs, driving and traffic safety. Basel: Birkhauser; 2009.

51. Verster JC, Kuerten Y, Olivier B, van Laar MW. The ACID-survey: methodology and design of an online survey to assess alcohol and recreational cocaine use and its consequences for traffic safety. The Open Addict J. 2009;3:24–31.

52. Degenhardt L, Dillon P, Duff C, Ross J. Driving, drug use behavior and risk perception of nightclub attendees in Victoria, Australia. Int J Drug Policy. 2006;17:41–6.

53. Riley SCE, James C, Gregory D, Dingle H, Cadger M. Patterns of recreational drug use at dance events in Edinburgh, Scotland. Addiction. 2001;96:1035–47.

54. Duff C, Rowland B. 'Rushing behind the wheel': Investigating the prevalence of 'drug driving' among club and rave patrons in Melbourne, Australia. Drugs Educ Prev Policy. 2006;13:299–312.

55. Neal J. Driving on recreational drugs: a qualitative investigation of experiences behind the wheel. Drugs Educ Prev Policy. 2001;8:315–25.

56. Matthews A, Bruno R, Johnston J, Black E, Degenhardt L, Dunn M. Factors associated with driving under the influence of alcohol and drugs among an Australian sample of regular ecstasy users. Drug Alcohol Depend. 2009;100:24–31.

57. Drummer OH, Gerostamoulos D, Chu M, Swann P, Boorman M, Cairns I. Drugs in oral fluid in randomly selected drivers. Forensic Sci Int. 2007;170:105–10.

58. Hausken AM, Skurtveit S, Christophersen AS. Characteristics of drivers testing positive for heroin or ecstasy in Norway. Traffic Inj Prev. 2004;5:107–11.

59. Drummer OH, Gerostamoulos J, Batziris H, Chu M, Caplehorn JRM, Robertson MD, et al. The incidence of drugs in drivers killed in Australian road traffic crashes. Forensic Sci Int. 2003; 134:154–62.

60. Cheng JYK, Chan DTW, Mok VKK. An epidemiological study on alcohol/drugs related fatal traffic crash cases of deceased drivers in Hong Kong between 1996 and 2000. Forensic Sci Int. 2005; 153:196–201.

61. Logan BK, Couper FJ. 3,4-methylenedioxymethamphetamine (MDMA, Ecstasy) and driving impairment. J Forensic Sci. 2001;46:1426–33.

62. Bost RO. 3,4-methylenedioxymethamphetamine (MDMA) and other amphetamine derivates. J Forensic Sci. 1988;33:576–87.

63. Tomaszewski C, Kirk M, Bingham E, Saltzman B, Cook R, Kullig K. Urine toxicology screens in drivers suspected of driving while impaired from drugs. J Toxicol Clin Toxicol. 1996;34:37–44.

64. Maes V, Charlier C, Grenez O, Verstraete A. Drugs and medicines that are suspected to have a detrimental impact on road user performance. (Deliverable D1,ROSITA). 1999. Ghent, Belgium: Rijks Universiteit Gent. Available at http://www.rosita.org/docs/rosita_d1.doc.

65. Cheng WC, Ng KM, Chan KK, Mok VKK, Cheung BKL. Roadside detection of impairment under the influence of ketamine—evaluation of ketamine impairment symptoms with reference to its concentration in oral fluid and urine. Forensic Sci Int. 2007;170:51–8.

66. Krystal JH, D'Souza DC, Karper LP, Bennett A, Abi-Dargham A, Abi-Saab D, et al. Interactive effects of subanesthetic ketamine and haloperidol in healthy humans. Psychopharmacology. 1999;145:193–204.

67. Morgan CJA, Mofeez A, Brandner B, Bromley L, Curran HV. Ketamine impairs response inhibition and is positively reinforcing in healthy volunteers: a dose–response study. Psychopharmacolgy. 2004;172:298–308.

68. Malhorta AK, Pinals DA, Weingartner H, Sirocco K, Missar CD, Pickar D, et al. NMDA receptor function and human cognition: the effects of ketamine in healthy volunteers. Neuropsychopharmacology. 1996;14:301–7.

69. Guilermain Y, Micallef J, Possamaï CA, Blin O, Hasbroucq T. N-methyl-d-aspartate receptors and information processing: human choice reaction time under a subanaesthetic dose of ketamine. Neurosci Lett. 2001;303:29–32.

70. Micallef J, Guilermain Y, Tardieu S, Hasbroucq T, Possamaï C, Jouve E, et al. Effects of subanesthetic doses of ketamine on sensorimotor information processing in healthy volunteers. Clin Neuropharmacol. 2002;25:101–6.

71. White PF, Way WL, Trecor AJ. Ketamine—its pharmacology and therapeutic uses. Anesthesiology. 1982;56:119–36.

72. Mozayani A. Ketamine—effects on human performance and behavior. Forensic Sci Rev. 2002;14:123–31.

73. Boorman M, Owens K. The Victorian legislative framework for the random testing drivers at the roadside for the presence of illicit drugs: an evaluation of the characteristics of drivers detected from 2004 to 2006. Traffic Inj Prev. 2009;10:16–22.

74. Schwilke EW, Sampaio Dos Santos MI, Logan BK. Changing patterns of drug and alcohol use in fatally injured drivers in Washington state. J Forensic Sci. 2006;51:1191–8.

75. Verschraagen M, Maes A, Ruiter B, Bosman IJ, Smink BE, Lusthof KJ. Post-mortem cases involving amphetamine-based drugs in the Netherlands Comparison with driving under the influence cases. Forensic Sci Int. 2007;170:163–70.

76. Crouch DJ, Birky MM, Gust SW, Rollins DE, Walsh JM, Moulden JV, et al. The prevalence of drugs in fatally injured truck drivers. J Forensic Sci. 1993;38:1342–53.

77. Labat L, Fontaine B, Delzenne C, Doublet A, Marek MC, Tellier D, Tonneau M, Lhermitte M, Frimat P. Prevalence of psychoactive substances in truck drivers in the Nord-Pas-de-Calais region (France). Forensic Sci Int. 2008;174:90–4.

78. Silber BY, Papafotiou K, Croft RJ, Ogden E, Swann P, Stough C. The effects of dexamphetamine on simulated driving performance. Psychopharmacology. 2005;179:536–43.

79. Miller MM, Hajdukovic R, Erman MK. Treatment of narcolepsy with methamphetamine. Sleep. 1993;16:306–17.

80. Gustavsen I, Mørland J, Bramness JG. Impairment related to blood amphetamine and/or methamphetamine concentrations in suspected drugged drivers. Accid Anal Prev. 2006;38:490–5.

81. Logan BK. Methamphetamine and driving impairment. J Forensic Sci. 1996;41:457–64.

82. Logan BK. Metamphetamine—effects on human performance and behavior. Forensic Sci Rev. 2002;14:134–51.

83. Del Rio CM, Alvarez FJ. Illegal drug taking and driving: patterns of drug taking among Spanish drivers. Drug Alcohol Depend. 1995;37:83–6.

84. Bennet ME, Walters ST, Miller JH, Woodall WG. Relationship of early inhalant use to substance use in college students. J Subst Abuse. 2000;12:227–40.

85. Korman M, Matthews RW, Lovitt R. Neuropsychological effects of abuse of inhalants. Percept Mot Skills. 1981;53:547–53.

86. Beckman NJ, Zackny JP, Walker DJ. Within subjects comparison of the subjective and psychomotor effects of a gaseous anesthetic and two volatile anesthetics in healthy volunteers. Drug Alcohol Depend. 2006;81:89–95.

87. Dinwiddie SH. Abuse of inhalants: a review. Addiction. 1994; 89:925–39.

88. Kurtzman TL, Otsuka KN, Wahl RA. Inhalant abuse by adolescents. J Adolesc Health. 2001;28:170–80.

89. Handelsman DJ, Gupta L. Prevalence and risk factors for anabolic-androgenic steroid abuse in Australian high-school students. Int J Androl. 1997;20:159–64.

90. Ellingrod VL, Perry PJ, Yates WR, MacIndoe JH, Watson G, Arndt S, et al. The effects of anabolic steroids on driving performance as assessed by the Iowa driving simulator. Am J Drug Alcohol Abuse. 1997;23:623–36.

91. Thiblin I, Petersson A. Pharmacoepidemiology of anabolic androgenic steroids: a review. Fundam Clin Pharmacol. 2004;19:24–44.

92. Hall RCW, Hall RCW, Chapman MJ. Psychiatric complications of anabolic steroid abuse. Psychosomatics. 2005;46:285–90.

93. McGabe SE, Brower KJ, West BT, Nelson TF, Wechsler H. Trends in non-medical use of anabolic steroids by U.S. college students: results from four national surveys. Drug Alcohol Depend. 2007;90:243–51.

94. Middleman AB, Faulkner AH, Woods E, Emans SJ, DuRant RH. High-risk behaviors among high school students in Massachusetts who use anabolic steroids. Pediatrics. 1995;96:268–72.

Medical Student and Physician Education in Substance Use Disorders

45

Stephen A. Wyatt and Bonnie B. Wilford

Abstract

Research consistently demonstrates that substance use disorders (SUDs) constitute a major public health problem in the USA and around the world. In fact, SUDs account for approximately one in four deaths in the USA each year and result in more lives lost, illness, and disability than any other preventable health condition (Hanson and Li, JAMA 289(8):1031–1032; 2003).

Persons with SUDs include those who use illicit drugs as well as those who use alcohol, prescription medications, or over-the-counter products in ways that vary from recommended practices. SUDs are conceptualized as occurring on a continuum that ranges from at-risk or hazardous use; through problematic or harmful use and abuse; and ultimately leading to dependence or addiction.

The general health care system in the USA offers an ideal opportunity to identify and treat persons afflicted with SUDs and thereby to reduce associated adverse health, family, and societal effects (Association for Medical Education and Research in Substance Abuse. Strategic plan for interdisciplinary faculty development: arming the nation's health professional workforce for a new approach to substance use disorders. Providence, RI: The Association; 2002). Physicians are particularly well positioned to intervene effectively with patients who have these disorders (National Institute on Drug Abuse. The economic costs of alcohol and drug abuse in the United States—1992. Rockville, MD: NIDA, National Institutes of Health; 1998).

Yet there is evidence that physicians are not adequately prepared to take advantage of this opportunity (Fiellin DA et al. The physician's role in caring for patients with substance use disorders: implications for medical education and training. In: Project mainstream: strategic plan for interdisciplinary faculty development: arming the nation's health professional workforce for a new approach to substance use disorders: part II. Discipline-specific recommendations for faculty development. Providence, RI: Association for Medical Education and Research in Substance Abuse; 2002). In a survey of 1,082 physicians that asked about screening practices regarding illicit drug use, 68% reported that they routinely screen

S.A. Wyatt, DO (✉)
Dual Diagnosis Program, Middlesex Hospital,
20 Jericho Drive, Old Lyme, CT 06371, USA
e-mail: WyattSA@sbcglobal.net

B.B. Wilford, MS
Coalition on Physician Education in Substance Use Disorders (COPE)
at Yale University School of Medicine, 210 Marlboro Avenue,
Suite 31, PMB 187, Easton, MD 21601, USA
e-mail: MedEdGroup@aol.com

J.C. Verster et al. (eds.), *Drug Abuse and Addiction in Medical Illness: Causes, Consequences and Treatment*,
DOI 10.1007/978-1-4614-3375-0_45, © Springer Science+Business Media, LLC 2012

patients, while 55% said they routinely offer referral to treatment to those patients who screen positive. However, 15% reported that they do not intervene, even when signs of SUD are apparent (Kessler et al., Arch Gen Psychiatry 51:8–18, 1994).

This chapter outlines the rationale for greater physician involvement in recognizing and treating patients with SUDs, describes core clinical competencies and didactic initiatives for all physicians, reviews current barriers to improved medical education about SUDs, and presents strategies for overcoming those barriers.

Learning Objectives
- Substance use disorders (SUDs)—which occur on a continuum ranging from risky use through abuse to addiction—account for one in four deaths in the USA each year and result in more lives lost, illness, and disability than any other preventable health condition.
- SUDs are preventable if risky behaviors are identified early and receive effective interventions. Addiction is a treatable disease of the brain.
- Given the significance of the problem and the demonstrated effectiveness of interventions, too little attention has been paid to educating primary care physicians and other health professionals to respond to the needs of the millions of individuals and families affected by SUDs.
- There is wide consensus as to specific steps that would improve teaching about SUDS at all levels of medical education—undergraduate, graduate, and continuing medical education.
- Obstacles to achieving improvements can be overcome through the application of strategies and the influence of external incentives like those cited in this chapter.

Issues that Need to Be Addressed by Future Research
There is an acute need for systematic evaluations of medical education about substance use disorders (SUDs). For example, a systematic examination of research funding [1] found that the majority of original medical education research published in 13 peer-reviewed journals was not formally funded. Moreover, research that *was* funded received substantially less funding than needed; i.e., funded studies received a median amount of $15,000 while their calculated median cost was $37,315. The authors pointed out that less than 0.04% of Federal spending on graduate medical education goes toward education research.

Introduction

Disorders related to unhealthy use of alcohol, tobacco, and other drugs are among the most serious public health problems in the world. Research consistently demonstrates that such substance use disorders (SUDs) constitute a major public health problem. Overall, SUDs account for approximately one in four deaths in the USA each year and result in more lives lost, illness, and disability than any other preventable health condition [1].

The problem is widespread. For example, estimates based on the National Survey on Drug Use and Health [2] show that in 2004, among Americans aged 12 or older, there were 19.1 million current users of illicit drugs, 121 million users of alcohol, and 70.3 million users of tobacco products. In addition, virtually all regular smokers are considered nicotine-dependent and or at great risk for becoming so.

Nor are the consequences for the public health or the public purse insignificant. In the USA, drug abuse was responsible for approximately 22,000 deaths in 2001 and $180.8 billion in total annual economic costs in 2002 [3]. Alcohol use in the USA is estimated to be responsible for 100,000 deaths annually and a health care cost of $185 billion [4]. Tobacco use, the leading underlying cause of death, results in 400,000 premature deaths annually.

Persons with SUDs include those who use illicit drugs as well as those who use alcohol, prescription medications, or over-the-counter products in ways that vary from recommended practices. SUDs are conceptualized as occurring on a continuum that ranges from at-risk or hazardous use; through problematic or harmful use and abuse; and ultimately leading to dependence or addiction. Any use of an illegal substance or tobacco is considered at-risk use. Problem drug users are those persons who have experienced drug-related harm yet continue to use. The criteria for addiction include loss of control, continued use despite adverse consequences, and evidence of physical dependence, although the criteria vary somewhat by drug class (see Table 45.1). For example, opioids often cause physical dependence when

Table 45.1 Diagnostic criteria for substance use disorders (SUDs)

The following criteria appear in the *Diagnostic and Statistical Manual of Mental Disorders, Fourth Edition, Text Revision (DSM-IV-TR)*, published by the American Psychiatric Association (APA 2000)

Criteria for substance abuse

A maladaptive pattern of substance use leading to clinically significant impairment or distress, as manifested by one (or more) of the following, occurring within a 12-month period:

1. Recurrent substance use resulting in a failure to fulfill major role obligations at work, school, or home (e.g., repeated absences or poor work performance related to substance use; substance-related absences, suspensions, or expulsions from school; neglect of children or household)
2. Recurrent use in situations in which it is physically hazardous (e.g., driving an automobile or operating a machine when impaired by substance use)
3. Recurrent substance-related legal problems (e.g., arrests for substance-related disorderly conduct)
4. Continued substance use despite having persistent or recurrent social or interpersonal problems caused or exacerbated by the effects of the substance (e.g., arguments with spouse about consequences of intoxication, physical fights)

The symptoms have never met the criteria for Substance Dependence for this class of substance

Criteria for substance dependence

A maladaptive pattern of substance use, leading to clinically significant impairment or distress, as manifested by three (or more) of the following, occurring at any time in the same 12-month period:

1. Tolerance, as defined by either of the following:
   a. A need for markedly increased amounts of the substance to achieve intoxication or desired effect
   b. Markedly diminished effect with continued use of the same amount of the substance
2. Withdrawal:
   a. The characteristic withdrawal syndrome for the substance
   b. The same (or closely related) substance is taken to relieve or avoid withdrawal symptoms
3. The substance is often taken in larger amounts or over a longer period than was intended
4. There is a persistent desire or unsuccessful efforts to cut down or control substance use
5. A great deal of time is spent in activities necessary to obtain the substance (e.g., visiting multiple doctors or driving long distances), use the substance (e.g., chain smoking), or recover from its effects
6. Important social, occupational, or recreational activities are given up or reduced because of substance use

The substance use is continued despite the knowledge of having a persistent or recurrent physical or psychological problem that is likely to have been caused or exacerbated by the substance (e.g., current cocaine use despite recognition of cocaine-induced depression or continued drinking despite recognition that an ulcer was made worse by alcohol consumption)

Source: American Psychiatric Association. *Diagnostic and Statistical Manual of Mental Disorders, Fourth Edition, Text Revision (DSM-IV-TR)*. Washington, DC: The Association, 2000

used therapeutically without any other evidence for addiction. Other drugs of abuse, such as hallucinogens and inhalants, do not appear to cause physical dependence at all, yet are considered addictive [5].

Further complicating the picture, evidence shows that the majority of health, family, and social problems related to alcohol and drug use in the USA—as in most countries of the world—occur in nondependent persons who are drinking and using drugs in excess of the recommended levels [6]. For example, most persons involved in fatal alcohol-related motor vehicle crashes are not alcoholics [7]. As a result, experts are beginning to advocate for the public health benefits of intervening with problem users, without waiting for addiction to develop [5, 8, 9]. This represents a significant shift in Federal policy and is supported by a considerable body of basic, clinical, and services research. However, it also demands changes in the way physicians and other health care professionals identify and address SUDs.

This chapter outlines the rationale for greater physician involvement in recognizing and treating patients with SUDs, describes core clinical competencies and didactic initiatives for all physicians, reviews current barriers to improved medical education about SUDs, and presents strategies for overcoming those barriers.

The Challenge of Teaching About Substance Use Disorders

Over the past decade, research has led to unprecedented advances in our understanding of SUDs. Investigators have identified the primary receptors for every major class of abused drug (including alcohol), identified their genetic codes, and cloned the receptors [10, 11]. They have mapped the locations of those receptors in the brain and determined the neurotransmitter systems involved [12]. Researchers have demonstrated the activation of these areas during addiction, withdrawal, and craving [13]; identified and separated the mechanisms underlying drug-seeking behavior and physical dependence [14]; and developed animal models for drug self-administration [15]. Most importantly, they have demonstrated that the mesolimbic dopamine system is the primary site of the dysfunction caused by abused drugs [16]. Outcomes studies have developed a documented body of knowledge regarding "what works" in the prevention and treatment of SUDs, as well as clear evidence that treatment of SUDs is at least as effective as treatment of other chronic medical disorders.

Such advances have provided a clear understanding that substance misuse and abuse are preventable behaviors and that addiction is a treatable disease of the brain. This paradigm shift provides unprecedented opportunities to achieve the goal of reducing the health and social consequences of substance misuse, abuse, and addiction, and to improve the care of those so afflicted.

Unfortunately, progress has not been so rapid or dramatic in another key area that holds tremendous potential: the education and training of the health care workforce. Far too little attention has been paid to educating primary care physicians and other health professionals to respond to the needs of the millions of individuals and families affected by SUDs. As a result, primary care physicians do not identify and diagnose alcohol, tobacco, and drug problems with the same acuity they bring to other medical disorders.

A significant body of research documents current shortcomings in medical education about SUDs:

- *Undergraduate medical education*: Overall, undergraduate medical education about SUDs is inadequate, inconsistently applied, and generally not viewed as a high priority [17]. For example, national surveys of medical schools have found widespread failures to offer or require training about SUDs [18, 19]. Only a minority of US medical schools have established Departments of Addiction Medicine, whose faculty can provide needed advocacy for teaching about SUDs as well as leadership in integrating such training into the curriculum across all 4 years of undergraduate medical education.
- *Graduate medical education*: Deficits in teaching about SUDs also are apparent in graduate education [20]. A study of 1,831 residency program directors [21] found that only 56% of residency programs required a curriculum in SUDs (ranging from 95% of psychiatric residencies to 32% of pediatric residencies). Other than psychiatry, only in internal and family medicine did more than half the programs require SUD training. The number of training hours required varied from 3 h in emergency medicine and OB/GYN to 12 h in family medicine.
- *Continuing medical education*: Multiple studies of continuing medical education about SUDs have reached similar conclusions: there are sufficient materials, policies and guidelines available from organized medical associations to underscore the responsibility of physicians for identifying and addressing patients' SUDs. However, the materials alone have proved insufficient to generate

substantial change in physician behavior and need to be supplemented by more effective approaches, including audit and feedback, financial incentives, and promulgation of guidelines [22–24].

Such shortcomings can be attributed in part to inadequate resources to conduct and scientifically evaluate medical education strategies. For example, a systematic examination of research funding [25] found that the majority of original medical education research published in 13 peer-reviewed journals was not formally funded. Moreover, research that *was* funded received substantially less funding than needed; e.g., funded studies received a median amount of $15,000 while their calculated median cost was $37,315. The authors pointed out that less than 0.04% of Federal spending on graduate medical education goes toward education research.

Why Is It Important to Reach Primary Care Physicians?

There is compelling evidence that the general health care system in the USA affords an ideal opportunity for the prevention and early identification of SUDs in children and adults, and thus a reduction in the associated adverse effects of SUDs on the health of individuals, families, and society. Multiple studies demonstrate that patients who have or are at risk for SUDs are commonly seen in clinical settings [26]. For example, an assessment of the 90-day prevalence of alcohol and drug use disorders in 22 primary care practices found that 9% of the patients screened were at-risk drinkers, 8% were problem drinkers, and 5% were alcohol-dependent [27].

Similarly, a study [28] of a sample of 1,419 patients in HMO primary care clinics found a prevalence of 7.5% for hazardous drinking and 3.2% for nonmedical drug use (with one in ten patients reporting one of the two problems)—rates that were similar to those for hypertension and diabetes. Compared with other patients, those at risk for or experiencing SUDs had higher rates of related medical problems (injury, hypertension), utilized services more often (1.5 times more primary care visits), and incurred higher costs per patient for services such as psychiatry, emergency department, and pharmacy. In another study, 7–20% of patients seen in outpatient settings, 30–40% of those in emergency departments, and 50% of trauma patients met the criteria for an alcohol use disorder [6].

Research also shows that physicians play an important role in their patients' health-related decisions. For example, reviews of brief interventions for alcohol and drug problems found that counseling by a primary care physician can be effective in changing the course of patients' harmful drinking [29, 30]. Smoking cessation research shows that a physician's advice to quit smoking is enough to convince many patients to undertake such an effort. And interventions by emergency physicians have been shown to reduce subsequent alcohol use and readmission for traumatic injuries [31], as well as drinking and driving, traffic violations, alcohol-related injuries, and alcohol-related problems among 18- and 19-year-olds [32].

Today, a goal of *Healthy People 2010* [33] is to reduce the incidence of SUDs so as to protect the health, safety, and quality of life for all children and adults. This involves preventing and reducing the adverse consequences of substance use and abuse, including deaths and injuries related to motor vehicle crashes; drug-induced deaths; drug-related hospital emergency department visits; drug-related violence; lost productivity; reduced adolescent and adult use of illicit substances and adolescent steroid and inhalant use; increasing the population of substance-free youth; and increasing access to treatment for substance abuse by closing the treatment gap. Earlier recognition of drug use, especially in children and adolescents and in populations at high risk for SUDs, may prevent progression from problem use or misuse to abuse and dependence.

There is a general consensus in the health care community that to achieve these goals, regular screening, early intervention (including the use of brief interventions and smoking cessation advice), and—where appropriate—referral for formal assessment and specialized treatment should be a routine part of primary care, even though many primary care physicians may not be comfortable in actually treating SUDs. In fact, when the US Preventive Services Task Force (USPSTF) systematically assessed the value of clinical preventive services for average-risk patients, it concluded that assessment and counseling of adolescents for drinking and drug use ranks among the 14 top-rated services that should be provided [34]. The Task Force also concluded that (a) physicians should be alert to the signs and symptoms of drug abuse in patients; (b) that affected patients should be referred to specialized treatment facilities; and (c) that all pregnant women should be advised of the potential adverse effects of alcohol and drug use on the developing fetus [35].

Recommended Content of Medical Education

Given the weight of evidence supporting intervention by primary care physicians to prevent, diagnose, and manage SUDs in their patients, what educational content and training experiences would best prepare them to execute this responsibility?

Undergraduate Medical Education

Medical school curricula need to be examined in terms of the multiple stages traversed by a medical student on the way to acquiring the knowledge and skills needed for the

good practice of medicine. Traditionally, the basic sciences—where SUD education would begin—have been taught in the first 2 years. However, recent changes in the way medical school curricula are organized suggest that no single teaching model is appropriate for all schools. At the same time, there is a wide agreement on the importance of establishing a basic foundation of knowledge in the preclinical years.

Certain basic texts also remain important to all medical education programs. A sampling of some of the classic textbooks reveals the presence of either specific sections or subsections identified as addiction-related or SUD-related materials interspersed throughout the texts [36–38]. However, it is not clear how much of this is studied throughout the basic science years. Studies to determine exactly what is covered thus are an important step in improving medical students' understanding of SUDs.

A variety of attempts have been made to establish a core curriculum for teaching about SUDs. Table 45.2 shows the outline of recommendations developed and/or endorsed by the American Medical Association [39, 40], the American Society of Addiction Medicine, the American Osteopathic Academy of Addiction Medicine [41], and the Association for Medical Education and Research in Substance Abuse [4].

Guidelines like those summarized in Table 45.2 can be helpful in establishing learning objectives for the didactic and clinical clerkship areas of study. Establishing well-articulated and accepted objectives within both the basic science and clinical faculty is essential in moving this initiative forward.

Providing adequate instruction about SUDs as part of undergraduate medical education requires the presence of an identifiable faculty member who can serve as a leader or advocate for or director of services and education. Ideally operating from a Department of Addiction Medicine, such an individual would be accountable for development, implementation, and maintenance of the didactic program, as well as establishments of clerkships that integrate SUD knowledge into practice. A demonstration of such integrated instruction is found at the Vanderbilt University School of Medicine, where a clearly identified faculty director leads the program in addiction medicine [42].

At many schools, however, a faculty leader and champion for SUD training would be difficult to find because of the relative scarcity of faculty who possess the requisite expertise. In such cases, the medical school should proactively sponsor a faculty development initiative and/or solicit the expertise from another institution.

Years 1 and 2

Once an individual or team is in place, their initial task would be to review what is being taught in the first 2 years. Individual

Table 45.2 Elements of a Core Curriculum for Undergraduate Medical Education

1. Screening, prevention, and brief intervention
   a. Students should know how and when to screen patients for substance use disorders
   b. They should know how to perform preventive counseling and brief interventions, as appropriate

2. Evaluation and management
   a. Students should understand the etiology, neurobiology, and epidemiology of substance use disorders
   b. They should be able to evaluate patients with substance use disorders and stage the disorder
   c. They should know when to refer such patients to specialized addiction services that match the patients' individual treatment needs
   d. They should be prepared to address the needs of special populations, such as adolescents and older adults

3. Co-occurring disorders
   a. Students should be able to identify and manage or appropriately refer patients with medical conditions and psychiatric disorders that co-occur with, or are complications of, substance use disorders

4. Legal and ethical issues
   a. Students should understand and be prepared to address the legal and ethical issues raised by the diagnosis and treatment of patients with substance use disorders

5. Prescriber education and the prevention of prescription drug abuse
   a. Students should understand and be prepared to address the clinical, legal, and ethical issues involved in prescribing medications with abuse potential
   b. They should know how to monitor patients for potential nonmedical use of such medications and how to address any indications of such nonmedical use

6. Impaired health professionals
   a. Students should be able to recognize substance use disorders in fellow physicians or other health professionals
   b. They should be able make appropriate referrals so as to protect patients and the public, while helping the impaired individual obtain treatment

Source: Adapted from multiple sources, particularly Fiellin DA, Butler R, D'Onofrio G, Brown RL, O'Connor PG. The physician's role in caring for patients with substance use disorders: Implications for medical education and training. In *Project Mainstream: Strategic Plan for Interdisciplinary Faculty Development: Arming the Nation's Health Professional Workforce for a New Approach to Substance Use Disorders: Part II. Discipline-Specific Recommendations for Faculty Development*. Providence, RI: Association for Medical Education and Research in Substance Abuse, 2002.

experts and commissions generally recommend that study of the basic sciences address the following topics:

- *Pharmacology*: The pharmacodynamics and pharmacokinetics of the most frequently abused substances (alcohol, tobacco, and prescription and illicit drugs) often are addressed in current curricula.
- *Physiology*: The physiologic response to alcohol, tobacco, and other drugs, as observed in animal and human models, should be addressed.
- *Pathology*: In pathology, the morbidity and mortality of drug and alcohol associated illnesses are often underrepresented. During the preclinical years, the Addiction Medicine program director can help to integrate an understanding of the role these substances play in the development of pathology in various organ systems.

The foregoing changes to the curriculum can be accomplished through careful review of the curriculum and establishment of specific learning objectives. An Addiction Medicine program director can be an advocate for increasing the time spent on such topics.

There is a need to accommodate the various ways in which the basic sciences are taught. For example, if instruction in the clinical areas of medicine—such as cardiology or neurology—is divided into discrete modules, then it would be advisable to create a module on SUDs. In other programs,

it might be more effective to adopt a disease- or system-focused approach. The paramount need is to review the instructional model used in each medical school and to develop or adapt the instruction about SUDs to fit that educational format. An Addiction Medicine program director would lead such a review process.

In most medical schools, introduction to the basic sciences is followed by exposure to training in how to conduct a clinical interview and physical examination. Schools vary in how they approach these important clinical skills, particularly in the amount of involvement by live patients. Some schools use trained actors or sophisticated computer simulations. An Addiction Medicine program director can play a role in advocating for patients with real or suspected SUDs to be included in this educational exercise, and then in evaluating the performance criteria. The program director also can assure that specific skills in screening and brief intervention for SUDs are included in the exercise.

Video has been used in creative ways to help medical students consider the difficulties confronting a patient with SUD. In some schools, faculty use feature films that dramatically depict many of the signs and symptoms of an addictive disease, and/or one of many scientific documentaries. Such visual presentations have proved effective in engaging students in discussions of both clinical and ethical issues.

They also present an opportunity to address the issue of stigma, which negatively affects patients' access to appropriate care.

The website of the Alcohol Medical Scholars Program (AMSP; see http://www.alcoholmedicalscholars.org/video-list.htm) contains a list of video programs dedicated to providing opportunities for young faculty interested in SUDs.

Another significant topic during the first 2 years of medical school is appropriate prescribing of controlled substances. This can reduce the potential for harm to future patients through inappropriate use or diversion of drugs [43]. It also may reduce the students' own vulnerability to enforcement and regulatory actions. Students can be taught how to appropriately screen patients and assess the risk of drug abuse and dependence. They also can learn to appreciate the complexities involved in prescribing controlled substances to a patient who is actively addicted or in recovery, while attending to adequate management of pain, anxiety, depression, comorbid mental illness, and other co-occurring conditions, as well as the laws and regulations that govern their use of such medications. Inappropriate prescribing by well-intentioned but ill-informed physicians has contributed to the Nation's problems with prescription drug abuse [44]. Careful instruction during the medical school years can help young physicians move confidently and knowledgeably into clinical practice.

An Addiction Medicine program director can facilitate inclusion of this topic in the curriculum at the point students complete their second year. The director also can coordinate consistent instruction by clinical faculty and house staff. This is important in light of evidence that students' attitudes toward SUD and prescribing practices are often negatively influenced by more senior physicians. [45] Prescribing practices have been described as being influenced in three ways [43]:

1. *Instrumental*: through critical analysis
2. *Command*: through a fear of external consequence
3. *Customary*: through the influence of general consensus among a peer group

Prescription practices are most strongly influenced by the customary mode, resulting in a situation in which use of medications is more often influenced by tradition than science [46]. This fact underscores the important but arduous task of attempting to change the attitudes of the more senior physician faculty through ongoing interaction and training by the Addiction Medicine program director and others.

The medical student's or young physician's personal vulnerability to SUDs should also be addressed during the first 2 years of medical school. Students and trainees need to acknowledge the occupational hazard posed by their own ready access to controlled substances. They also need to understand the preventive and remedial services available through physician health programs. The importance of addressing this subject is underscored by data showing that more than 7% of medical students and 30% of students'

family members had a history consistent with an SUD [47]. These influences not only increase their personal risk, but also lead them to minimize or stigmatize the degree of suffering encountered by patients with SUDs, which can negatively influence the care they offer their patients. Students may need close supervision and counseling to address this issue.

Years 3 and 4

In the third and fourth years of undergraduate education, medical students rotate through six clinical areas: family practice, internal medicine, surgery, pediatrics, psychiatry, and obstetrics/gynecology. These are taught through a combination of didactic presentations and supervised patient care, as students typically participate in discussions of inpatient cases, bedside teaching, case-based lectures, and small group discussions. Medical schools have the opportunity to adjust the opportunities for electives and selectives beyond these core areas.

Too often, teaching about SUDs is relegated to educational units on psychiatry but ignored in the other clinical areas. Psychiatry does play a major role in the identification and treatment of patients with SUDs and in addressing comorbid psychiatric disorders. Students need to be exposed to the appropriate use of psychotropic medications and psychotherapeutic techniques in the management of such patients.

There is, however, a critical need to integrate the core competencies regarding SUDs into all aspects of clinical medicine [48]. Strategies for achieving such integration include the following, using as an example the process known as SBIRT (screening, brief intervention, and referral to treatment; Table 45.3).

This information should be presented in didactic forum and/or through case discussions. Reinforcement of knowledge through clinical exposure is very effective in developing good clinical practice.

In addition to the foregoing, arrangements should be made for students to experience the support a recovering patient can receive through mutual support programs such as Alcoholics Anonymous (AA) or Narcotics Anonymous (NA). Many schools engage "recovery teachers" in the community to accompany students to open meetings, where students have an opportunity to witness individuals who are in long-term recovery and learn their stories first-hand. Volunteers from the community also can be invited to participate in didactic sessions to relate their struggles with the disease of addiction and which components of treatment they found most helpful. Students may welcome such an opportunity to ask questions about the experience of addiction.

Opportunities for direct contact with a person in recovery can help students see beyond the narrow window afforded by their interaction with hospitalized patients. As they become

Table 45.3 Integrated addiction medicine in core clinical rotations, years 3 and 4 of undergraduate medical education

1. Family medicine:
   a. Screening (esp. important in specialties with a high turnover of patients and thus a population with a potential high yield of positive results)
      i. Ask about use of tobacco, alcohol, and other drugs (prescription, over-the-counter, and illicit)
      ii. Learn to use validated screening tools such as the AUDIT [7], CAGE [8, 9], and DAST [10]
      iii. Use laboratory and clinical markers of SUDs
   b. Brief intervention and motivational interviewing
   c. Prescribing available medications to treat SUDs

2. Internal medicine:
   a. Screening:
      i. Ask about use of tobacco, alcohol, and other drugs (prescription, over-the-counter, and illicit)
      ii. Learn to use validated screening tools such as the AUDIT [7], CAGE [8, 9], and DAST [10]
      iii. Use laboratory and clinical markers of SUDs
   b. Brief intervention and motivational interviewing
   c. Clinical presentations of medical disorders associated with SUDs
   d. Management of medication-assisted withdrawal from alcohol, tobacco, and other drugs
   e. Treatment options for SUDs
   f. Appropriate prescribing of medications with abuse potential, including awareness of potential drug interactions

3. Surgery (the competencies recommended for internal medicine, as well as the following):
   a. Management of medication-assisted withdrawal from alcohol, tobacco, and other drugs
   b. Surgical risks and complications in persons with active SUDs
   c. Complications of anesthesia associated with SUDs
   d. Postoperative pain management in patients with active SUDs or in recovery

4. Obstetrics and gynecology (the competencies recommended for internal medicine, as well as the following):
   a. Evidence of sexual trauma
   b. Common issues in sexual and reproductive health
   c. Complications of maternal SUDs in the perinatal period
      i. Fetal alcohol syndrome
      ii. Neonatal abstinence syndrome secondary to opiate withdrawal
   d. Developmental issues in children exposed in utero to alcohol, tobacco, and other drugs

5. Pediatrics (the competencies recommended for internal medicine, as well as the following):
   a. Importance of prevention and early intervention in the pediatric population
   b. Complications of maternal SUDs in the perinatal period
      i. Fetal alcohol syndrome
      ii. Neonatal abstinence syndrome secondary to opiate withdrawal
   c. Developmental issues in children of families affected by SUDs

6. Psychiatry:
   a. Screening:
      i. Ask about use of tobacco, alcohol, and other drugs (prescription, over-the-counter, and illicit)
      ii. Learn to use validated screening tools such as the AUDIT [7], CAGE [8, 9], and DAST [10]
      iii. Use laboratory and clinical markers of SUDs
   b. Brief intervention and motivational interviewing
   c. Clinical presentations of psychiatric disorders associated with SUDs
   d. Management of medication-assisted withdrawal from alcohol, tobacco, and other drugs
   e. Treatment options for SUDs
   f. Appropriate prescribing of medications with abuse potential, including awareness of potential drug interactions

Source: Author

more knowledgeable about the process of recovery, students tend to let go of their negative attitudes toward addiction and caring for patients with SUDs. This, in turn, may stimulate their interest in more consistent screening, brief intervention, and referral to treatment.

Obstacles and Resources

An impediment to achievement of such integrated education has been the lack of funds to develop faculty who can serve as advocates for and leaders of teaching about SUDs. In fact, there are some funding mechanisms available through the National Institute on Drug Abuse and the National Institute on Alcohol Abuse and Alcoholism of the National Institutes of Health.

The American Academy of Family Physicians has been working to address faculty development through the efforts of the Society of Teachers of Family Medicine. Also, an interdisciplinary faculty development plan has been created by the Association for Medical Education and Research in Substance Abuse (AMERSA) through its Project Mainstream, which is supported by funds from the Health Resources and Services Administration (HRSA) and the Substance Abuse and Mental Health Services Administration (SAMSHA). Project Mainstream has formulated detailed recommendations for the content of health professions education and the development of multidisciplinary faculty who are knowledgeable about SUDs [4]. However, the support of medical schools is essential to make these accomplishments sustainable.

A relatively recent approach to faculty development involves use of the Internet, through which students can access resources worldwide, including case-based learning. Computer-assisted instruction (CAI) can facilitate the development of problem-solving skills. Computerized monitoring can lead to early detection of faulty reasoning patterns [49]. A consistent, high-quality message, related through an Internet presentation, can be discussed at a more intimate level by the local clinical instructor. Such a format has been shown to be successful on a limited scale [50], assuming the presence of clear goals, objectives, and expectations [51]. There is a need for the model to be expanded to larger objectives.

Students typically enter medical school with high ideals about their role as health care providers, and with a strong interest in prevention and health promotion [52]. In some medical schools, students have taken the lead in organizing forums, community activities, and publications designed to raise awareness of the incidence and influence of SUDs in health care. Notable among the organized groups is Health Professional Students for Substance Abuse Training (HPS-SAT). Among the group's activities are bringing physicians in training into contact with individuals in recovery, to help them achieve a more rounded perspective on the possibility and nature of recovery. Such exposure helps to advance trainees' understanding of the chronic disease model. Other projects involve training medical students to present prevention programs to middle-school students, thereby improving their understanding of the pressures facing young adolescents and reinforcing the role of physicians in preventing disease [53].

Projects like these require the support of the Association of American Colleges (AAMC) and the American Association of Colleges of Osteopathic Medicine (AACOM), as well as the Deans of the individual medical schools. Broad improvement in the content of undergraduate medical education can be reinforced through an increase in the number of questions relating to SUDs on medical licensure and specialty board examinations, through the support of the Federation of State Medical Boards, the National Board of Medical Examiners, and the National Board of Osteopathic Medical Examiners (Table 45.4).

Table 45.4 Strategies for integrating education about SUDs into medical school curricula

1. Establish administrative and funding sources to support a Department of Addiction Medicine and an Addiction Medicine program director to oversee and advocate for integration of SUD education into the curriculum and to serve as a role model for faculty development in all disciplines
2. Establish learning objectives related to SUDs, using a core competency model
3. Identify opportunities for didactic sessions within the first 2 years of undergraduate education
4. Integrate elements of training about SUDs throughout the medical school experience, using a multimodal presentation
5. Encourage and support medical student involvement in SBIRT, prevention, and health promotion projects in the community
6. Establish a uniform standard for the evaluation of medical students' knowledge about SUDs and skills related to screening and intervention [17]
7. Support research into and funding of studies of medical education about SUDs

Source: Adapted from Office of National Drug Control Policy. *Report of the Leadership Conference on Medical Education in Substance Abuse, December 1–2, 2004.* Washington, DC: ONDCP, Executive Office of the President, The White House, 2005

Graduate Medical Education

With stronger education about SUDs in medical schools, residents would enter training with heightened awareness of SUDs in the patients they see, as well as an awareness of the chronicity of SUDs and their prevalence within the various specialties. Given the current inadequate level of attention to SUDs in medical schools, however, most residents begin their training with limited knowledge in this area. For ill-prepared residents, the care of SUD patients often results in frustration by engendering a "helpless, hopeless" feeling, particularly if the patient is noncompliant and fails to make progress in treatment. This sets up a dynamic between the graduate physician and the patient who is without trust or respect, and thus is not conducive to a good outcome for the patient and the satisfying practice of medicine for the physician.

To avoid such problems, residents should be well schooled in the identification of SUDs and have the ability to intervene appropriately. They should be trained in techniques for screening and brief intervention (motivational interviewing) that are tailored to the ethnic and cultural populations with whom they practice. Studies of family practice residency training suggest that such an approach is possible and effective—it is the ability to sustain the gains through program consistency that remains elusive [54].

As with undergraduate medical education, the absence of faculty with expertise in SUDs is a problem in many residency training programs. Programs based in academic centers may have an advantage in this regard, in that they have opportunities to draw on experts in other specialties. Community-based programs, on the other hand, may need to designate an individual who is willing to undergo training to fill this role. As described in the beginning of the chapter there have been attempts to address this in the past and there are more underway. Three goals have been considered most important in these faculty development initiatives (a) cultivating research and scholarly knowledge; (b) disseminating knowledge into specialty areas of clinical medicine; and (c) improving the training of faculty. Faculty development can foster more positive attitudes, improved skills, and enhanced knowledge (ASK). This results in better doctors and more robust faculty development [55, 56].

Psychiatry has been notably successful in making training on SUDs part of the standard curriculum, leading to the establishment of fellowships, which feed faculty expertise. Family Medicine has also been active in developing stronger faculty expertise and curricula. However, such efforts have been difficult to sustain. Examples of successful programs are found at both Mercer University School of Medicine and Boston University Schools of Medicine and Public Health. Current efforts to establish an American Board of Addiction Medicine and to maintain the conjoint Board of Addiction Medicine offered by the American Osteopathic Association will help increase faculty expertise in the future.

Learning objectives and a didactic outline also need to be established (see Table 45.3). However, to be included in graduate medical education, this content will need to be represented on the respective specialty board examinations. In keeping with the number of patients with SUDs presenting in primary care settings, 10% of examination questions should be related to this topic. For this to happen, the support of leaders of the individual specialty groups is required. It is those individuals, with credibility within their specialty and the best perspective on how SUDs contribute to overall morbidity and mortality in their patient populations that are most likely to influence their colleagues to include training on SUDs in residency training curricula and specialty board examinations.

Continuing Medical Education

Continuing medical education can be effective in changing physicians' practice behaviors if it is framed correctly. Research shows that different teaching strategies are best suited to particular learning needs. For example, didactic lectures and textbooks are effective in transferring *data and information*. Supervised work and coaching support the development of *clinical skills*. Reflection and small group work facilitate the *transition to competence*. This is why CME that is effective in promoting change always involves multiple steps and modalities, delivered over time, and includes feedback as well as reminders in practice.

CME programs can contribute to changing existing clinical practice by finding effective ways to motivate physicians to seek, learn, and implement available evidence-based/informed practices on high-priority topics such as screening and brief intervention, and prescribing drugs with abuse potential.

Experts gathered at a 2006 National Leadership Conference on Medical Education in Substance Abuse, hosted by the Office of National Drug Control Policy (ONDCP) in the Executive Office of the President, reached consensus on the following strategies, which are designed to motivate physicians to seek, learn, and implement available evidence-based practices for identifying and managing SUDs [57].

1. Collaborate with organizations that can effectively reach the target audiences of physicians, such as the American Medical Association (AMA), the American Osteopathic Association (AOA), the Association of American Medical Colleges (AAMC), the Accreditation Council for Graduate Medical Education (ACGME), and the Accreditation Council on Continuing Medical Education (ACCME).
2. Identify and disseminate currently available CME programs that effectively address SUDs and increase awareness of their availability.
3. Establish and publicize an accessible information and referral resource or portal, such as a Web site, where physicians can identify and/or link to available CME programs addressing SUDs.
4. Encourage sponsors to develop CME programs that address substance use issues relevant to particular patient populations, such as children and adolescents, persons with co-occurring substance use and mental disorders, and diverse cultural groups. Explicitly address disparities in the burden of illness among various population groups.
5. Identify multiple conduits that can effectively reach physicians, such as live conferences, Internet-based activities, print journals and enduring materials, as well as public forums such as television, radio, and the Internet. Use these media to raise physicians' awareness of SUDs and CME courses about them, and to reduce stigma.

Implementing these changes in continuing medical education will require ongoing collaborative efforts. An encouraging start is represented by the activities of a new organization, the Coalition on Physician Education in Substance Use Disorders (COPE), sited at Yale University's School of Medicine [58]. COPE brings together leaders in medical education, specialty organizations, and representatives of Federal agencies in an umbrella group whose primary goals include facilitating the understanding and adoption of effective programs to educate physicians about SUDs.

Incentives to Change

Classic examples of successful initiatives to change the way physicians think about diseases include cancer and hypertension. Recent efforts to change physicians' attitudes toward depression and pain have met with some success. In each case, the goal was to eliminate beliefs that the conditions were hopeless and efforts to diagnose and treat them futile, and to replace those beliefs with a conviction that the conditions are both preventable and treatable and thus worthwhile objects of the physician's time and expertise.

Similar changes are needed to change physicians' beliefs about SUDs, and medical education can be part of the solution. SBIRT (screening, brief intervention, and referral to treatment) is a logical place to begin. Numerous studies have shown SBIRT to be effective and cost-effective [59–62], reflecting research showing that physicians have a strong influence on patients' motivation [63]. Widespread adoption of SBIRT depends on physicians' knowledge about and comfort in conducting screening and brief intervention, as well as their belief that it can be effective. However, as in the earlier initiatives around cancer and hypertension, consistent and meaningful change is not likely to occur until physicians are sufficiently motivated. Such motivation can be reinforced both through formal CME programs and through informal learning, as and when physicians see the improvements resulting from good care delivered by their colleagues. At that point, the standard of care will begin to rise and there may be greater interest in SBIRT throughout all medical specialties.

Financial incentives can also have an impact. The establishment in 2007 of ICD codes for SBIRT and their acceptance by Medicare, Medicaid plans, and private insurers sends a message that screening and brief intervention are legitimate practices worthy of reimbursement [64]. The ability to be reimbursed for SBIRT conducted in office settings has prompted many primary care physicians, psychiatrists, and pain medicine specialists to improve their knowledge of SUDs.

Enactment of Federal parity legislation in late 2008 provides further support for physician involvement in the care of patients with SUDs. By requiring health plans to reimburse such care at the same level of benefits as (or "at parity" with) benefits offered for other medical disorders, the new Federal law removes a major barrier to the delivery of care and provides another incentive for physicians to adjust their practices and further their education about SUDs.

A relatively new option for office-based practice involves the use of buprenorphine (Subutex™) or buprenorphine/ naloxone (Suboxone™) to treat opioid addiction. Physicians who meet Federal educational requirements and obtain a special waiver can use these medications to treat patients with opioid use disorders in the office setting. In fact, thousands already have qualified to do so. These physicians are supported by a mentoring network funded by the Substance Abuse and Mental Health Administration (SAMHSA), an agency of the US Department of Health and Human Services. The mentoring program gives practicing physicians an opportunity to speak directly with a physician who is experienced in the use of buprenorphine. The network, which is managed by the American Society of Addiction Medicine in collaboration with the American Osteopathic Academy of Addiction Medicine and the American Academy of Addiction Psychiatry, has proved to be an effective way to improve the care of patients with opioid addiction [65].

Advances in adoption of the electronic medical record afford opportunities to increase attention to SUDs [64]. For example, screening tools such as the AUDIT can be embedded in an electronic record, which then would prompt physicians to screen for SUDs at appropriate intervals. Electronic systems already are used to flag patients at risk for certain problems and a history of or documented vulnerability to SUDs can be added to the warnings. The electronic medical record thus has strong potential for promoting behavior change at all levels of practice, from the medical student to the practicing physician.

Beyond these positive influences, some mild discomfort may be necessary to drive a change in current standards of medical practice. Such stimuli may involve greater attention to SUDs in licensure and specialty board examinations, new requirements for registration with the Drug Enforcement Administration to prescribe or dispense controlled drugs, or new requirements for institutional accreditation by the Joint Commission on Accreditation of Healthcare Organizations, or JCAHO (something already seen with JCAHO's designation of pain as "the fifth vital sign") [64]. Other incentives might involve demands by third-party payers or government agencies for better identification and management of SUDs as the potential for significant cost savings becomes more widely understood.

Summary and Conclusions

The improvement of physician education about SUDs has important implications for health care and the public health. It is an area of medical care that, if addressed appropriately, could have a major impact on reducing the cost of health care and the degree of human suffering throughout the world [66].

To address the problem, medical schools should integrate teaching about SUDs across the basic science curriculum, as well as incorporating it in clinical rotations. Every medical school should have a program director who is knowledgeable about SUDs who can lead this effort and become a role model for younger faculty, residents, and students. Similar leadership is needed in graduate and continuing medical education.

Content areas that should be addressed at all levels of medical education include [67]:

1. Prevention of unhealthy/risky use of alcohol, tobacco, and other drugs (prescribed, over-the-counter, and illicit)
2. Routine screening and brief intervention (including motivational interviewing) for SUDs
3. Understanding addiction as a chronic disorder, marked by periods of remission and relapse
4. Recognizing evidence-based treatments for SUDs and setting up successful systems for referral
5. Addressing negative attitudes often associated with SUDs and the patients who have them
6. Strategies to assure safe and effective use of medications with abuse potential (controlled substances)
7. Risk factors for physician impairment, the availability of assistance through Physician Health Programs, and reporting requirements imposed by State and Federal regulations

A variety of private-sector initiatives to address these core competencies are currently under way [58, 64], some with support from government agencies. However, additional attention should be devoted to sustaining such initiatives, supporting educational research in the field, and building on initiatives that show the greatest promise of success.

Acknowledgments The research assistance of Mary A. Kelly, MSLS, is acknowledged with gratitude, as is the editorial assistance of Heather L. Talbert, MA.

References

References to Chapter

1. Hanson GR, Li TK. Public health implications of excessive alcohol consumption. Editorial. JAMA. 2003;289(8):1031–2.
2. Office of Applied Studies. Results from the 2005 National Survey on Drug Use and Health: national findings, NSDUH Series H-30 [DHHS Publication No. SMA 06-4194]. Rockville, MD: OAS, Substance Abuse and Mental Health Services Administration; 2006.
3. Office of National Drug Control Policy. National Drug Control Strategy of the United States. Washington, DC: Executive Office of the President, The White House; 2004.
4. Fiellin DA, Butler R, D'Onofrio G, Brown RL, O'Connor PG. The physician's role in caring for patients with substance use disorders: implications for medical education and training. In: Project mainstream: strategic plan for interdisciplinary faculty development: arming the nation's health professional workforce for a new approach to substance use disorders: part II. Discipline-specific recommendations for faculty development. Providence, RI: Association for Medical Education and Research in Substance Abuse; 2002.
5. Association for Medical Education and Research in Substance Abuse. Strategic plan for interdisciplinary faculty development: arming the nation's health professional workforce for a new approach to substance use disorders. Providence, RI: The Association; 2002.
6. Saitz R. Unhealthy alcohol use. N Engl J Med. 2005;352(56): 596–607.
7. World Health Organization. Public health problems caused by harmful use of alcohol. The World Health Report 2005; 22 Jan.
8. Grossberg PM, Brown DD, Fleming MF. Brief physician advice for high-risk drinking among young adults. Ann Fam Med. 2004;2(5):474–80.
9. Coffield AB, Maciosek MV, McGinnis JM, Harris JR, Caldwell MB, Teutsch SM, Atkins D, Richland JH, Haddix A. Priorities among recommended clinical preventive services. Am J Prev Med. 2001;21(1):1–9.
10. National Institute on Drug Abuse. Principles of drug addiction treatment: a research-based guide, [NIH Publication No. 00-4180]. Rockville, MD: NIDA, National Institutes of Health; 2000.
11. National Institute on Drug Abuse. The economic costs of alcohol and drug abuse in the United States–1992. Rockville, MD: NIDA, National Institutes of Health; 1998.
12. Cuff PA, Vanselow N, editors. Improving medical education: enhancing the behavioral and social science content of medical school curricula, Report of the Board on Neuroscience and Behavioral Health, Committee on Behavioral and Social Science in Medical School Curricula, Institute of Medicine of the National Academies of Science. Washington, DC: National Academies Press; 2004.
13. Volkow ND, Wang GJ, Fowler JS, Logan J, Hitzemann R, Ding YS, Pappas N, Shea C, Piscani K. Decreases in dopamine receptors but not in dopamine transporters in alcoholics. Alcohol Clin Exp Res. 1996;20(9):1594–8.
14. Maldonado R, Saiardi A, Valverde O, Samad TA, Roques BP, Borrelli E. Absence of opiate rewarding effects in mice lacking dopamine D2 receptors. Nature. 1997;388(6642):586–9.
15. Koob GF, Le Moal M. Drug addiction, dysregulation of reward, and allostasis. Review. Neuropsychopharmacology. 2001;24(2): 97–129.
16. Wise RA, Gingras MA, Amit Z. Influence of novel and habituated testing conditions on cocaine sensitization. Eur J Pharmacol. 1996;307(1):15–9.
17. Scott M, Parthasarathy S, Kohn C, et al. Adolescents with substance diagnoses in an HMO: factors associated with medical provider referrals to substance abuse and mental health treatment. Ment Health Serv Res. 2004;6(1):47–60.
18. Ferry LH, Grissino LM, Runfola PS. Tobacco dependence curricula in U.S. undergraduate medical education. JAMA. 1999;282(9): 825–9.
19. Montaldo NJ, Ferry LH, Stanhiser T. Tobacco dependence curricula in undergraduate osteopathic medical education. J Am Osteopath Assoc. 2004;104(8):317–23.
20. Hymowitz N, Schwab J, Eckholdt H. Pediatric residency training on tobacco. Pediatrics. 2001;108(1):E8.
21. Isaacson JH, Fleming MF, Kraus M, Kahn R, Mundt M. A national survey of training programs in SUD in residency programs. J Stud Alcohol. 2000;61:912–5.
22. Bauchner H, Simpson L, Chessare J. Changing physician behavior. Arch Dis Child. 2001;84:459–62.
23. Rivara FP, Tollefson S, Tesh E, et al. Screening trauma patients for alcohol problems: are insurance companies barriers? J Trauma. 2000;48(1):115–8.
24. Stimmel B, Cohen D, Colliver J, et al. An assessment of house staff's knowledge of alcohol and substance abuse utilizing standardized patients. Subst Abus. 2000;21(1):1–7.
25. Kahan M, Wilson L, Liu E, et al. Family medicine residents' beliefs, attitudes and performance with problem drinkers: a survey and simulated patient study. Subst Abus. 2004;25(1):43–51.

26. McDonald III AJ, Wang N, Camargo Jr CA. U.S. emergency department visits for alcohol-related diseases and injuries between 1992-2000. Arch Intern Med. 2004;164:531–7.

27. Manwell LB, Fleming MF, Johnson K, et al. Tobacco, alcohol, and drug use in a primary care sample: 90 day prevalence and associated factors. J Addict Dis. 1998;17(1):67–81.

28. Mertens JR, Weisner CM, Ray GT. Readmission among chemical dependency patients in private, outpatient treatment: patterns, correlates and role in long-term outcome. J Stud Alcohol. 2005; 66(6):842–7.

29. Bien TH, Miller WR, Tonigan JS. Brief interventions for alcohol problems: a review. Addiction. 1993;88:315–36.

30. Fleming MF, Manwell LB, Kraus M, Isaacson JH, Kahn R, Stauffacher EA. Who teaches residents about the prevention and treatment of substance use disorders? J Fam Pract. 1999;48(9):725–9.

31. Gentilello LM, Rivara FP, Donovan DM, et al. Alcohol interventions in a trauma center as a means of reducing the risk of injury recurrence. Ann Surg. 1999;230(4):473–80.

32. Monti PM, Colby SM, Barnett NP, Spirito A, Rohsenow DJ, Myers M, Woolard R, Lewander W. Brief intervention for harm reduction with alcohol-positive older adolescents in a hospital emergency department. J Consult Clin Psychol. 1999;67(6):989–94.

33. Institute of Medicine, Smedley BD, Syme SL, editors. Promoting health: intervention strategies from social and behavioral research, Committee on Capitalizing on Social Science and Behavioral Research to Improve the Public's Health, Division of Health Promotion and Disease Prevention, National Academy of Sciences. Washington, DC: National Academies Press; 2000.

34. Kaner EF, Wutzke S, Saunders JB, WHO Brief Intervention Study Group, et al. Impact of alcohol education and training on general practitioners' diagnostic and management skills: findings from a World Health Organization collaborative study. J Stud Alcohol. 2001;62(5):621–7.

35. U.S. Preventive Services Task Force. Guide to clinical preventive services, 2006, [AHRQ Publication No. 06-0588]. Rockville, MD: Agency for Healthcare Research and Quality; 2006.

36. Laurence L, Brunton LL, Lazo JS, Parker KL, editors. Goodman and Gilman's the pharmacological basis of therapeutics. 15th ed. New York, NY: McGraw-Hill; 2006. p. 591–613.

37. Kumar V, Fausto N, Abbas A. Robbins & Cotran Pathologic basis of disease. 7th ed. Philadelphia, PA: Elsevier; 2005. p. 419–42.

38. Fauci AS, Braunwald E, Kasper DL, Hauser SL, editors. Harrison's principles of internal medicine. 17th ed. New York, NY: McGraw-Hill; 2007. p. 2724–39.

39. American Medical Association. AMA guidelines for physician involvement in the care of substance-abusing patients (report of the Council on Scientific Affairs). Chicago, IL: The Association; 1979 (reaffirmed 1989, 1999).

40. American Medical Association. The status of education in substance use disorders in America's medical schools and residency programs (CME Report 11-A-07 of the Council on Medical Education). Chicago, IL: The Association; 2007.

41. Wyatt SA, Vilensky W, Manlandro Jr JJ, Dekker MA. Medical education in substance abuse: from student to practicing osteopathic physician. Review. J Am Osteopath Assoc. 2005;105(6 Suppl 3): ES18–25.

42. Burger MC, Spickard WA. Integrating substance abuse education in the medical student curriculum. Am J Med Sci. 1991;302:181–4.

43. Isaacson JH, Hopper JA, Alford DP, Parran T. Prescription drug use and abuse. Risk factors, red flags, and prevention strategies. Postgrad Med. 2005;118(1):19–26.

44. Compton WM, Volkow ND. Abuse of prescription drugs and the risk of addiction. Drug Alcohol Depend. 2006;83 Suppl 1:S4–7.

45. Fisher J, et al. Physicians and alcoholics: the effect of medical training on attitudes toward alcoholics. J Stud Alcohol. 1975;36:949–55.

46. Temin P. Taking your medicine: drug regulation in the United States. Cambridge, MA: Harvard University Press; 1980. p. 12–7.

47. Waller JA, Casey R. Teaching about substance abuse in medical school. Br J Addict. 1990;85:1451–5.

48. Labs SM. The Career Teacher Grant Program: alcohol and drug abuse education for the health professions. J Med Educ. 1981; 56(3):202–4.

49. Stevens RH, Najafi K. Artificial neural network comparison of expert and novice problem-solving strategy. In: Proceedings of the 18th annual symposium on computer application in medical care. Journal of the American Medical Informatics Association; 1994. p. 64–68.

50. Keane DR, Norman GR, Vickers J. The inadequacy of recent research on computer-assisted instruction. Acad Med. 1991;66:441–8.

51. Brown RL, Byrne K. Computer-assisted curriculum for medical students on early diagnosis of substance abuse. Fam Med. 1990;22:288–92.

52. Meakill RP, Lloyd MH. Disease prevention and health promotion: a study of medical students and teachers. Med Educ. 1996; 30:97–104.

53. Davis TC, George RB, Long S, Bates W, Morris G, Anderson J. Sophomore medical students as substance abuse prevention teachers. J La State Med Soc. 1994;146:275–8.

54. Seale JP, Shellenberger S, Tillery WK, Boltri JM, Vogel R, Barton B, et al. Implementing alcohol screening and intervention in a family medicine residency clinic: the healthy lifestyles project. Subst Abus. 2006;26(1):23–31.

55. Fleming M, Clark K, Davis A, et al. A national model of faculty development in addiction medicine. Acad Med. 1992;67:691–3.

56. Gelula MH. Addiction medicine: a place for faculty development. J Psychoactive Drugs. 1997;29(3):269–74.

57. Office of National Drug Control Policy. Report of the leadership conference on medical education in substance abuse, December 1–2, 2004. Washington, DC: ONDCP, Executive Office of the President, The White House; 2005.

58. Coalition on Physician Education in Substance Use Disorders (COPE) at Yale University School of Medicine. Mission Statement. Easton, MD: The Coalition; 2008.

59. Academic ED SBIRT Research Collaborative. The impact of screening, brief intervention, and referral for treatment on emergency department patients' alcohol use. Ann Emerg Med. 2007;50(6):699–710. 710.e1–710.e6.

60. U.S. Preventive Services Task Force. Screening and behavioral counseling interventions in primary care to reduce alcohol misuse: recommendation statement. American Family Physician; 2004. Accessed at http://www.aafp.org/afp/20040715/us.html.

61. Wilford BB. Briefing document on screening and brief intervention, Third national leadership conference on medical education in substance abuse, January 16, 2008. Washington, DC: Office of National Drug Control Policy, Executive Office of the President, The White House; 2008.

62. Fleming MF. Screening, assessment, and intervention for substance use disorders in general health care settings. In Project mainstream: strategic plan for interdisciplinary faculty development: arming the nation's health professional workforce for a new approach to substance use disorders; part i. evidence supporting the strategic plan. Providence, RI: Association for Medical Education and Research in Substance Abuse; 2002.

63. Madras BK, Compton WM, Avula D, Stegbauer T, Stein JB, Clark HW. Screening, brief intervention, referral to treatment (SBIRT) for illicit drug and alcohol use at multiple health care sites: comparison at intake and 6 months later. Drug Alcohol Depend. 2009; 99(1–3):280–95.

64. Office of National Drug Control Policy. Report of the third national leadership conference on medical education in substance abuse,

January 16, 2008. Washington, DC: ONDCP, Executive Office of the President, The White House; 2008.

65. American Society of Addiction Medicine. Physician clinical support system (PCSS): an educational resource for those treating patients with opioid dependence. Chevy Chase, MD: The Society; 2008. Accessed at http://www.pcssmentor.org.

66. Yoast RA, Wilford BB, Hayashi SW. Encouraging physicians to screen for and intervene in substance use disorders: obstacles and strategies for change. J Addict Dis. 2008;27(3):77–97.

67. Wyatt SA, Dekker MA. Improving physician and medical student education in substance use disorders. Review. J Am Osteopath Assoc. 2007;107(9 Suppl 5):ES27–38.

68. Kessler RC, McGonale KZ, Shanyang Z, et al. Lifetime and 12-month prevalence of DSM-III-R psychiatric disorders in the United States: results from the National Comorbidity Survey. Arch Gen Psychiatry. 1994;51:8–18.

References to Boxes

1. Reed DA, Kern DE, Levine RB, Wright SM. Costs and funding for published medical education research. JAMA. 2005;294(9): 1052–7.

School-based Alcohol and Other Drug Prevention

46

Nicola C. Newton, Patricia Conrod, Maree Teesson, and Fabrizio Faggiano

Introduction

The need to prevent the use of alcohol and other drugs is clearly highlighted by the high prevalence rates of these drugs by young people throughout the world and the significant associated harms [6, 8, 12, 82, 115, 123]. The detrimental effects of substance use are robust and include strains on forming and maintaining healthy relationships, disruption to educational and vocational paths, and hindrance to overall social development [37, 76, 155]. In addition, the burden of disease, social costs, and disability associated with this use are considerable [14, 38, 47]

The peak of this disability occurs in those aged 15–24 years and corresponds with the typical age of initiation of alcohol and drug use [1]. Early initiation to substance use is concerning as it is a strong risk factor for the later development of substance use disorders and co-morbid mental health problems [2, 15, 71, 75, 155]. To reduce the occurrence and cost of such problems, preventative interventions need to be initiated early before problems begin to cause disability, and vocational, educational and social harms [149].

Given that school-based drug prevention is the primary means by which drug education is delivered, it is essential to

N.C. Newton, Ph.D. (✉) • M. Teesson, Ph.D.
National Drug and Alcohol Research Centre, University of New South Wales, Randwick, NSW, 2052 Australia
e-mail: nickien@unsw.edu.au

P. Conrod, Ph.D.
National Addiction Centre, Institute of Psychiatry, King's College London, 4 Windsor Walk, Denmark Hill, London SE5 8AF, UK

Department of Psychiatry, Université de Montréal, CHU Hôpital Ste Justine, Montreal, Canada

F. Faggiano, Ph.D.
Department of Clinical and Experimental Medicine, Avogadro University, Via Solaroli 17, I-28100 Novara, Italy

focus on increasing programme efficacy. This chapter will review the evidence base and outline the common approaches to school-based drug prevention. It will then discuss the effective components of prevention programmes as well as the obstacles which commonly impede on program effectiveness.

Aetiology of Substance Use

Initiation of drug use by most adolescents is a result of social influences and rebellious behaviours that typically occur during the teenage years. As children move into adolescence they experience increased social, emotional and educational challenges [144]. This developmental progression coincides with periods of enhanced risk for drug use and access to addictive substances [114]. It has been suggested that the most promising route to effective prevention of adolescent substance use is to reduce risk factors and enhance protective factors to increase resistance [79, 150]. It is therefore important to identify and include risk and protective factors as central components when developing drug prevention programmes so that informed decisions can be made concerning the nature of interventions [148]. The evidence for risk and protective factors is reviewed below.

Risk and Protective Factors for Substance Use

Risk factors refer to individual characteristics, variables or hazards that *increase* the likelihood of an individual developing a disorder, in comparison to the random general population [3]. As the exposure to risk factors increases, so does the likelihood of developing substance misuse problems [117]. Protective factors are factors that *reduce* the likelihood of developing problem behaviour, by mediating or moderating the effect of exposure to risk factors [3].

J.C. Verster et al. (eds.), *Drug Abuse and Addiction in Medical Illness: Causes, Consequences and Treatment*,
DOI 10.1007/978-1-4614-3375-0_46, © Springer Science+Business Media, LLC 2012

There are numerous risk and protective factors which have been implicated in the development of substance use [30, 64, 79, 88, 150–152]. They can be divided into three main risk factor categories: (1) Genetic factors (predispositions to drug use); (2) Individual factors (characteristics within individuals and their interpersonal environments); and (3) Environmental/contextual factors (broad societal and cultural factors). The following pages summarise the risk and protective factors in the literature that have *strong* evidence to suggest they precede alcohol and drug misuse in adolescence [64, 79, 88, 150, 151]. The summary tables are based on those developed by Spooner et al. [150] and Vogl [163], and have been updated to reflect the most recent research.

Genetic Factors

Genetic factors play an important part in determining vulnerability to drug-seeking and addictive behaviour. Evidence including twin studies have shown robust genetic components in alcohol, cannabis, opiate, cocaine, and tobacco addictions, suggesting that a genetic predisposition to substance use problems and addictions are probable [79, 88, 90, 150, 165]. However, not all people who use drugs will become addicted. As such, it is likely that drug and alcohol problems occur due to an interaction between genetic predisposition and social and environmental factors, rather than genetic factors alone.

Individual and Interpersonal Factors

The individual and interpersonal factors which influence drug use are associated with personality, attitudes, beliefs and early childhood characteristics [79, 88, 138, 150, 151] Table 46.1 summarises the risk and protective factors associated with individual and interpersonal factors.

Environmental and Contextual Factors

Social influence is recognised to have a strong effect in determining behaviours in adolescents, including drug initiation of [10]. In particular the perception of drug use as a 'normal' behaviour, as well as the social acceptability and permissiveness, are good predictors of prevalence of use [161]. The major environmental factors which influence drug use pertain to peers [86, 122], family and society [79, 88, 150, 151]. Table 46.2 summarises the risk and protective factors associated with these environmental influences.

As outlined, the literature has identified a wide array of risk and protective factors for developing drug use. It is unclear however, which risk factors or combinations of risk factors are more pertinent in impacting on adolescents' drug use. What we do know is that a greater risk of drug dependence is correlated to a greater number of risk factors that persist and influence an individual over time [79, 88]. Therefore, drug use initiation is determined by a constellation

Table 46.1 Individual risk and protective factors for drug use

Risk factors	Protective factors

• Attitudes and beliefs:
  – Favourable attitudes to drug use
  – Low perceived risks of drug use
  – Low religiosity
• Personality characteristics which reflect alienation from societal values such as:
  – Rebelliousness
  – Non-conformity to traditional values and resistance to traditional authority
  – High tolerance for deviance
  – Strong need for independence
• Other personality characteristics
  – Sensation seeking
  – Adventurous personality
  – Low harm avoidance
• Behavioural and emotional issues:
  – Early and persistent aggression
  – Early conduct problems
  – Adolescent delinquency
  – Frequent drug use in late adolescence
	• Easy temperament in childhood
	• Social and emotional competence
	• Religious involvement
	• Shy and cautious temperament
	• Belief in natural order
	• Social problem-solving skills
	• Belief in own self-efficacy

of individual factors and social pressures, and can hardly be tackled by a single intervention. In terms of developing effective and efficient prevention programmes, it seems sensible to incorporate a multi-component approach to prevention aimed at reducing risks and enhancing protective factors, with interventions targeted both at the individual and societal level [79, 150]. In addition to taking into account the risk factors for substance use when developing effective prevention programmes, it is also necessary to determine the appropriate time at which prevention programmes are to be delivered.

When and Where Should Prevention Occur?

Adolescence and young adulthood coincide with the occurrence of critical developmental periods in terms of social and emotional wellbeing [144, 150]. It is a time when young people move toward independence and autonomy, decrease dependence on families and schools, and place more emphasis on acceptance by peers. For most young people, this progression to adulthood is positive. However, this transition is also the time when risk-taking behaviour is high and vulnerability to mental illness and substance use disorders is at its peak, which, if left untreated, can be lifelong and cause severe disability [1].

Coinciding with these social and emotional influences during the adolescent years is the ongoing development of

Table 46.2 Environmental risk and protective factors for drug use

Risk factors	Protective factors
Peers	*Peers*
• Relationship with peers who are involved in drug use • Perceived support for substance use by peers • Increased perception of friends' use of drugs • Rewards for antisocial behaviour • Gang involvement • Poor peer relationships and peer rejection	• Association with non-drug using peers
School	*School*
• School failure • Not completing secondary school—evidence is unclear as to whether this may be explained by earlier developmental influences • Low commitment to school	• Opportunities for pro-social involvement • Rewards for pro-social involvement • Antismoking school policies
Family	*Family*
• Attitude and drug behaviour: – Favourable parental attitudes to drug use – Parental alcohol and drug problems – Family history of anti-social behaviour • Poor family management and communication factors: – Poor family management – Parental rules pertaining to drug use – Inconsistent discipline strategies – High use of harsh discipline – High use of physical punishment – Negative communication patterns (e.g. blaming and criticism) • Family bonding and attachment factors: – Low attachment to parents – Low family bonding – Family breakdown – Child abuse and neglect – Parent adolescent conflict • Family structure: – Sole parent families—this factor appears to result from the association with lower economic status and high family conflict	• Good attachment to family in adolescence—i.e. high in caring and connectedness • Good parental supervision—being aware and in charge of what children are doing • Sharing of affection and communication with children • Parental interest in child activities • Minimal parental conflict • Opportunities for pro-social involvement • Rewards for pro-social involvement
Society	*Society*
• Extreme social disadvantage • Disorganisation and chaos in the community structure • Perceived and actual level of community drug use • Availability of drugs in the community • Low involvement in activities with adults in adolescence • Positive media portrayal of drug use • Laws and norms favourable to drug use • Low neighbourhood attachment • Personal transitions and mobility • Community transitions and mobility • Society labelling someone as a substance user after initial use	• Religious involvement • Opportunity for pro-social involvement • Rewards for pro-social involvement

the brain which continues well beyond childhood and adolescence [147, 154]. In particular, the prefrontal cortex (involved in judgement, decision-making and control of emotional responses) is one of the last areas of the brain to mature during late adolescence [66]. This can reduce an adolescents' ability to carry out intended and planned choices [89], and can exaggerate the brain's responses to immediate rewards [65].

Age of Initiation

The age of initiation to alcohol and other drug use has remained consistently low over the past decade [5, 6, 82, 92, 115]. This is of great concern because early use of substances is a strong risk factor for later development of substance use disorders, co-morbid mental health disorders and related harmful consequences [2, 15, 71, 75, 155]. Alcohol consumption initiated in early years, as opposed to adult years, has been associated with a greater risk of developing alcohol-related disorders (abuse and dependence), as well as related harms including serious problem behaviours such as violence and injuries [71, 75]. Research on cannabis has also shown that the earlier the age of initial use, the greater the chances are of becoming a regular user, developing a dependence, and in turn experiencing the related harms [15, 125]. And as for tobacco, more than 80% of smokers start smoking before 18 years.

In light of the above findings, it seems important that prevention programmes be introduced in the early adolescent years. Ideally, prevention should be implemented prior to initial exposure to drugs and before the social and emotional influences come into full effect to reduce the adverse impacts from drug use on the developing brain and reduce potential harms. Implementing programmes early will ensure young people are provided with the knowledge and skills they need to make responsible and informed decisions regarding their drug use [48].

For prevention to be effective it must be both relevant and developmentally appropriate [16, 50, 93, 101, 132]. It is argued that there are three periods during adolescence when the effects of school-based drug prevention interventions can be optimised: the inoculation phase, early relevance phase and the late relevance phase [80, 93]. The inoculation phase is the phase prior to initial drug experimentation. The early relevance phase occurs when most students are experiencing initial exposure to drugs. Finally, the late relevance phase is a phase when the prevalence of drug use increases and the context of use changes. Research has shown that there are a number of effective programmes which are implemented in the early relevance and late relevance phases [98]. These programmes are generally indicated programmes which target youth who have already started to use substances and experience related harms [124]. As the focus of the current chapter is on prevention rather than early intervention, these programmes will not be reviewed.

As the goal of most prevention programmes is to decrease the uptake of drugs and prevent the establishment of harmful patterns of use; the inoculation phase is considered the most appropriate phase to intervene. This allows us to inoculate students who may be at risk of the uptake of drugs prior to the initiation of drug use. In order to increase effectiveness, preventive interventions should aim to incorporate the school environment, drug policy, and family and community. Although such an holistic approach is conceptually sound, it is also resource intensive and not easily achievable [149]. School-based drug education alone is achievable and can be effective in appropriate conditions as discussed below.

School Is an Ideal Location for Prevention

School-based drug education offers numerous advantages over other prevention approaches such as family- or community-based interventions. Attending school is a mandatory requirement in most Western countries and it is at school where young people spend over a quarter of their waking lives [42]. Hence, schools offer a location where educators are able to reach large audiences at one time whilst keeping costs low [21, 22, 43, 69, 84, 142, 167].

Not only is school a place where peer interaction (a significant risk factor for drug use) is high, it also coincides with a time when young people are beginning to experiment or are exposed to drugs [6, 26, 141]. Therefore, schools provide a context to deliver preventive interventions before harmful use begins [16]. Evidence suggests that drug education is best taught in the context of sequential and developmentally appropriate stages, and the school health curriculum provides the ideal context to do this [9, 50, 101]. In addition, students have rated school-based programmes as significantly more effective than other forms of prevention, such as television advertisements and billboards, in preventing them from using drugs and encouraging them to seek help if they do have a problem [87]. Overall, school-based drug education is appealing to both students and educators because it offers both practical and economic advantages and can be tailored to different development stages [93].

Selective Versus Universal Prevention

There are two common approaches to school-based drug education: the 'selective approach' and the 'universal approach' [124]. The selective approach involves developing and delivering prevention programmes to target specific populations, such as individuals at greatest risk for developing substance use problems. Selective interventions have the advantage of allowing the focus of limited resources to be used on those most at need. They also address individual needs of homogeneous at risk groups and offer an opportunity to tailor interventions to the etiological processes implicated in different risk profiles [39, 41]. Selective prevention programmes are often overlooked due to their practical limitations. It is not only difficult to initially identify those individuals at greatest risk, but finding suitable, cost-effective ways to screen and deliver interventions can also be challenging [124]. However, in recent years we have seen the development of selective programmes such as 'Adventure' which are showing that these ethical and practical obstacles can be overcome [121].

The Adventure programme is a brief personality-targeted substance use preventive intervention for high-risk adolescents and is facilitated by trained teachers. It was modelled off the successful Preventure programme, which was the first selective school-based intervention shown to prevent growth in alcohol and substance misuse in adolescents [34, 39–41]. The Adventure programme addresses four personality risk factors for early-onset substance misuse and other risky behaviours: Sensation Seeking, Impulsivity, Anxiety Sensitivity and Negative Thinking [171]. The personality-targeted programme involves two 90-min group sessions which are carried out by two trained teachers: a facilitator and a co-facilitator. Early results from this trial found that high-risk students who received the intervention significantly decreased their average alcohol consumption, levels of binge-drinking and alcohol-related harms relative to the non-treatment group.

Universal prevention on the other hand is aimed at all students, regardless of their level of risk for drug and focus largely on teaching drug resistance skills [111]. Universal programmes offer the advantage of being delivered on large scales and as such, they have the potential ability to reduce substance use and harm to a greater audience [84, 104]. Importantly, universal prevention programmes avoid the risk of stigmatising individuals which is imperative, given the sensitive nature of drug use and risk [124]. Further, universal strategies of prevention offer specific advantages in relation to reducing the more common harms related to alcohol and tobacco use [88, 133].

Regardless of the approach, the effective components of school-based prevention programmes are the same. The remainder of this chapter will outline the common approaches to school-based drug prevention, discuss the effective components of programmes and discuss obstacles which commonly impede on programme effectiveness.

School-Based Alcohol and Drug Prevention

The development and evaluation of school-based prevention programmes intended to prevent substance use has significantly increased over the past few decades. The number of systematic reviews and meta-analyses examining the effectiveness of school-based drug prevention continues to grow. These reviews have consistently established that school-based prevention can result in significant increases in knowledge about substances and improved attitudes towards substance use [22, 27, 62, 77, 107, 135, 146, 157, 158]. However, they have not been able to consistently demonstrate the effectiveness of school-based drug prevention in reducing actual substance use [27, 168].

The following section reviews the literature surrounding school-based drug education. First, the different approaches to prevention are outlined, followed by the identification of the obstacles and effective principles that underlie successful drug education in schools. Together, these provide a solid foundation for developing effective school-based drug prevention.

Historically, approaches to school-based prevention can be divided into four main categories: (1) information dissemination approaches, (2) affective education approaches, (3) social influence approaches, and (4) comprehensive approaches [21, 26]. The least effective of these are the information and affective approaches, and for this reason they will only be briefly reviewed. The social influence and comprehensive approaches will be reviewed in more detail as research has shown them to be more effective.

Information Dissemination Approach

Early attempts to prevent drug use were based on teaching factual information to students about the adverse consequences of using drugs. This approach, known as the 'information dissemination approach' was based on the theory that, through information, students would develop negative attitudes towards, and abstain from using alcohol and other drugs [142]. In many cases, this approach relied on fear-arousal methods [26].

While results indicate that such programmes can increase knowledge and occasionally change attitudes towards drug use, evaluation studies and reviews have consistently shown this approach to be ineffective in reducing substance use [26, 51, 62, 77, 110]. Some studies have actually found this approach to increase drug use, possibly a reaction to enhanced curiosity about the drugs [22, 31].

There are a number of reasons which have been suggested as contributing to the ineffectiveness of the information dissemination approach. First, young people use drugs as a result of a multitude of risk and protective factors, not just their knowledge about the drug [110]. Therefore, increasing knowledge does not necessarily change behaviour. Further, information-based approaches are generally delivered in didactic, non-interactive ways. This method of delivery has been found to be ineffective in reducing drug use, regardless of the programme content [158, 159]. The findings that the information dissemination approach was unsuccessful led to the development of the affective-education approach to prevention.

Affective-Education Approach

The 'affective-education approach' to prevention attempts to prevent substance use by promoting affective development and focusing on increasing self-understanding and acceptance [153]. This is done through helping young people develop personal and social skills, and build self-esteem which in turn will foster them to make positive health decisions and avoid using drugs [26, 158, 159]. The components of affective-education programmes include decision-making and problem-solving activities, the teaching of skills to foster effective communication, assertiveness training, peer counselling and self-esteem building.

Affective-education interventions have been found to improve decision-making skills and drug-related knowledge more so than programmes which adopt an information dissemination approach to prevention [62]. However, when it comes to impacting on behaviour, the affective education approach has not been shown to decrease drug use [21, 26, 77, 158]. Reasons for this are similar to that of the 'information dissemination' approach. First, affective-education programmes are usually delivered using the ineffective didactic teaching method [158, 159]. Secondly, the majority of these programmes do not focus directly on drug use, but rather on enhancing general interpersonal skills. It is possible that students are unable to make the connection between these general skills and drug behaviour in order to reduce drug use [26].

Social Influence Approach

The 'social influence approach' to prevention was developed in the 1980s and is based on Bandura's [10] social learning theory and McGuire's [99, 100] social inoculation theory. The approach is derived from the belief that young people start to use drugs as a result of social and psychological pressure from peers, family and the media [57, 58]. This approach relies on the assumption that young people do not have sufficient skills and knowledge to recognise and resist such pressure. For that reason, the ultimate goal of the social influence programme is to teach young people to avoid using drugs by resisting external pressure and increasing coping skills [22]. These programmes are comprised of three important components, namely 'information', 'normative education' and 'drug resistance skills'.

Historically, one of the most prominent features of the social influence approach formulated by Evans [57] was psychological inoculation. The idea was that adolescents are first exposed to weak social influences to drink alcohol and use drugs, and as they grow, they are exposed to progressively stronger influences. It was thought that gradually exposing young people to pro-drug influences would build up a resistance to using drugs. In the early years, psychological inoculation was a prominent feature of the social influence approach [58]. Today, however, it is not seen as essential to its success and instead recent formulations of the social influence approach emphasise three major components: information, normative education and resistance-skills training [22]. The emphasis in the *information component* of the social influence approach for school-based drug prevention is to relay short-term rather than long-term consequences of drug use since this corresponds to the typical thinking style of young people [16].

The component of *normative education* arose in the 1970s when it was found that adolescents generally overestimate the prevalence of substance use in peers [63]. This overestimation can lead to the development of inaccurate normative expectations which can actually support drug use behaviour [22]. Therefore, an important aspect of the social influence approach to prevention is to correct these normative perceptions by providing students with the most current and accurate data, usually from large population-based surveys. Teaching normative education corrects students' misperceptions about the prevalence and acceptability of drug use by young people and can successfully deter the onset of alcohol, cannabis and tobacco use [22, 27, 43, 45, 78, 110].

The final assumption of the social influence approach is that adolescents use drugs largely because of pro-drug social influences from peers and the media. It is therefore important to provide students with the necessary skills to resist these social influences to use drugs. *Drug resistance-skills training* generally involves teaching students how to recognise, handle or avoid high-risk situations, increase students' awareness of media influences, and teach refusal skills training. The inclusion of resistance skills training in school-based prevention has been associated with enhanced effectiveness [22, 27]. However, in the absence of normative education, resistance-skills training has been found to be relatively ineffective and potentially iatrogenic [78]. A reason for this is that when students are provided with normative data and discover that drug use is not as widespread as is often assumed, it is easier for them to develop drug refusal strategies and to imagine the possibility of withstanding peer pressure [31]. As such, it may be the normative components of school-based prevention programmes that play a critical role in motivating students to utilise peer-resistance strategies and reduce drug use.

Until recently, the most well-documented, school-based drug prevention programme based on the social influence approach was the Drug Abuse Resistance Education (DARE) programme. The DARE programme is typically taught in the fifth grade (10 years of age) and what distinguishes the programme from others is that it is taught by police officers. Although some early studies found the programme to impact positively on drug-related attitudes, knowledge and behaviour, these studies have since been criticised for their weak or inadequate research methods [137]. More recently, studies with stronger designs and analysis methods have shown the DARE programme to have minimal or no impact on reducing drug use [17, 56, 136, 137]. The ineffectiveness of the DARE programme has been suggested to result from the instructional, non-interactive method of delivery by authority figures [159, 168].

Aside from the DARE programme, a considerable number of studies have examined the efficacy of other social influence programmes in preventing substance use. In contrast to the information and affective programmes, the social influence approach has been found to be effective in not only increasing knowledge and attitudes towards these drugs, but also importantly in reducing the use of these drugs [26, 43, 45, 62, 77, 102, 127, 135, 143, 146, 157–159, 168]. This success is thought to result from its effective components of normative education and resistance skills-training as discussed above [22, 68, 168].

Social influence programmes generally assume that young people use drugs as a result of peer influence and lack of resistance skills. However, they fail to take into account other factors which can influence drug use such as to deal with low self-esteem, depression or anxiety. The comprehensive programmes were designed to take such aetiological risk factors into account. This approach is also known as the competence enhancement approach to prevention [21, 26].

Comprehensive Approach

The final approach to school-based prevention is the 'comprehensive approach'. This approach is based on Bandura's [10] social learning theory and Jessor and Jessor [83] problem behaviour theory. The approach conceptualises drug use as a socially learned behaviour that results from the interplay of a variety of social factors (such as modelling and imitation) which influence personal factors (such as beliefs, attitudes and pro-drug cognitions) [22]. The comprehensive approach aims to combine components of the social influence approach with the teaching of generic self-management and social skills [21]. Teaching general personal and social skills in the absence of other components of the social influence approach such as resistance-skills training and normative education has only been found to have a minimal impact on drug use [33]. However, when elements of the social influence approach are included into the model, effects appear to be more robust [22]. The interactive delivery style of comprehensive programmes is essential to its success and generally involves class discussions, instruction and demonstration, group feedback and reinforcement, role-plays, and practice [26].

The most popular of the comprehensive programmes is the Life Skills Training (LST) model developed by Botvin [20]. The LST programme emphasises personal and social risks that underpin lifestyle and health behaviours and aims to teach students ways to avoid these. This is done by teaching decision-making and problem-solving skills, assertiveness training, skills to resist peer and media influences, techniques to communicate effectively and develop healthy personal relationships, ways to enhance one's self-esteem, and ways to manage stress and anxiety [22]. Various formats of the LST programme have been developed and evaluated, but the most common format consists of 15 lessons in Year 7, and 10 booster sessions over Years 8 and 9. Numerous studies testing the efficacy of the LST competence enhancement approach on alcohol and cannabis have found the programme to significantly reduce the use of these drugs [20, 24, 25, 27–29, 53, 61, 146]. Further, studies have also found that the LST programme can slow the rate of increase in substance use initiation [160].

However, these convincing results do not come without critique. In 2002, Gorman criticised the sampling and methodological aspects of the most prominent study reporting on the effectiveness of the LST programme. Specifically, he stated that the study conducted by [29] which involved a 6-year follow-up of the LST programme violated the fundamental principles of randomised controlled trials by restricting analysis to only a small subset, namely 7.5% of participants in the study [67]. Hence, the long-term effectiveness of the LST programme may be less conclusive than originally thought and caution should be used when making inferences about the robustness of such programmes in reducing substance use.

Recently new evidence comes from the evaluation of 'Unplugged', a school-based curriculum against youth substance use, based on the comprehensive social influence approach. The programme includes components such as normative education, the critical appraisal of the perception of prevalence of substance use among adolescents, and resistance skills to a more classical social influence approach [162]. The programme was packaged into standardised materials, translated into seven languages and evaluated within a multi-centre study in seven European countries: Belgium, Germany, Spain, Greece, Italy, Austria, and Sweden. The evaluation was conducted in the frame of the EU-DAP study, a randomised controlled community trial conducted between September 2004 and May 2006. At the first follow-up, 3 months after the end of the delivery, the programme showed a reduction of use of smoking and of cannabis, and a reduction of episodes of drunkenness [59]. At the 18-month follow-up, the effect on smoking faded, whereas the effect drunkenness and on cannabis use appear to survive [60].

In addition, a large study in the USA was conducted recently to evaluate the effectiveness of the Take Charge of Your Life (TCYL) programme, a comprehensive universal programme delivered by trained police facilitators of the DARE programme. Results from this study found an overall negative effect of the TCYL programme, with intervention students reporting an increase in their use of alcohol and cigarette use, and no differences between groups reported for cannabis use [145]. The authors are actively studying the effect of the intervention on mediators and modifiers in order to explain the reason for these disappointing findings; however, it appears that the more reasonable explanation is that the providers of the intervention were police, and that this could have reduced the possible effect of intervention among at-risk students.

In a series of meta-analyses, the comprehensive programmes have been found to have slightly higher effect sizes than social influence programmes in reducing alcohol and illicit drug use, but not significantly so [97, 158, 159]. In addition, a review of the literature for illicit drug use found that in comparison to the usual curricula, social influence and comprehensive programmes were generally effective in reducing the use of illicit drugs [62]. One strategy that has been found to improve the impact at the population level of both comprehensive and social influence programmes is to add a community-based component such as involvement from media or family and a change in the school system or policies [158]. This can contribute to change the normative belief of the population upon substance use, and de-normalise its use and abuse. Despite this, these programmes known as 'system-wide change programmes' or 'community prevention programmes' have a major disadvantage of being very costly and resource intensive therefore making them difficult to sustain [94].

What Makes Drug Education in Schools Effective?

As well as the different approaches to school-based prevention, there are certain components of prevention programmes that have been identified in the literature as contributing to their effectiveness. Research has attempted to summarise these characteristics into lists of 'effective principles for school drug education'. Although there does appear to be a large overlap between these lists, discrepancies still exist [9, 42, 50, 101, 106, 146]. The next section combines these reviews and identifies the evidence-informed principles which result in one prevention programme being more effective than another in reducing drug use.

Immediate Relevance
In line with the information component of the social influence approach to prevention, young people have a clear focus on the present and are more interested in the 'here and now' experience than in what the future holds [16, 113, 129]. In light of this, school-based prevention should have a practical and immediate relevance to students. This means that programmes have to address important aspects of the adolescent life, appreciated as directly useful, like the development of decision-making skills, or communication skills. Moreover, once confronted with knowledge dissemination, prevention efforts need to focus on the short-term rather than the long-term consequences of drug use, because it is the immediate health and social consequences of drug use that will impact directly on adolescent decision-making [50, 78, 106, 159].

Sequential Prevention and Booster Sessions
Given the changing phases of adolescent development, research has shown that drug education is best taught in the context of sequential and developmentally appropriate stages [9, 50, 101]. The target age groups have to be accurately considered and programmes have to be delivered before the start of the epidemic curve of the initiation of substance use. This is particularly true for programmes shown to act mainly on non-users population, producing a reduction of the frequency of first use [60]. Booster sessions are able to provide sequentially delivered messages which can be tailored to different developmental levels. A number of reviews have reported on the impact of booster sessions and additional follow-up components aimed at strengthening the effects of prevention programmes. All but one of these reviews have noted that the inclusion of booster sessions are beneficial [42]. Specifically,

research has demonstrated booster sessions to have the potential to cater for changes in developmental needs of an individual [143], increase programme effectiveness [22, 168], and maintain positive effects of a programme over time [26]. In contrast, one-off or stand-alone programmes have demonstrated few long-term effects [50].

Cultural Considerations
Programmes that are sensitive to the background and cultures of individuals have been found to be more effective and relevant to more young people [9, 50]. It is therefore important that school-based drug prevention address the values, beliefs and attitudes of the community and individual at hand [81, 106]. In addition, research has found that students are more likely to make responsible decisions about drugs when adult group and community groups demonstrate responsible practice and attitudes [9, 127].

Interactive Delivery of Programmes
Programmes with interactive delivery are those which engage students in role-plays, games, group discussions and activities to promote involvement and learning [50]. Reviews and meta-analyses have consistently found that, compared to didactic teaching techniques such as lectures, interactivity within school-based alcohol and cannabis prevention programmes increases their effectiveness in terms of impacting on knowledge, attitudes and use of these drugs [9, 27, 43, 45, 50, 61, 96, 101, 106, 109, 145, 146, 156–158]. Specifically, a comprehensive review by Tobler and Stratton [159] found interactive programmes to have effect sizes of approximately 0.20 compared to 0.02 for non-interactive programmes. Not only do evaluations favour interactive programmes, but students have also rated interactive programmes as significantly better than non-interactive programmes in encouraging them to talk about their feelings concerning substance use [87].

Peer Facilitated
Many studies have examined the effects of using peers versus teachers to deliver school-based prevention programmes. This strategy generally involves students electing 'liked or respected' peer leaders who are then trained to run certain aspects of the class [127]. The use of peer leaders has been found to be a popular and effective method of delivering drug education and reducing drug use potentially because peers are able to facilitate and support discussion with their fellow students [43, 45, 61, 70, 127, 168]. Although peer leaders offer a credible source to their target group, it is important they are selected and trained appropriately, and are supervised by the classroom teacher who will ultimately run the lesson and continue to play the central role in the classroom [9, 101, 106]. Moreover, in the age class interested in prevention interventions, given the young age of peers, correct and complete peer training is often difficult, and this can result in

a lack of outcome effect [62]. Caution should be taken when processes related to psychopathology are addressed as experienced facilitators are better skilled for such roles. Nevertheless, in these programmes, peer involvement during the interactive parts of the programme is still seen as critical.

Abstinence Versus Harm: Minimisation

Typically, school-based prevention programmes aimed at reducing substance use have adopted the abstinence-based approach [13]. This approach conveys a strict 'no-use' message regarding drug use and punishes the slightest deviation from the ideal [112]. The majority of studies in the USA continue to focus on abstinence-based outcomes; however, in countries which do not emphasise a strict no-use model, such as Australia, these outcomes may not be the best measure of efficacy [148].

Recently, we have seen a shift away from the abstinence-based approach to prevention, towards a more pragmatic approach referred to as 'informed choice' or harm minimisation [13, 133, 166]. This approach strives to not only reduce drug use, but also to minimise potential harm and problems resulting from the uninformed misuse of substances by fostering informed decision making and choices [170]. Over the past decade, this approach has become broadly accepted by educators, governments and schools alike [103]. Despite this acceptance, few school-based prevention programmes with an explicit harm-minimisation message exist [102, 105, 112, 118, 164]. Two prevention programmes which have been designed within a harm-minimisation framework are the SHAHRP programme [95] and the Climate Schools programme [118, 164]. The SHARP programme teaches resistance-skills training which is specific to minimising harms related to alcohol use and has demonstrated success in increasing knowledge and attitudes regarding alcohol, as well as decreasing alcohol use and related harm up to 2 years following the intervention [94, 96]. The Climate Schools programmes which are internet-based and adopt a harm-minimisation goal, have also demonstrated significant effects in reducing alcohol use and more recently in reducing frequency of cannabis use [118–120, 164]. To date, the Climate Schools cannabis trial was the first time a programme with an explicit harm-minimisation message has demonstrated success in reducing the use of an illicit drug. This area clearly warrants further research.

Effective Principles for School-Based Drug Prevention

As outlined above, many reviews and meta-analyses examining school-based prevention for substance use exist, although consistent findings are not clear [27, 62, 88, 106, 146, 157, 158]. Surprisingly, there appears to be no succinct or clear

Table 46.3 Effective principles of school-based prevention for substance use

- Be evidence-based and theory driven
- Acknowledge and target risk factors for substance use and psychopathology
- Present developmentally appropriate information
- Be implemented prior to harmful patterns of use are established
- Be part of a comprehensive health education curriculum
- Adopt a social influence or comprehensive approach to prevention and:
  - Provide resistance skills training
  - Incorporate normative education
- Make content of immediate relevance to students
- Make use of peer leadership, but keep teacher as the central role
- Address values, attitudes and behaviours of the individual and community
- Be sensitive to cultural characteristics of target audience
- Provide adequate initial coverage and continued follow-up in booster sessions
- Employ interactive teaching approaches
- Can be delivered within an overall framework of harm minimisation

summary of the factors in the literature which are consistently associated with effective drug prevention in schools. As such, Table 46.3 below attempts to summarise the 'effective principles' for school-based drug prevention [9, 42, 50, 101, 106].

Obstacles to Effective Drug Education in Schools

Although effective school-based prevention programmes do exist, there are also many barriers or 'obstacles' which can impede programme effectiveness [23, 52, 54, 85]. Arguably, the greatest obstacles to effective school-based drug prevention can be attributed to issues regarding implementation and dissemination of programmes [32, 35, 52, 55, 72, 126, 134].

Dissemination of Programmes

The dissemination of drug prevention programmes into schools is not always entirely successful [26, 27, 43]. Specifically, Ennett et al. [55] found that only 14% of schools in the United States implemented evidence-based programmes, i.e. programmes which incorporate correct content and delivery as identified in the literature as having the largest effect sizes in reducing drug use [158]. It is possible that because evidence-based programmes are rarely designed and packaged in ways that are competitive with commercial programmes and, once funded trials of prevention cease, schools do not have the motivation or sufficient resources to continue using such programmes [42, 44, 96, 167]. It could also be a result of the many challenges that arise when implementing prevention programmes into the classroom. This is known as 'implementation fidelity' [23, 26].

Implementation Fidelity

Implementation fidelity refers to adhering to, and implementing, a programme in the exact way it was designed to be [46]. A large study examining the implementation fidelity of substance use prevention programmes indicated that one-fifth of teachers reported not using a curriculum/programme guide at all, and only 15% reported following one very closely [130]. This is of great concern because research shows implementation fidelity is linked with the effectiveness of programmes. Specifically, programmes delivered with high fidelity lead to superior outcomes for students, and programmes delivered with poor fidelity lead to poorer outcomes for students [46, 54].

In schools, there are a number of potential barriers to fidelity which compromise programme efficacy. These relate predominately to inconsistent or incompetent delivery of programmes and include insufficient ongoing teacher training, inadequate resources, problems with adherence to existing guidelines, lack of support for teachers, insufficient time, classroom overcrowding and management, transient student populations and curriculum changes [23, 27, 32, 55, 130].

Given that teachers are the primary implementers of prevention programmes and that teacher training is associated with high fidelity [46], the lack of training and support for teachers to implement programmes is of considerable concern [126]. In a recent U.S.-based study, it was found that only 18% of schools reported training teachers in substance use prevention [167]. This is most likely because schools are unable or unwilling to provide training to teachers as a result of inadequate resources such as money and time [55].

When not given sufficient training and support, teachers may sense the need to adapt programmes to their specific school population [35, 55, 72]. In a review conducted by Ennett et al. [55], nearly 80% of teachers surveyed reported that they had previously adapted a prevention programme. Reasons for doing so included a personal preference in teaching style, and catering for specific needs of their class. Adaptation can be extremely detrimental to a programme since not only can it inadvertently remove the essential components of a programme, but it may even add components which can detract from the efficacy of the programme [131].

Increasing teacher education about the importance of prevention programmes and increasing monitoring of programmes have both been proposed as ways to improve adherence and thereby increase implementation fidelity [46, 130]. However, executing these methods is likely to be both timely and costly. Clearly, new innovative models are needed to overcome the obstacles to effective substance use prevention. To ensure that prevention programmes are successful, they must be simple and flexible, more user-friendly, appeal to students and teachers, and must not require extensive training or resource needs [26, 52]. Internet-based technology can address the limitations in the literature and offers a practical means of delivering evidence-based prevention whilst importantly assuring implementation fidelity.

Internet and Computer-Based Alcohol and Other Drug Prevention

Internet-based technology offers many advantages over traditional methods of delivering prevention programmes. Programmes delivered over the internet require minimal teacher training and input, guarantee complete and consistent delivery of the content of a programme, and are both feasible and scalable to meet the needs of large audiences. In addition, the internet offers a way of updating information with ease; therefore after, the initial development costs, internet-based resources offer a cost-effective means for delivering and disseminating prevention.

In comparison to traditional teaching methods, the use of computer technology in education has been shown to accelerate learning and improve educational achievement and outcomes [11, 18]. Computers also offer many educational advantages over traditional classroom settings [18], thereby allowing students to learn material at varied paces and providing them with immediate individual feedback. Furthermore, computers have the ability to engage and maintain student interest, and students themselves have reported they prefer to learn education via computers than by traditional teaching means [36]. Not only do computers and the internet appeal to young people and offer numerous educational advantages, they also offer advantages specific to drug prevention. The internet allows for the needs of students with different levels of drug use to be met, without the risk of labelling them [124], and allows students to learn information and skills with relative anonymity, which is important given the sensitive nature of drug use [19].

In recent years, promising research has been conducted into the development and evaluation of interventions delivered by computers or over the internet to reduce substance use in adolescents [19, 49, 73, 91, 118–120, 139, 140, 164]. Computer-based drug prevention programmes for adolescents generally involve young people navigating their way through simulated real-life situations involving characters and contexts to which they can relate [73, 139]. The current range of youth drug prevention programmes are both brief [49, 73] and intensive [74, 139, 140, 169] and have been designed for both universal [49, 73, 74, 139, 169] and targeted populations [19, 140]. From the evidence that exists, it appears that such programmes are both feasible and acceptable [19, 49, 73, 139, 140, 169]. In terms of efficacy, computerised drug prevention programmes for youth have been shown to increase knowledge [74, 91, 118–120, 164], decrease pro-drug attitudes [74, 139, 164, 169], increase drug resistance [49], increase anxiety management skills

[169] and decrease reported intention to use drugs [49, 73]. The evidence for behavioural change is more limited as most studies which have evaluated the efficacy of computer-based drug prevention programmes for youth have failed to collect behavioural measures [49, 73, 74]. From those that have collected measures of behavioural change, the results are promising.

A study conducted by the Body Awareness Resource Network (BARN) group tested the effectiveness of an interactive computer programme which delivered information to adolescents on important health issues including alcohol and drugs [19]. Results indicate that the programme was effective in slowing the progression of drug use from non-use through to problem use; however, only in a high-risk population [19]. In another cluster RCT by Schinke et al. [139], youth who completed a 10-session CD-ROM drug prevention programme had lower monthly rates of alcohol, tobacco and cannabis use than young people who did not receive the intervention. These results were sustained up until 3 years follow-up. A computerised smoking prevention programme for school students was also found to be effective in encouraging cessation in existing smokers and delaying onset in non-smokers [4]. Finally, an event-specific intervention for substance use which comprised of web-based personalised feedback was found to significantly decrease estimated alcohol concentration on participant's 21st birthday [116].

Delivering drug education using a computer-based resource is clearly both feasible and acceptable with young people. Recent evidence suggests that it may also be possible to deliver drug prevention programmes in the classroom. The Climate Schools programmes for drug prevention were designed to overcome factors which compromise programme efficacy. They are based on the effective harm-minimisation approach to prevention [95] and use cartoon storylines to engage and maintain student interest and involvement over time [139]. The programmes are designed to fit within the school health curriculum and are facilitated by the internet which guarantees complete and consistent delivery whilst ensuring high implementation fidelity. The findings from the evaluation of the Climate Schools drug prevention programmes provide evidence that such an innovative new platform for the delivery can increase knowledge, decrease positive attitudes and reduce the use of licit and illicit drugs in schools [118–120, 164].

Specifically, a cluster RCT in 16 schools found the Climate Schools: Alcohol Module to significantly increase alcohol-related knowledge, decrease alcohol-related harms, and decrease positive expectancies about alcohol up to 1 year following the intervention [164]. It was also found to reduce average alcohol consumption and frequency of binge drinking in female students [164]. The effectiveness of the Climate Schools: Alcohol Module has been validated in a separate RCT of 10 schools. Results from the trial indicate increased alcohol-related knowledge and decreased average alcohol consumption scores in students who received the intervention [164].

The Climate Schools: Alcohol and Cannabis course has been evaluated in a cluster RCT of 10 schools in Australia and found to increase alcohol and cannabis-related knowledge, decrease average alcohol consumption, decrease frequency of binge drinking and decrease frequency of cannabis use up to 1 year following the intervention [118, 119].

In addition, the delivery mode of both Climate Schools programmes was found to be acceptable to both students and teachers who rated the programme as enjoyable and superior to other drug prevention approaches.

In summary, research has demonstrated that computerised interventions can give rise to equivalent or even greater changes in desired outcomes than traditional drug intervention programmes. Although the majority of these studies have been delivered in non-school-based settings, the results attest to the effectiveness of using computers to deliver substance use interventions and, together with the numerous implementation advantages and high fidelity associated with computers, the internet offers a promising delivery method for school-based prevention.

School Policies

Several studies suggest that even at a lower level, changes in the environment can have an effect in setting norms and preventing substance use. Especially for smoking, schools can have strong influences on pupil's psychological and social outcomes. This could be the reason for the large inter-school variation in smoking prevalence often documented [7]. This effect seems to be mediated by teacher smoking. For example, a study on a random sample of Finnish schools showed that students exposed to a teacher smoking outdoors were at least 1.8 times more at risk to smoke than non-exposed students. This was true especially for girls [128]. Notably, changing the environment through school policies against smoking can have a positive effect. In a large survey carried out in UK, the prevalence of daily smoking in schools with a written policy stating that no pupils or teachers were allowed to smoke anywhere on the school premises, was 9.5% (6.1–12.9%), compared to schools without policy, where it was 30.1% (23.6–36.6%) [108].

Several interventions acting at the population level recognise the major pathway of change in norms setting and social influence. Recognising a common functioning pathway could allow strategy development aimed at tackling substance use by exploiting the positive interaction between interventions and poly-substance use, for example smoking and cannabis, in order to improve the strength and the success of prevention. It has been suggested that a comprehensive strategy integrating school-based interventions with the development of school policies against drug use, could reinforce the often short-lived effects of preventive interventions alone, especially for licit substances, such as tobacco and alcohol [60]. Future research may wish to examine the additive effects of school policies on existing school-based interventions.

Conclusions

Given that school based prevention is the primary means by which alcohol and other drug education is delivered, it is essential to focus on increasing programme efficacy. This chapter aimed to outline the ingredients of effective school-based substance use prevention programmes and to suggest ways to overcome common obstacles which can impede on programme success. According to the literature, ideally, preventive interventions should be based on either a social influence or comprehensive approach to prevention, should use interactive delivery techniques, be age and context appropriate, be taught in the context of sequential stages, and make use of peer leaders. Over the past decade, the array of school-based prevention programmes for alcohol and other drug use has significantly increased and programmes are starting to demonstrate effects in reducing actual substance use. Despite the existence of such programmes, many educators continue to implement programmes that have not been evaluated or which fail to show behaviour change. If the aim is to reduce substance use and the associated detrimental harms, it is imperative that schools and educators adopt only those programmes which are evidence-based and that future developments are driven from what we know works.

Acknowledgments This research was partially supported by funding from the European Community's 7th Framework Programme (FP7/2007-2013), Under Grant Agreement no 266813-Addictions and Lifestyle in Contemporary Europe - Reframing Addictions Project (ALICE-RAP), and the Alcohol Education and Rehabilitation Foundation, Australia.

References

1. Andrews G, Henderson S, Hall W. Prevalence, comorbidity, disability and service utilisation. Overview of the Australian National Mental Health Survey. Br J Psychiatry. 2001;178:145–53.
2. Anthony JC, Petronis KR. Early-onset drug use and risk of later drug problems. Drug Alcohol Depend. 1995;40(1):9–15.
3. Arthur M, Hawkins JD, Pollard JS, Catalano RF, Bajliono Jr AJ. Measuring risk and protective factors for substance use, delinquency, and other adolescent problem behaviours. The Communities That Care Survey. Eval Rev. 2002;26(6):575–601.
4. Ausems M, Mesters I, van Breukelen G, De Vries H. Short-term effects of a randomised computer-based out-of-school smoking prevention trial aimes at elementary school children. Prev Med. 2002;34:581–9.

5. Australian Institute of Health and Welfare. 2004 National drug strategy household survey: detailed findings. Canberra: AIHW; 2005.
6. Australian Institute of Health and Welfare. 2007 National drug strategy household survey: first results. Canberra: AIHW; 2008.
7. Aveyard P, Markham WA, Cheng KK. A methodological and substantive review of the evidence that schools cause pupils to smoke. Soc Sci Med. 2004;58:2253–65.
8. Babor T, Caetano R, Casswell S, Edwards G, Giesbrecht N, Graham K, et al. Alcohol: no ordinary commodity. New York: Oxford Medical Publications; 2003.
9. Ballard R, Gillespie A, Irwin R. Principles for drug education in schools: an initiative of the school development in health education project. Canberra: University of Canberra; 1994.
10. Bandura A. Social learning theory. Englewood Cliffs, NJ: Prentice Hall; 1977.
11. Barber JG. Computer-assisted drug prevention. J Subst Abuse Treat. 1990;7(2):125–31.
12. Bauman A, Phongsavan P. Epidemiology of substance use in adolescence: prevalence, trends and policy implications. Drug Alcohol Depend. 1999;55(3):187–207.
13. Beck J. 100 years of "just say no" versus "just say know". Re-evaluating drug education goals for the coming century. Eval Rev. 1998;22(1):15–45.
14. Begg S, Vos T, Barker B, Stevenson C, Stanley L, Lopez AD. The burden of disease and injury in Australia 2003. Canberra: AIHW; 2007.
15. Behrendt S, Wittchen H, Hofler M, Lieb R, Beesdo K. Transitions from first substance use to substance use disorders in adolescence: is early onset associated with a rapid escalation? Drug Alcohol Depend. 2009;99:68–78.
16. Berkowitz MW, Begun AL. Designing prevention programs: The developmental perspective. In: Sloboda Z, Bukoski WJ, editors. Handbook of drug abuse prevention: theory, science and practice. New York: Kluwer Academic/ Plenum Publishers; 2003.
17. Birkeland S, Murphy-Graham E, Weiss C. Good reasons for ignoring good evaluation: the case of the drug abuse resistance education (D.A.R.E.) program. Eval Program Plann. 2005;28(3):247–56.
18. Bosworth K. Application of computer technology to drug abuse prevention. In: Sloboda Z, Bukoski WJ, editors. Handbook of drug abuse prevention: theory, science and practice. New York: Kluwer Academic/ Plenum Publishers; 2003. p. 629–48.
19. Bosworth K, Gustafson D, Hawkins R. The BARN system: use and impact of adolescent health promotion via computers. Comput Hum Behav. 1994;10(4):467–82.
20. Botvin GJ. Preventing adolescent drug abuse through Life Skills Training: Theory, methods, and effectiveness. In: Crane J, editor. Social programs that work. New York: Russell Sage Foundation; 1998. p. 225–57.
21. Botvin GJ. Prevention in schools. In: Ammerman RT, Ott PJ, Tarter RE, editors. Prevention and societal impact of drug and alcohol abuse. Mahwah: Lawrence Erlbaum Associates; 1999. p. 281–305.
22. Botvin GJ. Preventing drug abuse in schools: social and competence enhancement approaches targeting individual-level etiologic factors. Addict Behav. 2000;25(6):887–97.
23. Botvin GJ. Advancing prevention science and practice: challenges, critical issues, and future directions. Prev Sci. 2004;5(1):69–72.
24. Botvin GJ, Baker E, Botvin EM, Filazzola AD, Millman RB. Prevention of alcohol misuse through the development of personal and social competence: a pilot study. J Stud Alcohol. 1984;45(6):550–2.
25. Botvin GJ, Baker E, Dusenbury L, Tortu S, et al. Preventing adolescent drug abuse through a multimodal cognitive-behavioral approach: results of a 3-year study. J Consult Clin Psychol. 1990;58(4):437–46.

26. Botvin GJ, Griffin KW. Drug abuse prevention curricula in schools. In: Sloboda Z, Bukoski WJ, editors. Handbook of drug abuse prevention: theory, science and practice. New York: Kluwer Academic/ Plenum Publishers; 2003. p. 45–74.

27. Botvin GJ, Griffin KW. School-based programmes to prevent alcohol, tobacco and other drug use. Int Rev Psychiatry. 2007;19(6): 607–15.

28. Botvin GJ, Griffin KW, Diaz T, Ifill-Williams M. Preventing binge drinking during early adolescence: one- and two-year follow-up of a school-based preventive intervention. Psychol Addict Behav. 2001;15(4):360–5.

29. Botvin GJ, Kantor LW. Preventing alcohol and tobacco use through life skills training. Alcohol Res Health. 2000;24(4):250–7.

30. Brook JS, Brook DW, Richter L, Whiteman M. Risk and protective factors of adolescent drug use: Implications for prevention programs. In: Sloboda Z, Bukoski WJ, editors. Handbook of drug abuse prevention: theory, science and practice. New York: Kluwer Academic/ Plenum Publishers; 2003.

31. Cahill H. Devising classroom drug education programs. In: Midford R, Munro G, editors. Drug education in schools: searching for the silver bullet. Melbourne: IP Communications; 2006.

32. Cahill H. Challenges in adopting evidence-based school drug education programmes. Drug Alcohol Rev. 2007;26:673–9.

33. Caplan M, Weissberg RP, Grober JS, Sivo P, Grady K, Jacoby C. Social competence promotion with inner-city and suburban young adolescents: effects of social adjustment and alcohol use. J Consult Clin Psychol. 1992;60:56–63.

34. Castellanos N, Conrod P (in press). Personality and substance misuse: evidence for a four factor model of vulnerability. In: Verster J, Brady K, Strain E, Galanter M, & Conrod PJ, editors. Drug abuse and addiction in medical illness. Vols. 1 & 2. New York: Humana/Spring Press.

35. Castro FG, Barrera Jr M, Martinez Jr CR. The cultural adaptation of prevention interventions: resolving tensions between fidelity and fit. Prev Sci. 2004;5(1):41–5.

36. Chambers M, Connor SL, McElhinney S. Substance use and young people: the potential of technology. J Psychiatr Ment Health Nurs. 2005;12:179–86.

37. Chikritzhs T, Pascal R. Under-age drinking among 14-17 year olds and related harms in Australia. Canberra: Australian Government Department of Health and Ageing; 2004.

38. Collins DJ, Lapsley HM. The costs of tobacco, alcohol and illicit drug abuse to Australian society in 2004/05. Canberra: Commonwealth of Australia; 2008.

39. Conrod P, Castellanos N, Mackie C. Personality-targeted intervention delay the growth of adolescent drinking and binge drinking. J Child Psychol Psychiatry. 2008;49(2):181–90.

40. Conrod P, Stewart SH, Comeau N, Maclean AM. Preventative efficacy of cognitive behavioural strategies matched to the motivational bases of alcohol misuse in at-risk youth. J Clin Child Adolesc Psychol. 2006;35:55–563.

41. Conrod PJ, Castellanos N, Strang J. Brief, personality-targeted coping skills interventions prolong survival as a non-drug user over a two-year period during adolescence. Arch Gen Psychiatry. 2010;67(1):85–93.

42. Cuijpers P. Effective ingredients of school-based drug prevention programs: a systematic review. Addict Behav. 2002;27(6): 1009–23.

43. Cuijpers P. Three decades of drug prevention research. Drugs Educ Prev Pol. 2003;10(1):6–20.

44. Cuijpers P, Jonkers R, Weerdt I, Jong A. The effects of drug abuse prevention at school: the 'Healthy School and Drugs' project. Addiction. 2002;97:67–73.

45. Cuipers P, Jonkers R, Weerdt I, Jong A. The effects of drug abuse prevention at school: the 'Healthy School and Drugs' project. Addiction. 2002;97:67–73.

46. Dane AV, Schneider BH. Program integrity in primary and early secondary intervention: are implementation effects out of control. Clin Psychol Rev. 1998;18(1):23–45.

47. Degenhardt L, Chiu W, Sampson N, Kessler RC, Anthony JC, Angermeyer M, et al. Toward a global view of alcohol, tobacco, cannabis, and cocaine use: findings from the WHO World Mental Health Surveys. PLoS Med. 2008;5(7):1053–67.

48. Dielman TE. School-based research on the prevention of adolescent alcohol use and misuse: Methodological issues and advances. In: Boyd GM, Howard J, Zucker RA, editors. Alcohol problems among adolescents: current directions in prevention research. Hillsdale: Lawrence Erlbaum Associates; 1995. p. 125–46.

49. Duncan TE, Duncan SC, Beauchamp N, Wells J, Ary D. Development and evaluation of an interactive CD-ROM refusal skills program to prevent youth substance use: 'refuse to use'. J Behav Med. 2000;23(1):59–72.

50. Dusenbury L, Falco M. Eleven components of effective drug abuse prevention curricula. J School Health. 1995;65(10):420–5.

51. Dusenbury L, Falco M. School-based drug abuse prevention strategies. In: Weissberg R, Gullotta T, Hampton R, Ryan B, Adams G, editors. Enhancing children's wellness. California: SAGE Publications; 1997. p. 47–75.

52. Dusenbury L, Hansen WB. Pursuing the course from research to practice. Prev Sci. 2004;5(1):55–9.

53. Eisen M, Zellman GL, Murray DM. Evaluating the Lions-Quest "Skills for Adolescence" drug education program. Second-year behavior outcomes. Addict Behav. 2003;28:883–97.

54. Elliott DS, Mihalic S. Issues in disseminating and replicating effective prevention programs. Prev Sci. 2004;5(1):47–53.

55. Ennett ST, Ringwalt CL, Thorne J, Rohrbach LA, Vincus A, Simons-Rudolph A, et al. A comparison of current practice in school-based substance use prevention programs with meta-analysis findings. Prev Sci. 2003;4(1 Mar):1–14.

56. Ennett ST, Rosenbaum DP, Flewelling RL, Bieler GS, et al. Long-term evaluation of drug abuse resistance education. Addict Behav. 1994;19(2):113–25.

57. Evans RI. Smoking in children: developing a social psychological strategy of deterrence. Prev Med. 1976;5:122–7.

58. Evans RI, Rozelle RM, Mittlemark MB, Hansen WB, Bane AL, Havis J. Deterring the onset of smoking in children: knowledge of immediate physiological effects an coping with peer pressure, media pressure, and parent modeling. J Appl Soc Psychol. 1978;8:126–35.

59. Faggiano F, Galanti MR, Bohrn K, Burkart G, Vigna-Taglianti FD, Cuomo L, et al. The effectiveness of a school-based substance abuse prevention program: EU-Dap cluster randomised controlled trial. Prev Med. 2008;47:537–43.

60. Faggiano F, Vigna-Taglianti FD, Burkart G, Bohrn K, Cuomo L, Gregori D, et al. The effectiveness of a school-based substance abuse prevention program: 18-month follow-up of the EU-Dap cluster randomized controlled trial. Drug Alcohol Depend. 2010;108:56–64.

61. Faggiano F, Vigna-Taglianti FD, Versino E, Zambon A, Borraccino A, Lemma P. School-based prevention for illicit drugs' use. Cochrane Database Syst Rev. 2005;(2).

62. Faggiano F, Vigna-Taglianti FD, Versino E, Zambon A, Borraccino A, Lemma P. School-based prevention for illicit drugs use: a systematic review. Prev Med. 2008;46(5):385–96.

63. Fishbein M. Consumer beliefs and behaviour with respect to cigarette smoking: a critical analysis of the public literature, Federal State Commission Report to Congress pursuant to the Public Health Cigarette Smoking Act of 1976. Washington DC: US Government Printing Office; 1977.

64. Frisher M, Crome I, Macleod J, Bloor R, Hickman M. Predictive factor for illicit drug use among young people: a literature review. United Kingdom: Research Development and Statistics Directorate, Home Office; 2007.

65. Galvan A, Hare TA, Parra CE, Penn J, Voss H, Glover G, et al. Earlier development of the accumbens relative to orbitofrontal cortex might underlie risk-taking behaviour in adolescents. J Neurosci. 2006;26:6885–92.

66. Gogtay N, Giedd JN, Lusk L, Hayashi KM, Greenstein D, Vaituzis AC, et al. Dynamic mapping of human cortical development during childhood through early adulthood. Proc Natl Acad Sci USA. 2004;101:8174–9.

67. Gorman DM. The "science" of drug and alcohol prevention: the case of the randomized trial of the Life Skills Training program. Int J Drug Pol. 2002;13(1):21–6.

68. Gorman DM. The best of practices, the worst of practices: the making of science-based primary prevention programs. Alcohol Drug Abuse. 2003;54(8):1087–9.

69. Gottfredson DC, Gottfredson GD, Skroban S. A multimodel school-based prevention demonstration. J Adolesc Res. 1996;11(1):97–115.

70. Gottfredson DC, Wilson DB. Characteristics of effective school-based substance abuse prevention. Prev Sci. 2003;4(1):27–38.

71. Grant J, Scherrer J, Lynskey M, Lyons MJ, Eisen S, Tsuang MY, et al. Adolescent alcohol use is a risk factor for adult alcohol and drug dependence: evidence from a twin design. Psychol Med. 2006;36(1):109–18.

72. Greenberg MT. Current and future challenges in school-based prevention: the researcher perspective. Prev Sci. 2004;5(1):5–13.

73. Gregor MA, Shope JT, Blow FC, Maio RF, Weber JE, Nypaver MM. Feasibility of using an interactive laptop program in the emergency department to prevent alcohol misuse among adolescents. Ann Emerg Med. 2003;42(2):276–84.

74. Gropper M. Computer integrated drug prevention: combining multi-media and social group work practices to teach inner city Israeli 6th graders how to say no to drugs. J Technol Hum Serv. 2002;20:49–65.

75. Gruber E, DiClements R, Anderson M, Lodico M. Early drinking onset and its association with alcohol use and problem behaviour in late adolescent. Prev Med. 1996;25:293–300.

76. Hall W, Degenhardt L, Lynskey M. The health and psychological effects of cannabis use. Canberra: National Drug Strategy; 2001.

77. Hansen WB. School-based substance abuse prevention: a review of the state of the art in curriculum, 1980-1990. Health Educ Res. 1992;7(3):403–30.

78. Hansen WB, Graham J. Preventing alcohol, marijuana, and cigarette use among adolescents: peer pressure resistance versus establishing conservative norms. Prev Med. 1991;20:414–30.

79. Hawkins JD, Catalano RF, Miller J. Risk and protective factors for alcohol and other drug problems in adolescence and early adulthood: implications for substance abuse prevention. Psychol Bull. 1992;112:64–105.

80. Hawks D, Scott K, McBride N. Prevention of psychoactive substance use: a selected review of what works in the area of prevention. Switzerland: WHO; 2002.

81. Hecht ML, Raup Krieger JL. The principle of cultural grounding in school-based substance abuse prevention. J Lang Soc Psychol. 2006;25(3):301–19.

82. Hibell B, Guttormsson U, Ahlström S, Balakireva O, Bjarnason T, Kokkevi A, et al. The 2007 ESPAD report: substance use among students in 35 European countries. Stockholm, Sweden: The European School Survey Project on Alcohol and Other Drugs; 2007.

83. Jessor R, Jessor SL. Problem behaviour and psychosocial development: a longitudinal study of youth. New York: Academic Press; 1977.

84. Jones L, Sumnall H, Burrell K, McVeigh J, Bellis MA. Universal drug prevention. Liverpool, UK: National Collaborating Centre for Drug Prevention; 2006.

85. Kaftarian S, Robinson E, Compton W, Watts Davis B, Valkow N. Blending prevention research and practice in schools: critical issues and suggestions. Prev Sci. 2004;5(1):1–3.

86. Kuntsche E, Delgrande Jordon M. Adolescent alcohol and cannabis use in relation to peer and school factors: results of multilevel analyses. Drug Alcohol Depend. 2006;84:167–74.

87. Lisnov L, Harding CG, Safer LA, Kavanagh J. Adolescents perceptions of substance abuse prevention strategies. Adolescence. 1998;33(130):301–11.

88. Loxley W, Toumbouruo JW, Stockwell T, Haines B, Scott K, Godfrey C, et al. The prevention of substance use, risk and harm in Australia: a review of the evidence. Canberra: Ministerial Council on Drug Strategy; 2004.

89. Luna B, Sweeney JA. The emergence of collaborative brain function: fMRI studies of the development of response inhibition. Ann NY Acad Sci. 2004;1021:296–309.

90. Lynskey M, Heath AC, Nelson AC. Genetic and environmental contributions to cannabis dependence in a National young adult twin sample. Psychol Med. 2002;32:195–207.

91. Marsch LA, Bickel WK, Badger GJ. Applying computer technology to substance abuse prevention science: results of a preliminary examination. J Child Adolesc Subst Abuse. 2007;16(2):69–94.

92. McAllister I. Alcohol consumption among adolescents and young adults. Canberra: Australian National University; 2003.

93. McBride N. A systematic review of school drug education. Health Educ Res. 2003;18(6):729–42.

94. McBride N, Farringdon F, Midford R, Meuleners L, Phillips M. Harm minimisation in school drug education: final results of the School Health and Alcohol Harm Reducation Project (SHAHRP). Addiction. 2004;99:278–91.

95. McBride N, Farringdon F, Muleners L, Midford R. School Health and Alcohol Harm Reduction Project: details of intervention development and research procedures. Perth, W.A.: National Drug Research Institute, Curtin University of Technology; 2006.

96. McBride N, Midford R, Farringdon F, Phillips M. Early results from a school alcohol harm minimization study: the School Health and Alcohol Harm Reduction Project. Addiction. 2000;95(7):1021–42.

97. McCambridge J. A case study of publication bias in an influential series of reviews of drug education. Drug Alcohol Rev. 2007;26:463–8.

98. McCambridge J, Strang J. The efficacy of single-session motivational interviewing in reducing drug consumption and perceptions of drug-related risk and harm among young people: results from a multi-site cluster randomized trial. Addiction. 2004;99:39–52.

99. McGuire WJ. Inducing resistance to persuasion: Some contemporary approaches. In: Berkowitz L, editor. Advances in experimental social psychology. New York: Academic Press; 1964. p. 192–227.

100. McGuire WJ. The nature of attitudes and attitude change. In: Lindzey G, Aronson E, editors. Handbook of social psychology. Reading, MA: Addison-Wesley; 1968. p. 136–341.

101. Meyer L, Cahill H. Principles for school drug education. Canberra: Australian Government Department of Education Science and Training; 2004.

102. Midford R. Does drug education work? Drug Alcohol Rev. 2000;19:441–6.

103. Midford R. Is Australia 'fair dinkum' about drug education in schools? Drug Alcohol Rev. 2007;26(4):421–7.

104. Midford R. Is this the path to effective prevention? Addiction. 2008;103(7):1169–70.

105. Midford R, McBride N, Munro G. Harn reduction in school drug education: developing an Australian approach. Drug Alcohol Rev. 1998;17(3):319–27.

106. Midford R, Munro G, McBride N, Snow P, Ladzinski U. Principles that underpin effective school-based drug education. J Drug Educ. 2002;32(4):363–86.

107. Midford R, Snow P, Lentin S. School-based illicit drug education programs: a critical review and analysis. Rockville, MD: National Drug Research Institute; 2001.

108. Moore L, Roberts C, Tudor-Smith C. School smoking policies and smoking prevalence among adolescents: multilevel analysis of cross-sectional data from Wales. Tob Control. 2001;10:117–23.

109. Morgenstern M, Wiborg G, Isensee B, Hanewinkel R. School-based alcohol education: results of a cluster-randomized controlled trial. Addiction. 2009;104:402–12.

110. Moskowitz JM. The primary prevention of alcohol problems: a critical review of the research literature. J Stud Alcohol. 1989;50(1):54–88.

111. Mrazek PJ, Haggerty RJ. Reducing risks for mental disorders: frontiers for prevention intervention research. Washington DC: National Academy Press; 1994.

112. Munro G, Midford R. 'Zero tolerance' and drug education in Australian schools. Drug Alcohol Rev. 2001;20:105–9.

113. Mussen PH, Conper JJ, Kagan J, editors. Child development and personality. 5th ed. New York: Harper and Row; 1979.

114. National Institute on Drug Abuse. Preventing drug abuse among children and adolescents. Bethesda, MD: National Institutes of Health; 2003.

115. National Institute on Drug Abuse. Monitoring the future: national results on adolescent drug use. Bethesda, MD: National Institutes of Health; 2008.

116. Neighbors C, Lee CM, Lewis MA, Fossos N, Walter T. Internet-based personalized feedback to reduce 21st-birthday drinking: a randomized controlled trial of an event-specific prevention intervention. J Consult Clin Psychol. 2009;77(1):51–63.

117. Newcomb MD. Identifying high-risk youth: Prevalence and patterns of adolescent drug abuse. In: Rahdert E, Czechowicz D, Amsei I, editors. Adolescent drug abuse: clinical assessment and therapeutic intervention. Rockville: National Institute on Drug Abuse; 1995. p. 7–38.

118. Newton N, Teesson M, Vogl L, Andrews G. Internet-based prevention for alcohol and cannabis use: final results of the Climate Schools course. Addiction. 2010;105(4):749–59.

119. Newton NC, Andrews G, Teesson M, Vogl LE. Delivering prevention for alcohol and cannabis using the internet: a cluster randomised controlled trial. Prev Med. 2009;48:579–84.

120. Newton NC, Vogl LE, Teesson M, Andrews G. CLIMATE Schools: alcohol module: cross-validation of a school-based prevention programme for alcohol misuse. Aust N Z J Psychiatry. 2009;43:201–7.

121. O'Leary-Barrett M, Mackie CJ, Castellanos-Ryan N, Al-Khudhairy N, Conrod PJ. Teacher-delivered personality-targeted interventions delay uptake of drinking and decrease risk of alcohol-related problems. J Am Acad Child Adolesc Psychiatry. 2010;49:954–63.

122. Oetting ER, Lynch RS. Peers and the prevention of adolescent drug use. In: Sloboda Z, Bukoski WJ, editors. Handbook of drug prevention: theory, science and practice. New York: Kluwer Academic/Plenum Publishers; 2003. p. 101–27.

123. Office of National Drug Control Policy. Marijuana: the greatest cause of illegal drug abuse. DC: Washington; 2008.

124. Offord DR. Selection of levels of prevention. Addict Behav. 2000;25(6):833–42.

125. Patton G, Coffey C, Lynskey MT, Reid S, Hemphill S, Carlin JB, et al. Trajectories of adolescent alcohol and cannabis use into young adulthood. Melbourne: Centre for Adolescent Health; 2007.

126. Pentz MA. Form follows function: designs for prevention effectiveness and diffusion research. Prev Sci. 2004;5(1):23–9.

127. Perry CL, Kelder SH. Models for effective prevention. J Adolesc Health. 1992;13(5):355–63.

128. Poulsen LH, Osler M, Roberts C, Due P, Damsgaard MT, Holstein BE. Exposure to teachers smoking and adolescent smoking behaviour: analysis of cross sectional data from Denmark. Tob Control. 2002;11:246–51.

129. Prensky M. Digital natives, digital immigrants. Lincoln: NCB University Press; 2001.

130. Ringwalt C, Ennett S, Johnson R, Rohrbach LA, Simons-Rudolph A, Vincus A, et al. Factors associated with fidelity to substance use prevention curriculum guides in the Nation's middle schools. Health Educ Behav. 2003;30(3):375–91.

131. Ringwalt C, Ennett S, Vincus A, Rohrbach LA, Simons-Rudolph A. Who's calling the shots? Decision-makers and the adoption of effective school-based substance use prevention curricula. J Drug Educ. 2004;34(1):19–31.

132. Roberts G, McCall D, Stevens Lavigne A, Anderson J, Paglia A, Bollenbach S, et al. Preventing substance use problems among young people: a compendium of best practices. Ottawa: Health Canada; 2001.

133. Roche AM, Evans KR, Stanton WR. Harm reducation: roads less travelled to the Holy Grail. Addiction. 1997;92(9).

134. Rohrbach LA, D'Onofrio CN, Backer TE, Montgomery SB. Diffusion of school-based substance abuse prevention programs. Am Behav Sci. 1996;39(7):919–34.

135. Roona MR, Streke AV, Ochshorn P, Marshall DM, Palmer AP. Identifying effective school-based substance abuse prevention interventions: background paper for Prevention 2000 Summit. NY: Albany; 2000.

136. Rosenbaum DP, Flewelling RL, Bailey SL, Ringwalt C. Cops in the classroom: a longitudinal evaluation of drug abuse resistance education (D.A.R.E). J Res Crime Delinq. 1994;31:3–31.

137. Rosenbaum DP, Hanson GS. Assessing the effects of school-based drug education: a six-year multilevel analysis of Project D.A.R.E. J Res Crime Delinq. 1998;35(4):381–412.

138. Scheier LM, Botvin GJ, Baker E. Risk and protective factors as predictors of adolescent alcohol involvement and transitions in alcohol use: a prospective analysis. J Stud Alcohol. 1997;58:652–67.

139. Schinke S, Schwinn TM, Noia JD, Cole KC. Reducing the risks of alcohol use among urban youth: three-year effects of a computer-based intervention with and without parent involvement. J Stud Alcohol. 2004;65:443–9.

140. Schinke S, Schwinn TM, Ozanian A. Alcohol prevention among high-risk youth: computer-based intervention. J Prev Interv Community. 2005;29:117–30.

141. Sharma M. Editorial: making effective alcohol education interventions for high schools. J Alcohol Drug Educ. 2006;50(2):1–4.

142. Shin C. A review of school-based drug prevention program evaluations in the 1990's. Am J Health Educ. 2001;32(3):139–47.

143. Shope JT, Copeland LA, Marcoux BC, Kamp ME. Effectiveness of a school-based substance abuse prevention program. J Drug Educ. 1996;26(4):323–37.

144. Simmons RG, Blyth D. Moving into adolescence: the impact of pubertal change and school context. New Brunswick: Transaction Publishers; 2008.

145. Sloboda Z, Stephens RC, Stephens PC, Grey SF, Teasdale B, Hawthorne RD, et al. The Adolescent Substance Abuse Prevention Study: a randomized field trial of a universal substance abuse prevention program. Drug Alcohol Depend. 2009;102(1–3):1–10.

146. Soole DW, Mazerolle L, Rombouts S. School based drug prevention: a systematic review of the effectiveness on illicit drug use, Drug Policy Modelling Project, Monograph 07. Sydney: Griffith University; 2005.

147. Sowell ER, Thompson PM, Toga AW. Mapping changes in the human cortex through out the span life. Neuroscientist. 2004;10: 372–92.

148. Spooner C, Hall W. Preventing drug misuse by young people: we need to do more than 'just say no'. Addiction. 2002;97(5):478–81.

149. Spooner C, Hall W. Public policy and the prevention of substance-use disorders. Curr Opin Psychiatr. 2002;15(3):235–9.

150. Spooner C, Mattick R, Howard J. The nature and treatment of adolescent substance abuse, Monograph No. 26. Sydney: National Drug and Alcohol Research Centre; 1996.

151. Stockwell T, Toumbouruo JW, Letcher P, Smart D, Sanson A, Bond L. Risk and protective factors for different intensities of adolescent substance use: when does the prevention paradox apply? Drug Alcohol Rev. 2004;23:67–77.

152. Swadi H. Individual risk factors for adolescent substance use. Drug Alcohol Depend. 1999;55:209–24.

153. Swisher JD. Prevention issues. In: Dupont RI, Goldstein A, O'Donnell J, editors. Handbook on drug abuse. Washington DC: National Institute on Drug Abuse; 1979. p. 49–62.

154. Tapert SF, Caldwell L, Burke C. Alcohol and the adolescent brain: human studies. Alcohol Res Health. 2005;28(4):205–12.

155. Teesson M, Degenhardt L, Hall W, Lynskey M, Toumbourou J, Patton G. Substance use and mental health in longitudinal perspective. In: Stockwall T, Grueneald P, Toumbourou J, Loxley W, editors. Preventing harmful substance use: the evidence base for policy and practice. Chichester: John Wiley and Sons; 2005.

156. Tobler NS. Lessons learned. J Prim Prev. 2000;20(4):261–74.

157. Tobler NS, Lassard T, Marshall D, Ochshorn P, Roona M. Effectiveness of school-based drug prevention programs for marijuana use. School Psychol Int. 1999;20:105–37.

158. Tobler NS, Roona MR, Ochshorn P, Marshall DG, Streke AV, Stackpole KM. School-based adolescent drug prevention programs: 1998 meta-analysis. J Prim Prev. 2000;20(4):275–336.

159. Tobler NS, Stratton HH. Effectiveness of school-based drug prevention programs: a meta-analysis of the research. J Prim Prev. 1997;18(1):71–128.

160. Trudeau L, Spoth R, Lillehoj C, Redmond C, Wickrama KAS. Effects of a preventive intervention on adolescent substance use initiation, expectancies and refusal intentions. Prev Sci. 2003;4(2):109–22.

161. Tyas SL, Pederson LL. Psychosocial factors related to adolescent smoking: a critical review of the literature. Tob Control. 1998;7:409–20.

162. Van Der Kreeft P, Wiborg G, Galanti MR, Siliquini R, Bohrn K, Scatigna M, et al. 'Unplugged': a new European school programme against substance abuse. Drugs Educ Prev Pol. 2009;16:167–81.

163. Vogl L. Climate Schools: alcohol module: the feasibility and efficacy of a universal school-based computerised prevention program for alcohol misuse and related harms. Sydney: University of New South Wales; 2007.

164. Vogl L, Teesson M, Andrews G, Bird K, Steadman B, Dillon P. A computerised harm minimisation prevention program for alcohol misuse and related harms: randomised controlled trial. Addiction. 2009;104:564–75.

165. Volkow ND, Li TK. Treating and preventing abuse, addiction, and their medical consequences. In: Tsuang MY, Stone WS, Lyons MJ, editors. Recognition and prevention of major mental and substance use disorders. Washington, DC: American Psychiatric Publishing Inc; 2007.

166. Weatherburn D. Dilemmas in harm minimization. Addiction. 2008;104:335–9.

167. Wenter DL, Ennett ST, Ribisl KM, Vincus AA, Rohrbach L, Ringwalt CL, et al. Comprehensiveness of substance use prevention programs in U.S. middle schools. J Adolesc Health. 2002;30(6):455–62.

168. White D, Pitts M. Review: educating young people about drugs: a systematic review. Addiction. 1998;93(10):1475–87.

169. Williams C, Griffin KW, Macaulay AP, West TL, Gronewold E. Efficacy of a drug prevention CD-ROM intervention for adolescents. Subst Use Misuse. 2005;40:869–78.

170. Wodak A. Harm reduction is now the mainstream global drug policy. Addiction. 2009;104:340–6.

171. Woicik PB, Conrod P, Stewart SH, Pihl RO. The Substance Use Risk Profile Scale: a scale measuring traits linked to reinforcement-specific substance use profiles. Addict Behav. 2009;32:1042–55.

Index

J.C. Verster et al. (eds.), *Drug Abuse and Addiction in Medical Illness: Causes, Consequences and Treatment,*
DOI 10.1007/978-1-4614-3375-0, © Springer Science+Business Media, LLC 2012

Printed by Publishers' Graphics LLC
ASO140417.15.19.4 20140417